New and Revised Nursing Diagnoses Approved at the 2007-2008 NANDA International Conference

Contamination
Moral Distress
Overflow Urinary Incontinence
Readiness for Enhanced Comfort
Readiness for Enhanced Decision Making
Readiness for Enhanced Hope
Readiness for Enhanced Immunization Status
Readiness for Enhanced Power
Readiness for Enhanced Self-Care
Risk for Acute Confusion
Risk for Contamination
Risk for Compromised Human Dignity
Risk for Impaired Liver Function
Risk for Unstable Blood Glucose
Stress Overload

REVISED NURSING DIAGNOSES, 2007-2008

Acute Confusion
Complicated Grieving (previously titled *"Dysfunctional Grieving"*)
Death Anxiety
Decisional Conflict
Delayed Surgical Recovery
Grieving (previously titled *"Anticipatory Grieving"*)
Latex Allergy Response
Impaired Bed Mobility
Impaired Transfer Ability
Impaired Urinary Elimination
Impaired Walking
Impaired Wheelchair Mobility
Ineffective Denial
Ineffective Infant Feeding Pattern
Ineffective Sexuality Pattern
Insomnia (previously titled "disturbed sleep pattern")
Risk for Complicated Grieving (previously titled "risk for dysfunctional grieving")
Risk for Latex Allergy
Risk for Loneliness
Risk for Perioperative Positioning Injury
Risk for Poisoning
Risk-Prone Health Behavior (previously titled "Impaired Adjustment")
Sexual Dysfunction
Stress Urinary Incontinence
Unilateral Neglect
Urge Urinary Incontinence

NURSING DIAGNOSIS MANUAL
Planning, Individualizing,
and Documenting Client Care

EDITION TWO

DATE DUE

OCT 0 9 2008	
NOV 2 0 2008	
NOV 1 7 2010	
DEC 0 3 2011	
MAR 1 9 2012	
JUL 0 9 2012	
Oct. 23, 2012	
JAN 2 9 2014	
FEB 1 2 2014	
Nov. 17, 2014	
OCT 2 6 2018	

NURSING DIAGNOSIS MANUAL

Planning, Individualizing,
and Documenting Client Care

EDITION TWO

MARILYNN E. DOENGES, APN, BC-RETIRED

Clinical Specialist—Adult Psychiatric/Mental Health Nursing, Retired Adjunct Faculty
Beth-El College of Nursing and Health Sciences, CU-Springs
Colorado Springs, Colorado

MARY FRANCES MOORHOUSE, RN, MSN, CRRN, LNC

Nurse Consultant, TNT-RN Enterprises, Adjunct Nursing Faculty
Pikes Peak Community College,
Colorado Springs, Colorado

ALICE C. MURR, RN, BSN

Legal Nurse Consultant, Telephone Triage Nurse
Collins, Mississippi

F.A. Davis Company • Philadelphia

F. A. Davis Company
1915 Arch Street
Philadelphia, PA 19103
www.fadavis.com

Printed in the United States of America

Last digit indicates print number: 10 9 8 7 6 5 4 3 2 1

Publisher, Nursing: Joanne Patzek DaCunha, RN, MSN
Director of Content Development: Darlene D. Pedersen
Project Editor: Meghan K. Ziegler, Padraic J. Maroney
Design and Illustrations Manager: Carolyn O'Brien

As new scientific information becomes available through basic and clinical research, recommended treatments and drug therapies undergo changes. The author(s) and publisher have done everything possible to make this book accurate, up to date, and in accord with accepted standards at the time of publication. The author(s), editors, and publisher are not responsible for errors or omissions or for consequences from application of the book, and make no warranty, expressed or implied, in regard to the contents of the book. Any practice described in this book should be applied by the reader in accordance with professional standards of care used in regard to the unique circumstances that may apply in each situation. The reader is advised always to check product information (package inserts) for changes and new information regarding dose and contraindications before administering any drug. Caution is especially urged when using new or infrequently ordered drugs.

Library of Congress Cataloging-in-Publication Data

Doenges, Marilynn E., 1922-
 Nursing diagnosis manual: planning, individualizing, and documenting client care / Marilynn E. Doenges, Mary Frances Moorhouse, Alice C. Murr. – 2nd ed.
     p. ; cm.
   Includes bibliographical references and index.
   ISBN-13: 978-0-8036-1859-6
   ISBN-10: 0-8036-1859-X
 1. Nursing diagnosis–Handbooks, manuals, etc. 2. Nursing assessment–Handbooks, manuals, etc. 3. Nursing–Planning–Handbooks, manuals, etc. I. Moorhouse, Mary Frances, 1947- II. Geissler-Murr, Alice, 1946- III. Title.
   [DNLM: 1. Nursing Diagnosis. 2. Nursing Records. 3. Patient Care Planning. WY 100.4 D649n 2008]
   RT48.6.D643 2008
   616.07'5–dc22

                                                                                                2007050302

To our spo, children, parents, and friends, who much of time have had to manage without us while wek and dream, as well as cope with our struggles and frutions.

The Doengamilies: the late Dean, Jim; Barbara and Bob Lanza; id, Monita, Matthew and Tyler; John, Holly, Nicole, arelsey; and the Daigle families: Nancy, Jim; Jennifer, Blon, Annabelle, Will & Henry Smith-Daigle, and Jonan, Kim, and Mandalyn JoAn.

The Moorhe family: Jan; Paul; Jason, Thenderlyn, Alexa, and Marabella.

In loving mory of Gwenyth Loughmiller Lynn, beloved aunt, impacted my life choices in significant ways. First she a teacher and taught me to read. Then she became a ne and planted in me the desire to follow in her footstepse co-authored nursing education materials still used ay at Kettering Medical Center. Here I am and she has gone on. I miss her and nursing will miss her too. *Alice*

To our FAD family, especially Bob Martone; and to Alan Sorkowitz whose support, 'acupressure' and encouragement were so vital to the completion of a project of this magnitude. And now Joanne DaCunha and Jennifer Kowalak who assisted us in meeting deadlines and completing this new edition.

To the nurses we are writing for, who daily face the challenge of meeting the needs of clients in varied settings and are looking for a practical way to organize and document this care. We believe that nursing diagnosis and these guides will help.

And to NANDA-I and the International nurses who are facilitating the development and dissemination of nursing diagnoses—we continue to champion your efforts and the work of promoting standardized languages.

Preface

The American Nurses Association (ANA) Social Policy Statement of 1980 was the first to define nursing as the diagnosis and treatment of human responses to actual and potential health problems. This definition, when combined with the ANA Standards of Practice, has provided impetus and support for the use of nursing diagnosis. Defining nursing and its effect on client care supports the growing awareness that nursing care is a key factor in client survival and in the maintenance, rehabilitative, and preventive aspects of healthcare. Changes and new developments in healthcare delivery in the last decade have given rise to the need for a common framework of communication to ensure continuity of care for the client moving between multiple healthcare settings and providers.

This book is designed to aid the student nurse and the practitioner in identifying interventions commonly associated with specific nursing diagnoses as proposed by NANDA International (formerly the North American Nursing Diagnosis Association). These interventions are the activities needed to implement and document care provided to the individual client and can be used in varied settings from acute to community/home care.

Chapter 1 presents a brief discussion of the nursing process and introduces the concept of evidence-based practice. Standardized nursing languages (SNLs) are discussed in Chapter 2 with a focus on NANDA-I (nursing diagnoses), NIC (interventions), and NOC (outcomes). NANDA-I has 187 diagnosis labels with definitions, defining characteristics, and related or risk factors used to define a client need or problem. NIC is a comprehensive standardized language providing 514 direct and indirect intervention labels with definitions and a list of activities a nurse might choose to carry out each intervention. NOC language provides 330 outcome labels with definitions, a set of indicators describing specific client, caregiver, family, or community states related to the outcome, and a 5-point Likert-type measurement scale that can demonstrate client progress even when outcomes are not fully met. Chapter 3 addresses the assessment process using a nursing framework for data collection such as the Diagnostic Divisions Assessment Tool.

A creative approach for developing and documenting the planning of care is demonstrated in Chapter 4. Mind or Concept Mapping is a new technique or learning tool provided to assist you in achieving a holistic view of your client, enhance your critical thinking skills, and facilitate the creative process of planning client care. For more in-depth information and inclusive plans of care related to specific medical/psychiatric conditions (with rationale and the application of the diagnoses), the nurse is referred to the larger work also published by the F. A. Davis Company: Nursing Care Plans: Guidelines for Individualizing Client Care Across the Lifespan, ed. 7 (Doenges, Moorhouse, & Murr, 2006) which includes psychiatric/mental health and maternal/ newborn plans of care on the CD-ROM accompanying the text.

Chapter 6 contains 850 disorders/health conditions reflecting all specialty areas with associated nursing diagnoses written as client problem/need statements to aide you in validating the assessment and diagnosis steps of the nursing process.

In Chapter 5, the heart of the book, all the nursing diagnoses are listed alphabetically for ease of reference and include the diagnoses accepted for use by NANDA-I through 2007. The alphabetization of diagnoses follows NANDA-I's own sequencing, whereby diagnoses are alphabetized first by their key term, which is capitalized.

Subordinate terminology or descriptors of the diagnosis are presented in lowercase words and are alphabetized secondarily to the key term (for example, chronic Pain is alphabetized under P, following acute Pain). Each approved diagnosis includes its definition and information divided into the NANDA-I categories of Related or Risk Factors and Defining Characteristics. Related/Risk Factors information reflects causative or contributing factors that can be useful for determining whether the diagnosis is applicable to a particular client. Defining Characteristics (signs and symptoms or cues) are listed as subjective and/or objective and are used to confirm actual diagnoses, aid in formulating outcomes, and provide additional data for choosing appropriate interventions. We have not deleted or altered NANDA-I's listings; however, on occasion, we have added to their definitions and suggested additional criteria to provide clarification and direction. These additions are denoted with brackets [].

NANDA-I nursing diagnosis labels are designed to be multiaxial with 7 axes or descriptors. An axis is defined as a dimension of the human response that is considered in the diagnostic process (see Appendix). Sometimes an axis may be included in the diagnostic concept, such as ineffective community Coping in which the unit of care (i.e., community) is named. Some are implicit, such as Activity Intolerance in which the individual is the unit of care. At times an axis may not be pertinent to a particular diagnosis and will not be a part of the nursing diagnosis label. For example, the time frame (e.g., acute, intermittent) or body part (e.g., cerebral, oral, skin) may not be relevant to each diagnostic situation.

Desired Outcomes/Evaluation Criteria are identified to assist you in formulating individual client outcomes and to support the evaluation process. Suggested NOC linkages to the nursing diagnosis are provided.

Nursing priorities are used to group the suggested interventions, which are primarily directed to adult care, although interventions designated as across the lifespan do include pediatric and geriatric considerations and are designated by an icon. In general, the interventions can be used in multiple settings—acute care, rehabilitation, community clinics, home care, or private practice. Most interventions are independent or nursing originated, however, some interventions are collaborative orders (e.g., medical, psychiatric), and you will need to determine when this is necessary and take the appropriate action. Icons are also used to differentiate collaborative interventions, diagnostic studies and medications, as well as transcultural considerations. All of these "specialized" interventions are presented with icons, rather than being broken out under separate headings, to maintain their sequence within the prioritization of all nursing interventions for the diagnosis. Although all defining characteristics are listed, interventions that address specialty areas outside the scope of this book are not routinely presented (e.g., obstetrics/pediatrics) except for diagnoses that are infancy-oriented, such as ineffective Breastfeeding, disorganized Infant Behavior, and risk for impaired parent/child Attachment. For example, when addressing deficient [isotonic] Fluid Volume (such as related to hemorrhage), the nurse is directed to stop blood loss; however, specific direction to perform fundal massage is not listed. Additionally, in support of evidence-based practice, rationales are provided for the interventions and references for these rationales are cited.

The inclusion of Documentation Focus suggestions is to remind you of the importance and necessity of recording the steps of the nursing process.

As noted, with few exceptions, we have presented NANDA-I's recommendations as formulated. We support the belief that practicing nurses and researchers need to study, use, and evaluate the diagnoses as presented. Nurses can be creative as they use the standardized language, redefining and sharing information as the diagnoses are used with individual clients. As new nursing diagnoses are developed, it is important that the data they encompass are added to assessment tools and current data base. As part of the process by clinicians, educators, and researchers across practice specialties and academic settings to define, test, and refine nursing diagnosis, nurses are encouraged to share insights and ideas with NANDA-I at the following address: NANDA International, 100 North 20th Street, 4th Floor, Philadelphia, PA 19103; e-mail: info@nanda.org

Marilynn E. Doenges
Mary Frances Moorhouse
Alice C. Murr

Contributors

Diane Bligh, RN, MS, CNS
Associate Professor, Nursing
Front Range Community College
Westminster, Colorado
   Co-author of Chapter 4: Concept Mapping to Create
   and Document the Plan of Care

Mary F. Johnston, RN, MSN
Program Director, Nursing
Front Range Community College
Westminster, Colorado
   Co-author of Chapter 4: Concept Mapping to Create
   and Document the Plan of Care

Sheila Marquez, RN, BSN, PNP
Executive Director
Vice President/Chief Operating Officer
The Colorado SIDS Program, Inc.

Denver, Colorado
   Contributor of Chapter 5 monograph on Risk for
   Sudden Infant Death Syndrome

Susan Moberly, RNC, BSN, ICCE (Deceased)
Childbirth Educator
Obstetric Nursing and Lactation Consultant
Colorado Springs, Colorado
   Contributor of Chapter 5 monographs related to
   Breastfeeding

Alma Mueller, RN, MEd
Retired Chair and Professor of Nursing
Front Range Community College
Westminster, Colorado
   Co-author of Chapter 4: Concept Mapping to Create
   and Document the Plan of Care

Contents

Chapter 1

The Nursing Process:
The Foundation of Quality Client Care

Defining the Profession

In the world of healthcare, nursing has long struggled to establish itself as a profession. Dictionary terms describe nursing as "a calling requiring specialized knowledge and often long and intensive academic preparation; a principal calling, vocation, or employment; the whole body of persons engaged in a calling."[1] Throughout the history of nursing, unfavorable stereotypes (based on the view of nursing as subservient and dependent on the medical profession) have negatively affected the view of nursing as an independent entity. In its early developmental years, nursing did not seek or have the means to control its own practice. Florence Nightingale, in discussing the nature of nursing in 1859, observed that "nursing has been limited to signify little more than the administration of medicines and the application of poultices."[2] Although this attitude may still persist to some degree, the nursing profession has defined what makes nursing unique and has identified a body of professional knowledge. As early as 1896, nurses in America banded together to seek standardization of educational programs and laws governing their practice. The task of nursing since that time has been to create descriptive terminology reflecting specific nursing functions and levels of competency.[3] Erickson, Tomlin, and Swain believe "nursing will thrive as a unique and valued profession when nurses present a theory and rationalistic model for their practice, correct misleading stereotypes, locate control with clients, and actively participate in processes for change."[4]

In the past several decades, more than a dozen prominent nursing scholars (e.g., Rogers, Parse, Henderson) have developed conceptualizations to define the nature of nursing. Because much of nursing is nonphenomenological or nonobservable, the nature of nursing cannot be explained using the usual parameters of scientific investigation. In her article, Kikuchi proposes that conceptualizations about nursing are philosophic in nature and as such are still testable.[5] As nursing research continues the work of establishing the profession as independent in its own right, the value of nursing goals is understood and the difference between nursing and other professions is being delineated. Nursing is now recognized as both a science and an art concerned with the physical, psychological, sociological, cultural, and spiritual concerns of the individual. The science of nursing is based on a broad theoretical framework; its art depends on the caring skills and abilities of the individual nurse. The importance of the nurse within the healthcare system is noted in many positive ways, and the profession of nursing is acknowledging the need for its practitioners to act professionally and be accountable for the care they provide.

Barely a century after Miss Nightingale noted that "the very elements of nursing are all but unknown," the American Nurses Association (ANA) developed their first Social Policy Statement in 1980, defining nursing as "the diagnosis and treatment of *human responses* to actual or potential health problems."[6] Human responses (defined as people's experiences with and responses to health, illness, and life events) are nursing's phenomena of concern. In 1995, this statement was revisited, updated, and titled "Nursing's Social Policy Statement." The new policy statement acknowledged that since the release of the original statement, "nursing has been influenced by many social and professional changes, as well as by the science of caring."[7]

The statement delineated four essential features of today's contemporary nursing practice:

1. Attention to the full range of human experiences and responses to health and illness without restriction to a problem-focused orientation
2. Integration of objective data with knowledge gained from an understanding of the client's or group's subjective experience
3. Application of scientific knowledge to the processes of diagnosis and treatment
4. Provision of a caring relationship that facilitates health and healing[7]

Thus, nursing's role includes promotion of health as well as performance of activities that contribute to recovery from or adjustment to illness. This is reflected in ANA's 2003 Nursing's Social Policy Statement, which recognizes nursing's full scope of care by defining nursing as "the protection, promotion, and optimization of health and abilities, prevention of illness and injury, alleviation of suffering through the diagnosis and treatment of human response, and advocacy in the care of individuals, families, communities, and populations."[21] Also, nurses support the right of clients to define their own health-related goals and to engage in care that reflects their personal values. Emphasis is placed on the mind-body-spirit connection with a holistic view of the individual as nurses facilitate the client's efforts in striving for growth and development.

In your readings, you will likely encounter other definitions of nursing. As your knowledge and experience develops, your definition of nursing may change to reflect your personal nursing philosophy, your focus on a particular care setting or population, or your specific role. For example, although the definition of nursing developed by Erickson, Tomlin, and Swain is more than 20 years old, it remains viable and timely because it incorporates the concepts noted previously with today's holistic approach to care. Their definition includes what nursing is, how it is accomplished, and the goals of nursing: "Nursing is the holistic helping of persons with their self-care activities in relation to their health. This is an interactive, interpersonal process that nurtures strengths to enable development, release, and channeling of resources for coping with one's circumstances and environment. The goal is to achieve a state of perceived optimum health and contentment."[4]

An understanding of human nature is certainly important in the development of a philosophy of nursing. Understanding that "needs motivate behavior" helps the nurse to determine the client's needs at a particular moment in time. Maslow's hierarchy of needs[20] provides a basis for understanding that unmet needs can interfere with an individual's holistic growth and may even result in physical/mental distress or illness. Other theorists have also studied how people are similar, providing the nurse with more information to help understand the client. For example, Erik Erikson's observations on the stages of psychological development suggest that the individual is a "work in progress" accomplishing age-specific maturational tasks throughout the life span. Piaget's cognitive stages address how thinking develops and how individuals adapt to and organize their environment intellectually.[4] However, in the end, the individual is the primary source of information about himself/herself. The nurse needs to listen with an open mind and empathic, unconditional acceptance to what the client is relating. Knowing how people are alike provides a basis to understanding human nature. However, each person is unique, and the nurse needs to look for the client's model of the world and how this relates to the client's own situation.

The nursing profession is further defined by fundamental philosophical beliefs that have been identified over time as essential to the practice of nursing and expanded by the Nursing's Social Policy Statement (ANA, 1995). These values and assumptions offer guidance to the nurse and need to be kept in mind to enhance the quality of nursing care provided:

- The client is a human being who has worth and dignity.
- Humans manifest an essential unity of mind/body/spirit.[7]
- There are basic human needs that must be met (Maslow's hierarchy).
- When these needs are not met, problems arise that may require intervention by another person until the individuals can resume responsibility for themselves.
- Human experience is contextually and culturally defined.[7]
- Health and illness are human experiences.[7]
- Clients have a right to quality health and nursing care delivered with interest, compassion, and competence with a focus on wellness and prevention.
- The presence of illness does not preclude health, nor does optimal health preclude illness.[7]
- The therapeutic nurse-client relationship is important in the nursing process and provision of individualized care.

Finally, the Code of Ethics for Nurses[8] addresses the need for nurses to respect human dignity, acknowledge the uniqueness of each client, and honor the client's right to privacy. The Code also calls on nurses to assume responsibility for individual nursing judgments and actions and for the delegation of nursing activities to others. Nurses are encouraged to maintain competence in nursing, contribute to the ongoing development of the profession, and participate in implementation and improvement of standards. This last goal can be accomplished by using the results of nursing research to engage in evidence-based nursing practice.

The roots of evidence-based practice lie in the efforts of many in the past. Hippocrates described the symptoms and course of illnesses and related them to the seasons, geographical area, and types of people associated with each. These hypotheses founded the rational approach to the understanding of disease. As knowledge grew and the germ theory of disease was accepted, epidemiology began to count disease events, leading to the establishment of a central government agency to collect and record data. This led to the posing of questions in the form of testable hypotheses, the collection of data to support or refute hypotheses, and the development of statistical tools to summarize numerical data.[9] The work of Pasteur and Koch expanded the understanding of causal relationships between bacterial causes of many diseases, leading to reducing illness and mortality.

Florence Nightingale used statistics to measure health, identify causes of mortality, evaluate health services, and reform institutions. After the Crimean War, she began organizing committees, assembling data, and preparing reports and hearings on how administrative inadequacies affected clients' health. Her work resulted in British Army Hospital and government reform in the interest of preventing death and disease. She became an honorary member of the American Statistical Association in 1874, and her papers were read at a National Social Science Congress in 1863 and at the nurses' congress of the Chicago World's Fair in 1893. The efforts of these pioneers laid the groundwork for the development of evidence-based practice.

Barnsteiner and Provost note "the current definition [of evidence-based practice] is the integration of best research evidence with clinical expertise and patient values"[10]—that is, both research and nonresearch components are combined to create evidence-based practice. Quantitative research is invaluable in measuring the effectiveness of nursing interventions while qualitative studies capture the preferences, attitudes, and values of healthcare consumers. However, the nurses' clinical judgment and individual client needs and perspectives must also be included. As nurses work to provide cost-effective care in the best setting for the client, "the most important [and challenging] requirement for practicing nurses in the 21st century will be to utilize [appropriate] evidence available to improve practice."[11]

Administering Nursing Care

Nursing leaders have identified a process that "combines the most desirable elements of the art of nursing with the most relevant elements of systems theory, using the scientific method."[12] This *nursing process* incorporates an interactive/interpersonal approach with a problem-solving and decision-making process that serves as a framework for the delivery of nursing care.[13–15]

The concept of nursing process was first introduced in the 1950s as a three-step process of assessment, planning, and evaluation based on the scientific method of observing, measuring, gathering data, and analyzing the findings. Years of study, use, and refinement have led nurses to expand the nursing process to five distinct steps that provide an efficient method of organizing thought processes for clinical decision making, problem-solving, and delivery of higher-quality, individualized client care. The nursing process now consists of

- *assessment* or the systematic collection of data relating to clients;
- *diagnosis/need identification* involving the analysis of collected data to identify the client's needs or problems;
- *planning,* which is a two-part process of identifying goals and the client's desired outcomes to address the assessed health and wellness needs along with the selection of appropriate nursing interventions to assist the client in attaining the outcomes;
- *implementation* or putting the plan of care into action; and
- *evaluation* by determining the client's progress toward attaining the identified outcomes, and the client's response to and effectiveness of the selected nursing interventions for the purpose of altering the plan as indicated.

Because these five steps are central to nursing actions in any setting, the nursing process is now included in the conceptual framework of nursing curricula and is accepted as part of the legal definition of nursing in the Nurse Practice Acts of most states.

When a client enters the healthcare system, whether as an inpatient, a clinic outpatient, or a home-care client, the nursing process steps are set into motion. The nurse collects data, identifies client needs (nursing diagnoses), establishes goals, creates measurable outcomes, and selects nursing interventions to assist the client in achieving these outcomes and goals. Finally, after the interventions have been implemented, the nurse evaluates the client's responses and the effectiveness of the plan of care in reaching the desired outcomes and goals to determine whether or not the needs or problems have been resolved and the client is ready to be discharged from the care setting. If the identified needs or problems remain unresolved, further assessment, additional nursing diagnoses, alteration of outcomes and goals, or changes of interventions are required.

Although we use the terms *assessment, diagnosis, planning, implementation,* and *evaluation* as separate, progressive steps, in reality they are interrelated. Together these steps form a continuous circle of thought and action, which recycles throughout the client's contact with the healthcare system. Figure 1–1 depicts a model for visualizing this process. You can see that the nursing process uses the nursing diagnosis (the clinical judgment product of critical thinking). Based on this judgment, nursing interventions are selected and implemented. Figure 1–1 also shows how the progressive steps of the nursing process create an understandable model of both the products and the processes of critical thinking contained within the nursing process. The model graphically emphasizes both the dynamic and cyclic characteristics of the nursing process.

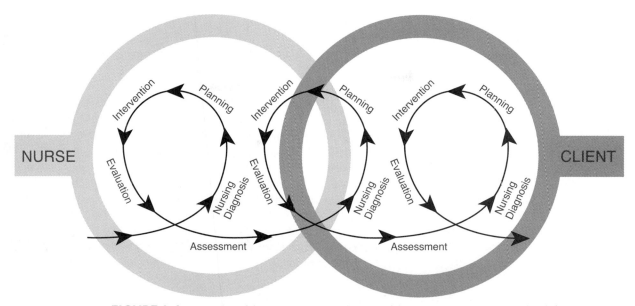

FIGURE 1–1 • Diagram of the nursing process. The steps of the nursing process are interrelated, forming a continuous circle of thought and action that is both dynamic and cyclic.

Application of the Nursing Process

The scientific method of problem-solving introduced in the previous section is used almost instinctively by most people, without conscious awareness.

> **FOR EXAMPLE** While studying for your semester finals, you snack on pepperoni pizza. After going to bed, you are awakened by a burning sensation in the center of your chest. You are young and in good health and note no other symptoms (assessment). You decide that your pain is the result of the spicy food you have eaten (diagnosis). You then determine that before you can return to sleep, you first need to relieve the discomfort with an over-the-counter preparation (planning). You take a liquid antacid for your discomfort (implementation). Within a few minutes, you note the burning sensation is relieved, and you return to bed without further concern (evaluation).

As you see, this is a process you routinely use to solve problems in your life that can be readily applied to client-care situations. You need only to learn the new terms describing the nursing process, rather than having to think about each step (assessment, diagnosis/need identification, planning, implementation, and evaluation) in an entirely new way.

To effectively use the nursing process, the nurse needs to possess and apply some basic abilities. Particularly important is a thorough knowledge of science and theory, not only as applied in nursing but also in other related disciplines such as medicine and psychology. Creativity is needed in the application of nursing knowledge as well as adaptability in handling change and the many unexpected happenings that occur. As a nurse, you must make a commitment to practice your profession in the best possible way, trusting in yourself and your ability to do your job well and displaying the necessary leadership to organize and supervise as your position requires. In addition, intelligence, well-developed interpersonal skills, and competent technical skills are essential.

FOR EXAMPLE A diabetic client's irritable behavior could be the result of low serum glucose or the effects of excessive caffeine intake. However, it could also arise from a sense of helplessness regarding life events. A single behavior may have varied causes. It is important that your nursing assessment skills identify the underlying etiology to provide appropriate care.

The practice responsibilities presented in the definitions of nursing and the nursing process are explained in detail in the publication *Nursing: Scope & Standards of Practice*.[16] The standards provide workable guidelines to ensure that the practice of nursing can be carried out by each nurse. Table 1–1 presents an abbreviated description of the standards of clinical practice. With the ultimate goal of quality healthcare, the effective use of the nursing process will result in a viable nursing-care system that is recognized and accepted as nursing's body of knowledge and that can be shared with other healthcare professionals.

TABLE 1–1

ANA STANDARDS OF NURSING PRACTICE

Standards of Practice
Describes a competent level of nursing care as demonstrated by the nursing process that encompasses all significant actions taken by the nurse in providing care and forms the foundation of clinical decision making.

1. Assessment: The registered nurse collects comprehensive data pertinent to the patient's health or situation.
2. Diagnosis: The registered nurse analyzes the assessment data to determine the diagnoses or issues.
3. Outcome Identification: The registered nurse identifies expected outcomes for a plan individualized to the patient or the situation.
4. Planning: The registered nurse develops a plan that prescribes strategies and alternatives to attain expected outcomes.
5. Implementation: The registered nurse implements the identified plan.
    a. Coordination of Care: The registered nurse coordinates care delivery.
    b. Health Teaching and Health Promotion: The registered nurse employs strategies to promote health and a safe environment.
    c. Consultation: The advanced practice registered nurse and the nursing role specialist provide consultation to influence the identified plan, enhance the abilities of others, and effect change.
    d. Prescriptive Authority and Treatment: The advanced practice registered nurse uses prescriptive authority, procedures, referrals, treatments, and therapies in accordance with state and federal laws and regulations.
6. Evaluation: The registered nurse evaluates progress toward attainment of outcomes.

Standards of Professional Performance
Describes roles expected of all professional nurses appropriate to their education, position, and practice setting.

7. Quality of Practice: The registered nurse systematically enhances the quality and effectiveness of nursing practice.
8. Education: The registered nurse attains knowledge and competency that reflects current nursing practice.
9. Professional Practice Evaluation: The registered nurse evaluates one's own nursing practice in relation to professional practice standards and guidelines, relevant statutes, rules, and regulations.
10. Collegiality: The registered nurse interacts with and contributes to the professional development of peers and colleagues.
11. Collaboration: The registered nurse collaborates with patient, family, and others in the conduct of nursing practice.
12. Ethics: The registered nurse integrates ethical provisions in all areas of practice.
13. Research: The registered nurse integrates research findings into practice.
14. Resource Utilization: The registered nurse considers factors related to safety, effectiveness, cost, and impact on practice in the planning and delivery of nursing services.
15. Leadership: The registered nurse provides leadership in the professional practice setting and the profession.

Source: American Nurses Association. (2004). *Nursing: Scope & Standards of Practice*. Silver Spring, MD: Nursesbooks.org.

Advantages of Using the Nursing Process

There are many advantages to the use of the nursing process:

- The nursing process provides an organizing framework for meeting the individual needs of the client, the client's family/significant other(s), and the community.
- The steps of the nursing process focus the nurse's attention on the "individual" human responses of a client/group to a given health situation, resulting in a holistic plan of care addressing the specific needs of the client/group.
- The nursing process provides an organized, systematic method of problem-solving (while still allowing for creative solutions) that may minimize dangerous errors or omissions in caregiving and avoid time-consuming repetition in care and documentation.
- The use of the nursing process promotes the active involvement of clients in their health-care, enhancing consumer satisfaction. Such participation increases clients' sense of control over what is happening to them, stimulates problem-solving, and promotes personal responsibility, all of which strengthen the client's commitment to achieving the identified goals.
- The use of the nursing process enables you as a nurse to have more control over your practice. This enhances the opportunity for you to use your knowledge, expertise, and intuition constructively and dynamically to increase the likelihood of a successful client outcome. This, in turn, promotes greater job satisfaction and your professional growth.
- The use of the nursing process provides a common language (nursing diagnosis) for practice, unifying the nursing profession. Using a system that clearly communicates the plan of care to coworkers and clients enhances continuity of care, promotes achievement of client goals, provides a vehicle for evaluation, and aids in the development of nursing standards. In addition, the structure of the process provides a format for documenting the client's response to all aspects of the planned care.
- The use of the nursing process provides a means of assessing nursing's economic contribution to client care. The nursing process supplies a vehicle for the quantitative and qualitative measurement of nursing care that meets the goal of cost-effectiveness and still promotes holistic care.

Summary

Nursing is continuing to evolve into a well-defined profession with a more clearly delineated definition and phenomena of concern. Fundamental philosophical beliefs and qualities have been identified that are important for the nurse to possess in order to provide quality care.

The nursing profession has developed a body of knowledge that contributes to the growth and well-being of the individual and the community, the prevention of illness, and the maintenance and/or restoration of health (or relief of pain/discomfort and provision of support when a return to health is not possible). The nursing process is the basis of all nursing actions and is the essence of nursing, providing a flexible, orderly, logical problem-solving approach for administering nursing care so that client (whether individual, community, or population) needs for such care are met comprehensively and effectively. It can be applied in any healthcare or educational setting, in any theoretical or conceptual framework, and within the context of any nursing philosophy.

Each step of the nursing process builds on and interacts with the other steps, ensuring an effective practice model. Inclusion of the standards of clinical nursing practice provides additional information to reinforce understanding and opportunities to apply knowledge.

Please note, the term *client* is used in this book rather than *patient* to reflect the philosophy that the individuals or groups you work with are legitimate members of the decision-making process with some degree of control over the planned regimen and as able, active participants in the planning and implementation of their care.[4]

Next, we will introduce the language described in the nursing process. This includes NANDA (formerly the North American Nursing Diagnosis Association) International Inc.'s classification of nursing diagnoses,[17] the Iowa Intervention and Outcome Projects: Nursing Intervention Classification (NIC),[18] and the Nursing Outcomes Classification (NOC).[19] NANDA, NIC, and NOC have combined their classification systems (NNN Alliance) to provide a comprehensive nursing language.

References

1. Merriam-Webster Online Dictionary. Available at www.m-w.com/dictionary.htm. Accessed on May 7, 2003.
2. Nightingale, F. (1859). *Notes on Nursing: What It Is and What It Is Not* (Facsimile edition). Philadelphia: J.B. Lippincott, 1946.
3. Jacobi, E. M. (1976). Foreword. In Flanigan, L. (ed.). *One Strong Voice: The Story of the American Nurses' Association*. Kansas City, MO: American Nurses' Association.
4. Erickson, H. C., Tomlin, E. M., Swain, M. A. P. (1983). *Modeling and Role-Modeling*. Englewood Cliffs, NJ: Prentice-Hall.
5. Kikuchi, J. F. (1999). Clarifying the nature of conceptualizations about nursing. *Canadian J Nurs Research*, 30(4), 115–128.
6. American Nurses Association. (1980). *Nursing: A Social Policy Statement*. Kansas City, MO: Author.
7. American Nurses Association. (1995). *Nursing's Social Policy Statement*. Washington, DC: American Nurses Publishing.
8. American Nurses Association. (2001). *Code of Ethics for Nurses*. Washington, DC: American Nurses Publishing.
9. Stolley, P. D., Lasky, T. (1995). *Investigating Disease Patterns: The Science of Epidemiology* (Scientific American Library, no. 57). New York: WH Freeman.
10. Barnsteiner, J., Provost, S. (2002). How to implement evidence-based practice: Some tried and true pointers. *Reflections on Nursing Leadership*, 28(2), 18.
11. Amarsi, Y. (2002). Evidence-based nursing: Perspective from Pakistan. *Reflections on Nursing Leasership*, 28(2), 28.
12. Shore, L. S. (1988). *Nursing Diagnosis: What It Is and How to Do It, a Programmed Text*. Richmond, VA: Medical College of Virginia Hospitals.
13. Peplau, H. E. (1952). *Interpersonal Relations in Nursing: A Conceptual Frame of Reference for Psychodynamic Nursing*. New York: Putnam.
14. King, L. (1971). *Toward a Theory for Nursing: General Concepts of Human Behavior*. New York: Wiley.
15. Yura, H., Walsh, M. B. (1988). *The Nursing Process: Assessing, Planning, Implementing, Evaluating*. 5th ed. Norwalk, CT: Appleton & Lange.
16. American Nurses Association. (2004). *Nursing: Scope and Standards of Practice*. Nursesbooks.org.
17. North American Nursing Diagnosis Association. (2001). *Nursing Diagnoses: Definitions & Classification*. Philadelphia: Author.
18. McCloskey, J. C., Bulecheck, G. M. (2000). *Nursing Interventions Classification (NIC)*. 3d ed. St. Louis, MO: Mosby.
19. Johnson, M., Maas, M., Moorhead, S. (2000). *Nursing Outcomes Classification (NOC)*. 2d ed. St. Louis, MO: Mosby.
20. Maslow, A. H. (1970). *Motivation and Personality*. 2d ed. New York: Harper & Row.
21. American Nurses Association. (2003). *Nursing's Social Policy Statement*. Washington, DC: Nursesbooks.org.

Chapter 2

The Language of Nursing: NANDA, NIC, NOC, and Other Standardized Nursing Languages

In this chapter, we will look at the process and progress of describing the work of nursing. At first glance, it seems a simple task. However, over many years, the profession has struggled with it. The struggle, in part, is a result of changes in healthcare delivery and financing, the expansion of nursing's role, and the dawning of the computer age. Gordon reminds us that classification system development parallels knowledge development in a discipline.[1] As theory development and research have begun to define nursing, it has become necessary for nursing to find a common language to describe what nursing is, what nursing does, and how to codify it. Thus, the terms "classification systems" and "standardized language" were born, and the work continues.

Changes in the healthcare system occur at an ever-increasing rate. One of these changes is the movement toward a paperless (computerized or electronic) client record. The use of electronic healthcare information systems is rapidly expanding, and the focus has shifted from its original uses—financial and personnel management functions—to the efficient documentation of the client encounter, whether that is a single office visit or a lengthy hospitalization. The move to electronic documentation is being fueled by changes in healthcare delivery and reimbursement as well as the advent of alternative healthcare settings (outpatient surgeries, home health, rehabilitation or subacute units, extended or long-term care facilities, etc.), all of which increase the need for a commonality of communication to ensure continuity of care for the client, who moves from one setting or level of care to another.

These changes in the business and documentation of healthcare require the industry to generate data about its operations and outcomes. Evaluation and improvement of provided services are important to the delivery of cost-effective client care. Therefore, providers and consumers interested in outcomes of care benefit from accurate documentation of the care provided and the client's response. With the use of language or terminology that can be coded, healthcare information can be recorded in terms that are universal and easily entered into an electronic database and that can generate meaningful reporting data about its operation and outcomes. In short, standardized language is required.

A standardized language contains formalized terms that have definitions and guidelines for use. For example, if the impact of nursing care on financial and clinical outcomes is to be analyzed, coding of this information is essential. While it has been relatively easy to code medical procedures, nursing is more of an enigma, because its work has not been so clearly defined.

Since the 1970s, nursing leaders have been working to define the profession of nursing and to develop a commonality of words describing practice (a framework of communication and documentation) so that nursing's contribution to healthcare is captured, is visible in healthcare databases, and is thereby recognized as essential. Therefore, the focus of the profession has been on the effort to classify tasks and to develop standardized nursing languages (SNLs) to better demonstrate what nursing is and what nursing does.

Around the world, nursing researchers continue their efforts to identify and label people's experiences with (and responses to) health and illness as they relate to the scope of nursing practice. The use of universal nursing terminology directs our focus to the central content and process of nursing care by identifying, naming, and standardizing the "what" and "how" of the work of nursing—including both direct and indirect activities. This wider application for a standardized language has spurred its development.

A recognized pioneer in SNL is NANDA International's (formerly North American Nursing Diagnosis Association) "nursing diagnosis."[2] Simply stated, a nursing diagnosis is defined as a clinical judgment about individual, family, or community responses to actual or potential health problems/life processes. Nursing diagnoses provide the basis for selecting nursing interventions to achieve outcomes for which the nurse is accountable.[3] NANDA-I nursing diagnoses currently include 188 labels with definitions, defining characteristics, and related or risk factors used to define a client need or problem. Once the client's need is defined, outcomes can be developed and nursing interventions chosen to achieve the desired outcomes.

The linkage of client problems or nursing diagnoses to specific nursing interventions and client outcomes has led to the development of several other SNLs, including Home Health Care Classification (HHCC;[4] now Clinical Care Classification),[12] Nursing Interventions Classification (NIC),[5] Nursing Outcomes Classification NOC),[6] Omaha System-Community Health Classification System (OS),[7] Patient Care Data Set (PCDS),[8] and Perioperative Nursing Data Set (PNDS).[9]

Whereas some of these languages (e.g., OS, PCDS, and PNDS) are designed for a specific client population, the NANDA, NIC, and NOC languages are comprehensively designed for use across systems and settings and at individual, family, and community or population levels.[10]

NIC is a comprehensive standardized language providing 514 direct and indirect intervention labels with definitions (Table 2–1). A list of activities a nurse might choose to carry out each intervention is also provided and can be modified as necessary to meet the specific needs of the client. These research-based interventions address general practice and specialty areas.

TABLE 2–1

NURSING INTERVENTIONS CLASSIFICATION LABELS

Abuse Protection Support	Acid-Base Monitoring
Abuse Protection Support: Child	Active Listening
Abuse Protection Support: Domestic Partner	Activity Therapy
Abuse Protection Support: Elder	Acupressure
Abuse Protection Support: Religious	Admission Care
Acid-Base Management	Airway Insertion and Stabilization
Acid-Base Management: Metabolic Acidosis	Airway Management
Acid-Base Management: Metabolic Alkalosis	Airway Suctioning
Acid-Base Management: Respiratory Acidosis	Allergy Management
Acid-Base Management: Respiratory Alkalosis	Amnioinfusion

Amputation Care
Analgesic Administration
Analgesic Administration: Intraspinal
Anaphylaxis Management
Anesthesia Administration
Anger Control Assistance
Animal-Assisted Therapy
Anticipatory Guidance
Anxiety Reduction
Area Restriction
Aromatherapy
Artificial Airway Management
Art Therapy
Aspiration Precautions
Assertiveness Training
Asthma Management
Attachment Promotion
Autogenic Training
Autotransfusion

Bathing
Bed Rest Care
Bedside Laboratory Testing
Behavior Management
Behavior Management: Overactivity/Inattention
Behavior Management: Self-Harm
Behavior Management: Sexual
Behavior Modification
Behavior Modification: Social Skills
Bibliotherapy
Biofeedback
Bioterrorism Preparedness
Birthing
Bladder Irrigation
Bleeding Precautions
Bleeding Reduction
Bleeding Reduction: Antepartum Uterus
Bleeding Reduction: Gastrointestinal
Bleeding Reduction: Nasal
Bleeding Reduction: Postpartum Uterus
Bleeding Reduction: Wound
Blood Products Administration
Body Image Enhancement
Body Mechanics Promotion
Bottle Feeding

Bowel Incontinence Care
Bowel Incontinence Care: Encopresis
Bowel Irrigation
Bowel Management
Bowel Training
Breast Examination
Breastfeeding Assistance

Calming Technique
Capillary Blood Sample
Cardiac Care
Cardiac Care: Acute
Cardiac Care: Rehabilitation
Cardiac Precautions
Caregiver Support
Care Management
Cast Care: Maintenance
Cast Care: Wet
Cerebral Edema Management
Cerebral Perfusion Promotion
Cesarean Section Care
Chemical Restraint
Chemotherapy Management
Chest Physiotherapy
Childbirth Preparation
Circulatory Care: Arterial Insufficiency
Circulatory Care: Mechanical Assist Device
Circulatory Care: Venous Insufficiency
Circulatory Precautions
Circumcision Care
Code Management
Cognitive Restructuring
Cognitive Stimulation
Communicable Disease Management
Communication Enhancement: Hearing Deficit
Communication Enhancement: Speech Deficit
Communication Enhancement: Visual Deficit
Community Disaster Preparedness
Community Health Development
Complex Relationship Building
Conflict Mediation
Constipation/Impaction Management
Consultation
Contact Lens Care
Controlled Substance Checking

continued

TABLE 2–1   *continued*

Coping Enhancement
Cost Containment
Cough Enhancement
Counseling
Crisis Intervention
Critical Path Development
Culture Brokerage
Cutaneous Stimulation

Decision-Making Support
Delegation
Delirium Management
Delusion Management
Dementia Management
Dementia Management: Bathing
Deposition/Testimony
Developmental Care
Developmental Enhancement: Adolescent
Developmental Enhancement: Child
Dialysis Access Maintenance
Diarrhea Management
Diet Staging
Discharge Planning
Distraction
Documentation
Dressing
Dying Care
Dysreflexia Management
Dysrhythmia Management

Ear Care
Eating Disorders Management
Electroconvulsive Therapy Management
Electrolyte Management
Electrolyte Management: Hypercalcemia
Electrolyte Management: Hyperkalemia
Electrolyte Management: Hypermagnesemia
Electrolyte Management: Hypernatremia
Electrolyte Management: Hyperphosphatemia
Electrolyte Management: Hypocalcemia
Electrolyte Management: Hypokalemia
Electrolyte Management: Hypomagnesemia
Electrolyte Management: Hyponatremia
Electrolyte Management: Hypophosphatemia

Electrolyte Monitoring
Electronic Fetal Monitoring: Antepartum
Electronic Fetal Monitoring: Intrapartum
Elopement Precautions
Embolus Care: Peripheral
Embolus Care: Pulmonary
Embolus Precautions
Emergency Care
Emergency Cart Checking
Emotional Support
Endotracheal Extubation
Energy Management
Enteral Tube Feeding
Environmental Management
Environmental Management: Attachment Process
Environmental Management: Comfort
Environmental Management: Community
Environmental Management: Home Preparation
Environmental Management: Safety
Environmental Management: Violence Prevention
Environmental Management: Worker Safety
Environmental Risk Protection
Examination Assistance
Exercise Promotion
Exercise Promotion: Strength Training
Exercise Promotion: Stretching
Exercise Therapy: Ambulation
Exercise Therapy: Balance
Exercise Therapy: Joint Mobility
Exercise Therapy: Muscle Control
Eye Care

Fall Prevention
Family Integrity Promotion
Family Integrity Promotion: Childbearing Family
Family Involvement Promotion
Family Mobilization
Family Planning: Contraception
Family Planning: Infertility
Family Planning: Unplanned Pregnancy
Family Presence Facilitation
Family Process Maintenance
Family Support
Family Therapy

Feeding
Fertility Preservation
Fever Treatment
Financial Resource Assistance
Fire-Setting Precautions
First Aid
Fiscal Resource Management
Flatulence Reduction
Fluid/Electrolyte Management
Fluid Management
Fluid Monitoring
Fluid Resuscitation
Foot Care
Forgiveness Facilitation

Gastrointestinal Intubation
Genetic Counseling
Grief Work Facilitation
Grief Work Facilitation: Perinatal Death
Guilt Work Facilitation

Hair Care
Hallucination Management
Healthcare Information Exchange
Health Education
Health Policy Monitoring
Health Screening
Health System Guidance
Heat/Cold Application
Heat Exposure Treatment
Hemodialysis Therapy
Hemodynamic Regulation
Hemofiltration Therapy
Hemorrhage Control
High-Risk Pregnancy Care
Home Maintenance Assistance
Hope Instillation
Hormone Replacement Therapy
Humor
Hyperglycemia Management
Hypervolemia Management
Hypnosis
Hypoglycemia Management
Hypothermia Treatment
Hypovolemia Management

Immunization/Vaccination Management
Impulse Control Training
Incident Reporting
Incision Site Care
Infant Care
Infection Control
Infection Control: Intraoperative
Infection Protection
Insurance Authorization
Intracranial Pressure (ICP) Monitoring
Intrapartal Care
Intrapartal Care: High-Risk Delivery
Intravenous (IV) Insertion
Intravenous (IV) Therapy
Invasive Hemodynamic Monitoring

Kangaroo Care

Labor Induction
Labor Suppression
Laboratory Data Interpretation
Lactation Counseling
Lactation Suppression
Laser Precautions
Latex Precautions
Learning Facilitation
Learning Readiness Enhancement
Leech Therapy
Limit Setting
Lower Extremity Monitoring

Malignant Hyperthermia Precautions
Mechanical Ventilation
Mechanical Ventilatory Weaning
Medication Administration
Medication Administration: Ear
Medication Administration: Enteral
Medication Administration: Eye
Medication Administration: Inhalation
Medication Administration: Interpleural
Medication Administration: Intradermal
Medication Administration: Intramuscular (IM)
Medication Administration: Intraosseous
Medication Administration: Intraspinal
Medication Administration: Intravenous (IV)

continued

TABLE 2–1   *continued*

Medication Administration: Nasal

Medication Administration: Oral

Medication Administration: Rectal

Medication Administration: Skin

Medication Administration: Subcutaneous

Medication Administration: Vaginal

Medication Administration: Ventricular Reservoir

Medication Management

Medication Prescribing

Meditation Facilitation

Memory Training

Milieu Therapy

Mood Management

Multidisciplinary Care Conference

Music Therapy

Mutual Goal Setting

Nail Care

Nausea Management

Neurologic Monitoring

Newborn Care

Newborn Monitoring

Nonnutritive Sucking

Normalization Promotion

Nutrition Management

Nutrition Therapy

Nutritional Counseling

Nutritional Monitoring

Oral Health Maintenance

Oral Health Promotion

Oral Health Restoration

Order Transcription

Organ Procurement

Ostomy Care

Oxygen Therapy

Pain Management

Parent Education: Adolescent

Parent Education: Childbearing Family

Parent Education: Infant

Parenting Promotion

Pass Facilitation

Patient Contracting

Patient-Controlled Analgesia (PCA) Assistance

Patient Rights Protection

Peer Review

Pelvic Muscle Exercise

Perineal Care

Peripheral Sensation Management

Peripherally Inserted Central (PIC) Catheter Care

Peritoneal Dialysis Therapy

Pessary Management

Phlebotomy: Arterial Blood Sample

Phlebotomy: Blood Unit Acquisition

Phlebotomy: Cannulated Vessel

Phlebotomy: Venous Blood Sample

Phototherapy: Mood/Sleep Regulation

Phototherapy: Neonate

Physical Restraint

Physician Support

Pneumatic Tourniquet Precautions

Positioning

Positioning: Intraoperative

Positioning: Neurologic

Positioning: Wheelchair

Postanesthesia Care

Postmortem Care

Postpartal Care

Preceptor: Employee

Preceptor: Student

Preconception Counseling

Pregnancy Termination Care

Premenstrual Syndrome (PMS) Management

Prenatal Care

Preoperative Coordination

Preparatory Sensory Information

Presence

Pressure Management

Pressure Ulcer Care

Pressure Ulcer Prevention

Product Evaluation

Program Development

Progressive Muscle Relaxation

Prompted Voiding

Prosthesis Care

Pruritus Management

Quality Monitoring

Radiation Therapy Management
Rape-Trauma Treatment
Reality Orientation
Recreation Therapy
Rectal Prolapse Management
Referral
Religious Addiction Prevention
Religious Ritual Enhancement
Relocation Stress Reduction
Reminiscence Therapy
Reproductive Technology Management
Research Data Collection
Resiliency Promotion
Respiratory Monitoring
Respite Care
Resuscitation
Resuscitation: Fetus
Resuscitation: Neonate
Risk Identification
Risk Identification: Childbearing Family
Risk Identification: Genetic
Role Enhancement

Seclusion
Security Enhancement
Seduction Management
Seizure Management
Seizure Precautions
Self-Awareness Enhancement
Self-Care Assistance
Self-Care Assistance: Bathing/Hygiene
Self-Care Assistance: Dressing/Grooming
Self-Care Assistance: Feeding
Self-Care Assistance: IADL
Self-Care Assistance: Toileting
Self-Care Assistance: Transfer
Self-Esteem Enhancement
Self-Hypnosis Facilitation
Self-Modification Assistance
Self-Responsibility Facilitation
Sexual Counseling
Shift Report

Shock Management
Shock Management: Cardiac
Shock Management: Vasogenic
Shock Management: Volume
Shock Prevention
Sibling Support
Simple Guided Imagery
Simple Massage
Simple Relaxation Therapy
Skin Care: Donor Site
Skin Care: Graft Site
Skin Care: Topical Treatments
Skin Surveillance
Sleep Enhancement
Smoking Cessation Assistance
Socialization Enhancement
Specimen Management
Spiritual Growth Facilitation
Spiritual Support
Splinting
Sports-Injury Prevention: Youth
Staff Development
Staff Supervision
Subarachnoid Hemorrhage Precautions
Substance Use Prevention
Substance Use Treatment
Substance Use Treatment: Alcohol Withdrawal
Substance Use Treatment: Drug Withdrawal
Substance Use Treatment: Overdose
Suicide Prevention
Supply Management
Support Group
Support System Enhancement
Surgical Assistance
Surgical Precautions
Surgical Preparation
Surveillance
Surveillance: Community
Surveillance: Late Pregnancy
Surveillance: Remote Electronic
Surveillance: Safety
Sustenance Support
Suturing
Swallowing Therapy

continued

TABLE 2–1 *continued*

Teaching: Disease Process

Teaching: Foot Care

Teaching: Group

Teaching: Individual

Teaching: Infant Nutrition

Teaching: Infant Safety

Teaching: Infant Stimulation

Teaching: Preoperative

Teaching: Prescribed Activity/Exercise

Teaching: Prescribed Diet

Teaching: Prescribed Medication

Teaching: Procedure/Treatment

Teaching: Psychomotor Skill

Teaching: Safe Sex

Teaching: Sexuality

Teaching: Toddler Nutrition

Teaching: Toddler Safety

Teaching: Toilet Training

Technology Management

Telephone Consultation

Telephone Follow-Up

Temperature Regulation

Temperature Regulation: Intraoperative

Temporary Pacemaker Management

Therapeutic Play

Therapeutic Touch

Therapy Group

Total Parenteral Nutrition (TPN) Administration

Touch

Traction/Immobilization Care

Transcutaneous Electrical Nerve Stimulation (TENS)

Transport

Trauma Therapy: Child

Triage: Disaster

Triage: Emergency Center

Triage: Telephone

Truth Telling

Tube Care

Tube Care: Chest

Tube Care: Gastrointestinal

Tube Care: Umbilical Line

Tube Care: Urinary

Tube Care: Ventriculostomy/Lumbar Drain

Ultrasonography: Limited Obstetric

Unilateral Neglect Management

Urinary Bladder Training

Urinary Catheterization

Urinary Catheterization: Intermittent

Urinary Elimination Management

Urinary Habit Training

Urinary Incontinence Care

Urinary Incontinence Care: Enuresis

Urinary Retention Care

Values Clarification

Vehicle Safety Promotion

Venous Access Device (VAD) Maintenance

Ventilation Assistance

Visitation Facilitation

Vital Signs Monitoring

Vomiting Management

Weight Gain Assistance

Weight Management

Weight Reduction Assistance

Wound Care

Wound Care: Closed Drainage

Wound Irrigation

Source: Dochterman, J., Bulecheck, G. (2004). *Nursing Interventions Classifications (NIC)*. 4th ed. St. Louis: Mosby.

NOC is also a comprehensive standardized language providing 330 outcome labels (Table 2–2) with definitions; a set of indicators describing specific client, caregiver, family, or community states related to the outcome; and a 5-point Likert-type measurement scale that facilitates tracking clients across care settings and that can demonstrate client progress even when outcomes are not fully met. The outcomes are research-based and are applicable in all care settings and clinical specialties.

TABLE 2–2

NURSING OUTCOMES CLASSIFICATION LABELS

Abuse Cessation

Abuse Protection

Abuse Recovery Status

Abuse Recovery: Emotional

Abuse Recovery: Financial

Abuse Recovery: Physical

Abuse Recovery: Sexual

Abusive Behavior Self-Restraint

Acceptance: Health Status

Activity Tolerance

Adaptation to Physical Disability

Adherence Behavior

Agression Self-Control

Allergic Response: Localized

Allergic Response: Systemic

Ambulation

Ambulation: Wheelchair

Anxiety Level

Anxiety Self-Control

Appetite

Aspiration Prevention

Asthma Self-Management

Balance

Blood Coagulation

Blood Glucose Level

Blood Loss Severity

Blood Transfusion Reaction

Body Image

Body Mechanics Performance

Body Positioning: Self-Initiated

Bone Healing

Bowel Continence

Bowel Elimination

Breastfeeding Establishment: Infant

Breastfeeding Establishment: Maternal

Breastfeeding Maintenance

Breastfeeding Weaning

Cardiac Disease Self-Management

Cardiac Pump Effectiveness

Caregiver Adaptation to Patient Institutionalization

Caregiver Emotional Health

Caregiver Home Care Readiness

Caregiver Lifestyle Disruption

Caregiver-Patient Relationship

Caregiver Performance: Direct Care

Caregiver Performance: Indirect Care

Caregiver Physical Health

Caregiver Stressors

Caregiver Well-Being

Caregiving Endurance Potential

Child Adaptation to Hospitalization

Child Development: 1 Month

Child Development: 2 Months

Child Development: 4 Months

Child Development: 6 Months

Child Development: 12 Months

Child Development: 2 Years

Child Development: 3 Years

Child Development: 4 Years

Child Development: Preschool

Child Development: Middle Childhood

Child Development: Adolescence

Circulation Status

Client Satisfaction: Access to Care Resources

Client Satisfaction: Caring

Client Satisfaction: Communication

Client Satisfaction: Continuity of Care

Client Satisfaction: Cultural Needs Fulfillment

Client Satisfaction: Functional Assistance

Client Satisfaction: Physical Care

Client Satisfaction: Physical Environment

Client Satisfaction: Protection of Rights

Client Satisfaction: Psychological Care

Client Satisfaction: Safety

Client Satisfaction: Symptom Control

Client Satisfaction: Teaching

Client Satisfaction: Technical Aspects of Care

Cognition

Cognitive Orientation

Comfortable Death

Comfort Level

Communication

continued

TABLE 2–2   *continued*

Communication: Expressive
Communication: Receptive
Community Competence
Community Disaster Readiness
Community Health Status
Community Health Status: Immunity
Community Risk Control: Chronic Disease
Community Risk Control: Communicable Disease
Community Risk Control: Lead Exposure
Community Risk Control: Violence
Community Violence Level
Compliance Behavior
Concentration
Coordinated Movement
Coping

Decision-Making
Depression Level
Depression Self-Control
Diabetes Self-Management
Dignified Life Closure
Discharge Readiness: Independent Living
Discharge Readiness: Supported Living
Distorted Thought Self-Control

Electrolyte and Acid/Base Balance
Endurance
Energy Conservation

Fall Prevention Behavior
Falls Occurrence
Family Coping
Family Functioning
Family Health Status
Family Integrity
Family Normalization
Family Participation in Professional Care
Family Physical Environment
Family Resiliency
Family Social Climate
Family Support During Treatment
Fear Level
Fear Level: Child
Fear Self-Control
Fetal Status: Antepartum

Fetal Status: Intrapartum
Fluid Balance
Fluid Overload Severity

Grief Resolution
Growth

Health Beliefs
Health Beliefs: Perceived Ability to Perform
Health Beliefs: Perceived Control
Health Beliefs: Perceived Resources
Health Beliefs: Perceived Threat
Health Orientation
Health-Promoting Behavior
Health-Seeking Behavior
Hearing Compensation Behavior
Hemodialysis Access
Hope
Hydration
Hyperactivity Level

Identity
Immobility Consequences: Physiological
Immobility Consequences: Psycho-Cognitive
Immune Hypersensitivity Response
Immune Status
Immunization Behavior
Impulse Self-Control
Infection Severity
Infection Severity: Newborn
Information Processing

Joint Movement: Ankle
Joint Movement: Elbow
Joint Movement: Fingers
Joint Movement: Hip
Joint Movement: Knee
Joint Movement: Neck
Joint Movement: Passive
Joint Movement: Shoulder
Joint Movement: Spine
Joint Movement: Wrist

Kidney Function
Knowledge: Body Mechanics
Knowledge: Breastfeeding

Knowledge: Cardiac Disease Management
Knowledge: Child Physical Safety
Knowledge: Conception Prevention
Knowledge: Diabetes Management
Knowledge: Diet
Knowledge: Disease Process
Knowledge: Energy Conservation
Knowledge: Fall Prevention
Knowledge: Fertility Promotion
Knowledge: Health Behavior
Knowledge: Health Promotion
Knowledge: Health Resources
Knowledge: Illness Care
Knowledge: Infant Care
Knowledge: Infection Control
Knowledge: Labor and Delivery
Knowledge: Medication
Knowledge: Ostomy Care
Knowledge: Parenting
Knowledge: Personal Safety
Knowledge: Postpartum Maternal Health
Knowledge: Preconception Maternal Health
Knowledge: Pregnancy
Knowledge: Prescribed Activity
Knowledge: Sexual Functioning
Knowledge: Substance Abuse Control
Knowledge: Treatment Procedure(s)
Knowledge: Treatment Regimen

Leisure Participation
Loneliness Severity

Maternal Status: Antepartum
Maternal Status: Intrapartum
Maternal Status: Postpartum
Mechanical Ventilation Response: Adult
Mechanical Ventilation Weaning Response: Adult
Medication Response
Memory
Mobility
Mood Equilibrium
Motivation

Nausea and Vomiting Control
Nausea and Vomiting: Disruptive Effects
Nausea and Vomiting Severity
Neglect Cessation

Neglect Recovery
Neurological Status
Neurological Status: Autonomic
Neurological Status: Central Motor Control
Neurological Status: Consciousness
Neurological Status: Cranial Sensory/Motor Function
Neurological Status: Spinal Sensory/Motor Function
Newborn Adaptation
Nutritional Status
Nutritional Status: Biochemical Measures
Nutritional Status: Energy
Nutritional Status: Food & Fluid Intake
Nutritional Status: Nutrient Intake

Oral Hygiene
Ostomy Self-Care

Pain: Adverse Psychological Response
Pain Control
Pain: Disruptive Effects
Pain Level
Parent-Infant Attachment
Parenting: Adolescent Physical Safety
Parenting: Early/Middle Childhood Physical Safety
Parenting: Infant/Toddler Physical Safety
Parenting Performance
Parenting: Psychological Safety
Participation in Healthcare Decisions
Personal Autonomy
Personal Health Status
Personal Safety Behavior
Personal Well-Being
Physical Aging
Physical Fitness
Physical Injury Severity
Physical Maturation: Female
Physical Maturation: Male
Play Participation
Post Procedure Recovery Status
Prenatal Health Behavior
Preterm Infant Organization
Psychomotor Energy
Psychosocial Adjustment: Life Change

Quality of Life

Respiratory Status: Airway Patency
Respiratory Status: Gas Exchange

continued

TABLE 2–2 *continued*

Respiratory Status: Ventilation
Rest
Risk Control
Risk Control: Alcohol Use
Risk Control: Cancer
Risk Control: Cardiovascular Health
Risk Control: Drug Use
Risk Control: Hearing Impairment
Risk Control: Sexually Transmitted Diseases (STD)
Risk Control: Tobacco Use
Risk Control: Unintended Pregnancy
Risk Control: Visual Impairment
Risk Detection
Role Performance

Safe Home Environment
Seizure Control
Self-Care Status
Self-Care: Activities of Daily Living (ADL)
Self-Care: Bathing
Self-Care: Dressing
Self-Care: Eating
Self-Care: Hygiene
Self-Care: Instrumental Activities of Daily Living (IADL)
Self-Care: Non-Parenteral Medications
Self-Care: Oral Hygiene
Self-Care: Parenteral Medication
Self-Care: Toileting
Self-Direction of Care
Self-Esteem
Self-Mutilation Restraint
Sensory Function Status
Sensory Function: Cutaneous
Sensory Function: Hearing
Sensory Function: Proprioception
Sensory Function: Taste and Smell
Sensory Function: Vision
Sexual Functioning
Sexual Identity
Skeletal Function
Sleep

Social Interaction Skills
Social Involvement
Social Support
Spiritual Health
Stress Level
Student Health Status
Substance Addiction: Consequences
Suffering Severity
Suicide Self-Restraint
Swallowing Status
Swallowing Status: Esophageal Phase
Swallowing Status: Oral Phase
Swallowing Status: Pharyngeal Phase
Symptom Control
Symptom Severity
Symptom Severity: Perimenopause
Symptom Severity: Premenstrual Syndrome
Systemic Toxic Clearance: Dialysis

Thermoregulation
Thermoregulation: Newborn
Tissue Integrity: Skin and Mucous Membranes
Tissue Perfusion: Abdominal Organs
Tissue Perfusion: Cardiac
Tissue Perfusion: Cerebral
Tissue Perfusion: Peripheral
Tissue Perfusion: Pulmonary
Transfer Performance
Treatment Behavior: Illness or Injury

Urinary Continence
Urinary Elimination

Vision Compensation Behavior
Vital Signs

Weight: Body Mass
Weight Control
Will to Live
Wound Healing: Primary Intention
Wound Healing: Secondary Intention

Source: Moorhead, S., Johnson, M., Maas, M. (Eds). (2004). *Nursing Outcomes Classifications (NOC)*. 3d ed. St. Louis: Mosby.

In addition, NIC and NOC have been linked to the Omaha System problems, to resident assessment protocols (RAPs) used in extended/long-term care settings, and to NANDA-I. This last linkage created the NANDA, NIC, NOC (NNN) Taxonomy of Nursing Practice. The combination of NANDA-I nursing diagnoses, NOC outcomes, and NIC interventions in a common unifying structure provides a comprehensive nursing language recognized by the American Nurses Association (ANA) and is coded in the Systematized Nomenclature of Medicine (SNOMED) in support of the electronic client record.

Having an SNL entered into international coded terminology allows nursing to describe the care received by the client and to document the effects of that care on client outcomes, and it facilitates the comparison of nursing care across worldwide settings and diverse databases. In addition, it supports research by comparing client care delivered by nurses with that delivered by other providers, which is essential if nursing's contribution is to be recognized and nurses are to be reimbursed for the care they provide.

Today, 13 versions of SNLs are recognized by the ANA and have been submitted to the National Library of Medicine for inclusion in the Unified Medical Language System Metathesaurus. The Metathesaurus provides a uniform, integrated distribution format from over 100 biomedical vocabularies and classifications (the majority in English and some in multiple languages), and it links many different names for the same concepts, establishing new relationships between terms from different source vocabularies.

Indexing of the entire medical record supports disease management activities (including decision support systems), research, and analysis of outcomes for quality improvement for all healthcare disciplines. Coding also supports telehealth (the use of telecommunications technology to provide medical information and healthcare services over distance) and facilitates access to healthcare data across care settings and different computer systems.

So, to those who stated, "Nursing will thrive as a unique and valued profession when nurses present a theory and rationalistic model for their practice . . . and actively participate in processes for change,"[11] we answer, "We are actively participating in processes for change, and as a profession, we will continue."

References

1. Gordon, M. (1998). Nursing nomenclature and classification system development. Online Journal of Issues in Nursing. Available at: http://nursingworld.org/ojin/tpc7/tpc7_1.htm. Accessed 2004.
2. NANDA International. (2003). *Nursing Diagnoses: Definitions & Classifications 2003–2004*. Philadelphia: Author.
3. Carroll-Johnson, R. M. (Ed). (1991). *Classification of Nursing Diagnoses: Proceedings of the Ninth Conference*. Philadelphia: J. B. Lippincott.
4. Saba, V. K. (1994). *Home Health Care Classification (HHCC) of Nursing Diagnoses and Interventions*. (Revised). Washington, DC: Author.
5. McCloskey, J. C., Bulechek, G. M. (Eds). (2004). *Nursing Interventions Classification (NIC)*. 4th ed. St. Louis, MO: Mosby.
6. Moorhead, S., Johnson, M., Maas, M. (Eds). (2004). *Nursing Outcomes Classification (NOC)*. 3d ed. St. Louis, MO: Mosby.
7. Martin, K. S., Scheet, N. J. (Eds). (1992). *The Omaha System: Applications for Community Health Nursing*. Philadelphia: W. B. Saunders.
8. Ozboldt, J. G. (1996). From minimum data to maximum impact: Using clinical data to strengthen patient care. *Advanced Practice Nursing Quarterly*, 1, 62–69.
9. Beyea, S. (2002). *Perioperative Nursing Data Set (PNDS)*. 2d ed. Denver: AORN.
10. Johnson, M., Bulechek, G., Dochterman, J. M., Maas, M., Moorhead, S. (Eds). (2001). *Nursing Diagnoses, Outcomes, and Interventions: NANDA, NOC, and NIC Linkages*. St. Louis, MO: Mosby.
11. Erickson, H. C., Tomlin, E. M., Swain, M. A. P. (1983). *Modeling and Role-Modeling*. Englewood Cliffs, NJ: Prentice-Hall.
12. Saba, V. K. (2007). *Clinical Care Classification (CCC) System Manual: A Guide to Nursing Documentation*. New York: Springer.

Chapter 3

The Assessment Process: Developing the Client Database

The *Nursing: Scope & Standard of Practice*[1] addresses the assessment process. The standard stipulates that the data-collection process is systematic and ongoing. The nurse collects client health data from the client, significant others, and healthcare providers when appropriate. The priority of the data-collection activities is determined by the client's immediate condition or needs. Pertinent data are collected using appropriate assessment techniques and instruments. Relevant data are documented in a retrievable form.

The Client Database

The assessment step of the nursing process is focused on eliciting a profile of the client that allows the nurse to identify client problems or needs and corresponding nursing diagnoses, to plan care, to implement interventions, and to evaluate outcomes. This profile, or *client database,* supplies a sense of the client's overall health status, providing a picture of the client's physical, psychological, sociocultural, spiritual, cognitive, and developmental levels; economic status; functional abilities; and lifestyle. It is a combination of data gathered from the history-taking interview (a method of obtaining SUBJECTIVE information by talking with the client or significant other(s) and listening to their responses), from the physical examination (a "hands-on" means of obtaining OBJECTIVE information), and from the results of laboratory/diagnostic studies. To be more specific, subjective data are what the client/significant others perceive and report, and objective data are what the nurse observes and gathers from other sources.

Assessment involves three basic activities:

- Systematically gathering data
- Organizing or clustering the data collected
- Documenting the data in a retrievable format

Gathering Data—The Interview

Information in the client database is obtained primarily from the client (who is the most important source) and then from family members/significant others (secondary sources), as appropriate, through conversation and by observation during a structured interview. Clearly, the interview involves more than simply exchanging and processing data. Nonverbal communication is as important as the client's choice of words in providing the data. The ability to collect data that are meaningful to the client's health concerns depends heavily on the nurse's knowledge base; on the choice and sequence of questions; and on the ability to give meaning to the client's responses, integrate the data gathered, and prioritize the resulting information. Insight into the nature and behavior of the client is essential as well.

The nurse's initial responsibility is to observe, collect, and record data without drawing conclusions or making judgments/assumptions. Self-awareness is a crucial factor in the interaction, because perceptions, judgments, and assumptions can easily color the assessment findings unless they are recognized.

The quality of a history improves with experience with the interviewing process. Tips for obtaining a meaningful history include the following:

- Be a good listener.
- Listen carefully and attentively for whole thoughts and ideas, not merely isolated facts.
- Use skills of active listening, silence, and acceptance to provide ample time for the person to respond. Be as objective as possible.
- Identify only the client's or significant others' contributions to the history.

The interview question is the major tool used to acquire information. How the question is phrased is a skill that is important in obtaining the desired results and in getting the information necessary to make accurate nursing diagnoses. Note: Some questioning strategies to avoid include closed-ended and leading questions, probing, and agreeing or disagreeing that implies the client is "right" or "wrong." It is important to remember, too, that the client has the right to refuse to answer any question at all, no matter how reasonably phrased.

Nine effective data-collection questioning techniques include the following:

1. Open-ended questions allow clients maximum freedom to respond in their own way, impose no limitations on how the question may be answered, and can produce considerable information.
2. Hypothetical questions pose a situation and ask the client how it might be handled.
3. Reflecting or "mirroring responses" are useful techniques in getting at underlying meanings that might not be verbalized clearly.
4. Focusing consists of eye contact (within cultural limits), body posture, and verbal responses.
5. Giving broad openings encourages the client to take the initiative in what is to be discussed.
6. Offering general leads encourages the client to continue.
7. Exploring pursues a topic in more depth.
8. Verbalizing the implied gives voice to what has been suggested.
9. Encouraging evaluation helps clients to consider the quality of their own experiences.

The client's medical diagnosis can provide a starting point for gathering data. Knowledge of the anatomy and physiology of the specific disease process/severity of the condition also helps in choosing and prioritizing precise portions of the assessment. For example, when examining a client with severe chest pain, it may be wise to evaluate the pain and the cardiovascular system in a focused assessment before addressing other areas, possibly at a later time. Likewise, the duration and length of any assessment depend on circumstances such as the client's condition and the situation's urgency.

The data collected about the client or significant others contain a vast amount of information, some of which may be repetitious. However, some of it will be valuable for eliciting information that was not recalled or volunteered previously. Enough material needs to be noted in the history so that a complete picture is presented, and yet not so much that the information will not be read or used.

Gathering Data—The Physical Examination

The physical examination is performed to gather objective information and serves as a screening device. Four common methods used during the physical examination are inspection, palpation, percussion, and auscultation. These techniques incorporate the senses of sight, hearing, touch, and smell. For the data collected during the physical examination to be meaningful, it is vital to know the normal physical and emotional characteristics of humans well enough to be able to recognize deviations. To gain as much information as possible from the assessment procedure, the same format should be used each time a physical examination is performed to lessen the possibility of omissions.

Gathering Data—Laboratory Tests/Diagnostic Procedures

Laboratory and other diagnostic studies are a part of the information-gathering stage providing supportive evidence. These studies aid in the management, maintenance, and restoration of health. In reviewing and interpreting laboratory tests, it is important to remember that the origin of the test material does not always correlate to an organ or body system (e.g., a urine test to detect the presence of bilirubin and urobilinogen could indicate liver disease, biliary obstruction, or hemolytic disease). In some cases, the results of a test are *nonspecific,* because they indicate only a disorder or abnormality and not the location of the cause of the problem (e.g., an elevated erythrocyte sedimentation rate suggests the presence but not the location of an inflammatory process).

In evaluating laboratory tests, it is advisable to consider which medications (e.g., heparin, promethazine) are being administered to the client, including over-the-counter and herbal supplements (e.g., vitamin E), because these have the potential to alter, blur, or falsify results, creating a misleading diagnostic picture.

Documenting and Clustering the Data

Data gathered during the interview and physical examination, and from other records/sources are organized and recorded in a concise, systematic way and clustered into similar categories. Various formats have been used to accomplish this, including a review of body systems. This approach has been utilized by both medicine and nursing for many years but was initially developed to aid the physician in making medical diagnoses. Currently, nursing is developing and fine-tuning its own tools for recording and clustering data. Several nursing models available to guide data collection include Doenges and Moorhouse Diagnostic Divisions (Table 3–1),[2,3] Gordon's Functional Health Patterns,[4] and Guzzetta's Clinical Assessment Tool.[5]

The use of a nursing model as a framework for data collection (rather than a body-systems approach [assessing the heart, moving on to the lungs] or the commonly known head-to-toe approach) has the advantage of focusing data collection on the nurse's phenomena of concern—the human responses to health and illness.[6] This facilitates the identification and validation of *nursing* diagnosis labels to describe the data accurately.

Reviewing and Validating Findings

The nurse's initial responsibility is to observe, collect, and record data without drawing conclusions or making judgments/assumptions. Self-awareness is a crucial factor in this

TABLE 3–1

GENERAL ASSESSMENT TOOL

This is a suggested guideline/tool applicable in most care settings for creating a client database. It provides a nursing focus (Doenges & Moorhouse's Diagnostic Divisions of Nursing Diagnoses) that will facilitate planning client care. Although the sections are alphabetized here for ease of presentation, they can be prioritized or rearranged to meet individual needs.

Adult Medical/Surgical Assessment Tool
General Information
Name:_____ Age:_____ DOB:_____ Gender:_____ Race:_____

Admission Date:_____ Time:_____ From:_____

Reason for this visit/admission (primary concern):_____

Source of Information:_____ Reliability (1–4 with 4 = very reliable):_____

Activity/Rest
Subjective (Reports)
Occupation:_____ Able to participate in usual activities/hobbies:_____

Leisure time/diversional activities:_____

Ambulatory:_____ Gait (describe):_____ Activity level (sedentary to very active):_____

Daily exercise (type):_____

Changes in muscle mass/tone/strength:_____

History of problems/limitations imposed by condition (e.g., immobility, weakness, breathlessness, fatigue):_____

Feelings (e.g., exhaustion, restlessness, boredom, dissatisfaction):_____

Developmental factors (e.g., delayed/age):_____

Sleep: Hours:_____ Naps:_____ Aids:_____ Insomnia:_____ Related to:_____

Difficulty falling asleep:_____ Difficulty staying asleep:_____

Rested on awakening:_____ Excessive grogginess:_____ Bedtime rituals:_____

Relaxation techniques:_____ Sleeps on more than one pillow:_____

Use of oxygen (type):_____ When used:_____

Medications or herbals for/affecting sleep:_____

Objective (Exhibits)
Observed response to activity: Heart rate:_____ Rhythm (reg/irreg):_____

Blood pressure:_____ Respiratory rate:_____ Pulse oximetry:_____

Mental status (e.g., cognitive impairment, withdrawn/lethargic):_____

Neuromuscular assessment: Muscle mass/tone:_____ Posture (e.g., normal, stooped, curved spine):_____

Tremors (location):_____ ROM:_____

Strength:_____ Deformity:_____

Mobility aids (list):_____

Circulation
Subjective (Reports)
History of/treatment for: High blood pressure:_____ Brain injury:_____ Stroke:_____

Heart condition/surgery:_____ Rheumatic fever:_____ Palpitations:_____ Syncope:_____

Claudication:_____ Ankle/leg edema:_____ Blood clots:_____ Bleeding tendencies:_____

Dysreflexia episodes(describe):_____

Slow healing (describe):_____

Extremities: Numbness (location):_____ Tingling (location):_____

Cough (describe)/hemoptysis:_____

Change in frequency/amount of urine:_____

Medications/herbals:_____

Objective (Exhibits)

Color (e.g., pale, cyanotic, jaundiced, mottled, ruddy): Skin:_____ Mucous membranes:_____

Lips:_____ Nailbeds:_____ Conjunctiva:_____ Sclera:_____

Skin moisture: (e.g., dry, diaphoretic):_____

BP: (R & L): Lying:_____ Sitting:_____ Standing:_____

Pulse pressure:_____ Auscultatory gap:_____

Pulses (Palpated 1–4 strength): Carotid:____ Temporal:____ Jugular:____ Radial:____ Femoral:____ Popliteal:____

Posttibial:_____ Dorsalis pedis:_____

Cardiac (palpation): Thrill:_____ Heaves:_____

Heart sounds (auscultation): Rate:_____ Rhythm:_____ Quality:_____ Friction rub:_____

Murmur (describe location/sounds):_____

Vascular bruit (location):_____ Jugular vein distention:_____

Breath sounds (describe location & sounds):_____

Extremities: Temperature:_____ Color:_____ Capillary refill (1–3 sec):_____

Homan's sign (+ or –):_____ Varicosities (location):_____ Nail abnormalities:_____

Edema (+1 to +4):_____ Distribution/quality of hair:_____

Trophic skin changes:_____

Ego Integrity

Subjective (Reports)

Relationship status:_____

Expressed concerns (e.g., financial, relationships, recent or anticipated lifestyle or role
changes):_____

Stress factors:_____ Usual ways of handling stress:_____

Expression of feelings of: Anger:_____ Anxiety:_____ Fear:_____ Grief:_____

Helplessness:_____ Hopelessness:_____ Powerlessness:_____

Cultural factors/ethnic ties:_____

Religious affiliation:_____ Active/practicing:_____ Practices prayer/meditation:_____

Religious/Spiritual concerns:_____ Desires clergy visit:_____

Expression of sense of connectedness/harmony with self and others:_____

Medications/herbals:_____

Objective (Exhibits)

Emotional status (check those that apply):

Calm:____ Anxious:____ Angry:____ Withdrawn:____ Fearful:____ Irritable:____ Restive:____ Euphoric:____

Observed body language:_____

Observed physiological responses (e.g., crying, change in voice quality/volume):_____

Changes in energy field: Temperature:_____ Color:_____ Distribution:_____ Movement:_____

Sounds:_____

Elimination

Subjective (Reports)

Usual bowel elimination pattern and character of stool (e.g., hard, soft, liquid):_____

Stool color (e.g., brown, black, yellow, clay-colored, tarry):_____ Last BM and character of stool:_____

History of bleeding:_____ Hemorrhoids/fistula:_____

Constipation (acute/chronic):_____ Diarrhea (acute/chronic):_____ Bowel incontinence:_____

continued

TABLE 3–1   *continued*

Laxative use:_____ How often:_____ Enema/suppository:_____ How often:_____
Usual voiding pattern and character of urine:_____
Difficulty voiding:_____ Urgency:_____ Frequency:_____ Retention:_____ Bladder spasms:_____ Pain/burning:_____
Urinary incontinence (type & time of day usually occurs):_____
History of kidney/bladder disease:_____
Diuretic use:_____ Other medications/herbals:_____

Objective (Exhibits)
Abdomen (palpation): Soft/firm:_____ Tenderness/pain (quadrant location):_____
Distention:_____ Palpable mass:_____ Size/girth:_____
CVA tenderness:_____
Abdomen (auscultation): Bowel sounds (location/type):_____
Bladder palpable:_____ Residual (per scan):_____ Overflow voiding:_____
Rectal sphincter tone (describe):_____ Hemorrhoids/fistulas:_____
Stool in rectum:_____ Impaction:_____ Occult blood: (+ or –):_____
Presence/use of catheter or continence devices:_____
Ostomy appliances (describe appliance and location):_____

Food/Fluid
Subjective (Reports)
Usual diet (type):_____ Calorie/carbohydrate/protein/fat-g/day:_____
# of meals daily:_____ Snacks (# daily, time consumed, & type):_____
Last meal consumed/content:_____
Food preferences:_____ Food allergies/intolerances:_____
Cultural or religious food preparation concerns/prohibitions:_____
Usual appetite:_____ Change in appetite:_____
Usual weight:_____ Unexpected/undesired weight loss or gain:_____
Nausea/vomiting:_____ Related to?_____ Heartburn/indigestion:_____ Related to?_____
Relieved by?_____
Chewing/swallowing problems:_____ Gag/swallow reflex (present):_____
Facial injury/surgery:_____ Stroke/other neurological deficit:_____
Teeth: Normal:_____ Dentures (full/partial):_____ Loose/absent teeth:_____ Sore mouth/gums:_____
Dental hygiene practices:_____ Professional dental care/frequency:_____
Diabetes/type:_____ Controlled with diet/pills/insulin:_____
Vitamin/food supplement use:_____ Medications/herbals:_____

Objective (Exhibits)
Current weight:_____ Height:_____ Body build:_____ Body fat %:_____
Skin turgor (e.g., firm, supple, dehydrated):_____ Mucous membranes (moist/dry):_____
Edema (describe): Generalized:_____ Dependent:_____ Feet/ankles:_____
Periorbital:_____ Abdominal/ascites:_____
Jugular vein distention:_____
Breath sounds (auscultation)/location: Normal:_____ Faint/distant:_____
Crackles:_____ Wheezes:_____
Condition of teeth/gums:_____ Appearance of tongue:_____ Mucous membranes:_____
Abdomen: Bowel sounds (quadrant location/type):_____ Hernia/masses:_____
Urine S/A or Chemstix:_____ Serum glucose (Glucometer):_____

Hygiene
Subjective (Reports)
Ability to carry out activities of daily living: Independent/dependent (level 1 [no assistance needed] to level 4 [completely dependent]): _____

Mobility: _____ Needs assistance (describe): _____ Assistance provided by: _____

Equipment/prosthetic devices required: _____

Feeding: _____ Needs assistance (describe): _____ Assistive devices: _____

Hygiene: _____ Needs assistance (describe): _____ Preferred time of personal care/bath: _____

Dressing/grooming: _____ Needs assistance (describe): _____

Toileting: _____ Needs assistance with (describe): _____

Objective (Exhibits)
General appearance: Manner of dress: _____ Grooming/personal habits: _____

Condition of hair/scalp: _____

Body odor: _____ Presence of vermin (e.g., lice, scabies): _____

Neurosensory
Subjective (Reports)
History of brain injury, trauma, stroke (residual effects): _____

Fainting spells/dizziness: _____ Headaches (location/type/frequency): _____

Tingling/numbness/weakness (location): _____

Seizures: _____ History/onset: _____ Type (e.g., generalized, partial): _____ Frequency: _____ Aura (describe): _____ Postictal state: _____ How controlled: _____

Vision loss/changes: _____ Glasses/contacts: _____ Last exam: _____

Glaucoma: _____ Cataract: _____ Eye surgery (type/date): _____

Hearing loss: _____ Sudden or gradual: _____ Hearing aids: _____ Last exam: _____

Sense of smell (changes): _____ Epistaxis: _____

Sense of taste (changes): _____

Other: _____

Objective (Exhibits)
Mental status (note duration of change):

Oriented/disoriented: Time: _____ Place: _____ Person: _____ Situation: _____

Check all that apply: Alert: __ Drowsy: __ Lethargic: __ Stuporous: __ Comatose: __ Cooperative: __ Follows commands: _____ Agitated/Restless: _____ Combative: _____

Delusions (describe): _____ Hallucinations (describe): _____

Affect (describe): _____ Speech: _____

Memory: Recent: _____ Remote: _____

Pupil shape: _____ Size/reaction: R/L: _____ Accommodation: _____

Facial droop: _____ Swallowing: _____

Handgrasp/release, R/L: _____ Deep tendon reflexes (present/absent/location): _____

Coordination: _____ Balance: _____ Walking: _____

Tremors: _____ Posturing: _____ Paralysis (L/R): _____

Pain/Discomfort
Subjective (Reports)
Primary focus: Location: _____ Intensity (use pain scale or pictures): _____ Quality (e.g., stabbing, aching, burning): _____ Radiation: _____ Frequency: _____ Duration: _____

Precipitating/aggravating factors: _____

continued

TABLE 3–1   *continued*

How relieved (including nonpharmaceuticals/therapies):_____

Associated symptoms (e.g., nausea, sleep problems, photosensitivity):_____

Effect on daily activities:_____ Relationships:_____ Job:_____ Enjoyment of life:_____

Additional pain focus/describe:_____

Cultural expectations regarding pain perception and expression:_____

Objective (Exhibits)

Facial grimacing:____ Guarding affected area:____ Posturing:____ Behaviors:_____ Narrowed focus:_____

Emotional response (e.g., crying, withdrawal, anger):_____

Vital sign changes (acute pain): BP:_____ Pulse:_____ Respirations:_____

Respiration

Subjective (Reports)

Dyspnea/related to:_____ Precipitating factors:_____ Relieving factors:_____

Airway clearance (e.g., spontaneous/device):_____

Cough/describe (e.g., hard, persistent, croupy):_____ Produces sputum (describe

color/character):_____ Requires suctioning:_____

History of (year): Bronchitis:_____ Asthma:_____ Emphysema:_____ Tuberculosis:___ Recurrent pneumonia:____

Exposure to noxious fumes/allergens, infectious agents/diseases, poisons:_____

Smoker:_____ packs/day:_____ # of pack years:_____ Cigar use:_____

Use of respiratory aids:_____ Oxygen (type & frequency):_____

Medications/herbals:_____

Objective (Exhibits)

Respirations (spontaneous/assisted):____ Rate:_____ Depth:_____ Chest excursion (e.g., equal/symmetrical):____

Use of accessory muscles:_____ Nasal flaring:_____ Fremitus:_____

Breath sounds (describe):_____ Egophony:_____

Skin/mucous membrane color (e.g., pale, cyanotic):_____ Clubbing of fingers:_____

Sputum characteristics:_____

Mentation (e.g., calm, anxious, restless):_____

Pulse oximetry:_____

Safety

Subjective (Reports)

Allergies/sensitivity (medications, foods, environment, latex):_____

Type of reaction:_____

Blood transfusion/number:_____ Date:_____ Reaction (describe):_____

Exposure to infectious diseases (e.g., measles, influenza, pink eye):_____

Exposure to pollution, toxins, poisons/pesticides, radiation (describe reactions):_____

Geographic areas lived in/recent travel:_____

Immunization history/date: Tetanus:_____ MMR:_____ Polio:_____ Hepatitis:_____ Pneumonia:_____

Influenza:_____ HPV:_____

Altered/suppressed immune system (list cause):_____

History of sexually transmitted disease (date/type):_____ Testing:_____

High-risk behaviors (specify):_____

Uses seat belt regularly:_____ Uses helmets/other safety devices:_____

Workplace safety/health issues (describe):_____ Occupation:_____ Currently working:_____

Rate working:_____ conditions (e.g., safety, noise, heating, water, ventilation, etc.):_____

History of accidental injuries:_____ Fractures/dislocations:_____

Arthritis/unstable joints:_____ Back problems:_____

Skin problems (e.g., rashes, lesions, moles, breast lumps, enlarged nodes)/describe:_____

Delayed healing (describe):_____

Cognitive limitations (e.g., disorientation, confusion):_____

Sensory limitations (e.g., impaired vision/hearing, detecting heat/cold, taste, smell, touch):_____

Prosthesis:_____ Ambulatory devices:_____

Violence (episodes or tendencies):_____

Objective (Exhibits)

Body temperature/method (e.g., oral, rectal, tympanic):_____

Skin integrity (mark location on diagram): Scars:_____ Rashes:_____ Lacerations:_____ Ulcerations:_____

Bruises:_____ Blisters:_____ Drainage:_____ Burns (degree/% of body surface):_____

Musculoskeletal: General strength:_____ Muscle tone:_____ Gait:_____ ROM:_____ Paresthesia/paralysis:_____

Results of testing (e.g., cultures, immune function, TB, hepatitis):_____

Sexuality (Component of Social Interaction)

Subjective (Reports)

Sexually active:_____ Monogamous/Committed relationship:_____ Use of condoms:_____

Birth control method:_____

Sexual concerns/difficulties:_____ Recent change in frequency/interest:_____

Pain/discomfort:_____

Objective (Exhibits)

Comfort level with subject matter:_____

Female: Subjective (Reports)

Menstruation: Age at menarche:____ Length of cycle:____ Duration:____ Number of pads/tampons used/day:____

Last menstrual period:_____ Bleeding between periods:_____

Menopausal:_____ Last period:_____ Hysterectomy (type/date):_____

Problems with: Hot flashes:_____ Vaginal lubrication:_____ Vaginal discharge:_____

Other related surgeries (type and date):_____

Infertility concerns:_____ Type of therapy:_____

Pregnant now:_____ Para:_____ Gravida:_____ Due date:_____

Practices breast self-examination:_____ Last mammogram:_____ Last Pap smear/results:_____

Hormonal therapy:_____ Supplemental calcium:_____ Other medications/herbals:_____

continued

TABLE 3–1 *continued*

Objective (Exhibits)

Breast examination:_____

Genitalia:_____ Warts/lesions:_____ Vaginal bleeding/discharge:_____

STD test results:_____

Male: Subjective (Reports)

Penis: Circumcised:_____ Lesions/discharge:_____ Vasectomy:_____

Prostate disorder:_____

Practice self-exam: Breast:_____ Testicles:_____

Last proctoscopic/prostate examination:_____ Last PSA:_____

Medications/herbals:

Objective (Exhibits)

Genitalia: Penis:_____ Warts/lesions:_____ Bleeding/discharge:_____ Testicles (e.g., descended, lumps):_____

Prostate:_____

Breast examination:_____

STD test results:_____ PSA:_____

Social Interactions

Subjective (Reports)

Relationship status: Single:_____ Married:_____ Living with partner:_____ Divorced:_____ Widowed:_____

Years in relationship:_____ Perception of relationship:_____ Concerns/stresses:_____

Role within family structure:_____ Number/age of children:_____

Individuals living in home:_____ Caregiver (to whom & how long):_____

Extended family/availability:_____ Other support person(s):_____

Perception of relationship with family members:_____

Ethnic/cultural affiliation:_____ Strength of ethnic identity:_____ Lives in ethnic community:_____

Feelings of (describe): Mistrust:_____ Rejection:_____ Unhappiness:_____

Loneliness/isolation:_____

Problems related to illness/condition:_____

Difficulties with communication (e.g., speech, another language, brain injury):_____

Use of communication aids (list):_____ Requires interpreter:_____

Genogram: (complete on separate form)

Objective (Exhibits)

Communication/speech: Clear:_____ Slurred:_____ Unintelligible:_____ Aphasic:_____

Unusual speech pattern/impairment:_____ Laryngectomy present:_____

Use of speech/communication aids:_____

Verbal/nonverbal communication with family/SO(s):_____

Family interaction (behavioral) pattern:_____

Teaching/Learning

Subjective (Reports)

Communication: Dominant language (specify):_____ Second language:_____

Literate (reading/writing):_____

Education level:_____ Learning disabilities (specify):_____ Cognitive limitations:_____

Culture/ethnicity:_____ Where born:_____ If immigrant, how long in this country:_____

Health and illness beliefs/practices/customs:_____

Which family member makes healthcare decisions/is spokesperson for client: _____

Presence of Advance Directives: _____ Code status: _____ Durable Medical Power of Attorney: _____

Designee: _____

Health goals: _____

Current health problem: _____ Client understanding of problem: _____

Special healthcare concerns (e.g., impact of religious/cultural practices, healthcare decisions, family involvement): _____

Familial risk factors (indicate relationship): Diabetes: _____ Thyroid (specify): _____ Tuberculosis: _____

Heart disease: _____ Stroke: _____ High BP: _____ Epilepsy/seizures: _____ Kidney disease: _____ Cancer: _____

Mental illness/depression: _____ Other: _____

Prescribed medications (list each separately):

Drug: _____ Dose: _____ Times (circle last dose): _____

Take regularly: _____ Purpose: _____ Side effects/problems: _____

Nonprescription drugs/frequency:

OTC drugs: _____ Vitamins: _____ Herbals: _____ Street drugs: _____

Alcohol (amount/frequency): _____ Tobacco: _____ Smokeless tobacco: _____

Admitting diagnosis per provider: _____

Reason for hospitalization (or visit) per client: _____

History of current problem/concern: _____

Client expectations of this hospitalization (or visit): _____

Will admission cause any lifestyle changes (describe): _____

Previous illnesses and/or hospitalizations/surgeries: _____

Evidence of failure to improve: _____

Last complete physical examination: _____

Discharge Plan Considerations

Projected length of stay (hours/days): _____ Anticipated date of discharge: _____

Date information obtained: _____ Source: _____

Resources available: Persons: _____ Financial: _____ Community supports: _____

Groups: _____

Areas that may require alteration/assistance: Food preparation: _____ Shopping: _____ Transportation: _____

Ambulation: _____ Self-care (specify): _____ Socialization: _____ Medication/IV therapy: _____ Treatments: ____

Wound care: _____ Supplies: _____

Homemaker/maintenance (specify): _____ Physical layout of home (specify): _____

Anticipated changes in living situation after discharge: _____

Living facility other than home (specify): _____

Referrals (date/source/services): Social services: _____ Rehab services: _____

Dietary: _____ Home care: _____ Resp/O$_2$: _____ Equipment: _____ Supplies: _____

Other: _____

interaction, because perceptions, judgments, and assumptions can easily color the assessment findings.

Validation is an ongoing process that occurs during the data-collection phase and upon its completion, when the data are reviewed and compared. The nurse should review the data to be sure that the recordings are factual, to identify errors of omission, and to compare the objective and subjective data for congruencies or inconsistencies that require additional investigation or a more focused assessment. Data that are grossly abnormal are rechecked, and any temporary factors that may affect the data are identified/noted. Validation is particularly important when the data are conflicting, when the data's source may be unreliable, or when serious harm to the client could result from any inaccuracies. Validating the information can avoid the possibility of making wrong inferences or conclusions that could result in inaccurate nursing diagnoses, incorrect outcomes, or inappropriate nursing actions. This can be done by sharing the assumptions with the individuals involved (e.g., client, significant other/family) and having them verify the accuracy of those conclusions. Sharing pertinent data with other healthcare professionals, such as the physician, dietician, or physical therapist can aid in collaborative planning of care. Data given in confidence should not be shared with other individuals (unless withholding that information would hinder appropriate evaluation or care of the client).

Summary

The assessment step of the nursing process emphasizes and should provide a holistic view of the client. The generalized assessment done during the overall data-gathering creates a profile of the client. A focused, or more detailed, assessment may be warranted given the client's condition or emergent time constraints, or it may be done to obtain more information about a specific issue that needs expansion or clarification. Both types of assessments provide important data that complement each other. A successfully completed assessment creates a picture of clients' states of wellness, their response to health concerns or problems, and individual risk factors—this is the foundation for identifying appropriate nursing diagnoses, developing client outcomes, and choosing relevant interventions necessary for providing individualized care.

References

1. American Nurses Association. (2004). *Nursing: Scope & Standards of Practice.* Silver Spring, MD: Nursesbooks.org.
2. Doenges, M. E., Moorhouse, M. F., Geissler-Murr, A. C. (2008). *Nurse's Pocket Guide: Diagnoses, Interventions, and Rationales.* 11th ed. Philadelphia: F.A. Davis.
3. Doenges, M. E., Moorhouse, M. F., Geissler-Murr, A. C. (2006). *Nursing Care Plans: Guidelines for Individualizing Patient Care.* 7th ed. Philadelphia: F.A. Davis.
4. Gordon, M. (1994). *Nursing Diagnosis: Process and Application.* 3d ed. St. Louis, MO: Mosby.
5. Guzzetta, C. E., et al. (1989). *Clinical Assessment Tools for Use with Nursing Diagnoses.* St. Louis, MO: Mosby.
6. American Nurses Association. (1995). *Nursing's Social Policy Statement.* Washington, DC: Author.

Chapter 4

Concept Mapping to Create and Document the Plan of Care

The plan of care may be recorded on a single page or in a multiple-page format, with one page for each nursing diagnosis or client diagnostic statement. The format for documenting the plan of care is determined by agency policy. As a practicing professional, you might use a computer with a plan-of-care database, preprinted standardized care plan forms, or clinical pathways. Whichever form you use, the plan of care enables visualization of the nursing process and must reflect the basic nursing standards of care; personal client data; nonroutine care; and qualifiers for interventions and outcomes, such as time, frequency, or amount.

As students, you are asked to develop plans of care that often contain more detail than what you see in the hospital plans of care. This is to help you learn how to apply the nursing process and create individualized client care plans. However, even though much time and energy may be spent focusing on filling the columns of traditional clinical care plan forms, some students never develop a holistic view of their clients and fail to visualize how each client need interacts with other identified needs. A new technique or learning tool has been developed to assist you in visualizing the linkages, to enhance your critical thinking skills, and to facilitate the creative process of planning client care.

Concept Mapping Client Care

Have you ever asked yourself whether you are more right-brained or left-brained? Those who naturally use their left brains are more linear in their thinking. Right-brain thinkers see more in pictures and illustrations. It is best for nurses to use the whole brain (right and left) when thinking about providing the broad scope of nursing care to clients.

No More Columns!

Traditional nursing care plans are linear—that is, they are designed in columns. They speak almost exclusively to the left brain. The traditional nursing care plan is organized according to the nursing process, which guides us in problem-solving the nursing care we give. However, the linear nature of the traditional plan does not facilitate interconnecting data from one "row" to another or between parts in a column. Concept mapping allows us to show the interconnections between various client symptoms, interventions, or problems as they impact each other.

You can keep the parts that are great about traditional care plans (problem-solving and categorizing) but change the linear/columnar nature of the plan to a design that uses the whole brain—bringing left-brained, linear problem-solving together with the freewheeling, interconnected, creative right brain. Joining concept mapping and care planning enables you to create a whole picture of a client with all the interconnections identified.

There are several diverse and innovative ways to mind map or to concept map nursing care plans.[1] The examples in this chapter use mind mapping and require placing the client at the center, with all ideas on one page (for a whole picture); the examples also use color-coding and creative energy.[2,3] When doing a large mapped plan of care, a light posterboard is often used so that all ideas fit on one page.

Components of a Concept Map

Tony Buzan developed the idea of concept mapping, a way to depict how ideas about a main subject are related. Mapping represents graphically the relationships and interrelationships of ideas and concepts.[4] It fosters and encourages critical thinking through brainstorming about a particular subject.

Instead of starting at the top of the page, concept mapping starts in the page's center. The main concept of our thinking goes in this center stage place.

From that central thought, simply begin thinking of other main ideas that relate to the central topic. These ideas radiate out from the central idea likes spokes of a wheel (see subsequent discussion); however, they do not have to be added in a balanced manner; the "wheel" does not have to be round.

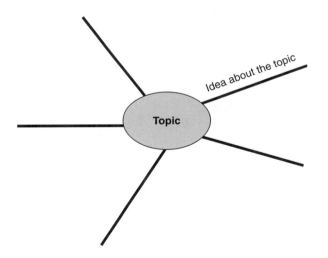

You will generate further ideas related to each spoke (see subsequent discussion); and your mind will race with even more ideas from those thoughts, which can be represented through pictures or words.

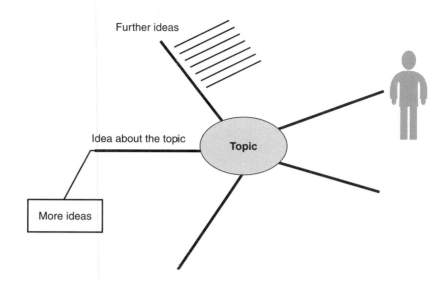

As you think of new ideas, write them down immediately. This may require going back and forth from one area of the page to another. Writing your concept map by hand allows you to move faster. Avoid using a computer to generate a map because this hinders the fast-paced process. You can group different concepts together by color-coding or by placement on the page (see subsequent discussion).

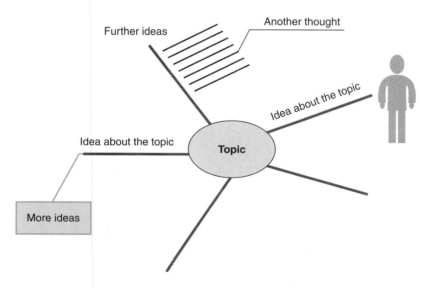

As you see connections and interconnections between groups of ideas, use arrows or lines to connect those concepts (refer to the dotted lines). You can also add defining phrases that explain how the interconnected thoughts relate to one another, as in the following figure.

Some left-brain thinkers find it very difficult to start their ideas in the middle of a page. If you are this type of thinker, try starting at the top of the page (see subsequent discussion), but you must still represent your ideas in illustration form, not in paragraphs.

Concept maps created by different people look different. They are unique to the mind's eye picture so don't expect your map to be the same as someone else's.

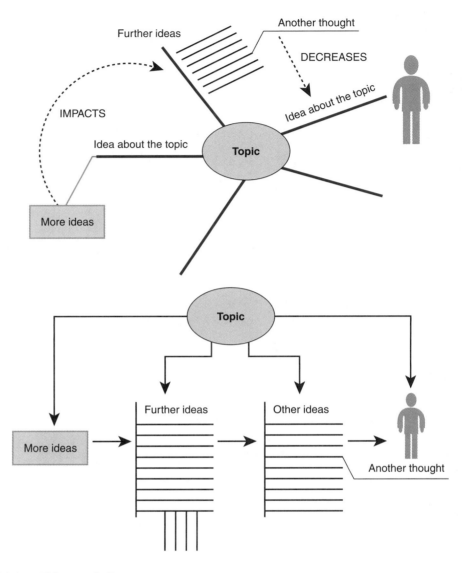

Concept Mapping a Plan of Care

Concept mapping is an exciting alternative format for illustrating a written plan of care. A mapped care plan will look very different from traditional plans of care, which are usually completed on linear forms.

To begin mapping a client plan of care, you must begin with the central topic—the client. Now you are thinking like a nurse. Create a shape that signifies "client" to you and place that at your map's center. If your hand just can't start at the center, then put the shape at the top. This will help you remember that the client is the focus of your plan, not the medical diagnosis or condition. All other pieces of the map will be connected in some manner to the client. Many different pieces of information about the client can be connected directly to the client. For example, each of the following pieces of critical client data could stem from the center:

- Seventy-eight-year-old widower
- No family in the state

- Obese
- Medical diagnosis of recurrent community-acquired pneumonia

Now, you must do a bit of thinking about how you think. To create the rest of your map, ask yourself how *you* plan client care. For example, which of these items do you see first or think of first as the basis for your plan: the clustered assessment data, nursing diagnoses, or outcomes? Whichever piece you choose becomes your first layer of connections. Suppose when thinking about a plan of care for a female client with heart failure, you think first in terms of all the nursing diagnoses about that woman and her condition. Your map would start with the diagnoses featured as the first "branches," each one being listed separately in some way on the map.

Completing the map then becomes a matter of adding the rest of the pieces of the plan using the nursing process and your own way of thinking/planning as your guide. If you began your map using nursing diagnoses, you might think, "What signs and symptoms or data support these diagnoses?" Then, you would connect clusters of supporting data to the related nursing diagnosis. Or you might think, "What client outcomes am I trying to achieve when I address this nursing diagnosis?" In that case, you would next connect client outcomes (or NOC labels) to the nursing diagnoses.

To keep your map clear, as suggested previously, use different colors and maybe a different shape/spoke/line for each piece of the care plan that you are adding. For example:

- Red for signs and symptoms (to signify danger)
- Yellow for nursing diagnoses (for "stop and think what this is")
- Green for nursing interventions/NIC labels (for "go")
- Blue (or some other color) for outcomes/NOC labels

When all the pieces of the nursing process are represented, each "branch" of the map is complete. There should be a nursing diagnosis (supported by subjective and objective assessment data), nursing interventions, desired client outcome(s), and any evaluation data, all connected in a manner that shows there is a relationship between them.

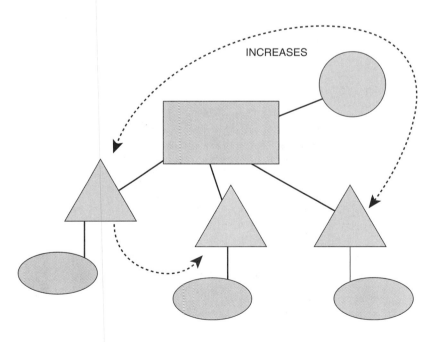

It is critical to understand that there is no preset order for the pieces, because one cluster is not more or less important than another (or one is not "subsumed" under another). It is important, however, that those pieces within a branch be in the same order in each branch.

So, you might ask, how is this different than writing out information in a linear manner? What makes mapping so special? One of the things you may have discovered about caring for clients is that the care you deliver is very interconnected. Taking care of one problem often results in the simultaneous correction of another. For example, if you resolve a fluid volume problem in a client with heart failure, you will also positively impact the client's gas exchange and decrease his or her anxiety. These kinds of interconnections cannot be shown on linear

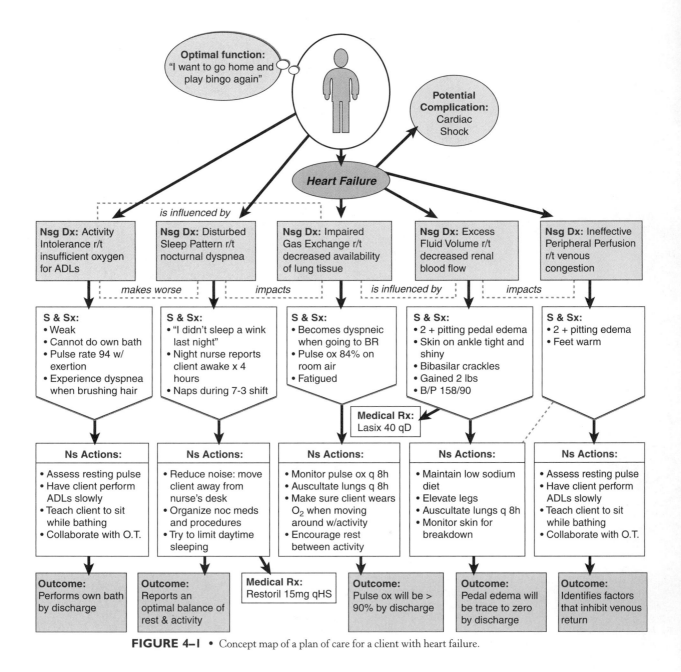

FIGURE 4–I • Concept map of a plan of care for a client with heart failure.

plans of care, yet they are what practicing nurses see in their mind's eye all the time. These interconnections can be represented on a map with arrows or dotted or dashed lines that tie related ideas together. Then, defining phrases that explain the nature of the interconnection can be added to further clarify the relationship, as shown in Figure 4–1.

In addition to the pieces of the nursing process, there are other components of care that can be illustrated on a map. Nurses have certain responsibilities when clients have diagnostic tests (such as an angiography or a bronchoscopy). These tests can be connected to the appropriate piece of your map, along with the correct nursing interventions related to those tests. Another item to be added would be potential complications (collaborative problems).

Taking your clients' needs one step further, try asking every client you have (medical, surgical, or otherwise), "What is the most important thing to you now in relation to why you are here?" Obtaining this information builds an alliance between you and your client, and together you can work toward that desired outcome. Add it to your map and see how your plan of care becomes more client-centered (refer to Fig. 4–2).

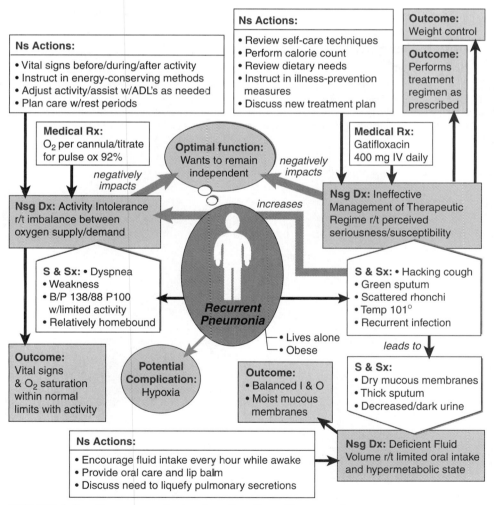

FIGURE 4–2 • Concept map of a plan of care for a client with pneumonia.

Summary

Concept maps allow you to do something that is different and creative. They require you to think (and learn), make connections, and use colors and shapes. They help you to focus on the client; and having the map on one page helps you to understand the "whole picture" better. Concept maps also help you to become better organized and to develop your own unique approach to "thinking like a nurse" much sooner.

A student who had written many traditional plans of care in her previous nursing program wrote the following about concept-mapped care plans:

Concept mapping is painting a picture using colors of the rainbow on blank paper to tell the story of your client using "NANDA" nursing diagnoses and the nursing process. Previously, I was a student in prison (my mind) who hated the words "CARE PLAN," writing page after page in narrative form. It was laborious to do and boring to read. There was no life or heartbeat.

Concept mapping opened the prison doors, and my care plan took on human form with a VOICE, a beating HEART, and COLOR while still incorporating the nursing process and standardized nursing language. My mind now took on the professional thought process that NANDA, NIC, and NOC were created to facilitate nursing; however, the magic was in concept mapping, which removed all my fears, and the client became a beautiful painting with a heartbeat.

References

1. Schuster, P. (2002). *Concept Mapping: A Critical-Thinking Approach to Care Planning.* Philadelphia: F. A. Davis.
2. Mueller, A., Johnston, M., Bligh, D. (2001). Mind-mapped care plans, a remarkable alternative to traditional nursing care plans. *Nurse Educator,* 26(2), 75–80.
3. Mueller, A., Johnston, M., Bligh, D. (2002). Viewpoint: Joining mind mapping and care planning to enhance student critical thinking and achieve holistic nursing care. *Nursing Diagnosis: The International Journal of Nursing Language and Classification,* 13(1).
4. Buzan T. (1995). *The MindMap Book.* 2d ed. London: BBC Books.

Chapter 5

Nursing Diagnoses in Alphabetical Order

Activity Intolerance [specify level]

Definition: Insufficient physiological or psychological energy to endure or complete required or desired daily activities

RELATED FACTORS
Generalized weakness
Sedentary lifestyle
Bedrest/immobility
Imbalance between oxygen supply and demand, [anemia]
[Cognitive deficits/emotional status; secondary to underlying disease process/depression]
[Pain, vertigo, dysrhythmias, extreme stress]

DEFINING CHARACTERISTICS

Subjective
Verbal report of fatigue/weakness
Exertional discomfort/dyspnea
[Verbalizes no desire and/or lack of interest in activity]

Objective
Abnormal heart rate/blood pressure response to activity
Electrocardiographic changes reflecting arrhythmias/or ischemia
[Pallor, cyanosis]

FUNCTIONAL LEVEL CLASSIFICATION (GORDON, 1987):
Level I: Walk, regular pace, on level indefinitely; one flight or more but more short of breath than normally
Level II: Walk one city block [or] 500 ft on level; climb one flight slowly without stopping
Level III: Walk no more than 50 ft on level without stopping; unable to climb one flight of stairs without stopping
Level IV: Dyspnea and fatigue at rest

Information that appears in brackets has been added by the authors to clarify and enhance the use of the nursing diagnoses.

ACTIVITY INTOLERANCE [specify level]

Sample Clinical Applications: Anemias, angina, aortic stenosis, bronchitis, emphysema, diabetes mellitus, dysmenorrhea, heart failure, human immunodeficiency virus/acquired immunodeficiency disease (HIV/AIDS), labor/preterm labor, leukemias, mitral stenosis, obesity, pain, pericarditis, peripheral vascular disease, rheumatic fever, thrombocytopenia, tuberculosis, uterine bleeding

DESIRED OUTCOMES/EVALUATION CRITERIA
Sample NOC linkages:
Activity Tolerance: Physiological response to energy-consuming movements with daily activities
Energy Conservation: Personal actions to manage energy for initiating and sustaining activity
Endurance: Capacity to sustain activity

Client Will (Include Specific Time Frame)

- Identify negative factors affecting activity tolerance and eliminate or reduce their effects when possible.
- Use identified techniques to enhance activity tolerance.
- Participate in necessary/desired activities.
- Report measurable increase in activity tolerance.
- Demonstrate a decrease in physiological signs of intolerance (e.g., pulse, respirations, and blood pressure remain within client's usual range).

ACTIONS/INTERVENTIONS

Sample NIC linkages:
Activity Therapy: Prescription of and assistance with specific physical, cognitive, social, and spiritual activities to increase the range, frequency, or duration of an individual's (or group's) activity
Energy Management: Regulating energy use to treat or prevent fatigue and optimize function
Exercise Promotion: Facilitation of regular physical activity to maintain or advance to a higher level of fitness and health

NURSING PRIORITY NO. 1 To identify causative/precipitating factors:

- Note presence of acute or chronic illness, such as heart failure, hypothyroidism, diabetes mellitus, AIDS, cancers, acute and chronic pain, etc. *Many factors cause or contribute to fatigue, but acitivity intolerance implies that the client cannot endure or adapt to increased energy or oxygen demands caused by an actvity.*[1,8,9]
- Assess cardiopulmonary response to physical activity by measuring vital signs, noting heart rate/regularity, respiratory rate/work of breathing, and blood pressure before, during, and after activity. Note progression/accelerating degree of fatigue. *Dramatic changes in heart rate and rhythm, changes in usual blood pressure, and progressively worsening fatigue result from imbalance of oxygen supply and demand. These changes are potentially greater in the frail, elderly population.*[1–3,10,11]
- Note treatment-related factors such as side effects/interactions of medications. *Can influence presence and degree of fatigue.*
- Determine if client is receiving medications such as vasodilators, diuretics, or beta-blockers. Orthostatic hypotension can occur with activity because of medication effects (vasodilation), fluid shifts (diuresis), or compromised cardiac pumping function.[4]

◉ Cultural ◉ Collaborative 🏠 Community/Home Care ␀ Diagnostic Studies ∞ Pediatric/Geriatric/Lifespan ♿ Medications

- Note client reports of difficulty accomplishing tasks or desired activities. Evaluate current limitations/degree of deficit in light of usual status and what the client perceives causes, exacerbates, and helps the problem. *Provides comparative baseline and influences choice of interventions and may reveal causes that the client is unaware of affecting energy, such as sleep deprivation, smoking, poor diet, depression, or lack of support.*[2,10,11]
- Ascertain ability to sit, stand, and move about as desired. Note degree of assistance necessary, and/or use of assistive equipment. *Helps to differentiate between problems relating to movement and problems with oxygen supply and demand characterized by fatigue and weakness.*[2,8,9,11]
- Identify activity needs versus desires (e.g., client barely able to walk upstairs but states would like to play racquetball). *Assists caregiver in dealing with reality of situation, as well as the feasibility of goals client wants to achieve when developing activity plan.*[4]
- Assess emotional/psychological factors affecting the current situation. *Stress and/or depression may be exacerbating the effects of an illness, or depression may be the result of therapy/limitations.*

NURSING PRIORITY NO. 2 To assist client to deal with contributing factors and manage activities within individual limits:

- Monitor vital signs, before and during activity, watching for changes in blood pressure, heart and respiratory rate, as well as postactivity vital sign response. *Vital signs increase during activity and should return to baseline within 5 to 7 minutes after activity if response to activity is normal.*[1]
- Observe respiratory rate, noting breathing pattern, breath sounds, skin color, and mental status. *Pallor and/or cyanosis, presence of respiratory distress, or confusion may be indicative of need for oxygen during activities, especially if respiratory infection or compromise is present.*[4]
- Plan care with rest periods between activities *to reduce fatigue.*
- Assist with self-care activities. Adjust activities/reduce intensity level, or discontinue activities that cause undesired physiological changes. *Prevents overexertion.*
- Increase exercise/activity levels gradually; encourage stopping to rest for 3 minutes during a 10-minute walk, sitting down instead of standing to brush hair, etc. *Methods of conserving energy.*
- Encourage expression of feelings contributing to/resulting from condition. Provide positive atmosphere while acknowledging difficulty of the situation for the client. *Helps to minimize frustration, rechannel energy.*
- Involve client/significant others (SOs) in planning of activities as much as possible. *May give client opportunity to perform desired/essential activities during periods of peak energy.*
- Assist with activities and provide/monitor client's use of assistive devices. *Enables client to maintain mobility while protecting from injury.*
- Promote comfort measures and provide for relief of pain *to enhance client's ability and desire to participate in activities.*[9,11] (Refer to NDs acute Pain, chronic Pain.)
- Provide referral to collaborative disciplines such as exercise physiologist, psychological counseling/therapy, occupational/physical therapy, and recreation/leisure specialists. *May be needed to develop individually appropriate therapeutic regimens.*
- Prepare for/assist with and monitor effects of exercise testing. *May be performed to determine degree of oxygen desaturation and/or hypoxemia that occurs with exertion, or to optimize titration of supplemental oxygen when used.*[5,8]
- Implement graded exercise/rehabilitation program under direct medical supervision. *Gradual increase in activity avoids excessive myocardial workload/excessive oxygen demand.*[4]

• Administer supplemental oxygen, medications, prepare for surgery, as indicated. *Type of therapy or medication is dependent on the underlying condition and might include medications (such as antiarryhthmics) or surgery (e.g., stents or CABG) to improve myocardial perfusion and systemic circulation. Other treatments might include iron preparations or blood transfusion to treat severe anemia, or use of oxygen and bronchodilators to improve respiratory function.*[6,7]

NURSING PRIORITY NO. 3 To promote wellness (Teaching/Discharge Considerations):

• Review expectations of client/SO(s)/providers and explore conflicts/differences. *Helps to establish goals and to reach agreement for the most effective plan.*

• Assist/direct client/SO to plan for progressive increase of activity level aiming for maximal activity within the client's ability. *Promotes improved or more normal activity level, stamina, and conditioning.*

• Instruct client/SOs in monitoring response to activity and in recognizing signs/symptoms that indicate need to alter activity level. *Assists in self-management of condition and in understanding of reportable problems.*[8,9]

• Give client information that provides evidence of daily/weekly progress *to sustain motivation.*

• Assist client to learn and demonstrate appropriate safety measures *to prevent injuries.*

• Provide information about proper nutrition to meet metabolic and energy needs, obtaining or maintaining normal body weight. *Energy is improved when nutrients are sufficient to meet metabolic demands.*[1]

• Encourage client to use relaxation techniques such as visualization/guided imagery as appropriate. *Useful in maintaining positive attitude and enhancing sense of well-being.*

• Encourage participation in recreation/social activities and hobbies appropriate for situation. (Refer to ND deficient Diversional Activity.)

• Monitor laboratory values (such as for anemia) and pulse oximetry.

DOCUMENTATION FOCUS

Assessment/Reassessment

• Level of activity as noted in Functional Level Classification.
• Causative/precipitating factors.
• Client reports of difficulty/change.

Planning

• Plan of care and who is involved in planning.

Implementation/Evaluation

• Response to interventions/teaching and actions performed.
• Implemented changes to plan of care based on assessment/reassessment findings.
• Teaching plan and response/understanding of teaching plan.
• Attainment/progress toward desired outcome(s).

Discharge Planning

• Referrals to other resources.
• Long-term needs and who is responsible for actions.

⊕ Cultural   Collaborative   🏠 Community/Home Care   Diagnostic Studies   ∞ Pediatric/Geriatric/Lifespan   Medications

References

1. Cox, H. C., et al. (2002). *Clinical Applications of Nursing Diagnosis: Adult, Child, Womens's, Psychiatric, Gerontic, and Home Health Considerations.* 4th ed. Philadelphia: F. A. Davis, pp. 231–237.
2. Blair, K. A. (1999). Immobility and activity intolerance in older adults. In Stanley, M., Beare, P. G. (eds). *Gerontological Nursing: A Health Promotion/Protection Approach.* 2d ed. Philadelphia: F.A. Davis, pp. 193–202.
3. Gordon, M. (2002). *Manual of Nursing Diagnosis.* 10th ed. St. Louis, MO: Mosby, p. 223.
4. Hypertension: Severe; Heart failure: Chronic; Myocardial infarction; and Pneumonia: Microbial. In Doenges, M. E., Moorhouse, M. F., Geissler-Murr, A. C. (2002). *Nursing Care Plans: Guidelines for Individualizing Patient Care.* 6th ed. Philadelphia: F. A. Davis, pp. 37, 51, 75, 133.
5. Exercise testing for evaluation of hypoxemia and/or desaturation. (2001). Revision & update. *Resp Care,* 46(5), 514–522.
6. Gibbons, R. J., et al. (1999). ACC/AHA/ACP-ASIM: Guidelines for the management of patients with chronic stable angina: A report of the American College of Cardiology/American Heart Association Task Force on Practice Guidelines. *J Am Coll Cardiol,* 33(7), 2092.
7. Congestive heart failure in adults. (2002). Bloomington, MN: Institute for Clinical Systems Improvement (ICSI).
8. Michael, K. M., Allen, J. K., Macko, R. E. (2006). Fatigue after stroke: Relationship to mobility, fitness, ambulatory activity, social support, and falls efficacy. *Rehabilitation Nursing,* 31(5), 210–217.
9. Graf, C. (2006). Functional decline in hospitalized older adults. *AJN,* 106(1), 58–67. 10. Perry, A. (2005). Quality of life. *Rehab Management,* 18(7), 18–21.
11. Hurr, H. K., Park, S. M., Kim, S. S., et al. (2005). Activity intolerance and impaired physical mobility in elders. *Int J of Nursing Terminologies and Classifications,* 16(3–4), 47–53.

risk for Activity Intolerance

Definition: At risk of experiencing insufficient physiological or psychological energy to endure or complete required or desired daily activities

RISK FACTORS
History of previous intolerance
Presence of circulatory/respiratory problems, [dysrhythmias]
Deconditioned status; [aging]
Inexperience with the activity
[Diagnosis of progressive disease state/debilitating condition, anemia]
[Verbalized reluctance/inability to perform expected activity]
NOTE: A risk diagnosis is not evidenced by signs and symptoms as the problem has not occurred; rather, nursing interventions are directed at prevention.

Sample Clinical Applications: Anemias, angina aortic stenosis, bronchitis, emphysema, dysmenorrhea, heart failure, HIV/AIDS, labor/preterm labor, leukemias, mitral stenosis, obesity, pain, pericarditis, peripheral vascular disease, rheumatic fever, thrombocytopenia, tuberculosis, uterine bleeding

DESIRED OUTCOMES/EVALUATION CRITERIA
Sample NOC linkages:
Endurance: Capacity to sustain activity
Energy Conservation: Personal actions to manage energy for initiating and sustaining activity
Circulation Status: Unobstructed, unidirectional blood flow at an appropriate pressure through large vessels of the systemic and pulmonary circuits

Client Will (Include Specific Time Frame)

• Verbalize understanding of potential loss of ability in relation to existing condition.
• Participate in conditioning/rehabilitation program to enhance ability to perform.

- Identify alternative ways to maintain desired activity level (e.g., if weather is bad, walking in a shopping mall could be an option).
- Identify conditions/symptoms that require medical reevaluation.

ACTIONS/INTERVENTIONS

Sample NIC linkages:

Energy Management: Regulating energy use to treat or prevent fatigue and optimize function

Exercise Promotion: Facilitation of regular physical activity to maintain or advance to a higher level of fitness and health

Pain Management: Alleviation of pain or a reduction in pain to a level of comfort that is acceptable to the client

NURSING PRIORITY NO. 1 To assess factors affecting current situation:

- Note presence of medical diagnosis and/or therapeutic regimens (e.g., AIDS, COPD, cancer, heart failure/other cardiac problems, anemia, multiple medications/treatment modalities, extensive surgical interventions, musculoskeletal trauma, neurological disorders) *that have potential for interfering with client's ability to perform at a desired level of activity. Note: Many factors cause or contribute to fatigue, but activity intolerance implies that the individual cannot endure or adapt to increased energy or oxygen demands caused by an actvity.*[1]
- Ask client/SO about usual level of energy *to identify potential problems and/or client's/SO's perception of client's energy and ability to perform needed/desired activities.*
- Identify factors (e.g., age, functional decline, painful conditions, breathing problems, client resistive to efforts; vision or hearing impairments, climate, or weather; unsafe areas to exercise; need for mobility assistance, etc.) *that could block/affect desired level of activity.*
- Determine current activity level and physical condition with observation, exercise tolerance testing, use of functional level classification system (e.g., Gordon's), as appropriate. *Provides baseline for comparison and opportunity to track changes.*

NURSING PRIORITY NO. 2 To develop/investigate alternative ways to remain active within the limits of the disabling condition/situation:

- Implement physical therapy/exercise program in conjunction with the client and other team members such as a physical and/or occupational therapist, exercise/rehabilitation physiologist. *Collaborative program with short-term achievable goals enhances likelihood of success and may motivate client to adopt a lifestyle of physical exercise for enhancement of health.*[2]
- Promote/implement conditioning program and support inclusion in exercise/activity groups to prevent/limit deterioration.
- Instruct client in proper performance of unfamiliar activities and/or alternate ways of doing familiar activities *to learn methods of conserving energy and promote safety in performing activities.*

NURSING PRIORITY NO. 3 To promote wellness (Teaching/Discharge Considerations):

- Discuss with client/SO relationship of illness/debilitating condition to inability to perform desired activity(ies). *Understanding these relationships can help with acceptance of limitations or reveal opportunity for changes of practical value.*[1–5]

   Cultural Collaborative Community/Home Care Diagnostic Studies Pediatric/Geriatric/Lifespan Medications

• Provide information regarding factors, such as smoking when one has respiratory problems, weight management, lack of motivation/interest in exercise. *Education is essential to encourage modification of potential interferences to activity.*[3,4]

 • Assist client/SO(s) with planning for changes that may become necessary (e.g., shifting of family responsibilities, use of supplemental oxygen to improve client's ability to participate in desired activities). *Anticipatory guidance facilitates adaptation if symptoms occur.*[3,4] (Refer to ND Activity Intolerance.)

• Identify and discuss symptoms for which client needs to seek medical assistance/ evaluation, *providing for timely intervention.*[3]

• Refer to appropriate sources for assistance (e.g., smoking cessation, dietary counseling) and/or equipment, as needed, *to sustain or improve activity level and to promote client safety.*

DOCUMENTATION FOCUS

Assessment/Reassessment

• Identified/potential risk factors for individual.
• Current level of activity tolerance and blocks to activity.

Planning

• Treatment options, including physical therapy/exercise program, other assistive therapies and devices.
• Lifestyle changes that are planned, who is to be responsible for each action, and monitoring methods.

Implementation/Evaluation

• Responses to interventions/teaching and actions performed.
• Attainment/progress toward desired outcome(s).
• Modification of plan of care.

Discharge Planning

• Referrals for medical assistance/evaluation.

References

1. Cox, H. C., et al. (2002). *Clinical Applications of Nursing Diagnosis: Adult, Child, Womens's, Psychiatric, Gerontic, and Home Health Considerations.* 4th ed. Philadelphia: F. A. Davis, pp. 231–237.
2. Blair, K. A. (1999). Immobility and activity intolerance in older adults. In Stanley, M., Beare, P. G. (eds). *Gerontological Nursing: A Health Promotion/Protection Approach.* 2d ed. Philadelphia: F. A. Davis, pp. 193–202.
3. Congestive heart failure in adults. (2002). Bloomington, MN: Institute for Clinical Systems Improvement (ICSI).
4. Meleski, D. D. (2002). Families with chronically ill children. *AJN,* 102(5), 47.
5. Borroso, J. (2002). HIV-related fatigue. *AJN,* 102(5), 83.

ineffective Airway Clearance

Definition: Inability to clear secretions or obstructions from the respiratory tract to maintain a clear airway

RELATED FACTORS

Environmental
Smoking; secondhand smoke; smoke inhalation

Obstructed airway
Retained secretions; secretions in the bronchi; exudate in the alveoli; excessive mucus; airway spasm; foreign body in airway; presence of artificial airway

Physiological
Chronic obstructive pulmonary disease (COPD); asthma; allergic airways; hyperplasia of the bronchial walls
Neuromuscular dysfunction
Infection

DEFINING CHARACTERISTICS

Subjective
Dyspnea

Objective
Diminished/adventitious breath sounds [rales, crackles, rhonchi, wheezes]
Cough, ineffective/absent; excessive sputum
Changes in respiratory rate and rhythm
Difficulty vocalizing
Wide-eyed; restlessness
Orthopnea
Cyanosis

Sample Clinical Applications: COPD, pneumonia, influenza, acute respiratory distress syndrome (ARDS), cancer of lung/head and neck, congestive heart failure (CHF), cystic fibrosis, neuromuscular diseases, inhalation injuries

DESIRED OUTCOMES/EVALUATION CRITERIA
Sample NOC linkages:
Respiratory Status: Airway Patency: Open, clear tracheobronchial passages for air exchange
Aspiration Control: Personal actions to prevent the passage of fluid and solid particles into the lung
Cognition: Ability to execute complex mental processes

Client Will (Include Specific Time Frame)

- Maintain airway patency.
- Expectorate/clear secretions readily.
- Demonstrate absence/reduction of congestion with breath sounds clear, respirations noiseless, improved oxygen exchange (e.g., absence of cyanosis, ABG results within client norms).
- Verbalize understanding of cause(s) and therapeutic management regimen.
- Demonstrate behaviors to improve or maintain clear airway.
- Identify potential complications and how to initiate appropriate preventive or corrective actions.

Cultural   Collaborative   Community/Home Care   Diagnostic Studies   Pediatric/Geriatric/Lifespan   Medications

ACTIONS/INTERVENTIONS

Sample NIC linkages:

Airway Management: Facilitation of patency of air passages

Respiratory Monitoring: Collection and analysis of patient data to ensure airway patency and adequate gas exchange

Cough Enhancement: Promotion of deep inhalation by the patient with subsequent generation of high intrathoracic pressures and compression of underlying lung parenchyma for the forceful expulsion of air

NURSING PRIORITY NO. I To maintain adequate, patent airway:

- Identify client populations at risk. *Persons with impaired ciliary function (e.g., cystic fibrosis, status post-heart-lung transplantation); those with excessive or abnormal mucus production (e.g., asthma, emphysema, pneumonia, dehydration, bronchiectasis, mechanical ventilation); those with impaired cough function (e.g., neuromuscular diseases, such as muscular dystrophy; neuromotor conditions, such as cerebral palsy, spinal cord injury); those with swallowing abnormalities (e.g., poststroke, seizures, head/neck cancer, coma/sedation, tracheostomy, facial burns/trauma/surgery); those who are immobile (e.g., sedated individual, frail elderly, developmental delay); infant/child (e.g., feeding intolerance, abdominal distention, and emotional stressors that may compromise airway) are all at risk for problems with maintenance of open airways.*[1,2]
- Assess level of consciousness/cognition and ability to protect own airway. *Information essential for identifying potential for airway problems, providing baseline level of care needed, and influencing choice of interventions.*
- Evaluate respiratory rate/depth and breath sounds. *Tachypnea is usually present to some degree and may be pronounced during respiratory stress. Respirations may be shallow. Some degree of bronchospasm is present with obstruction in airways and may/may not be manifested in adventitious breath sounds, such as scattered moist crackles (bronchitis), faint sounds with expiratory wheezes (emphysema), or absent breath sounds (severe asthma).*[2]
- Position head appropriate for age and condition/disorder. *Repositioning head may, at times, be all that is needed to open or maintain open airway in at-rest or compromised individual, such as one with sleep apnea.*
- ∞ Insert oral airway, using correct size for adult or child, when indicated. Have appropriate emergency equipment at bedside (such as tracheostomy equipment, ambu-bag, suction apparatus) *to restore or maintain an effective airway.*[3,4]
- Evaluate amount and type of secretions being produced. *Excessive and/or sticky mucus can make it difficult to maintain effective airways, especially if client has impaired cough function, is very young or elderly, is developmentally delayed, has restrictive or obstructive lung disease, or is mechanically ventilated.*[5]
- Note ability/effectiveness of cough. *Cough function may be weak or ineffective in diseases and conditions such as extremes in age (e.g., premature infant or elderly), cerebral palsy, muscular dystrophy, spinal cord injury, brain injury, postsurgery, and/or mechanical ventilation due to mechanisms affecting muscles of throat, chest, and lungs.*[5,6]
- ∞ Suction (nasal/tracheal/oral), when indicated, using correct-size catheter and suction timing for child or adult *to clear airway when secretions are blocking airways, client is unable to clear airway by coughing, cough is ineffective, infant is unable to take oral feedings because of secretions, or ventilated client is showing desaturation of oxygen by oximetry or ABGs.*[2,5,7]

- Assist with/prepare for appropriate testing (e.g., pulmonary function/sleep studies) *to identify causative/precipitating factors.*
- Assist with procedures (e.g., bronchoscopy, tracheostomy) *to clear/maintain open airway.*
- Keep environment free of smoke, dust, and feather pillows according to individual situation. *Precipitators of allergic type of respiratory reactions that can trigger/exacerbate acute episode.*[3]

NURSING PRIORITY NO. 2 To mobilize secretions:

- Elevate head of the bed/change position, as needed. *Elevation/upright position facilitates respiratory function by use of gravity; however, the client in severe distress will seek position of comfort.*[3]
- Position appropriately (e.g., head of bed elevated, side-to-side) and discourage use of oil-based products around nose *to prevent vomiting with aspiration into lungs.* (Refer to NDs risk for Aspiration, impaired Swallowing.)
- Encourage/instruct in deep-breathing and directed-coughing exercises; teach (presurgically) and reinforce (postsurgically) breathing and coughing while splinting incision *to maximize cough effort, lung expansion, and drainage, and to reduce pain impairment.*
- Mobilize client as soon as possible. *Reduces risk or effects of atelectasis, enhancing lung expansion and drainage of different lung segments.*[5]
- Administer analgesics, as indicated. *Analgesics may be needed to improve cough effort when pain is inhibiting. Note: Overmedication, especially with opioids, can depress respirations and cough effort.*
- Administer medications (e.g., expectorants, anti-inflammatory agents, bronchodilators, and mucolytic agents), as indicated, *to relax smooth respiratory musculature, reduce airway edema, and mobilize secretions.*[8]
- Increase fluid intake to at least 2000 mL/day within cardiac tolerance (may require IV in acutely ill, hospitalized client). Encourage/provide warm versus cold liquids, as appropriate. *Warm hydration can help liquefy viscous secretions and improve secretion clearance. Note: Individuals with compromised cardiac function may develop symptoms of CHF (crackles, edema, weight gain).*[4,5]
- Provide ultrasonic nebulizer/room humidifier, as needed, *to deliver supplemental humidification, helping to reduce viscosity of secretions.*
- Assist with use of respiratory devices and treatments (e.g., intermittent positive-pressure breathing [IPPB], incentive spirometer [IS], positive expiratory pressure [PEP] mask, mechanical ventilation, oscillatory airway device [flutter], assisted and directed cough techniques, etc.). *Various therapies/modalities may be required to maintain adequate airways, improve respiratory function and gas exchange.* (Refer to NDs ineffective Breathing Pattern, impaired Gas Exchange, impaired spontaneous Ventilation.)[3,11]
- Perform/assist client in learning airway clearance techniques, particularly when airway congestion is a chronic/long-term condition. *Numerous techniques may be used, including (but not limited to) postural drainage and percussion (CPT), flutter devices, high-frequency chest compression with an inflatable vest, intrapulmonary percussive ventilation administered by a percussinator, and active cycle breathing (ACB), as indicated. Many of these techniques are the result of research in treatments of cystic fibrosis and muscular dystrophy as well as other chronic lung diseases.*[9]

NURSING PRIORITY NO. 3 To assess changes, note complications:

- Auscultate breath sounds, noting changes in air movement *to ascertain current status/effects of treatments to clear airways.*

- Monitor vital signs, noting blood pressure/pulse changes. Observe for increased respiratory rate, restlessness/anxiety, and use of accessory muscles for breathing, *suggesting advancing respiratory distress.*
- Monitor/document serial chest radiographs, ABGs, pulse oximetry readings. *Identifies baseline status, influences interventions, and monitors progress of condition and/or treatment response.*
- Evaluate changes in sleep pattern, noting insomnia or daytime somnolence. *May be evidence of nighttime airway incompetence or sleep apnea.* (Refer to ND Insomnia.)
- Document response to drug therapy and/or development of adverse reactions or side effects with antimicrobial agents, steroids, expectorants, bronchodilators. *Pharmacological therapy is used to prevent and control symptoms, reduce severity of exacerbations, and improve health status. The choice of medications depends on availability of the medication and the client's decision making about medication regimen and response to any given medication.*[10]
- Observe for signs/symptoms of infection (e.g., increased dyspnea, onset of fever, increase in sputum volume, change in color or character) *to identify infectious process/promote timely intervention.*[10]
- Obtain sputum specimen, preferably before antimicrobial therapy is initiated, *to verify appropriateness of therapy. Note: The presence of purulent sputum during an exacerbation of symptoms is a sufficient indication for starting antibiotic therapy, but a sputum culture and antibiogram (antibiotic sensitivity) may be done if the illness is not responding to the initial antibiotic.*[10]

NURSING PRIORITY NO. 4 To promote wellness (Teaching/Discharge Considerations):

- Assess client's/caregiver's knowledge of contributing causes, treatment plan, specific medications, and therapeutic procedures *to determine educational needs.*
- Provide information about the necessity of raising and expectorating secretions versus swallowing them, *to note changes in color and amount.*
- Identify signs/symptoms to be reported to primary care provider. *Prompt evaluation and intervention is required to prevent/treat infection.*
- Demonstrate/assist client/SO in performing specific airway clearance techniques (e.g., forced expiratory breathing [also called "huffing"] or respiratory muscle strength training, chest percussion), if indicated.[11]
- Review breathing exercises, effective coughing techniques, and use of adjunct devices (e.g., IPPB or incentive spirometry) in preoperative teaching *to facilitate postoperative recovery, reduce risk of pneumonia.*
- Instruct client/SO/caregiver in use of inhalers and other respiratory drugs. Include expected effects and information regarding possible side effects and interactions of respiratory drugs with other medications/OTC/herbals. Discuss symptoms requiring medical follow-up. *Client is often taking multiple medications that have similar side effects and potential for interactions. It is important to understand the difference between nuisance side effects (such as fast heartbeat after albuterol inhaler) and adverse effects (such as chest pain, hallucinations, or uncontrolled cardiac arrhythmia).*[9]
- Encourage/provide opportunities for rest; limit activities to level of respiratory tolerance. *Prevents/diminishes fatigue associated with underlying condition or efforts to clear airways.*
- Urge reduction/cessation of smoking. *Smoking is known to increase production of mucus and to paralyze (or cause loss of) cilia needed to move secretions to clear airway and improve lung function.*[10]

• Refer to appropriate support groups (e.g., stop-smoking clinic, COPD exercise group, weight reduction, American Lung Association, Cystic Fibrosis Foundation, Muscular Dystrophy Association).

 • Instruct in use of nocturnal positive pressure airflow for treatment of sleep apnea. (Refer to NDs Insomnia, Sleep Deprivation.)

DOCUMENTATION FOCUS

Assessment/Reassessment

• Related factors for individual client.
• Breath sounds, presence/character of secretions, use of accessory muscles for breathing.
• Character of cough/sputum.

Planning

• Plan of care and who is involved in planning.
• Teaching plan.

Implementation/Evaluation

• Client's response to interventions/teaching and actions performed.
• Attainment/progress toward desired outcome(s).
• Modifications to plan of care.

Discharge Planning

• Long-term needs and who is responsible for actions to be taken.
• Specific referrals made.

References

1. Impaired Airway Clearance: Information for Patients and Information for Health Plans: The Vest Airway Clearance System. Advanced Respiratory, Inc., 2002. Available at www.abivest.com.
2. Seay, S. J., Gay, S. L., Strauss, M. (2002). Tracheostomy emergencies. *AJN*, 102(3), 59.
3. Doenges, M. E., Moorhouse, M. F., Geissler-Murr, A. C. (2002). *Nursing Care Plans: Guidelines for Individualizing Patient Care.* 6th ed. Philadelphia: F. A. Davis, pp. 118–120.
4. Cox, H. C., et al. (2002). *Clinical Applications of Nursing Diagnosis: Adult, Child, Psychiatric, Gerontic, and Home Health Considerations.* 4th ed. Philadelphia: F. A. Davis, pp. 244–249.
5. Fink, J. B., Hess D. R. (2002). Secretion clearance techniques. In Hess, D. R. et al., (eds). *Respiratory Care: Principles and Practices.* Philadelphia: W. B. Saunders.
6. Blair, K. A. (1999). The aging pulmonary system. In Stanley, M., Beare, P. G. (eds). *Gerontological Nursing.* 2d ed. Philadelphia: F. A. Davis.
7. (1996). Suctioning of the patient in the home. American Association for Respiratory Care (AARC) Clinical Practice Guidelines. *Respir Care,* 41(7), 647–653.
8. Deglin, J. H., Vallerand, A. H. (2003). *Davis's Drug Guide for Nurses.* 8th ed. Bronchodilators: Pharmacolgic Profile G56. Philadelphia: F. A. Davis.
9. Yngsdal-Krenz, R. (Spring 1999). Airway Clearance Techniques. Center Focus, newsletter of the University of Wisconsin, Madison.
10. Global strategy for the diagnosis, management, and prevention of chronic obstructive pulmonary disease. Developers: World Health Organization (WHO); National Heart, Lung and Blood Institute (NHLBI); Global Imitative for Chronic Obstructive Lung Disease (GOLD). National Guideline Clearinghouse, May 2001. Available at www.ngc.com.
11. McCool, F. D., Rosen, M. J. (2006). Nonpharmacologic airway clearance therapies. *Chest,* 129, 250S–259S.

latex Allergy Response

Definition: A hypersensitive reaction to natural latex rubber products

RELATED FACTORS
Hypersensitivity to natural latex rubber protein

DEFINING CHARACTERISTICS

Subjective
Life-threatening reactions occurring <1 hour after exposure to latex proteins:
Tightness in chest; [feeling breathless]
Gastrointestinal characteristics: Abdominal pain; nausea
Orofacial characteristics: Itching of the eyes; nasal/facial/oral itching; nasal congestion
Generalized characteristics: Generalized discomfort; increasing complaints of total body warmth
Type IV reactions occurring >1 hour after exposure to latex protein:
Discomfort reaction to additives such as thiurams and carbamates

Objective
Life-threatening reactions occurring <1 hour after exposure to latex proteins:
Contact urticaria progressing to generalized symptoms
Edema of the lips/tongue/uvula/throat
Dyspnea; wheezing; bronchospasm; respiratory arrest
Hypotension; syncope; cardiac arrest
Orofacial characteristics: Edema of sclera/eyelids; erythema/tearing of the eyes; nasal facial/erythema; rhinorrhea
Generalized characteristics: Flushing; generalized edema; restlessness
Type IV reactions occurring >1 hour after exposure to latex protein:
Eczema; irritation; redness

Sample Clinical Applications: Multiple allergies, neural tube defects (e.g., spina bifida, myelomeningoceles), multiple surgeries at early age, chronic urological conditions (e.g., neurogenic bladder, exstrophy of bladder), spinal cord trauma

DESIRED OUTCOMES/EVALUATION CRITERIA
Sample NOC linkages:
Immune Hypersensitivity Control: Extent to which inappropriate immune responses are suppressed
Symptom Severity: Extent of perceived adverse changes in physical, emotional, and social functioning
Knowledge: Treatment Regimen: Extent of understanding conveyed about a specific treatment regimen

Client Will (Include Specific Time Frame)

• Be free of signs of hypersensitive response.
• Verbalize understanding of individual risks/responsibilities in avoiding exposure.
• Identify signs/symptoms requiring prompt intervention.

ACTIONS/INTERVENTIONS

Sample NIC linkages:

Latex Precautions: Reducing the risk of a systemic reaction to latex

Allergy Management: Identification, treatment, and prevention of allergic responses to food, medications, insect bites, contrast material, blood, or other substances

Environmental Risk Protection: Preventing and detecting disease and injury in populations at risk from environmental hazards

NURSING PRIORITY NO. 1 To assess contributing factors:

- Identify persons in high-risk categories such as those with history of certain food allergies (e.g., banana, avocado, chestnut, kiwi, papaya, peach, nectarine), prior allergies, asthma, and skin conditions (e.g., eczema and other dermatitis), those occupationally exposed to latex products (e.g., healthcare workers, police/firefighters, emergency medical technicians [EMTs], food handlers, hairdressers, cleaning staff, factory workers in plants that manufacture latex-containing products), those with neural tube defects (e.g., spina bifida) or congenital urological conditions requiring frequent surgeries and/or catheterizations (e.g., extrophy of the bladder). *Note: The most severe reactions tend to occur with latex proteins contacting internal tissues during invasive procedures and when they touch mucous membranes of the mouth, vagina, urethra, or rectum.*[9,10,11,13]
- Question new client regarding latex allergy upon admission to healthcare facility, especially when procedures are anticipated (e.g., laboratory, emergency department, operating room, wound care management, one-day surgery, dentist). *Basic safety information to help healthcare providers prevent/prepare for safe environment for client and themselves while providing care.*[2,4,7]
- Discuss history of exposure: client works in environment where latex is manufactured or latex gloves are used frequently; child was blowing up balloons (may be an acute reaction to the powder); use of condoms (may affect either partner); individual requires frequent catheterizations. *Finding cause of reaction may be simple or complex but often requires diligent investigation and history-taking from multiple sources.*
- Administer or note presence of positive skin-prick test (SPT), when performed. *Sensitive, specific, and rapid test but should be used with caution in persons with suspected sensitivity, as it carries risk of anaphylaxis.*[10]
- Perform challenge/patch test, if appropriate, *to identify specific allergens in client with known type IV hypersensitivity.*
- Note response to radioallergosorbent test (RAST) or enzyme-linked latex-specific IgE (ELISA). *Performed to measure the quantity of IgE antibodies in serum after exposure to specific antigens and has generally replaced skin tests and provocation tests, which are inconvenient, often painful, and/or hazardous to the client.*[1,11]

NURSING PRIORITY NO. 2 To take measures to reduce/limit allergic response/avoid exposure to allergens:

- Ascertain client's current symptoms, noting rash, hives, itching, eye symptoms, edema, diarrhea, nausea, and feeling of faintness. *Baseline for determining where the client is along a continuum of symptoms so that appropriate treatments can be initiated.*
- Determine time since exposure (e.g., immediate or delayed onset such as 24 to 48 hours).
- Assess skin (usually hands but may be anywhere) for dry, crusty, hard bumps, horizontal cracks caused by irritation from chemicals used in/on the latex item (e.g., latex or powder

Cultural Collaborative Community/Home Care Diagnostic Studies Pediatric/Geriatric/Lifespan Medications

used in latex gloves, condoms, etc.). *Dry itchy rash (contact irritation) is the most common response and is not a true allergic reaction but can progress to a delayed type of allergic contact dermatitis with oozing blisters and spread in a way similar to poison ivy.*[2-5,12]

- Assist with treatment of contact dermatitis/type IV reaction:
  Wash affected skin with mild soap and water.
  Wash hands between glove changes and after each glove removal.
  Avoid oil-based salves or lotions when using latex gloves.
  Consider application of topical steroid ointment.
  Inform client that the most common cause is latex gloves but that many other products contain latex and could aggravate condition.
- Monitor closely for signs of systemic reactions (e.g., difficulty breathing or swallowing; wheezing; hoarseness; stridor; hypotension; tremors; chest pain; tachycardia; dysrhythmias; edema of face, eyelids, lips, tongue, and mucous membranes). *Type IV response can progress to type I anaphylaxis.*
- Note behavior such as agitation, restlessness, and expressions of fearfulness, in the presence of above listed symptoms. *Indicative of severe allergic response that can result in anaphylactic reaction and lead to respiratory/cardiac arrest.*[6]
- Administer treatment, as appropriate, if severe/life-threatening reaction occurs:
  Stop treatment or procedure, if needed.
  Support airway and administer 100% oxygen or mechanical ventilation, if needed.
  Administer emergency medications and treatments per protocol (e.g., antihistamines, epinephrine, corticosteroids, and IV fluids).
- Educate care providers in ways to prevent inadvertent exposure (e.g., post latex precaution signs in client's room, document allergy to latex in chart, routinely monitor client's environment for latex-containing products and remove them promptly) and in emergency treatment measures should they be needed.
- Ascertain that latex-safe environment (e.g., surgery/hospital room) and products are available according to recommended facility guidelines and standards, including equipment and supplies, (e.g., powder-free, low-protein latex products) and latex-free items (e.g., gloves, syringes, catheters, tubings, tape, thermometers, electrodes, oxygen cannulas, underpads, storage bags, diapers, feeding nipples, etc.), as appropriate.[2,9,10,13]
- Notify physicians, colleagues, and medical products suppliers of condition (e.g., pharmacy *so that medications can be prepared in latex-free environment*, home-care oxygen company *to provide latex-free cannulas*).
- Encourage client to wear medical ID bracelet *to alert providers to condition if client is unresponsive.*[3,4,7]

NURSING PRIORITY NO. 3 To promote wellness (Teaching/Learning):

- Instruct in signs of reaction and emergency treatment needs. *Reactions range from skin irritation to anaphylaxis. Reaction may be gradual but progressive, affecting multiple body systems, or may be sudden, requiring lifesaving treatment. Allergy can result in chronic illness, disability, career loss, hardship, and death. There is no cure except complete avoidance of latex*
- Emphasize the critical importance of taking immediate action for type I reaction *to limit life-threatening symptoms.*
- Demonstrate procedure and recommend client carry auto-injectable epinephrine *to provide timely emergency treatment, as needed.*
- Emphasize necessity of informing all new care providers of hypersensitivity *to reduce preventable exposures.*

🏠 • Instruct client/family/SO that latex exposure occurs through contact with skin or mucous membrane, by inhalation, parenteral injection, or wound inoculation.

• Instuct client/SO(s) to survey and routinely monitor environment for latex-containing products, and replace as needed.

🏠 • Provide printed lists or Web sites for identifying common household products that may contain latex (e.g, carpet backing, hoses, rubber grip utensils, diapers, undergarments, shoes, toys, pacifiers, computer mouse pad, erasers, rubber bands, and much more) and where to obtain latex-free products and supplies.[4,7]

🏠 • Provide resource and assistance numbers for emergencies. *When allergy is suspected or the potential for allergy exists, protection must begin with identification and removal of possible sources of latex.*

🏠 • Provide worksite review/recommendations to prevent exposure. *Latex allergy can be a disabling occupational disease. Education about the problem promotes prevention of allergic reaction, facilitates timely intervention, and helps nurse to protect clients, latex-sensitive colleagues, and themselves.*[3,4]

⊛ • Recommend full medical workup for client presenting with hand dermatitis, especially if job tasks include use of latex.[8]

⊛ • Contact suppliers to verify that latex-free equipment, products, and supplies are available, including (but not limited to) low-allergen/powder-free synthetic gloves, airways, masks, stethoscope tubings, IV tubing, tape, thermometers, urinary catheters, stomach and intestinal tubes, electrodes, oxygen cannulas, pencil erasers, wrist name bands, and rubber bands.[7]

🏠 • Ascertain that procedures are in place to identify and resolve problems with medical devices relevant to allergic reactions or glove performance.[4]

🏠 • Refer to resources, including but not limited to ALERT (Allergy to Latex Education & Resource Team, Inc.), Latex Allergy News, Spina Bifida Association, National Institute for Occupational Safety and Health (NIOSH), Kendall's Healthcare Products [Web site], Hudson RCI [Web site]), *for further information about common latex products in the home, latex-free products, and assistance.*

DOCUMENTATION FOCUS

Assessment/Reassessment

• Assessment findings/pertinent history of contact with latex products/frequency of exposure.
• Type/extent of symptoms.

Planning

• Plan of care and interventions and who is involved in planning.
• Teaching plan.

Implementation/Evaluation

• Response to interventions/teaching and actions performed.
• Attainment/progress toward desired outcome(s).
• Modifications to plan of care.

Discharge Planning

• Discharge needs/referrals made, additional resources available.

🌐 Cultural ⊛ Collaborative 🏠 Community/Home Care ✏ Diagnostic Studies ∞ Pediatric/Geriatric/Lifespan 💊 Medications

References

1. Cavanaugh, B. M. (1999). *Nurse's Manual of Diagnostic Tests.* 3d ed. Philadelphia: F. A. Davis.
2. Latex Allergy: Protect yourself, protect your patients. Nursing World: Workplace Issues: Occupational Safety and Health. ANA pub No.WP-7, 1996.
3. Preventing Allergic Reactions to Natural Rubber Latex in the Workplace, National Institutes for Occupational Safety and Health (NIOSH) Alert. June 1997. DHHS (NIOSH) Pub No. 97–135.
4. ANA Position Statement: Latex Allergy [online]. Effective September 1997. Available at www.nursingworld.org.
5. Truscott, W., Roley, L. (1995). Glove-associated reactions: Addressing an increasing concern. *Dermatol Nurs,* 7(5), 283.
6. Urticaria and angioedema. In Sommers, M. S. Johnson, S. A. (eds). (1997). *Davis's Manual of Nursing Therapeutics for Diseases and Disorders.* Philadelphia: F. A. Davis.
7. AANA Latex Protocol. Certified Registered Nurse Anesthetists (CRNA), American Association of Nurse Anesthetists. Developed 1993, Revised and Approved July 1998. Available at www.aana.com.
8. Worthington, K., Wilburn, S. (2001). Latex allergy: What's the facility's responsibility and what's yours? *AJN,* 101(7), 88.
9. Klotter, J. (2006). Latex allergy prevention. Townsend Letter for Doctors and Patients, May 1, 2006.
10. Behrman, A. J., Howarth, M. (2005). Latex allergy. Article for Emedicine Web site. Retrieved February 2007 at www.emedicime.com/emerg/topic814.htm.
11. Allery testing. Article for Lab Tests Online. Retrieved February 2007 at www.labtestsonline.
12. Haines, C. (2006). Learning about allergies to latex. Article for WebMD Web site. Retrieved February 2007 at www.webmd.com/content/pages/10/1625.htm.
13. AORN Latex Guideline: 2004 standards, recommended practices, and guidelines. *AORN J,* 79(3), 653–672.

risk for latex Allergy Response

Definition: Risk of hypersenitivity to natural latex rubber products

RISK FACTORS
History of reactions to latex
Allergies to bananas, avocados, tropical fruits, kiwi, chestnuts, poinsettia plants
History of allergies and asthma
Professions with daily exposure to latex
Multiple surgical procedures, especially from infancy
NOTE: A risk diagnosis is not evidenced by signs and symptoms, as the problem has not occurred and nursing interventions are directed at prevention.

Sample Clinical Applications: Multiple allergies, neural tube defects (e.g., spina bifida, myelomeningoceles), multiple surgeries at early age, chronic urological conditions (e.g., neurogenic bladder, exstrophy of bladder), spinal cord trauma

DESIRED OUTCOMES/EVALUATION CRITERIA
Sample NOC linkages:
Immune Hypersensitivity Response: Severity of inappropriate immune responses
Risk Control: Personal actions to prevent, eliminate, or reduce modifiable health threats
Knowledge: Health Behavior: Extent of understanding conveyed about the promotion and protection of health

Client Will (Include Specific Time Frame)
- Identify and correct potential risk factors in the environment.
- Demonstrate appropriate lifestyle changes to reduce risk of exposure.
- Identify resources to assist in promoting a safe environment.
- Recognize need for/seek assistance to limit response/complications.

ACTIONS/INTERVENTIONS

Sample NIC linkages:
Latex Precautions: Reducing the risk of a systemic reaction to latex
Allergy Management: Identification, treatment, and prevention of allergic responses to food, medications, insect bites, contrast material, blood, or other substances
Risk Identification: Analysis of potential risk factors, determination of health risks, and prioritization of risk-reduction strategies for an individual or group

NURSING PRIORITY NO. 1 To assess causative/contributing factors:

- Identify persons in high-risk categories such as those with history of certain food allergies (e.g., banana, avocado, chestnut, kiwi, papya, peach, nectarine); asthma; skin conditions (e.g., eczema); those occupationally exposed to latex products (e.g., healthcare workers, police/firefighters, emergency medical technicians [EMTs], food handlers, hairdressers, cleaning staff, factory workers in plants that manufacture latex-containing products); those with neural tube defects (e.g., spina bifida) or congenital urological conditions requiring frequent surgeries and/or catheterizations (e.g., extrophy of the bladder). *Note: The most severe reactions tend to occur with latex proteins contacting internal tissues during invasive procedures and when they touch mucous membranes of the mouth, vagina, urethra, or rectum.*[5–7]
- Question client regarding latex allergy upon admission to healthcare facility, especially when procedures are anticipated (e.g., laboratory, emergency department, operating room, wound care management, one-day surgery, dentist). *Current information indicates that natural latex is found in thousands of medical supplies; however, many manufacturers are now using synthetic SB latex. These products have not been associated with allergic reactions, even among individuals that are sensitive to natural latex.*[1]

NURSING PRIORITY NO. 2 To assist in correcting factors that could lead to latex allergy:

- Ascertain that facilities have established policies and procedures. *Promotes awareness in the workplace to address safety and reduce risk to workers and client.*[3]
- Create latex-safe environments in care setting (e.g., substitute nonlatex products, such as natural rubber gloves, PCV IV tubing, latex-free tape, thermometers, electrodes, oxygen cannulas, etc.). *Reduces risk of exposure.*[8,9]
- Promote good skin care when latex gloves may be preferred/required for barrier protection (e.g., in specific disease conditions such as HIV or during surgery). Use powder-free gloves, wash hands immediately after glove removal; refrain from use of oil-based hand cream. *Reduces dermal and respiratory exposure to latex proteins that bind to the powder in gloves.*[10]
- Discuss necessity of avoiding latex exposure. Recommend/assist client/family to survey environment and remove any medical or household products containing latex. *Avoidance of latex is the only way to prevent the allergy.*[2]
- Provide worksite review/recommendations to prevent exposure. *Latex allergy can be a disabling occupational disease. Education about the problem promotes prevention of allergic reaction, facilitates timely intervention, and helps nurse to protect clients, latex-sensitive colleagues, and themselves.*[1,4]

NURSING PRIORITY NO. 3 To promote wellness (Teaching/Discharge Considerations):

- Instruct client/care providers about types of potential reactions. *Reaction may be gradual and progressive (e.g., irritant contact rash with gloves); can be progressive, affecting multiple body systems; or may be sudden and anaphylactic requiring lifesaving treatment.*[1,3]

- Identify measures to take if reactions occur and ways to avoid exposure to latex products *to reduce risk of injury.* (Refer to ND latex Allergy Response.)
- Refer to allergist for testing as appropriate. *Testing may include challenge test with latex gloves, skin patch test, or blood test for IgE.*
- Encourage client to wear medical ID bracelet and emphasize importance of informing all new care providers of hypersensitivity *to reduce preventable exposures.*[1,4]
- Refer to resources (e.g., Latex Allergy News, National Institute for Occupational Safety and Health [NIOSH], Kendall's Healthcare Products [Web site], Hudson RCI [Web site]) *for further information about common latex products in the home, latex-free products, and assistance.*

DOCUMENTATION FOCUS

Assessment/Reassessment

- Assessment findings, pertinent history of contact with latex products, and frequency of exposure.

Planning

- Plan of care and who is involved in planning.
- Teaching plan.

Implementation/Evaluation

- Response to interventions/teaching and actions performed.
- Attainment/progress toward desired outcome(s).
- Modifications to plan of care.

Discharge Planning

- Long-term needs and who is responsible for actions to be taken.
- Specific referrals made.

References

1. American Nurses Association (ANA) Position Statement: Latex Allergy [online]. Effective September 1997. Available at www.nursingworld.org.
2. Statement on natural latex allergies and SB latex. Occupational Hazards. Retrieved February 11, 2003. Available at www.occupationalhazards.com.
3. Latex Allergy: Protect yourself, protect your patients. Nursing World: Workplace Issues: Occupational Safety and Health. ANA Pub No. WP-7, 1996.
4. Preventing allergic reactions to natural rubber in the workplace. National Institutes for Occupational Safety and Health (NIOSH) Alert. DHHS Pub No. 97–135, June 1997.
5. Klotter, J. (2006). Latex allergy prevention. Townsend Letter for Doctors and Patients, May 1, 2006.
6. Behrman, A. J., Howarth, M. (2005). Latex allergy. Article for Emedicine Web site. Retrieved February 2007. Available at www.emedicine.com/emerg/topic814.htm.
7. Haines, C. (2006). Learning about allergies to latex. Article for WebMD Web site. Retrieved February 2007. Available at www.webmd.com/allergies/guide/latex-allergies.
8. AORN latex guideline: 2004 standards, recommended practices, and guidelines. *AORN J*, 79(3), 653–672.
9. Molnlycke Health Care, US, LLC. (2006). Latex-safe is best gloving practice against latex allergy. PR Newswire. Retrieved February 2007. Available at www.biogellatexsafe.com/downloads/yahoo_finance_latex-safe.doc.

10. Centers for Disease Control and Prevention. (2000-2007). Latex allergy prevention. Article for National Institute for Occupational Safety and Health (NIOSH) Web site. Retrieved February 2007. Available at www.cdc.gov/niosh/98-113.html.

Anxiety [specify level: mild, moderate, severe, panic]

Definition: Vague uneasy feeling of discomfort or dread accompanied by an autonomic response (the source often nonspecific or unknown to the individual); a feeling of apprehension caused by anticipation of danger. It is an alerting signal that warns of impending danger and enables the individual to take measures to deal with threat.

RELATED FACTORS

Unconscious conflict about essential [beliefs]/goals and values of life
Situational/maturational crises
Stress
Familial association/heredity
Interpersonal transmission/contagion
Threat to self-concept [perceived or actual]; [unconscious conflict]
Threat of death [perceived or actual]
Threat to or change in health status [progressive/debilitating disease, terminal illness], interaction patterns, role function/status, environment [safety], economic status
Unmet needs
Exposure to toxins
Substance abuse
[Positive or negative self-talk]
[Physiological factors, such as hyperthyroidism, pulmonary embolism, dysrhythmias, pheochromocytoma, drug therapy including steroids]

DEFINING CHARACTERISTICS

Subjective
Behavioral
Expressed concerns due to change in life events; insomnia
Affective
Regretful; scared; rattled; distressed; apprehensive; uncertainty; fearful; feelings of inadequacy; jittery; worried; painful/persistent increased helplessness; [sense of impending doom]; [hopelessness]
Cognitive
Fear of unspecific consequences; awareness of physiological symptoms
Physiological
Shakiness
Sympathetic
Dry mouth, heart pounding; weakness; respiratory difficulties; anorexia; diarrhea
Parasympathetic
Tingling in extremeties; nausea; abdominal pain; diarrhea; urinary frequency/hesitancy; faintness; fatigue; sleep disturbance; [chest, back, neck pain]

Objective
Behavioral
Poor eye contact, glancing about, scanning and vigilance, extraneous movement [e.g., foot shuffling, hand/arm movements, rocking motion]; fidgeting; restlessness; diminished productivity; [crying/tearfulness]; [pacing/purposeless activity], [immobility]

Cultural   Collaborative   Community/Home Care   Diagnostic Studies   Pediatric/Geriatric/Lifespan   Medications

Affective
Increased wariness; focus on self; irritability; overexcited; anguish
Cognitive
Preoccupation; impaired attention; difficulty concentrating; forgetfulness; diminished ability to problem-solve; diminished learning ability; rumination; tendency to blame others; blocking of thought; confusion; decreased perceptual field
Physiological
Voice quivering; trembling/hand tremors; increased tension, facial tension, increased perspiration
Sympathetic
Cardiovascular excitation; facial flushing; superficial vasoconstriction; increased pulse/respiration; increased blood pressure; pupil dilation; twitching, increased reflexes
Parasympathetic
Urinary urgency; decreased blood pressure/pulse

Sample Clinical Applications: Major life changes/events, hospital admissions/surgery, cancer, hyperthyroidism, drug intoxication/abuse, mental health disorders

DESIRED OUTCOMES/EVALUATION CRITERIA
Sample NOC linkages:
Anxiety Self-Control: Personal actions to eliminate or reduce feelings of apprehension, tension, or uneasiness from an unidentifiable source
Coping: Personal actions to manage stressors that tax an individual's resources
Impulse Self-Control: Self-restraint of compulsive or impulsive behaviors

Client Will (Include Specific Time Frame)

- Appear relaxed and report anxiety is reduced to a manageable level.
- Verbalize awareness of feelings of anxiety.
- Identify healthy ways to deal with and express anxiety.
- Demonstrate problem-solving skills.
- Use resources/support systems effectively.

ACTIONS/INTERVENTIONS

Sample NIC linkages:
Anxiety Reduction: Minimizing apprehension, dread, foreboding, or uneasiness related to an unidentified source or anticipated danger
Dementia Management: Provision of a modified environment for the patient who is experiencing a chronic confusional state
Calming Technique: Reducing anxiety in patient experiencing acute distress

NURSING PRIORITY NO. 1. To assess level of anxiety:

- Review familial/physiological factors, such as genetic depressive factors, psychiatric illness; active medical conditions (e.g., thyroid problems, metabolic imbalances, cardiopulmonary disease, anemia, dysrhythmias); recent/ongoing stressors (e.g., family member illness/death, spousal conflict/abuse, loss of job). *These factors can cause/exacerbate anxiety/anxiety disorders.*[7,13,14]

- Determine current prescribed medication regimen and recent drug history of prescribed or OTC medications (e.g., steroids, thyroid preparations, weight-loss pills, caffeine. *Can heighten feelings/sense of anxiety.*[13,14]
- Identify client's perception of the threat represented by the situation. *Distorted perceptions of the situation may magnify feelings. Understanding client's point of view promotes a more accurate plan of care.*[2]
- Note cultural factors that may influence anxiety. *Individual responses are influenced by the cultural values/beliefs and culturally learned patterns of family of origin. (For example, Arab-Americans are very expressive about feelings, whereas Chinese are more reticent).*[4] *Biological factors may also be involved.*[3]
- Monitor physical responses; for example, palpitations/rapid pulse, repetitive movements, pacing. *Changes in vital signs may suggest degree of anxiety client is experiencing or reflect the impact of physiological factors such as endocrine imbalances, medication effect.*[1,7]
- Observe behavior indicative of anxiety, *which can be a clue to the client's level of anxiety:*

   Mild
   Alert, more aware of environment, attention focused on environment and immediate events.
   Restless, irritable, wakeful, reports of insomnia.
   Motivated to deal with existing problems in this state.
   Moderate
   Perception narrower, concentration increased and able to ignore distractions in dealing with problem(s).
   Voice quivers or changes pitch.
   Trembling, increased pulse/respirations.
   Severe
   Range of perception is reduced; anxiety interferes with effective functioning.
   Preoccupied with feelings of discomfort/sense of impending doom.
   Increased pulse/respirations with reports of dizziness, tingling sensations, headache, and so forth.
   Panic
   Ability to concentrate is disrupted; behavior is disintegrated; client distorts the situation and does not have realistic perceptions of what is happening.
   May be experiencing terror or confusion or be unable to speak or move (paralyzed with fear).

- Note own feelings of anxiety or uneasiness. *Feelings of anxiety are circular, and those in contact with the client may find themselves feeling more anxious.*[3]
- Note use of drugs (including alcohol), insomnia, or excessive sleeping, and limited/avoidance of interactions with others, *which may be behavioral indicators of use of drugs/withdrawal to deal with problems.*[5]
- Review results of diagnostic tests (e.g., drug screens, cardiac testing, complete blood count, chemistry panel), *which can point to physiological sources of anxiety.*
- Review coping skills used in past. *Can determine those that might be helpful in current circumstances.*[6]

NURSING PRIORITY NO. 2 To assist client to identify feelings and begin to deal with problems:

- Establish a therapeutic relationship, conveying empathy and unconditional positive regard. *Enables client to become comfortable and to begin looking at feelings and dealing with situation.*[3]
- Be available to client for listening and talking. *Establishes rapport, promotes expression of feelings, and helps client/SO look at realities of the illness/treatment without confronting issues they are not ready to deal with.*[3]

Cultural   Collaborative   Community/Home Care   Diagnostic Studies   Pediatric/Geriatric/Lifespan   Medications

- Encourage client to acknowledge and to express feelings—for example, crying (sadness), laughing (fear, denial), swearing (fear, anger), and using Active-listening, reflection. *Often acknowledging feelings enables client to accept and deal more appropriately with situation, thus relieving anxiety.*[8]
- Assist client to develop self-awareness of verbal and nonverbal behaviors. *Becoming aware helps client to control these behaviors and begin to deal with issues that are causing anxiety.*[9]
- Clarify meaning of feelings/actions by providing feedback and checking meaning with the client. *Validates meaning and ensures accuracy of communication.*[10]
- Acknowledge anxiety/fear. Do not deny or reassure client that everything will be all right. *Validates reality of feelings. False reassurances may be interpreted as lack of understanding or honesty, further isolating client.*[3]
- Be aware of defense mechanisms being used (e.g., denial, regression, and so forth). *Use of defense mechanisms may be helpful coping mechanisms initially. However, continued use of such mechanisms diverts the energy that the client needs for healing, thus delaying the client from focusing and dealing with his actual problems.*[6]
- Identify coping skills the individual is using currently, such as anger, daydreaming, forgetfulness, eating, smoking, or lack of problem-solving. *These may be useful for the moment but may eventually interfere with resolution of current situation.*[6]
- Provide accurate information about the situation. *Helps client to identify what is reality based and provides opportunity for client to feel reassured.*[11]
- ∞ If the client is a child, be truthful, avoid bribing, and provide physical contact (e.g., hugging, rocking). *Soothes fears and provides assurance. Children need to recognize that their feelings are not different from others.*[5]

NURSING PRIORITY NO. 3 To provide measures to comfort and aid client to handle problematic situations:

- Provide comfort measures (e.g., calm/quiet environment, soft music, warm bath, back rub: Therapeutic Touch). *Aids in meeting basic human need, decreasing sense of isolation and assisting client to feel less anxious. Therapeutic Touch requires the nurse to have specific knowledge and experience to use the hands to correct energy field disturbances by redirecting human energies to help or heal.*[3,11]
- ∞ Modify procedures, as necessary (e.g., substitute oral for intramuscular medications, combine blood draws/use fingerstick method). *Limits degree of stress, avoids overwhelming child or anxious adult.*[2]
- ∞ Manage environmental factors, such as harsh lighting and high traffic flow, excessive noise. *May be confusing/stressful to older individuals. Managing these factors can lessen anxiety, especially when client is in strange and unusual circumstances.*[2]
- Discuss the use of music and accommodate client's preferences. *Promotes calming atmosphere, helping to alleviate anxiety.*[3]
- Accept client as is. *The client may need to be where he or she is at this point in time, such as in denial after receiving the diagnosis of a terminal illness.*[3]
- Allow the behavior to belong to the client; do not respond personally. *Reacting personally can escalate the situation, promoting a nontherapeutic situation and increasing anxiety.*[1]
- Assist client to use anxiety for coping with the situation if helpful. *Moderate anxiety heightens awareness and can help client to focus on dealing with problems.*[9]
- Encourage awareness of negative self-talk and discuss replacing with positive statements, such as using "can" instead of "can't," etc. *Negative self-talk promotes feelings of anxiety and self-doubt. Becoming aware and replacing these thoughts can enhance sense of self-worth and reduce anxiety.*[9]

PANIC STATE

- Stay with client, maintaining a calm, confident manner. *Presence communicates caring and helps client to calm down.*[1]
- Speak in brief statements using simple words. *Client is not able to comprehend complex information at this time.*[1]
- Provide for nonthreatening, consistent environment/atmosphere. Minimize stimuli and monitor visitors and interactions with others. *Lessens effect of transmission of anxious feelings.*[1]
- Set limits on inappropriate behavior and help client to develop acceptable ways of dealing with anxiety.
- Provide safe controls/environment until client regains control. *Behavior may result in damage or injury that client will regret when control is regained, diminishing sense of self-worth.*[1]
- Gradually increase activities/involvement with others as anxiety is decreased. *Promotes sense of normalcy, helps control feelings of anxiety.*[1]
- Use cognitive therapy to focus on/correct faulty catastrophic interpretations of physical symptoms. *For example, thoughts of dying increase anxiety and feelings of panic. Controlling these thoughts allows client to look at situation more realistically and begin to deal appropriately with what is happening.*[1]
- Administer antianxiety agents/sedatives, as ordered. *Appropriate medication can be helpful in enabling the client to regain control.*[1]

NURSING PRIORITY NO. 4 To promote wellness (Teaching/Discharge Considerations):

- Assist client to identify/deal with precipitating factors and learn new methods of coping with disabling anxiety. *Lessens possibility of repeat episodes.*[9]
- Review happenings, thoughts, and feelings preceding the anxiety attack. *Identifies factors that led to onset of attack, promoting opportunity to prevent recurrences.*[2]
- Identify actions/activities the client has previously used to cope successfully when feeling nervous/anxious. *Realizing that individual already has coping skills that can be applied in current and future situations can empower client.*[2]
- List helpful resources/people, including available "hotline" or crisis managers. *Provides ongoing/timely support.*[2]
- Encourage client to develop a regular exercise/activity program. *May be helpful in reducing level of anxiety by relieving tension and has been shown to raise endorphin levels to enhance sense of well-being.*[2]
- Assist in developing skills (e.g., awareness of negative thoughts, saying "Stop" and substituting a positive thought). *Eliminating negative self-talk can lead to feelings of positive self-esteem. (Note: Mild phobias seem to respond better to behavioral therapy.)*[10]
- Review such strategies as role-playing, use of visualizations to practice anticipated events, prayer/meditation. *These activities can help the client practice behaviors in a safe/supportive environment, enabling individual to manage anxiety-provoking situations.*[10]
- Review medication regimen and possible interactions, especially with OTC drugs/alcohol, herbal products. *Enhances understanding of reason for medication and can avoid untoward/harmful reactions from incompatible drugs.*[12]
- Discuss appropriate drug substitutions or changes in dosage or time of dose. *Ensures proper dosage and avoids untoward side effects. This is especially important in the elderly, who are particularly susceptible to multidrug complications.*[12]
- Refer to physician for drug management program/alteration of prescription regimen. *Drugs that often cause symptoms of anxiety include aminophylline/theophylline, anticholinergics, dopamine, levodopa, salicylates, and steroids. Monitoring provides opportunity to correct possible undesirable effects of these drugs.*[12]

• Refer to individual and/or group therapy, as appropriate. *May be useful to help client deal with chronic anxiety states.*[2]

DOCUMENTATION FOCUS

Assessment/Reassessment

- Level of anxiety and precipitating/aggravating factors.
- Description of feelings (expressed and displayed).
- Awareness/ability to recognize and express feelings.
- Related substance use, if present.

Planning

- Treatment plan and individual responsibility for specific activities.
- Teaching plan.

Implementation/Evaluation

- Client involvement and response to interventions/teaching and actions performed.
- Attainment/progress toward desired outcome(s).
- Modifications to plan of care.

Discharge Planning

- Referrals and follow-up plan.
- Specific referrals made.

References

1. Doenges, M., Moorhouse, M., Murr, A. (2002). *Nursing Care Plans, Guidelines for Individualizing Patient Care.* 6th ed. Philadelphia: F. A. Davis.
2. Doenges, M., Townsend, M., Moorhouse, M. (1993). *Psychiatric Care Plans: Guidelines for Individualizing Care.* 3d ed. Philadelphia: F. A. Davis.
3. Townsend, M. (2003). *Psychiatric Mental Health Nursing: Concepts of Care.* 4th ed. Philadelphia: F. A. Davis.
4. Lipson, J. G., Dibble, S. L., Minarik, P. A. (1996). *Culture & Nursing Care: A Pocket Guide. School of Nursing.* San Francisco: UCSF Nursing Press.
5. National Institute of Mental Health. (2000). Anxiety Disorders, NIH Publication No. 00-3879. Rockville, MD: Author. Available at www.nimh.nih.gov.anxiety/anxiety.cfm.
6. Stuart, G. W. (2001). Anxiety responses and anxiety disorders. In Stuart, G. W., Laraia, M. T. (eds). *Principles and Practice of Psychiatric Nursing.* 7th ed. St. Louis, MO: Mosby.
7. Kunert, P. K. (2002). Stress and adaptation. In Porth, C. M. (ed). *Pathophysiology: Concepts of Altered Health States.* Philadelphia: Lippincott.
8. Moller, M. D., Murphy, M. F. (1998). *Recovering from Psychosis: A Wellness Approach.* Nine Mile Falls, WA: Psychiatric Rehabilitation Nurses Inc.
9. Bohrer, G. J. (March 18, 2002). Anxiety, emotional and physical discomfort. *NurseWeek* (Mountain West edition), 3(1), 21–22.
10. Burns, D. D. (1999). *Feeling Good: The New Mood Therapy.* New York: Avon.
11. Krieger, D. O. (1979). *The Therapeutic Touch: How to Use Your Hands to Heal.* Englewood Cliffs, NJ: Prentice Hall.
12. Townsend, M. (2001). Nursing Diagnoses in Psychiatric Nursing: Care Plans and Psychotropic Medications. 5th ed. Philadelphia: F. A. Davis.
13. Murphy, K. (2005). Anxiety: When is it too much? *Nursing Made Incredibly Easy!* 3(5), 22–31.
14. Lamemeh, T., Shah, A. M., Hsu, K. (2006). Anxiety. Article for Emedicine Web site. Retrieved January 2007. Available at www.emedicine.com/emerg/topic35.htm.

death Anxiety

Definition: Vague uneasy feeling of discomfort or dread generated by perceptions of a real or imagined threat to one's existence

RELATED FACTORS

Anticipating pain; suffering; adverse consequences of general anesthesia; impact of death on others

Confronting reality of terminal disease; experiencing dying process; perceived proximity of death

Discussions on topic of death; observations related to death; near-death experience

Uncertainty of prognosis; nonacceptance of own mortality

Uncertainty about the existance of a higher power; life after death; an encounter with a higher power

DEFINING CHARACTERISTICS

Subjective

Fear of developing a terminal illness; the process of dying; pain/suffering related to dying; loss of mental/[physical] abilities when dying; premature death; prolonged dying

Negative thoughts related to death and dying

Feeling powerlessness over dying

Worrying about the impact of one's death on significant others; [about meeting one's creator or feeling doubtful about the existence of God or higher being]

Concerns of overworking the caregiver

Sample Clinical Applications: Chronic debilitating health conditions, cancer, hospital admission, impending major surgery

DESIRED OUTCOMES/EVALUATION CRITERIA

Sample NOC linkages:

Dignified Life Closure: Personal actions to maintain control during approaching end of life

Fear Self-Control: Personal actions to eliminate or reduce disabling feelings of apprehension, tension, or uneasiness from an identifiable source

Acceptance: Health Status: Reconciliation to significant change in health circumstances

Client Will (Include Specific Time Frame)

- Identify and express feelings (e.g., sadness, guilt, fear) freely/effectively.
- Look toward/plan for the future one day at a time.
- Formulate a plan dealing with individual concerns and eventualities of dying.

ACTIONS/INTERVENTIONS

Sample NIC linkages:

Dying Care: Promotion of physical comfort and psychological peace in the final phase of life

Spiritual Support: Assisting the patient to feel balance and connection with a greater power

Grief Work Facilitation: Assistance with the resolution of a significant loss

Cultural · Collaborative · Community/Home Care · Diagnostic Studies · Pediatric/Geriatric/Lifespan · Medications

NURSING PRIORITY NO. 1 To assess causative/contributing factors:

- Determine how client sees self in usual lifestyle role functioning and determine perception and meaning of anticipated loss to him or her and SO(s). *Provides information that can be compared to changes that are occurring. Understanding these factors are helpful for planning.*[1]
- Ascertain current knowledge of situation. *Identifies misconceptions, lack of information, and other pertinent issues and determines accuracy of knowledge. Death may not be anticipated by healthcare providers in current situation.*[1]
- Determine client's role in family constellation. Observe patterns of communication in family and response of family/SO to client's situation and concerns. *In addition to identifying areas of need/concern, this also reveals strengths useful in addressing the current concerns.*[3]
- Assess impact of client reports of subjective experiences and experience with death (or exposure to death); for example, witnessed violent death or, as a child, viewed body in casket, and so forth. *Identifies possible feelings that may be affecting current situation, thus promoting accurate planning.*[2]
- Identify cultural factors/expectations and impact on current situation/feelings. *These factors affect client attitude toward events and impending loss. For instance, in Russia, the head of the family is informed first of the impending death, as they may not want the client to know so he or she will have a peaceful death. Many cultures prefer to keep the client at home instead of in a nursing home or hospital. Growth of the hospice movement in the United States provides palliative care and comfort during the client's final days in any setting.*[4]
- Note age, physical/mental condition, complexity of therapeutic regimen. *May affect ability to handle current situation. Younger people may handle stress of illness in more positive ways. Older people may be more accepting of possibility of death. Individuals of any age will deal with situation in own way, depending on diagnosis, condition, expectations, situation.*[1,8]
- Determine ability to manage own self-care, end-of-life and other affairs, awareness/use of available resources. *Information will be necessary for determining needs, planning care.*[1,8]
- Observe behavior indicative of the level of anxiety present (mild to panic). *The level of anxiety affects client's/SO's ability to process information/participate in activities.*[5]
- Note use of drugs (including alcohol), presence of insomnia, excessive sleeping, avoidance of interactions with others. *Indicators of withdrawal and need for intervention to deal with symptoms and help client deal realistically with diagnosis/illness.*[6]
- Determine sense of futility, feelings of hopelessness, helplessness, lack of motivation to help self. *Indicators of depression and need for early intervention to help client acknowledge and deal with impending death.*[7,8]
- Listen for expressions of inability to find meaning in life or suicidal ideation. *Signs of depression indicating need for referral to therapist/psychiatrist and possible pharmacological treatment to help client deal with terminal illness/situation.*[7]

NURSING PRIORITY NO. 2 To assist client to deal with situation:

- Provide open and trusting relationship. *Promotes opportunity to explore feelings about impending death.*[2]
- Make time for nonjudgmental discussion of philosophical issues/questions about spiritual impact of illness/situation. *Can help client clarify own position on these issues.*[3]
- Respect client desire/request not to talk. Provide hope within parameters of the individual situation. *Promotes open environment that encourages client to talk freely about thoughts and feelings. Client may not be ready to talk about situation/concerns about death or may be denying reality of what is happening.*[1,8]

Nursing Diagnoses in Alphabetical Order

- Encourage expressions of feelings (anger, fear, sadness, etc.). Acknowledge anxiety/fear. Do not deny or reassure client that everything will be all right. Be honest when answering questions/providing information. *Enhances trust and therapeutic relationship.*[2]
- Use therapeutic communication skills of Active-listening. *Technique acknowledges reality of feelings and encourages client to find own solutions.*[2]
- Provide information about normalcy of feelings and individual grief reaction. *Most individuals question their reactions and whether they are normal or not, and information can provide reassurance for individual.*[3] (Refer to ND Grieving.)
- Identify coping skills currently used and how effective they are. Be aware of defense mechanisms being used by the client. *Provides a starting point to plan care and assists client to acknowledge reality and deal more effectively with what is happening.*[3]
- Review life experiences of loss, noting client strengths and successes. *Provides opportunity to identify and use previously successful skills.*[2]
- Provide calm, peaceful setting and privacy, as appropriate. *Promotes relaxation and enhances ability to deal with situation.*[1,8]
- Include family in discussions and decision making, as appropriate. *Involved family members can provide support and ideas for problem-solving.*[7]
- Note client's religious/spiritual orientation, involvement in religious/church activities, presence of conflicts regarding spiritual beliefs. *May benefit by referral to appropriate resource to help client resolve these issues, if desired.*[7]
- Assist client to engage in spiritual growth activities, experience prayer/meditation and forgiveness to heal past hurts. Provide information that anger with God is a normal part of the grief process. *May reduce feelings of guilt/conflict, allowing client to move forward toward resolution.*[1]
- Refer to therapists, spiritual advisors, or counselors, as appropriate. *Promotes facilitation of grief work.*[1]
- Refer to community agencies/resources. *Assists client/SO in planning for eventualities (legal issues, funeral plans, etc.).*[1]

NURSING PRIORITY NO. 3. To promote independence:

- Support client's efforts to develop realistic steps to put plans into action. *Provides sense of control over situation in which client does not have much control.*[1]
- Direct client's thoughts beyond present state, encouraging client to try to enjoy each day and look to the future, as appropriate. *Being in the moment can help client enjoy this time rather than dwelling on what is ahead.*[1]
- Provide opportunities for client to make simple decisions. *Enhances sense of control.*[1]
- Develop individual plan using client's locus of control. *Incorporating locus of control (internal or external) enhances success of plan by enabling client/family to manage situation more effectively.*[2]
- Treat expressed decisions and desires with respect and convey to others, as appropriate. *Expresses regard for the individual and enhances sense of control in situation that is not controllable.*[1]
- Assist with completion of Advance Directives and cardiopulmonary resuscitation (CPR) instructions. *Provides opportunity for client to understand options and express desires.*[1]
- Refer to palliative, hospice, or end-of-life care resources, as appropriate. *Provides support and assistance to client and SO/family through potentially complex and difficult process. Choice of type of care is dependent on timing of care (e.g., palliative care interfaces with curative treatment, which hospice does not allow).*[1]

🌐 Cultural 🅐 Collaborative 🏠 Community/Home Care 🧪 Diagnostic Studies ∞ Pediatric/Geriatric/Lifespan 💊 Medications

DOCUMENTATION FOCUS

Assessment/Reassessment

- Assessment findings, including client's fears and signs/symptoms being exhibited.
- Responses/actions of family/SOs.
- Availability/use of resources.

Planning

- Plan of care and who is involved in planning.

Implementation/Evaluation

- Client's response to interventions/teaching and actions performed.
- Attainment/progress toward desired outcome(s).
- Modifications to plan of care.

Discharge Planning

- Identified needs and who is responsible for actions to be taken.
- Specific referrals made.

References

1. Doenges, M., Moorhouse, M., Murr, A. C. (2002). *Nursing Care Plans, Guidelines for Individualizing Patient Care.* 6th ed. Philadelphia: F. A. Davis.
2. Doenges, M., Townsend, M., Moorhouse, M. (1998). *Psychiatric Care Plans: Guidelines for Individualizing Care.* 3d ed. Philadelphia: F. A. Davis.
3. Townsend, M. (2003). *Psychiatric Mental Health Nursing: Concepts of Care.* 4th ed. Philadelphia: F. A. Davis.
4. Lipson, J. G., Dibble. S. L., Minarik, P. A. (1996). *Culture & Nursing Care: A Pocket Guide.* San Francisco: School of Nursing, UCSF Nursing Press.
5. Doenges, M., Moorhouse, M., Murr, A. C. (2004). *Nurse's Pocket Guide Diagnoses, Interventions, and Rationales.* 9th ed. Philadelphia: F. A. Davis.
6. Bruera, E., et al. (1995). The frequency of alcoholism among patients with pain due to terminal cancer. *J Pain Symptom Manage*, 10(8), 599–603.
7. Paice, J. (2002). Managing psychological conditions in palliative care. *AJN*, 102(11), 36–43.
8. Kouch, M. (2006). Managing symptoms for a "good death." *Nursing2006*, 36(11), 58–63.

risk for Aspiration

Definition: At risk for entry of gastrointestinal secretions, oropharyngeal secretions, or [exogenous food] solids or fluids into tracheobronchial passages [due to dysfunction or absence of normal protective mechanisms]

RISK FACTORS

Reduced level of consciousness [sedation/anesthesia]

Depressed cough/gag reflexes

Impaired swallowing [inability of the epiglottis and true vocal cords to close off trachea]

Facial/oral/neck surgery or trauma, wired jaws, [congenital malformations]

Situation hindering elevation of upper body [weakness, paralysis]

Incompetent lower esophageal sphincter [hiatal hernia or other esophageal disease affecting stomach valve function], delayed gastric emptying, decreased gastrointestinal motility, increased intragastric pressure, increased gastric residual

Presence of tracheostomy or endotracheal (ET) tube [inadequate or overinflation of tracheostomy/ET tube cuff]

[Presence of] gastrointestinal tubes, tube feedings/medication administration

NOTE: A risk diagnosis is not evidenced by signs and symptoms, as the problem has not occurred; rather, nursing interventions are directed at prevention.

Sample Clinical Applications: Surgery, vomiting/bulimia nervosa, presence of nasogastric tube, brain injury, spinal cord injury, enteral feedings

DESIRED OUTCOMES/EVALUATION CRITERIA

Sample NOC linkages:

Risk Control: Personal actions to prevent, eliminate, or reduce modifiable health threats

Neurological Status: Ability of the peripheral and central nervous system to receive, process, and respond to internal and external stimuli

Respiratory Status: Airway Patency: Open, clear tracheobronchial passages for air exchange

Client Will (Include Specific Time Frame)

- Experience no aspiration as evidenced by noiseless respirations, clear breath sounds; clear, odorless secretions.
- Identify causative/risk factors.
- Demonstrate techniques to prevent and/or correct aspiration.

ACTIONS/INTERVENTIONS

Sample NIC linkages:

Aspiration Precautions: Prevention or minimization of risk factors in the patient at risk for aspiration

Artificial Airway Management: Maintenance of endotracheal and tracheostomy tubes and prevention of complications associated with their use

Postanesthesia Care: Monitoring and management of the patient who has recently undergone general or regional anesthesia

NURSING PRIORITY NO. 1   To assess causative/contributing factors:

- Identify at-risk client according to condition/disease process as listed in Risk Factors *to determine when more active observation and/or interventions may be required.*
- Assess for age-related risk factors, potentiating risk of aspiration (e.g., premature infant, elderly infirm).[13]
- Note level of consciousness/awareness of surroundings, cognitive impairment. *Aspiration is common in comatose clients, owing to inability to cough, to swallow well, and/or presence of artifical airway/mechanical ventilation and tube feedings.*[1]
- Evaluate neuromuscular dysfunction, if present, noting muscle groups involved, degree of impairment, and whether acute or of a progressive nature (e.g., stroke, cerebral palsy, Parkinson's disease, Guillain-Barré syndrome, amyotrophic lateral sclerosis [ALS], psychiatric client following electric shock therapy). *May result in temporary or chronic/progressive impairment of protective muscle functions.*[12]
- Assess client's ability to swallow, strength of gag/cough reflex, and evaluate amount/consistency of secretions. *Helps to determine presence/effectiveness of protective mechanisms.*

- Observe for neck and facial edema; for example, client with head/neck surgery, tracheal/bronchial injury (upper torso burns, inhalation/chemical injury). *Problems with swallowing and maintenance of airways can be expected in this client and the potential is high for aspiration and aspiration pneumonia.*
- Assess amount and consistency of respiratory secretions, breath sounds, and rate/depth of respirations as well as client's coughing and swallowing abilities. *Helps differentiate the potential cause for risk of aspiration. The major pathophysiological dysfunction is the inability of the epiglottis and true vocal cords to move to close the trachea (e.g., changes in the structures themselves or because messages to the brain are absent, decreased, or impaired). Problems with coughing (clearing airways) and swallowing (pooling of saliva, liquids) increase risk of aspiration and respiratory complications.*[2–4]
- Auscultate lung sounds periodically (especially in client who is coughing frequently or not coughing at all; ventilator client being tube-fed, immediately following extubation) and observe chest radiographs *to determine presence of aspirated food or secretions and "silent aspiration."*[5]
- Evaluate for/note presence of gastrointestinal pathology and motility disorders. *Nausea with vomiting (associated with metabolic disorders, following surgery, certain medications) and gastroesophageal reflux disease (GERD) can be a cause for aspiration.*[3,6]
- Note administration of enteral feedings, which may be initiated when oral nutrition is not possible, such as in head injury, stroke/other neurological disorders, head and neck surgery, esophageal obstruction, and discontinuous gastrointestinal tract. *Potential exists for regurgitation and aspiration, even with proper tube placement, necessitating the need for clients at high risk for aspiration associated with nasogastroenteral feedings to be evaluated for enteral feedings into the jejunum.*[7]
- Ascertain lifestyle habits (e.g., chronic use of alcohol and drugs, alcohol intoxication, tobacco, and other CNS suppressant drugs). *Can affect awareness as well as impair gag and swallow mechanisms.*[5]
- Assist with/review diagnostic studies (e.g., video-fluoroscopy or fiber-optic endoscopy) *that may be done to assess for presence/degree of impairment.*[12]

NURSING PRIORITY NO. 2 To assist in correcting factors that can lead to aspiration:

- Place client in proper position for age and condition/disease affecting airways. Adult and child should be upright for meals or placed on right side to decrease likelihood of drainage into trachea rather than esophagus to reduce reflux and to improve gastric emptying.[2] Prone position may provide shorter gastric emptying time and decreased incidence of regurgitation and subsequent aspiration in premature infants.[8]
- Encourage client to cough, as able, to clear secretions. *May simply need to be reminded or encouraged to cough, such as might occur in elderly person with delayed gag reflex or in postoperative, sedated client.*[2]
- Provide close monitoring for use of oxygen masks in clients at risk for vomiting. Refrain from using oxygen mask for comatose individuals.
- Keep wire cutters/scissors with client at all times when jaws are wired/banded *to facilitate clearing airway in emergencies.*
- Assist with postural drainage and other respiratory therapies *to mobilize thickened secretions that may interfere with swallowing.*
- In client requiring suctioning to manage secretions.[2,9,10,15]
  Maintain operational suction equipment at bedside/chairside.
  Suction (oral cavity, nose, and ET/tracheostomy tube), as needed, using correct size of catheter and timing for adult or child *to clear secretions in client with more frequent or*

congested-sounding cough; presence of coarse rhonchi and expiratory wheezing (audible with or without auscultation); visible secretions, increased peak pressures during volume-cycled ventilation; indication from client that suctioning is necessary; suspected aspiration of gastric or upper airway secretions; or otherwise unexplained increases in shortness of breath, respiratory rate, or heart rate.

Avoid triggering gag mechanism when performing suction or mouth care.

Avoid keeping client supine/flat when on mechanical ventilation (especially when also receiving enteral feedings). *Supine positioning and enteral feeding have been shown to be independent risk factors for the development of aspiration pneumonia.*

- For a verified swallowing problem:[3,5,12-14]

Provide a rest period prior to feeding time. *Rested person may have less difficulty with swallowing.*

Elevate client to highest or best possible position for eating and drinking.

Feed slowly, and instruct client to take small bites and to chew thoroughly.

Vary placement of food in client's mouth according to type of deficit (e.g., place food in right side of mouth if facial weakness present on left side). Use semisolid/soft foods that stick together/form a bolus (e.g., casseroles, puddings, stews), *which aids swallowing effort by improving client's ability to manipulate food with the tongue.*

Avoid pureed foods and mucus-producing foods (milk).

Determine food and liquid viscosity best tolerated by client. Add thickening agent to liquids, as appropriate. *Some individuals may swallow thickened liquids better than thin liquids.*

Offer very warm or very cold liquids *to activate temperature receptors in the mouth that help to stimulate swallowing.*

Avoid washing solids down with liquids *to prevent bolus of food pushing down too rapidly, increasing risk of aspiration.*

Provide oral medications in elixir form or crush, if appropriate. Have client self-medicate when possible. Time medications to coincide with meals when possible.

Refer to physician/speech therapist *for medical/surgical interventions or specific exercises to strengthen muscles and techniques to enhance swallowing.*

- When feeding tube is in place:[3,11,15]

Note radiograph and/or measurement of aspirate pH following placement of feeding tube *to verify correct position.*

Ask client about feeling of fullness and/or measure residuals just prior to feeding and several hours after feeding, when appropriate, *to prevent overfeeding.*

Elevate head of bed 30 degrees during and for at least 30 minutes after bolus feedings.

Add food coloring (per protocol) to feeding *to identify regurgitation.*

Determine best position for infant/child (e.g., with the head of bed elevated 30 degrees and infant propped on right side after feeding). *Upper airway patency is facilitated by upright position, and turning to right side decreases likelihood of drainage into trachea.*

Provide oral medications in elixir form or crush, if appropriate.

Minimize use of sedatives/hypnotics when possible. *Agents can impair coughing and swallowing.*

NURSING PRIORITY NO. 3 To promote wellness (Teaching/Discharge Considerations):

- Review individual risk or potentiating factors with client/care provider.
- Provide information about the effects of aspiration on the lungs. *Note: Severe coughing and cyanosis associated with eating or drinking and voice change after swallowing indicates onset of respiratory symptoms associated with aspiration and requires intervention for actual presence of aspiration.*[13,14]

🌐 Cultural   Ⓐ Collaborative   🏠 Community/Home Care   ✏️ Diagnostic Studies   ∞ Pediatric/Geriatric/Lifespan   💊 Medications

- Instruct in safety concerns when feeding orally or tube feeding. (Refer to ND impaired Swallowing.)
- Train client to suction self or train family members in suction techniques (especially if client has constant or copious oral secretions) *to enhance safety/self-sufficiency.*
- Instruct individual/family member to avoid/limit activities after eating that increase intra-abdominal pressure (straining, strenuous exercise, tight/constrictive clothing). *May slow digestion/increase risk of regurgitation.*

DOCUMENTATION FOCUS

Assessment/Reassessment

- Assessment findings/conditions that could lead to problems of aspiration.
- Verification of tube placement, observations of physical findings.

Planning

- Interventions to prevent aspiration or reduce risk factors and who is involved in the planning.
- Teaching plan.

Implementation/Evaluation

- Client's responses to interventions/teaching and actions performed.
- Foods/fluids client handles with ease/difficulty.
- Amount/frequency of intake.
- Attainment/progress toward desired outcome(s).
- Modifications to plan of care.

Discharge Planning

- Long-term needs and who is responsible for actions to be taken.

References

1. Dimancescu, M. D. (Fall 1989). Aspiration pneumonia. Coma Recovery Institute, Newsletter.
2. Cox, H. C., et al. (2002). *Clinical Applications of Nursing Diagnosis: Adult, Child, Women's Psychiatric, Gerontic, and Home Health Considerations.* 4th ed. Philadelphia: F.A. Davis.
3. Altered nutritional status. Clinical Practice Guidelines. American Medical Directors Association (AMDA). December 2002. Available at www.amda.com.
4. American Gastroenterological Association. (1999). Medical position statement: Management of oropharyngeal dysphagia. 116(2), 452.
5. Galvan, T. J. (2001). Dysphagia: Going down and staying down. *AJN*, 101(1), 37.
6. Clinical consensus statement: Managing cough as a defense mechanism and as a symptom. (Quick Reference Guide for Clinicians). Northbrook, IL: American College of Chest Physicians, 1998.
7. Practice management guidelines for nutritional support of the trauma patient. Eastern Association for the Surgery of Trauma (EAST). March 1998. EAST Web site.
8. Apnea of prematurity. Clinical Practice Guideline, National Association of Neonatal Nurses (NANN), February 1999.
9. Removal of the endotracheal tube. The ARC Clinical Practice Guidelines. American Association for Respiratory Care (ARC), April 1999. Available at www.aarc.org.
10. Suctioning of the patient in the home. The ARC Clinical Practice Guidelines. American Association for Respiratory Care (ARC), April 1999. Available at www.aarc.org.
11. Metheny, N. A., Titler, M. G. (2001). Assessing placement of feeding tubes. *AJN*, 101(5), 36.
12. Bowman, A., Breiner, J. E., Doerschug, K. C., et al. (2005). Implementation of an evidence-based feeding protocol and aspiration risk reduction algorithm. *Crit Care Nurse Quarterly*, 28(4), 324–333.

13. Goldstein, L. B. (January 2006). Cough and aspiration of food and liquids due to oral-pharyngeal dysphagia: AACP evidence-based clinical practice guidelines. *Chest*.
14. Metheny, N. A. (April 2006). Preventing aspiration in older adults with dysphagia. (Try this: Best Practices in Nursing Care to Older Adults). *MedSurg Nursing*.
15. McClave, S. A., Lukan, J. K., Lowen, J. A., et.al. (2005). Poor validity of residual volumes as a marker for risk of aspiration in critically ill patients. *Crit Care Medicine*, 33(2), 324–330.

risk for impaired parent/child Attachment

Definition: Disruption of the interactive process between parent/SO and child/infant that fosters the development of a protective and nurturing reciprocal relationship

RISK FACTORS
Inability of parents to meet personal needs
Anxiety associated with the parent role; [parents who themselves experienced altered attachment]
Premature infant/ill infant/child who is unable to effectively initiate parental contact due to altered behavioral organization; parental conflict due to altered behavioral organization
Separation; physical barriers; lack of privacy
Substance abuse
[Difficult pregnancy and/or birth (actual or perceived)]
[Uncertainty of paternity; conception as a result of rape/sexual abuse]
NOTE: A risk diagnosis is not evidenced by signs and symptoms, as the problem has not occurred; rather, nursing interventions are directed at prevention.

Sample Clinical Applications: Prematurity, genetic/congenital conditions, autism, attention deficit disorder, developmental delay (parent or child), substance abuse (parent), bipolar disorder (parent)

DESIRED OUTCOMES/EVALUATION CRITERIA
Sample NOC linkages:
Parent-Infant Attachment: Parent and infant behaviors that demonstrate an enduring affectionate bond
Parenting Performance: Parental actions to provide a child a nurturing and constructive physical, emotional, and social environment
Child Development: [specify age group]: Milestones of physical, cognitive, and psychosocial progression by [specify] months/years of age

Parent Will (Include Specific Time Frame)

- Identify and prioritize family strengths and needs.
- Exhibit nurturant and protective behaviors toward child.
- Identify and use resources to meet needs of family members.
- Demonstrate techniques to enhance behavioral organization of the infant/child.
- Engage in mutually satisfying interactions with child.

ACTIONS/INTERVENTIONS

Sample NIC linkages:
Attachment Promotion: Facilitation of the development of the parent-infant relationship

Cultural   Collaborative   Community/Home Care   Diagnostic Studies   Pediatric/Geriatric/Lifespan   Medications

Parenting Promotion: Providing parenting information, support, and coordination of comprehensive services to high-risk families

Environmental Management: Attachment Process: Manipulation of the patient's surroundings to facilitate the development of the parent-infant relationship

NURSING PRIORITY NO. 1 To identify causative/contributing factors:

- Interview parents, noting their perception of situation, individual concerns. *Identifies problem areas/strengths to formulate appropriate plans to change situation that is currently creating problems for the parents.*[8]

- Assess parent/child interactions. *Identifies relationships, communication skills, and feelings about one another. The way in which a parent responds to a child and how the child responds to the parent largely determines how the child develops. Identifying the way in which this family responds to one another is crucial in determining the need for and type of interventions required.*[8]

- Ascertain availability/use of resources to include extended family, support groups, and financial. *Lack of support from or presence of extended family, lack of involvement in groups such as church or specific resources such as La Leche League and financial stresses can affect family negatively, interfering with ability to deal effectively with parenting responsibilites. Parents need support from both inside and outside of the family.*[9,12]

- Determine emotional and behavioral problems of the child. *Attachment-disordered children are unable to give and receive love and affection, defy parental rules and authority, and are physically and emotionally abusive, creating ongoing stress and turmoil in the family and in future relationships.*[12]

- Evaluate parents' ability to provide protective environment, participate in reciprocal relationship. *Parents may be immature, may be substance abusers, or may be mentally ill and unable or unwilling to assume the task of parenting. The ways in which the parent responds to the child is critical to the child's development, and interventions need to be directed at helping the parents to deal with own issues and learn positive parenting skills.*[1,7]

- Note attachment behaviors between parent and child(ren), recognizing cultural background. *For example, lack of eye contact and touching may indicate bonding problems. Behaviors such as eye-to-eye contact, use of en face position, talking to the infant in a high-pitched voice are indicative of attachment behaviors in American culture but may not be appropriate in another culture. Failure to bond effectively is thought to affect subsequent parent-child interaction.*[4,5]

- Assess parenting skill level, considering intellectual, emotional, and physical strengths and limitations. Identifies areas of need for further education, skill training, and factors that might interfere with ability to assimilate new information.[1,2]

NURSING PRIORITY NO. 2 To enhance behavioral organization of infant/child:

- Identify infant's strengths and vulnerabilities. *Each child is born with his or her own temperament that affects interactions with caregivers, and when these are known, actions can be taken to assist parents/caregivers to parent appropriately.*[2,7,11]

- Educate parents regarding child growth and development, addressing parental perceptions. *Parents often have misconceptions about the abilities of their children, and providing correct information clarifies expectations and is more realistic.*[6]

- Assist parents in modifying the environment. *The environment can be changed to provide appropriate stimulation; for example, to diminish stimulation before bedtime, to simplify when the environment is too complex to handle, and to provide life space where the child can play unrestricted, resulting in freedom for the child to meet his or her needs.*[2,7] (Refer to ND readiness for enhanced organized Infant Behavior.)

∞ • Model caregiving techniques that best support behavioral organization, such as attachment parenting. *Recognizing that the child deserves to have his or her needs taken seriously and responding to those needs in a loving fashion promotes trust, and children learn to model their behavior after what they have seen the parents do.*[9,11]

∞ • Respond consistently with nurturance to infant/child. *Babies come wired with an ability to signal their needs by crying, and when parents respond to these signals, they develop a sensitivity that in turn develops parental intuition, providing the infant with gratification of their needs and trust in their environment.*[10]

NURSING PRIORITY NO. 3 To enhance best functioning of parents:

🏠 • Develop therapeutic nurse-client relationship. Provide a consistently warm, nurturant, and nonjudgmental environment. *Parents are often surprised to find that a tiny infant can cause so many changes in their lives and need help to adjust to this new experience. The warm caring relationship of the nurse can help with this adjustment and provide the information and empathy they need at this time.*[1]

🏠 • Assist parents in identifying and prioritizing family strengths and needs. *Promotes positive attitude by looking at what they already do well and using those skills to address needs.*[2]

🏠 • Support and guide parents in process of assessing resources. *Outside support is important at this time, and making sure that parents receive the help they need will help them in this adjustment period.*[12]

∞ • Involve parents in activities with the infant/child that they can accomplish successfully. *Activities such as Baby Gymboree and baby yoga enable the parents to get to know their child and themselves, enhancing their confidence and self-concept.*[12]

🏠 • Recognize and provide positive feedback for nurturant and protective parenting behaviors. *Using I-messages to let parents know their behaviors are effective reinforces continuation of desired behaviors and promotes feelings of confidence in their abilities.*[2,12]

NURSING PRIORITY NO. 4 To support parent/child attachment during separation:

• Provide parents with telephone contact as appropriate. *Knowing there is someone they can call if they have problems provides a sense of security.*[3]

• Establish a routine time for daily phone calls/initiate calls as indicated when child is hospitalized. *Provides sense of consistency and control; allows for planning of other activities so parents can maintain contact and get information on a regular basis.*[1]

🔗 • Minimize number of professionals on team with whom parents must have contact. *Parents begin to know the individuals they are dealing with on a regular basis, fostering trust in these relationships and providing opportunities for modeling and learning.*[3]

• Invite parents to use Ronald McDonald House or provide them with a listing of a variety of local accommodations, restaurants. *When child is hospitalized out of town, parents need to have a place to stay so they can have ready access to the hospital and be able to rest and refresh from time to time.*[3]

• Arrange for parents to receive photos, progress reports from the child. *Provides information and comfort as the child progresses, allowing the parents to continue to have hope for a positive resolution.*[3]

• Suggest parents provide a photo and/or audiotape of themselves for the child. *Provides a connection during the separation, sustaining attachment between parent and child.*[1]

- Consider use of contract with parents. *Clearly communicating expectations of both family and staff serves as a reminder of what each person has committed to and serves as a tool to evaluate whether expectations are being maintained.*[3]
- Suggest parents keep a journal of infant/child progress. *Serves as a reminder of the progress that is being made, especially when they become discouraged and believe infant/child is "never" going to be better.*[3]
- Provide "homelike" environment for situations requiring supervision of visits. *An environment that is comfortable supports the family as they work toward resolving conflicts and promotes a sense of hopefulness, enabling them to experience success when family is involved with a legal situation.*[12]

NURSING PRIORITY NO. 5 To promote wellness (Teaching/Discharge Considerations):

- Refer to addiction counseling/treatment, individual counseling, or family therapies as indicated. *May need additional assistance when situation is complicated by drug abuse (including alcohol), mental illness, disruptions in caregiving, parents who are burned out with caring for child with attachment or other difficulties.*[12,13]
- Identify services for transportation, financial resources, housing, and so forth. *Assistance with these needs can help families focus on therapeutic regimen and on issues of parenting to improve family dynamics.*[9]
- Develop support systems appropriate to situation (e.g., extended family, friends, social worker). *Depending on individual situation, support from extended family, friends, social worker, or therapist can assist family to deal with attachment disorders.*[10]
- Explore community resources (e.g., church affiliations, volunteer groups, day/respite care). *Church affiliations, volunteer groups, day/respite care can help parents who are overwhelmed with care of a child with attachment or other disorder.*[12]

DOCUMENTATION FOCUS

Assessment/Reassessment

- Identified behaviors of both parents and child.
- Specific risk factors, individual perceptions/concerns.
- Interactions between parent and child.

Planning

- Plan of care and who is involved in planning.
- Teaching plan.

Implementation/Evaluation

- Parents'/child's responses to interventions/teaching and actions performed.
- Attainment/progress toward desired outcomes.
- Modifications to plan of care.

Discharge Planning

- Long-term needs and who is responsible.
- Plan for home visits to support parents and to ensure infant/child safety and well-being.
- Specific referrals made.

References

1. Townsend, M. C. (2006). *Psychiatric Mental Health Nursing, Concepts of Care in Evidence-Based Practice.* 5th ed. Philadelphia, FA Davis
2. Gordon, T. (2000). *Parent Effectiveness Training.* (Updated edition). New York: Three Rivers Press.
3. Cox, H. C. et al. (2002). *Clinical Applications of Nursing Diagnosis: Adult, Child, Women's, Psychiatric, Gerontic, and Home Health Considerations.* 4th ed. Philadelphia: F.A. Davis
4. Lipson, J. G. Dibble, S. L., Minarik, P. A. (1996). *Culture & Nursing Care. A Pocket Guide.* San Francisco: UCSF Nursing Press.
5. Doenges, M. E., Townsend, M. C., Moorhouse, M. F. (1998). *Psychiatric Care Plans Guidelines for Individualizing Care.* 3d ed. Philadelphia, F. A. Davis.
6. Gordon, T. (1989). *Teaching Children Self-Discipline: At Home and at School.* New York: Random House.
7. Gordon, T. (2000). *Family Effectiveness Training Video.* Solana Beach, CA: Gordon Training Intnl.
8. Doenges, M. E., Moorhouse, M. F., Murr, A. C. (2008). Nurse's Pocket Guide Diagnoses, Interventions and Rationales. 11th ed. Philadelphia, F. A. Davis.
9. Henningsen, M. (1996). *Attachment Disorder: Theory, Parenting and Therapy.* Evergreen, CO: Evergreen Family Counseling Center.
10. Sears, W. (1999). Attachment Parenting: A Style That Works. Excerpted from Nighttime Parenting: How to Get Your Baby and Child to Sleep (La Leche International Book, revised edition). NY, NY: Plume.
11. Hunt, J. What Is Attachment Parenting? The Natural Child Project. Available at www.naturalchild.com/jan.hunt/attachment parenting.html. Accessed February 2004.
12. Corrective Attachment Parenting. Evergreen, CO: Evergreen Psychotherapy Center Attachment Treatment and Training Institute.
13. London, M. L., et al. (2007). *Maternal & Child Nursing Care.* New Jersey: Pearson Prentice Hall.

Autonomic Dysreflexia

Definition: Life-threatening, uninhibited sympathetic response of the nervous system to a noxious stimulus after a spinal cord injury (SCI) at T7 or above

RELATED FACTORS
Bladder or bowel distention; [catheter insertion, obstruction, irrigation]
Skin irritation
Deficient client and caregiver knowledge
[Sexual excitation; menstruation; pregnancy; labor and delivery]
[Environmental temperature extremes]

DEFINING CHARACTERISTICS

Subjective
Headache (a diffuse pain in different portions of the head and not confined to any nerve distribution area)
Paresthesia, chilling, blurred vision, chest pain, metallic taste in mouth, nasal congestion

Objective
Paroxysmal hypertension (sudden periodic elevated blood pressure in which systolic pressure >140 mm Hg and diastolic >90 mm Hg)
Bradycardia or tachycardia
Diaphoresis (above the injury), red splotches on skin (above the injury), pallor (below the injury)
Horner's syndrome [contraction of the pupil, partial ptosis of the eyelid, enophthalmos and sometimes loss of sweating over the affected side of the face]; conjunctival congestion
Pilomotor reflex [gooseflesh formation when skin is cooled]

Sample Clinical Applications: Spinal cord injury

Cultural   Collaborative   Community/Home Care   Diagnostic Studies   Pediatric/Geriatric/Lifespan   Medications

DESIRED OUTCOMES/EVALUATION CRITERIA

Sample NOC linkages:

Neurological Status: Autonomic: Ability of the autonomic nervous system to coordinate visceral and homeostatic function

Knowledge: Disease Process: Extent of understanding conveyed about a specific disease process

Symptom Severity: Severity of perceived adverse changes in physical, emotional, and social functioning

Client/Caregiver Will (Include Specific Time Frame)

- Identify risk factors.
- Recognize signs/symptoms of syndrome.
- Demonstrate corrective techniques.
- Experience no episodes of dysreflexia or will seek medical intervention in a timely manner.

ACTIONS/INTERVENTIONS

Sample NIC linkages:

Dysreflexia Management: Prevention and elimination of stimuli that cause hyperactive reflexes and inappropriate autonomic responses in a patient with a cervical or high thoracic cord lesion

Urinary Elimination Management [or] Bowel Management: Maintenance of an optimum urinary elimination pattern/establishment and maintenance of a regular pattern of bowel elimination

Anxiety Reduction: Minimizing apprehension, dread, foreboding, or uneasiness related to an unidentified source or anticipated danger

NURSING PRIORITY NO. 1 To assess precipitating risk factors.[1–3,7–9]

- Monitor for bladder distention, presence of bladder spasms/stones, or infection. *The most common stimulus for autonomic dysreflexia (AD) is bladder irritation or overstretch associated with urinary retention or infection; blocked catheter; overfilled collection bag; or noncompliance with intermittent catheterization.*
- Evaluate for bowel distention, fecal impaction, and problems with bowel management program. *Bowel irritation or overstretch is associated with constipation or impaction; digital stimulation, suppository/enema use during bowel program; hemorrhoids/fissures; and/or infection of gastrointestinal tract, such as might occur with ulcers or appendicitis.*
- Observe skin/tissue pressure areas, especially following prolonged sitting. *Skin/tissue irritants include direct pressure (e.g., object in chair or shoe, leg straps, abdominal support, orthotics; wounds (e.g., bruise, abrasion, lacerations, pressure ulcer); ingrown toenail; tight clothing; or sunburn/other burn.*
- Inquire about sexual activity and/or determine if reproductive issues are involved. *Overstimulation/vibration, sexual intercourse/ejaculation, scrotal compression, menstrual cramps, and/or pregnancy (especially labor and delivery) are known stimulants.*
- Inform client/care providers of additional precipitators during course of care. *Client is prone to physical conditions/treatments (e.g., intolerance to temperature extremes; deep vein thrombosis [DVT]; kidney stones; fractures/other trauma, surgical, dental, and diagnostic procedures) any of which can precipitate AD.*
- Monitor environmental temperature for extremes/drafts, *which can precipitate episode.*

NURSING PRIORITY NO. 2 To provide for early detection and immediate intervention:

- Investigate associated complaints/syndrome of symptoms (e.g., severe pounding headache, [blood pressure may be >200/100 mm Hg], chest pain, irregular heart rate/dysrhythmias, blurred vision, nausea, facial flushing, metallic taste, or severe anxiety; or minimal symptoms or expressed complaints in presence of significantly elevated blood pressure-silent AD]). *Body's reaction to misinterpreted sensations from below the injury site, resulting in an autonomic reflex, can cause blood vessels to constrict and increase blood pressure. This is a potentially life-threatening condition, requiring immediate and correct action.*[1–3,7,8]

- Note onset of crying, irritability, or somnolence in infant or child (*may present with nonspecific symptoms; may not be able to verbalize discomforts*).[1]

- Locate/eliminate causative stimulus, moving in stepwise fashion. (Cause can be anything that would normally cause pain or discomfort below level of injury.)[1–8]

  Assess for bladder distention (*most common cause of AD*):

  Empty bladder by voiding or catheterization-applying local anesthetic ointment *to prevent exacerbation of AD by procedure.*

  Ascertain that urine is free-flowing if Foley or suprapubic catheter is in place, empty drainage bag, straighten tubing if kinked, and lower drainage bag if it is higher than bladder.

  Irrigate gently or change catheter, if not draining freely.

  Note color, character, and odor of urine; obtain specimen for culture as indicated (*infection can cause AD*).

  Check for distended bowel (*if urinary problem is not causing AD*):

  Perform digital stimulation, checking for constipation/impacted stool. (If symptoms first appear while performing digital stimulation, stop procedure.)

  Apply local anesthetic ointment to rectum; remove impaction after symptoms subside *to remove causative problem without causing additional symptoms.*

  Check for skin pressure/irritation (*if bowel problem is not causing AD*):

  Perform a pressure release if sitting.

  Check for tight clothing, straps, belts.

  Note whether pressure sore has developed or changed.

  Observe for bruising, signs of infection.

  Check for ingrown toenail or other injury to skin, tissue (e.g., burns, sunburn) or fractured bones.

  Check for other possible causes (*if skin pressure is not causing AD*):

  Menstrual cramps, sexual activity, labor and delivery.

  Abdominal conditions (e.g., colitis, ulcer).

  Environmental temperature extremes.

- Take steps to reduce blood pressure, *thereby reducing potential for stroke (primary concern)*:[1–8]

  Elevate head of bed immediately, or place in sitting position with legs hanging down. *Lowers blood pressure by pooling of blood in legs.*

  Loosen any clothing or restrictive devices. *May allow pooling of blood in abdomen and lower extremities.*

  Monitor vital signs frequently during acute episode. (*Blood pressure may fluctuate quickly due to impaired autonomic regulation.*) Continue to monitor blood pressure at intervals during procedures to remove cause of AD and after acute episodic symptoms subside *to evaluate effectiveness of interventions and antihypertensives.*

  Administer medications, as indicated. *If an episode is particularly severe or persists after removal of suspected cause, antihypertensive medications with rapid onset and short duration*

⊕ Cultural ⊗ Collaborative 🏠 Community/Home Care ⬱ Diagnostic Studies ∞ Pediatric/Geriatric/Lifespan 🔋 Medications *(such as nifedipine, hydralazine, clonidine) may be used to block excessive autonomic nerve transmission, normalize heart rate, and reduce hypertension.*[1,4]

Carefully adjust dosage of antihypertensive medications for child, elderly person, and pregnant woman. *Prevents complications, such as systemic hypotension or seizure activity, and maintains blood pressure within optimal range.*[1]

NURSING PRIORITY NO. 3 To promote wellness (Teaching/Discharge Considerations):

- Discuss with client/caregivers warning signs of AD, as listed previously. Be aware of client's communication abilities. *AD can occur at any age from infant to very old, and the individual may not be able to verbalize a pounding headache, which is often the first symptom during onset of AD.*[1,8]

- Ascertain that client/caregivers understand ways to avoid onset or treat syndrome as noted previously. Provide information card and instruct/reinforce teaching, as needed, regarding:[1,2,5–8]

  Maintaining indwelling catheter by keeping tubing free of kinks, bag empty and situated below bladder level, and checking daily for deposits (bladder grit) inside catheter.

  Performing intermittent catheterization as often as necessary *to prevent overfilling/ distention.*

  Monitoring for adequate spontaneous voiding, noting frequency and amount.

  Maintaining a regular and effective bowel evacuation program.

  Performing routine skin assessments.

  Monitoring all systems for signs of infection and reporting promptly *for timely medical treatment.*

  Scheduling routine medical evaluations.

- Instruct family member/caregiver in proper blood pressure monitoring and discuss plan for monitoring hypertension during acute episodes. *A spinal cord-injured client's (both adult and child) baseline blood pressure is lower than that of a noninjured person, thus necessitating frequent measurements during acute episodes.*

- Review proper use/administration of medications, when used. *Client may have medication(s) both for emergent situations and/or prevention of AD, and if so, should receive medication instructions as well as symptoms to report for immediate or emergent care, when blood pressure is not responsive.*[1,8]

- Refer for/advise treatment of sexual and reproductive concerns, as indicated.[9]

- Recommend wearing Medic Alert bracelet/necklace and carrying information card about signs/symptoms of AD and usual methods of treatment. *Provides vital information in emergency.*

- Assist client/family in identifying emergency referrals (e.g., physician, rehabilitation nurse/home-care supervisor). Place telephone number(s) in prominent place.

DOCUMENTATION FOCUS

Assessment/Reassessment

- Individual findings, noting previous episodes, precipitating factors, and individual signs/symptoms.

Planning

- Plan of care and who is involved in planning.
- Teaching plan.

Implementation/Evaluation

- Client's responses to interventions and actions performed, understanding of teaching.
- Attainment/progress toward desired outcome(s).
- Modifications to plan of care.

Discharge Planning

- Long-term needs and who is responsible for actions to be taken.

References

1. Acute management of autonomic dysreflexia: Individuals with spinal cord injury presenting to health-care facilities. Paralyzed Veterans of America/Consortium for Spinal Cord Medicine. Washington DC, Paralyzed Veterans of America (PVA) July 2001. Retrieved September 2003 at www.pva.org.
2. Acuff, M. (2005). Autonomic dysreflexia: What it is, what it does, and what to do if you experience it. The Missouri Model Spinal Cord Injury System. Columbia, MO: University of Missouri-Columbia, School of Health Professions.
3. Christopher & Dana Reeve Paralysis Resource Center: Health: Autonomic Dysreflexia. Retrieved January 2007 at www.paralysis.org/site/c.erJMJUOxFmH/b.1338071/k.5E45/Autonomic_Dysreflexia.htm.
4. Deglan, J. H., Vallerand, A. H. (2003). *Davis's Drug Guide for Nurses.* 8th ed. Philadelphia: F. A. Davis.
5. Other complications of spinal cord injury: Autonomic dysreflexia (hyperreflexia) treatment. RehabTeamSite. Available at www.calder.med.miami.edu.
6. SCI Complications Resource: National Spinal Cord Injury Association (NSCIA). Update January 2003. Available at www.spinalcord.org.
7. Compagnolo, D. I. (2006). Autonomic dysreflexia in spinal cord injury. Article for Emedicine Web site. Retrieved January 2007 at www.emedicine.com/pmr/topic217.htm.
8. Cody, T., Zieroff. (2005). Automonic dysreflexia. Article for Northeast Rehabilitation Health Network. Retrieved January 2007 at www.northeastrehab.com/Articles/dysreflexia.htm.
9. Ducharme, S. (2000). Sexuality and spinal cord injury. Article for Paraplegia News. Reprint available at www.stanleyducharme.com/resources/sex_spinalcord_injury.htm.

risk for Autonomic Dysreflexia

Definition: At risk for life-threatening, uninhibited response of the sympathetic nervous system post-spinal shock, in an individual with a spinal cord injury [SCI] or lesion at T6 or above (has been demonstrated in clients with injuries at T7 and T8)

RISK FACTORS

An injury at T6 or above or a lesion at T6 or above AND at least one of the following noxious stimuli:

Musculoskeletal-Integumentary Stimuli

Cutaneous stimulations (e.g., pressure ulcer, ingrown toenail, dressing, burns, rash); sunburns; wounds

Pressure over bony prominences/genitalia; range-of-motion exercises; spasms

Fractures; heterotrophic bone

Gastrointestinal Stimuli

Constipation; difficult passage of feces; fecal impaction; bowel distention; hemorrhoids

Digital stimulation; suppositories; enemas

GI system pathology; esophageal reflux; gastric ulcers; gallstones

🌐 Cultural   Ⓒ Collaborative   🏠 Community/Home Care   Diagnostic Studies   ∞ Pediatric/Geriatric/Lifespan   Medications

Urological Stimuli
Bladder distention/spasm
Detrusor sphincter dyssynergia
Catheterization; instrumentation; surgery
Urinary tract infection; cystitis; urethritis; epididymitis; calculi

Regulatory Stimuli
Temperature fluctuations; extreme environmental temperatures

Situational Stimuli
Positioning; surgical [diagnostic] procedure
Constrictive clothing (e.g., straps, stockings, shoes)
Drug reactions (e.g., decongestants, sympathomimetics, vasoconstrictors); opioid
    withdrawal

Neurological Stimuli
Painful/irritating stimuli below the level of injury

Cardiac/Pulmonary Problems
Pulmonary emboli; deep-vein thrombosis

Reproductive Stimuli
Sexual intercourse; ejaculation; [vibrator overstimulation; scrotal compression]
Menstruation; pregnancy; labor and delivery; ovarian cyst

NOTE: A risk diagnosis is not evidenced by signs and symptoms, as the problem has not
    occurred; rather, nursing interventions are directed at prevention.

Sample Clinical Applications: Spinal cord injury

DESIRED OUTCOMES/EVALUATION CRITERIA
Sample NOC linkages:
Risk Control: Personal actions to prevent, eliminate, or reduce modifiable health threats
Knowledge: Disease Process: Extent of understanding conveyed about a specific disease process
Caregiver Home-Care Readiness: Extent of preparedness of a caregiver to assume respon-
    sibility for the healthcare of a family member in the home

Client Will (Include Specific Time Frame)

- Identify risk factors present.
- Demonstrate preventive/corrective techniques.
- Be free of episodes of dysreflexia.

ACTIONS/INTERVENTIONS

Sample NIC linkages:
Dysreflexia Management: Prevention and elimination of stimuli that cause hyperactive
    reflexes and inappropriate autonomic responses in a patient with a cervical or high thoracic
    cord lesion

Surveillance: Purposeful and ongoing acquisition, interpretation, and synthesis of patient data for clinical decision making

Medication Management: Facilitation of safe and effective use of prescription and over-the-counter drugs

NURSING PRIORITY NO. 1 To assess risk factors present:

- Monitor for potential precipitating factors, including urological (e.g., bladder distention, urinary tract infections, kidney stones); gastrointestinal (e.g., bowel overdistention, hemorrhoids, digital stimulation); cutaneous (e.g., pressure ulcers, extreme external temperatures, dressing changes); reproductive (e.g., sexual activity, menstruation, pregnancy/delivery); and miscellaneous (e.g., pulmonary emboli, drug reaction, deep-vein thrombosis).[1,2,6,7]

NURSING PRIORITY NO. 2 To prevent occurrence:

- Monitor vital signs routinely, noting changes in blood pressure, heart rate, and temperature, especially during times of physical stress *to identify trends and intervene in a timely manner. The baseline blood pressure in spinal cord-injured clients (adult and child) is lower than general population; therefore, an elevation of >15 mm Hg above baseline may be indicative of autonomic dysreflexia (AD).*[1,2,6,7]
- Instruct all caregivers in regularly timed/safe bowel and bladder/catheter care and in interventions for long-term prevention of skin stress/breakdown (e.g., appropriate padding for skin and tissues, proper positioning with frequent pressure-relief actions, routine foot/toenail care) *to reduce risk of AD episode.*[1-7]
- Instruct client/caregivers in additional preventive interventions (e.g., temperature control; checking frequently for tight clothes/leg straps; sunburn/other burn prevention).[1-7]
- Administer antihypertensive medications, as indicated. *At-risk client may be placed on routine "maintenance dose," such as when noxious stimuli cannot be removed (e.g., presence of chronic sacral pressure ulcer, fracture, or acute postoperative pain).*[1]
- Refer to ND Autonomic Dysreflexia.

NURSING PRIORITY NO. 3 To promote wellness (Teaching/Discharge Considerations):

- Review warning signs of AD with client/caregiver (e.g., sudden, severe pounding headache; flushed, red face; increased blood pressure/acute hypertension; nasal congestion; anxiety; blurred vision; metallic taste in mouth; sweating and/or flushing above the level of SCI, goose bumps; bradycardia, cardiac irregularities). *AD can develop rapidly (in minutes), thus requiring quick intervention.*
- Be aware of client's communication abilities. *AD can occur at any age, from infant to very old, and the individual may not be able to verbalize a pounding headache, which is often the first symptom during onset of AD.*[1]
- Ascertain that client/caregivers understand ways to avoid onset of syndrome. Provide information card and instruct/reinforce teaching, as needed, regarding the following:[1-7]
  Keeping indwelling catheter free of kinks, keeping bag empty and situated below bladder level, and checking daily for deposits (bladder grit) inside catheter.
  Catheterizing as often as necessary *to prevent overfilling.*
  Monitoring voiding patterns for adequate frequency and amount.
  Performing regular bowel evacuation program.
  Performing routine skin assessments.

🌐 Cultural   Ⓐ Collaborative   🏠 Community/Home Care   🧪 Diagnostic Studies   ∞ Pediatric/Geriatric/Lifespan   💊 Medications

Monitoring all systems for signs/symptoms of infection and reporting promptly *for timely medical treatment.*

- Instruct family member/caregivers in proper blood pressure monitoring.
- Review use/administration of medications, when used. *Some clients are on medications routinely, and if so, should receive instructions for routine administration as well as symptoms to report for immediate or emergent care, when blood pressure is not responsive.*[1,6]
- Emphasize importance of regularly scheduled medical evaluations *to monitor status, identify developing problems.*
- Recommend wearing Medic Alert bracelet/necklace with information card about signs/symptoms of AD and usual methods of treatment. *Provides vital information in emergencies.*
- Assist client/family in identifying emergency referrals (e.g., physician, rehabilitation nurse/home-care supervisor). Place telephone number(s) in prominent place.

DOCUMENTATION FOCUS

Assessment/Reassessment

- Individual findings, noting previous episodes, precipitating factors, and individual signs/symptoms.

Planning

- Plan of care and who is involved in planning.
- Teaching plan.

Implementation/Evaluation

- Client's responses to interventions and actions performed, understanding of teaching.
- Attainment/progress toward desired outcome(s).
- Modifications to plan of care.

Discharge Planning

- Long-term needs and who is responsible for actions to be taken.

References

1. Acute management of autonomic dysreflexia: Individuals with spinal cord injury presenting to health-care facilities. (2001). Paralyzed Veterans of America/Consortium for Spinal Cord Medicine. Washington DC: Paralyzed Veterans of America (PVA). Retrieved September 2003 at www.pva.org.
2. Acuff, M. (2005). Autonomic dysreflexia: What it is, what it does, and what to do if you experience it. The Missouri Model Spinal Cord Injury System. Columbia, MO: University of Missouri-Columbia, School of Health Professions.
3. Christopher and Dana Reeve Paralysis Resource Center: Health: Autonomic Dysreflexia. Retrieved 2002 at www.paralysis.org/site/c.erJMJUOxFmH/b.1338071/k.5E45/Autonomic_Dysreflexia.htm.
4. Other complications of spinal cord injury: Autonomic dysreflexia (hyperreflexia) treatment. RehabTeam Site. Available at www.calder.med.miami.edu.
5. SCI Complications Resource: National Spinal Cord Injury Association (NSCIA). Update January 2003. Available at www.spinalcord.org.
6. Compagnolo, D. I. (2006). Autonomic dysreflexia in spinal cord injury. Article for Emedicine Web site. Retrieved January 2007 at www.emedicine.com/pmr/topic217.htm.
7. Cody, T., Zieroff. (2005). Automonic Dysreflexia. Article for Northeast Rehabilitation Health Network. Retrieved January 2007 at www.northeastrehab.com/Articles/dysreflexia.htm.

risk-prone health Behavior

Definition: Inability to modify lifestyle/behavior in a manner consistent with a change in health status

RELATED FACTORS

Inadequate comprehension; low self-efficacy
Multiple stressors
Inadequate social support; low socioeconomic status
Negative attitude toward healthcare

DEFINING CHARACTERISTICS

Subjective
Minimizes health status change
Fails to achieve optimal sense of control

Objective
Fails to take action that prevents health problems
Demonstrates nonacceptance of health status change

Sample Clinical Applications: New diagnosis/life changes for client, Alzheimer's disease, brain injury, personality or psychotic disorders, postpartum depression/psychosis, substance use/abuse

DESIRED OUTCOMES/EVALUATION CRITERIA

Sample NOC linkages:
Acceptance: Health Status: Reconciliation to significant change in health circumstances
Psychosocial Adjustment: Life Change: Adaptive psychosocial response of an individual to a significant life change
Treatment Behavior: Illness or Injury: Personal actions to palliate or eliminate pathology

Client Will (Include Specific Time Frame)

- Demonstrate increasing interest/participation in self-care.
- Develop ability to assume responsibility for personal needs when possible.
- Identify stress situations leading to difficulties in adapting to change in health status and specific actions for dealing with them.
- Initiate lifestyle changes that will permit adaptation to present life situations.
- Identify and use appropriate support systems.

ACTIONS/INTERVENTIONS

Sample NIC linkages:
Coping Enhancement: Assisting a patient to adapt to perceived stressors, changes, or threats that interfere with meeting life demands and roles
Counseling: Use of an interactive helping process focusing on the needs, problems, or feelings of the patient and significant others to enhance or support coping, problem-solving, and interpersonal relationships
Teaching: Disease Process: Assisting the patient to understand information related to a specific disease process

Cultural   Collaborative   Community/Home Care   Diagnostic Studies   Pediatric/Geriatric/Lifespan   Medications

NURSING PRIORITY NO. 1 To assess degree of impaired function:

- Perform a physical and/or psychosocial assessment. *Determines the extent of the limitation(s) of the present condition.*[1]
- Listen to the client's perception of inability/reluctance to adapt to situations that are occurring at present. *Perceptions are reality to the client and need to be identified so they may be addressed and dealt with.*[3]
- Survey (with the client) past and present significant support systems (family, church, groups, and organizations). *Identifies helpful resources that may be needed in current situation/change in health status.*[2]
- Explore the expressions of emotions signifying impaired adjustment by client/SO(s). *Overwhelming anxiety, fear, anger, worry, passive or active denial can be experienced by the client who is having difficulty adjusting to change in health, feared diagnosis.*[4]
- Note child's interaction with parent/care provider. *Interactions can be indicative of problems when family is dealing with major health problems and change in family functioning. Development of coping behaviors is limited at this age, and primary caregivers provide support for the child and serve as role models.*[5]
- Determine whether child displays problems with school performance, withdraws from family/peers, or demonstrates aggressive behavior toward others/self. *Indicators of poor coping and need for specific interventions to help child deal with own health issues or what is happening in the family.*[6]

NURSING PRIORITY NO. 2 To identify the causative/contributing factors relating to the impaired adjustment:

- Listen to client's perception of the factors leading to the present dilemma, noting onset, duration, presence/absence of physical complaints, social withdrawal. *Change often creates a feeling of disequilibrium, and the individual may respond with fears that are irrational or unfounded. Client may benefit from feedback that corrects misperceptions about how life will be with the change in health status.*[7]
- Identify possible cultural beliefs/values influencing client's response to change. *Different cultures deal with change of health issues, such as cancer, chronic obstructive pulmonary disease, diabetes mellitus, in different ways (i.e., Native Americans may believe they should be sick, quiet, and stoic; Chinese are often passive and expect the family to care for the client; Americans may be assertive and direct their care more frequently).*[14]
- Assess affective climate within family system and how it determines family members' response to adjustment to major health challenge. *Families who are high-strung and nervous may interfere with client's dealing with illness in a rational manner while those who are more sedate and phlegmatic may be more helpful to the client in accepting the current circumstances.*[2]
- Determine lack of/inability to use available resources. *The high degree of anxiety that usually accompanies a major lifestyle change often interferes with ability to deal with problems created by the change or loss. Helping client learn to use these resources enables him or her to take control of own illness.*[8]
- Discuss normalcy of anger as life is being changed and encourage channeling anger to healthy activities. *The increased energy of anger can be used to accomplish other tasks and enhance feelings of self-esteem.*[2]
- Review available documentation and resources to determine actual life experiences (e.g., medical records, statements of SOs, consultants' notes). *In situations of great stress, physical or emotional, the client may not accurately assess occurrences leading to the present situation.*[9]

NURSING PRIORITY NO. 3 To assist client in coping/dealing with impairment:

- Organize a team conference (including client and ancillary services). *Individuals who are involved and knowledgeable can focus on the contributing factors that are affecting client's adjustment to the current situation and can plan for management as indicated.*[11]
- Explain disease process/causative factors and prognosis as appropriate, promote questioning, and provide written/other materials. *Enhances understanding, clarifies information, and provides opportunity to review information at individual's leisure.*[10]
- Share information with adolescent's peers with client's permission and involvement when illness/injury affects body image. *Peers are primary support for this age group, and sharing information promotes understanding and compassion.*[5]
- Provide an open environment encouraging communication. *Supports expression of feelings concerning impaired function so they can be dealt with realistically.*[2]
- Use therapeutic communication skills (Active-listening, acknowledgment, silence, I-statements). *Promotes open relationship in which client can explore possibilities and solutions for changing lifestyle situation.*[15]
- Acknowledge client's efforts to adjust: "You have done your best." *Avoids feelings of blame/guilt and defensive response.*[12]
- Discuss/evaluate resources that have been useful to the client in adapting to changes in other life situations. *Vocational rehabilitation, employment experiences, psychosocial support services may be useful in current situation.*[12]
- Develop a plan of action with client to meet immediate needs (e.g., physical safety and hygiene, emotional support of professionals and SOs) and assist in implementation of the plan. *Provides a starting point to deal with current situation for moving ahead with plan for adjusting to change in life circumstances and for evaluation of progress toward goals.*[13]
- Reinforce structure in daily life. Include exercise as part of routine. *Routines help the client focus. Exercise improves sense of wellness and enhances immune response.*[10]
- Review with client coping skills used in previous life situations and role changes. *Identifies the strengths that may be used to facilitate adaptation to change or loss that has occurred.*[8]
- Refine/develop new coping strategies as appropriate. *Strengthens skills for dealing with change in health/lifestyle.*[10]
- Identify and problem-solve with the client frustrations in daily care. *Focusing on the smaller factors of concern gives the individual the ability to perceive the impaired function from a less-threatening perspective (one-step-at-a-time concept). Also promotes sense of control over situation.*[10]
- Involve SO(s) in long-range planning for emotional, psychological, physical, and social needs. *Change that is occurring when illness is long-term/permanent indicates that lifestyle changes will need to be made and dealt with on an ongoing basis, which may be difficult for client and family to adjust to.*[14]
- Refer for individual/family counseling, as indicated. *May need additional assistance to cope with current situation.*[13]

NURSING PRIORITY NO. 4 To promote wellness (Teaching/Discharge Considerations):

- Identify strengths the client perceives in present life situation. Keep focus on the present. *Unknowns of the future may be too overwhelming when diagnosis/injury means permanent changes in lifestyle/management.*[13]
- Assist SOs to learn methods of managing present needs. (Refer to NDs specific to client's deficits.) *Promotes internal locus of control and helps develop plan for long-term needs reflecting changes required by illness/changes in health status.*[2]

Cultural   Collaborative   Community/Home Care   Diagnostic Studies   Pediatric/Geriatric/Lifespan   Medications

- Pace and time learning sessions to meet client's needs, providing for feedback during and after learning experiences (e.g., self-catheterization, range-of-motion exercises, wound care, therapeutic communication). *Promotes skill and enhances retention, thereby improving confidence.*[1]
- Refer to other resources in the long-range plan of care. *Occupational therapy, vocational rehabilitation may be useful for making indicated changes in life, assisting with adjustment to new situation, as needed.*[2]
- Assist client/SO(s) to see appropriate alternatives and potential changes in locus of control. *Often major change in health status results in loss of sense of control, and client needs to begin to look at possibilities for managing illness and what abilities can make life go on in a positive manner.*[10]

DOCUMENTATION FOCUS

Assessment/Reassessment

- Reasons for/degree of impairment.
- Client's/SO(s) perception of the situation.
- Effect of behavior on health status/condition.

Planning

- Plan for adjustments and interventions for achieving the plan and who is involved.
- Teaching plan.

Implementation/Evaluation

- Client responses to the interventions/teaching and actions performed.
- Attainment/progress toward desired outcome(s).
- Modifications to plan of care.

Discharge Planning

- Resources that are available for the client and SO(s) and referrals that are made.

References

1. Doenges, M. E., Moorhouse, M. F., Geissler-Murr, A. C. (2002). *Nursing Care Plans: Guidelines for Individualizing Patient Care.* 6th ed. Philadelphia: F. A. Davis.
2. Doenges, M. E., Townsend, M. C., Moorhouse, M. F. (1998). *Psychiatric Care Plans: Guidelines for Individualizing Care.* 3d ed. Philadelphia: F. A. Davis.
3. Locher, J., et al. (2002). Effects of age and casual attribution to aging on health-related behaviors associated with urinary incontinence in older women. *Gerontologist,* 42(4), 515–521.
4. Cox, H., et al. (2002). *Clinical Applications of Nursing Diagnoses.* 4th ed. Philadelphia: F. A. Davis.
5. Pinhas-Hamiel, O., Dolan, L. M., et al. (1996). Increased incidence of non-insulin-dependent diabetes mellitus among adolescents. *J Pediatr,* 128(8), 608.
6. Deckelbaum, R. J., Williams, C. L. (2001). Childhood obesity: The health issue. *Obesity Res,* 9(5) 239s.
7. Badger, J. M. (2001). Burns: The psychological aspect. *AJN,* 101(11), 38-41.
8. Bartol, T. (2002). Putting a patient with diabetes in the driver's seat. *Nursing2002,* 32(2), 53–55.
9. Konigova, R. (1992). The psychological problems of burned patients. The Rudy Hermans Lecture 1991. *Burns,* 18(3), 189–199.
10. Townsend, M. C. (2006). *Psychiatric Mental Health Nursing: Concepts of Care.* 3d ed. Philadelphia: F. A. Davis.
11. Konstam, M., et al. (1994). Heart failure: Evaluation and care of patients with left-ventricular systolic dysfunction. Rockville (MD): Agency for Health Care Policy and Research; Clinical Practice Guideline No. 11. AHCPR Pub. No 94–0612. Available at www.gerweb.com/HeartDSS/hpract.htm.

12. Rolland, J. S. (1994). *Families, Illness, and Disability.* New York: HarperCollins.
13. Wright, L.M., Leahey, M. (1987). *Families and Chronic Illness.* Springhouse, PA: Springhouse.
14. Lipson, J., Dibble, S., Minarik, P. (1996). *Culture & Nursing Care: A Pocket Guide.* San Francisco: UCSF Nursing Press, School of Nursing, University of California.
15. Gordon, T. (2000). *Parent Effectiveness Training.* Updated edition. New York: Three Rivers Press.

disturbed Body Image

Definition: Confusion [and/or dissatisfaction] in mental picture of one's physical self

RELATED FACTORS

Biophysical; illness; trauma; injury; surgery; [mutilation, pregnancy]
Illness treatment [change caused by biochemical agents (drugs), dependence on machine]
Psychosocial
Cultural; spiritual
Cognitive; perceptual
Developmental changes; [maturational changes]
[Significance of body part or functioning with regard to age, gender, developmental level, or basic human needs]

DEFINING CHARACTERISTICS

Subjective
Verbalization of feelings that reflect an altered view of one's body (e.g., appearance, structure, function)
Verbalization of perceptions that reflect an altered view of one's body in appearance
Verbalization of change in lifestyle
Fear of rejection/reaction by others
Focus on past strength/function/appearance
Negative feelings about body (e.g., feelings of helplessness, hopelessness, or powerlessness); [depersonalization/grandiosity]
Preoccupation with change/loss
Refusal to verify actual change
Emphasis on remaining strengths; heightened achievement
Personalization of part/loss by name
Depersonalization of part/loss by impersonal pronouns

Objective
Behaviors of acknowledgment of one's body; avoidance of one's body; monitoring one's body
Nonverbal response to actual/perceived change in body (e.g., appearance, structure, function)
Missing body part
Actual change in structure/function
Not looking at/not touching body part
Trauma to nonfunctioning part
Change in ability to estimate spatial relationship of body to environment
Extension of body boundary to incorporate environmental objects
Intentional/unintentional hiding/overexposing of body part
Change in social involvement
[Aggression; low frustration tolerance level]

Cultural Collaborative Community/Home Care Diagnostic Studies Pediatric/Geriatric/Lifespan Medications

Sample Clinical Applications: Eating disorders (anorexia/bulimia nervosa), traumatic injuries, amputation, ostomies, aging process, arthritis, pregnancy, chronic renal failure/dialysis, burns

DESIRED OUTCOMES/EVALUATION CRITERIA
Sample NOC linkages:
Body Image: Positive perception of own appearance and body functions
Self-Esteem: Personal judgment of self-worth
Distorted Thought Control: Self-restraint of disruption in perception, thought processes, and thought content

Client Will (Include Specific Time Frames)

• Verbalize acceptance of self in situation (e.g., chronic progressive disease, amputee, decreased independence, weight as is, effects of therapeutic regimen).
• Verbalize relief of anxiety and adaptation to actual/altered body image.
• Verbalize understanding of body changes.
• Recognize and incorporate body image change into self-concept in accurate manner without negating self-esteem.
• Seek information and actively pursue growth.
• Acknowledge self as an individual who has responsibility for self.
• Use adaptive devices/prosthesis appropriately.

ACTIONS/INTERVENTIONS

Sample NIC linkages:
Body Image Enhancement: Improving a patient's conscious and unconscious perceptions and attitudes toward his/her body
Developmental Enhancement: Adolescent: Facilitating optimal physical, cognitive, social, and emotional growth of individuals during the transition from childhood to adulthood
Self-Esteem Enhancement: Assisting a patient to increase his/her personal judgment of self-worth

NURSING PRIORITY NO. I To assess causative/contributing factors:

• Discuss pathophysiology present or situation affecting the individual and refer to additional NDs, as appropriate. For example, when alteration in body image is related to neurological deficit (e.g., stroke), refer to ND unilateral Neglect; for presence of severe, ongoing pain, refer to ND chronic Pain; or in loss of sexual desire/ability, refer to ND Sexual Dysfunction.
• Determine whether condition is permanent/no hope for resolution. (May be associated with other NDs such as Self-Esteem [specify] or risk for impaired parent/infant/child Attachment when child is affected.) *Identifies appropriate interventions based on reality of situation and need to plan for long- or short-term prognosis. There is always something that can be done to enhance acceptance, and it is important to hold out the possibility of living a good life with the disability.*[1]
• Assess mental/physical influence of illness/condition on the client's emotional state (e.g., diseases of the endocrine system, use of steroid therapy, and so forth). *Some diseases can*

have a profound effect on one's emotions and need to be considered in the evaluation and treatment of the individual's behavior and reaction to the current situation.[1,9]

- Evaluate level of client's knowledge of and anxiety related to situation. Observe emotional changes. *Provides information about starting point for providing information about illness. Emotional changes may indicate level of anxiety and need for intervention to lower anxiety before learning can take place.*[1]
- Recognize behavior indicative of overt preoccupation with body and its processes. *May interfere with ability to engage in therapy and indicate need to provide interventions to deal with concern before beginning therapy.*[2,3]
- Assume all individuals are sensitive to changes in appearance, but avoid stereotyping. *Not all individuals react to body changes in the same way, and it is important to determine how this person is reacting to changes.*[2,3]
- Have client describe self, noting what is positive and what is negative. Be aware of how client believes others see self. *Identifies self-image and whether there is a discrepancy between own view and how client believes others see him or her, which may have an effect on how client perceives changes that have occurred.*[3,4]
- ∞ Discuss meaning of loss/change to client. *A small (seemingly trivial) loss may have a big impact (such as the use of a urinary catheter or enema for bowel continence). A change in function (such as immobility) may be more difficult for some to deal with than a change in appearance. Permanent facial scarring of child may be difficult for parents to accept.*[1]
- ∞ Use developmentally appropriate communication techniques for determining exact expression of body image in child (e.g., puppet play or constructive dialogue for toddler). *Developmental capacity must guide interaction to gain accurate information.*[4]
- Note signs of grieving/indicators of severe or prolonged depression. *May require evaluation of need for counseling or medications.*[3]
- 🌐 Determine ethnic background and cultural/religious perceptions and considerations. *Understanding how these factors affect the individual in this situation and how they may influence how individual deals with what has happened is necessary to develop appropriate interventions.*[5]
- Identify social aspects of illness/disease. *Sexually transmitted diseases, sterility, chronic conditions such as vitiligo or multiple sclerosis may affect how client views self and functions in social settings and how others view them.*[2,8]
- Observe interaction of client with SO(s). *Distortions in body image may be unconsciously reinforced by family members, or secondary gain issues may interfere with progress.*[2,8]

NURSING PRIORITY NO. 2. To determine coping abilities and skills:

- Assess client's current level of adaptation and progress. *Client may have already adapted somewhat, and information provides starting point for developing plan of care.*[2]
- Listen to client's comments and note responses to the situation. *Different situations are upsetting to different people, depending on individual coping skills, severity of the perceived changes in body image, and past experiences with similar illnesses/conditions.*[2–4,8]
- Note withdrawn behavior and the use of denial. *May be normal response to situation or may be indicative of mental illness (e.g., depression, schizophrenia).*[6] (Refer to ND ineffective Denial.)
- 💊 Note dependence on prescription medications or use of addictive substances/alcohol. *May reflect dysfunctional coping as client turns to use of these substances to avoid dealing with changes that are occurring to body or ability to function in their accustomed manner.*[4]
- Identify previously used coping strategies and effectiveness. *Familiar coping strategies can be used to begin adaptation to current situation.*[2]

• Determine individual/family/community resources. *Can provide efficient assistance and support to enable the client to adapt to changing circumstances.*[4]

NURSING PRIORITY NO. 3 To assist client and SO(s) to deal with/accept issues of self-concept related to body image:

- Establish therapeutic nurse-client relationship. *Conveys an attitude of caring and develops a sense of trust in which client can discuss concerns and find answers to issues confronting him or her in new situation*[4,8]
- Visit client frequently and acknowledge the individual as someone who is worthwhile. *Provides opportunities for listening to concerns and questions to promote dealing positively with individual situation and change in body image.*[1]
- Assist in correcting underlying problems when possible. *Promotes optimal healing/ adaptation to individual situation (i.e., amputation, presence of colostomy, mastectomy, and impotence).*[1]
- Provide assistance with self-care needs/measures, as necessary, while promoting individual abilities/independence. *Client needs support to achieve the goal of independence and positive return to managing own life.*[4]
- Work with client's self-concept without moral judgments regarding client's efforts or progress (e.g., "You should be progressing faster; you're weak/lazy/not trying hard enough"). *Such statements diminish self-esteem and are counterproductive to progress. Positive reinforcement encourages client to continue efforts/strive for improvement.*[2,8]
- Discuss concerns about fear of mutilation, prognosis, and rejection when client is facing surgery or potentially poor outcome of procedure/illness. *Addresses realities and provides emotional support to enable client to be ready to deal with whatever the outcome may be.*[1]
- Acknowledge and accept feelings of dependency, grief, and hostility. *Conveys a message of understanding.*[1]
- Encourage verbalization of anticipated conflicts *to enhance handling of potential situations. Provides an opportunity to imagine and practice how different situations can be dealt with, thus promoting confidence.*[4]
- Encourage client and SO(s) to communicate feelings to each other and discuss situation openly. *Enhances relationship, improving sense of self-worth and sense of support.*[2]
- Alert staff to be cognizant of own facial expressions and other nonverbal behaviors. *Important to convey acceptance and not revulsion, especially when the client's appearance is affected. Clients are very sensitive to reactions of those around them, and negative reactions will affect self-esteem and may retard adaptation to situation.*[1]
- Encourage family members to treat client normally and not as an invalid. *Helps client return to own routine and begin to gain confidence in ability to manage own life.*[1]
- Encourage client to look at/touch affected body part *to begin to incorporate changes into body image. Acceptance will enhance self-esteem and enable client to move forward in a positive manner.*[1,7]
- Allow client to use denial without participating (e.g., client may at first refuse to look at a colostomy; the nurse says, "I am going to change your colostomy now" and proceeds with the task). *Provides individual time to adapt to situation.*[4,9]
- Set limits on maladaptive behavior; assist client to identify positive behaviors. *Self-esteem will be damaged if client is allowed to continue behaviors that are destructive or not helpful, and adaptation to new image will be delayed.*[4,10]
- Provide accurate information, as desired/requested. Reinforce previously given information. *Accurate knowledge helps client make better decisions for the future.*[4]

- Discuss the availability of prosthetics, reconstructive surgery, and physical/occupational therapy or other referrals, as dictated by individual situation. *Provides hope that situation is not impossible and the future does not look so bleak.*[1,7,8]
- Help client to select and use clothing/makeup *to minimize body changes and enhance appearance.*[1]
- Discuss reasons for infectious isolation and procedures when used, and make time to sit down and talk/listen to client while in the room. *Promotes understanding and decreases sense of isolation/loneliness.*[1]

NURSING PRIORITY NO. 4 To promote wellness (Teaching/Discharge Considerations):

- Begin counseling/other therapies (e.g., biofeedback/relaxation) as soon as possible. *Provides early/ongoing sources of support to promote rehabilitation in a timely manner.*[1]
- Provide information at client's level of acceptance and in small segments. *Allows for easier assimilation.*[1,2,7]
- Clarify misconceptions and reinforce explanations given by other health team members. *Ensures client is hearing factual information to make the best decisions for own situation.*[1,2,7]
- Include client in decision-making process and problem-solving activities. *Promotes adherence to decisions and plans that are made.*[1]
- Assist client to incorporate therapeutic regimen into activities of daily living (ADLs) (e.g., specific exercises, housework activities). *Promotes continuation of program by helping client see that progress can be made within own daily activities.*[1]
- Identify/plan for alterations to home and work environment/activities when necessary. *Accommodates individual needs and supports independence.*[1,9]
- Assist client in learning strategies for dealing with feelings/venting emotions. *Helps individual move toward healing and optimal recuperation.*[1,2]
- Offer positive reinforcement for efforts made (e.g., wearing makeup, using prosthetic device). *Client needs to hear that what he or she is doing is helping.*[1,9]
- Refer to appropriate support groups. *May need additional help to adjust to new situation and life changes.*[1]

DOCUMENTATION FOCUS

Assessment/Reassessment

- Observations, presence of maladaptive behaviors, emotional changes, stage of grieving, level of independence.
- Physical wounds, dressings; use of life-support-type machine (e.g., ventilator, dialysis machine).
- Meaning of loss/change to client.
- Support systems available (e.g., SOs, friends, groups).

Planning

- Plan of care and who is involved in planning.
- Teaching plan.

Implementation/Evaluation

- Client's response to interventions/teaching and actions performed.
- Attainment/progress toward desired outcome(s).

Cultural · Collaborative · Community/Home Care · Diagnostic Studies · Pediatric/Geriatric/Lifespan · Medications

• Modifications of plan of care.

Discharge Planning

• Long-term needs and who is responsible for actions.
• Specific referrals made (e.g., rehabilitation center, community resources).

References

1. Doenges, M., Moorhouse, M., Murr, A. (2002). *Nursing Care Plans, Guidelines for Individualizing Patient Care.* 6th ed. Philadelphia: F. A. Davis.
2. Doenges, M., Townsend, M., Moorhouse, M. (1998). *Psychiatric Care Plans: Guidelines for Individualizing Care.* 3d ed. Philadelphia: F. A. Davis.
3. Townsend, M. (2003). *Psychiatric Mental Health Nursing: Concepts of Care.* 4th ed. Philadelphia: F. A. Davis.
4. Cox, H., Hinz, M., Lubno, M. A., Newfield, S., Scott-Tilley, D., Slater, M., Sridaromont, K. (2002). *Clinical Applications of Nursing Diagnosis: Adult, Child, Women's Psychiatric, Gerontic and Home Health Considerations.* 4th ed. Philadelphia: F. A. Davis.
5. Lipson, J. G., Dibble, S. L., Minarik, P. A. (1996). *Culture & Nursing Care: A Pocket Guide.* School of Nursing. San Francisco: UCSF Nursing Press.
6. Townsend, M. (2001). *Nursing Diagnoses in Psychiatric Nursing: Care Plans and Psychotropic Medications.* 5th ed. Philadelphia: F. A. Davis.
7. Aacovou, I. (2004). The role of the nurse in the rehabilitation of patients with radical changes in body image due to burn injuries. Psychiatric Department, Makarios Hospital, Nicosia, Cyprus.
8. Breakey, J. W. (1997). Body image: The inner mirror. *Journal of Prosthetics and Orthotics*, 9(3), 107.
9. Kater, K. (2006). Building healthy body esteem in a body toxic world. Retrieved June 2007 at bodyimagehealth.org.
10. Reasoner, R. The true meaning of self-esteem Retrieved June 2007 at www.self-esteem-nase.org/ whatisselfesteem.shtml. http://www.self-esteem-NASE.org

risk for imbalanced Body Temperature

Definition: At risk for failure to maintain body temperature within normal range

RISK FACTORS

Extremes of age/weight

Exposure to cold/cool or warm/hot environments; inappropriate clothing for environmental temperature

Dehydration

Inactivity; vigorous activity

Medications causing vasoconstriction/vasodilation; sedation; [use or overdose of certain drugs or exposure to anesthesia]

Illness/trauma affecting temperature regulation [e.g., infections, systemic or localized; neoplasms, tumors; collagen/vascular disease]; altered metabolic rate

NOTE: A risk diagnosis is not evidenced by signs and symptoms, as the problem has not occurred; rather, nursing interventions are directed at prevention.

Sample Clinical Applications: Any infectious process, surgical procedures, brain injuries, hypo/hyperthyroidism, prematurity

DESIRED OUTCOMES/EVALUATION CRITERIA

Sample NOC linkages:

Risk Control: Personal actions to prevent, eliminate, or reduce modifiable health threats

Infection Severity: Severity of infection and associated symptoms

Hydration: Adequate water in the intracellular and extracellular compartments of the body

---

Client Will (Include Specific Time Frame)

- Maintain body temperature within normal range.
- Verbalize understanding of individual risk factors and appropriate interventions.
- Demonstrate behaviors for monitoring and maintaining appropriate body temperature.

ACTIONS/INTERVENTIONS

Sample NIC linkages:

Fever Treatment: Management of a patient with hyperpyrexia caused by nonenvironmental factors

Temperature Regulation: Attaining or maintaining body temperature within a normal range

Temperature Regulation: Intraoperative: Attaining or maintaining desired intraoperative body temperature

NURSING PRIORITY NO. 1   To identify causative/risk factors present:

- Note presence of condition that can affect body's heat production and heat dissipation (e.g., spinal cord injury; burns or skin diseases; endocrine disorders; neurological disorders, such as parkinsonism; kidney disease; being significantly overweight or underweight).[3,4,7,8]
- Determine if present illness/condition results from exposure to environmental factors, surgery, infection, or trauma. *Helps to determine the scope of interventions that may be needed (e.g., simple addition of warm blankets after surgery or hypothermia therapy following brain trauma).*[1]
- Monitor laboratory values (e.g., tests indicative of infection, thyroid/other endocrine tests, drug screens) *to identify potential internal causes of temperature imbalances.*
- Note client's age (e.g., premature neonate, young child, or aging individual), *as it can directly impact ability to maintain/regulate body temperature and respond to changes in environment.*[2]
- Assess nutritional status *to determine metabolism effect on body temperature and to identify foods or nutrient deficits that affect metabolism.*[1,2]

NURSING PRIORITY NO. 2   To prevent occurrence of temperature alteration:

- Monitor temperature regularly (e.g., q 1–4 hr) measuring core body temperature, whenever needed to observe this vital sign. *Traditionally, temperature measurements have been taken orally (good in alert, oriented adult), rectally (accurate but not always easy to obtain), or axillary (readings may be lower than core temperature), with each site offering advantages and disadvantages in terms of accuracy and safety. Newer technologies allow temperatures to be instantly and accurately measured. Tympanic temperature measurement is the most noninvasive way to measure core temperature, as blood is supplied to the tympanic membrane by the carotid artery. This method is preferred by healthcare providers and parents, although some pediatricians may still prefer rectal temperature measurements in sick newborns or infants.*[3]
- Maintain comfortable ambient environment *to reduce risk of body-temperature alterations.*[1,2,4,6,7]
  Provide environmental heating/cooling measures, as needed, such as space heater or air conditioner/fans.
  Ascertain that cooling and warming equipment and supplies are available during/following procedures and surgery.

🌐 Cultural   🅐 Collaborative   🏠 Community/Home Care   🧪 Diagnostic Studies   ∞ Pediatric/Geriatric/Lifespan   💊 Medications

- Dress or discuss with client/caregivers dressing appropriately[6–8]
  Wear layers of clothing *that can be removed or added, as needed.* Wear hat and gloves in cold weather, wear light, loose protective clothing in hot weather, and wear water-resistant outer gear *to protect from wet weather chill.*
- Cover infant's head with knit cap, use layers of lightweight blankets. Place newborn infant under radiant warmer. Teach parents to dress infant appropriately for weather and home environment. *Newborns/infants can have temperature instability with heat loss greatest through head and by evaporation and convection.*[5]
- Maintain adequate fluid intake. Offer cool or warm liquids, as appropriate. *Hydration assists in maintaining normal body temperature.*[1,2,4,7,8]
- Restore/maintain core temperature within client's normal range. (If temperature is below or above normal range, or parameters defined by physician, refer to NDs Hypothermia or Hyperthermia for additional interventions.)
- Recommend lifestyle changes, such as cessation of substance use, normalization of body weight, nutritious meals, or regular exercise *to maximize metabolism and general health.*[1,2]
- Refer at-risk persons to appropriate community resources (e.g., home care, social services, Foster Adult Care, housing agencies) *to provide assistance to meet individual needs.*[1]

NURSING PRIORITY NO. 3 To promote wellness (Teaching/Discharge Considerations):

- Review potential problem/individual risk factors with client/SO(s).
- Discuss effects of age and gender with client/caregiver, as appropriate. *Older/debilitated persons, infants, and young children typically feel more comfortable in higher ambient temperatures. Women notice feeling cool quicker than men, which may be related to body size or to differences in metabolism and the rate that blood flows to extremities to regulate body temperature.*[6,7]
- Instruct in measures to protect from identified risk factors. *Provides understanding for ways in managing lifestyle and environment (e.g., adding or removing clothing; adding/removing heat sources; evaluating home/shelter for ability to manage heat and cold; addressing nutritional and hydration status) and enhances self-care abilities.*[6]
- Review client's medications for possible thermoregulatory side effects (e.g., diuretics, certain sedatives and antipsychotic agents, some heart and blood pressure medications, or anesthesia).[1,2,7,8]
- Discuss with client using sympathomimetics (e.g., cocaine, methamphetamines) the effects of drug on body-temperature regulation.[1,2,7,8]
- Identify ways to prevent accidental thermoregulation problems. *For example, hypothermia can result from overzealous cooling to reduce fever, or maintaining too warm an environment when client has lost the ability to perspire can lead to hyperthermia.*

DOCUMENTATION FOCUS

Assessment/Reassessment

- Identified individual causative/risk factors.
- Record of core temperature, initially and PRN.
- Results of diagnostic studies/laboratory tests.

Planning

- Plan of care and who is involved in planning.
- Teaching plan, including best ambient temperature and ways to prevent hypothermia or hyperthermia.

Implementation/Evaluation

- Response to interventions/teaching and actions performed.
- Attainment/progress toward desired outcome(s).
- Modifications to plan of care.

Discharge Planning

- Long-term need and who is responsible for actions.
- Specific referrals made.

References

1. Surgical Intervention. In Doenges, M. E., Moorhouse, M. F., Geissler-Murr, A. C. (2002). *Nursing Care Plans: Guidelines for Individualizing Patient Care.* 6th ed. Philadelphia: F. A. Davis.
2. Cox, H. C., et al. (2002). *Clinical Applications of Nursing Diagnosis: Adult, Child, Women's, Psychiatric, Gerontic, and Home Health Considerations.* 4th ed. Philadelphia: F. A. Davis.
3. Nicoll, L. H. (2002). Heat in motion: Evaluating and managing temperature. *Nursing2002*, 32(5), s1–s12.
4. American Academy of Pediatrics: Section on Anesthesiology. (1999). Guidelines for the pediatric perioperative anesthesia environment. Pediatrics. 103(2), 512–515.
5. Early discharge of the term newborn. (1999). Guideline from National Association of Neonatal Nurses. Glenview, IL. Retrieved from National Guideline Clearinghouse Web site at www.guideline.gov.
6. Beattie, S. (2006). In from the cold. *RN* 69(11), 22–27.
7. Lien, C. A. (no date). Thermoregulation in the elderly. Syllabus on Geriatric Anesthesiology. American Society of Anesthesiologists Web site. Retrieved January 2007 at www.asahq.org/clinical/geriatrics/thermo.htm.
8. Hoppe, J., Sinert, R. (2006). Heat exhaustion and heatstroke. Article for Emedicine Web site. Retrieved March 2007 at www.emedicine.com/emerg/topic/236.htm.

Bowel Incontinence

Definition: Change in normal bowel habits characterized by involuntary passage of stool

RELATED FACTORS

Toileting self-care deficit; environmental factors (e.g., inaccessible bathroom); impaired cognition; immobility

Dietary habits; medications; laxative abuse

Stress

Colorectal lesions; impaired reservoir capacity

Incomplete emptying of bowel; impaction; chronic diarrhea

General decline in muscle tone; abnormally high abdominal/intestinal pressure

Rectal sphincter abnormality; loss of rectal sphincter control; lower/upper motor nerve damage

DEFINING CHARACTERISTICS

Subjective

Recognizes rectal fullness but reports inability to expel formed stool

Urgency; inability to delay defecation

Self-report of inability to feel rectal fullness

Objective

Constant dribbling of soft stool

Cultural ⬤ Collaborative ⬤ Community/Home Care 🏠 Diagnostic Studies ∞ Pediatric/Geriatric/Lifespan Medications

Fecal staining of clothing and/or bedding
Fecal odor
Red perianal skin
Inability to recognize/inattention to urge to defecate

Sample Clinical Applications: Hemorrhoids, rectal prolapse, anal/gynecological surgery, childbirth injuries/uterine prolapse, spinal cord injury, stroke, multiple sclerosis, ulcerative colitis, dementia

DESIRED OUTCOMES/EVALUATION CRITERIA
Sample NOC linkages:
Bowel Continence: Control of passage of stool from the bowel
Bowel Elimination: Formation and evacuation of stool
Neurological Status: Ability of the peripheral and central nervous system to receive, process, and respond to internal and external stimuli

Client Will (Include Specific Time Frame)
- Verbalize understanding of causative/controlling factors.
- Identify individually appropriate interventions.
- Participate in therapeutic regimen to control incontinence.
- Establish/maintain as regular a pattern of bowel functioning as possible.

ACTIONS/INTERVENTIONS

Sample NIC linkages:
Bowel Incontinence Care: Promotion of bowel continence and maintenance of perineal skin integrity
Bowel Incontinence Care: Encopresis: Promotion of bowel continence in children
Bowel Training: Assisting the patient to train the bowel to evacuate at specific intervals

NURSING PRIORITY NO. 1 To assess causative/contributing factors:

- Identify pathophysiological conditions present (e.g., multiple sclerosis, acute/chronic cognitive impairments, spinal cord injury, stroke, ileus, ulcerative colitis).
- Determine historical aspects of incontinence with preceding/precipitating factors. *Common causes include (1) structural changes in the sphincter muscle (e.g., hemorrhoids, rectal prolapse, anal or gynecological surgery, childbirth injuries); (2) injuries to sensory nerves (e.g., spinal cord injury, trauma, stroke, tumor, radiation therapy, multiple sclerosis); (3) strong-urge diarrhea (e.g., ulcerative colitis, Crohn's disease, infectious diarrhea); (4) dementia (e.g., acute or chronic cognitive impairment, not necessarily related to sphincter control); (5) result of toxins (e.g., salmonella); and (6) effects of improper diet or type/rate of enteral feedings.*[1–6,8]
- Note client's age and gender. *Constipation from holding stool is more common in children. Bowel incontinence is more common in children and elderly adults (difficulty responding to urge in a timely manner, problems walking or undoing zippers); more common in boys than girls, but more common in elderly women than elderly men.*[1–6]
- Review medication regimen, including OTC drugs. *Laxative abuse, drugs with side effects of diarrhea (e.g., antibiotics) or constipation (e.g., sedatives, hypnotics, opioids, muscle relaxants) may impact bowel control.*
- Assist with/perform physical evaluation. Palpate abdomen for masses and auscultate for presence/location and characteristics of bowel sounds.

- Review diagnostic studies. *Pelvic and/or anal ultrasound may be used to identify structural abnormalities; endoscopy, to visualize lower gastrointestinal tract; manometry, to measure pressure and strength of anal muscles; and nerve studies, to check for nerve damage. Blood tests and stool cultures may be done to identify presence of bacteria and toxins.*[1,2,3,5,7]

NURSING PRIORITY NO. 2 To determine current pattern of elimination:

- Ascertain timing and characteristic aspects of incontinent occurrence, noting preceding/precipitating events. *Helps to identify patterns or worsening trends. Interventions are different for sudden acute accident than for chronic long-term incontinence problems. Person may have passive incontinence, in which person is unaware that stool is being passed (related to poorly functioning sphincter muscle), or urge incontinence, in which person is aware but unable to prevent passage of stool (sphincter muscle normal). Problem may have been present for a long time, either because of client/caregiver sense of embarrassment or failure to realize that effective treatment may be available.*[2,5]
- Determine stool characteristics, including consistency (may be liquid, hard formed, or hard at first and then soft), amount (may be a small amount of liquid or entire solid bowel movement), and frequency. *Provides information that can help differentiate type of incontinence present and provides comparative baseline for response to interventions.*[4,6]
- Note where bowel accidents occur and what client is experiencing at the time. *Changes in usual routines or surrounding environment, general health condition, addition of emotional stressors, such as new baby in the home or increased confusion in dementia client, can cause or exacerbate incontinence behaviors.*[5]

NURSING PRIORITY NO. 3 To promote control/management of incontinence:

- Assist in treatment of underlying factors (e.g., as listed in Related Factors and Defining Characteristics sections). *While incontinence is a symptom and not a disease, appropriate treatment can often correct the problem or at least improve the client's quality of life.*[2]
- Administer medications, as indicated: stool softeners/bulk formers and laxatives *may be used when cause is constipation;* antidiarrheals, including cholinergics, *may be used to decrease intestinal secretions and bowel motility if diarrhea is cause for incontinence.*[1,2,4]
- Establish toileting program as early as possible *to maximize success of program and preserve comfort and self-esteem*[1–6]

  Take client to the bathroom/place on commode or bedpan at specified intervals, taking into consideration individual needs and incontinence patterns.

  Use the same type of facility for toileting as much as possible.

  Make sure bathroom is safe for impaired person (good lighting, support rails, good height for getting onto and up from stool).

  Provide time and privacy for elimination.

  Demonstrate techniques/assist client/caregiver to practice contracting abdominal muscles, leaning forward on commode *to increase intra-abdominal pressure during defecation,* and left to right abdominal massage *to stimulate peristalsis.*
- Encourage and instruct client/caregiver in providing diet high in natural bulk/fiber, with fruits, vegetables, and grains and reduced fatty foods. Identify/eliminate problem foods *to avoid diarrhea, constipation, or gas formation.*[2,4,6]
- Adjust enteral feedings and/or change formula, as indicated, *to reduce diarrhea effect.*[4]
- Encourage adequate fluid intake (at least 2000 mL/d) within client's need and tolerance, including fruit juices *to help manage constipation.* Encourage warm fluids after meals *to promote intestinal motility.* Avoid caffeine and alcohol *to reduce diarrhea.*[4,6]

⊕ Cultural Ⓐ Collaborative 🏠 Community/Home Care ✏ Diagnostic Studies ∞ Pediatric/Geriatric/Lifespan 💊 Medications

- Recommend walking and regular exercise program, pelvic floor exercises, and biofeedback, as individually indicated, *to improve abdominal and pelvic muscles and strengthen rectal sphincter tone.*[2,4,6]
- Encourage/provide perineal care with frequent gentle cleansing and use of emollients after incontinent stools *to reduce excoriation of skin.*[7]
- Provide incontinence aids/pads until control is obtained. Change pads frequently *to reduce incidence of skin rashes/breakdown.*[7]
- Refer to ND Diarrhea *if incontinence is due to uncontrolled diarrhea;* ND Constipation *if incontinence is due to impaction.*

NURSING PRIORITY NO. 4 To promote wellness (Teaching/Discharge Considerations):

- Review and encourage continuation of successful interventions as individually identified.
- Instruct in use of suppositories or laxatives or stool softeners, when indicated, *to stimulate timed defecation.*
- Identify foods (e.g., daily bran muffins or prunes) *that promote bowel regularity.* Recommend avoidance of problem foods dependent on individual reactions.
- Refer client/caregivers to outside resources when condition is long-term or chronic *to obtain care assistance and emotional support and respite.*
- Encourage scheduling of social activities within time frame of bowel program, as indicated (e.g., avoid a 4-hour excursion with no access to appropriate facilities if bowel program requires toileting every 3 hours) *to maximize social functioning and success of bowel program.*

DOCUMENTATION FOCUS

Assessment/Reassessment

- Current and previous pattern of elimination/physical findings, character of stool, actions tried.

Planning

- Plan of care and who is involved in planning.
- Teaching plan.

Implementation/Evaluation

- Client's/caregiver's responses to interventions/teaching and actions performed.
- Changes in pattern of elimination, characteristics of stool.
- Attainment/progress toward desired outcome(s).
- Modifications to plan of care.

Discharge Planning

- Identified long-term needs, noting who is responsible for each action.
- Specific bowel program at time of discharge.

References

1. Whitehead, W. E. (2002). Understanding fecal incontinence. Patient Information Page. Chapel Hill, NC: The UNC School of Medicine Center for functional GI and Motility Disorders Web site. Available at www.med.unc.edu/medicine/fgidc/understanding_fecal_incontinence.pdf.
2. What is bowel incontinence? Cleveland Clinic Health System, May 2001. Available at http://cms.clevelandclinic.org/digestivedisease/body.cfm?id=84.
3. Bowel incontinence. Patient Brochure. (1996). Arlington Heights, IL: American Society of Colon and Rectal Surgeons.
4. Doenges, M. E., Moorhouse, M. F., Geissler-Murr, A. C. (2002). Spinal cord injury (acute rehabilitative phase). In: *Nursing Care Plans: Guidelines for Individualizing Patient Care.* 6th ed. Philadelphia: F. A. Davis, p. 276.

5. Monicken, D. Special care problems, part 5: Bowel incontinence. In: What to do? A Guide for Families Caring for Persons with Dementia-Related Diseases. Geriatric Research. Minneapolis, MN: Education and Clinical Center (GRECC) of the Dept of Veterans Affairs Medical Center.
6. Cox, H. C., et al. (2002). *Clinical Applications of Nursing Diagnosis: Adult. Child, Women's, Psychiatric, Gerontic, and Home Health Considerations.* 4th ed. Philadelphia: F. A. Davis.
7. Gray, M., Bliss, D. Z., Doughty, D. B., et al. (2007). Incontinence-associated dermatitis: A consensus. *J Wound, Ostomy and Continence Nursing,* 34(1), 45–54.
8. Lehrer, J. K. (2006). Bowel incontinence. Article for MedlinePlus, a service of National Library of Medicine and National Institutes of Health. Retrieved January 2007 at www.nlm.nih.gov/medlineplus/ency/article/003135.htm.

effective Breastfeeding [Learning Need]*

Definition: Mother-infant dyad/family exhibits adequate proficiency and satisfaction with breastfeeding process

RELATED FACTORS
Basic breastfeeding knowledge
Normal [maternal] breast structure
Normal infant oral structure
Infant gestational age greater than 34 weeks
Support sources [available]
Maternal confidence

DEFINING CHARACTERISTICS

Subjective
Maternal verbalization of satisfaction with the breastfeeding process

Objective
Mother able to position infant at breast to promote a successful latch-on response
Infant is content after feedings
Regular and sustained suckling/swallowing at the breast [e.g., 8 to 10 times/24 hr]
Appropriate infant weight patterns for age
Effective mother/infant communication patterns [infant cues, maternal interpretation and response]
Signs/symptoms of oxytocin release (letdown or milk-ejection reflex)
Adequate infant elimination patterns for age [stools soft; more than six wet diapers/day of unconcentrated urine]
Eagerness of infant to nurse [breastfeed]

Sample Clinical Applications: Wellness diagnosis associated with pre/postnatal client

DESIRED OUTCOMES/EVALUATION CRITERIA
Sample NOC linkages:
Breastfeeding Establishment: Infant: Infant attachment to and sucking from the mother's breast for nourishment during the first 2 to 3 weeks
Breastfeeding Establishment: Maternal: Maternal establishment of proper attachment of an infant to and sucking from the breast for nourishment during the first 2 to 3 weeks of breastfeeding

---

*This is difficult to address, because the Related Factors and Defining Characteristics are in fact the outcome/evaluation criteria that would be desired. We believe that normal breastfeeding behaviors need to be learned and supported, with interventions directed at learning activities for enhancement.

🌐 Cultural   Ⓐ Collaborative   🏠 Community/Home Care   ⟋ Diagnostic Studies   ∞ Pediatric/Geriatric/Lifespan   💊 Medications

Breastfeeding Maintenance: Continuation of breastfeeding for nourishment of an infant/toddler

Client Will (Include Specific Time Frame)

- Verbalize understanding of breastfeeding techniques.
- Demonstrate effective techniques for breastfeeding.
- Demonstrate family involvement and support.
- Attend classes/read appropriate materials/access resources as necessary.

ACTIONS/INTERVENTIONS

Sample NIC linkages:

Lactation Counseling: Use of an interactive helping process to assist in maintenance of successful breastfeeding

Anticipatory Guidance: Preparation of patient for an anticipated developmental and/or situational crisis

Teaching: Infant Nutrition: Instruction on nutrition and feeding practices during the first year of life

NURSING PRIORITY NO. 1 To assess individual learning needs:

- Assess mother's knowledge and previous experience with breastfeeding. *Provides information for developing plan of care. Accurate knowledge and previous experience can lead to a positive breastfeeding experience.*[1]
- Note culture and society influences regarding infant feeding (breast/bottle-feeding), lactation process, letdown techniques, maternal food preferences. *In Western cultures, the breast has taken on a sexual connotation and some mothers may be embarrassed to breastfeed. While breastfeeding may be accepted, in some cultures certain beliefs may affect specific feeding practices (e.g., in Mexican American, Navajo, Filipino, and Vietnamese cultures, colostrum is not offered to the newborn; breastfeeding begins only after the milk flow is established).*[3]
- Note incorrect myths/misunderstandings especially in teenage mothers *who are more likely to have limited knowledge and concerns about body image issues.*[6]
- Monitor effectiveness of current breastfeeding efforts. *Determining the actions client is taking provides information about measures that may enhance efforts to be successful in endeavor.*[1]
- Determine support systems available to mother/family. *Presence of adequate support can provide encouragement to mother who may be feeling nervous and unsure about new role.*[1,6]

NURSING PRIORITY NO. 2 To promote effective breastfeeding behaviors:

- Initiate breastfeeding within first hours after birth. *The time of the first feeding is determined by the infant's physiological and behavioral cues. Throughout the first 2 hours after birth, the infant is usually alert and ready to nurse. Early feedings are of great benefit to mother and infant, because oxytocin release is stimulated, helping to expel the placenta and prevent excessive maternal blood loss; the infant receives the immunological protection of colostrum; peristalsis is stimulated; lactation is accelerated; and maternal-infant bonding is enhanced.*[2]
- Demonstrate how to support and position infant and use of aides (e.g., infant sling, nursing footstool/pillows). *The mother should be made as comfortable as possible and given specific instructions for positioning self and baby depending on the type of birth (e.g., cesarean section or vaginal).*[1,5]

- Observe mother's return demonstration. *Provides practice and the opportunity to correct misunderstandings and add additional information to promote optimal experience for breastfeeding.*[1]
- Keep infant with mother for unrestricted breastfeeding duration and frequency. *Rooming-in offers opportunity for spontaneous encounters for the family to practice handling skills and increase confidence in own ability. It also encourages feeding in response to cues from the baby.*[1]
- Encourage skin-to-skin contact.
- 🏠 Encourage mother to follow a well-balanced diet containing an extra 500 calories/day and to drink at least 2000 to 3000 mL of fluid/day. *There is an increased need for maternal energy, protein, minerals, and vitamins, as well as increased fluid intake during lactation to restore what the mother loses in secreting milk to provide adequate nutrients for the nourishment of the infant and to protect the mother's own stores.*[4]
- Provide information, as needed, in support of breastfeeding. *Having adequate information about the nutritional, psychological, immunological advantages, contraindications, and disadvantages of breastfeeding helps the parents to make a decision that is best for the family. Many mothers indicate that if they had had adequate information, they would have chosen breastfeeding.*[1]
- 🏠 Discuss early infant feeding cues (e.g., rooting, lip smacking, sucking fingers/hand) versus late cue of crying. *Early recognition of infant hunger promotes timely/more rewarding feeding experience for infant and mother.*[6]
- 🏠 Discuss/demonstrate breastfeeding aids (e.g., infant sling, nursing footstool/pillows, breast pumps) *to enhance comfort.*[5]
- 🏠 Promote peer counseling for teen mothers. *Provides positive role model teen can relate to and feel comfortable discussing concerns/feelings.*[6]

NURSING PRIORITY NO. 3. To enhance optimum wellness (Teaching/Discharge Considerations):

- 🏠 Provide for follow-up contact/home visit 48 hours after discharge; repeat visit, as necessary. *Provides opportunity to assess adequacy of home situation and breastfeeding efforts as well as support and assistance with problem-solving, if needed.*[1]
- 🏠 Recommend monitoring number of infant's wet diapers (at least six wet diapers in 24 hrs suggests adequate hydration). *Often mothers who are breastfeeding worry about whether infant is getting adequate nutrition, because they cannot measure the amount of milk being received, and having this information can allay these fears.*[1]
- Encourage mother/other family members to express feelings/concerns, and Active-listen *to determine nature of concerns. Identifying the concerns of the parents promotes problem-solving and alleviation of worries and fears. When individuals do not express these concerns, they can become frustrated, which can interfere with successful breastfeeding.*[1]
- 🏠 Educate father/SO about benefits of breastfeeding and how to manage common lactation challenges. *Enlisting support of father/SO is associated with higher ratio of successful breastfeeding at 6 months.*[8]
- 🏠 Review techniques for expression and storage of breast milk to help sustain breastfeeding activity. *Having this information enables the mother to successfully manage continuation of breastfeeding while engaging in activities outside the home for specified periods of time.*[1]
- 🏠 Explain changes in feeding needs/frequency. *Growth spurts require increased intake/more feedings by infant.*[5]
- Review normal nursing behaviors of older breastfeeding infants/toddlers.[5]
- 🏠 Discuss importance of delaying introduction of solid foods until infant is at least 4 months, preferably 6 months old. *Note:* American Academy of Pediatrics now recommends delaying solids until at least 6 months.[5]

🌐 Cultural   Ⓐ Collaborative   🏠 Community/Home Care   ⬎ Diagnostic Studies   ∞ Pediatric/Geriatric/Lifespan   🔖 Medications

- Recommend avoidance of specific medications/substances (e.g., estrogen-containing contraceptives, bromocriptine, nicotine, alcohol) *known to decrease milk supply. Note: Small amounts of alcohol have not been shown to be detrimental.*[6,7]
- Stress importance of client notifying healthcare providers/dentists/pharmacists of breast-feeding status.
- Problem-solve return-to-work issues or periodic infant care requiring bottle/supplemental feeding. *Enables mothers who need/desire to return to work (for economic or personal reasons) or who simply want to attend activities without the infant to deal with these issues, thus allowing more freedom while maintaining adequate breastfeeding.*[1]
- Recommend using expressed breast milk instead of formula or at least partial breastfeeding for as long as mother and child are satisfied.[6]
- Refer to support groups, such as La Leche League, as indicated. *While the father or SO is the most important support person in Western society, family support systems may be lacking information about other support systems/groups.*[1]
- Refer to ND ineffective Breastfeeding for more specific information, as appropriate.

DOCUMENTATION FOCUS

Assessment/Reassessment

- Identified assessment factors (maternal and infant).
- Number of daily wet diapers and periodic weight.

Planning

- Plan of care/interventions and who is involved in the planning.
- Teaching plan.

Implementation/Evaluation

- Mother's response to interventions/teaching plan and actions performed.
- Effectiveness of infant's efforts to feed.
- Attainment/progress toward desired outcome(s).
- Modifications to plan of care.

Discharge Planning

- Long-term needs/referrals and who is responsible for follow-up actions.

References

1. Ladewig, P., London, M., Moberly, S., Olds, S. (2002). *Contemporary Maternal-Newborn Care.* 5th ed. Upper Saddle River, NJ: Prentice Hall.
2. Riodan, J., Auerbach, K. (1993). *Breastfeeding and Human Lactation.* Boston: Jones & Bartlett.
3. Lipson, J., Dibble, S., Minarik, P. (1996). *Culture & Nursing Care: A Pocket Guide.* UCSF Nursing Press.
4. Lowdermilk, D., Perry, S., Bobak, I. (2001). *Maternity & Women's Health Care.* 6th ed. St. Louis, MO: Mosby.
5. American Academy of Pediatrics: Ten steps to support parents' choice to breastfeed their baby. Revised May 2003. Accessed February 2007 at www.aap.org/breastfeeding/tenSteps.pdf.
6. American Academy of Family Physicians: Breastfeeding (position paper). Accessed February 2007 at www.aafp.org/online/en/home/policy/policies/b/breastfeedingpositionpaper.html.
7. Callen, J., Pinelli, J. (2005). A review of the literature examining the benefits and challenges, incidence and duration, and barriers to breastfeeding in preterm infants *Adv Neonatal Care,* 5(2), 72–88. Accessed February 2007 at www.medscape.com/viewarticle/502591.
8. Pisacane, A., Continisio, G., et al. (2005). A controlled trial of the father's role in breastfeeding promotion. *Pediatrics,* 116(4), e494–e498. Accessed February 2007 at www.sidsalliance.org/research/Fathers%20Role%20in%20Successful%20Breastfeeding.pdf.

ineffective Breastfeeding

Definition: Dissatisfaction or difficulty a mother, infant, or child experiences with the breastfeeding process

RELATED FACTORS

Prematurity; infant anomaly; poor infant sucking reflex

Infant receiving [numerous or repeated] supplemental feedings with artificial nipple

Maternal anxiety/ambivalence

Knowledge deficit

Previous history of breastfeeding failure

Interruption in breastfeeding

Nonsupportive partner/family

Maternal breast anomaly; previous breast surgery; [physical discomfort during feeding]

DEFINING CHARACTERISTICS

Subjective

Unsatisfactory breastfeeding process

Persistence of sore nipples beyond the first week of breastfeeding

Insufficient emptying of each breast per feeding

Inadequate/perceived inadequate milk supply

Objective

Observable signs of inadequate infant intake [decrease in number of wet diapers, inappropriate weight loss/or inadequate gain]

Nonsustained/insufficient opportunity for suckling at the breast; infant inability [failure] to latch onto maternal breast correctly

Infant arching/crying at the breast; resistant latching on

Infant exhibiting fussiness/crying within the first hour after breastfeeding; unresponsive to other comfort measures

No observable signs of oxytocin release

Sample Clinical Applications: Prematurity, cleft lip/palate, child abuse/neglect, failure to thrive, diseases of the breast

DESIRED OUTCOMES/EVALUATION CRITERIA

Sample NOC linkages: Knowledge:

Knowledge: Breastfeeding: Extent of understanding conveyed about lactation and nourishment of infant through breastfeeding

Breastfeeding Establishment: Maternal [or] Infant: Maternal establishment of proper attachment of an infant to and sucking from the breast for nourishment during the first 3 weeks of breastfeeding/infant attachment to and sucking from the mother's breast for nourishment during the first 3 weeks of breastfeeding

Breastfeeding Maintenance: Continuation of breastfeeding for nourishment of an infant/toddler

Client Will (Include Specific Time Frame)

- Verbalize understanding of causative/contributing factors.
- Demonstrate techniques to improve/enhance breastfeeding experience.
- Assume responsibility for effective breastfeeding.

Cultural   Collaborative   Community/Home Care   Diagnostic Studies   Pediatric/Geriatric/Lifespan   Medications

- Achieve mutually satisfactory breastfeeding regimen with infant content after feedings and gaining weight appropriately.

ACTIONS/INTERVENTIONS

Sample NIC linkages:

Lactation Counseling: Use of an interactive helping process to assist in maintenance of successful breastfeeding

Breastfeeding Assistance: Preparing a new mother to breastfeed her infant

Support Group: Use of a group environment to provide emotional support and health-related information for members

NURSING PRIORITY NO. 1   To identify maternal causative/contributing factors:

- Assess client knowledge about breastfeeding and extent of instruction previously received. *Provides baseline information for identifying needs and developing plan of care.*[1,7]
- Encourage discussion of current/previous breastfeeding experience(s). *Identifies current needs and problems encountered to develop a plan of care.*[5]
- Note previous unsatisfactory experience (including self or others). *Often unsolved problems and stories told by others may cause doubt about chance for success.*[1]
- Perform physical assessment, noting appearance of breasts/nipples, marked asymmetry of breasts, obvious inverted or flat nipples, minimal or no breast enlargement during pregnancy. *Identifies existing problems that may interfere with successful breastfeeding experience and provides opportunity to correct them when possible.*[1,7]
- Determine whether lactation failure is primary (i.e., maternal prolactin deficiency/serum prolactin levels, inadequate mammary gland tissue, breast surgery that has damaged the nipple, areola enervation) or secondary (i.e., sore nipples, severe engorgement, plugged milk ducts, mastitis, inhibition of letdown reflex, maternal/infant separation with disruption of feedings). *Primary failure may be irremedial and alternate plans need to be made. Secondary failure can be remedied so breastfeeding efforts can be successful.*[5] *Note: Overweight women and obese women are 2.5 times and 3.6 times, respectively, less successful in initiating breastfeeding than the general population.*[9]
- Note history of pregnancy, labor, and delivery (vaginal or cesarean section), other recent or current surgery, preexisting medical problems (e.g., diabetes mellitus, seizure disorder, cardiac diseases, or presence of disabilities), or if client is adoptive mother. *While some conditions may preclude breastfeeding and alternate plans need to be made, others will need specific plans for monitoring and treatment to ensure successful breastfeeding.*[5]
- Identify maternal support systems and presence and response of SO(s), extended family, and friends. *Infant's father and maternal grandmother (in addition to caring healthcare providers) are important factors in whether breastfeeding is successful.*[8] *Having sufficient support enhances opportunity for a successful breastfeeding experience. Negative attitudes and comments interfere with efforts and may cause client to abandon attempt to breastfeed.*[5]
- Ascertain mother's age, number of children at home, and need to return to work. *These factors may have a detrimental effect on desire to breastfeed. Immaturity may influence mother to avoid breastfeeding, believing that it will be inconvenient, or cause her to be insensitive to the infant's needs. The stress of the responsibility of other children or the need to return to work can affect the ability to manage effective breastfeeding; mother will need support and information to be successful.*[6]

🏠 • Determine maternal feelings (e.g., fear/anxiety, ambivalence, depression). *Indicators of underlying emotional state that may suggest need for intervention and referral.*[1]

🌐 • Ascertain cultural expectations/conflicts about breastfeeding and beliefs/practices regarding lactation, letdown techniques, maternal food preferences. *Understanding impact of culture and idiosyncrasies of specific feeding practices is important to determine the effect on infant feeding. The practice may be different but not inferior. For example, in many cultures, such as Mexican American, Navajo, and Vietnamese, colostrum is not offered to the newborn. Intervention is only necessary if the practice/belief is harmful to the infant.*[1,3,8]

∞ • Note incorrect myths/misunderstandings especially in teenage mothers *who are more likely to have limited knowledge and more concerns about body-image issues.*[8]

NURSING PRIORITY NO. 2 To assess infant causative/contributing factors:

🏠 • Determine suckling problems or infant anomaly (e.g., cleft palate). *These factors indicate need for interventions directed at correcting individual situation. Conditions such as cleft palate need evaluation for correction and individualized instruction in holding infant upright and using special nipple or feeding device.*[1,2]

• Note prematurity. *Degree of prematurity will dictate type of interventions needed to deal with situation. Infant may be put to breast if sufficiently developed, or mother may pump breast and the breast milk given via gavage.*[2]

🏠 • Review feeding schedule to note increased demand for feeding (at least eight times/day, taking both breasts at each feeding for more than 15 minutes on each side) or use of supplements with artificial nipple. *Provides opportunity to evaluate infant's growth, determine whether sufficient nourishment is provided, and make adjustments as needed.*[2]

🏠 • Evaluate observable signs of inadequate infant intake. *Baby latches onto mother's nipples with sustained suckling but minimal audible swallowing/gulping noted, infant arching and crying at the breasts with resistance to latching on, decreased urinary output/frequency of stools, inadequate weight gain indicate need for evaluation and intervention.*[1,7]

🏠 • Determine whether baby is content after feeding or exhibits fussiness and crying within the first hour after breastfeeding. *Suggests unsatisfactory breastfeeding process.*[1]

🏠 • Note any correlation between maternal ingestion of certain foods and "colicky" response of infant. *Some foods may seem to result in reaction by the infant and identification and elimination may correct the problem.*[2]

NURSING PRIORITY NO. 3. To assist mother to develop skills of adequate breastfeeding:

🏠 • Provide emotional support to mother. Use 1:1 instruction with each feeding during hospital stay/clinic visit. *New mothers say they would like more support, encouragement, and practical information, especially when they are discharged early. Contact during each feeding provides the opportunity to develop nurse-client relationship in which these goals can be attained.*[1] *Note: Adoptive mothers choosing to breastfeed will require more supportive instruction from a lactation consultant to assist with induced lactation techniques.*[8]

• Inform mother about early infant feeding cues (e.g., rooting, lip smacking, sucking fingers/hand) versus late cue of crying. *New mothers may not be aware that these behaviors indicate hunger and may not respond appropriately. Early recognition of infant hunger promotes timely/more rewarding feeding experience for infant and mother.*[1,8]

• Recommend avoidance or overuse of supplemental feedings and pacifiers (unless specifically indicated). *These can lessen infant's desire to breastfeed. The shape of the mouth and lips and the sucking mechanism is different for breast and bottle, and the infant may be confused by the difference, causing interference in the breastfeeding process/increase risk of early weaning.*

Note: Adoptive mothers may not develop a full breast milk supply, necessitating supplemental feedings.[1,8]

- Restrict use of breast shields (i.e., only temporarily to help draw the nipple out), then place baby directly on nipple. *These have been found to contribute to lactation failures. Shields prevent the infant's mouth from coming into contact with the mother's nipple, which is necessary for continued release of prolactin (promoting milk production) and can interfere with or prevent establishment of adequate milk supply. However, temporary use of shield may be beneficial in the presence of severe nipple cracking.*[6]

- Discuss/demonstrate breastfeeding aids (e.g., infant sling, nursing footstool/pillows) and suggest using a variety of nursing positions *to find the most comfortable for mother and infant. Positions particularly helpful for "plus-sized" women or those with large breasts include the "football" hold, with infant's head to mother's breast and body curved around behind her, or lying down to nurse.*[10]

- Encourage frequent rest periods, sharing household/child-care duties. *The new mother may feel overwhelmed with taking care of infant and carrying out other household duties; having assistance can limit fatigue and facilitate relaxation at feeding times.*[6]

- Suggest abstinence/restriction of tobacco, caffeine, alcohol, drugs, and excess sugar, as appropriate. *May affect milk production/letdown reflex or be passed on to the infant.*[1]

- Promote early management of breastfeeding problems. *Dealing with problems in a timely manner will promote successful breastfeeding.*[1,7]

For example:

Engorgement: Apply heat or cool applications to the breasts, massage from chest wall down to nipple; use synthetic oxytocin nasal spray to enhance letdown reflex; soothe "fussy baby" before latching on the breast, properly position baby on breast/nipple; alternate the side on which baby starts nursing; nurse round the clock or pump with piston-type electric breast pump with bilateral collection chambers at least 8 to 12 times/day.

Sore nipples: Wear 100% cotton fabrics, do not use soap/alcohol/drying agents on nipples, avoid use of nipple shields or nursing pads that contain plastic; cleanse and then air dry, use thin layers of lanolin (if mother/baby not sensitive to wool); provide exposure to sunlight/sunlamps with extreme caution; administer mild pain reliever as appropriate, apply ice before nursing; soak with warm water before attaching infant to soften nipple and remove dried milk, begin with least sore side or begin with hand expression to establish letdown reflex, properly position infant on breast/nipple, and use a variety of nursing positions.

Clogged ducts: Use larger bra or extender to avoid pressure on site; use moist or dry heat, gently massage from above plug down to nipple; nurse infant, hand express, or pump after massage; nurse more often on affected side.

Inhibited letdown: Use relaxation techniques before nursing (e.g., maintain quiet atmosphere, assume position of comfort, massage, apply heat to breasts, have beverage available); develop a routine for nursing, concentrate on infant; administer synthetic oxytocin nasal spray as appropriate.

Mastitis: Promote bedrest (with infant) for several days; administer antibiotics; provide warm, moist heat before and during nursing; empty breasts completely, continuing to nurse baby at least 8 to 12 times/day, or pumping breasts for 24 hours, then resuming breastfeeding as appropriate.

- Demonstrate use of electric piston-type breast pump with bilateral collection chamber when necessary to maintain or increase milk supply. *The need to use a pump to store milk for feedings while the mother is away (i.e., going back to work, or simply to allow time away from the infant) demands some degree of proficiency in the use of the pump.*[1]

NURSING PRIORITY NO. 4 To condition infant to breastfeed:

- Scent breast pad with breast milk and leave in bed with infant along with mother's photograph when separated from mother for medical purposes (e.g., prematurity).
- Increase skin-to-skin contact.
- Provide practice times at breast.
- Express small amounts of milk into baby's mouth.
- Have mother pump breast after feeding to enhance milk production.
- Use supplemental nutrition system cautiously when necessary.
- Identify special interventions for feeding in presence of cleft lip/palate. These measures promote optimal interaction between mother and infant and provide adequate nourishment for the infant, enhancing successful breastfeeding.[1]

NURSING PRIORITY NO. 5 To promote wellness (Teaching/Discharge Considerations):

- Schedule follow-up visits with healthcare provider 48 hours after hospital discharge and 2 weeks after birth. *Provides opportunity to evaluate milk intake/breastfeeding process and adequacy of home situation.*[2]
- Recommend monitoring number of infant's wet diapers. *At least six wet diapers a day suggests adequate hydration and provides reassurance that infant is receiving sufficient intake.*[6]
- Weigh infant at least every third day initially as indicated and record. *Provides record of appropriate weight gain verifying adequacy of nutritional intake or indicates need for evaluation of insufficient weight gain.*[1]
- Educate father/SO about benefits of breastfeeding and how to manage common lactation challenges. *Enlisting support of father/SO is associated with higher ratio of successful breastfeeding at 6 months.*[11]
- Discuss with spouse/SO mother's need for rest, relaxation, and time together with spouse and with other children as appropriate. *Promotes understanding of mother's needs and cooperation with incorporation of new member into family. Spouse and children feel included when they have time alone with mother and are more willing to allow mother time with infant and for herself.*[4]
- Promote peer counseling for teen mothers. *Provides positive role model that teen can relate to and feel comfortable discussing concerns/feelings.*[8]
- Discuss importance of adequate nutrition/fluid intake, prenatal vitamins, or other vitamin/mineral supplements, such as vitamin C, as indicated. *During lactation, there is an increased need for energy, and supplementation of protein, minerals, and vitamins is necessary to provide nourishment for the infant and to protect mother's stores, along with extra fluid intake. Alternating different types of fluid, water, juices, decaffeinated tea, and milk can help mother promote sufficient intake. Beer or wine are not recommended for increasing lactation.*[4]
- Address specific problems (e.g., suckling problems, prematurity/anomalies). *Individualized planning can enhance mother's understanding and ability to manage situation.*[1,7]
- Inform mother that the return of menses varies in nursing mothers and usually averages 3 to 36 weeks with ovulation returning in 17 to 28 weeks. *Return of menstruation does not affect breastfeeding, and breastfeeding is not a reliable method of birth control.*[1]
- Refer to support groups (e.g., La Leche League, parenting support groups, stress reduction, or other community resources as indicated). *Provides information and visible support for ensuring an effective outcome.*[5]
- Provide bibliotherapy/appropriate Web sites for further information. *Additional resources to assist mother and family learn and apply new skills.*[1]

🌐 Cultural ⊛ Collaborative 🏠 Community/Home Care ✎ Diagnostic Studies ∞ Pediatric/Geriatric/Lifespan 💊 Medications

DOCUMENTATION FOCUS

Assessment/Reassessment

• Identified assessment factors, both maternal and infant (e.g., is engorgement present, is infant demonstrating adequate weight gain without supplementation).

Planning

• Plan of care/interventions and who is involved in planning.
• Teaching plan.

Implementation/Evaluation

• Mother's/infant's responses to interventions/teaching and actions performed.
• Changes in infant's weight.
• Attainment/progress toward desired outcome(s).
• Modifications to plan of care.

Discharge Planning

• Referrals that have been made and mother's choice of participation.

References

1. Ladewig, P., London, M., Moberly, S., Olds, S. (2002). *Contemporary Maternal-Newborn Nursing Care.* 5th ed. Upper Saddle River, NJ: Prentice Hall.
2. Riodan, J., Auerbach, K. (1993). *Breastfeeding and Human Lactation.* Boston: Jones & Bartlett.
3. Lipson, J., Dibble, S., Minarik, P. (1996). *Culture & Nursing Care: A Pocket Guide.* San Francisco: UCSF Nursing Press.
4. Lowdermilk, D., Perry, S., Bobak, I. (2001). *Maternal & Women's Health Care.* 6th ed. St. Louis, MO: Mosby.
5. Doenges, M., Moorhouse, M. (1999). *Maternal/Newborn Plans of Care Guidelines for Individualizing Care.* 3d ed. Philadelphia: F. A. Davis.
6. Phillips, C. (1996). *Family-Centered Maternity and Newborn Care.* 4th ed. St. Louis, MO: Mosby.
7. London, M., Ladewig, P., Ball, J., Bindler, R. (2003). *Maternal-Newborn and Child Nursing: Family Centered Care.* Upper Saddle River, NJ: Prentice Hall.
8. American Academy of Family Physicians: Breastfeeding (Position paper). Accessed February 2007 at www.aafp.org/online/en/home/policy/policies/b/breastfeedingpositionpaper.html.
9. Oddy, W.H., Li, J., Landsborough, L., Kendall, G. E., Henderson, S., Downie, J. (2006). The association of maternal overweight and obesity with breastfeeding duration. *Journal of Pediatrics,* 149(2), 185–191.
10. American Academy of Pediatrics: Ten steps to support parents' choice to breastfeed their baby. Revised May 2003. Accessed February 2007 at www.aap.org/breastfeeding/tenSteps.pdf.
11. Pisacane, A., Continisio, G., et al. (2005). A controlled trial of the father's role in breastfeeding promotion. *Pediatrics,* 116(4), e494–e498. Accessed February 2007 at www.sidsalliance.org/research/Fathers%20Role%20in%20Successful%20Breastfeeding.pdf.

interrupted Breastfeeding

Definition: Break in the continuity of the breastfeeding process as a result of inability or inadvisability to put baby to breast for feeding

RELATED FACTORS
Maternal/infant illness
Prematurity
Maternal employment

Contraindications to breastfeeding [e.g., drugs, true breast milk jaundice]
Need to abruptly wean infant

DEFINING CHARACTERISTICS

Subjective
Infant receives no nourishment at the breast for some or all of feedings
Maternal desire to maintain breastfeeding for infant/child's nutritional needs
Maternal desire to provide/eventually provide breast milk for infant/child's nutritional needs
Lack of knowledge regarding expression/storage of breast milk

Objective
Separation of mother and infant

Sample Clinical Applications: Prematurity, postpartum depression, conditions requiring hospitalization of infant or mother, occasionally maternal medication/drug use

DESIRED OUTCOMES/EVALUATION CRITERIA
Sample NOC linkages:
Knowledge: Breastfeeding: Extent of understanding conveyed about lactation and nourishment of infant through breastfeeding
Breastfeeding Maintenance: Continuation of breastfeeding for nourishment of an infant/toddler
Parent-Infant Attachment: Parent and infant behaviors that demonstrate an enduring affectionate bond

Client Will (Include Specific Time Frame)
• Identify and demonstrate techniques to sustain lactation until breastfeeding is reinitiated.
• Achieve mutually satisfactory feeding regimen with infant content after feedings and gaining weight appropriately.
• Achieve weaning and cessation of lactation, if desired or necessary.

ACTIONS/INTERVENTIONS

Sample NIC linkages:
Lactation Counseling: Use of an interactive helping process to assist in maintenance of successful breastfeeding
Emotional Support: Provision of reassurance, acceptance, and encouragement during times of stress
Bottle-Feeding: Preparation and administration of fluids to an infant via a bottle

NURSING PRIORITY NO. 1 To identify causative/contributing factors:

• Assess client knowledge and perceptions about breastfeeding and extent of instruction that has been given. *Provides baseline information to develop plan of care for individual situation.*[1,8]
∞ • Note incorrect myths/misunderstandings especially in teenage mothers *who are more likely to have limited knowledge and concerns about body-image issues.*[9]
• Encourage discussion of current/previous breastfeeding experience(s). *Useful for determining efforts needed to continue breastfeeding, if desired, while circumstances interrupting process are resolved, if possible.*[2]

🌐 Cultural 🅐 Collaborative 🏠 Community/Home Care ✏ Diagnostic Studies ∞ Pediatric/Geriatric/Lifespan 💊 Medications

- Ascertain cultural expectations/conflicts. *The dominant culture in America has sexualized women's breasts, and mother may be embarrassed by breastfeeding or mate may not want mother to breastfeed. Mother may believe her independence will be curtailed by breastfeeding. Some cultures, such as Arab American, may believe that modernization means giving up breastfeeding.*[1,3]
- Determine support systems available to mother/family. *Infant's father and maternal grandmother in addition to caring healthcare providers are important factors in whether breastfeeding is successful/sustained.*[9]
- Identify factors necessitating interruption or, occasionally, cessation of breastfeeding (e.g., maternal illness, drug use) or desire/need to wean infant. *In general, infants with chronic diseases benefit from breastfeeding, and only a few maternal infections (e.g., HIV, active/untreated tuberculosis for initial 2 weeks of multidrug therapy, active herpes simplex of the breasts, development of chickenpox within 5 days prior to delivery or 2 days after delivery) are hazardous to breastfeeding infants. In addition, use of antiretroviral medications/chemotherapy agents or maternal substance abuse usually requires weaning of infant. Exposure to radiation therapy requires interruption of breastfeeding for length of time radioactivity is known to be present in breast milk and is therefore dependent on agent used. (However, feedings with stored breast milk may be an option.)*[1, 8–11]
- Determine maternal responsibilities, routines, and scheduled activities. *Caretaking of siblings, employment in/out of home, work/school schedules of family members may affect ability to visit hospitalized infant when this is the reason for mother/infant separation.*[6,7]

NURSING PRIORITY NO. 2 To assist mother to maintain breastfeeding, as desired:

- Provide information, as needed, regarding need/decision to interrupt breastfeeding.
- Give emotional support to mother and accept decision regarding cessation/continuation of breastfeeding. *Many women are ambivalent about breastfeeding, and providing information about the pros and cons of both breast- and bottle-feeding along with support for the mother's/couple's decision will promote a positive experience.*[1,8]
- Promote peer counseling for teen mothers. *Provides positive role model teen can relate to and feel comfortable discussing concerns/feelings.*[9]
- Educate father/SO about benefits of breastfeeding and how to manage common lactation challenges. *Enlisting support of father/SO is associated with higher ratio of successful breastfeeding at 6 months.*[12]
- Discuss/demonstrate use of breastfeeding aids (e.g., infant sling, nursing footstool/pillows, manual and/or electric piston-type breast pump). *Enhances comfort and relaxation for breastfeeding. When circumstances dictate that mother and infant are separated for a time, whether by illness, prematurity, or returning to work, the milk supply can be maintained by use of the pump. Storing the milk for future use enables the infant to continue to receive the value of breast milk. Learning the correct technique is important for successful use of the pump.*[1,4,13,15]
- Review techniques for storage/use of expressed breast milk. *Provides safety and optimal nutrition, promoting continuation of the breastfeeding process.*[1]
- Determine if a routine visiting schedule or advance warning can be provided. *When infant remains in the hospital or when working mother continues to nurse, it helps to make preparations so that infant will be hungry/ready to feed when the mother arrives. A sleepy baby can be gently played with to arouse him or her, clothing can be loosened, exposing infant to room air, or if infant is hungry and upset, a calm voice and gentle rocking can calm the infant and prepare him or her to nurse.*[1]
- Provide privacy/calm surroundings when mother breastfeeds in hospital/work setting.
- Problem-solve return-to-work issues or periodic infant care requiring bottle/supplemental feeding.[14,15]

🏠 • Recommend using expressed breast milk instead of formula or at least partial breastfeeding for as long as mother and child are satisfied. *Prevents temporary interruption in breastfeeding, decreasing the risk of premature weaning.*[13,15]

NURSING PRIORITY NO. 3 To promote successful infant feeding:

🏠 • Recommend/provide for infant sucking on a regular basis, especially if gavage feedings are part of the therapeutic regimen. *Reinforces that feeding time is pleasurable and enhances digestion.*[1]

🏠 • Explain anticipated changes in feeding needs/frequency. *Growth spurts require increased intake/more feedings by infant.*[13]

🏠 • Discuss proper use and choice of supplemental nutrition and alternate feeding methods (e.g., bottle/syringe). *If infant is not receiving sufficient nourishment, whether by mother's choice to reduce number of feedings (e.g., returning to work) or necessity (specific maternal illness/medication use), other means for supplementing intake must be taken, and mother needs to be given information regarding method chosen.*[1]

🏠 • Review safety precautions when bottle-feeding is necessary/chosen. *Identifying importance of proper flow of formula from nipple, frequency of burping, holding bottle instead of propping, techniques of formula preparation, and sterilization techniques are necessary for successful bottle-feeding.*[1]

NURSING PRIORITY NO. 4 To promote wellness (Teaching/Discharge Considerations):

🏠 • Encourage mother to obtain adequate rest, maintain fluid and nutritional intake, and schedule breast pumping every 3 hours while awake, as indicated. *Sustains adequate milk production and enhances breastfeeding process when mother and infant are separated for any reason.*[1,8]

🏠 • Suggest abstinence/restriction of tobacco, caffeine, alcohol, drugs, and excess sugar, as appropriate, when breastfeeding is reinitiated. *These substances may affect milk production/letdown reflex or may be passed on to the infant.*[1]

🏠 • Identify other means of nurturing/strengthening infant attachment. *Activities that provide comfort, consolation, and play activities help mother become comfortable with handling infant, thus enhancing relationship.*[7,15]

Ⓐ 🏠 • Refer to support groups (e.g., La Leche League, Lact-Aid) or community resources (e.g., public health nurse, lactation specialist, WIC program). *Additional support may provide assistance and education to promote a successful outcome. WIC and other federal programs support breastfeeding through education and enhanced nutritional intake.*[5,15]

🏠 • Promote use of bibliotherapy/appropriate Web sites. *Provides an additional source of information.*[5]

NURSING PRIORITY NO. 5 To assist mother in weaning process, when desired:

🏠 • Discuss reducing frequency of daily feedings/breast pumping by one every 2 to 3 days. *Preferred method of weaning, if circumstance permits, to reduce problems associated with engorgement.*[16,17]

🏠 • Encourage wearing a snug, well-fitting bra, but refrain from binding breasts, *because of increased risk of clogged milk ducts and inflammation.*[15,16]

🏠 • Recommend expressing some milk from breasts regularly each day over a 1- to 3-week period, if necessary, *to reduce discomfort associated with engorgement until milk production decreases.*[16,17]

🌐 Cultural Ⓐ Collaborative 🏠 Community/Home Care 🧪 Diagnostic Studies ∞ Pediatric/Geriatric/Lifespan 💊 Medications

- Suggest holding infant differently during bottle-feeding/interactions *to prevent infant rooting for breast, and limit stimulation of nipples.*
- Discuss use of ibuprofen/acetaminophen *for discomfort during weaning process.*[8]
- Suggest use of ice packs to breast tissue (not nipples) for 15 to 20 minutes at least four times a day *to help reduce swelling during sudden weaning.*[17]

DOCUMENTATION FOCUS

Assessment/Reassessment

- Baseline findings maternal/infant factors.
- Reason for interruption/cessation of breastfeeding.
- Number of wet diapers daily/periodic weight.

Planning

- Method of feeding chosen.
- Plan of care and who is involved in planning.
- Teaching plan.

Implementation/Evaluation

- Maternal response to interventions/teaching and actions performed.
- Infant's response to feeding and method.
- Whether infant appears satisfied or still seems to be hungry.
- Attainment/progress toward desired outcome(s).
- Modifications to plan of care.

Discharge Planning

- Referrals, plan for follow-up, and who is responsible.
- Specific referrals made.

References

1. Ladewig, P., London, M., Moberly, S., Olds, S. (2002). *Contemporary Maternal-Newborn Nursing Care.* Upper Saddle River, NJ: Prentice Hall.
2. Riodan J., Auerbach K. (1993). *Breastfeeding and Human Lactation.* Boston: Jones & Bartlett.
3. Lipson, J., Dibble, S., Minarik, P. (1996). *Culture & Nursing Care: A Pocket Guide.* San Francisco: UCSF Nursing Press.
4. Lowdermilk, D., Perry, S., Bobak, I. (2001). *Maternity and Woman's Health Care.* 6th ed. St. Louis, MO: Mosby.
5. Doenges, M., Moorhouse, M. (1999). *Maternal/Newborn Plans of Care Guidelines for Individualizing Care.* 3d ed. Philadelphia: F. A. Davis.
6. Phillips, C. (1996). *Family-Centered Maternity and Newborn Care.* 4th ed. St. Louis, MO: Mosby.
7. Cox, H., Hinz, M., Lubno, M., Newfield, S., Ridenour, N., Slater, M., Sridaromont, K. (2002). *Clinical Applications of Nursing Diagnosis: Adult, Child, Women's, Psychiatric, Gerontic and Home Health Considerations.* 4th ed. Philadelphia: F. A. Davis.
8. London, M., Ladewig, P., Ball, J., Bindler, R. (2003). *Maternal-Newborn and Child Nursing: Family Centered Care.* Upper Saddle River, NJ: Prentice Hall.
9. American Academy of Family Physicians: Breastfeeding (Position paper). Accessed February 2007 at www.aafp.org/online/en/home/policy/policies/b/breastfeedingpositionpaper.html.
10. Centers for Disease Control and Prevention: When should a mother avoid breastfeeding. August 2006. Accessed February 2007 at www.cdc.gov/breastfeeding/disease/contraindicators.htm.
11. Breastfeeding guidelines following radiopharmaceutical administration. Accessed February 2007 at http://nuclearpharmacy.uams.edu/resources/breastfeeding.asp.

ineffective BREATHING PATTERN

12. Pisacane, A., Continisio, G., et al. (2005). A controlled trial of the father's role in breastfeeding promotion. *Pediatrics*, 116(4), e494–e498. Accessed February 2007 at www.sidsalliance.org/research/Fathers%20Role%20in%20Successful%20Breastfeeding.pdf.
13. American Academy of Pediatrics: Ten steps to support parents' choice to breastfeed their baby. Revised May 2003. Accessed February 2007 at www.aap.org/breastfeeding/tenSteps.pdf.
14. Coping with breastfeeding challenges. U.S. Department of Health & Human Services—womenshealth.gov, August 2005. Accessed February 2007 at www.4woman.gov/Breastfeeding/index.cfm?page=229.
15. Bouchez, C. (2006). Breastfeeding 101: Tips for new mothers. Retrieved July 2007 at www.webmd.com/solutions/sc/breastfeeding-101.
16. Children's Hospitals and Clinics of Minnesota. (2005). Retrieved July 2007 at www.noah-health.org/en/pregnancy/feeding/breastfeeding/weaning.html.
17. University Hospitals of Cleveland. (1998). Retrieved July 2007 at www.breastfeedingbasics.org/pi/pi-175.pdf.

ineffective Breathing Pattern

Definition: Inspiration and/or expiration that does not provide adequate ventilation

RELATED FACTORS
Neuromuscular dysfunction; spinal cord injury; neurological immaturity
Musculoskeletal impairment; bony/chest wall deformity
Anxiety; [panic attacks]
Pain
Perception/cognitive impairment
Fatigue; [deconditioning]; respiratory muscle fatigue
Body position; obesity
Hyperventilation; hypoventilation syndrome; [alteration of client's normal O_2:CO_2 ratio (e.g., lung diseases, pulmonary hypertension, airway obstruction, O_2 therapy in COPD)]

DEFINING CHARACTERISTICS

Subjective
[Feeling breathless]

Objective
Dyspnea; orthopnea
Bradypnea; tachypnea
Alterations in depth of breathing
Timing ratio; prolonged expiration phases; pursed-lip breathing
Decreased minute ventilation/vital capacity
Decreased inspiratory/expiratory pressure
Use of accessory muscles to breathe; assumption of three-point position
Altered chest excursion; [paradoxical breathing patterns]
Nasal flaring; [grunting]
Increased anterior-posterior diameter

Sample Clinical Applications: Chronic obstructive pulmonary disease (COPD), emphysema, asthma, pneumonia, chest trauma/surgery, SCI, Guillain-Barré syndrome, cystic fibrosis, drug/alcohol toxicity

DESIRED OUTCOMES/EVALUATION CRITERIA
Sample NOC linkages:
Respiratory Status: Ventilation: Movement of air in and out of the lungs

Cultural Collaborative Community/Home Care Diagnostic Studies Pediatric/Geriatric/Lifespan Medications

Respiratory Status: Airway Patency: Open, clear tracheobronchial passages for air exchange

Asthma Self-Management: Personal actions to reverse inflammatory condition resulting in bronchial constriction of the airways

Client Will (Include Specific Time Frame)

- Establish a normal/effective respiratory pattern.
- Be free of cyanosis and other signs/symptoms of hypoxia with ABGs within client's normal/acceptable range.
- Verbalize awareness of causative factors and initiate needed lifestyle changes.
- Demonstrate appropriate coping behaviors.

ACTIONS/INTERVENTIONS

Sample NIC linkages:

Ventilation Assistance: Promotion of an optimal spontaneous breathing pattern that maximizes oxygen and carbon dioxide exchange in the lungs

Airway Management: Facilitation of patency of air passages

Respiratory Monitoring: Collection and analysis of patient data to ensure airway patency and adequate gas exchange

NURSING PRIORITY NO. 1 To identify etiology/precipitating factors:

- Identify age and ethnic group of client that may be at increased risk. *Respiratory ailments in general are increased in infants and children with neuromuscular disorders, the frail elderly, and persons living in highly polluted environments.[1,2] Smoking (and potential for smoking-related disorders) is prevalent among such groups as Appalachians, African Americans, Chinese men, Latinos, and Arabs.[3,4] People most at risk for infectious pneumonias include the very young and frail elderly, those suffering from chronic respiratory or circulatory problems, those with compromised immune systems from congenital deficiencies, AIDS, cancers, and cancer therapies.[2,5]*
- Ascertain if client has history of underlying or new conditions with potential for breathing problems (e.g., asthma, other acute or chronic respiratory diseases, neuromuscular disorders, heart disease, sepsis, burns, acute chest or brain trauma). *Important in pointing to cause for current problems.[6]*
- Assess for pregnancy, other abdominal distention and muscle guarding. *Distended abdomen and muscle tension can impede diaphragmatic excursion and reduce lung expansion.[8]*
- Note current symptoms and how they relate to past history. *Assessing current illness, including history of (1) onset and duration of symptoms; (2) how they are similar to/different from past symptoms; (3) precipitating, relieving, and exacerbating factors; and (4) exposures (e.g., environmental toxins, alcohol/other drugs, source of infection) may help in selecting the correct diagnosis.*
- Note emotional state. *Gasping, crying, anxiety, irritability, struggling, look of fear, report of tingling lips/fingers, withdrawal, and self-focus are responses often associated with respiratory distress. Emotional changes can accompany a condition or precipitate or aggravate ineffective breathing patterns.[6–9]*
- Evaluate client's respiratory status:
   Note rate and depth of respirations, counting for 1 full minute, if rate is irregular. *Rate may be greater or less than usual. In infants and younger children, rate increases dramatically*

relative to anxiety, crying, fever, or disease. Depth may be difficult to evaluate but is usually described as shallow, normal, or deep.[7,8]

Note client's reports/perceptions of breathing ease. *Client may report a range of symptoms (e.g., air hunger, shortness of breath with speaking, activity, or at rest) and demonstrate wide range of signs (e.g., tachypnea, gasping, wheezing, coughing).*

 Observe characteristics of breathing pattern. *May note use of accessory muscles for breathing, sternal retractions (infants and young children) nasal flaring, pursed-lip breathing. Client may change position in effort to breathe easier. Irregular patterns may be pathological (e.g., prolonged expiration, periods of apnea, obvious agonal breathing) with pronounced alterations in conditions such as severe asthma attack, brainstem damage, or impending respiratory failure.*[6,7]

Auscultate and percuss chest, describing presence, absence, and character of breath sounds. *Air should be moving freely through air passages (differs from ineffective airway clearance), but ventilatory effort is insufficient to bring in enough oxygen or to exchange sufficient amounts of carbon dioxide. Abnormal breath sounds are indicative of numerous problems (e.g., obstruction by foreign object, hypoventilation such as might occur with chest or spinal cord injury, atelectasis, or presence of secretions, improper endotracheal tube placement, collapsed lung) and must be evaluated and reported for further intervention.*[8,9]

Observe chest size, shape, and symmetry of movement. *Changes in movement of chest wall (such as might occur with chest trauma, chest wall deformities) can impair breathing patterns.*

Note color of skin and mucous membranes. *If pallor, duskiness, and/or cyanosis are present, supplemental oxygen and/or other interventions may be required.* (Refer to ND impaired Gas Exchange.)

Note presence and character of cough. *Cough function may be weak or ineffective in diseases and conditions such as extremes in age (e.g., premature infant or elderly), cerebral palsy, muscular dystrophy, SCI, brain injury, after surgery, and/or mechanical ventilation due to mechanisms affecting muscles of throat, chest, and lungs. Cough that is persistent and constant can interfere with breathing (such as can occur with asthma, acute bronchitis, cystic fibrosis, croup, whooping cough).*[1,6–10] (Refer to ND ineffective Airway Clearance.)

- Assess client's awareness and cognition. *Affects ability to manage own airway and cooperate with interventions such as controlling breathing and managing secretions.*[2,8,9]
- Assist with/monitor results of diagnostic testing (e.g., pulmonary/cardiac function studies, neuromuscular evaluation, sleep studies) *to diagnose presence/severity of lung diseases and degree of respiratory compromise.*
- Review chest radiographs and laboratory data (e.g., arterial blood gases [ABGs], pulse oximetry at rest and activity, drug screens, white blood cell count, blood and sputum culture tests for viruses and bacteria).

NURSING PRIORITY NO. 2 To provide for relief of causative factors promoting ease of breathing:[6–12]

- Assist in treatment of underlying conditions, administering medications and therapies as ordered.
- Suction airway to clear secretions as needed. (Refer to ND impaired Airway Clearance for additional interventions.)
- Maintain emergency equipment in readily accessible location, and include age/size appropriate airway/ET/trach tubes (e.g., infant, child, adolescent, or adult).
- Administer oxygen (by cannula, mask, mechanical ventilation) at lowest concentration needed (per ABGs, pulse oximetry) *for underlying pulmonary condition and current respiratory problem.*[13,14] (Refer to ND impaired Gas Exchange for additional interventions.)

🌐 Cultural   Ⓐ Collaborative   🏠 Community/Home Care   ✏ Diagnostic Studies   ∞ Pediatric/Geriatric/Lifespan   💊 Medications

- Elevate head of bed, or have client sit up in chair; support with pillows *to prevent slumping and promote rest*; or place in position of comfort, as appropriate, *to promote maximal inspiration*. In ventilated client, place in prone position for short periods when indicated *to improve pulmonary perfusion and increase oxygen diffusion*.
- Reposition client frequently *to enhance respiratory effort and ventilation of all lung segments, especially if immobility is a factor*.
- Encourage early ambulation, using assistive devices, as individually indicated *to prevent onset or reduce severity of respiratory complications*.
- Direct client in breathing efforts as needed. Encourage slower/deeper respirations, use of pursed-lip technique, *to assist client in "taking control" of the situation, especially when condition is associated with anxiety and air hunger*.
- Coach client in effective coughing techniques. Place in appropriate position for clearing airways. Splint rib cage/surgical incisions as appropriate. Medicate for pain, as indicated. *Promotes breathing that is more effective and airway management when client is guarding, as might occur with chest, rib cage, or abdominal injuries or surgeries*. (Refer to NDs acute Pain; chronic Pain for additional interventions.)
- Provide and assist with use of respiratory therapy adjuncts such as spirometry.
- Maintain calm attitude while working with client/SOs. Provide quiet environment, instruct/reinforce client in the use of relaxation techniques, and administer antianxiety medications as indicated *to reduce intensity of anxiety/deal with fear that may be present*. (Refer to NDs Fear; Anxiety for additional interventions.)
- Avoid overfeeding, such as might occur with young infant or client on tube feedings. *Abdominal distention can interfere with breathing as well as increase risk of aspiration*.
- Assist with bronchoscopy or chest tube insertion as indicated.

NURSING PRIORITY NO. 3 To promote wellness (Teaching/Discharge Considerations):

- Review with client/SO the type of respiratory condition, treatments, rehabilitation measures, and quality-of-life issues. *Many conditions with impaired breathing are associated with chronic conditions that require lifetime management*.[9]
- Teach/reinforce breathing retraining. *Education may include many measures, such as conscious control of respiratory rate, effective use of accessory muscles, breathing exercises (diaphragmatic, abdominal breathing, inspiratory resistive, and pursed-lip), assistive devices such as rocking bed*.[6]
- Discuss relationship of smoking to respiratory function. Stress importance of smoking cessation and smoke-free environment.
- Encourage client/SO(s) to develop a plan for smoking cessation. Provide appropriate referrals.
- Encourage self-assessment and symptom management:[6–12]
  Use of equipment to identify respiratory decompensation, such as peak flow meter.
  Appropriate use of oxygen (dosage, route, and safety factors).
   Medication regimen, including actions, side effects, and potential interactions of medications, over-the-counter (OTC) drugs, vitamins, and herbal supplements.
  Adhere to home treatments such as metered-dose inhalers (MDIs), compressor, nebulizer, chest physiotherapies.
  Dietary patterns and needs; access to foods and nutrients supportive of health and breathing.
  Management of personal environment, including stress reduction, rest and sleep, social events, travel, and recreation issues.
  Avoidance of known irritants, allergens, and sick persons.
  Immunizations against influenza and pneumonia.

Early intervention when respiratory symptoms occur, and what symptoms require reporting to medical providers, seeking emergency care.

- Discuss benefits of exercise for endurance, muscle strengthening, and flexibility training *to improve general health and respiratory muscle function.*

 • Refer to physical therapy and rehabilitation resources as indicated.[13]

- Review energy conservation techniques (e.g., sitting instead of standing to wash dishes, pacing activities, taking short rest periods between activities) *to limit fatigue and improve endurance.*

- Review environmental factors (e.g., exposure to dust, high pollen counts, severe weather, perfumes, animal dander, household chemicals, fumes, second-hand smoke; insufficient home support for safe care, etc.) *that may require avoidance/modification of lifestyle or environment to limit inpact on client's breathing.*[13,14,15]

- Reinforce instruction in proper use and safety concerns for home oxygen therapy, and/or use of respirator/diaphragmatic stimulator, rocking bed, apnea monitor, when used. *Protects client's safety, especially when used in the very young, fragile elderly, or when cognitive or neuromuscular impairment present.*

- Discuss impact of respiratory condition on occupational performance, as well as work environment issues that affect client.

- Provide referrals as indicated by individual situation. *May include a wide variety of services and providers, including support groups, comprehensive rehabilitation program, occupational nurse, oxygen and DME companies for supplies, home health services, occupational and physical therapy, transportation, assisted/alternate living facilities, local and national Lung Association chapters, and Web sites for educational materials.*

DOCUMENTATION FOCUS

Assessment/Reassessment
- Relevant history of problem.
- Respiratory pattern, breath sounds, use of accessory muscles.
- Laboratory values.
- Use of respiratory supports, ventilator settings, and so forth.

Planning
- Plan of care/interventions and who is involved in the planning.
- Teaching plan.

Implementation/Evaluation
- Response to interventions/teaching, actions performed, and treatment regimen.
- Mastery of skills, level of independence.
- Attainment/progress toward desired outcome(s).
- Modifications to plan of care.

Discharge Planning
- Long-term needs, including appropriate referrals and action taken, available resources.
- Specific referrals provided.

References

1. Evidence-Based Clinical Practice Guideline of Community-Acquired Pneumonia in Children 60 days to 17 years of age. (2000). Cincinnati Children's Hospital Medical Center. HPCE@chmcc.org.

2. Stanley, M., Beare, P. G. (1999). *Gerontological Nursing: A Health Promotion/Protection Approach.* 2d ed. Philadelphia: F. A. Davis.
3. Lung Disease in Minorities in 1999. Focus Asthma. Available at www.stateoftheair.org.
4. Purnell, L. D., Paulanka, B. J. (1998). *Transcultural Health Care: A Culturally Competent Approach.* Philadelphia: F. A. Davis.
5. Minority Lung Disease Data—Major Acute Infections: Influenza and Pneumonia. American Lung Association: State of the Air 2002. Available at www.stateoftheair.org.
6. Global strategy for the diagnosis, management, and prevention of chronic obstructive pulmonary disease. Global Initiative for Chronic Obstructive Lung Disease (GOLD), World Health Organization, National Heart, Lung, and Blood Institute, 2001, National Guideline Clearinghouse [NGC 2205].
7. Engel, J. (2002). *Mosby's Pocket Guide to Pediatric Assessment.* 4th ed. St Louis, MO: Mosby.
8. Cox, H. C., et al. (2002). *Clinical Applications of Nursing Diagnosis: Adult, Child, Women's, Gerontic, and Home Health Considerations.* 4th ed. Philadelphia: F. A. Davis, pp. 256–261.
9. Doenges, M. E., Moorhouse, M. F., Geissler-Murr, A. C. (2002). *Nursing Care Plans: Guidelines for Individualizing Patient Care.* 6th ed. Philadelphia: F. A. Davis, p. 167.
10. Irwin, R. S., et al. (1998). Managing cough as a defense mechanism and as a symptom: A clinical reference guide. Northbrook, IL: American College of Chest Physicians (ACCP).
11. Marion, B. S. (2001). A turn for the better: "Prone positioning" of patients with ARDS. *AJN,* 101(5), 26–33.
12. Pulmonary Rehabilitation. American Association for Respiratory Care (AARC): Clinical Practice Guideline. National Guideline Clearinghouse [NGC: 2437] 2002.
13. Bauldoff, G. S., Diaz, P. T. (2006). Improving outcomes for COPD patients. The Nurse Practitioner. *American Journal of Primary Care,* 31(8), 26–43.
14. Pruitt, B. (2006). Weaning patients from mechanical ventilation. *Nursing2006,* 36 (9), 36–41.
15. Saglimbeni, A. J. (2005). Exercise-induced asthma. Article for Emedicine Web site. Retrieved January 2007 at www.emedicine.com/SPORTS/topic155.htm.

decreased Cardiac Output

Definition: Inadequate blood pumped by the heart to meet the metabolic demands of the body. [Note: In a hypermetabolic state, although cardiac output may be within normal range, it may still be inadequate to meet the needs of the body's tissues. Cardiac output and tissue perfusion are interrelated, although there are differences. When cardiac output is decreased, tissue perfusion problems will develop; however, tissue perfusion problems can exist without decreased cardiac output.]

RELATED FACTORS

Altered heart rate/rhythm [conduction]

Altered stroke volume: Altered preload [e.g., decreased venous return]; altered afterload [e.g., systemic vascular resistance]; altered contractility [e.g., ventricular-septal rupture, ventricular aneurysm, papillary muscle rupture, valvular disease]

DEFINING CHARACTERISTICS

Subjective
Altered heart rate/rhythm: Palpitations
Altered preload: Fatigue
Altered afterload: [Feeling breathless]
Altered contractility: Orthopnea/paroxysmal nocturnal dyspnea [PND]
Behavioral/emotional: Anxiety

Objective
Altered heart rate/rhythm: [Dys]arrhythmias (tachycardia, bradycardia); EKG [ECG] changes

Altered preload: Jugular vein distention (JVD); edema; weight gain; increased/decreased central venous pressure (CVP); increased/decreased pulmonary artery wedge pressure (PAWP); murmurs

Altered afterload: Dyspnea; clammy skin; skin [and mucous membrane] color changes [cyanosis, pallor]; prolonged capillary refill; decreased peripheral pulses; variations in blood pressure readings; increased/decreased systemic vascular resistance (SVR); increased/decreased pulmonary vascular resistance (PVR); oliguria; [anuria]

Altered contractility: Crackles; cough; decreased cardiac output/cardiac index; decreased ejection fraction; decreased stroke volume index (SVI)/left ventricular stroke work index (LVSWI); S3 or S4 sounds [gallop rhythm]

Behavioral/emotional: Restlessness

Sample Clinical Applications: Myocardial infarction, CHF, valvular heart disease, dysrhythmias, cardiomyopathy, cardiac contusions/trauma, pericarditis, ventricular aneurysm

DESIRED OUTCOMES/EVALUATION CRITERIA
Sample NOC linkages:

Cardiac Pump Effectiveness: Adequacy of blood volume ejected from the left ventricle to support systemic perfusion pressure

Circulation Status: Unobstructed, unidirectional blood flow at an appropriate pressure through large vessels of the systemic and pulmonary circuits

Energy Conservation: Personal actions to manage energy for initiating and sustaining activity

Client Will (Include Specific Time Frame)

- Display hemodynamic stability (e.g., blood pressure, cardiac output, urinary output, peripheral pulses).
- Report/demonstrate decreased episodes of dyspnea, angina, and dysrhythmias.
- Demonstrate an increase in activity tolerance.
- Verbalize knowledge of the disease process, individual risk factors, and treatment plan.
- Participate in activities that reduce the workload of the heart (e.g., stress management or therapeutic medication regimen program, weight reduction, balanced activity/rest plan, proper use of supplemental oxygen, cessation of smoking).
- Identify signs of cardiac decompensation, alter activities, and seek help appropriately.

ACTIONS/INTERVENTIONS

Sample NIC linkages:

Hemodynamic Regulation: Optimization of heart rate, preload, afterload, and contractility

Cardiac Care: Limitation of complications resulting from an imbalance between myocardial oxygen supply and demand for a patient with symptoms of impaired cardiac function

Circulatory Care: Mechanical Assist Devices: Temporary support of the circulation through the use of mechanical devices or pumps

NURSING PRIORITY NO. 1 To identify causative/contributing factors:

- Review clients at risk as noted in Related Factors and Defining Characteristics. *In addition to individuals obviously at risk with known cardiac problems, there is a potential for cardiac output problems in persons with trauma, hemorrhage, alcohol and other drug intoxication/ chronic use/overdose; pregnant women with hypertensive states; individuals with chronic renal failure; with brainstem trauma, or spinal cord injuries at T8 or above.*[1]

🌐 Cultural 👥 Collaborative 🏠 Community/Home Care 🔬 Diagnostic Studies ∞ Pediatric/Geriatric/Lifespan 💊 Medications

- Be aware of age and ethnic-related cardiovascular considerations. *In infants, failure to thrive with poor ability to suck and feed can be indications of heart problems. Children with poor cardiac function are tachypneic, exercise-intolerant, and may have episodes of syncope because of restricted ventricular outflow (such as might occur with aortic stenosis or abnormal vasomotor tone).[2,3] When in the supine position, pregnant women incur decreased vascular return during the second and third trimesters, potentially compromising cardiac output.[4] Contractile force is naturally decreased in the elderly with reduced ability to increase cardiac output in response to increased demand. Also, arteries are stiffer, veins more dilated, and heart valves less competent, often resulting in systemic hypertension and blood pooling.[5] Heart failure may affect as many as 1 in 10 elderly people.[6] Generally, higher-risk populations include African Americans (because of higher incidence of hypertension, obesity, and diabetes mellitus) and Latinos (higher incidence of obesity and diabetes mellitus).[7]*

- Review diagnostic studies, including/not limited to: chest radiograph, cardiac stress testing, ECG, echocardiogram, cardiac output/ventricular ejection studies, and heart scan/catheterization. *For example, EGG may show previous or evolving MI, left ventricular hypertrophy, and valvular stenosis. Ventricular function studies with ejection fraction <40% is indicative of systolic dysfunction, and cardiac output <4 L/m is indicative of heart failure. Additional cardiac studies (e.g., radionuclide scans or catheterization) may be indicated to assess left ventricular function, valvular function, and coronary circulation. Chest radiography may show enlarged heart, pulmonary infiltrates.[8–10,14,15]*

- Review laboratory data, including/not limited to complete blood cell (CBC) count, electrolytes, arterial blood gases (ABGs), cardiac enzymes; kidney, thyroid, and liver function studies; cultures (e.g., blood/wound/secretions), bleeding and coagulation studies *to identify imbalances, disease processes, and effects of interventions.[1,8]*

NURSING PRIORITY NO. 2 To assess degree of debilitation:

- Assess for signs of poor ventricular function or impending cardiac failure/shock:[1–5,9]
  Client reports/evidence of extreme fatigue, intolerance for activity, sudden or progressive weight gain, swelling of extremities, and progressive shortness of breath.
  Client reports chest pain. *May indicate evolving heart attack; can also accompany congestive heart failure. Chest pain may be atypical in women experiencing an MI and is often atypical in the elderly owing to altered pain perception.*
  Mental status changes. *Confusion, agitation, decreased cognition and coma may occur due to decreased brain perfusion.*
  Changes in heart rate/rhythm: Tachycardia at rest, bradycardia, atrial fibrillation, or multiple dysrhythmias may be noted. *Heart irritability is common, reflecting conduction defects and/or ischemia.*
  Heart sounds may be distant, with irregular rhythms; murmurs-systolic (*valvular stenosis and shunting*) and diastolic (*aortic or pulmonary insufficiency*) or gallop rhythm (S3, S4) noted *when heart failure is present and ventricles are stiff.*
  Peripheral pulses may be weak and thready, *reflecting hypotension, vasoconstriction, shunting, and venous congestion.*
  Changes in skin color, moisture, temperature, and capillary refill time. *Pallor or cyanosis, cool moist skin, and slow capillary refill time may be present because of peripheral vasoconstriction and decreased oxygen saturation. Note: Children with chronic heart failure and adults with COPD often show clubbing of fingertips.*
  Blood pressure changes. *Hypertension may be chronic or blood pressure elevated initially in client with impending cardiogenic, hypovolemic, or septic shock. Later, as cardiac output decreases, profound hypotension can be present, often with narrowed pulse pressure.*

Breath sounds may reveal bilateral crackles and wheezing *associated with congestion. Respiratory distress/failure often occurs as shock progresses.*

Edema with neck vein distention is often present, and pitting edema is noted in extremities and dependent portions of body *because of impaired venous return.* Other veins in trunk and extremities can be prominent, *owing to venous congestion.*

 Urinary output may be decreased or absent *reflecting poor perfusion of kidneys. Note: Output <30 mL/hr (adult) or <10 mL/hr (child) indicates inadequate renal perfusion.*

NURSING PRIORITY NO. 3 To minimize/correct causative factors, maximize cardiac output:

Acute/severe phase[1–3,9–12,14,17]

- Keep client on bed or chair rest in position of comfort. In congestive state, semi-Fowler's position is preferred. May raise legs 20 to 30 degrees in shock situation. *Decreases oxygen consumption/demand, reducing myocardial workload and risk of decomposition.*

- Administer supplemental oxygen, as indicated (by cannula, mask, ET/trach tube with mechanical ventilation) *to improve cardiac function by increasing available oxygen and reducing oxygen consumption. Critically ill client may be on ventilator to support cardiopulmonary function.*[14]

- Monitor vital signs frequently *to evaluate response to treatments and activities.* Perform periodic hemodynamic measurements, as indicated (e.g., arterial, central venous pressure [CVP], pulmonary artery wedge pressure [PAWP], and left atrial pressures; cardiac output/cardiac index and oxygen saturation). *These measurements (via central line monitoring) are commonly used in the critically ill to provide continuous, accurate assessment of cardiac function and response to inotropic and vasoactive medications that affect cardiac contractility and systemic circulation (preload and afterload).*[17]

- Monitor cardiac rhythm continuously *to note changes, and evaluate effectiveness of medications and devices (e.g., implanted pacemaker/defibrillator).*

- Administer or restrict fluids, as indicated. *Replacement of blood and large amounts of IV fluids may be needed if low output state is due to hypovolemia.* Use infusion pumps for IVs *to monitor IV rates closely to prevent bolus or exacerbation of fluid overload.*

- Assess hourly or periodic urinary output and daily weight, noting 24-hr total fluid balance *to evaluate kidney function and effects of interventions, as well as to allow for timely alterations in therapeutic regimen.*

- Administer medications as indicated (e.g., inotropic drugs *to enhance cardiac contractility,* antiarrhythmics *to improve cardiac output,* diuretics *to reduce congestion by improving urinary output,* vasopressors, and/or dilators as indicated *to manage systemic effects of vasoconstriction and low cardiac output;* pain medications and antianxiety agents *to reduce oxygen demand and myocardial workload;* anticoagulants *to improve blood flow and prevent thromboemboli).*

- Note reports of anorexia/nausea and limit/withhold oral intake as indicated. *Symptoms may be systemic reaction to low cardiac output, visceral congestion, or reaction to medications or pain.*

- Assist with preparations for/monitor response to support procedures/devices as indicated (e.g., cardioversion, pacemaker, angioplasty, coronary artery bypass-graft [CABG] or valve replacement, intra-aortic balloon pump [IABP], left ventricular assist device [LVAD]). *Any number of interventions may be required to correct a condition causing heart failure or to support a failing heart during recovery from myocardial infarction, while awaiting transplantation or for long-term management of chronic heart failure.*

- Promote rest *to reduce catecholamine-induced stress response and cardiac workload:*[1,13,17] Decrease stimuli, providing quiet environment.

🌐 Cultural 🅐 Collaborative 🏠 Community/Home Care ⬲ Diagnostic Studies ∞ Pediatric/Geriatric/Lifespan 💊 Medications

Schedule activities/assessments *to maximize sleep periods.*

Assist with or perform self-care activities for client.

Avoid the use of restraints whenever possible, especially if client is confused.

Use sedation and analgesics, as indicated, with caution *to achieve desired rest state without compromising hemodynamic responses.*

Postacute/chronic phase[1]

- Provide for adequate rest, positioning client for maximum comfort.
- Encourage changing positions slowly, dangling legs before standing *to reduce risk of orthostatic hypotension.*
- Increase activity levels gradually as permitted by individual condition, noting vital sign response to activity.
- Administer medications, as appropriate, and monitor cardiac responses.
- Encourage relaxation techniques *to reduce anxiety, muscle tension.*
- Refer for nutritional needs assessment and management *to provide for supportive nutrition while meeting diet restrictions (e.g., IV nutrition [TPN], sodium-restricted or other type diet with frequent small feedings).*
- Monitor intake/output and calculate 24-hour fluid balance. Provide/restrict fluids, as indicated, *to maximize cardiac output and improve tissue perfusion.*[17]

NURSING PRIORITY NO. 4 To enhance safety/prevent complications:[1,4,16,17]

- Wash hands before and after client contact, maintain aseptic technique during invasive procedures, and provide site care, as indicated, *to prevent nosocomial infection.* (Refer to ND risk for Infection for additional interventions.)
- Provide antipyretics/fever control actions as indicated. Adjust ambient environmental temperature *to maintain body temperature in near-normal range.*
- Maintain patency of invasive intravascular monitoring/infusion lines and tape connections *to prevent exsanguination or air embolus.*
- Minimize activities that can elicit Valsalva response (e.g., rectal straining, vomiting, spasmodic coughing with suctioning, prolonged breath-holding during pushing stage of labor) and encourage client to breathe deeply in/out during activities that increase risk of Valsalva effect. *Valsalva response to breath-holding causes increased intrathoracic pressure, reducing cardiac output and blood pressure.*[16]
- Avoid prolonged sitting position for all clients, and supine position for sleep/exercise for gravid clients (second/third trimesters) *to maximize vascular return.*[4,17]
- Elevate legs when in sitting position and edematous extremities when at rest. Apply antiembolic hose or sequential compression devices when indicated, being sure they are individually fitted and appropriately applied. *Limits venous stasis, improves venous return, and reduces risk of thrombophlebitis.* (Refer to ND ineffective Tissue Perfusion for additional interventions.)
- Provide skin care, special bed or mattress (e.g., air, water, gel, foam) and assist with frequent position changes *to prevent the development of pressure sores.*
- Provide psychological support *to reduce anxiety and its adverse effects on cardiac function:*
  Maintain calm attitude and limit stressful stimuli.
  Provide/encourage use of relaxation techniques, such as massage therapy, soothing music, or quiet activities.
  Promote visits from family/SO(s) *to provide positive social interaction.*
  Provide information about testing procedures and client participation.
  Explain limitations imposed by condition and dietary and fluid restrictions.
  Share information about positive signs of improvement.

NURSING PRIORITY NO. 5 To promote wellness (Teaching/Discharge Considerations):[1,13,18]

🏠 • Provide information to clients/caregivers on individual condition, therapies, and expected outcomes. Use various forms of teaching according to client needs, desires, and learning style.

♒ • Direct client and/or caregivers to resources for emergency assistance, financial help, durable medical supplies, and psychosocial support and respite, especially when client has impaired functional capabilities or requires supporting equipment (such as pacemaker, LVAD, or 24-hour oxygen).

♒ • Emphasize importance of regular medical follow-up care *to monitor client's condition and response to treatment and provide most effective care.*

💊 • Educate client/caregivers about drug regimen, including indications, dose and dosing schedules, potential adverse side effects, or drug/drug interactions. *Client is often on multiple medications, which can be difficult to manage, thus increasing potential that medications can be missed or incorrectly used.*

💊 • Emphasize reporting of adverse/side effects of medications *so that adjustments can be made in dosing or another class of medication considered.*

♒ • Discuss significant signs/symptoms that need to be reported to healthcare provider, such as *unrelieved or increased chest pain, dyspnea, fever, swelling of ankles, and sudden unexplained cough—these are all "danger signs" that require immediate evaluation and possible change of usual therapies.*[18]

🏠 • Teach home monitoring of weight, pulse, and blood pressure, as appropriate, *to detect change and allow for timely intervention.*

💊 • Recommend annual influenza vaccination.

🏠 • Discuss individual's particular risk factors (e.g., smoking, stress, obesity, recent MI) and specific resources for assistance (e.g., written information sheets, direction to helpful Web sites, formalized rehabilitation programs, and home interventions) for management of identified factors for:

Smoking cessation

Stress management techniques

Energy conservation techniques

Nutrition education regarding needs (e.g., to improve general health status, reduce or gain weight, lower blood fat levels, manage sodium, etc.)

Exercise/activity plan *to systematically increase endurance*

• Refer to NDs Activity Intolerance, deficient Diversional Activity, ineffective Coping, compromised family Coping, Sexual Dysfunction, acute/chronic Pain, imbalanced Nutrition (specify), deficient/excess Fluid Volume, as indicated.

DOCUMENTATION FOCUS

Assessment/Reassessment

• Baseline and subsequent findings and individual hemodynamic parameters, heart and breath sounds, ECG pattern, presence/strength of peripheral pulses, skin/tissue status, renal output, and mentation.

Planning

• Plan of care and who is involved in planning.
• Teaching plan.

🌐 Cultural ♒ Collaborative 🏠 Community/Home Care 🧪 Diagnostic Studies ∞ Pediatric/Geriatric/Lifespan 💊 Medications

Implementation/Evaluation

- Client's responses to interventions/teaching and actions performed.
- Status and disposition at discharge.
- Attainment/progress toward desired outcome(s).
- Modifications to plan of care.

Discharge Planning

- Discharge considerations and who will be responsible for carrying out individual actions.
- Long-term needs.
- Specific referrals made.

References

1. Doenges, M. E., Moorhouse, M. F., Geissler-Murr, A. C. (2002). *Nursing Care Plans: Guidelines for Individualizing Patient Care*. 6th ed. Philadelphia: F. A. Davis.
2. Cox, H. C., et al. (2002). *Clinical Applications of Nursing Diagnosis: Adult, Child, Women's Psychiatric, Gerontic, and Home Health Considerations*. 4th ed. Philadelphia: F. A. Davis, pp. 262–269.
3. Pathophysiologic interpretation of cardiac symptoms and signs. Pediatric Cardiology for Parents and Patients, Rush Children's Heart Center, Chicago, IL. Available at www.rchc.rush.edu/rmawebfiles/HP.htm.
4. Ladewig, P., London, M., Moberly, S., Olds, S. (2002). *Contemporary Maternal-Newborn Nursing Care*. 5th ed. Upper Saddle River, NJ: Prentice Hall.
5. Stanley, M., Beare, P. G. (1999). Gerontological Nursing: A Health Promotion/Protection Approach. 2d ed. Philadelphia: F. A. Davis.
6. Heidenreich, P. A., Ruggerico, C. M., Massie, B. M. (2000). Effect of a home-based monitoring system on hospitalization and resource use for patients with heart failure. Pilot study supported by Agency for Healthcare Research and Quality (National Research Service Award Training Grant T32 HS00028). Available at www.ahrq.gov.
7. Purnell, L. D., Paulanka, B. J. (1998). *Transcultural Health Care: A Culturally Competent Approach*. Philadelphia: F. A. Davis.
8. Cavanaugh, B. M. (1999). *Nurse's Manual of Laboratory and Diagnostic Tests*. 3d ed. Philadelphia: F. A. Davis, pp. 654–659.
9. Heart failure. Clinical Practice Guideline. (2002). Columbia, MD: American Medical Directors Association (AMDA), NGC: 2529.
10. The pharmacologic management of chronic heart failure. (2001). Washington, DC: Department of Veterans Affairs (U.S.), Veterans Health Administration (VHA).
11. Bond, A. E., et al. (2003). The left ventricular assist device, *AJN*, 103(1), 33–40.
12. Gawlinski, A., McAtee, M. E. (May 2002). Biventricular pacing: New treatment for patients with heart failure: Important nursing implications. *AJN Suppl. Critical Care Update* 102(5), 4–7.
13. Clinical Practice Guidelines: Cardiac Rehabilitation Guidelines. Cosponsored by the National Heart, Lung, and Blood Institute and Agency for Healthcare Policy and Research (AHCPR), October 1995. Available at www.ahrq.gov.
14. Brandler, E. S., Sinert, R., Hostetler, M. A. (2006). Shock, cardiogenic. Article for Emedicine Web site. Retrieved January 2007 at www.emedicine.com/emerg/topic530.htm.
15. Olade, R., Safi, A., Kesari, S. (2006). Cardiac catheterization (left heart). Article for Emedicine Web site. Retrieved January 2007 at www.emedicine.com/emerg/topic2958.htm.
16. Bernardi, L., Saviolo, R., Sodick, D. H. (May 1, 1989). Do hemodynamic responses to the Valsalva maneuver reflect myocardial dysfunction? *Chest*.
17. Cheever, K. H. (2005). An overview of pulmonary arterial hypertension: Risks, pathogensis, clinical manifestations, and management. *J Cardiovascular Nursing*, 20(2), 108–116.
18. Purgason, K. (2006). Broken hearts: Differentiating stress-induced cardiomyopathy from acute myocardial infarction in the patient presenting with acute coronary syndrome. *Dimensions in Crit Care Nursing*, 25(6), 247–253.

Caregiver Role Strain

Definition: Difficulty in performing caregiver role

RELATED FACTORS

Care receiver health status
Illness severity/chronicity
Unpredictability of illness course; instability of care receiver's health
Increasing care needs; dependency
Problem behaviors; psychological or cognitive problems
Addiction; codependency

Caregiving activities
Discharge of family member to home with significant care needs [e.g., premature
 birth/congenital defect, frail elder poststroke]
Unpredictability of care situation; 24-hour care responsibilities; amount/complexity of
 activities; years of caregiving
Ongoing changes in activities

Caregiver health status
Physical problems; psychological/cognitive problems
Inability to fulfill one's own/others' expectations; unrealistic expectations of self
Marginal coping patterns
Addiction; codependency

Socioeconomic
Competing role commitments
Alienation/isolation from others
Insufficient recreation

Caregiver–care receiver relationship
Unrealistic expectations of caregiver by care receiver
History of poor relationship
Mental status of elder inhibits conversation
Presence of abuse/violence

Family processes
History of marginal family coping/family dysfunction

Resources
Inadequate physical environment for providing care (e.g., housing, temperature, safety)
Inadequate equipment for providing care; inadequate transportation
Insufficient finances
Inexperience with caregiving; insufficient time; physical energy; emotional strength; lack
 of support
Lack of caregiver privacy
Deficient knowledge about/difficulty accessing community resources; inadequate
 community services (e.g., respite services, recreational resources)
Formal/informal assistance; formal/informal support
Caregiver is not developmentally ready for caregiver role

⊕ Cultural 🅐 Collaborative 🏠 Community/Home Care 🧪 Diagnostic Studies ∞ Pediatric/Geriatric/Lifespan 💊 Medications

Subjective

Caregiving activities

Apprehension about possible institutionalization of care receiver; the future regarding care receiver's health/caregiver's ability to provide care; care receiver's care if caregiver unable to provide care

Caregiver health status—physical

GI upset; weight change

Headaches; fatigue; rash

Hypertension; cardiovascular disease; diabetes

Caregiver health status—emotional

Feeling depressed; anger; stress; frustration; increased nervousness

Disturbed sleep

Lack of time to meet personal needs

Caregiver health status—socioeconomic

Changes in leisure activities; refuses career advancement

Caregiver—care receiver relationship

Difficulty watching care receiver go through the illness

Grief/uncertainty regarding changed relationship with care receiver

Family processes—caregiving activities

Concerns about family members

Objective

Caregiving activities

Difficulty performing/completing required tasks

Preoccupation with care routine

Dysfunctional change in caregiving activities

Caregiver health status—emotional

Impatience; increased emotional lability; somatization

Impaired individual coping

Caregiver health status—socioeconomic

Low work productivity; withdraws from social life

Family processes

Family conflict

[NOTE: The presence of this problem may encompass other numerous problems/high-risk concerns, such as deficient Diversional Activity, Insomnia, Fatigue, Anxiety, ineffective Coping, compromised family Coping, and disabled family Coping, decisional Conflict, ineffective Denial, Grieving, Hopelessness, Powerlessness, Spiritual Distress, ineffective Health Maintenance, impaired Home Maintenance, ineffective Sexuality Pattern, readiness for enhanced family Coping, interrupted Family Processes, Social Isolation. Careful attention to data-gathering will identify and clarify the client's specific needs, which can then be coordinated under this single diagnostic label.]

Sample Clinical Applications: Chronic conditions (e.g., severe brain injury, spinal cord injury, severe developmental delay), progressive debilitating conditions (e.g., muscular dystrophy, multiple sclerosis, dementia/Alzheimer's disease, end-stage COPD, renal failure/dialysis), substance abuse, end-of-life care, psychiatric conditions (e.g., schizophrenia, personality disorders)

DESIRED OUTCOMES/EVALUATION CRITERIA

Sample NOC linkages:

Caregiver Lifestyle Disruption: Severity of disturbances in the lifestyle of a family member due to caregiving

Caregiver Stressors: Severity of biopsychosocial pressure on a family care provider caring for another over an extended period of time

Caregiver Well-Being: Extent of positive perception of primary care provider's health status and life circumstances

Caregiver Will (Include Specific Time Frame)

- Identify resources within self to deal with situation.
- Provide opportunity for care receiver to deal with situation in own way.
- Express more realistic understanding and expectations of the care receiver.
- Demonstrate behavior/lifestyle changes to cope with or resolve problematic factors.
- Report improved general well-being, ability to deal with situation.

ACTIONS/INTERVENTIONS

Sample NIC linkages:

Caregiver Support: Provision of the necessary information, advocacy, and support to facilitate primary patient care by someone other than a healthcare professional

Family Involvement Promotion: Facilitating family participation in the emotional and physical care of the patient

Parenting Promotion: Providing parenting information, support, and coordination of comprehensive services to high-risk families

NURSING PRIORITY NO. 1 To assess degree of impaired function:

- Inquire about/observe physical condition of care receiver and surroundings as appropriate. *Important to determine factors that may indicate problems that can interfere with ability to continue caregiving.*[4]
- Assess caregiver's current state of functioning (e.g., hours of sleep, nutritional intake, personal appearance, demeanor). *Provides basis for determining needs that indicate caregiver is having difficulty dealing with role.*[4]
- Determine use of prescription/over-the-counter (OTC)/illicit drugs, alcohol. *Caregiver may turn to using these substances to deal with situation.*[1]
- Identify safety issues concerning caregiver and receiver. *The stress and anxiety of caregiving situations can lead to inattention, and by identifying these issues, an opportunity is provided to correct problems before injury occurs.*[1]
- Assess current actions of caregiver and how they are received by care receiver. *Caregiver may be trying to be helpful but is not perceived as helpful; may be too protective or may have unrealistic expectations of care receiver's abilities, which can lead to misunderstanding and conflict.*[4]
- Note choice/frequency of social involvement and recreational activities. *Caregiver needs to take time away from situation to maintain own sense of self and ability to continue in role.*[1]

- Determine use/effectiveness of resources and support systems. *May not be aware of what is available or may need help in using them to the best advantage.*[4]

NURSING PRIORITY NO. 2 To identify the causative/contributing factors relating to the impairment:

- Note presence of high-risk situations. *Elderly client with total self-care dependence or caregiver with several small children with one child requiring extensive assistance due to physical condition/developmental delays may necessitate role reversal resulting in added stress or placing excessive demands on parenting skills.*[4]
- Determine current knowledge of the situation, noting misconceptions, lack of information. *May interfere with caregiver/care receiver's response to situation.*[2]
- Identify relationship of caregiver to care receiver (e.g., spouse/lover, parent/child, sibling, friend). *Close relationships may make it more difficult to remain separate when caring for care receiver.*[2]
- Ascertain proximity of caregiver to care receiver. *Caregiver could be living in the home of care receiver (e.g., spouse or parent of disabled child), or could be adult child stopping by to check on elderly parent each day, providing support, food preparation/shopping, assistance in emergencies. Note: There is added stress in maintaining own life and responsibilities when caregiver has to travel some distance to provide care.*[4,10]
- Note physical/mental condition, complexity of therapeutic regimen of care receiver. *Caregiving activities can be complex, requiring hands-on care, problem-solving skills, clinical judgment, organizational and communication skills that can tax the caregiver, increasing likelihood of burnout.*[7,10]
- Determine caregiver's level of involvement in/preparedness for the reponsibilities of caring for the client and anticipated length of care. *Information needed to develop plan of care that takes into consideration who will provide care, timing, and any other factors to maintain coverage for situation.*[4]
- Ascertain physical/emotional health and developmental level/abilities and additional responsibilities of caregiver (e.g., job, raising family, etc.). *Provides clues to potential stressors and possible supportive interventions.*[1,10,11]
- Assess caregiver as appropriate using tool such as Burden Interview or Caregiver Reaction Assessment *to further determine caregiver's stressors and abilities providing additional information to aid in planning.*[17,18]
- Identify individual cultural factors and impact on caregiver. *Helps clarify expectations of caregiver/receiver, family, and community. Many cultures, such as Native American, Cuban, believe strongly in keeping care receiver in the home and caring for them.*[5]
- Identify presence/degree of conflict between caregiver/care receiver/family. *Stressful situations can exacerbate underlying feelings of anger and resentment, resulting in difficulty managing caregiving needs.*[2]
- Determine preillness/current behaviors that may be interfering with the care/recovery of the care receiver. *Underlying personality of care receiver may create situation in which old conflicts interfere with current treatment regimen.*[2]
- Note codependency needs/enabling behaviors of caregiver. *These behaviors can interfere with competent caregiving and contribute to caregiver burnout.*[2]

NURSING PRIORITY NO. 3 To assist caregiver to identify feelings and begin to deal with problems:

- Establish a therapeutic relationship, conveying empathy and unconditional positive regard. *A compassionate approach blending the nurse's expertise in healthcare with the caregiver's first-hand knowledge of the care receiver can provide encouragement, especially in a long-term difficult situation.*[2,10,12]

🏠 • Acknowledge difficulty of the situation for the caregiver/family. *Research shows that the two greatest predictors of caregiver's strain are poor health and the feeling that there is no choice but to take on additional responsibilities.*[10]

• Discuss caregiver's view of and concerns about situation. *Important to identify issues so planning and solutions can be developed.*[7]

• Encourage caregiver to acknowledge and express negative feelings. Discuss normalcy of the reactions without using false reassurance. *There are no bad feelings, and individual needs to understand that all are acceptable to be expressed, dealt with, but not acted on in the situation.*[2]

• Discuss caregiver's/family members' life goals, perceptions, and expectations of self. *Clarifies unrealistic thinking and identifies potential areas of flexibility or compromise.*[4]

🏠 • Discuss caregiver's perception of impact of and ability to handle role changes necessitated by situation. *May not initially realize the changes that will be encountered as situation develops, and it helps to identify and plan for changes before they arise.*[1]

NURSING PRIORITY NO. 4 To enhance caregiver's ability to deal with current situation:

• Identify strengths of caregiver and care receiver. *Bringing these to the individual's awareness promotes positive thinking and helps with problem-solving to deal more effectively with circumstances.*[4]

🏠 • Discuss strategies to coordinate caregiving tasks and other responsibilities (e.g., employment, care of children/dependents, housekeeping activities). *Managing these tasks will reduce the stress associated with performing the activities of daily living.*[1]

🅐 • Facilitate family conference to share information and develop plan for involvement in care activities as appropriate. *Involving everyone promotes sense of control/ownership of plan and willingness to follow through on responsibilities.*[1]

🅐 • Identify classes or needed specialists (e.g., first aid/cardiopulmonary resuscitation classes, enterostomal/physical therapist). *Provides information needed to manage tasks of caregiving more effectively, giving individuals more sense of control.*[1]

🅐 • Determine need for/sources of additional resources (e.g., financial, legal, respite care, educational, social, spiritual). *Can help to resolve problems that arise in the course of caregiving that are out of the knowledge/abilities of the individual. Solving these issues can relieve caregiver of anxiety and concern.*[4,13]

🏠 • Provide information or demonstrate techniques for dealing with acting out/violent or disoriented behavior. *Presence of dementia necessitates learning these techniques/skills to enhance safety of caregiver and receiver.*[2]

🅐 • Identify equipment needs/resources, adaptive aids. *Enhances the independence and safety of the care receiver and makes the task of caregiving easier.*[1]

🅐 • Provide contact person/case manager to partner with care provider(s) in coordinating care, providing physical/social support, and to assist with problem-solving as needed/desired. *Promotes more effective caregiving, thereby preventing burnout.*[2,10,14]

NURSING PRIORITY NO. 5 To promote wellness (Teaching/Discharge Considerations):

🏠 • Advocate for/assist caregiver to plan for/implement changes that may be necessary (e.g., home-care providers, adult day care, eventual placement in long-term care facility). *As caregiving tasks become more difficult, other options need to be considered, and planning ahead can promote acceptance of necessary changes.*[8,11,15]

🌐 Cultural 🅐 Collaborative 🏠 Community/Home Care ⚗ Diagnostic Studies ∞ Pediatric/Geriatric/Lifespan 💊 Medications

- Encourage attention to own needs (e.g., eating and sleeping regularly, setting realistic goals, talking with trusted friend, periodic respite from caregiving), accepting own feelings/frustrations and limitations, and being realistic about loved one's condition. *Supports and enhances caregiver's general well-being and coping ability.*[15,16]
- Review signs of burnout (e.g., emotional/physical exhaustion, changes in appetite and sleep, withdrawal from friends/family/life interests). *Recognition of developing problem allows for timely intervention.*
- Discuss/demonstrate stress management techniques and importance of self-nurturing (e.g., pursuing self-development interests, hobbies, social activities, spiritual enrichment). *Being involved in activities such as these can prevent caregiver burnout.*[4,15]
- Encourage involvement in caregiver support group. *Having others to share concerns and fears is therapeutic, provides ideas for different ways to manage problems, helping caregivers deal more effectively with the situation.*[1]
- Refer to classes/other therapies as indicated. *Provides additional information as needed.*[1]
- Identify available 12-step program when indicated to provide tools *to deal with enabling/codependent behaviors that impair level of function. Provides a more structured environment to learn how to deal with problems of caregiving situation.*[2]
- Refer to counseling or psychotherapy as needed. *Intensive treatment may be needed in very stressful situations.*[2]
- Provide bibliotherapy of appropriate references/Web sites for self-paced learning and encourage discussion of information. *Further information can help individuals understand what is happening and manage more effectively.*[9]

DOCUMENTATION FOCUS

Assessment/Reassessment

- Assessment findings, functional level/degree of impairment, caregiver's understanding/perception of situation.
- Identified risk factors.

Planning

- Plan of care and individual responsibility for specific activities.
- Needed resources, including type and source of assistive devices/durable equipment.
- Teaching plan.

Implementation/Evaluation

- Caregiver's/receiver's response to interventions/teaching and actions performed.
- Identification of inner resources, behavior/lifestyle changes to be made.
- Attainment/progress toward desired outcome(s).
- Modifications to plan of care.

Discharge Planning

- Plan for continuation/follow-through of needed changes.
- Referrals for assistance/evaluation.

References

1. Doenges, M., Moorhouse, M., Murr, A. (2002). *Nursing Care Plans, Guidelines for Individualizing Patient Care.* 6th ed. Philadelphia: F. A. Davis.

2. Doenges, M., Townsend, M., Moorhouse, M. (1998). *Psychiatric Care Plans: Guidelines for Individualizing Care.* 3d ed. Philadelphia: F. A. Davis.

4. Cox, H., Hinz, M., Lubno, M. A., Newfield, S., Scott-Tilley, D., Slater, M., Sridaromont, K. (2002). *Clinical Applications of Nursing Diagnosis: Adult, Child, Women's Psychiatric, Gernontic and Home Health Considerations.* 4th ed. Philadelphia: F. A. Davis.

5. Lipson, J. G., Dibble, S. L., Minarik, P. A. (1996). *Culture & Nursing Care: A Pocket Guide.* San Francisco: School of Nursing, UCSF Nursing Press.

7. Hareven, T. K., Adams, K. J. (eds). (1982). *Aging and Life Course Transitions: An Interdisciplinary Perspective.* New York: Guilford.

8. Liken, M. A. (2001). Caregivers in crisis: Moving a relative with Alzheimer's to assisted living. *Clin Nurs Res,* 10(1), 53–69.

9. Liken, M. A. Experiences of family caregivers of a relative with Alzheimer's disease. *J Psychosoc Nurs,* 39(12), 33–37.

10. Schumacher, K., Beck, C. A., Marren, J. M. (2006). Family caregivers: Caring for older adults, working with their families. *AJN,* 106(8), 40–49.

11. Weiss, B. (2005). When a family member requires your care. *RN* 68(4), 63–65.

12. O'Donnell, R. P., Rosenbaum, P., Walter, B. J., et al. (2005). The health and well-being of caregivers of children with cerebral palsy. *Pediatrics,* 115(6), e626–e636.

13. Spurlock, W. R. (2005). Spiritual well-being and caregiver burden in Alzheimer's caregivers. *Geriatr Nurs,* 26(3), 154–161.

14. Travis, S. (2006). "Caring for you, caring for me": A ten-year caregiver educational initiative of the Rosalynn Carter Institute for Human Development. Health and Social Work, May 1, 2006.

15. Haines, C. (2005). Heart failure: Recognizing caregiver burnout. Article for WebMD. Retrieved February 2007 at www.webmd.com/content/Article/51/40695.htm.

16. Boyles, S. (2005). Spouse caregivers most likely to be abusive. Article for WebMD. Retrieved February 2007 at www.webmd.com/content/Article/100/105831.htm.

17. Given C. W., Given, B., Stommel, M., et al. (1992). The caregiver reaction assessment (CRA) for caregivers to persons with chronic physical and mental impairments. *Research in Nursing & Health,* 15, 271–283.

18. Zarit S. H., Todd, P. A., Zarit, J. M. (1986). Subjective burden of husbands and wives as caregivers: A longitudinal study. *Gerontologist,* 26, 260–266.

risk for Caregiver Role Strain

Definition: Caregiver is vulnerable for felt difficulty in performing the family caregiver role

RISK FACTORS

Illness severity of the care receiver; psychological or cognitive problems in care receiver; addiction or codependency

Discharge of family member with significant home-care needs; premature birth/congenital defect

Unpredictable illness course or instability in the care receiver's health

Duration of caregiving required; inexperience with caregiving; complexity/amount of caregiving tasks; caregiver's competing role commitments

Caregiver health impairment

Caregiver is female/spouse

Caregiver not developmentally ready for caregiver role [e.g., a young adult needing to provide care for middle-aged parent]; developmental delay or retardation of the care receiver or caregiver

Presence of situational stressors that normally affect families (e.g., significant loss, disaster or crisis, economic vulnerability, major life events [such as birth, hospitalization, leaving home, returning home, marriage, divorce, change in employment, retirement, death])

Inadequate physical environment for providing care (e.g., housing, transportation, community services, equipment)

Cultural Collaborative Community/Home Care Diagnostic Studies Pediatric/Geriatric/Lifespan Medications

Family/caregiver isolation

Lack of respite/recreation for caregiver

Marginal family adaptation or dysfunction prior to the caregiving situation

Marginal caregiver's coping patterns

Past history of poor relationship between caregiver and care receiver

Care receiver exhibits deviant, bizarre behavior

Presence of abuse or violence

NOTE: A risk diagnosis is not evidenced by signs and symptoms, as the problem has not occurred; rather, nursing interventions are directed at prevention.

Sample Clinical Applications: Chronic conditions (e.g., severe brain injury, SCI, severe developmental delay), progressive debilitating conditions (e.g., muscular dystrophy, multiple sclerosis, dementia/Alzheimer's disease, end-stage COPD, renal failure/ dialysis), substance abuse, end-of-life care, psychiatric conditions (e.g., schizophrenia, personality disorders)

DESIRED OUTCOMES/EVALUATION CRITERIA

Sample NOC linkages:

Caregiver Home Care Readiness: Extent of preparedness of a caregiver to assume responsibility for the healthcare of a family member in the home

Caregiving Endurance Potential: Factors that promote family care provider continuance over an extended period of time

Family Resiliency: Capacity of the family system to successfully adapt and function competently following significant adversity or crisis

---

Caregiver Will (Include Specific Time Frame)

• Identify individual risk factors and appropriate interventions.

• Demonstrate/initiate behaviors or lifestyle changes to prevent development of impaired function.

• Use available resources appropriately.

• Report satisfaction with current situation.

ACTIONS/INTERVENTIONS

Sample NIC linkages:

Caregiver Support: Provision of the necessary information, advocacy, and support to facilitate primary patient care by someone other than a healthcare professional

Family Support: Promotion of family values, interests, and goals

Parenting Promotion: Providing parenting information, support, and coordination of comprehensive services to high-risk families

NURSING PRIORITY NO. 1 To assess factors affecting current situation:

∞ • Note presence of high-risk situations (e.g., elderly client with total self-care dependence or several small children with one child requiring extensive assistance due to physical condition/developmental delays). *May necessitate role reversal resulting in added stress or place excessive demands on parenting skills. Identification of high-risk situations can help in planning and resolving problems before they can become unmanageable.*[1]

🏠 • Identify relationship and proximity of caregiver to care receiver (e.g., spouse/lover, parent/child, friend). *There is added stress in maintaining own life and responsibilities when caregiver has to travel some distance to provide care.[4] Close relationships may create problems of codependency and identification that can be counterproductive to caregiving.[3]*

• Determine current knowledge of the situation, noting misconceptions, lack of information. *May interfere with caregiver/care receiver's response to situation.[2]*

• Compare caregiver's and receiver's view of situation. *Different views need to be openly expressed so each person understands how other sees situation.[1]*

🏠 • Note therapeutic regimen and physical/mental condition of care receiver to ascertain potential areas of need (e.g., teaching, direct care support, respite). *Knowledge of these factors is necessary for planning adequate care for the individual. Plans for additional help my be necessary to prevent caregiver role strain.[1]*

🏠 • Determine caregiver's level of responsibility, involvement in, and anticipated length of care. *Information that may indicate level of stress that may be anticipated for the situation. Progressive debilitation taxes caregiver and may alter ability to meet client/own needs.[1]*

🌐 • Identify individual cultural factors and impact on caregiver. *Helps clarify expectations of caregiver/receiver, family, and community. Many cultures, such as Native American, Cuban, believe strongly in keeping care receiver in the home and caring for them.[5]*

🏠 • Ascertain caregiver's physical/emotional health and developmental level/abilities, as well as additional responsibilities of caregiver (e.g., job, raising family, etc.). *Provides information indicative of ability of the individual to take on the task of caregiver, as well as clues to potential stressors and possible supportive interventions.[4,11,12]*

• Assess caregiver as appropriate using tool such as Burden Interview or Caregiver Reaction Assessment *to further determine caregiver's stressors and abilities providing additional information to aid in planning.[6,7]*

• Identify strengths/weaknesses of caregiver and care receiver. *Caregiver may not be aware of demands that will be expected. Knowing these factors helps to determine how to use them to advantage in planning and delivering care.*

🏠 • Note any codependency needs of caregiver and plan for dealing appropriately with them. *Can contribute to burnout unless identified and dealt with.[2]*

🏠 • Verify safety of caregiver/receiver. *Identifying and correcting unsafe situations is crucial so both individuals can be assured of safety in dealing with difficult situation.[2]*

🏠 • Determine available supports and resources currently used. *Helpful to identify if they are being used effectively.[4]*

NURSING PRIORITY NO. 2 To enhance caregiver's ability to deal with current situation:

🏠 • Establish a therapeutic relationship, conveying empathy and unconditional positive regard. *Promotes positive environment in which needs and concerns can be discussed and proactive solutions identified.[2]*

🏠 • Discuss strategies to coordinate care and other responsibilities (e.g., employment, care of children/dependents, housekeeping activities). *Such planning can prevent chaos and resultant burnout.[8]*

🅐 • Facilitate family conference as appropriate to share information and develop plan for involvement in care activities. *When everyone is involved and listened to, each person is more likely to carry out his or her responsibilities.[4]*

🅐 • Refer to classes and/or specialists (e.g., first aid/CPR classes, enterostomal/physical therapist) for special training as indicated. *Additional information that can help individuals involved feel more competent and able to deal with situation more effectively.[1]*

• Identify additional resources to include financial, legal, respite care. *Can help to resolve problems that arise in the course of caregiving that are out of the knowledge/abilities of the individual. Solving these issues can relieve caregiver of associated anxiety and concern.*[4]

• Identify equipment needs/resources, adaptive aids. *Enhances the independence and safety of the care receiver and reduces chances for untoward incidents.*[1]

• Identify contact person/case manager as needed to coordinate care, provide support, assist with problem-solving. *Assistance with planning minimizes problems that could arise.*[10]

• Provide information or demonstrate techniques for dealing with acting out/violent or disoriented behavior. *Planning ways to deal with these behaviors before they occur promotes safety and enhances positive outcomes.*[2]

• Assist caregiver to recognize codependent behaviors (i.e., doing things for others that others are able to do for themselves) and how these behaviors affect the situation. *Provides options for changing behaviors in ways that enhance the caregiving situation.*[2]

NURSING PRIORITY NO. 3 To promote wellness (Teaching/Discharge Considerations):

• Review signs of burnout (e.g., emotional/physical exhaustion, changes in appetite and sleep, withdrawal from friends/family/life interests). *Recognition of developing problem allows for timely intervention.*[13]

• Discuss/demonstrate stress management techniques and importance of self-nurturing (e.g., meeting personal needs, pursuing self-development interests, hobbies, social activities, spiritual enrichment). *Improves/maintains quality of life for caregiver. May provide care provider with options to protect self.*[4,6,13]

• Encourage involvement in caregiver/other specific support group(s). *Opportunity to be with others in similar situations, and discussing different ways to handle problems helps caregiver deal with difficult role in positive ways.*[3]

• Provide bibliotherapy of appropriate references/Web sites and encourage discussion of information. *Promotes retention of new information that can help caregiver manage more effectively.*[3]

• Advocate for/assist caregiver to plan for and implement changes that may become necessary for the care receiver (e.g., home-care providers, eventual placement in long-term care facility, use of palliative/hospice services). *Getting information and thinking about possibilities will help with decision making. As caregiving tasks become more difficult, other options need to be considered, and planning ahead can promote acceptance of necessary changes.*[8,12,13]

• Refer to classes/therapists as indicated. *May need additional support and information.*[3]

• Identify available 12-step program when indicated to provide tools *to deal with codependent behaviors that impair level of function. Provides a more structured environment to learn how to deal with problems of caregiving situation in positive ways.*[1,2]

• Refer to counseling or psychotherapy as needed. *May need additional help to resolve issues that are interfering with caregiving responsibilities.*[4]

DOCUMENTATION FOCUS

Assessment/Reassessment

• Identified risk factors and caregiver perceptions of situation.
• Reactions of care receiver/family.

Planning

• Treatment plan and individual responsibility for specific activities.
• Teaching plan.

Implementation/Evaluation

• Caregiver/receiver response to interventions/teaching and actions performed.
• Attainment/progress toward desired outcome(s).
• Modifications to plan of care.

Discharge Planning

• Long-term needs and who is responsible for actions to be taken.
• Specific referrals provided for assistance/evaluation.

References

1. Doenges, M., Moorhouse, M., Murr, A. (2002). *Nursing Care Plans, Guidelines for Individualizing Patient Care.* 6th ed. Philadelphia: F. A. Davis.
2. Doenges, M., Townsend, M., Moorhouse, M. (1998). *Psychiatric Care Plans: Guidelines for Individualizing Care.* 3d ed. Philadelphia: F. A. Davis.
3. Townsend, M. (2003). *Psychiatric Mental Health Nursing: Concepts of Care.* 4th ed. Philadelphia: F. A. Davis.
4. Cox, H., Hinz, M., Lubno, M. A., Newfield, S., Scott-Tilley, D., Slater, M., Sridaromont, K. (2002). *Clinical Applications of Nursing Diagnosis: Adult, Child, Women's Psychiatric, Gernontic and Home Health Considerations.* 4th ed. Philadelphia: F. A. Davis.
5. Lipson, J. G., Dibble, S. L., Minarik, P. A. (1996). *Culture & Nursing Care: A Pocket Guide.* San Francisco: School of Nursing, UCSF Nursing Press.
6. Given C. W., Given, B., Stommel, M., et al. (1992). The caregiver reaction assessment (CRA) for caregivers to persons with chronic physical and mental impairments. *Research in Nursing & Health*, 15, 271–83.
7. Zarit, S. H., Todd, P. A., Zarit, J. M. (1986). Subjective burden of husbands and wives as caregivers: A longitudinal study. *Gerontologist*, 26, 260–266.
8. Liken, M. A. (2001). Caregivers in crisis: Moving a relative with Alzheimer's to assisted living. *Clin Nurs Res,* 10(1), 53–69.
9. Liken, M. A. (2001b). Experiences of family caregivers of a relative with Alzheimer's disease. *J Psychosoc Nurs*, 39(12), 33–37.
10. Halper, J., et. al. (2000). Multiple Sclerosis: Best Practices in Nursing Care (monograph). Columbia, MD: Medicalliance.
11. Schumacher, K., Beck, C. A., Marren, J. M. (2006). Family caregivers: Caring for older adults, working with their families. *AJN*, 106(8), 40–49.
12. Weiss, B. (2005). When a family member requires your care. *RN*, 68(4), 63–65.
13. Haines, C. (2005). Heart failure: Recognizing caregiver burnout. Article for WebMD. Retrieved February 2007 at www.webmd.com/content/Article/51/40695.htm.

readiness for enhanced Comfort

Definition: A pattern of ease, relief, and transcendence in physical, psychospiritual, environmental, or social dimensions that can be strengthened

RELATED FACTORS
To be developed by nurse researchers and submitted to NANDA

DEFINING CHARACTERISTICS

Subjective
Expresses desire to enhance comfort/feeling of contentment

Cultural 　Collaborative 　Community/Home Care 　Diagnostic Studies 　Pediatric/Geriatric/Lifespan 　Medications

Expresses desire to enhance relaxation
Expresses desire to enhance resolution of complaints

Objective
[Appears relaxed/calm]
[Participates in comfort measures of choice]

Sample Clinical Applications: Presence of chronic physical or psychological conditions, or any individual seeking improved quality of life

DESIRED OUTCOMES/EVALUATION CRITERIA
Sample NOC linkages:
Comfort Level: Extent of positive perception of physical and psychological ease
Personal Well-Being: Extent of positive perception of one's health and life circumstances
Quality of Life: Extent of positive perception of current life circumstances

Client Will (Include Specific Time Frame)

- Verbalize sense of comfort/contentment.
- Demonstrate behaviors of optimal level of ease.
- Participate in desirable and realistic health-seeking behaviors.

ACTIONS/INTERVENTIONS

Sample NIC linkages:
Self-Modification Assistance: Reinforcement of self-directed change initiated by the patient to achieve personally important goals
Simple Relaxation Therapy: Use of techniques to encourage and elicit relaxation for the purpose of decreasing undesirable signs and symptoms such as pain, muscle tension, or anxiety
Self-Awareness Enhancement: Exploration and understanding of patient's thoughts, feelings, motivations, and behaviors

NURSING PRIORITY NO. 1 To determine current level of comfort/motivation for growth:

- Determine the type of comfort client is experiencing: (1) relief—as from pain; (2) ease—a state of calm or contentment; or (3) transcendence—state in which one rises above one's problems or pain.[1]
- Note cultural/religious beliefs and values that impact perceptions of comfort.
- Ascertain motivation/expectations for change. *Motivation to improve and high expectations can encourage client to make changes that will improve his or her life. However, presence of external locus of control or unrealistic expectations may hamper efforts.*
- Discuss concerns with client and Active-listen to identify underlying issues (e.g., physical or emotional stressors, or external factors such as environmental surroundings, social interactions) that could impact client's ability to control own well-being. *Helps to determine client's level of satisfaction with current situation and readiness for change.*
- Establish context(s) in which comfort is realized: (1) physical—pertaining to bodily sensations; (2) psychospiritual—pertaining to internal awareness of self and meaning in one's life; relationship to a higher order or being; (3) environmental—pertaining to external surroundings,

conditions, and influences; (4) sociocultural—pertaining to interpersonal, family, and societal relationships:[1]

Physical

- Verify that client is managing pain and pain components effectively. *Success in this arena usually addresses other issues/emotions (e.g., fear, loneliness, anxiety, noxious stimuli, anger).*[1]
- Ascertain what is used/required for comfort or rest (e.g., head of bed up/down, music on/off, white noise, rocking motion, certain person or thing).[2]

Psychospiritual

- Determine how psychological and spiritual indicators overlap (e.g., meaningfulness, faith, identity, self-esteem) for client in enhancing comfort.[1]
- Ascertain that client/SO has received desired support regarding spiritual enrichment, including prayer/meditation/access to spiritual counselor of choice.[3]

Environmental

- Determine that client's environment respects privacy and provides natural lighting and readily accessible view to outdoors (*an aspect that can be manipulated to enhance comfort*).[1,3]

Social

- Ascertain meaning of comfort in context of interpersonal, family, cultural values and societal relationships.[4]
- Validate client/SO understanding of client's situation and ongoing methods of managing condition, as appropriate or desired by client. *Considers client/family needs in this area and shows appreciation for their desires.*[4]

NURSING PRIORITY NO. 2 To assist client in developing plan to improve comfort:

- Review knowledge base and note coping skills that have been used previously to change behavior/promote well-being. *Brings these to client's awareness and promotes use in current situation.*[8]
- Acknowledge client's strengths in present situation and build on in planning for future.

Physical

- Collaborate in treating/managing medical conditions involving oxygenation, elimination, mobility, cognitive abilities, electrolyte balance, thermoregulation, hydration *to promote physical stability.*[2,5,6]
- Work with client to prevent pain, nausea, itching, thirst, other physical discomforts.
- Suggest parent be present during procedures *to comfort child.*
- Provide age-appropriate comfort measures (e.g., back rub, change of position, cuddling, use of heat/cold) *to provide nonpharmacological pain management.*
- Review interventions/activities to promote ease such as Therapeutic Touch (TT), biofeedback, self-hypnosis, guided imagery, breathing exercises, play therapy, and humor *to promote relaxation and refocus attention.*
- Assist client to use and modify medication regimen *to make best use of pharmacological pain management.*
- Assist client/SO(s) to develop plan for activity and exercise within individual ability, emphasizing necessity of allowing sufficient time to finish activities.

🌐 Cultural   🅐 Collaborative   🏠 Community/Home Care   ✏ Diagnostic Studies   ∞ Pediatric/Geriatric/Lifespan   💊 Medications

- Maintain open/flexible visitation with client's desired persons.
- Encourage/plan care to allow individually adequate rest periods *to prevent fatigue.* Schedule activities for periods when client has the most energy *to maximize participation.*
- Discuss routines to promote restful sleep.

Psychospiritual

- Interact with client in therapeutic manner. *The nurse could be the most important comfort intervention for meeting client's needs. For example, assuring client that nausea can be treated successfully with both pharmacological and nonpharmacological methods may be more effective than simply administering an antiemetic without reassurance and comforting presence.*[7]
- Encourage verbalization of feelings and make time for listening/interacting.
- Identify ways (e.g., meditation, sharing oneself with others, being out in nature/garden, other spiritual activities) to achieve connectedness or harmony with self, others, nature, higher power.
- Establish realistic activity goals with client. *Enhances commitment to promoting optimal outcomes.*
- Involve client/SO(s) in schedule planning and decisions about timing and spacing of treatments *to promote relaxation/reduce sense of boredom.*
- Encourage client to do whatever possible (e.g., self-care, sit up in chair, walk). *Enhances self-esteem and independence.*
- Use distraction with music, chatting/texting with family/friends, watching TV, playing video/computer games *to limit dwelling on/transcend unpleasant sensations and situations.*
- Encourage client to develop assertiveness skills, prioritizing goals/activities, and to make use of beneficial coping behaviors. *Promotes sense of control and improves self-esteem.*
- Offer/identify opportunities for client to participate in experiences that enhance control and independence.

Environmental

- Provide quiet environment, calm activities.
- Provide for periodic changes in the personal surroundings when client is confined. Use the individual's input in creating the changes (e.g., seasonal bulletin boards, color changes, rearranging furniture, pictures).
- Suggest activities, such as bird feeders/baths for bird-watching, a garden in a window box/terrarium, or a fishbowl/aquarium, *to stimulate observation as well as involvement and participation in activity.*

Social

- Encourage age-appropriate diversional activities (e.g., TV/radio, playtime, socialization/outings with others).
- Avoid overstimulation/understimulation (cognitive and sensory).
- Make appropriate referrals to available support groups, hobby clubs, or service organizations.

NURSING PRIORITY NO. 3 To promote optimum wellness (Teaching/Discharge Considerations):

- Provide information about conditions/health risk factors or concerns in desired format (e.g., pictures, TV programs, articles, handouts, audio/visual materials, classes, group discussions, Web sites, and other databases), as appropriate. *Use of multiple modalities enhances acquisition/retention of information and gives client choices for accessing and applying information.*

Physical

- Promote overall health measures (e.g., nutrition, adequate fluid intake, appropriate vitamin/iron supplementation).
- Discuss potential complications and possible need for medical follow-up or alternative therapies. *Timely recognition and intervention can promote wellness.*
- Assist client/SO(s) to identify and acquire necessary equipment (e.g., lifts, commode chair, safety grab bars, personal hygiene supplies) to meet individual needs.

Psychospiritual

- Collaborate with others when client expresses interest in lessons, counseling, coaching, or mentoring to meet/enhance emotional and spiritual comfort.
- Promote/encourage client's contributions toward meeting realistic goals.
- Encourage client to take time to be introspective in the search for contentment/transcendence.

Environmental

- Create a compassionate, supportive, and therapeutic environment that incorporates client's cultural and age/developmental factors.
- Correct environmental hazards that could influence safety/negatively affect comfort.
- Arrange for home visit/evaluation, as needed.
- Discuss long-term plan for taking care of environmental needs.

Social

- Advocate for growth-promoting environment in conflict situations and consider issues from client/family perspective.
- Support client/SO access to resources (e.g., knowledge and skills, financial resources/assistance, personal/psychological support, social systems).

DOCUMENTATION FOCUS

Assessment/Reassessment

- Individual findings, including client's description of current status/situation.
- Motivation and expectations for change.
- Pertinent cultural/religious beliefs and values.
- Medication use/nonpharmacological measures.

Planning

- Plan of care/interventions and who is involved in planning.
- Teaching plan.

Implementation/Evaluation

- Responses to interventions/teaching and actions performed.
- Attainment/progress toward desired outcome(s).
- Modifications to plan of care.

Discharge Planning

- Long-term needs and who is responsible for actions to be taken.
- Specific referrals made.

   Cultural   Collaborative   Community/Home Care   Diagnostic Studies   Pediatric/Geriatric/Lifespan   Medications

References:

1. Kolcaba, K. Y., Fisher, E. M. (1996). A holistic perspective on comfort care as an advance directive. *Crit Care Nurs Quarterly,* 18(4), 66–67.
2. Kolcaba, K., DiMarco, M. A. (2005).Comfort theory and its application to pediatric nursing. *Pediatr Nurse,* 31(3), 187–194.
3. Barclay, L., Lie, D. (2007). New guidelines issued for family support in patient-centered ICU. CME/CE for Medscape Web site. Retrieved February 2007 at www.medscape/viewarticle/551738.
4. Malinowski, A., Stamler, L. L. (2002). Comfort: Exploration of the concept in nursing. *Journal of Advanced Nursing,* 39(6), 599–606.
5. Kolcaba, K. (2006). FAQs (Frequently Asked Questions). On the Comfort Line. Web site devoted to the Concept of Comfort in Nursing. Retrieved February 2007 at www.thecomfortline.com/FAQ.htm.
6. Kaplow, R. (February 2003). AACN synergy model for patient care: A framework to optimize outcomes. *Crit Care Nurse Suppl,* 27–30.
7. Wilson, L., Kolcaba, K. (2004). Practical application of comfort theory in the perianesthesia setting. *J of Perianesthesia Nursing Online.* Retrieved February 2007 at www.aspan.org/JOPAN/comfot_theory.htm.
8. Townsend, M. C. (2003). *Psychiatric Mental Health Nursing Concepts of Care.* 4th ed. Philadelphia: F. A. Davis.

impaired verbal Communication

Definition: Decreased, delayed, or absent ability to receive, process, transmit, and use a system of symbols

RELATED FACTORS

Decrease in circulation to brain, brain tumor

Anatomical deficit (e.g., cleft palate, alteration of the neurovascular visual system, auditory system, or phonatory apparatus)

Difference related to developmental age

Physical barrier (tracheostomy, intubation)

Physiological conditions [e.g., dyspnea]; alteration of central nervous system (CNS); weakening of the musculoskeletal system

Psychological barriers (e.g., psychosis, lack of stimuli); emotional conditions [depression, panic, anger]; stress

Environmental barriers

Cultural difference

Lack of information

Side effects of medication

Alteration of self-esteem/self-concept

Altered perceptions

Absence of SO(s)

DEFINING CHARACTERISTICS

Subjective
[Reports of difficulty expressing self]

Objective
Inability to speak dominant language

Speaks/verbalizes with difficulty; stuttering; slurring

Does not/cannot speak; willful refusal to speak

Difficulty forming words/sentences (e.g., aphonia, dyslalia, dysarthria)

Difficulty expressing thoughts verbally (e.g., aphasia, dysphasia, apraxia, dyslexia)

Inappropriate verbalization, [incessant, loose association of ideas; flight of ideas]
Difficulty in comprehending/maintaining usual communication pattern
Absence of eye contact/difficulty in selective attending; partial/total visual deficit
Inability/difficulty in use of facial/body expressions
Dyspnea
Disorientation to person/space/time
[Inability to modulate speech]
[Message inappropriate to content]
[Use of nonverbal cues (e.g., pleading eyes, gestures, turning away)]
[Frustration, anger, hostility]

Sample Clinical Applications: Brain injury/stroke, facial trauma, head/neck cancer, radical neck surgery/laryngectomy, cleft lip/palate, dementia, Tourette's syndrome, autism, schizophrenia

DESIRED OUTCOMES/EVALUATION CRITERIA
Sample NOC linkages:
Communication: Reception, interpretation, and expression of spoken, written, and nonverbal messages
Communication: Expressive: Expression of meaningful verbal or nonverbal messages
Information Processing: Ability to acquire, organize, and use information

Client Will (Include Specific Time Frame)
- Verbalize or indicate an understanding of the communication difficulty and plans for ways of handling.
- Establish method of communication in which needs can be expressed.
- Participate in therapeutic communication (e.g., using silence, acceptance, restating reflecting, Active-listening, and I-messages).
- Demonstrate congruent verbal and nonverbal communication.
- Use resources appropriately.

ACTIONS/INTERVENTIONS

Sample NIC linkages:
Communication Enhancement: Speech Deficit: Assistance in accepting and learning alternative methods for living with impaired speech
Communication Enhancement: Hearing Deficit: Assistance in accepting and learning alternative methods for living with diminished hearing
Active Listening: Attending closely to and attaching significance to a patient's verbal and nonverbal messages

NURSING PRIORITY NO. I To assess causative/contributing factors:

- Identify physiological/neurological conditions impacting speech such as severe shortness of breath, cleft palate, facial trauma, neuromuscular weakness, stroke, brain tumors/ infections, dementia, brain trauma, deafness/hard of hearing.
- Review results of diagnostic studies (e.g., speech/language and hearing evaluations, neurological testing/brain function studies—such as electroencephalogram [EEG], computed tomography [CT] scan, psychological evaluations) *to assess/delineate underlying conditions affecting verbal communication.*

Cultural Collaborative Community/Home Care Diagnostic Studies Pediatric/Geriatric/Lifespan Medications

- Note new onset or diagnosis of deficits that will progress/permanently affect speech.
- Note presence of physical barriers, including tracheostomy/intubation, wired jaws; or problem resulting in failure of voice production or "problem voice" (*pitch, loudness, or quality calls attention to voice rather than what speaker is saying as might occur with electronic voice box or "talking valves" when tracheostomy in place*).[7,8]

∞ • Determine age/developmental considerations: (1) child too young for language or has developmental delays affecting speech and language skills/comprehension; (2) autism or other mental impairments; (3) older client doesn't or isn't able to speak, verbalizes with difficulty, has difficulty hearing or comprehending language or concepts.[1–3]

- Obtain history of hearing/speech-related pathophysiology or trauma (e.g., cleft lip/palate, traumatic brain injury/shaken baby syndrome, frequent ear infections affecting hearing, or sensorineural changes associated with aging, etc.).
- Identify dominant language spoken. *Knowing the language spoken and fluency in English is important to understanding. While some individuals may be fluent in English, they may still have limited understanding of the language, especially the language of health professionals, and may have difficulty answering questions, describing symptoms, or following directions.*[17]

🌐 • Ascertain whether client is recent immigrant/country of origin and what cultural, ethnic group client identifies as own (e.g., *recent immigrant may identify with home country and its people, beliefs, and healthcare practices*).[6]

🌐 • Determine cultural factors affecting communication such as beliefs concerning touch and eye contact (*certain cultures may prohibit client from speaking directly to healthcare provider; some Native Americans, Appalachians, or young African Americans may interpret direct eye contact as disrespectful, impolite, an invasion of privacy, or aggressive; Latinos, Arabs, and Asians may shout and gesture when excited;*[4] *silence and tone of voice has various meanings, and slang words can cause confusion/misunderstandings*);[5] and conditions/factors of high prevalence in certain groups/populations (*e.g., middle-ear infection high among Native Americans with potential for hearing deficits*).

- Identify environmental barriers: recent or chronic exposure to hazardous noise in home, job, recreation, and healthcare setting (e.g., rock music, jackhammer, snowmobile, lawn mower, truck traffic/busy highway, heavy equipment, medical equipment). *Noise not only affects hearing, but it also increases blood pressure and breathing rate, can have negative cardiovascular effects, disturbs digestion, increases fatigue, causes irritability, and reduces attention to tasks.*[9]
- Investigate client reports of problems such as constantly raising voice to be heard, can't hear someone 2 feet away, conversation in room sounds muffled/dull, too much energy required to listen, or pain/ringing in ears after exposure to noise.[9]
- Determine if client with communication impairment has a speech or language problem, or both. *Language is a code made up of rules (e.g., what words mean, how to make new words, combine words, and what combinations work in what situations). When a person cannot understand the language code, there is a receptive problem. When a speech problem is present, the language code can be correct, but words might be garbled, person may stutter, or there may be problems with voice. Language and speech problems can exist together or by themselves.*[10]
- Determine presence of psychological/emotional barriers: history/presence of psychiatric conditions (e.g., manic-depressive illness, schizoid/affective behavior); high level of anxiety, frustration, or fear; presence of angry, hostile behavior. Note effect on speech and communication.[1,4]
- Identify information barriers such as lack of knowledge/need of information or misunderstanding of terms related to client's medical conditions, procedures, treatments, and equipment.[4]
- Assess level of understanding in a sensitive manner. *Individual may be reluctant to say they don't understand or may be embarrassed to ask for help. Head nodding and smiles do not always mean comprehension.*[17]

NURSING PRIORITY NO. 2 To assist client to establish a means of communication to express needs, wants, ideas, and questions:

- Ascertain that you have client's attention before communicating.
- Establish rapport with client, initiate eye contact, shake hands, address by preferred name, meet family members present; ask simple questions, smile, engage in brief social conversation if appropriate. *Helps establish a trusting relationship with client/family, demonstrating caring about the client as a person.*[2–4,19]
- Advise other care providers of client's communication deficits (e.g., deafness, aphasia, mechanical ventilations strategies) and needed means of communication (e.g., writing pad, signing, yes/no responses, gestures, picture board, etc.) *to minimize client's frustration and promote understanding.*[20]
- Provide/encourage use of glasses, hearing aids, dentures, electronic speech devices as needed to maximize sensory perception and improve speech patterns.[2,4]
- Maintain a calm, unhurried manner, sit at client's eye level if possible. Provide sufficient time for client to respond. *Sitting down conveys that nurse has time and interest in communicating.*
- Pay attention to speaker. Be an active listener.
- Begin conversation with elderly individual with casual and familiar topics (e.g., weather, happenings with family members) *to convey interest and stimulate conversation and reminiscence.*[2,15]
- Reduce environmental distractions and background noise (e.g., close the door, turn down the radio/television).[15,21,22]
- Refrain from shouting when directing speech to confused, deaf, or hearing-impaired client. Speak slowly and clearly, pitching voice low *to increase likelihood of being understood.*[2,16,21,22]
- Be honest and let speaker know when you have difficulty understanding. Repeat part of message that you do understand, *so speaker doesn't have to repeat entire message.*[11]
- Clarify type and special features of aphasia, when present. *Aphasia is a temporary, permanent, or progressive impairment of language, affecting production or comprehension of speech and the ability to read or write. Some people with aphasia have problems primarily with expressive language (what is said), others with receptive language (what is understood). Aphasia can also be global (person understands almost nothing that is said, and says little or nothing).*[4,11]
- Note diagnosis of apraxia (*impairment in carrying out purposeful movements affecting rhythm and timing of speech*), dysarthria (*language code can be correct but the right body parts do not move at the right time to produce the right message*), or dementia (*defect is in decline in mental functions, including memory, attention, intellect, and personality*) to help clarify individual needs, appropriate interventions.[11,12]
- Determine meaning of words used by the client and congruency of communication and nonverbal messages.
- Evaluate the meaning of words that are used/needed to describe aspects of healthcare (e.g., pain) and ascertain how to communicate important concepts.[5]
- Observe body language, eye movements, and behavioral clues. *For example, when pain is present, client may react with tears, grimacing, stiff posture, turning away, angry outbursts.*[14]
- Use confrontation skills, when appropriate, within an established nurse-client relationship *to clarify discrepancies between verbal and nonverbal cues.*[4,16]
- Point to objects or demonstrate desired actions when client has difficulty with language. *Speaker's own body language can be used to assist client's understanding.*
- Validate meaning of nonverbal communication; do not make assumptions, *because they may be wrong.* Be honest; if you do not understand, seek assistance from others.[19]
- Work with confused, brain-injured, mentally disabled or sensory-deprived client *to correctly interpret his or her environment.* Establish understanding/convey to others meaning of

symbolic speech *to reduce frustration.* Teach basic signs such as "eat," "toilet," "more," "finished" *to communicate basic needs.*[4,16]

- Provide reality orientation by responding with simple, straightforward, honest statements. Associate words with objects using repetition and redundancy *to improve communication patterns.*[2,4,16]
- Assess psychological response to communication impairment, willingness to find alternate means of communication.
- Identify family member who can speak for client and who is the family decision maker regarding healthcare decisions.[5,17]
- Note SO/parent/caregiver's speech patterns and interactive manner of communicating with client, including gestures.[21]
- Obtain interpreter with language or signing abilities and preferably with medical knowledge when needed. *Federal law mandates that interpretation services be made available. Trained, professional interpreter who translates precisely and possesses a basic understanding of medical terminology and healthcare ethics is preferred (over a family member) to enhance client and provider interactions.*[6,18]
- Evaluate ability to read/write and musculoskeletal status, including manual dexterity (e.g., ability to hold a pen and write); and need/desire for pictures or written communications and instructions as part of treatment plan.
- Plan for/provide alternative methods of communication:[2–4,18]
  Provide pad and pencil, slate board *when client able to write but cannot speak.*
  Use letter/picture board *when client can't write and picture concepts are understandable to both parties.*
  Establish hand/eye signals *when client can understand language but cannot speak or has physical barrier to writing.*
  Remove isolation mask *when client is deaf and reads lips.*
  Obtain/provide access to typewriter/computer *if communication impairment is long-standing/or client is used to this method.*
- Consider form of communication when placing IV. *IV positioned in hand/wrist may limit ability to write or sign.*
- Answer call bell promptly. Anticipate needs and avoid leaving client alone with no way to summon assistance. *Reduces fear, conveys caring to client, and protects nurse from problems associated with failure to provide due care.*[13]
- Refer for appropriate therapies/support services. *Client and family may have multiple needs (e.g., sources for further examinations and rehabilitation services, local community/national support groups and services for disabled, financial assistance with obtaining necessary aids for improving communication).*[4,13]

NURSING PRIORITY NO. 3 To promote wellness (Teaching/Discharge Considerations):

- Encourage family presence and use of touch. Involve them in plan of care as much as possible. *Enhances participation and commitment to plan, assists in normalizing family role patterns, and provides support and encouragement when learning new patterns of communicating.*[4]
- Review information about condition, prognosis, and treatment with client/SO(s), reinforcing that loss of speech does not imply loss of intelligence.
- Teach client and family the needed techniques for communication, whether it be speech/language techniques or alternate modes of communicating. Encourage family to involve client in family activities using enhanced communication techniques. *Reduces stress of difficult situation and promotes earlier return to more normal life patterns.*[4]

- Assess family for possible role changes resulting from client's impairment. Discuss methods of dealing with impairment.
- Use and assist client/SOs to learn therapeutic communication skills of acknowledgment, Active-listening, and I-messages. *Improves general communication skills, emphasizes acceptance, and conveys respect.*
- Discuss ways to provide environmental stimuli as appropriate *to maintain contact with reality; or reduce environmental stimuli/noise. Unwanted sound affects physical health, increases fatigue, reduces attention to tasks, and makes speech communication more difficult.*[9,15]
- Refer to appropriate resources (e.g., speech/language therapist, support groups [e.g., stroke club], individual/family and/or psychiatric counseling) *to address long-term needs, enhance coping skills.*
- Refer to NDs ineffective Coping, disabled family Coping, Anxiety, Fear for additional interventions.

DOCUMENTATION FOCUS

Assessment/Reassessment

- Assessment findings/pertinent history information (i.e., physical/psychological/cultural concerns).
- Meaning of nonverbal cues, level of anxiety client exhibits.

Planning

- Plan of care and interventions (e.g., type of alternative communication/translator).
- Teaching plan.

Implementation/Evaluation

- Response to interventions/teaching and actions performed.
- Attainment of/progress toward desired outcomes.
- Modifications to plan of care.

Discharge Planning

- Discharge needs/referrals made, additional resources available.

References

1. Szymanski, L., King, B. (1999). Practice parameters for the assessment and treatment of children, adolescents, and adults with mental retardation and comorbid mental disorders. American Academy of Child and Adolescent Psychiatry (AACAP) Working Group on Quality Issues. *J Am Acad Child Adolesc Psychiatry*, 38(12 suppl).
2. Stanley, M., Beare, P. G. (1999). Gerontological Nursing: A Health Promotion Approach. 2d ed. Philadelphia: F. A. Davis.
3. Cox, H. C., et al. (2002). *Clinical Applications of Nursing Diagnosis: Adult, Child, Women's, Psychiatric, Gerontic, and Home Health Considerations.* 4th ed. Philadelphia: F. A. Davis.
4. Doenges, M. E., Moorhouse, M. F., Geissler-Murr, A. C. (2002). *Nurse's Pocket Guide: Diagnoses, Interventions, and Rationales.* 8th ed. Philadelphia: F. A. Davis, pp. 134–138.
5. Purnell, L., Paulanka, B. (1998). *Transcultural Health Care: A Culturally Diverse Approach.* 2d ed. Philadelphia: F. A. Davis.
6. Enslein, J., et al. (2002). Evidence-based protocol. Interpreter facilitation for persons with limited English proficiency. University of Iowa Gerontological Nursing Interventions Research Center. Retrieved September 2003 from National Guidelines Clearinghouse. Available at www.guideline.gov/browse/gawithdrawn.aspx?st=U.

Cultural Collaborative Community/Home Care Diagnostic Studies Pediatric/Geriatric/Lifespan Medications

7. Questions/Answers about Voice Problems. (Information sheet). Retrieved September 2003 from American Speech-Language-Hearing Association (ASHA). Available at www.asha.org.
8. Speech for Patients with Tracheostomies or Ventilators. (Information sheet). Retrieved September 2003 from American Speech-Language-Hearing Association (ASHA). Available at www.asha.org.
9. Noise. Retrieved September 2003 from American Speech-Language-Hearing Association (ASHA). Available at www.asha.org.
10. What Is Language? What Is Speech? Retrieved September 2003 from American Speech-Language-Hearing Association (ASHA). Available at www.asha.org.
11. Aphasia Fact Sheet. (Revised June 1999). Retrieved September 2003 from National Aphasia Association (NAA). Available at www.aphasia.org.
12. Understanding Primary Progressive Aphasia. (Revised January 2001). Retrieved September 2003 from National Aphasia Association. Available at www.aphasia.org.
13. Doenges, M. E., Moorhouse, M. F., Geissler-Murr, A. C. (2002). *Nursing Care Plans: Guidelines for Individualizing Patient Care.* 6th ed. Philadelphia: F. A. Davis.
14. Hahn, J. (1999). Cueing in to patient language. *Reflections,* 25(1), 8–11.
15. Tip Sheet: "I can hear, but I can't understand what's being said." (2000). Retrieved September 2003 from American Speech-Language-Hearing Association (ASHA). Available at www.asha.org.
16. Research Dissemination Core: Acute Confusion/Delirium. (1998). Iowa City, IA: University of Iowa Gerontological Nursing Interventions Research Center.
17. Lipson, J. G., Dibble, S. L., Minarik, P. A. (1996). *Culture & Nursing Care: A Pocket Guide.* San Francisco: UCSF Nursing Press.
18. Harquez-Rebello, M. C., Tornel-Costa M. C. (1997) Design of a non-verbal method of communication using cartoons. *Rev Neurol,* 25(148), 2027–2045.
19. No author listed. (2005) Understanding transcultural nursing. *Nursing 2005,* 35(1), 14–23. Supplement Career Directory.
20. Jacobs, D. H.(2005). Aphasia. Article for Emedicine Web site. Retrieved February 2007 at www.emedicine.com/NEURO/topic437.htm.
21. Wallhagen, M. I., Pettengill, E., Whiteside, M. (2006). Sensory impairment in older adults part 1: Hearing loss. *AJN,* 106(10), 40–49.
22. Sommer, K. D., Sommer, N. W. (2002). When your patient is hearing impaired. *RN,* 65(12), 28–32.

readiness for enhanced Communication

Definition: A pattern of exchanging information and ideas with others that is sufficient for meeting one's needs and life goals, and can be strengthened

RELATED FACTORS
To be developed by nurse researchers and submitted to NANDA

DEFINING CHARACTERISTICS

Subjective
Expresses willingness to enhance communication
Expresses thoughts/feelings
Expresses satisfaction with ability to share information/ideas with others

Objective
Able to speak/write a language
Forms words, phrases, sentences
Uses/interprets nonverbal cues appropriately

Sample Clinical Applications: Brain injury/stroke, head/neck cancer, facial trauma, cleft lip/palate, Tourette's syndrome, autism, foreign-born individual communicating in second language

DESIRED OUTCOMES/EVALUATION CRITERIA
Sample NOC Linkages:
Communication: Reception, interpretation, and expression of spoken, written, and nonverbal messages
Information Processing: Ability to acquire, organize, and use information

Client/SO/Caregiver Will (Include Specific Time Frame)

- Verbalize or indicate an understanding of the communication process.
- Identify ways to improve communication.

ACTIONS/INTERVENTIONS

Sample NIC Linkages:
Communication Enhancement: Speech Deficit: Assistance in accepting and learning alternative methods for living with impaired speech
Communication Enhancement: Hearing Deficit: Assistance in accepting and learning alternative methods for living with diminished hearing
Active Listening: Attending closely to and attaching significance to a patient's verbal and nonverbal messages

NURSING PRIORITY NO. 1 Assess how client is managing communication and potential difficulties:

- Identify circumstances that result in client's desire to improve communication. *Many factors are involved in communication, and identifying specific needs/expectations helps in developing realistic goals and determining likelihood of success.*
- Ascertain motivation/expectations for change. *Motivation to improve and high expectations can encourage client to make changes that will improve his or her life. However, presence of external locus of control or unrealistic expectations may hamper efforts.*
- Evaluate mental status. *Disorientation, psychotic conditions may be affecting speech and the communication of thoughts, needs, and desires.*
- Determine client's developmental level of speech and language comprehension. *Provides baseline information for developing plan for improvement.*
- Determine ability to read/write preferred language. *Evaluating grasp of language as well as musculoskeletal states, including manual dexterity (e.g., ability to hold a pen and write) provides information about nature of client's situation. Educational plan can address language skills. Neuromuscular deficits require individual physical/occupational therapeutic program to improve.*
- Determine country of origin, dominant language, whether client is recent immigrant, and what cultural/ethnic group client identifies as own. *Recent immigrant may identify with home country and its people, language, beliefs, and healthcare practices affecting desire to learn language skills and ability to improve interactions in new country.*[1]
- Ascertain if interpreter is needed/desired. *Law mandates that interpretation services be made available. Trained, professional interpreter who translates precisely and possesses a basic understanding of medical terminology and healthcare ethics is preferred over family member to enhance client and provider interaction and sharing of information.*[1]
- Determine comfort level in expression of feelings and concepts in nonproficient language. *Concern about language skills can impact perception of own ability to communicate effectively.*

🌐 Cultural 🅐 Collaborative 🏠 Community/Home Care 🧪 Diagnostic Studies ∞ Pediatric/Geriatric/Lifespan 💊 Medications

- Note any physical challenges to effective communication (e.g., hearing impairment, talking tracheostomy apparatus, wired jaws) or physiological/neurological conditions (e.g., severe shortness of breath, neuromuscular weakness, stroke, brain trauma, deafness, cleft palate, facial trauma). *Client may be dealing with speech/language comprehension or have voice production problems (pitch, loudness or quality). which calls attention to voice rather than what speaker is saying. These barriers may need to be addressed to enable client to improve communication skills.*[2,3]
- Clarify meaning of words used by the client to describe important aspects of life and health/well-being (e.g., pain, sorrow, anxiety). *Words can easily be misinterpreted when sender and receiver have different ideas about their meanings. This can affect the way both client and caregivers communicate important concepts. Restating what one has heard can clarify whether an expressed statement has been understood or misinterpreted.*[4]
- Determine presence of emotional lability/frequency of unstable behaviors. *Emotional/psychiatric issues can affect communication and interfere with understanding.*
- Evaluate congruency of verbal and nonverbal messages. *Communication is enhanced when verbal and nonverbal messages are congruent.*[5]
- Determine lack of knowledge or misunderstanding of terms related to client's specific situation. *Indicators of need for additional information, clarification to help client improve ability to communicate.*
- Evaluate need/desire for pictures or written communications and instructions as part of treatment plan. *Alternative methods of communication can help client feel understood and promote feelings of satisfaction with interaction.*

NURSING PRIORITY NO. 2 To improve client's ability to communicate thoughts, needs, and ideas:

- Maintain a calm, unhurried manner. Provide sufficient time for client to respond. *An atmosphere in which client is free to speak without fear of criticism provides the opportunity to explore all the issues involved in making decisions to improve communication skills.*[10]
- Pay attention to speaker. Be an active listener. *The use of Active-listening communicates acceptance and respect for the client, establishing trust and promoting openness and honest expression. It communicates a belief that the client is a capable and competent person.*
- Sit down, maintain eye contact, preferably at client's level, and spend time with the client. *Conveys message that the nurse has time and interest in communicating.*[10]
- Encourage client to express feelings/clarify meaning of nonverbal clues. *Client may be reluctant to share presence of/dissatisfaction with events.*
- Help client identify and learn to avoid use of nontherapeutic communication. *These barriers are recognized as detriments to open communication, and learning to avoid them maximizes the effectiveness of communication between client and others.*
- Obtain interpreter with language or signing abilities as needed. *May be needed to enhance understanding of words and language concepts to ascertain that interpretation of communication is accurate.*[6,10]
- Encourage use of pad and pencil, slate board, letter/picture board when interacting or to interface in new situations, as indicated. *When client has physical impairments that interfere with spoken communication, alternate means can provide concepts that are understandable to both parties.*[4,10]
- Obtain/provide access to voice-enabled computer. *Use of these devices may be more helpful when communication challenges are long-standing or when client is used to using them.*[1]
- Respect client's cultural communication needs. *Different cultures can dictate beliefs of what is normal or abnormal, (i.e., in some cultures, eye-to-eye contact is considered disrespectful,*

---

impolite, or an invasion of privacy; silence and tone of voice have various meanings, and slang words can cause confusion).[4]

- Provide/encourage use of glasses, hearing aids, dentures, electronic speech devices, as needed. *These devices maximize sensory perception and can improve understanding and enhance speech patterns.*[7]
- Reduce distractions and background noises (e.g., close the door, turn down the radio/television). *A distracting environment can interfere with communication, limiting attention to tasks, and makes speech and communication more difficult. Reducing noise can help both parties hear clearly, improving understanding.*[8]
- Associate words with objects using repetition and redundancy, point to objects, or demonstrate desired actions. *Speaker's own body language can be used to enhance client's understanding when neurological conditions result in difficulty understanding language.*[9]
- Use confrontation skills carefully when appropriate, within an established nurse-client relationship. *Can be used to clarify discrepancies between verbal and nonverbal cues, enabling client to look at areas that may require change.*[10]

NURSING PRIORITY NO. 3 To promote optimum communication:

- Discuss with family/SO and other caregivers effective ways in which the client communicates. *Identifying positive aspects of current communication skills enables family members to learn and move forward in desire to enhance ways of interacting.*[10]
- Encourage client and family to familiarize themselves/use new/developing communication technologies. *Enhances family relationships and promotes self-esteem for all members, as they are able to communicate regardless of problems (e.g., progressive neurological disorder) that could interfere with ability to interact.*[10]
- Reinforce client's/SO's learning and use of therapeutic communication skills of acknowledgment, Active-listening, and I-messages. *Improves general communication skills, emphasizes acceptance, and conveys respect, enabling family relationships to improve.*
- Refer to appropriate resources (e.g., speech therapist, language classes, individual/family or psychiatric counseling). *May need further assistance to overcome challeges as family reaches toward desired goal of enhanced communication.*

DOCUMENTATION FOCUS

Assessment/Reassessment

- Assessment findings/pertinent history information (i.e., physical/psychological/cultural concerns).
- Meaning of nonverbal cues, level of anxiety client exhibits.
- Motivation and expectations for change.

Planning

- Plan of care and interventions (e.g., type of alternative communication/translator).
- Teaching plan.

Implementation/Evaluation

- Progress toward desired outcome(s).
- Modifications to plan of care.

⊕ Cultural Ⓐ Collaborative 🏠 Community/Home Care ⟋ Diagnostic Studies ∞ Pediatric/Geriatric/Lifespan 💊 Medications

Discharge Planning

• Discharge needs/referrals made, additional resources available.

References

1. Enslein, J., et al. (2002). Evidence-based protocol. Interpreter facilitation for persons with limited English proficiency. University of Iowa Gerontological Nursing Interventions Research Center. Retrieved September 2003 from National Guidelines Clearinghouse. Available at www.guideline.gov/browse/gawithdrawn.aspx?st=U.
2. Questions/Answers about Voice Problems. (Information sheet). Retrieved September 2003 from American Speech-Language-Hearing Association (ASHA). Available at www.asha.org.
3. Speech for Patients with Tracheostomies or Ventilators. (Information sheet). Retrieved September 2003 from American Speech-Language-Hearing Association (ASHA). Available at www.asha.org.
4. Purnell, L., Paulanka, B. (1998). *Transcultural Health Care: A Culturally Diverse Approach.* 2d ed. Philadelphia: F. A. Davis.
5. Hahn, J. (1999). Cueing in to client language. *Reflections,* 25(1), 8–11.
6. What Is Language? What Is Speech? Retrieved September 2003 from American Speech-Language-Hearing Association (ASHA). Available at www.asha.org.
7. Stanley, M., Beare, P. G. (1999). *Gerontological Nursing: A Health Promotion Approach.* 2d ed. Philadelphia: F. A. Davis.
8. Noise. (Information sheet.) Retrieved September 2003 from American Speech-Language-Hearing Association (ASHA). Available at www.asha.org.
9. Acute confusion/delirium. (1998). Research Dissemination Core, University of Iowa Gerontological Nursing Interventions Research Center. Iowa City, IA.
10. Cox, H. C., et al. (2002). *Clinical Applications of Nursing Diagnosis: Adult, Child, Women's, Psychiatric, Gerontic, and Home Health Considerations.* 4th ed. Philadelphia: F. A. Davis.

decisional Conflict [specify]

Definition: Uncertainty about course of action to be taken when choice among competing actions involves risk, loss, or challenge to values and beliefs

RELATED FACTORS

Unclear personal values/beliefs; perceived threat to value system
Lack of experience or interference with decision making
Lack of relevant information, multiple or divergent sources of information
Moral obligations that require performing/not performing actions
Moral principles/rules/values that support mutually inconsistent courses of action
Support system deficit
[Age, developmental state]
[Family system, sociocultural factors]
[Cognitive, emotional, behavioral level of functioning]

DEFINING CHARACTERISTICS

Subjective

Verbalizes uncertainty about choices; undesired consequences of alternative actions being considered
Verbalizes feeling of distress while attempting a decision
Questions moral principles/rules/values or personal values/beliefs while attempting a decision

Objective

Vacillates between alternative choices; delayed decision making

Self-focusing

Physical signs of distress or tension (e.g., increased heart rate, increased muscle tension, restlessness, etc.)

Sample Clinical Applications: Therapeutic options with undesired side effects (e.g., amputation, visible scarring)/conflicting with belief system (e.g., blood transfusion, termination of pregnancy), chronic disease states, dementia/Alzheimer's disease, terminal/end-of-life situations

DESIRED OUTCOMES/EVALUATION CRITERIA

Sample NOC linkages:

Decision Making: Ability to choose between two or more alternatives

Health Beliefs: Personal convictions that influence health behaviors

Psychosocial Adjustment: Life Change: Psychosocial adaptation of an individual to a life change

Client Will (Include Specific Time Frame)

- Verbalize awareness of positive and negative aspect of choices/alternative actions.
- Acknowledge/ventilate feelings of anxiety and distress associated with choice/related to making difficult decision.
- Identify personal values and beliefs concerning issues.
- Make decision(s) and express satisfaction with choices.
- Meet psychological needs as evidenced by appropriate expression of feelings, identification of options, and use of resources.
- Display relaxed manner/calm demeanor, free of physical signs of distress.

ACTIONS/INTERVENTIONS

Sample NIC linkages:

Decision-Making Support: Providing information and support for a person who is making a decision regarding healthcare

Values Clarification: Assisting another to clarify patient's own values in order to facilitate effective decision making

Coping Enhancement: Assisting a patient to adapt to perceived stressors, changes, or threats that interfere with meeting life demands and roles

NURSING PRIORITY NO. 1 To assess causative/contributing factors:

- Determine usual ability to manage own affairs. Clarify who has legal right to intervene on behalf of child/developmentally delayed adult (e.g., parent, other relative or court-appointed guardian/advocate). *Family disruption/conflicts can complicate decision-making process. All adults have the right to make their own decisions unless a legal court has ruled the individual is incompetent and a guardian appointed.*[4]
- Note expressions of indecision, dependence on others, availability/involvement of support persons (e.g., lack of/conflicting advice). *Care providers need to be sensitive to the physical, cognitive, and emotional effects of illness on decision-making capabilities and whether the individual wants to be involved in making the decision.*[6]
- Ascertain dependency of other(s) on client and/or issues of codependency. *Influence of others may lead client to make decision that is not what is really wanted or in his or her best interest.*[1]

Cultural Collaborative Community/Home Care Diagnostic Studies Pediatric/Geriatric/Lifespan Medications

- Active-listen/identify reason for indecisiveness. *Helps client to clarify problem and begin looking for resolution. May talk about uncertainty—and alternative choices that can lead to risky, uncertain outcomes—and the need to make value judgments about losses versus the gains.*[2,6]
- Identify cultural values/beliefs or moral obligations/principles that may be creating conflict for client and complicating decision-making process. *These issues must be addressed before client can be at peace with the decision that is made.*[5]
- Determine effectiveness of current problem-solving techniques. *Provides information about client's ability to make decisions that are needed/desired.*[1]
- Note presence/intensity of physical signs of anxiety (e.g., increased heart rate, muscle tension). *Client may be conflicted about the decision that is required and may need help to deal with anxiety to begin to deal with reality of situation. Different treatment decisions may have more uncertainty and generate more conflict in client.*[2,6]
- Listen for expressions of inability to find meaning in life/reason for living, feelings of futility, or alienation from God and others around them. (Refer to ND Spiritual Distress, as indicated.) *May need to talk about reasons for feelings of alienation to resolve concerns and may engage in questioning about own values.*[6,7]
- Review information client has to support the decision to be made. *Inaccurate/incomplete information and misinterpretations complicate the process and may result in a poor outcome.*[8,9]

NURSING PRIORITY NO. 2 To assist client to develop/effectively use problem-solving skills:

- Promote safe and hopeful environment, as needed. *Client needs to be protected and supported while he or she regains inner control.*[8]
- Encourage verbalization of conflicts/concerns. *Helps client to clarify these issues so he or she can come to a resolution of the situation.*[8,9]
- Accept verbal expressions of anger/guilt. Set limits on maladaptive behavior. *Verbalization of feelings enables client to sift through feelings and begin to deal with situation. Behavior that is inappropriate is not helpful for dealing with the situation and will lead to feelings of guilt and low self-worth.*[2]
- Clarify and prioritize individual goals, noting where the subject of the "conflict" falls on this scale. *Helps to identify importance of problems client is addressing, enabling realistic problem-solving.*[2]
- Identify strengths and use of positive coping skills (e.g., use of relaxation techniques, willingness to express feelings). *Helpful for developing solutions to current situation.*[1]
- Identify positive aspects of this experience and assist client to view it as a learning opportunity. *Reframing the situation can help the client see things in a different light, enabling client to develop new and creative solutions.*[1]
- Correct misperceptions client may have and provide factual information, as needed. *Promotes understanding and enables client to make better decisions for own situation.*[1,6]
- Provide opportunities for client to make simple decisions regarding self-care and other daily activities. Accept choice not to do so. Advance complexity of choices, as tolerated. *Acceptance of what client wants to do, with gentle encouragement to progress, enhances self-esteem and ability to try more. Providing individualized decision support can help the client move to more difficult decisions.*[1,6]
- Encourage child to make developmentally appropriate decisions concerning own care. *Fosters child's sense of self-worth and enhances ability to learn/exercise coping skills.*[4]
- Discuss time considerations, setting time line for small steps and considering consequences related to not making/postponing specific decisions to facilitate resolution of conflict. *When time is a factor in making a decision, these strategies can promote movement toward solution.*[4]

- Have client list some alternatives to present situation or decisions, using a brainstorming process. Include family in this activity, as indicated (e.g., placement of parent in long-term care facility, use of intervention process with addicted member). Refer to NDs interrupted Family Processes; dysfunctional Family Processes: alcoholism; compromised family Coping; Moral Distress. *Involving family and looking at different options can promote successful resolution of decision to be made.*[8,9]
- Practice use of problem-solving process with current situation/decision. *Promotes identification of different possibilities that may not have been thought of otherwise.*[1]
- Discuss/clarify spiritual concerns, accepting client's values in a nonjudgmental manner. *Client will be willing to consider own situation when accepted as an individual of worth.*[5]

NURSING PRIORITY NO. 3 To promote wellness (Teaching/Discharge Considerations):

- Promote opportunities for using conflict-resolution skills, identifying steps as client does each one. *Learning this process can help to solve current dilemma and provide the person with skills they can use in the future.*[3]
- Provide positive feedback for efforts and progress noted. *Client needs to hear he or she is doing well, and feedback promotes continuation of efforts.*[2]
- Encourage involvement of family/SO(s), as desired/available. *Provides support for the client and facilitates resolution.*[10]
- Support client for decisions made, especially if consequences are unexpected/difficult to cope with. *Positive feedback promotes feelings of success even when difficult situations occur/outcome is less than desired.*[10]
- Encourage attendance at stress-reduction/assertiveness classes. *Learning these skills can help client achieve lowered stress level that can promote ability to make decisions.*[4]
- Refer to other resources, as necessary (e.g., clergy, psychiatric clinical nurse specialist/psychiatrist, family/marital therapist, addiction support groups). *May need this additional help to deal with complicated problems and facilitate problem-solving and decision making.*[2]

DOCUMENTATION FOCUS

Assessment/Reassessment

- Assessment findings/behavioral responses, degree of impairment in lifestyle functioning.
- Individuals involved in the conflict.
- Personal values/beliefs.

Planning

- Plan of care/interventions and who is involved in the planning process.
- Teaching plan.

Implementation/Evaluation

- Client's and involved individual's responses to interventions/teaching and actions performed.
- Ability to express feelings, identify options; use of resources.
- Attainment/progress toward desired outcome(s).
- Modifications to plan of care.

Discharge Planning

- Long-term needs/referrals, actions to be taken, and who is responsible for doing.
- Specific referrals made.

Cultural Collaborative Community/Home Care Diagnostic Studies Pediatric/Geriatric/Lifespan Medications

References

1. Doenges, M., Moorhouse, M., Murr, A. (2002). *Nursing Care Plans, Guidelines for Individualizing Patient Care.* 6th ed. Philadelphia: F. A. Davis.
2. Doenges, M., Townsend, M., Moorhouse, M. (1998). *Psychiatric Care Plans: Guidelines for Individualizing Care.* 3d ed. Philadelphia: F. A. Davis.
3. Townsend, M. (2003). *Psychiatric Mental Health Nursing: Concepts of Care.* 4th ed. Philadelphia: F. A. Davis.
4. Cox, H., Hinz, M., Lubno, M. A., Newfield, S., Scott-Tilley, D., Slater, M., Sridaromont, K. (2002). *Clinical Applications of Nursing Diagnosis: Adult, Child, Women's Psychiatric, Gerontic and Home Health Considerations.* 4th ed. Philadelphia: F. A. Davis.
5. Lipson, J. G., Dibble, S. L., Minarik, P. A. (1996). *Culture & Nursing Care: A Pocket Guide.* San Francisco: School of Nursing, UCSF Nursing Press.
6. Llewelllyn-Thomas, H. (2004). Helping Patients Make Health Care Decisions. Evaluative Clinical Sciences Dartmouth Medical School. Retrieved July 2007 at www.dartmouthatlas.org/atlases/DecisionSupport.pdf.
7. Hareven, T. K., Adams, K. J. (eds). (1982). *Aging and Life Course Transitions: An Interdisciplinary Perspective.* New York: Guilford.
8. Liken, M. A. (2001). Caregivers in crisis: Moving a relative with Alzheimer's to assisted living. *Clin Nurs Res,* 10(1), 53–69.
9. Liken, M. A. (2001). Experiences of family caregivers of a relative with Alzheimer's disease. *J Psychosoc Nurs,* 39(12), 33–37.
10. Halper, J., et. al. Multiple sclerosis: Best practices in nursing care (monograph). Columbia, MD: Medicallance.

parental role Conflict

Definition: Parent experience of role confusion and conflict in response to crisis

RELATED FACTORS

Separation from child due to chronic illness [or disability]

Intimidation with invasive modalities (e.g., intubation); restrictive modalities (e.g., isolation); specialized care centers

Home care of a child with special needs [e.g., apnea monitoring, postural drainage, hyperalimentation]

Change in marital status, [conflicts of the role of the single parent]

Interruptions of family life due to home-care regimen (e.g., treatments, caregivers, lack of respite)

DEFINING CHARACTERISTICS

Subjective

Parent(s) express(es) concerns/feeling of inadequacy to provide for child's needs (e.g., physical and emotional)

Parent(s) express(es) concerns about changes in parental role; about family (e.g., functioning, communication, health)

Express(es) concern about perceived loss of control over decisions relating to their child

Verbalize(s) feelings of guilt/frustration; anxiety; fear

[Verbalizes concern about role conflict of wanting to date while having responsibility of child care]

Objective

Demonstrates disruption in caretaking routines

Reluctant to participate in usual caretaking activities even with encouragement and support

Sample Clinical Applications: Prematurity, genetic/congenital conditions, chronic illness (parent/child)

DESIRED OUTCOMES/EVALUATION CRITERIA
Sample NOC linkages:
Parenting: Provision of an environment that promotes optimum growth and development of dependent children
Role Performance: Congruence of an individual's role behavior with role expectations
Caregiver Home-Care Readiness: Preparedness to assume responsibility for the healthcare of a family member or significant other in the home

Parent(s) Will (Include Specific Time Frame)

- Verbalize understanding of situation and expected parent's/child's role.
- Express feelings about child's illness/situation and effect on family life.
- Demonstrate appropriate behaviors concerning parenting role.
- Assume caretaking activities, as appropriate.
- Handle family disruptions effectively.

ACTIONS/INTERVENTIONS

Sample NIC linkages:
Parenting Promotion: Providing parenting information, support, and coordination of comprehensive services to high-risk families
Role Enhancement: Assisting a patient, significant other, or family to improve relationships by clarifying and supplementing specific role behaviors
Family Process Maintenance: Minimization of family process disruption effects

NURSING PRIORITY NO. 1 To assess causative/contributory factors:

- Assess individual situation and parent's perception of/concern about what is happening and expectations of self as caregiver. *Identifies needs of the family to deal realistically with the current situation and what interventions are necessary to work toward identified goals.*[5]
- Note parental status, including age and maturity, stability of relationship, single parent, other responsibilities. *Young parents may lack the necessary maturity to deal with unexpected illness of infant or child. Single parent may feel overwhelmed in trying to balance work and caretaking responsibilities. Increasing numbers of elderly individuals who were expecting retirement and a simpler life are providing full-time care for young grandchildren whose parents are unavailable or unable to provide care.*[1]
- Ascertain parent's understanding of child's developmental stage and expectations for the future to identify misconceptions/strengths. *Parents often have no information regarding developmental stages and have unrealistic expectation of abilities of the child. Identifying what the parents know and providing information can help them deal more realistically with the situation.*[1]
- Note coping skills currently used by each individual as well as how problems have been dealt with in the past. *Provides basis for comparison and reference for client's coping abilities in current situation.*[1]
- Determine use of substances (e.g., alcohol, other drugs, including prescription medications). *May interfere with individual's ability to cope/problem-solve and manage current illness/situation and indicates need for additional interventions.*[8]
- Determine availability/use of resources, including extended family, support groups, and financial. *Factors that may affect ability to manage illness, unexpected expenses/caregiving, etc.*[1]

• Perform testing such as Parent-Child Relationship Inventory (PCRI) for further evaluation as indicated. *Provides information on which to develop plan of care and appropriate interventions.*[1]
• Determine cultural/religious influences on parenting expectations of self and child, sense of success/failure. *Parenting is one of the most important jobs an individual will have and one for which they are least prepared. Family of origin practices and beliefs will influence parents in how they parent, and this information is crucial to developing a plan of care that meets their needs.*[4]

NURSING PRIORITY NO. 2 To assist parents to deal with current crisis:

• Encourage free verbal expression of feelings (including negative feelings of anger and hostility), setting limits on inappropriate behavior. *Verbalization of feelings enables parent(s) to sift through situation and begin to deal with reality of what is happening. Behavior that is inappropriate is not helpful for dealing with the situation and will lead to feelings of guilt and low self-worth.*[2]
• Acknowledge difficulty of situation and normalcy of feeling overwhelmed and helpless. Encourage contact with parents who experienced similar situation with child and had positive outcome. *Parents feel listened to when feelings are acknowledged, and hearing how other parents have dealt with situation can give them hope.*[2]
• Provide information in an honest and forthright manner at level of understanding of the client, including technical information when appropriate. *Helping client understand what is happening corrects misconceptions and helps to make decisions that meet individual needs.*[3]
• Promote parental involvement in decision making and care as much as possible/desired. *When family members are involved in the process, it enhances their sense of control and they are more likely to follow through on plans that have been made.*[2]
• Encourage interaction/facilitate communication between parent(s) and child. *Sometimes people who find themselves in difficult/distressful situations tend to withdraw because they do not know what to do. Encouraging these interactions enables them to connect with one another to facilitate dealing with situation.*[2]
• Discuss problems of attachment disorder when diagnosed in child who has been adopted. *Children who have been adopted often suffer from problems of believing they will not be loved, and parents need to learn reasons behind problems as well as skills to deal with them.*[9,10]
• Promote use of assertiveness, relaxation skills. *Providing information and helping individuals learn these skills will help them to deal more effectively with situation/crisis.*[6]
• Instruct parent in proper administration of medications/treatments as indicated. *May need to be involved in care, and knowing how to do these activities enhances their sense of control and comfort in their ability to handle situation.*[5]
• Provide for/encourage use of respite care, parent time off. *Parents may believe they are being "selfish" if they take time out for themselves, that they have to remain with the child. However, parents are important, children are important, and the family is important, and when parents take time for themselves, it enhances their emotional well-being and promotes ability to deal with ongoing situation.*[7,11]
• Help single parent distinguish between parent love and partner love. *New focus of parent's attention/love may result in neglect of relationship with child. Attention needs to be given to both individuals for the relationships to flourish.*[9]

NURSING PRIORITY NO. 3 To promote wellness (Teaching/Discharge Considerations):

• Provide anticipatory guidance relevant to the situation/long-term expectations of the illness. *Encourages making plans for future needs, provides feelings of hope, and promotes sense of control over difficult situation.*[3]

🏠 • Encourage parents to set realistic and mutually agreed-on goals. *As family members work together, they can feel empowered and are more apt to follow through on decisions that they have been involved in making.*[2,12]

🏠 • Discuss infant attachment behaviors such as breastfeeding on cue, co-sleeping, and baby-wearing (carrying baby around on chest/back) as appropriate. *Dealing with ill child/home-care pressures can strain the bond between parent/child. Activities such as these encourage secure relationships.*[12]

🏠 • Provide/identify learning opportunities specific to needs. *Activities such as parenting classes, information about equipment use, and methods of troubleshooting can enhance knowledge and ability to deal with situation.*[3]

⊛ • Refer to community resources, as appropriate (e.g., visiting nurse, respite care, social services, psychiatric care/family therapy, well-baby clinics, special needs support services). *Provides additional assistance, as needed, to handle individual situation/illness.*[5]

• Refer to ND impaired Parenting for additional interventions.

DOCUMENTATION FOCUS

Assessment/Reassessment

• Findings, including specifics of individual situation/parental concerns, perceptions, expectations.

Planning

• Plan of care and who is involved in the planning.
• Teaching plan.

Implementation/Evaluation

• Parent's responses to interventions/teaching and actions performed.
• Attainment/progress toward desired outcome(s).
• Modifications to plan of care.

Discharge Planning

• Long-term needs and who is responsible for each action to be taken.
• Specific referrals made.

References

1. Townsend, M. C. (2003). *Psychiatric Mental Health Nursing Concepts of Care.* 4th ed. Philadelphia: F. A. Davis.
2. Gordon, T. (2000). *Parent Effectiveness Training.* (Updated ed). New York: Three Rivers Press.
3. Cox, H. C., et al. (2002). *Clinical Applications of Nursing Diagnosis: Adult, Child, Women's, Psychiatric, Gerontic, and Home Health Considerations.* 4th ed. Philadelphia: F. A. Davis.
4. Lipson, J. G., Dibble, S. L., Minarik, P. A. (1996). *Culture & Nursing Care: A Pocket Guide.* San Francisco: UCSF Nursing Press.
5. Doenges, M. E., Townsend, M. C., Moorhouse, M. F. (1998). *Psychiatric Care Plans Guidelines for Individualizing Care.* 3d ed. Philadelphia: F. A. Davis.
6. Gordon, T. (1989). *Teaching Children Self-Discipline: At Home and At School.* New York: Random House.
7. Gordon, T. (2000). *Family Effectiveness Training Video.* Solana Beach, CA: Gordon Training Intn'l.
8. Townsend, M. (2001). Nursing Diagnoses in Psychiatric Nursing: Care Plans and Psychotropic Medications. 5th ed. Philadelphia: F. A. Davis.
9. Pickhardt, C. (2002). Role Conflict of the Single Parent. Adoption Media, LLC.
10. Breazeale, T. (2001). Attachment Parenting: A Practical Approach for the Reduction of Attachment Disorders and the Promotion of Emotionally Secure Children. A Master's Thesis Submitted to the Faculty of Bethel College.

🌐 Cultural   ⊛ Collaborative   🏠 Community/Home Care   🧪 Diagnostic Studies   ∞ Pediatric/Geriatric/Lifespan   💊 Medications

11. Walant, K. (September 2000). A little self-care goes a long way. *Attachment Parenting International News.* Retrieved July 2007 at http://attachmentparenting.org/artselfcare.shtml.
12. Sands, S. (September 1, 2004). Some call it alternative parenting; they call it traditional. *Gazette.* Retrieved July 2007 at http://attachmentparenting.org/gazettearticle.shtml.

acute Confusion

Definition: Abrupt onset of reversible disturbances of consciousness, attention, cognition, and perception that develop over a short period of time

RELATED FACTORS

Alcohol abuse; drug abuse; [medication reaction/interaction; anesthesia/surgery; metabolic imbalances]

Fluctuation in sleep-wake cycle

Over 60 years of age

Delirium [including febrile epilepticum (following or instead of an epileptic attack), toxic and traumatic]

Dementia

[Exacerbation of a chronic illness, hypoxemia]

[Severe pain]

DEFINING CHARACTERISTICS

Subjective

Hallucinations [visual/auditory]

[Exaggerated emotional responses]

Objective

Fluctuation in cognition/level of consciousness

Fluctuation in psychomotor activity [tremors, body movement]

Increased agitation/restlessness

Misperceptions, [inappropriate responses]

Lack of motivation to initiate/follow through with purposeful behavior

Lack of motivation to initiate/follow through with goal-directed behavior

Sample Clinical Applications: Brain injury/stroke, respiratory conditions with hypoxia, medication adverse reactions, drug/alcohol intoxication, hyperthermia/infectious processes, malnutrition/eating disorders, fluid and electrolyte imbalances, chemical exposure

DESIRED OUTCOMES/EVALUATION CRITERIA

Sample NOC linkages:

Cognition: Ability to execute complex mental processes

Information Processing: Ability to acquire, organize, and use information

Distorted Thought Self-Control: Self-restraint of disruption in perception, thought processes, and thought content

Client Will (Include Specific Time Frame)

• Regain/maintain usual reality orientation and level of consciousness.
• Verbalize understanding of causative factors when known.
• Initiate lifestyle/behavior changes to prevent or minimize recurrence of problem.

ACTIONS/INTERVENTIONS

Sample NIC linkages:

Delirium Management: Provision of a safe and therapeutic environment for the patient who is experiencing an acute confusional state

Reality Orientation: Promotions of patient's awareness of personal identity, time, and environment

Surveillance: Safety: Purposeful and ongoing collection and analysis of information about the client and the environment for use in promoting and maintaining patient safety

NURSING PRIORITY NO. 1 To assess causative/contributing factors:

- Identify factors present such as recent trauma/fall; use of large numbers of medications/polypharmacy; intoxication, substance use/abuse; history/current seizure activity, episodes of fever/pain, presence of acute infection (especially urinary tract infection in elderly client), exposure to toxic substances, traumatic events; person with dememtia experiencing sudden change in environment/unfamiliar surroundings or people. *Acute confusion is a symptom associated with numerous causes (e.g., hypoxia, abnormal metabolic conditions, ingestion of toxins or medications, electrolyte abnormalities, sepsis/systemic infections, nutritional deficiencies, endocrine disorders, CNS infections/other neurological pathology, acute psychiatric disorders). Note: Elderly persons may be more affected by toxic or metabolic insults than younger people.*[1,11,12]
- Assess mental status. *Typical symptoms of delirium include anxiety, disorientation, tremors, hallucinations, delusions, and incoherence. Onset is usually sudden, developing over a few hours or days.*[2]
- Evaluate vital signs. *Signs of poor tissue perfusion (i.e., hypotension, tachycardia, tachypnea, or fever) may identify underlying cardiovascular or infectious cause for mental status changes.*[2]
- Determine current medications/drug use (especially antianxiety agents, barbiturates, lithium, methyldopa, disulfiram, cocaine, alcohol, amphetamines, hallucinogens, opiates). *Use, misuse, overdose, and withdrawal of many drugs is associated with high risk of confusion, disorientation, and delirium.*[1,11]
- Investigate possibility of alcohol/illicit drug withdrawal or medication interactions. *Noncompliance with regimen, sudden discontinuation or overuse of substances, and certain drug combinations increase risk of toxic reactions and adverse reactions/interactions.*[1,2,12]
- Evaluate for exacerbation of psychiatric conditions (e.g., mood disorder, dissociative disorders, dementia). *Identification of the presence of mental illness provides opportunity for correct treatment and medication.*[10,11]
- Assess diet/nutritional status to identify possible deficiencies of essential nutrients and vitamins. *Failure to eat (forgetfulness or lack of food) can lead to deficiencies (e.g., vitamin B_{12}, folate, thiamine, iron) that could affect mental status.*[2,11]
- Evaluate sleep/rest status, noting deprivation/oversleeping. *Discomfort, worry, and lack of sleep and rest can cause/exacerbate confusion.* (Refer to ND Insomnia, as appropriate.)
- Monitor laboratory values (e.g., CBC, blood cultures, oxygen saturation, electrolytes, thyroid, ammonia levels, liver function studies, serum glucose, urinalysis, toxicology, and drug levels [including peak/trough, as appropriate]).[1–7,11]
- Review results of diagnostic studies (e.g., brain scans/imaging studies, EEG, lumbar puncture/CSF studies).[11]

NURSING PRIORITY NO. 2 To determine degree of impairment:

- Talk with client/SOs to determine client's physical, functional, cognitive, and behavioral baseline, observed changes, and onset/precipitator of changes *to understand and clarify the current situation.*[1]

- Collaborate with medical and psychiatric providers *to evaluate extent of impairment in orientation, attention span, ability to follow directions, send/receive communication, appropriateness of response.*[1]
- Note occurrence/timing of agitation, hallucinations, and violent behaviors (*e.g., delirium may occur as early as 1 or 2 days after last drink in an alcoholic; or "sundown syndrome" may occur in ICU, with client oriented during daylight hours but confused during night*).[1,3]
- Determine threat to safety of client/others. *Delirium can cause client to become verbally and physically aggressive, resulting in behavior threatening to safety of self and others.*

NURSING PRIORITY NO. 3 To maximize level of function, prevent further deterioration:

- Assist with treatment of underlying problem (e.g., establish/maintain normal fluid and electrolyte balance and oxygenation; treat infectious process or pain; detoxify from alcohol and other drugs; provide psychological interventions, etc.).[1–7,9,11,12,14]
- Monitor/adjust medication regimen and note response. Determine which medications can be changed or eliminated when polypharmacy, side effects, or adverse reactions are determined to be associated with current condition.
- Implement helpful communication measures, such as:[1–7,9,11,14]
Use short simple sentences. Speak slowly and clearly.
Call client by name and identify yourself at each contact.
Tell client what you want done, not what to do.
Orient client to surroundings, staff, and necessary activities as often as needed.
Acknowledge client's fears and feelings. *Confusion can be very frightening, especially when client knows thinking is not normal.*
Listen to what client says and try to identify message/emotion or need being communicated.
Limit choices and decisions until client is able to make them.
Give simple directions. Allow sufficient time for client to respond, to communicate, and to make decisions.
Present reality concisely and briefly and avoid challenging illogical thinking. *Defensive reactions may result.*
Refer to ND impaired verbal Communication for additional interventions.
- Manage environment, using the following measures:[1–7,9 11,14]
Provide undisturbed rest periods. Eliminate extraneous noise/stimuli. *Preventing overstimulation can help client relax and can result in reduced level of confusion.*[10]
Provide calm and comfortable environment with good lighting. Encourage client to use vision/hearing aids, when needed, *to reduce disorientation and discomfort from sensory overload or deprivation.*
Observe client on regular basis, informing client of this schedule.
Provide adequate supervision (may need one-to-one during severe episode); remove harmful objects from environment; provide siderails, seizure precautions; place call bell and position needed items within reach/clear traffic paths; ambulate with devices to meet client's safety needs.
Provide clear feedback on appropriate and inappropriate behavior.
Remove client from situation; provide time-out, seclusion, as indicated, *for protection of client/others.*
Encourage family/SO(s) to participate in reorientation and provide ongoing normal life input (e.g., current news and family happenings). Provide normal levels of essential sensory/tactile stimulation—include personal items/pictures. *Client may respond positively to well-known person and familiar items.*
- Note behavior that may be indicative of potential for violence and take appropriate actions to prevent injury to client/caregiver. (Refer to NDs risk for self-/other-directed Violence.)

- Administer medication cautiously to control restlessness, agitation, and hallucinations. *In acute confusion, the short-term goal is to calm the person down quickly. Sedation with conventional antipsychotic agent (e.g., haloperidol, lorazepam) may be used, although many other medications can be used, depending on the underlying cause of the delirium.*[1,5–7]
- Assist with treatment of alcohol/drug intoxication and/or withdrawal, as indicated.[11,12,14]
- Avoid/limit use of restraints. *May worsen agitation, increase likelihood of untoward complications/injury.*[5,12]
- Mobilize elderly client (especially after orthopedic injury) as soon as possible. *Older person with low level of activity prior to crisis is at particular risk for acute confusion and may fare better when out of bed.*[4,14]
- Establish and maintain elimination patterns. *Disruption of elimination may be a cause for confusion, or changes in elimination may also be a symptom of acute confusion.*[5]
- Consult with psychiatric clinical nurse specialist or psychiatrist for additional interventions related to disruptive behaviors, psychosis, and unresolved symptoms.
- Refer to NDs disturbed Thought Processes and disturbed Sensory Perception for additional interventions.

NURSING PRIORITY NO. 4 To promote wellness (Teaching/Discharge Considerations):

- Explain reason for confusion, if known. *Acute confusion usually subsides over time as client recovers from underlying cause or adjusts to situation, but can be frightening to client/SO. Information about cause and treatment to improve condition may be helpful in managing sense of fear and powerlessness.*[13,14]
- Educate SO/caregivers to monitor client at home for sudden change in cognition and behavior. *An acute change is a classic presentation of delirium and should be considered a medical emergency. Early intervention can often prevent long-term complications.*[8]
- Discuss need for ongoing medical review of client's medications to limit possibility of misuse and/or potential for dangerous side effects/interactions. *Medications are frequent precipitant of acute confusion, especially in very young or old.*[8,9]
- Stress importance of keeping vision/hearing aids in good repair *to improve client's interpretation of environmental stimuli and communication.*
- Provide appropriate referrals. *Additional assistance may be required for client with confusion (e.g., cognitive retraining, substance abuse support groups, medication monitoring program, Meals on Wheels, home health, and adult day care).*[1]

DOCUMENTATION FOCUS

Assessment/Reassessment

- Nature, duration, frequency of problem.
- Current and previous level of function, effect on independence/lifestyle (including safety concerns).

Planning

- Plan of care and who is involved in planning.
- Teaching plan.

Implementation/Evaluation

- Response to interventions and actions performed.
- Attainment/progress toward desired outcomes.
- Modifications to plan of care.

Discharge Planning

• Long-term needs and who is responsible for actions to be taken.
• Available resources and specific referrals.

References

1. Doenges, M. E., Moorhouse, M. F., Geissler-Murr, A. C. (2002). *Nurse's Pocket Guide: Diagnoses, Interventions and Rationales.* 8th ed. Philadelphia: F. A. Davis, pp 142–145.
2. Altered mental states. (1998). Columbia, MD: American Medical Directors Association (AMDA). Available at the AMDA Web site: www.amda.com.
3. Stanley, M., Bear, P. G. (1999). Gerontological Nursing: A Health Promotion/Protection Approach. 2d ed. Philadelphia: F.A Davis, pp. 342–349.
4. Matthiesen, V., et al. (1994). Acute confusion: Nursing intervention in older patients, *Orthop Nurs*, 13, 25.
5. Rapp, C. (1997). Acute confusion/delirium, Iowa Veterans Affairs Nursing Research Consortium: Iowa City: University of Iowa.
6. American Psychiatric Association. (1999). Practice guideline for the treatment of patients with delirium. *Am J Psychiatry*, 156(5 Suppl), 1–20.
7. Expert Consensus Guideline Series: Agitation in older persons with dementia: A guide for families and care-givers. Available at www.psychguides.com/gahe.php.
8. Ackley, B. J., Ladwig, G.B. (2002). *Nursing Diagnosis Handbook: A Guide to Planning Care.* 5th ed. St Louis, MO: Mosby.
9. Cox, H. C., et al. (2002). *Clinical Applications of Nursing Diagnosis: Adult, Child, Women's, Psychiatric, Gerontic and Home Health Considerations.* 4th ed. Philadelphia: F. A. Davis, pp. 391–397.
10. Doenges, M. E., Townsend, M. C., Moorhouse. M. F. (1999). *Psychiatric Care Plans Guidelines for Individualizing Care.* 3d ed. Philadelphia: F. A. Davis.
11. Jacobs, D. H. (2006). Confusional states and acute memory disorders. Article for Emedicine Web site. Retrieved January 2007 at www.emedicine.com/neuro/topic435.htm.
12. Jenninngs-Ingle, S.(2007). The sobering facts about alcohol withdrawal syndrome. *Nursing Made Incredibly Easy!* 5(1), 50–60.
13. McCaffrey, R, Rozzano L. (2006). The effect of music on pain and acute confusion in older adults undergoing hip and knee surgery. *Holistic Nursing Practice*, 20(5), 218–224.
14. Naylor, M. D., Stephens, C., Bowles, K. H., et al. (2005). Cognitively impaired older adults. *AJN*, 105(2), 52–61.

risk for acute Confusion

Definition: At risk for reversible disturbances of consciousness, attention, cognition, and perception that develop over a short period of time

RELATED FACTORS
Alcohol use; substance abuse
Infection; urinary retention
Pain
Fluctuation in sleep-wake cycle
Medication/drugs: Anesthesia; anticholinergics; diphenhydramine; opioids; psychoactive drugs; multiple medications
Metabolic abnormalities: Decreased hemoglobin; electrolyte imbalances; dehydration; increased BUN/creatinine; azotemia; malnutrition
Decreased mobility; decreased restraints
History of stroke; impaired cognition; dementia; sensory deprivation
Over 50 years of age; male gender
Note: Signs and symptoms do not evidence a risk diagnosis, as the problem has not occurred; rather, nursing interventions are directed at prevention.
Sample Clinical Applications: Brain injury/stroke, respiratory conditions with hypoxia, medication adverse reactions.

DESIRED OUTCOMES/EVALUATION CRITERIA
Sample NOC linkages:
Cognition: Ability to execute complex mental processes
Information Processing: Ability to acquire, organize, and use information
Risk Control: Personal actions to prevent, eliminate, or reduce modifiable health threats

Client Will (Include Specific Time Frame)

- Maintain usual level of consciousness and cognition.
- Verbalize understanding of individual cause/risk factor(s).
- Engage in activities/interventions to prevent/reduce risk of confusion.

ACTIONS/INTERVENTIONS

Sample NIC linkages:
Reality Orientation: Promotions of patient's awareness of personal identity, time, and environment
Teaching: Disease Process: Assisting the patient to understand information related to a specific disease process
Surveillance: Safety: Purposeful and ongoing collection and analysis of information about the patient and the environment for use in promoting and maintaining patient safety

NURSING PRIORITY NO. 1   To assess causative/contributing factors:

- Identify risk factors present such as recent trauma/fall; use of large numbers of medications/polypharmacy; substance use/abuse; history/current seizures; episodes of fever/pain/acute infection; exposure to toxic substances; traumatic events in client/SO life; person with dementia experiencing sudden change in environment/unfamiliar surroundings or people; exacerbation of psychiatric conditions (e.g., mood disorder, dissociative disorders). *Individuals are at risk of developing confusion associated with numerous causes (e.g., hypoxia, abnormal metabolic conditions, ingestion of toxins or medications, electrolyte abnormalities, sepsis/systemic infections, nutritional deficiencies, endocrine disorders, CNS infections/other neurological pathology, acute psychiatric disorders). Note: Elderly persons may be more prone to confusion as a result of toxic or metabolic insults than youger people.*[1–5]
- Evaluate vital signs for indicators of poor tissue perfusion (i.e., hypotension, tachycardia, tachypnea), *which can decrease perfusion to the brain, resulting in confusion.*
- Determine current medication regimen/drug use—especially antianxiety agents, barbiturates, lithium, methyldopa, disulfiram, cocaine, alcohol, amphetamines, hallucinogens, and opiates, *which are associated with high risk of confusion;* and OTC medications, such as Benadryl and Tylenol PM, *which can cause an exaggerated response (including sundowner syndrome) in elderly individuals.* Note schedule of use (e.g., cimetidine + antacid, digoxin + diuretics). *Combinations can increase risk of adverse reactions/interactions, thus affecting mental status.*[2–5]
- Determine client's mobility and functional level. *Conditions/situations that limit client's mobility and independence potentiate prospect of acute confusional state.*
- Ascertain life events (e.g., death of spouse/other family member, absence of known care provider, move from lifelong home, catastrophic natural disaster) *that can affect client's perceptions, attention, and concetration.*[3]
- Assess diet/nutritional status *to identify possible deficiencies of essential nutrients and vitamins that could affect mental status.*[2,5]

Cultural   Collaborative   Community/Home Care   Diagnostic Studies   Pediatric/Geriatric/Lifespan   Medications

- Evaluate sleep/rest status, noting deprivation/oversleeping. *Discomfort, worry, and lack of sleep and rest can cause/exacerbate confusion.* (Refer to NDs Insomnia, Sleep Deprivation, as appropriate.)

- Monitor laboratory values as indicated (e.g., CBC, blood cultures; oxygen saturation, electrolytes, thyroid, ammonia levels, liver function studies, serum glucose, urinalysis, toxicology, and drug levels [including peak/trough as appropriate]) *to identify imbalances that have potential for causing cofusion.*[1,2,5]

NURSING PRIORITY NO. 2 To reduce/correct existing risk factors:

- Assist with treatment of underlying problem (e.g., drug intoxication/substance abuse, infectious processes, hypoxemia, biochemical imbalances, nutritional deficits, pain management) *to reduce potential for confusion.*[1,2,5]
- Monitor/adjust medication regimen and note response. *May identify medications that can be changed or eliminated in client prone to adverse or exaggerated responses to medications (including confusion).*[1,2,5]
- Provide normal levels of essential sensory/tactile stimulation—include personal items/pictures, desired music, activities, and contacts. Encourage family/SO(s) to participate in orientation by providing ongoing input (e.g., current news and family happenings).[1,2]
- Maintain calm environment and eliminate extraneous noise/stimuli *to prevent overstimulation.*
- Encourage client to use vision/hearing aids/other adaptive equipment when needed *to assist client in interpretation of environment and communication.*
- Promote early ambulation acitvities *to enhance well-being and reduce effects of prolonged bedrest/inactivity.*[1]

NURSING PRIORITY NO. 3 To promote wellness (Teaching/Discharge Considerations):

- Assist with treatment of underlying medical conditions, and/or management of risk factors *to reduce/limit potential for conditions associated with confusion.*[1,2,5]
- Discuss need for ongoing medical review of client's medications *to limit possibility of misuse or potential for dangerous side effects/interactions.*[1]
- Review ways to maximize sleep (e.g., prefered bedtime rituals, comfortable room temperature, bedding/pillows; eliminate or reduce extraneous noise/stimuli, and interruptions) *to prevent confusional state caused by sleep deprivation.*[1]
- Provide appropriate referrals (e.g., medication monitoring program, nutritionist, substance abuse treatment, support groups, home health, and adult day care).[1,2]

DOCUMENTATION FOCUS

Assessment/Reassessment

- Existing conditions/risk factors for individual.
- Current level of function, effect on independence and ability to meet own needs, including food/fluid intake and medication use.

Planning

- Plan of care and who is involved in planning.
- Teaching plan.

Implementation/Evaluation

- Response to interventions and actions performed.

- Attainment/progress toward desired outcomes.
- Modifications to plan of care.

Discharge Planning

- Long-term needs and who is responsible for actions to be taken.
- Available resources and specific referrals.

References

1. Acute Confusion. In Doenges, M. E., Moorhouse, M. F., Geissler-Murr, A. C. (2005). *Nursing Diagnosis Manual: Planning, Individualizing and Documentation Client Care.* Philadelphia: F. A. Davis, pp. 150–154.
2. Jacobs, D. H. (2006). Confusional states and acute memory disorders. Article for Emedicine Web site. Retrieved January 2007 at www.emedicine.com/neuro/topic435.htm.
3. Naylor, M. D., Stephens, C., Bowles, K. H., et al. (2005). Cognitively impaired older adults. *AJN*, 105(2), 52–61.
4. Jenninngs-Ingle, S.(2007). The sobering facts about alcohol withdrawal syndrome. *Nursing Made Incredibly Easy!* 5(1), 50–60.
5. Clinical Practice Guideline: Altered mental states. (1998). Columbia, MD: American Medical Directors Association (AMDA). 2004 update. Available at www.ngc.org/summary/summary.aspx?doc_id=1804.

chronic Confusion

Definition: Irreversible, long-standing, and/or progressive deterioration of intellect and personality characterized by decreased ability to interpret environmental stimuli; decreased capacity for intellectual thought processes; and manifested by disturbances of memory, orientation, and behavior

RELATED FACTORS

Alzheimer's disease [dementia of the Alzheimer's type]
Korsakoff's psychosis
Multi-infarct dementia
Cerebral vascular attack
Head injury

DEFINING CHARACTERISTICS

Objective

Clinical evidence of organic impairment
Altered interpretation
Altered response to stimuli
Progressive/long-standing cognitive impairment
No change in level of consciousness
Impaired socialization
Impaired short-term/long-term memory
Altered personality

Sample Clinical Applications: Brain injury/stroke, dementia/Alzheimer's disease, medication adverse reactions, drug/alcohol abuse, malnutrition/eating disorders, chemical exposure

DESIRED OUTCOME/EVALUATION CRITERIA
Sample NOC linkages:
Physical Injury Severity: Severity of injuries from accidents and trauma
Cognitive Orientation: Ability to identify person, place, and time accurately

🌐 Cultural   ⚛ Collaborative   🏠 Community/Home Care   ✏ Diagnostic Studies   ∞ Pediatric/Geriatric/Lifespan   💊 Medications

Client Will (Include Specific Time Frame)

- Remain safe and free from harm.
- Maintain usual level of orientation.

Family/SO Will (Include Specific Time Frame)

- Verbalize understanding of disease process/prognosis and client's needs.
- Identify/participate in interventions to deal effectively with situation.
- Provide for maximal independence while meeting safety needs of client.

Knowledge: Disease Process: Extent of understanding conveyed about a specific disease process

ACTIONS/INTERVENTIONS

Sample NIC linkages:

Dementia Management: Provision of a modified environment for the patient who is experiencing a chronic confusional state

Calming Technique: Reducing anxiety in patient experiencing acute distress

Surveillance: Purposeful and ongoing acquisition, interpretation, and synthesis of patient data for clinical decision making

NURSING PRIORITY NO. 1 To assess degree of impairment:

- Determine the underlying cause for chronic confusion, as noted in Related Factors. *Helps to sort out possible causes and likelihood for improvement, as well as helping to identify potentially useful interventions and therapies.*[1]
- Review/evaluate responses on diagnostic examinations (e.g., cognitive, functional capacity, behavior, memory impairments, reality orientation, attention span, quality of life). *A combination of tests (e.g., Confusion Assessment Method [CAM], Mini-Mental State Examination [MMSE], Alzheimer's Disease Assessment Scale [ADAS-cog], Brief Dementia Severity Rating Scale [BDSRS], Neuropsychiatric Inventory [NPI], Functional Assessment Questionnaire [FAQ], Clinical Global Impression of Change (CGIC)]) is often needed to complete an evaluation of client's overall condition relating to chronic/irreversible condition.*[2,8]
- Talk with SO(s) regarding baseline behaviors, length of time since onset/progression of problem, their perception of prognosis, and other pertinent information and concerns for client. *The client's SO/primary caregiver is an invaluable and essential source of information, regarding history and current situation, as both cognitive and behavioral symptoms tend to change over time and are often variable from day to day. If history reveals a gradual and insidious decline over months to years and if memory loss is a prominent part of the confusion, dementia is likely. Conditions that permanently damage brain structure and tissue (e.g., vascular, traumatic, infectious or demyelinating conditions) can lead to dementia in person of any age.*[1–4,9,10]
- Obtain information regarding recent changes or disruptions in client's health or routine. *Decline in physical health or disruption in daily living situation (e.g., hospitalization, change in medications, or moving to new home) can exacerbate agitation or bring on acute confusion.* (Refer to ND acute Confusion.)
- Evaluate client's response to primary care providers as well as receptiveness to interventions. *Awareness of these dynamics is helpful for evaluation of ongoing needs for both client and caregiver as client becomes increasingly dependent on caregivers or resistant to interventions.*

- Determine client and caregiver anxiety level in relation to situation. Note behavior that may be indicative of potential for violence. *The diagnosis of irreversible condition, the organic brain changes, and the day-to-day problems of living with it causes great stress and can potentiate violence.*[3]

NURSING PRIORITY NO. 2 To limit effects of deterioration/maximize level of function:

- Monitor for treatable conditions (e.g., depression, infections, malnutrition, electrolyte imbalances, and adverse medication reactions) *that may contribute to or exacerbate distress, discomfort, and agitation.*[1-6]
- Implement behavioral and environmental management interventions to promote orientation, provide opportunity for client interaction using current cognitive skills, and preserve client's dignity and safety:[2-6]

  Ascertain interventions previously used/tried and evaluate effectiveness.

  Provide calm environment, eliminate extraneous noise/stimuli *that may increase client's level of agitation/confusion.*

  Introduce yourself at each contact, if needed. Call client by preferred name.

  Use touch judiciously. Tell client what is being done before touching *to reduce sense of surprise/negative reaction.*

  Be supportive and sensitive to fears, misperceived threats, and frustration with expressing what is wanted.

  Be open and honest when discussing client's disease, abilities, and prognosis.

  Maintain continuity of caregivers and care routines as much as possible.

  Use positive statements, offer guided choices between two options.

  Avoid speaking in loud voice, crowding, restraining, shaming, demanding, or condescending actions toward client.

  Set limits on acting-out behavior *for safety of client/others.*

  Remove from stressors and agitation triggers or danger; move client to quieter place; offer privacy.

  Simplify client's tasks and routines *to reduce agitation associated with multiple options/demands.*

  Provide for/assist with daily care activities, including bathing, dressing, grooming, toileting, exercise. *Client may "forget" how to perform ADLs.*

  Monitor and assist with meeting nutritional needs, feeding and fluid intake; monitor weight. Provide finger food if client has problems with eating utensils or is unable to sit to eat.

  Assist with toileting and perineal care, as needed. Provide incontinence supplies.

  Allow adequate rest between stimulating events.

  Use lighting and visual aids *to reduce confusion.*

  Encourage family/SO(s) to provide ongoing orientation/input to include current news and family happenings.

  Maintain reality-oriented relationship/environment (clocks, calendars, personal items, seasonal decorations).

  Encourage participation in resocialization groups.

  Allow client to reminisce/exist in own reality if not detrimental to well-being.

  Avoid challenging illogical thinking because defensive reactions may result.

  Provide appropriate safety measures. *Client who is confused needs close supervision. Measures, such as use of identification bracelet and alarms on unlocked exits; lockup of toxic substances and medication; supervision of outdoor activities and wandering; removal of car or car keys; and lowered temperature on hot water tank can prevent injuries.*[5]

Cultural Collaborative Community/Home Care Diagnostic Studies Pediatric/Geriatric/Lifespan Medications

- Avoid use of restraints as much as possible. Use vest (instead of wrist) restraints when required. Provide pants with hip pad insert. *Although restraints can prevent falls, they can increase client's agitation and distress, resulting in injury or even death.*[10,11]
 • Administer medications (e.g., antidepressants, anxiolytics, antipsychotics), as ordered, at lowest possible therapeutic dose. Monitor for expected and/or adverse responses, side effects, and interactions. *May be used to manage symptoms of psychosis and aggressive behavior but need to be used cautiously.*[5]
- Implement complementary therapies (e.g., music therapy, hand massage, Therapeutic Touch—if touch is tolerated—aromatherapy, bright-light treatment), as ordered/desired. *Use of alternative therapies can be calming and provide relaxation, thus allowing care to be provided with less difficulty.*[7]
- Refer to NDs acute Confusion, impaired Memory, disturbed Thought Processes, impared verbal Communication for additional interventions.

NURSING PRIORITY NO. 3 To assist SO(s) to develop coping strategies:

- Determine family dynamics, cultural values, resources, availability, and willingness to participate in meeting client's needs. Evaluate SO's attention to own needs, including health status, grieving process, and respite. *Primary caregiver and other members of family will suffer from the stress that accompanies caregiving and will require ongoing information and support.*
- Discuss caregiver burden, if appropriate. Provide educational materials and list of available resources, help lines, Web sites, etc., as desired, *to assist SO(s) in dealing and coping with long-term care issues.*[5,11] (Refer to NDs Caregiver Role Strain, risk for Caregiver Role Strain.)
- Involve SO(s) in care and discharge planning. Maintain frequent interactions with SOs *in order to relay information, to change care strategies, try different responses, or implement other problem-solving solutions.*[6]
- Identify appropriate community resources (e.g., Alzheimer's Disease and Related Disorders Association [ADRDA], stroke or other brain injury support groups, senior support groups, respite care, clergy, social services, therapists, attorney services for advance directives, and durable power of attorney) *to provide support for client and SOs and assist with problem-solving.*[5]

NURSING PRIORITY NO. 4 To promote wellness (Teaching/Discharge Considerations):

- Discuss how client's condition may progress, ongoing age-appropriate treatment needs, and appropriate follow-up. *Intermittent evaluations are needed to determine client's general health, any deterioration in cognitive function, or required adjustment in medication regimen to help the client maintain the highest possible level of functioning.*[6]
- Review medications with SO/caregiver(s), including dosage, route, action, expected and reportable side effects, and potential drug interactions *to prevent/limit complications associated with multiple psychiatric and CNS medications.*[5]
- Develop plan of care with family to meet client's and SO's individual needs. *The individual plan is dependent on cultural and belief patterns as well as family (personal, emotional, and financial) resources.*[6]
- Instruct SO/caregivers to share information about client's condition, functional status, and medications whenever encountering new providers. *Clients often have multiple doctors, each of whom may prescribe medications with potential for adverse effects and overmedication.*[7]
- Provide appropriate referrals (e.g., Meals on Wheels, adult day care, home-care agency, nursing home placement, respite care for family member). *May need additional assistance to maintain the client in the home setting or make arrangements for placement if necessary.*[6]

Assessment/Reassessment

• Individual findings, including current level of function and rate of anticipated changes.

Planning

• Plan of care and who is involved in planning.

Implementation/Evaluation

• Response to interventions and actions performed.
• Attainment/progress toward desired outcomes.
• Modifications to plan of care.

Discharge Planning

• Long-term needs/referrals and who is responsible for actions to be taken.
• Available resources, specific referrals made.

References

1. Bostwick, J. M. (2000). The many faces of confusion: Timing and collateral history often holds the key to diagnosis. *Postgrad Med,* 108(6), 60–72.
2. About Alzheimer's. Physicians and Care Professionals, Various Educational Materials. Alzheimer's Disease and Related Disorders Association (ADRDA) 2003. Available at www.alz.org.
3. Doenges, M. E., Moorhouse, M. F., Geissler-Murr, A. C. (2002). *Nurse's Pocket Guide: Diagnoses, Interventions, and Rationales.* 8th ed. Philadelphia: F. A. Davis, pp. 145–147.
4. Expert Consensus Guideline Series: Agitation in older persons with dementia: A guide for families and caregivers. Expert Knowledge Systems, LLC. Ross Editorial Services, April 1998. Available at www.psychguides.com/gahe.php.
5. Sommers, M. S., Johnson, S.A. (1997). Alzheimer's disease and delirium/dementia. In *Davis's Manual of Nursing Therapeutics for Diseases and Disorders.* Philadelphia: F. A. Davis.
6. Kovach, C. R., Wilson, S. A. (1999). Dementia in older adults. In Stanley, M., Beare P. G. (eds), *Gerontologic Nursing: A Health Promotion/Protection Approach.* 2d ed. Philadelphia: F. A. Davis.
7. Burns, A., Byrne, J., Ballard, C. (2002). Sensory stimulation in dementia: An effective option for managing behavioral problems. *BMJ,* 325, 1312–1313. Summarized on Dementia Center Health and Age Web site: www.healthandage.com.
8. Naylor, M. D., Stephens, C., Bowles, K. H., et al. (2005). Cognitively impaired older adults. *AJN,* 105(2), 52–61.
9. Borbasi, S., Jones, J., Lockwood, C., et al. (2006). Health professionals' perspective of providing care to people with dementia in the acute setting: Toward better practice. *Geriatric Nursing,* 27(5), 300–308.
10. Jacobs, D. H. (2006). Confusional states and acute memory disorders. Article for Emedicine Web site. Retrieved January 2007 at www.emedicine.com/neuro/topic435.htm.
11. Naylor, M. D., Stephens, C., Bowles, K. H., et al. (2005). Cognitively impaired older adults. *AJN,* 105(2), 52–61.

Constipation

Definition: Decrease in normal frequency of defecation accompanied by difficult or incomplete passage of stool and/or passage of excessively hard, dry stool

RELATED FACTORS

Functional

Irregular defecation habits; inadequate toileting (e.g., timeliness, positioning for defecation, privacy)

Insufficient physical activity; abdominal muscle weakness
Recent environmental changes
Habitual denial/ignoring of urge to defecate

Psychological
Emotional stress; depression; mental confusion

Pharmacological
Antilipemic agents; laxative overdose; calcium carbonate; aluminum-containing antacids; nonsteroidal anti-inflammatory agents; opiates; anticholinergics; diuretics; iron salts; phenothiazines; sedatives; sympathomimetics; bismuth salts; antidepressants; calcium channel blockers; anticonvulsants

Mechanical
Hemorrhoids; pregnancy; obesity
Rectal abscess/ulcer/prolapse; rectal anal fissures/strictures; rectocele
Prostate enlargement; postsurgical obstruction
Neurological impairment; Hirschsprung's disease; tumors
Electrolyte imbalance

Physiological
Poor eating habits; change in usual foods/eating patterns; insufficient fiber/fluid intake; dehydration
Inadequate dentition/oral hygiene
Decreased motility of gastrointestinal tract

DEFINING CHARACTERISTICS

Subjective
Change in bowel pattern; unable to pass stool; decreased frequency; decreased volume of stool
Increased abdominal pressure; feeling of rectal fullness/pressure
Abdominal pain; pain with defecation; nausea; vomiting; headache; indigestion; generalized fatigue

Objective
Hard, formed stool
Straining with defecation
Hypoactive/hyperactive bowel sounds; borborygmi
Distended abdomen; abdominal tenderness with/without palpable muscle resistance; palpable abdominal/rectal mass
Percussed abdominal dullness
Presence of soft pastelike stool in rectum; oozing liquid stool; bright red blood with stool
Severe flatus; anorexia
Atypical presentations in older adults (e.g., change in mental status, urinary incontinence, unexplained falls, elevated body temperature)

Sample Clinical Applications: Abdominal surgeries, hemorrhoids/anal lesions, irritable bowel syndrome, diverticulitis, spinal cord injury, multiple sclerosis, enteral/parenteral feedings, hypothyroidism, iron deficiency anemia, uremia/renal dialysis, Alzheimer's disease/dementia

DESIRED OUTCOMES/EVALUATION CRITERIA
Sample NOC linkages:
Bowel Elimination: Formation and evacuation of stool
Nutritional Status: Nutrient Intake: Adequacy of usual pattern of nutrient intake
Self-Care: Nonparenteral medications: Ability to administer oral and topical medications to meet therapeutic goals independently with or without assistive device

Client Will (Include Specific Time Frame)

- Establish/regain normal pattern of bowel functioning.
- Verbalize understanding of etiology and appropriate interventions/solutions for individual situation.
- Demonstrate behaviors or lifestyle changes to prevent recurrence of problem.
- Participate in bowel program, as indicated.

ACTIONS/INTERVENTIONS

Sample NIC linkages:
Constipation/Impaction Management: Prevention and alleviation of constipation/impaction
Bowel Management: Establishment and maintenance of a regular pattern of bowel elimination
Ostomy Care: Maintenance of elimination through a stoma and care of surrounding tissue

NURSING PRIORITY NO. 1   To identify causative/contributing factors:

- Review medical/surgical history *for conditions commonly associated with constipation, including problems with colon or rectum (e.g., obstruction, scar tissue/stricture, diverticulitis, irritable bowel syndrome, tumors, anal fissure), metabolic or endocrine disorders (e.g., diabetes mellitus, hypothyroidism, uremia), limited physical activity (e.g., bedrest, poor mobility, chronic disability), chronic pain problems (especially when client is on pain medications), pregnancy and childbirth, recent abdominal or perianal surgery, and neurological disorders (e.g., Parkinson's disease, multiple sclerosis, spinal cord abnormalities).*[1,2,4,5,7–12]

∞ - Note client's age. *Constipation is more likely to occur in individuals older than 55 years of age*[1,13] *but can occur in any age from infant to elderly. A bottle-fed infant is more prone to constipation than breastfed infant, especially when formula contains iron.*[2,5] *Toddlers are at risk because of developmental factors (e.g., too young, too interested in other things, rigid schedule during potty training), and children and adolescents are at risk because of unwillingness to take break from play, poor eating and fluid intake habits, and withholding because of perceived lack of privacy.*[3] *Many older adults experience constipation as a result of duller nerve sensations, incomplete emptying of the bowel, or failing to attend to signals to defecate.*[4]

- Review daily dietary regimen, noting if diet is deficient in fiber. *Imbalanced nutrition influences the amount and consistency of feces.*[2] *Inadequate dietary fiber (vegetable, fruits, and whole grains) and highly processed foods contribute to poor intestinal function.*[1,4,5,8]

- Assess general oral/dental health. *Dental problems can impact dietary intake (e.g., loss of teeth can force individuals to eat soft foods, mostly lacking in fiber).*[1,4]

- Determine fluid intake to note deficits. *Most individuals do not drink enough fluids, even when healthy, reducing the speed at which stool moves through the colon. Active fluid loss through sweating, vomiting, diarrhea, or bleeding can greatly increase chances for constipation.*[1,2,4,5,7-10]

- Evaluate medication/drug usage *for agents that could slow passage of stool and cause/exacerbate constipation (e.g., narcotic pain relievers, antidepressants, anticonvulsants, aluminum-containing antacids, chemotherapy, iron, contrast media, steroids).*[1,2,4,5,7-11]
- Note energy/activity level and exercise pattern. *Lack of physical activity or regular exercise is often a factor in constipation.*[1-4,7,8,10,13]
- Identify areas of life changes/stressors. *Factors such as pregnancy, travel, traumas, changes in personal relationships, occupational factors, or financial concerns can cause or exacerbate constipation.*[7,10]
- Determine access to bathroom, privacy, and ability to perform self-care activities.
- Investigate reports of pain with defecation. *Hemorrhoids, fissures, skin breakdown, or other abnormal findings may be hindering passage of stool or causing client to hold stool.*[1,5-8]
- Discuss laxative/enema use. Note signs/reports of laxative abuse/overuse of stimulant laxatives. *This is most common among older adults preoccupied with having daily bowel movement.*[5,7,13]
- Auscultate abdomen for presence, location, and characteristics of bowel sounds *reflecting bowel activity.*
- Palpate abdomen for hardness, distention, and masses, *indicating possible obstruction or retention of stool.*
- Perform digital rectal examination, as indicated, *to evaluate rectal tone and detect tenderness, blood, or fecal impaction.*
- Assist with medical workup (e.g., x-rays, abdominal imaging, colonoscopy/proctosigmoidoscopy, colonic transit studies, stool sample tests) *for identification of possible causative factors.*[11-13]

NURSING PRIORITY NO. 2 To determine usual pattern of elimination:

- Discuss customary elimination habits (e.g., normal urge time [client unable to eliminate unless in own home, passing hard stool after prolonged effort, and anal pain]). *Helps to identify/clarify client's perception of problem. For example, constipation has been defined as not only infrequent stools (less than three per week), but also straining with bowel movements, hard stools, unproductive urges, and feeling of incomplete evacuation.*[8]
- Ascertain presence of associated symptoms. *Bloating, abdominal pain, loss of appetite, and feeling of being unwell often accompany constipation and are present between infrequent stools.*[8]
- Note factors that usually stimulate bowel activity and any interferences present. *Client may describe having to sit in a particular position or needing to apply perineal pressure or digital stimulation to start stool. Interferences can include not wanting to use a particular facility or not wanting to interrupt play or an activity.*[8]

NURSING PRIORITY NO. 3 To assess current pattern of elimination:

- Note color, odor, consistency, amount, and frequency of stool following each bowel movement during assessment phase. *Provides a baseline for comparison, promoting recognition of changes. If usual number of weekly bowel movements is decreased, stool is hard formed, or client is straining, constipation is likely present.*[2,10]
- Ascertain duration of current problem and client's degree of concern. *Long-standing condition that client has "lived with" may not cause undue concern, while an acute postsurgical constipation can cause great distress. Client's response may/may not be congruent with the severity of condition.*[10]
- Note interventions client has tried to relieve current situation (e.g., dietary supplements/fiber pills, laxatives, suppositories, enemas), and document success/lack of effectiveness.

NURSING PRIORITY NO. 4 To facilitate return to usual/acceptable pattern of elimination:

 • Review client's current medication regime with physician *to determine if drugs contributing to constipation can be discontinued or changed.*

• Promote lifestyle changes:[1–10]

Instruct in/encourage balanced fiber and bulk in diet (e.g., fruits, vegetables, and whole grains) and fiber supplements (e.g., wheat bran, psyllium) *to improve consistency of stool and enhance passage through colon. Note: Improvement in elimination as a result of dietary changes takes time and is not a treatmemt for acute constipation.*[11]

Limit foods with little or no fiber (e.g., ice cream, cheese, meat, and processed foods)

Promote adequate fluid intake, including water, high-fiber fruit, and vegetable juices. Suggest drinking warm, stimulating fluids (e.g., decaffeinated coffee, hot water, tea) *to promote moist/soft stool and facilitate passage of stool.*

Encourage daily activity/exercise within limits of individual ability *to stimulate contractions of the intestines.*

Encourage client to not ignore urge. Provide privacy and routinely scheduled time for defecation (bathroom or commode preferable to bedpan) *to promote psychological readiness and comfort.*

• Administer medications, as indicated: stool softeners (*to provide moisture to stool*), mild stimulants (*to cause rhythmic muscle contractions*), lubricants (*to enable stool to move more easily*), saline or hyperosmolar laxatives (*to draw water into colon*), or bulk-forming agents (*to absorb water in intestine*), as prescribed, or routinely when appropriate (e.g., client receiving opiates, decreased level of activity/immobility).[1–3,7–10]

• Administer enemas/suppositories, as indicated. Digitally remove impacted stool, when necessary, after applying lubricant/anesthetic ointment to anus *to soften impaction and decrease rectal pain.*[7,8]

• Provide sitz bath before stools *to relax sphincter* and after stools *for soothing effect to rectal area.*[5,10]

• Establish bowel program *to provide predictable and effective elimination and reduce evacuation problems when long-term or permanent bowel dysfunction is present (such as with spinal cord injury).* Include dietary and fluid management, abdominal massage, Valsalva maneuver, deep breathing, ingestion of warm fluids, digital stimulation, and medications/enemas, use of particular position for defecation.[9,10]

• Support/assist with treatment of underlying medical cause where appropriate (e.g., surgery to repair rectal prolapse, thyroid treatment) *to improve body and bowel function.*[1–10]

NURSING PRIORITY NO. 5 To promote wellness (Teaching/Discharge Considerations):[1,8,10]

• Discuss client's particular anatomy and physiology of bowel and acceptable variations in elimination.[1,8,10]

• Provide information and resources to client/SO about relationship of diet, exercise, fluid, and appropriate use of laxatives, as indicated.[1,8,10]

• Provide social and emotional support *to help client manage actual or potential disabilities associated with long-term bowel management.* Discuss rationale for and encourage continuation of successful interventions.[1,8,10]

• Encourage client to maintain elimination diary, if appropriate, *to facilitate monitoring of long-term problem and choice of interventions.*[1,8,10]

• Design bowel management program to be easily replicated in home and community setting.[1,8,10]

• Identify specific actions to be taken if problem does not resolve *to promote timely intervention, thereby enhancing client's independence.*[1,8,10]

DOCUMENTATION FOCUS

Assessment/Reassessment

- Usual and current bowel pattern, duration of the problem, and individual contributing factors.
- Characteristics of stool.
- Underlying dynamics.

Planning

- Plan of care/interventions and changes in lifestyle that are necessary to correct individual situation, and who is involved in planning.
- Teaching plan.

Implementation/Evaluation

- Responses to interventions/teaching and actions performed.
- Change in bowel pattern, character of stool.
- Attainment/progress toward desired outcomes.
- Modifications to plan of care.

Discharge Planning

- Individual long-term needs, noting who is responsible for actions to be taken.
- Recommendations for follow-up care.
- Specific referrals made.

References

1. Hert, M., Huseboe, J. (1998). Management of constipation. University of Iowa Gerontological Nursing Interventions Research Center, Research Dissemination Core. Iowa City (IA). [NGC: 543]. Retrieved from National Guideline Clearinghouse. Available at www.guideline.gov.
2. Cox, H. C., et al. (2002). *Clinical Applications of Nursing Diagnosis: Adult, Child, Women's Psychiatric, Gerontic, and Home Health Considerations*. 3d ed. Philadelphia: F. A. Davis, pp. 192–205.
3. Streeter, B. L. (2002). Teenage constipation: A case study. *Gastroenterol Nurs* 25(6), 253–256.
4. Stanley, M. (1999). The aging gastrointestinal system, with nutritional considerations. In Stanley, M., Beare, P. G. (eds). *Gerontological Nursing: A Health Promotion/Protection Approach*. 7th ed. Philadelphia: F. A. Davis, pp. 180–181.
5. Constipation in Children. NIH Publication No. 02–4633, October 2001, National Digestive Diseases Information Clearinghouse (NDDIC), Bethesda, MD. Available at http://digestive.niddk.nih.gov/ddiseases/pubs/constipationchild/index.htm.
6. Functional constipation and soiling in children. University of Michigan Medical Center. Ann Arbor, 1997. [NCG 1011]. Available at www.guideline.gov/summary/summary.aspx?ss=15&doc_id=4113&nbr=3158.
7. Constipation. NIH Publication No. 95–2754, July 1995. National Digestive Diseases Information Clearinghouse (NDDIC), Bethesda MD. Available at http://nddic@info.niddk.nih.gov.
8. Locke, G. R., Pemberton, J. H., Phillips, S. F. (2000). American Gastroenterological Association: Medical position statement: Guidelines on constipation. *Gastroenterology*, 119(6), 1761–1766.
9. Neurogenic bowel management in adults with spinal cord injury. (1998). Paralyzed Veterans of America, Consortium for Spinal Cord Medicine: Clinical Practice Guidelines. Washington, DC.
10. Doenges, M. E., Moorhouse, M. F., Geissler-Murr, A. C. (2002). *Nurse's Pocket Guide: Diagnoses, Interventions, and Rationales*. 8th ed. Philadelphia: F. A. Davis, p. 151.
11. Marks, J. W. (2006). Constipation. Article for MedicineNet Web site. Retrieved January 2007 at www.medicinenet.com.
12. Holson, D., Gathers, S. (2006). Constipation. Article for eMedicine Web site. Retrieved January 2007 at www.emedicine.com/emerg/topic111.htm.
13. Aazer, S. A. (2005). Constipation in adults. Article for eMedicineHealth Web site. Retrieved January 2007 at www.emedicinehealth/com.

perceived Constipation

Definition: Self-diagnosis of constipation and abuse of laxatives, enemas, and suppositories to ensure a daily bowel movement

RELATED FACTORS
Cultural/family health beliefs
Faulty appraisal [long-term expectations/habits]
Impaired thought processes

DEFINING CHARACTERISTICS

Subjective
Expectation of a daily bowel movement
Expected passage of stool at same time every day
Overuse of laxatives/enemas/suppositories

Sample Clinical Applications: Irritable bowel, confused states/dementia, hypochondriasis

DESIRED OUTCOMES/EVALUATION CRITERIA
Sample NOC linkages:
Health Beliefs: Personal convictions that influence health behaviors
Bowel Elimination: Formation and evacuation of stool
Knowledge: Health Behavior: Extent of understanding conveyed about the promotion and protection of health

Client Will (Include Specific Time Frame)

- Verbalize understanding of physiology of bowel function.
- Identify acceptable interventions to promote adequate bowel function.
- Decrease reliance on laxatives/enemas.
- Establish individually appropriate pattern of elimination.

ACTIONS/INTERVENTIONS

Sample NIC linkages:
Bowel Management: Establishment and maintenance of a regular pattern of bowel elimination
Counseling: Use of an interactive helping process focusing on the needs, problems, or feelings of the patient and SOs to enhance or support coping, problem-solving, and interpersonal relationships
Medication Management: Facilitation of safe and effective use of prescription and over-the-counter drugs

NURSING PRIORITY NO. 1 To identify factors affecting individual beliefs:

- Determine client's understanding of a "normal" bowel pattern. Compare with client's current bowel functioning. *Helps to identify areas for discussion or intervention. For example, what is considered "normal" varies with the individual, cultural, and familial factors with differences in expectations and dietary habits.*[1] *In addition, individuals can think they are constipated when, in fact, their bowel movments are regular and soft, possibly revealing a problem with thought processes/perception. Some people believe they are constipated, or irregular, if they do not have a*

Cultural · Collaborative · Community/Home Care · Diagnostic Studies · Pediatric/Geriatric/Lifespan · Medications

bowel movement every day because of ideas instilled from childhood.[2] The elderly client may believe that laxatives or purgatives are necessary for elimination, when in fact the problem may be long-standing habits (e.g., insufficient fluids, lack of exercise and/or fiber in the diet).[3]

- Discuss client's use/frequency of laxatives. *Perceived constipation typically results in self-medicating with various laxatives. Although laxatives may correct the acute problem, chronic use leads to habituation, requiring ever-increasing doses that result in drug dependency and, ultimately, a hypotonic laxative colon.[5]*

- Identify interventions used by client to correct perceived problem *to establish needed changes/interventions or points for discussion/teaching.*

NURSING PRIORITY NO. 2 To promote wellness (Teaching/Discharge Considerations):

- Discuss the following with client/SO/caregiver (*to clarify issues regarding actual and perceived bowel functioning, and to provide support during behavior modification/bowel retraining*):[3,4]

  Review anatomy and physiology of bowel function and acceptable variations in elimination.

  Identify detrimental effects of habitual laxative/enema use and discuss alternatives.

  Provide information about relationship of diet, hydration, and exercise to improved elimination.

  Encourage client to maintain elimination calendar or diary, if appropriate.

  Provide support by Active-listening and discussing client's concerns/fears.

  Provide social and emotional support *to help client manage actual or potential disabilities associated with long-term bowel management.*

  Encourage use of stress-reduction activities/refocusing of attention while client works to establish individually appropriate pattern.

- Offer educational materials/resources for client/SO to peruse at home *to assist them in making informed decisions regarding constipation and management options.*

- Refer to ND Constipation for additional interventions, as appropriate.

DOCUMENTATION FOCUS

Assessment/Reassessment

- Assessment findings/client's perceptions of the problem.
- Current bowel pattern, stool characteristics.

Planning

- Plan of care/interventions and who is involved in the planning.
- Teaching plan.

Implementation/Evaluation

- Client's responses to interventions/teaching and actions performed.
- Changes in bowel pattern, character of stool.
- Attainment/progress toward desired outcome(s).
- Modifications to plan of care.

Discharge Planning

- Referral for follow-up care.

References

1. Pieken, S. R. (1999). Constipation. In *Gastrointestinal Health*. New York: HarperCollins.

2. Constipation. HIH Publication No. 95–2745, July 1995. Bethesda, MD: National Digestive Diseases Information Clearinghouse (NDDIC).
3. Stanley, M. (1999). The aging gastrointestinal system with nutritional considerations. In Stanley, M., Beare, P. G. (eds). *Gerontological Nursing: A Health Promotion/Protection Approach.* 7th ed. Philadelphia: F. A. Davis, pp. 180–181.
4. Hert, M., Huseboe, J. (1998). Management of constipation. Iowa City (IA): University of Iowa Gerontological Nursing Interventions Research Center, Research Dissemination Core:[NGC 543]. Accessed June 2003. Available at www.guideline.gov/browse/gawithdrawn.aspx?st=U.
5. Brasson, M. D. (2007). Constipation. Article for Emedicine Web site. Retrieved June 2007 at www.emedicine.com/med/topic2833.htm.

risk for Constipation

Definition: At risk for a decrease in normal frequency of defecation accompanied by difficult or incomplete passage of stool and/or passage of excessively hard, dry stool

RISK FACTORS

Functional
Irregular defecation habits; inadequate toileting (e.g., timeliness, positioning for defecation, privacy)
Insufficient physical activity, abdominal muscle weakness
Recent environmental changes
Habitual denial/ignoring of urge to defecate

Psychological
Emotional stress, depression, mental confusion

Physiological
Change in usual foods/eating patterns, insufficient fiber/fluid intake, dehydration, poor eating habits
Inadequate dentition/oral hygiene
Decreased motility of gastrointestinal tract

Pharmacological
Phenothiazines; nonsteroidal anti-inflammatory agents; sedatives; aluminum-containing antacids; laxative overuse; bismuth salts; iron salts; anticholinergics; antidepressants; anticonvulsants; antilipemic agents; calcium channel blockers; calcium carbonate; diuretics; sympathomimetics; opiates

Mechanical
Hemorrhoids, pregnancy; obesity
Rectal abscess/ulcer, anal stricture/fissures, rectal prolapse, rectocele
Prostate enlargement, postsurgical obstruction
Neurological impairment; Hirschsprung's disease; tumors
Electrolyte imbalance
NOTE: A risk diagnosis is not evidenced by signs and symptoms, as the problem has not occurred; rather, nursing interventions are directed at prevention.

Sample Clinical Applications: Abdominal surgeries, hemorrhoids/anal lesions, irritable bowel syndrome, diverticulitis, spinal cord injury, multiple sclerosis, enteral/parenteral

Cultural   Collaborative   Community/Home Care   Diagnostic Studies   Pediatric/Geriatric/Lifespan   Medications

feedings, hypothyroidism, iron deficiency anemia, uremia/renal dialysis, Alzheimer's disease/dementia

DESIRED OUTCOMES/EVALUATION CRITERIA
Sample NOC linkages:
Bowel Elimination: Formation and evacuation of stool
Risk Control: Personal actions to prevent, eliminate, or reduce modifiable health threats
Knowledge: Medication: Extent of understanding conveyed about the safe use of medication

Client/Caregiver Will (Include Specific Time Frame)

- Maintain effective pattern of bowel functioning.
- Verbalize understanding of risk factors and appropriate interventions/solutions related to individual situation.
- Demonstrate behaviors or lifestyle changes to prevent developing problem.

ACTIONS/INTERVENTIONS

Sample NIC linkages:
Constipation/Impaction Management: Prevention and alleviation of constipation/impaction
Bowel Management: Establishment and maintenance of a regular pattern of bowel elimination
Medication Management: Facilitation of safe and effective use of prescription and OTC drugs

NURSING PRIORITY NO. 1 To identify individual risk factors/needs:

- Review medical/surgical history *for conditions commonly associated with constipation, including problems with colon or rectum (e.g., obstruction, scar tissue/stricture, diverticulitis, irritable bowel syndrome, tumors, anal fissure), metabolic or endocrine disorders (e.g., diabetes mellitus, hypothyroidism, uremia), limited physical activity (e.g., bedrest, poor mobility, chronic disability), chronic pain problems (especially when client is on pain medications), pregnancy and childbirth, recent abdominal or perianal surgery, neurological disorders (e.g., Parkinson's, multiple sclerosis, spinal cord abnormalities).*[1,2,4–11]
- ∞ Note client's age. *Constipation is more likely to occur in individuals older than 55 years of age[1] but can occur in any age from infant to elderly. A bottle-fed infant is more prone to constipation than breastfed infant, especially when formula contains iron.[2,5] Toddlers are at risk because of developmental factors (e.g., too young, too interested in other things, rigid schedule during potty training), and children and adolescents are at risk because of unwillingness to take break from play, poor eating and fluid intake habits, and withholding because of perceived lack of privacy.[3] Many older adults experience constipation as a result of duller nerve sensations, incomplete emptying of the bowel, or failing to attend to signals to defecate.[4]*
- Discuss usual elimination pattern and use of laxatives *to establish baseline and identify possible areas for intervention/instruction.*
- Ascertain client's beliefs and practices about bowel elimination, such as "must have a bowel movement every day or I need an enema." *These factors reflect familial or cultural thinking about elimination, which affect client's lifetime patterns.*
- Review daily dietary regimen. *Imbalanced nutrition influences the amount and consistency of feces.[2] Inadequate dietary fiber (vegetable, fruits, and whole grains) highly processed foods contribute to poor intestinal function.*[1,4,6]

- Assess general oral/dental health. *Dental problems can impact dietary intake (e.g., loss of teeth can force individuals to eat soft foods, mostly lacking in fiber).*[1,4]
- Determine fluid intake *to note deficits. Most individuals do not drink enough fluids, even when healthy, reducing the speed at which stool moves through the colon. Active fluid loss through sweating, vomiting, diarrhea, or bleeding can greatly increase chances for constipation.*[1,2,4,5,8]
- Evaluate medication/drug usage *for agents that could slow passage of stool and increase risk of constipation (e.g., narcotic pain relievers, antidepressants, anticonvulsants, aluminum-containing antacids, chemotherapy, iron, contrast media, steroids).*[1,2,4–8]
- Note energy/activity level and exercise pattern. *Lack of physical activity or regular exercise is often a factor in constipation.*[1–6,8]
- Identify areas of life changes/stressors. *Factors such as pregnancy, travel, traumas, and changes in personal relationships, occupational factors, or financial concerns can cause or exacerbate constipation.*[5,8]
- Auscultate abdomen for presence, location, and characteristics of bowel sounds *reflecting bowel activity.*

NURSING PRIORITY NO. 2 To facilitate normal bowel function:

- Promote healthy lifestyle for elimination:[1–11]
    Instruct in/encourage balanced fiber and bulk (e.g., fruits, vegetbles, and whole grains) in diet and fiber supplements (e.g., wheat bran, psyllium) *to improve consistency of stool and facilitate passage through colon.*
    Limit foods with little or no fiber (e.g., ice cream, cheese, meat, and processed foods).
    Promote adequate fluid intake, including water, high-fiber fruit and vegetable juices. Suggest drinking warm, stimulating fluids (e.g., decaffeinated coffee, hot water, tea) *to promote moist/soft stool and increase rate of passage.*
    Encourage daily activity/exercise within limits of individual ability to stimulate contractions of the intestines.
    Encourage client to not ignore urge. Provide privacy and routinely scheduled time for defecation (bathroom or commode preferable to bedpan) to promote psychological readiness and comfort.
- Administer medications (stool softeners, mild stimulants, or bulk-forming agents) prn and/or routinely when appropriate *to prevent constipation (e.g., client taking pain medications, especially opiates, or who is inactive, immobile, or unconscious).*[11]

NURSING PRIORITY NO. 3 Promote wellness (Teaching/Discharge Considerations):

- Discuss physiology and acceptable variations in elimination. *May help reduce concerns/anxiety about situation.*[1,6,8]
- Review individual risk factors/potential problems and specific interventions for prevention of constipation.[1,6,8]
- Encourage/support treatment of underlying medical causes where appropriate *to improve organ function, including the bowel.*[1,6,8]
- Educate client/SO about safe and risky practices for managing constipation. *Information can assist client to make beneficial choices when need arises.*[1,6,8]
- Encourage client to maintain elimination diary if appropriate *to help monitor bowel pattern.*[1,6,8]
- Discuss client's current medication regime with physician *to determime if drugs that may contribute to constipation can be discontinued or changed.*[11]
- Refer to NDs Constipation; perceived Constipation for additional interventions as appropriate.

DOCUMENTATION FOCUS

Assessment/Reassessment

- Current bowel pattern, characteristics of stool, medications.

Planning

- Plan of care and who is involved in planning.
- Teaching plan.

Implementation/Evaluation

- Responses to interventions/teaching and actions performed.
- Attainment/progress toward desired outcomes.
- Modifications to plan of care.

Discharge Planning

- Individual long-term needs, noting who is responsible for actions to be taken.
- Specific referrals made.

References

1. Hert, M., Huseboe, J. (1998). Management of constipation. University of Iowa Gerontological Nursing Interventions Research Center, Research Dissemination Core. Iowa City (IA). [NGC: 543]. Retrieved from National Guideline Clearinghouse. Available at www.guideline.gov.
2. Cox, H. C., et al. (2002). *Clinical Applications of Nursing Diagnosis: Adult, Child, Women's Psychiatric, Gerontic, and Home Health Considerations*. 3d ed. Philadelphia: F. A. Davis, pp. 192–205.
3. Streeter, B. L. (2002). Teenage constipation: A case study. *Gastroenterol Nurs*, 25(6), 253–256.
4. Stanley, M. (1999). The Aging Gastrointestinal System, with Nutritional Considerations. In Stanley, M., Beare, P. G. *Gerontological Nursing: A Health Promotion/Protection Approach*. 7th ed. Philadelphia: F. A. Davis, pp. 180–181.
5. Constipation. NIH Publication no. 95-2754, July 1995. National Digestive Diseases Information Clearinghouse (NDDIC), Bethesda, MD. Contact: nddic@info.niddk.nih.gov.
6. Locke, G. R., Pemberton, J. H., Phillips, S. F. (2000). American Gastroenterological Association: Medical position statement: Guidelines on constipation. *Gastroenterology*, 119(6), 1761–1766.
7. Neurogenic bowel management in adults with spinal cord injury. (1998). Paralyzed Veterans of America, Consortium for Spinal Cord Medicine: Clinical Practice Guidelines. Washington, DC.
8. Doenges, M. E., Moorhouse, M. F., Geissler-Murr, A. C. (2002). *Nurse's Pocket Guide: Diagnoses, Interventions, and Rationales*. 8th ed. Philadelphia: F. A. Davis, p. 151.
9. Marks, J. W. (2006). Constipation. Article for MedicineNet Web site. Retrieved January 2007 at www.medicinenet.com.
10. Holson, D., Gathers, S. (2006). Constipation. Article for eMedicine Web site. Retrieved January 2007 at www.emedicine.com/emerg/topic111.htm.
11. Wooten, J. M. (2006) OTC laxatives aren't all the same. Available on RNweb. http://rnweb.com/rnweb/author/authorDetail.jsp?id=6733.

Contamination

Definition: Exposure to environmental contaminants in doses sufficient to cause adverse health effects

RELATED FACTORS

External

Chemical contamination of food/water; presence of atmospheric pollutants

---

Inadequate municipal services (trash removal, sewage treatment facilities)

Geographic area (living in area where high level of contaminants exist)

Playing in outdoor areas where environmental contaminants are used

Personal/household hygiene practices

Living in poverty (increases potential for multiple exposure, lack of access to healthcare, and poor diet)

Use of environmental contaminants in the home (e.g., pesticides, chemicals, environmental tobacco smoke)

Lack of breakdown of contaminants once indoors (breakdown is inhibited without sun and rain exposure)

Flooring surface (carpeted surfaces hold contaminant residue more than hard floor surfaces)

Flaking, peeling paint/plaster in presence of young children

Paint, lacquer, in poorly ventilated areas/without effective protection

Inappropriate use/lack of protective clothing

Unprotected contact with heavy metals or chemicals (e.g., arsenic, chromium, lead)

Exposure to radiation (occupation in radiography, employment in nuclear industries and electrical generating plants, living near nuclear industries and electrical generation plants)

Exposure to disaster (natural or man-made); exposure to bioterrorism

---

Internal

Age (children less than 5 years, older adults); gestational age during exposure; developmental characteristics of children

Female gender; pregnancy

Nutritional factors (e.g., obesity, vitamin and mineral deficiencies)

Preexisting disease states; smoking

Concomitant exposure; previous exposures

DEFINING CHARACTERISTICS

(Defining characteristics are dependent on the causative agent. Agents cause a variety of individual organ responses as well as systemic responses.)

Subjective/Objective

Pesticides: (Major categories of pesticides: insecticides, herbicides, fungicides, antimicrobials, rodenticides; major pesticides: organophosphates, carbamates, organochlorines, pyrethrum, arsenic, glycophosphates, bipyridyis, chlorophenoxy)

Dermatological/gastrointestinal/neurological/pulmonary/renal effects of pesticide

Chemicals: (Major chemical agents: petroleum-based agents, anticholinesterases; type I agents act on proximal tracheobronchial portion of the respiratory tract, type II agents act on alveoli, type III agents produce systemic effects)

Dermatological/gastrointestinal/immunological/neurological/pulmonary/renal effects of chemical exposure

Biologicals: Dermatological/gastrointestinal/neurological/pulmonary/renal effects of exposure to biologicals (toxins from living organisms [bacteria, viruses, fungi])

Pollution: (Major locations: air, water, soil; major agents: asbestos, radon, tobacco [smoke], heavy metal, lead, noise, exhaust)

Neurological/pulmonary effects of pollution exposure

Waste: (Categories of waste: trash, raw sewage, industrial waste)

Dermatological/gastrointestinal/hepatic/pulmonary effects of waste exposure

Radiation: (Categories: Internal—ingestion of radioactive material [e.g., food/water contamination]; external—exposure through direct contact with radioactive material)

Immunological/genetic/neurological/oncological effects of radiation exposure

---

🌐 Cultural Ⓐ Collaborative 🏠 Community/Home Care ⚗ Diagnostic Studies ∞ Pediatric/Geriatric/Lifespan 💊 Medications

Sample Clinical Applications: *E. coli* infection, plague, hantavirus, asthma, botulism, cholera, lead or other heavy metal poisoning, chemical burns, asbestosis, carbon monoxide poisoning, radiation sickness

DESIRED OUTCOMES/EVALUATION CRITERIA

Sample NOC linkages:

Symptom Severity: Severity of perceived adverse changes in physical, emotional, and social functioning

Knowledge: Personal Safety: Extent of understanding conveyed about prevention of unintentional injuries

Risk Control: Personal actions to prevent, eliminate, or reduce modifiable health threats

Client Will (Include Specific Time Frame)

- Be free of injury.
- Verbalize understanding of individual factors that contributed to injury and plans for correcting situation(s) where possible.
- Modify environment, as indicated, to enhance safety.

Sample NOC linkages:

Community Health Status: General state of well-being of a community or population

Community Risk Control: Lead Exposure: Community actions to reduce lead exposure and poisoning

Community Disaster Readiness: Community preparedness to respond to a natural or man-made calamitous event

Client/Community Will (Include Specific Time Frame)

- Identify hazards that led to exposure/contamination.
- Correct environmental hazards, as identified.
- Demonstrate necessary actions to promote community safety.

ACTIONS/INTERVENTIONS

In reviewing this ND, it is apparent there is overlap with other diagnoses. We have chosen to present generalized interventions. Although there are commonalities to Contamination situations, we suggest that the reader refer to other primary diagnoses, as indicated, such as ineffective Airway Clearance, ineffective Breathing Pattern, impaired Gas Exchange, ineffective Home Maintenance, risk for Infection, risk for Injury, risk for Poisoning, impaired/risk for impaired Skin Integrity, Suffocation, ineffective Tissue Perfusion, and Trauma.

Sample NIC linkages:

Risk Identification: Analyzing potential risk factors, determining health risks, and prioritizing risk-reduction strategies for an individual or group

Community Health Development: Assisting members of a community to identify a community's health concerns, moblize resources, and implement solutions

Environmental Risk Protection: Preventing and detecting disease and injury in populations at risk from environmental hazards

NURSING PRIORITY NO. 1 To evaluate degree/source of exposure:

- Ascertain (1) type of contaminant(s) to which client has been exposed (e.g., chemical, biological, air pollutant); (2) manner of exposure (e.g., inhalation, ingestion, topical);

(3) whether exposure was accidental or intentional; and (4) immediate/delayed reactions. *Determines course of action to be taken by all emergency/other care providers. Note: Intentional exposure to hazardous materials requires notification of law enforcement for further investigation and possible prosecution.*[1-6]

∞ • Note age and gender. *Children (less than 5 years of age) are at greater risk for adverse effects from exposure to contaminants because (1) smaller body size causes them to receive a more concentrated "dose" than adults; (2) they spend more time outside than most adults, increasing exposure to air and soil pollutants; (3) young children spend more time on the floor, increasing exposure to toxins in carpets and low cupboards;(4) they consume more water and food per pound than adults, increasing their body-weight-to-toxin ratio; and (5) development of fetal/infant and young children's organ systems can be disrupted. Older adults have a normal decline in function of immune, integumentary, cardiac, renal, hepatic, and pulmonary systems, an increase in adipose tissue mass, and a decline in lean body mass. Females in general have a greater proportion of body fat, increasing the chance of accumulating more lipid soluble toxins than men.*[1-6]

• Ascertain geographic location (e.g., home/work) where exposure occurred. *Individual and/or community intervention may be needed to modify/correct problem.*

• Note socioeconomic status/availability and use of resources. *Living in poverty increases potential for multiple exposures, delayed/lack of access to healthcare, and poor general health potentially increasing the severity of adverse effects of exposure.*[6]

• Determine factors associated with particular contaminant:

  Pesticides: Determine if client has ingested contaminated foods (e.g., fruits, vegetables, commercially raised meats) or inhaled agent (e.g., aerosol bug sprays, in vicinity of crop spraying).[2,3,9]

  Chemicals: Ascertain if client uses environmental contaminants in the home or at work (e.g., pesticides, chemicals, chlorine household cleaners) and fails to use/inappropriately uses protective clothing.[2,3,9]

  Pollution Air/Water: Determine if client has been exposed/is sensitive to atmospheric pollutants (e.g., radon, benzene [from gasoline], carbon monoxide, automobile emissions [numerous chemicals], chlorofluorocarbons [refrigerants, solvents], ozone/smog, particles [acids, organic chemicals, particles in smoke], commercial plants [e.g., pulp and paper mills]).[7]

  Investigate possibility of home-based exposure to air pollution—carbon monoxide (e.g., poor ventilation, especially in the winter months [poor heating systems/use of charcoal grill indoors, car left running in garage]; cigarette/cigar smoke indoors; ozone (spends a lot of time outdoors such as playing children, adults participating in moderate to strenuous work or recreational activities).[7]

  Biologicals: Determine if client may have been exposed to biological agents (bacteria, viruses, fungi) or bacterial toxins (e.g., botulinum, ricin). *Exposure occurring as a result of an act of terrorism would be rare; however, individuals may be exposed to bacterial agents or toxins through contaminated/poorly prepared foods.*

  Waste: Determine if client lives in area where trash/garbage accumulates or is exposed to raw sewage or industrial wastes that can contaminate soil and water.

  Radiation: Ascertain if client/household member experienced accidental exposure (e.g., occupation in radiography, living near/working in nuclear industries, or electrical generating plants).

• Observe for signs and symptoms of infective agent and sepsis, such as fatigue, malaise, headache, fever, chills, diaphoresis, skin rash, and altered level of consciousness. *Initial symptoms of some diseases may mimic influenza and be misdiagnosed if healthcare providers do not maintain an index of suspicion.*

Cultural   Collaborative   Community/Home Care   Diagnostic Studies   Pediatric/Geriatric/Lifespan   Medications

- Note presence and degree of chemical burns and initial treatment provided.
- Obtain/assist with diagnostic studies, as indicated. *Provides information about type and degree of exposure/organ involvement or damage.*
- Identify psychological response (e.g., anger, shock, acute anxiety, confusion, denial) to accidental or mass exposure incident. *Although these are normal responses, they may recycle repeatedly and result in post-trauma syndrome if not dealt with adequately.*
- Alert proper authorities to presence/exposure to contamination, as appropriate. *Depending on agent, there may be reporting requirements to local/state/national agencies such as the local health department and Centers for Disease Control and Prevention (CDC).*

NURSING PRIORITY NO. 2 To assist in treating effects of exposure:

- Implement a coordinated decontamination plan (e.g., removal of clothing, showering with soap and water), when indicated, following consultation with medical toxicologist, hazardous materials team, industrial hygiene, and safety officer *to prevent further harm to client and to protect healthcare providers.*[8]
- Insure availablity of/use personal protective equipment (PPE) (e.g., high-efficiency particulate air [HEPA] filter masks, special garments, and barrier materials, including gloves/face shield) *to protect from exposure to biological, chemical, and radioactive hazards.*[10]
- Provide for isolation or group/cohort individuals with same diagnosis/exposure, as resources require. *Limited resources may dictate open wardlike environment; however, the need to control spread of infection still exists. Only plague, smallpox, and viral hemorrhagic fevers require more than standard infection control precautions.*
- Provide/assist with therapeutic interventions, as individually appropriate. *Specific needs of the client and the level of care available at a given time/location determine response.*
- Refer pregnant client for individually appropriate diagnostic procedures/screenings. *Helpful in determining effects of teratogenic exposure on fetus allowing for informed choices/preparations.*[14]
- Screen breast milk in lactating client following radiation exposure. *Depending on type and amount of exposure, breastfeeding may need to be briefly interrupted or occasionally terminated.*[12,13]
- Cooperate with/refer to appropriate agencies (e.g., the Centers for Disease Control and Prevention [CDC]; U.S. Army Medical Research Institute of Infectious Diseases [USAMRIID]; Federal Emergency Management Agency [FEMA]; Department of Health and Human Services [DHHS]; Office of Emergency Preparedness [OEP]; and Environmental Protection Agency [EPA]) *to prepare for and manage mass casualty incidents.*[9,10]

NURSING PRIORITY NO. 3 To promote wellness (Teaching/Discharge Considerations):

Client/Caregiver

- Identify individual safety needs and injury/illness prevention in home, community, and work setting.
- Install carbon monoxide monitors and a radon detector in home, as appropriate.
- Review individual nutritional needs, appropriate exercise program, and need for rest. *Essentials for well-being and recovery.*
- Repair/replace/correct unsafe household items/situations (e.g., storage of solvents in soda bottles, flaking/peeling paint or plaster, filtering unsafe tap water).
- Stress importance of supervising infant/child or individuals with cognitive limitations.

- 🏠 • Encourage removal of/cleaning of carpeted floors, especially for small children and persons with respiratory conditions. *Carpets hold up to 100 times as much fine particle material as a bare floor and can contain metals, pesticides.*[1]
- 🏠 • Identify commericial cleaning resources, if appropriate, *for safe cleaning of contaminated articles/surfaces.*
- 🏠 • Install dehumidifier in damp areas *to retard growth of molds.*[1]
- 🏠 • Encourage timely cleaning/replacement of air filters on furnace and air-conditioning unit. *Good ventilation cuts down on indoor air pollution from carpets, machines, paints, solvents, cleaning materials, and pesticides.*
- 🏠 • Discuss protective actions for specific "bad air" days (e.g., limiting /avoiding outdoor activities), especially in sensitive groups (e.g., children who are active outdoors, adults involved in moderate or strenuous outdoor activities, persons with respiratory diseases).[6]
- 🏠 • Review effects of secondhand smoke and importance of refraining from smoking in home/car where others are likely to be exposed.
- 🏠 • Recommend periodic inspection of well water/tap water *to identify possible contaminants.*
- 🏠 • Encourage client/caregiver to develop a personal/family disaster plan; to gather needed supplies to provide for self/family during a community emergncy; and to learn how specific public health threats might affect client and actions *to reduce the risk to health and safety.*
- 🏠 • Instruct client to always refer to local authorities and health experts for specific up-to-date information for community and to follow their advice.
- 🔗 • Refer to counselor/support groups for ongoing assistance in dealing with traumatic incident/aftereffects of exposure.
- 🏠 • Provide bibliotherapy/written resources and appropriate Web sites *for later review and self-paced learning.*
- 🔗 • Refer to smoking cessation program, as needed.

Community

- 🏠 • Promote community education programs in different modalities/languages/cultures and educational levels geared *to increasing awareness of safety measures and resources available to individuals/community.*
- 🏠 • Review pertinent job-related health department/OSHA regulations.
- 🏠 • Refer to resources that provide information about air quality (e.g., pollen index, "bad air days").
- 🏠 • Encourage community members/groups to engage in problem-solving activities.
- 🔗 • Verify presence/participate in developing a comprehensive disaster plan for the community that includes a chain of command, equipment, communication, training, decontamination area(s), and safety and security plans *to ensure an effective response to any emergency (e.g., flood, toxic spill, infectious disease outbreak, radiation release).*[11]

DOCUMENTATION FOCUS

Assessment/Reassessment

- • Details of specific exposure, including location and circumstances.
- • Client's/caregiver's understanding of individual risks/safety concerns.

Planning

- • Plan of care and who is involved in planning.
- • Teaching plan.

🌐 Cultural   🔗 Collaborative   🏠 Community/Home Care   Diagnostic Studies   ∞ Pediatric/Geriatric/Lifespan   Medications

Implementation/Evaluation
- Individual responses to interventions/teaching and actions performed.
- Specific actions and changes that are made.
- Attainment/progress toward desired outcome(s).
- Modifications to plan of care.

Discharge Planning
- Long-range plans for discharge needs, lifestyle and community changes, and who is responsible for actions to be taken.
- Specific referrals made.

References

1. McElgunn, V. (1990). Environmental hazards and child health and development: Advances in research and policy. Presentation in the Linking Research to Practice: Second Canadian Forum Proceedings Report and published by the Canadian Child Care Federation. Retrieved February 2007 at www.cfc-efc.ca/cccf.
2. No author listed. (1999). Chemical toxins safety. Fact sheet for Resources for Child Care Givers. All Family Resources Web site. Retrieved February 2007 at. http://familymanagement.com/childcare/facility/chemical.toxins.safety.html.
3. Rajen, M. (2006). Toxins everywhere. Article for *New Straits Times*. Retrieved February 2007 at www.redorbit.com/news/health/786618/toxins_everywhere/index.html.
4. Stabin, M. G., Breitz, H. (2000). Breast milk secretion of radiopharmaceuticals; mechanisms, findings, and radiation dosimetry. *J Nuclear Med*, 41(5), 863–873.
5. Environmental Protection Agency. (1998). The EPA Children's Evironmental Health Yearbook, Chapter 1. United States Department of Health and Human Services. Washington, DC.
6. Wilkinson, R., Marmot, M. (2003). *Social Determinants of Health: The Solid Facts.* 2d ed. World Health Organization.
7. No author listed. (1999). Smog—Who does it hurt? What you need to know about ozone and your health. Public information brochure. United States Environmental Protection Agency. Washington, DC.
8. Jagminas, L. (2005). CBRN-Evaluation of a biological warfare victim. Article for Emedicine Web site. Retrieved February 2007 at www.emedicine.com/emerg/topic891.htm.
9. Jagminas, L., Erdman, D. P. (2006). CBRNE—Chemical decontamination. Article for Emedicine Web site. Retrieved February 2007 at www.emedicine.com/emerg/topic893.htm.
10. Arnold, J. L. (2006). Personal protective equipment. Article for patient education, eMedicineHealth Web site. Retrieved February 2007 at www.emedicinehealth.com.
11. Bauer, J., Steinhauer, R. (2002). A readied response: The emergency plan. *RN*, 65(6), 40.
12. Centers for Disease Control and Prevention: When should a mother avoid breastfeeding. August 2006. Accessed February2007 at www.cdc.gov/breastfeeding/disease/contraindicators.htm.
13. Breastfeeding guidelines following radiopharmaceutical administration. Accessed February 2007 at http://nuclearpharmacy.uams.edu/resources/breastfeeding.asp.
14. American Academy of Family Physicians: Breastfeeding (Position paper). Accessed February 2007 at www.aafp.org/online/en/home/policy/policies/b/breastfeedingpositionpaper.html.

risk for Contamination

Definition: Accentuated risk of exposure to environmental contaminants in doses sufficient to cause adverse health effects

RISK FACTORS

External
Chemical contamination of food/water; presence of atmospheric pollutants
Inadequate municipal services (trash removal, sewage treatment facilities)

Geographic area (living in area where high level of contaminants exist)

Playing in outdoor areas where environmental contaminants are used

Personal/household hygiene practices

Living in poverty (increases potential for multiple exposure, lack of access to healthcare, and poor diet)

Use of environmental contaminants in the home (e.g., pesticides, chemicals, environmental tobacco smoke)

Lack of breakdown of contaminants once indoors (breakdown is inhibited without sun and rain exposure)

Flooring surface (carpeted surfaces hold contaminant residue more than hard floor surfaces)

Flaking, peeling paint/plaster in presence of young children

Paint, lacquer, etc., in poorly ventilated areas/without effective protection

Inappropriate use/lack of protective clothing

Unprotected contact with heavy metals or chemicals (e.g., arsenic, chromium, lead)

Exposure to radiation (occupation in radiography, employment in nuclear industries and electrical generating plants, living near nuclear industries and electrical generation plants)

Exposure to disaster (natural or man-made); exposure to bioterrorism

Internal

Age (children less than 5 years, older adults); gestational age during exposure; developmental characteristics of children

Female gender; pregnancy

Nutritional factors (e.g., obesity, vitamin and mineral deficiencies)

Preexisting disease states; smoking

Concomitant exposure; previous exposures

NOTE: A risk diagnosis is not evidenced by signs and symptoms, as the problem has not occurred; rather, nursing interventions are directed at prevention.

Sample Clinical Applications: E. coli infection, plague, hantavirus, asthma, botulism, cholera, lead or other heavy metal poisoning, chemical burns, asbestosis, carbon monoxide poisoning, radiation sickness

DESIRED OUTCOMES/EVALUATION CRITERIA

Sample NOC linkages:

Knowledge: Personal Safety: Extent of understanding conveyed about prevention of unintentional injuries

Risk Control: Personal actions to prevent, eliminate, or reduce modifiable health threats

Client Will (Include Specific Time Frame)

• Verbalize understanding of individual factors that contribute to possibility of injury and take steps to correct situation(s).

• Demonstrate behaviors, lifestyle changes to reduce risk factors and protect self from injury.

• Modify environment as indicated to enhance safety.

• Be free of injury.

• Support community activities for disaster preparedness.

Sample NOC linkages:

Community Health Status: General state of well-being of a community or population

Community Risk Control: Lead Exposure: Community actions to reduce lead exposure and poisoning

⊕ Cultural   🅐 Collaborative   🏠 Community/Home Care   ⚗ Diagnostic Studies   ∞ Pediatric/Geriatric/Lifespan   💊 Medications

Community Disaster Readiness: Community preparedness to respond to a natural or man-made calamitous event

---

Community Will (Include Specific Time Frame)

• Identify hazards that could lead to exposure/contamination.
• Correct environmental hazards as identified.
• Demonstrate necessary actions to promote community safety/disaster preparedness.

ACTIONS/INTERVENTIONS

Sample NIC linkages:

Risk Identification: Analysis of potential risk factors, determination of health risks, and prioritization of risk-reduction strategies for an individual or group

Community Health Development: Assisting members of a community to identify a community's health concerns, moblize resources, and implement solutions

Environmental Risk Protection: Preventing and detecting disease and injury in populations at risk from environmental hazards

NURSING PRIORITY NO. 1 To evaluate degree/source of risk inherent in the home/community/work site:

• Ascertain type of contaminant(s) and exposure routes posing a potential hazard to client or community (e.g., air/soil/water pollutants, food source, chemical, biological, radiation) as listed in Risk Factors. *Determines course of action to be taken by client/community/care providers.*
• Note age and gender of client/community base (e.g., community health clinic serving primarily poor children or elderly; school near large industrial plant, family living in smog-prone area). *Young children, frail elderly, and females have been found to be at higher risk for effects of exposure to toxins.*[1,2] *(Refer to ND Contamination.)*
• Ascertain client's geographic location at home/work (e.g., lives where crop spraying is routine; works in nuclear plant; contract worker/soldier returning from combat area). *Individual and/or community intervention may be needed to reduce risks of accidental/intentional exposures.*
• Note socioeconomic status/availability and use of resources. *Living in poverty increases the potential for multiple exposures, delayed/lack of access to healthcare, and poor general health.*[3]
• Determine client's/SO's understanding of potential risk and appropriate protective measures.

NURSING PRIORITY NO. 2 To assist client to reduce or correct individual risk factors:

• Assist client to develop plan to address individual safety needs and injury/illness prevention in home, community, and work setting.
• Repair/replace/correct unsafe household items/situations (e.g., flaking/peeling paint or plaster, filtering unsafe tap water).
• Review effects of secondhand smoke and importance of refraining from smoking in home/car *where others are likely to be exposed.*
• Encourage removal/cleaning of carpeted floors, especially for small children, persons with respiratory conditions. *Carpets hold up to 100 times as much fine particle material as a bare floor and can contain metals, pesticides.*[1]
• Encourage timely cleaning/replacement of air filters on furnace and air-conditioning unit. *Good ventilation cuts down on indoor air pollution from carpets, machines, paints, solvents, cleaning materials, and pesticides.*

• Recommend periodic inspection of well water/tap water *to identify possible contaminants.*

• Encourage client to install carbon monoxide monitors and a radon detector in home as appropriate.

• Recommend placing dehumidifier in damp areas *to retard growth of molds.*

• Review proper handling of household chemicals:[4,5]

Read chemical labels *to be aware of primary hazards (especially in commonly used household cleaning/gardening products).*

Follow directions printed on product label (e.g., avoid use of certain chemicals on food preparation surfaces, refrain from spraying garden chemicals on windy days).

Choose least hazardous products for the job, preferably multiuse products *to reduce number of different chemicals used/stored.* Use products labeled "nontoxic" wherever possible.

Use form of chemical that most reduces risk of exposure (e.g., cream instead of liquid or aerosol).

Wear protective clothing, gloves, and safety glasses when using chemicals. Avoid mixing chemicals at all times, and use in well-ventilated areas.

Store chemicals in locked cabinets. Keep chemicals in original labeled containers and do not pour into other containers.

 Place safety stickers on chemicals *to warn children of harmful contents.*

• Review proper food-handling/storage/cooking techniques.

• Stress importance of pregnant or lactating women following fish/wildlife consumption guidelines provided by state/U.S. territorial or Native American tribes. *Ingestion of non-commercial fish/wildlife can be a significant source of pollutants.*[8]

NURSING PRIORITY NO. 3 To promote wellness (Teaching/Discharge Considerations):

Home

• Discuss general safety concerns with client/SO.

• Stress importance of supervising infant/child or individuals with cognitive limitations.

• Post emergency and poison control numbers in a visible location.

• Encourage learning CPR and first aid.

• Discuss protective actions for specific "bad air" days (e.g., limiting /avoiding outdoor activities).

• Review pertinent job-related safety regulations. Stress necessity of wearing appropriate protective equipment.

• Encourage client/caregiver develop a personal/family disaster plan, to gather needed supplies to provide for self/family during a community emergncy; to learn how specific public health threats might affect client and actions to promote preparedness and reduce the risk to health and safety.

• Provide information/refer to appropriate resourses about potential toxic hazards and protective measures. Provide bibliotherapy/written resources and appropriate Web sites *for client review and self-paced learning.*

• Refer to smoking cessation program as needed.

Community

• Promote education programs geared toward increasing awareness of safety measures and resources available to individuals/community.

• Review pertinent job-related health department/OSHA regulations to safeguard the workplace and the community.

🏠 • Verify presence/participate in developing a comprehensive disaster plan for the community that includes a chain of command, equipment, communication, training, decontamination area(s), safety and security plans *to ensure an effective response to any emergency (e.g., flood, toxic spill, infectious disease outbreak, radiation release).*[6]

• Refer to appropriate agencies (e.g., Centers for Disease Control and Prevention [CDC], U.S. Army Medical Research Institute of Infectious Diseases [USAMRIID]; Federal Emergency Management Agency [FEMA]; Department of Health and Human Services [DHHS], Office of Emergency Preparedness [OEP]; Environmental Protection Agency [EPA]) *to prepare for and manage mass casualty incidents.*[7]

DOCUMENTATION FOCUS

Assessment/Reassessment

• Client's/caregiver's understanding of individual risks/safety concerns.

Planning

• Plan of care and who is involved in planning.
• Teaching plan.

Implementation/Evaluation

• Individual responses to interventions/teaching and actions performed.
• Specific actions and changes that are made.
• Attainment/progress toward desired outcome(s).
• Modifications to plan of care.

Discharge Planning

• Long-range plans, lifestyle and community changes, and who is responsible for actions to be taken.
• Specific referrals made.

References

1. McElgunn, V. (1990). Environmental hazards and child health and development: Advances in research and policy. Presentation in the Linking Research to Practice: Second Canadian Forum Proceedings Report and published by the Canadian Child Care Federation. Retrieved February 2007 at www.cfc-efc.ca/cccf.
2. Evironmental Protection Agency. (1998). The EPA Children's Evironmental Health Yearbook, Chapter 1. United States Department of Health and Human Services. Washington, DC.
3. Wilkinson, R., Marmot, M. (2003). *Social Determinants of Health: The Solid Facts.* 2d ed. World Health Organization.
4. Rajen, M. (2006). Toxins everywhere. Article for *New Straits Times.* Retrieved February 2007 at www.redorbit.com/news/health/786618/toxins_everywhere/index.html.
5. No author listed. (1999). Chemical toxins safety. Fact sheet for Resources for Child Care Givers. All Family Resources Web site. Retrieved February 2007 at http://familymanagement.com/childcare/facility/chemical.toxins.safety.html.
6. Bauer, J., Steinhauer, R. (2002). A readied response: The emergency plan. *RN*, 65(6), 40.
7. Jagminas, L., Erdman, D. P. (2006). CBRNE-Chemical decontamination. Article for Emedicine Web site. Retrieved February 2007 at www.emedicime.com/emerg/topic893.htm.
8. American Academy of Family Physicians: Breastfeeding (Position paper). Accessed February 2007 at www.aafp.org/online/en/home/policy/policies/b/breastfeedingpositionpaper.html.

compromised family Coping

Definition: Usually supportive primary person (family member or close friend [SO]) provides insufficient, ineffective, or compromised support, comfort, assistance, or encouragement that may be needed by the client to manage or master adaptive tasks related to his or her health challenge

RELATED FACTORS

Coexisting situations affecting the significant person

Developmental/situational crises the significant person may be facing

Prolonged disease [or disability progression] that exhausts the supportive capacity of SO(s)

Exhaustion of supportive capacity of significant people

Inadequate/incorrect understanding of information by a primary person

Lack of reciprocal support; little support provided by client, in turn, for primary person; [unrealistic expectations of client/SO(s) or each other]

Temporary preoccupation by a significant person

Temporary family disorganization/role changes

[Lack of mutual decision-making skills]

[Diverse coalitions of family members]

DEFINING CHARACTERISTICS

Subjective

Client expresses a complaint/concern about significant other's response to health problem

SO expresses an inadequate knowledge base/understanding, which interferes with effective supportive behaviors

SO describes preoccupation with personal reaction (e.g., fear, anticipatory grief, guilt, anxiety) to client's need

---

Objective

SO attempts assistive/supportive behaviors with less-than-satisfactory results

SO displays protective behavior disproportionate to the client's abilities/need for autonomy

SO enters into limited personal communication with client

SO withdraws from client

[SO displays sudden outbursts of emotions/emotional lability or interferes with necessary nursing/medical interventions]

Sample Clinical Applications: Chronic conditions (e.g., COPD, AIDS, Alzheimer's disease, pain, renal failure), substance abuse, cancer, depression, hypochondriasis

DESIRED OUTCOMES/EVALUATION CRITERIA

Sample NOC linkages:

Family Coping: Family actions to manage stressors that tax family resources

Family Normalization: Capacity of the family system to maintain routines and develop strategies for optimal functioning when a member has a chronic illness or disability

Family Social Climate: Supportive milieu as characterized by family member relationships and goals

---

Family Will (Include Specific Time Frame)

- Identify/verbalize resources within themselves to deal with the situation.
- Interact appropriately with the client, providing support and assistance, as indicated.
- Provide opportunity for client to deal with situation in own way.
- Verbalize knowledge and understanding of illness/disability/disease.

Cultural · Collaborative · Community/Home Care · Diagnostic Studies · Pediatric/Geriatric/Lifespan · Medications

- Express feelings honestly.
- Identify need for outside support and seek such.

ACTIONS/INTERVENTIONS

Sample NIC linkages:

Family Involvement Promotion: Facilitating family participation in the emotional and physical care of the patient

Family Support: Promotion of family values, interests, and goals

Family Mobilization: Utilization of family strengths to influence patient's health in a positive direction

NURSING PRIORITY NO. 1 To assess causative/contributing factors:

- Identify underlying situation(s) that may contribute to the inability of family to provide needed assistance to the client. *Circumstances may have preceded the illness and now have a significant effect (e.g., client had a heart attack during sexual activity, mate is afraid of repeating).*[1]
- Note cultural factors related to family relationships that may be involved in problems of caring for member who is ill. *Family composition and structure, methods of decision making, and gender issues and expectations will affect how family deals with stress of illness/negative prognosis. Depending on role the client has in the family, such as mother or father, other members may have difficulty assuming authoritative role and managing the family.*[6]
- Note the length of illness, such as cancer, multiple sclerosis, and/or other long-term situations that may exist. *Chronic/unresolved illness, accompanied by changes in role performance/responsibility, often exhausts supportive capacity and coping abilities of SO/family.*[1]
- Assess information available to and understood by the family/SO(s). *Access to and understanding of information regarding the specific illness/condition and treatment and prognosis is essential to family cooperation and care of the client.*[2,3]
- Discuss family perceptions of situation. *Expectations of client and family members may/may not be realistic and may interfere with ability to cope with situation.*[1]
- Identify role of the client in family and how illness has changed the family organization. *Illness affects how client performs usual functions in the family and affects how others in the family take over those responsibilities. These changes may result in dysfunctional behaviors, anger, hostility, and hopelessness.*[1]
- Note other factors, besides the client's illness, that are affecting abilities of family members to provide needed support. *Individual members' preoccupation with own needs/concerns can interfere with providing needed care/support for stresses of long-term illness. Additionally, caregivers may incur decrease or loss of income/risk of losing own health insurance if they alter their work hours to care for client.*[1]

NURSING PRIORITY NO. 2 To assist family to reactivate/develop skills to deal with current situation:

- Listen to client's/SO's comments, remarks, and expression of concern(s). Note nonverbal behaviors and responses and congruency. *Provides information and promotes understanding of client's view of the illness and needs related to current situation.*[1]
- Encourage family members to verbalize feelings openly/clearly. *Promotes understanding of feelings in relationship to current events and helps them to hear what other person is saying, leading to more appropriate interactions.*[5]

- Discuss underlying reasons for client's behavior. *Helps family/SO understand and accept/deal with client behaviors that may be triggered by emotional or physical effects of illness.*[4]
- Assist the family and client to understand "who owns the problem" and who is responsible for resolution. Avoid placing blame or guilt. *When these boundaries are defined, each individual can begin to take care of own self and stop taking care of others in inappropriate ways.*[3,4]
- Encourage client and family to develop problem-solving skills to deal with the situation. *Use of these skills enables each member of the family to identify what he or she sees as the problem to be dealt with and contribute ideas for solutions that are acceptable to them, promoting more effective interactions among the family members.*[4]

NURSING PRIORITY NO. 3 To promote wellness (Teaching/Discharge Considerations):

- Provide information for family/SO(s) about specific illness/condition. *Promotes better understanding of need for following therapeutic regimen to provide maximum benefit.*[8]
- Involve client and family in planning care as often as possible. *When family members are knowledgeable and understand needs, commitment to plan is enhanced.*[7,8]
- Promote assistance of family in providing client care, as appropriate. *Identifies ways of demonstrating support while maintaining client's independence (e.g., providing favorite foods, engaging in diversional activities).*[5]
- Refer to appropriate resources for assistance, as indicated (e.g., counseling, psychotherapy, financial, spiritual). *May need additional help, and getting to the appropriate resource provides accurate help for individual situation (e.g., family counseling, financial planning).*[7,8]
- Refer to NDs Anxiety, death Anxiety, ineffective Coping, readiness for enhanced family Coping, disabled family Coping, Fear, Grieving, as appropriate.

DOCUMENTATION FOCUS

Assessment/Reassessment

- Assessment findings, including current/past coping behaviors, emotional response to situation/stressors, support systems available.

Planning

- Plan of care, who is involved in planning and areas of responsibility.
- Teaching plan.

Implementation/Evaluation

- Responses of family members/client to interventions/teaching and actions performed.
- Attainment/progress toward desired outcome(s).
- Modifications to plan of care.

Discharge Planning

- Long-range plan and who is responsible for actions.
- Specific referrals made.

References

1. Doenges, M., Moorhouse, M., Geissler-Murr, A. (2002). *Nursing Care Plans Guidelines for Individualizing Patient Care.* 6th ed. Philadelphia: F. A. Davis.
2. Bluman, I. G., et al. (1999). Attitudes, knowledge, and risk perceptions of women with breast and/or ovarian cancer considering testing for BRCA1 and BRCA2. *J Clin Oncol,* 17(3), 1040–1046.

Cultural   Collaborative   Community/Home Care   Diagnostic Studies   Pediatric/Geriatric/Lifespan   Medications

3. Doenges, M., Townsend, M., Moorhouse, M. (1998). Psychiatric Care Plans: Guidelines for Individualizing Care. 3d ed. Philadelphia: F. A. Davis.
4. Townsend, M. (2006). *Psychiatric Mental Health Nursing: Concepts of Care*. 5th ed. Philadelphia: F. A. Davis.
5. Cox, H., Hinz, M., Lubno, M. A., Newfield, S., Ridenour, N., Slater, M., Sridaromont, K. (2002). *Clinical Applications of Nursing Diagnosis: Adult, Child, Women's, Psychiatric, Gerontic and Home Health Considerations*. 4th ed. Philadelphia: F. A. Davis.
6. Lipson, J. G., Dibble, S. L., Minarik, P. A. (1996). *Culture & Nursing Care: A Pocket Guide.* San Francisco: School of Nursing, UCSF Nursing Press.
7. Haeven, T. K., Adams, K. J. (eds). (1982). Aging and life course transitions: An interdisciplinary perspective. New York: Guilford.
8. Ammon, S. (2001). Managing patients with heart failure. *AJN*, 101(12), 34–40.

defensive Coping

Definition: Repeated projection of falsely positive self-evaluation based on a self-protective pattern that defends against underlying perceived threats to positive self-regard

RELATED FACTORS
To be developed by nurse researchers and submitted to NANDA
[Refer to ND ineffective Coping]

DEFINING CHARACTERISTICS

Subjective
Denial of obvious problems/weaknesses
Projection of blame/responsibility
Hypersensitive to slight/criticism
Grandiosity
Rationalizes failures
[Refuses or rejects assistance]

Objective
Superior attitude toward others
Difficulty establishing/maintaining relationships; [avoidance of intimacy]
Hostile laughter; ridicule of others; [aggressive behavior]
Difficulty in perception of reality/reality testing
Lack of follow-through in treatment/therapy
Lack of participation in treatment/therapy
[Attention-seeking behavior]

Sample Clinical Applications: Eating disorders, substance abuse, chronic illness, bipolar/adjustment/dissociative disorders

DESIRED OUTCOMES/EVALUATION CRITERIA
Sample NOC linkages:
Self-Esteem: Personal judgment of self-worth
Coping: Actions to manage stressors that tax an individual's resources
Social Interaction Skills: An individual's use of effective interaction behaviors

Client Will (Include Specific Time Frame)
- Verbalize understanding of own problems/stressors.
- Identify areas of concern/problems.

- Demonstrate acceptance of responsibility for own actions, successes, and failures.
- Participate in treatment program/therapy.
- Maintain involvement in relationships.

ACTIONS/INTERVENTIONS

Sample NIC linkages:

Self-Awareness Enhancement: Assisting a patient to explore and understand his or her thoughts, feelings, motivations, and behaviors

Coping Enhancement: Assisting a patient to adapt to perceived stressors, changes, or threats that interfere with meeting life demands and roles

Counseling: Use of an interactive helping process focusing on the needs, problems, or feelings of the patient and significant others to enhance or support coping, problem-solving, and interpersonal relationships

NURSING PRIORITY NO. 1 To determine degree of impairment:

- Assess ability to comprehend current situation, developmental level of functioning. *Crucial to planning care for this individual. Client will have difficulty functioning in these circumstances.*[1]
- Determine level of anxiety and effectiveness of current coping mechanisms. *Severe anxiety will interfere with ability to cope, and client will need to assess what is working and develop new ways to deal with current situation.*[2]
- Perform/review results of testing, such as Taylor Manifest Anxiety Scale (I-MAS) and Marlowe-Crowne Social Desirability Scale (MCSDS), as indicated. *Helps to identify coping styles, enabling more accurate therapeutic interventions.*
- Determine coping mechanisms used (e.g., projection, avoidance, rationalization) and purpose of coping strategy (e.g., may mask low self-esteem). *Provides information about how these behaviors affect current situation.*[3]
- Assist client to identify/consider need to address problem differently. *Until client is willing to consider different approaches to dealing with situation, little progress can be expected.*[1]
- Describe all aspects of the problem through the use of therapeutic communication skills such as Active-listening. *Provides an opportunity for the client to clarify the situation and begin to look at options for problem-solving.*[2]
- Observe interactions with others. *Noting difficulties/ability to establish satisfactory relationships can provide clues to client behaviors that interfere with interactions with others.*[2]
- Note expressions of grandiosity in the face of contrary evidence (e.g., "I'm going to buy a new car" when the individual has no job or available finances). *Evidence of distorted thinking and possibility of mental illness.*[3]
- Assess physical condition. *Defensive coping style has been connected with physical well-being and illnesses, especially chronic health concerns (e.g., CHF, diabetes, chronic fatigue syndrome).*[5]

NURSING PRIORITY NO. 2 To assist client to deal with current situation:

- Provide explanation of the rules of the treatment program and discuss consequences of lack of cooperation. Encourage client participation in setting of consequences and agreement to them. *Promotes understanding and possibility of cooperation on the part of the client, especially when they have been involved in the decisions.*[2]
- Set limits on manipulative behavior; be consistent in enforcing consequences when rules are broken and limits tested. *Providing clear information and following through on identified consequences reduces the ability to manipulate staff/therapist and environment.*[3]

Cultural Collaborative Community/Home Care Diagnostic Studies Pediatric/Geriatric/Lifespan Medications

- Develop therapeutic relationship to enable client to test new behaviors in a safe environment. Use positive, nonjudgmental approach and "I" language. *Promotes sense of self-esteem and enhances sense of control.*[1]
- Encourage control in all situations possible; include client in decisions and planning. *Preserves autonomy, enabling realization of sense of self-worth.*[1]
- Acknowledge individual strengths and incorporate awareness of personal assets/strengths in plan. *Promotes use of positive coping behaviors and progress toward effective solutions.*[4]
- Convey attitude of acceptance and respect (unconditional positive regard). *Avoids threatening client's self-concept, preserving existing self-esteem.*[2]
- Encourage identification and expression of feelings. *Provides opportunity for client to learn about and accept self and feelings as normal.*[2]
- Provide/encourage use of healthy outlets for release of hostile feelings (e.g., punching bags, pounding boards). Involve in outdoor recreation program when available. *Promotes acceptable expression of these feelings, which, when unexpressed, can lead to development of undesirable behaviors and make situation worse.*[4]
- Provide opportunities for client to interact with others in a positive manner. *Promotes self-esteem and encourages client to learn how to develop/enhance relationships.*[4]
- Assist client with problem-solving process. Identify and discuss responses to situation, maladaptive coping skills. Suggest alternative responses to situation. *Helps client select more adaptive strategies for coping.*[2]
- Use confrontation judiciously *to help client begin to identify defense mechanisms (e.g., denial/projection) that are hindering development of satisfying relationships.*[2]
- Assist with treatments for physical illnesses as appropriate. *Taking care of physical self will enable client to deal with emotional and psychological issues more effectively.*[4]

NURSING PRIORITY NO. 3 To promote wellness (Teaching/Discharge Considerations):

- Use cognitive-behavioral therapy. *Helps change negative thinking patterns when rigidly held beliefs are used by client to defend the individual against low self-esteem.*[3]
- Encourage client to learn/use relaxation techniques, guided imagery, and positive affirmation of self. *Enables client to incorporate and practice new behaviors to deal with stressors and view/respond to situation in a more realistic and positive manner.*[4]
- Promote involvement in activities/classes. *Client can practice new skills, develop new relationships, and learn new and positive ways of interacting with others.*[1]
- Refer to additional resources (e.g., substance rehabilitation, family/marital therapy), as indicated. *Can be useful in making desired changes and developing new coping skills.*[2]
- Refer to ND ineffective Coping for additional interventions.

DOCUMENTATION FOCUS

Assessment/Reassessment

- Assessment findings/presenting behaviors.
- Client perception of the present situation and usual coping methods/degree of impairment.
- Health concerns.

Planning

- Plan of care and interventions and who is involved in development of the plan.
- Teaching plan.

Implementation/Evaluation

- Response to interventions/teaching and actions performed.
- Attainment/progress toward desired outcome(s).
- Modifications to plan of care.

Discharge Planning

- Referrals and follow-up programming.

References

1. Doenges, M., Moorhouse, M., Murr, A. (2004). *Nursing Care Plans, Guidelines for Individualizing Patient Care.* 7th ed. Philadelphia: F. A. Davis.
2. Doenges, M., Townsend, M., Moorhouse, M. (1998). *Psychiatric Care Plans: Guidelines for Individualizing Care.* 3d ed. Philadelphia: F. A. Davis.
3. Townsend, M. (2006). *Psychiatric Mental Health Nursing: Concepts of Care.* 5th ed. Philadelphia: F. A. Davis.
4. Cox, H., Hinz, M., Lubno, M. A., Newfield, S., Ridenour, N., Slater, M., Sridaromont, K. (2002). *Clinical Applications of Nursing Diagnosis: Adult, Child, Women's Psychiatric, Gerontic and Home Health Considerations.* 4th ed. Philadelphia: F. A. Davis.
5. Creswell, C., Chalder, T. (2001). Defensive coping styles in chronic fatigue syndrome. *J Psychosomatic Research,* 51(4), 607–610.

disabled family Coping

Definition: Behavior of significant person (family member or other primary person) that disables his or her capacities and the client's capacity to effectively address tasks essential to either person's adaptation to the health challenge

RELATED FACTORS

Significant person with chronically unexpressed feelings (e.g., guilt, anxiety, hostility, despair)

Dissonant coping styles for dealing with adaptive tasks by the significant person and client among significant people

Highly ambivalent family relationships

Arbitrary handling of family's resistance to treatment [that tends to solidify defensiveness as it fails to deal adequately with underlying anxiety]

[High-risk family situations, such as single or adolescent parent, abusive relationship, substance abuse, acute/chronic disabilities, member with terminal illness]

DEFINING CHARACTERISTICS

Subjective

[Expresses despair regarding family reactions/lack of involvement]

Objective

Psychosomaticism

Intolerance; rejection; abandonment; desertion; agitation; aggression; hostility; depression

Carrying on usual routines without regard for client's needs; disregarding client's needs

Neglectful care of the client in regard to basic human needs/illness treatment

Neglectful relationships with other family members.

Family behaviors that are detrimental to well-being

Distortion of reality regarding the client's health problem

⊕ Cultural   Ⓐ Collaborative   🏠 Community/Home Care   Diagnostic Studies   ∞ Pediatric/Geriatric/Lifespan   Medications

Impaired restructuring of a meaningful life for self, impaired individualization, prolonged overconcern for client

Taking on illness signs of client

Client's development of dependence

Sample Clinical Applications: Chronic conditions (e.g., COPD, AIDS, Alzheimer's disease, chronic pain, renal failure, brain/spinal cord injury), substance abuse, cancer, genetic conditions (e.g., Down syndrome, sickle cell disease, Huntington's disease), depression, hypochondriasis

DESIRED OUTCOMES/EVALUATION CRITERIA

Sample NOC linkages:

Family Normalization: Capacity of the family system to maintain routines and develop strategies for optimal functioning when a member has a chronic illness or disability

Family Coping: Family actions to manage stressors that tax family resources

Family Social Climate: Supportive milieu as characterized by family member relationships and goals

Family Will (Include Specific Time Frame)

- Verbalize more realistic understanding and expectations of the client.
- Visit/contact client regularly.
- Participate positively in care of client, within limits of family's abilities and client's needs.
- Express feelings and expectations openly and honestly as appropriate.

ACTIONS/INTERVENTIONS

Sample NIC linkages:

Family Therapy: Assisting family members to move their family toward a more productive way of living

Family Support: Promotion of family values, interests, and goals

Family Involvement Promotion: Facilitating family participation in the emotional and physical care of the patient

NURSING PRIORITY NO. 1 To assess causative/contributing factors:

- Ascertain preillness behaviors/interactions of the family. *Provides comparative baseline for developing plan of care and determining interventions needed.*[4,8]
- Identify current behaviors of the family members (e.g., withdrawal-not visiting, brief visits, or ignoring client when visiting; anger and hostility toward client and others; ways of touching between family members, expressions of guilt). *Indicators of extent of problems existing within family. Relationships among family members before and after current illness affect ability to deal with problems of caretaking and lengthy illness.*[1,8]
- Discuss family perceptions of situation. *Expectations of client and family members may/may not be realistic and may interfere with ability to deal with situation.*[6]
- Note cultural factors related to family relationships that may be involved in problems of caring for member who is ill. *Family composition and structure, methods of decision making, gender issues, and expectations will affect how family perceives situation and deals with stress of illness, negative prognosis.*[7]

- Note other factors that may be stressful for the family (e.g., financial difficulties or lack of community support, as when illness occurs when out of town). *Appropriate referrals can be made to provide information and assistance as needed. If not addressed, these problems can lead to caregiver burnout and compassion fatigue.*[6]
- Determine readiness of family members to be involved with care of the client. *Family members are involved in their lives, jobs, and families and may find it difficult to manage tasks necessary for helping with care of the client.*[5,6]

NURSING PRIORITY NO. 2 To provide assistance to enable family to deal with the current situation:

- Establish rapport with family members who are available. *Promotes therapeutic relationship and support for problem-solving solutions.*[1]
- Acknowledge difficulty of the situation for the family. *Communicates understanding of family's feelings and can reduce blaming and guilt feelings.*[2]
- Active-listen to concerns, note both overconcern/lack of concern. *Identifies accuracy of client's information and measure of concern, which may interfere with ability to resolve situation.*[2]
- Allow free expression of feelings, including frustration, anger, hostility, and hopelessness while placing limits on acting out/inappropriate behaviors. *Provides opportunity to identify accuracy and validate appropriateness of feelings. Limits/minimizes risk of violent behavior.*[4]
- Give accurate information to SO(s) from the beginning. *Establishes trust and promotes opportunity for clarification and correction of misunderstandings.*[4]
- Act as liaison between family and healthcare providers. *Establishes single contact to provide explanations and clarify treatment plan, enhancing reliability of information.*[4]
- Provide brief, simple explanations about use and alarms when equipment (such as a ventilator) is required. Identify appropriate professional(s) for continued support/problem-solving. *Having information and ready access to appropriate resources can reduce feelings of helplessness and promote sense of control.*[1]
- Provide time for private interaction between client and family/significant other(s). *Individuals need to talk about what is happening and process new and frightening information to learn to deal with situation/diagnosis within family relationships.*[3]
- Accompany family when they visit client. *Being available for questions, concerns, and support promotes trusting relationship in which family feels free to learn all they can about situation/diagnosis.*[3]
- Assist SO(s) to initiate therapeutic communication with client. *Learning to use new methods of communication (Active-listening and I-messages) can enhance relationships and promote effective problem-solving for the family.*[3]
- Include SO(s) in the plan of care. Provide instruction/demonstrate necessary skills. *Promotes family's ability to provide care and develop a sense of control over difficult situation.*[3,5]
- Refer client to protective services as necessitated by risk of physical harm/neglect. *Removing client from home enhances individual safety. May reduce stress on family to allow opportunity for therapeutic intervention.*[3]

NURSING PRIORITY NO. 3 To promote wellness (Teaching/Discharge Considerations):

- Assist family to identify coping skills being used and how these skills are/are not helping them deal with situation. *When family members know this information, they can begin to enhance those skills that are more effective in promoting healthy family functioning in difficult times.*[3]
- Answer family's questions patiently and honestly. Reinforce information provided by other providers. *Continues trusting relationship with family members and promotes understanding of the situation/prognosis so family members can deal more effectively with what is happening.*[1]

🌐 Cultural 🔄 Collaborative 🏠 Community/Home Care 🔬 Diagnostic Studies ∞ Pediatric/Geriatric/Lifespan 💊 Medications

- Reframe negative expressions into positive whenever possible. *A positive frame contributes to supportive interactions and can lead to better outcomes.*[2]
- Respect family needs for withdrawal and intervene judiciously. *Situation may be overwhelming, and time away can be beneficial to continued participation. A brief respite can refresh family members who are serving as caregivers and permit renewed ability to manage situation.*[1]
- Encourage family to deal with the situation in small increments rather than trying to deal with the whole picture. *Reduces likelihood of individual being overwhelmed by possibilities that may face them in potentially disabling or fatal outcomes.*[1]
- Assist the family to identify familiar things that would be helpful to the client (e.g., a family picture on the wall), especially when hospitalized for long time, such as in hospice or long-term care. *Reinforces/maintains orientation and provides a sense of home and family for client.*[1,5]
- Refer family to appropriate resources as needed (e.g., family therapy, financial counseling, spiritual advisor). *May need additional help to deal with difficult situation/illness.*[6]
- Refer to ND Grieving as appropriate.

DOCUMENTATION FOCUS

Assessment/Reassessment

- Assessment findings, current/past behaviors, including family members who are directly involved and support systems available.
- Emotional response(s) to situation/stressors.
- Specific health/therapy challenges.

Planning

- Plan of care/interventions and who is involved in planning.
- Teaching plan.

Implementation/Evaluation

- Responses of individuals to interventions/teaching and actions performed.
- Attainment/progress toward desired outcome(s).
- Modifications to plan of care.

Discharge Planning

- Ongoing needs/resources/other follow-up recommendations and who is responsible for actions.
- Specific referrals made.

References

1. Doenges, M., Moorhouse, M., Murr, A. (2002). *Nursing Care Plans, Guidelines for Individualizing Patient Care.* 6th ed. Philadelphia: F. A. Davis.
2. Doenges, M., Townsend, M., Moorhouse, M. (1998). *Psychiatric Care Plans: Guidelines for Individualizing Care.* 3d ed. Philadelphia: F. A. Davis.
3. Townsend, M. (2003). *Psychiatric Mental Health Nursing: Concepts of Care.* 4th ed. Philadelphia: F. A. Davis.
4. Cox, H., Hinz, M., Lubno, M. A., Newfield, S., Ridenour, N., Slater, M., Sridaromont, K. (2002). *Clinical Applications of Nursing Diagnosis: Adult, Child, Women's Psychiatric Gerontic and Home Health Considerations.* 4th ed. Philadelphia: F. A. Davis.
5. Hareven, T. K., Adams, K. J. (eds). (1982). *Aging and Life Course Transitions. An Interdisciplinary Perspective.* New York: Guilford.
6. Sims, D. D. (1993). *If I Could Just See Hope, Finding Your Way Through Grief.* Louisville, KY: Grief Inc.

7. Lipson, J. G., Dibble, S. L., Minarik, P. A. (1996). *Culture & Nursing Care: A Pocket Guide.* San Francisco: School of Nursing, UCSF Nursing Press.
8. No Author. (2002). Defensive Functioning Scale, Brandies University Psychological Counseling Center. Retrieved July 2007 at www.brandeis.edu/pcc/coping.html.

ineffective Coping

Definition: Inability to form a valid appraisal of the stressors, inadequate choices of practiced responses, or inability to use available resources

RELATED FACTORS

Situational/maturational crises

High degree of threat

Inadequate opportunity to prepare for stressor; disturbance in pattern of appraisal of threat

Inadequate level of confidence in ability to cope; inadequate level of perception of control; uncertainty

Inadequate resources available; inadequate social support created by characteristics of relationships

Disturbance in pattern of tension release

Inability to conserve adaptive energies

Gender differences in coping strategies

[Work overload, too many deadlines]

[Impairment of nervous system; cognitive/sensory/perceptual impairment, memory loss]

[Severe/chronic pain]

DEFINING CHARACTERISTICS

Subjective

Verbalization of inability to cope/ask for help

Sleep disturbance; fatigue

Abuse of chemical agents

[Reports of muscular/emotional tension, lack of appetite]

Objective

Lack of goal-directed behavior/resolution of problem, including inability to attend to and difficulty with organizing information; [lack of assertive behavior]

Use of forms of coping that impede adaptive behavior [including inappropriate use of defense mechanisms, verbal manipulation]

Inadequate problem-solving

Inability to meet role expectations/basic needs [including skipping meals, little or no exercise, no time for self/no vacations]

Decreased use of social support

Poor concentration

Change in usual communication patterns

High illness rate [including high blood pressure, ulcers, irritable bowel, frequent headaches/neckaches]

Risk taking

Destructive behavior toward self [including overeating, excessive smoking/drinking, overuse of prescribed/OTC medications, illicit drug use]; destructive behavior toward self

[Behavioral changes (e.g., impatience, frustration, irritability, discouragement)]

Cultural   Collaborative   Community/Home Care   Diagnostic Studies   Pediatric/Geriatric/Lifespan   Medications

Sample Clinical Applications: New diagnosis of major illness, chronic conditions, major depression, substance abuse, eating disorders, bipolar disorder, social anxiety disorder, pregnancy/parenting

DESIRED OUTCOMES/EVALUATION CRITERIA

Sample NOC linkages:

Coping: Personal actions to manage stressors that tax an individual's resources

Impulse Self-Control: Self-restraint of compulsive or impulsive behaviors

Decision Making: Ability to make judgments and choose between two or more alternatives

Client Will (Include Specific Time Frame)

- Assess the current situation accurately.
- Identify ineffective coping behaviors and consequences.
- Verbalize awareness of own coping abilities.
- Verbalize feelings congruent with behavior.
- Meet psychological needs as evidenced by appropriate expression of feelings, identification of options, and use of resources.

ACTIONS/INTERVENTIONS

Sample NIC linkages:

Coping Enhancement: Assisting a patient to adapt to perceived stressors, changes, or threats that interfere with meeting life demands and roles

Decision-Making Support: Providing information and support for a person who is making a decision regarding healthcare

Impulse Control Training: Assisting the patient to mediate impulsive behavior through application of problem-solving strategies to social and interpersonal situations

NURSING PRIORITY NO. 1 To determine degree of impairment:

- Identify individual stressors (e.g., family, social, work environment, life changes or nursing/healthcare management). *Helps define problem(s), providing a starting point for intervention.*[1]
- Evaluate ability to understand events, provide realistic appraisal of situation. *Necessary information for developing workable plan of care.*[2]
- Identify developmental level of functioning. *People tend to regress to a lower developmental stage during illness/crisis, and recognition of client's level enables more appropriate interventions to be implemented.*[2]
- Assess current functional capacity and note how it is affecting the individual's coping ability. *Promotes identification of strategies that will be helpful in current situation.*[4]
- Determine alcohol intake, drug use, smoking habits, sleeping and eating patterns. *Substance abuse impairs ability to deal with what is happening in current situation. Identification of impaired sleeping and eating patterns provides clues to extent of anxiety and impaired coping.*[2,3,16]
- Ascertain impact of illness on sexual needs/relationship. *Illnesses, medications, and many treatment regimens can affect sexual functioning, further stressing coping ability.*[2,3]
- Assess level of anxiety and coping on an ongoing basis. *Identifies changes in ability to cope and worsening of ability to understand at an early stage where intervention can be most effective.*[4]
- Note speech and communication patterns. Be aware of negative/catastrophizing thinking. *Identifies existing problems and assesses ability to understand situation/communicate needs.*[7,15]

- Observe and describe behavior in objective terms. Validate observations. *Promotes accuracy and assures correctness of conclusions to arrive at the best possible solutions.*[7]

NURSING PRIORITY NO. 2 To assess coping abilities and skills:

- Ascertain client's understanding of current situation and its impact on life and work. *Client may not understand situation, and being aware of these factors is necessary to planning care and identifying appropriate interventions.*[8]
- Active-listen and identify client's perceptions of what is happening/effectiveness of coping techniques. *Reflecting client's thoughts can provide a forum for understanding perceptions in relation to reality for planning care and determining accuracy of interventions needed.*[2,3]
- Discuss cultural background and whether some beliefs from family may contribute to difficulties coping with situation. *Family of origin can have a positive or negative effect on individual's ability to deal with stressful situations.*[5]
- Evaluate client's decision-making ability. *When ability to make decisions is impaired by illness or treatment regimen, it is important to take this into consideration when planning care to maximize participation and positive outcomes.*[9]
- Determine previous methods of dealing with life problems. *Identifies successful techniques that can be used in current situation. Often client is preoccupied by current concerns and does not think about previous successful skills.*[8]

NURSING PRIORITY NO. 3 To assist client to deal with current situation:

- Call client by name. Ascertain how client prefers to be addressed. *Using client's name enhances sense of self and promotes individuality/self-esteem.*[2]
- Encourage communication with staff/SOs. *Developing positive interactions between staff, SO(s) and client ensures that everyone has the same understanding.*[8]
- Use reality orientation (e.g., clocks, calendars, bulletin boards) and make frequent references to time, place as indicated. Place needed/familiar objects within sight for visual cues. *Often client can be disoriented by changes in routine, anxiety about illness and treatment regimens, and these measures help the client maintain orientation and a sense of reality.*[9]
- Provide for continuity of care with same personnel taking care of the client as often as possible. *Developing relationships with same caregivers promotes trust and enables client to discuss concerns and fears freely.*[9]
- Explain disease process/procedures/events in a simple, concise manner. *Devoting time for listening may help client to express emotions, grasp situation, and feel more in control.*[10]
- Discuss use of medications as needed. *Short-term use of antianxiety medication or antidepressants may be helpful for lifting mood and encouraging individual to develop new coping skills.*[6]
- Provide for a quiet environment/position equipment out of view as much as possible. *Anxiety is increased by noisy surroundings.*[8]
- Schedule activities so periods of rest alternate with nursing care. Increase activity slowly. *Client is weakened by illness and failure to cope with situation. Ensuring rest can promote ability to cope.*[8]
- Assist client in use of diversion, recreation, relaxation techniques. *Learning new skills can be helpful for reducing stress and will be useful in the future as the client learns to cope more successfully.*[8]
- Stress positive body responses to medical conditions, but do not negate the seriousness of the situation (e.g., stable blood pressure during gastric bleed or improved body posture in depressed client). *Acknowledging the reality of the illness while accurately stating the facts can provide hope and encouragement.*[8]

🌐 Cultural 🔄 Collaborative 🏠 Community/Home Care 🧪 Diagnostic Studies ∞ Pediatric/Geriatric/Lifespan 💊 Medications

- Encourage client to try new coping behaviors and gradually master situation. *Practicing new ways of dealing with what is happening leads to being more comfortable and can promote a positive outcome as client relaxes and handles illness and treatment regimen more successfully.*[9]
- Confront client when behavior is inappropriate, pointing out difference between words and actions. *Provides external locus of control, enhancing safety while client learns self-control.*[2]
- Assist in dealing with change in concept of body image as appropriate. (Refer to ND disturbed Body Image.) *New view of self may be negative, and client needs to incorporate change in a positive manner to enhance self-image.*[11]

NURSING PRIORITY NO. 4 To provide for meeting psychological needs:

- Treat the client with courtesy and respect. Converse at client's level, providing meaningful conversation while performing care. *Enhances therapeutic relationship.*[2]
- Take advantage of teachable moments. *Individuals learn best and are open to new information when they feel accepted and are in a comfortable environment.*[11]
- Allow client to react in own way without judgment by staff/caregivers. Provide support and diversion as indicated. *Unconditional positive regard and support promotes acceptance, enabling client to deal with difficult situation in a positive way.*[8]
- Encourage verbalization of fears and anxieties and expression of feelings of denial, depression, and anger. *Free expression allows for dealing with these feelings, and when the client knows that these are normal reactions, he or she can deal with them better.*[11]
- Help client to learn how to substitute positive thoughts for negative ones (i.e., "I can do this; I am in charge of myself"). *The mind plays a significant role in one's response to stressors, and negative thoughts can actually increase the impact of the stressor.*[15]
- Provide opportunity for expression of sexual concerns. *Important aspect of person that may be difficult to express. Providing an opening for discussion by asking sensitive questions allows client to talk about concerns.*[11]
- Help client to set limits on acting-out behaviors and learn ways to express emotions in an acceptable manner. *Enables client to gain sense of self-esteem, promoting internal locus of control.*[2]

NURSING PRIORITY NO. 5 To promote wellness (Teaching/Discharge Considerations):

- Give updated/additional information needed about events, cause (if known), and potential course of illness as soon as possible. *Knowledge helps reduce anxiety/fear, allows client to deal with reality.*[8]
- Provide and encourage an atmosphere of realistic hope. *Promotes optimistic outlook, energizing client to address situation. Client needs to hear positive things while undergoing difficult circumstances.*[8]
- Give information about purposes and side effects of medications/treatments. *Client feels included, promotes sense of control, enabling client to cope with situation in a more positive manner.*[8]
- Stress importance of follow-up care. *Checkups verify that regimen is being followed accurately and that healing is progressing to promote a satisfactory outcome.*[8]
- Encourage and support client in evaluating lifestyle, occupation, and leisure activities. *Helps client to look at difficult areas that may contribute to anxiety and ability to cope, to make changes gradually without undue/debilitating anxiety.*[8,16]
- Discuss effects of stressors (e.g., family, social, work environment, or nursing/healthcare management) and ways to deal with them. *Addressing these factors will enable client to develop strategies to make changes needed to promote wellness.*[8]

- 🏠 • Provide for gradual implementation and continuation of necessary behavior/lifestyle changes. *Change is difficult, and beginning slowly enhances commitment to plan.*[8]
- 🏠 • Discuss/review anticipated procedures and client concerns, as well as postoperative expectations when surgery is recommended. *Knowledge allays fears and helps client to understand procedures and treatments and expected results. When client has prior information about what to expect during postoperative course, he or she will remain calm, anxiety will be reduced, and client will cope more effectively with situation.*[11,14]
- 🔗 • Refer to outside resources and professional therapy as indicated/ordered. *May be necessary to assist with long-term improvement.*[11]
- 🏠 • Determine need/desire for religious representative/spiritual counselor and facilitate arrangements for visit. *Spiritual needs are an integral part of being human, and determining and meeting individual preferences helps client deal with concerns/desires for discussion/assistance in this area.*[12]
- 🔗 • Provide information/consultation as indicated for sexual concerns. Provide privacy when client is not in home. *Individuals are sexual beings and concerns about role in family/relationship, ability to function are often not readily expressed. Discussion opens opportunity for clarification and understanding, and helps to meet need for intimacy.*[11]
- • Refer to other NDs as indicated (e.g., Anxiety, impaired verbal Communication, acute/chronic Pain, risk for self-/other-directed Violence). *Provides further assistance in area of identified need.*[13]

DOCUMENTATION FOCUS

Assessment/Reassessment

- Baseline findings, degree of impairment, and client's perceptions of situation.
- Coping abilities and previous ways of dealing with life problems.

Planning

- Plan of care/interventions and who is involved in planning.
- Teaching plan.

Implementation/Evaluation

- Client's responses to interventions/teaching and actions performed.
- Medication dose, time, and client's response.
- Attainment/progress toward desired outcome(s).
- Modifications to plan of care.

Discharge Planning

- Long-term needs and actions to be taken.
- Support systems available, specific referrals made, and who is responsible for actions to be taken.

References

1. Doenges, M., Moorhouse, M., Murr, A. (2002). *Nursing Care Plans, Guidelines for Individualizing Patient Care.* 6th ed. Philadelphia: F. A. Davis.
2. Doenges, M., Townsend, M., Moorhouse, M. (1998). *Psychiatric Care Plans: Guidelines for Individualizing Care.* 3d ed. Philadelphia: F. A. Davis.
3. Townsend, M. (2003). *Psychiatric Mental Health Nursing: Concepts of Care.* 4th ed. Philadelphia: F. A. Davis.

4. Cox, H., Hinz, M., Lubno, M. A., Newfield, S., Ridenour, N., Slater, M., Sridaromont, K. (2002). *Clinical Applications of Nursing Diagnosis: Adult, Child, Women's Psychiatric, Gerontic and Home Health Considerations.* 3d ed. Philadelphia: F. A. Davis.
5. Lipson, J. G., Dibble, S. L., Minarik, P. A. (1996). *Culture & Nursing Care: A Pocket Guide.* San Francisco: School of Nursing, UCSF Nursing Press.
6. Townsend, M. (2001). *Nursing Diagnoses in Psychiatric Nursing: Care Plans and Psychotropic Medications.* 5th ed. Philadelphia: F. A. Davis.
7. Haeven, T. K., Adams, K. J. (eds). (1982). *Aging and Life Course Transitions: An Interdisciplinary Perspective.* New York: Guilford.
8. Cherif, M., Younis, E. I. (2000). Liver transplantation. *Clin Fam Prac,* 2(1), 117.
9. Liken, M. A. (2001b). Caregivers in crisis: Moving a relative with Alzheimer's to assisted living. *Clin Nurs Res,* 10(1), 53–69.
10. HIV/AIDS Treatment Information Service. (2001). Guidelines for the use of antiretroviral agents in HIV-infected adults and adolescents. Available at www.hivatis.org/guidelines/adult/aug13_01/pdf/aaaug 13s.pdf (9 Nov. 2001).
11. Tan, G., Waldman, K., Bostick, R. (Winter 2002). Psychosocial issues, sexuality, and Cancer. *Sexuality Disabil,* 20(4), 297–318.
12. Geiter, H. (2002). The spiritual side of nursing. *RN,* 65(5), 43–44.
13. Doenges, M., Moorhouse, M., Murr, A. (2004). *Nurse's Pocket Guide Diagnoses, Interventions, and Rationales.* 9th ed. Philadelphia: F. A. Davis.
14. Dispatcher stress—actively coping with stress. Retrieved July 2007 at www.headsets911.com/activecoping.htm.
15. Coping with stress (2000). Retrieved July 2007 at www.hubbynet.com/stresscoping.htm.
16. Franke, J. (1999). Stress, burnout, and addiction. *Texas Medicine* 95(3), 43–52.

ineffective community Coping

Definition: Pattern of community activities for adaptation and problem-solving that is unsatisfactory for meeting the demands or needs of the community

RELATED FACTORS
Deficits in community social support services/resources
Inadequate resources for problem-solving
Ineffective/nonexistent community systems (e.g., lack of emergency medical system, transportation system, or disaster planning systems)
Natural/man-made disasters

DEFINING CHARACTERISTICS

Subjective
Community does not meet its own expectations
Expressed vulnerability; community powerlessness
Stressors perceived as excessive

Objective
Deficits of community participation
Excessive community conflicts
High illness rates
Increased social problems (e.g., homicide, vandalism, arson, terrorism, robbery, infanticide, abuse, divorce, unemployment, poverty, militancy, mental illness)

Sample Clinical Applications: High rate of illness/injury/violence in community

DESIRED OUTCOMES/EVALUATION CRITERIA
Sample NOC linkages:

Community Competence: Capacity of a community to collectively problem-solve to achieve goals

Community Health Status: General state of well-being of a community or population

Community Disaster Readiness: Community preparedness to respond to a natural or man-made calamitous event

Community Will (Include Specific Time Frame)

- Recognize negative and positive factors affecting community's ability to meet its demands or needs.
- Identify alternatives to inappropriate activities for adaptation/problem-solving.
- Report a measurable increase in necessary/desired activities to improve community functioning.

ACTIONS/INTERVENTIONS

Sample NIC linkages:

Community Health Development: Facilitating members of a community to identify a community's health concerns, mobilize resources, and implement solutions

Environmental Management: Community: Monitoring and influencing of the physical, social, cultural, economic, and political conditions that affect the health of groups and communities

Community Disaster Preparedness: Preparing for an effective response to a large-scale disaster

NURSING PRIORITY NO. 1 To identify causative or precipitating factors:

- Evaluate community activities as related to meeting collective needs within the community itself and between the community and the larger society. *Determines what activities are currently available and what needs are not being met, either by the local or county/state entities. Provides information on which to base the steps needed to begin planning for desired changes.*[1]
- Note community reports of community functioning (e.g., immunization status, transportation, water supply, financing), including areas of weakness or conflict. *Community is responsible for identifying needed changes for possible action.*[1]
- Identify effects of Related Factors on community activities. Note immediate needs (e.g., healthcare, food, shelter, funds). *Provides a baseline to determine community needs, and identifying factors that are pertinent to the community allows community to deal with current concerns.*[1,5]
- Plan for the possibility of a disaster when determined by current circumstances. *In relation to threats, terrorist activities, and natural disasters, actions need to be coordinated between the local and the larger community.*[5]
- Determine availability and use of resources. *Helpful to begin planning to correct deficiencies that have been identified. Sometimes even though resources are available, they are not being used appropriately or fully.*[2]
- Identify unmet demands or needs of the community. *Determining where the deficiencies are is a crucial step to beginning to make an accurate plan for correction. Sometimes elected bodies see the problems differently from the general population and conflict can arise; therefore, it is important for communication to resolve the issues that are in question.*[2]

Cultural Collaborative Community/Home Care Diagnostic Studies Pediatric/Geriatric/Lifespan Medications

NURSING PRIORITY NO. 2 To assist the community to reactivate/develop skills to deal with needs:

- Determine community *strengths. Promotes understanding of ways in which community is already meeting identified needs, and once identified, they can be built on to develop plan to improve community.*[1]
- Identify and prioritize community goals. *Goals enable the identification of actions to direct the changes that are needed to improve the community. Prioritizing enables actions to be taken in order of importance.*[1]
- Encourage community members/groups to engage in problem-solving activities. *Individuals who are involved in the problem-solving process and make a commitment to the solutions have an investment and are more apt to follow through on their commitments.*[3]
- Develop a plan jointly with community to deal with deficits in support. *Working together will enhance efforts and help to meet identified goals.*[3]

NURSING PRIORITY NO. 3 To promote wellness as related to community health:

- Create plans managing interactions within the community itself and between the community and the larger society. *These activities will meet collective needs.*[1]
- Assist the community to form partnerships within the community and between the community and the larger society. *Promotes long-term development of the community to deal with current and future problems.*[1]
- Provide channels for dissemination of information to the community as a whole—for example, print media; radio/television reports and community bulletin boards; speakers' bureau; reports to committees, councils, advisory boards on file and accessible to the public. *Having information readily available for everyone provides opportunity for all members of the community to know what is being planned and have input into the planning. Keeping community informed promotes understanding of needs and plans and probability of follow-through to successful outcomes.*[1]
- Make information available in different modalities and geared to differing educational levels and cultural/ethnic populations of the community. *Assures understanding by all members of the community and promotes cooperation with planning and follow-through.*[1]
- Seek out and evaluate underserved populations, including the homeless. *These members of the community deserve to be helped to become productive citizens and be involved in the changes that are occurring.*[3]
- Work with community members to identify lifestyle changes that can be made to meet the goals identified to improve the community deficits. *Changing lifestyles can promote a sense of power and encourage members to become involved in improving their community.*[4]

DOCUMENTATION FOCUS

Assessment/Reassessment

- Assessment findings, including perception of community members regarding problems.
- Availability of resources.

Planning

- Plan of care and who is involved in planning.
- Teaching plan.

Implementation/Evaluation

- Response of community entities to plan/interventions and actions performed.
- Attainment/progress toward desired outcome(s).
- Modifications to plan of care.

Discharge Planning

- Long-range plans and who is responsible for actions to be taken.

References

1. Higgs, Z. R., Gustafson, D. (1985). *Community as a Client: Assessment and Diagnosis*. Philadelphia: F. A. Davis.
2. Hunt, R. (1998). Community-based nursing. *AJN*, 98(10), 44.
3. Schaeder, C., et al. (1997). Community nursing organizations: A new frontier. *AJN*, 97(1), 63.
4. Lai, S. C., Cohen, M. N. (1999). Promoting lifestyle changes. *AJN*, 99(4), 63.
5. Doenges, M., Moorhouse, M., Geissler-Murr, A. (2002). Nursing Care Plans Guidelines for Individualizing Patient Care. 6th ed. Philadelphia: F. A. Davis.

readiness for enhanced Coping

Definition: A pattern of cognitive and behavioral efforts to manage demands that is sufficient for well-being and can be strengthened

RELATED FACTORS
To be developed by nurse researchers and submitted to NANDA

DEFINING CHARACTERISTICS

Subjective
Defines stressors as manageable
Seeks social support/knowledge of new strategies
Acknowledges power
Acknowledges possible environmental changes

Objective
Uses a broad range of problem-oriented/emotion-oriented strategies
Uses spiritual resources

Sample Clinical Applications: Chronic health conditions (e.g., asthma, diabetes mellitus, arthritis, systemic lupus, multiple sclerosis, AIDS), mental health concerns (e.g., seasonal affective disorder, attention deficit disorder, Down syndrome)

DESIRED OUTCOMES/EVALUATION CRITERIA
Sample NOC linkages:
Coping: Personal actions to manage stressors that tax an individual's resources
Quality of Life: Extent of positive perception of current life circumstances
Hope: Optimism that is personally satisfying and life-supporting

Client Will (Include Specific Time Frame)

- Assess current situation accurately.

Cultural   Collaborative   Community/Home Care   Diagnostic Studies   Pediatric/Geriatric/Lifespan   Medications

- Identify effective coping behaviors currently being used.
- Verbalize feelings congruent with behavior.
- Meet psychological needs as evidenced by appropriate expression of feelings, identification of options, and use of resources.

ACTIONS/INTERVENTIONS

Sample NIC linkages:

Coping Enhancement: Assisting a patient to adapt to perceived stressors, changes, or threats that interfere with meeting life demands and roles

Self-Awareness Enhancement: Assisting a patient to explore and understand his or her thoughts, feelings, motivations, and behaviors

Teaching: Individual: Planning, implementation, and evaluation of a teaching program designed to address a patient's particular needs

NURSING PRIORITY NO. 1   To determine needs and desire for improvement:

- Evaluate client's understanding of situation and ability to provide realistic appraisal of situation. *Provides information about client's perception, cognitive ability, and whether the client is aware of the facts of the situation, which reveals essential information for planning care.*[1]
- Determine stressors that may be affecting client. *Accurate identification of situation that client is dealing with provides information for planning interventions to enhance coping abilities.*[1]
- Ascertain motivation/expectations for change. *Motivation to improve and high expectations can encourage client to make changes that will improve his or her life. However, presence of external locus of control or unrealistic expectations may hamper efforts.*
- Identify social supports available to client. *Available support systems, such as family/friends, can provide client with ability to handle current stressful events, and "talking it out" with an empathic listener will help client move forward to enhance coping skills.*[1]
- Review coping strategies client is aware of and currently using. *The desire to improve one's coping ability is based on an awareness of the status of the stressful situation.*[1]
- Determine use of alcohol/other drugs and smoking habits during times of stress. *Recognition of potential for substituting these actions or old habits to deal with anxiety increases individual's awareness of opportunity to choose new ways to cope with life stressors.*[2]
- Assess level of anxiety and coping on an ongoing basis. *Provides baseline to develop plan of care to improve coping abilities.*[2]
- Note speech and communication patterns. *Assesses ability to understand and provides information necessary to help client make progress in desire to enhance coping abilities.*[2]
- Evaluate client's decision-making ability. *Understanding client's ability provides a starting point for developing plan and determining what information client needs to develop more effective coping skills.*[1]

NURSING PRIORITY NO. 2   To assist client to develop enhanced coping skills:

- Active-listen and clarify client's perceptions of current status. *Reflecting client's statements and thoughts can provide a forum for understanding perceptions in relation to reality for planning care and determining accuracy of interventions needed.*[3]
- Review previous methods of dealing with life problems. *Enables client to identify successful techniques used in the past, promoting feelings of confidence in own ability.*[2]

🏠 • Discuss desire to improve ability to manage stressors of life. *Understanding client's decision to seek new information to enhance life will help client determine what is needed to learn new coping skills.*[1]

🏠 • Discuss understanding of concept of knowing what can and cannot be changed. *Acceptance of reality that some things cannot be changed allows client to focus energies on dealing with things that can be changed.*[1]

🏠 • Help client strengthen problem-solving skills. *Learning the process for problem-solving will promote successful resolution of potentially stressful situations that arise.*[4]

NURSING PRIORITY NO. 3 To promote optimal well-being (Teaching/Learning Considerations):

🏠 • Discuss predisposing factors related to any individual's response to stress. *Understanding that genetic influences, past experiences, and existing conditions determine whether a person's response is adaptive or maladaptive will give client a base on which to continue to learn what is needed to improve life.*[1]

🏠 • Encourage client to develop a stress-management program. *An individualized program of relaxation, meditation, etc., enhances sense of balance in life and strengthens client's ability to manage challenging situations.*[1]

🏠 • Recommend involvement in activities of interest, such as exercise/sports, music, and art. *Individuals must decide for themselves what coping strategies are adaptive for them. Most people find enjoyment and relaxation in these kinds of activities.*[1]

🏠 • Discuss possibility of doing volunteer work in an area of the client's choosing. *Many individuals report satisfaction in giving of themselves—involvement with caring for others/pets, and client may find sense of fulfillment in service to others.*[1]

🏠 • Refer to classes and/or reading material/Web sites, as appropriate. *May be helpful to further learning and pursuing goal of enhanced coping ability.*[1]

DOCUMENTATION FOCUS

Assessment/Reassessment

• Baseline information, client's perception of need to enhance abilities.
• Coping abilities and previous ways of dealing with life problems.
• Motivation and expectation for change.

Planning

• Plan of care/interventions and who is involved in planning.
• Teaching plan.

Implementation/Evaluation

• Client's responses to interventions/teaching and actions performed.
• Attainment/progress toward desired outcome(s).
• Modifications to plan of care.

Discharge Planning

• Long-term needs and actions to be taken.
• Support systems available, specific referrals made, and who is responsible for actions to be taken.

⊕ Cultural Ⓐ Collaborative 🏠 Community/Home Care ✎ Diagnostic Studies ∞ Pediatric/Geriatric/Lifespan ⬤ Medications

References

1. Townsend, M. (2003). *Psychiatric Mental Health Nursing Concepts of Care.* 4th ed. Philadelphia: F. A. Davis.
2. Doenges, M. E., Moorhouse, M. F., Murr, A. C. (2004). *Nurse's Pocket Guide Diagnoses, Interventions, and Rationales.* 9th ed. Philadelphia: F. A. Davis.
3. Doenges, M., Townsend, M., Moorhouse, M. (1998). *Psychiatric Care Plans: Guidelines for Individualizing Care.* 3d ed. Philadelphia: F. A. Davis.
4. Gordon, T. (2000). Parent Effectiveness Training. (Updated edition). New York: Three Rivers Press.

readiness for enhanced community Coping

Definition: Pattern of community activities for adaptation and problem-solving that is satisfactory for meeting the demands or needs of the community but can be improved for management of current and future problems/stressors

RELATED FACTORS
Social supports available
Resources available for problem-solving
Sense of power to manage stressors

DEFINING CHARACTERISTICS
One or more characteristics that indicate effective coping

Subjective
Agreement that community is responsible for stress management

Objective
Active planning by community for predicted stressors
Active problem-solving by community when faced with issues
Positive communication among community members
Positive communication between community/aggregates and larger community
Programs available for recreation/relaxation
Resources sufficient for managing stressors

Sample Clinical Applications: Reducing rates of illness/injury/violence

DESIRED OUTCOMES/EVALUATION CRITERIA
Sample NOC linkages:
Community Competence: Capacity of a community to collectively problem-solve to achieve goals
Community Health Status: General state of well-being of a community or population
Community Disaster Readiness: Community preparedness to respond to a natural or man-made calamitous event

Community Will (Include Specific Time Frame)

• Identify positive and negative factors affecting management of current and future problems/stressors.
• Have an established plan in place to deal with identified problems/stressors.
• Describe management of challenges in characteristics that indicate effective coping.
• Report a measurable increase in ability to deal with problems/stressors.

ACTIONS/INTERVENTIONS

Sample NIC linkages:

Program Development: Planning, implementing, and evaluating a coordinated set of activities designed to enhance wellness, or to prevent, reduce, or eliminate one or more health problems of a group or community

Environmental Management: Community: Monitoring and influencing of the physical, social, cultural, economic, and political conditions that affect the health of groups and communities

Health Policy Monitoring: Surveillance and influence of government and organization regulations, rules, and standards that affect nursing systems and practices to ensure quality care of patients

NURSING PRIORITY NO. 1 To determine existence of and deficits or weaknesses in management of current and future problems/stressors:

- Review community plan for dealing with problems/stressors, untoward events such as natural disaster/terrorist activity. *Provides a baseline for comparisons of preparedness with other communities and developing plan to address concerns.*[5]
- Assess effects of Related Factors on management of problems/stressors. *Identifying social supports available and awareness of the power of the community can enhance the plans needed to improve the community.*[1]
- Identify limitations in current pattern of community activities, such as transportation, water needs, and roads. *Recognition of the factors that can be improved through adaptation and problem-solving will make it easier for the community to proceed with planning to make necessary improvements.*[4]
- Evaluate community activities as related to management of problems/stressors within the community itself and between the community and the larger society. *Disasters occurring in the community or in the country affect the local community and need to be recognized and addressed.*[5]

NURSING PRIORITY NO. 2 To assist the community in adaptation and problem-solving for management of current and future needs/stressors:

- Define and discuss current needs and anticipated or projected concerns. *Agreement on scope/parameters of needs is essential for effective planning.*[2]
- Determine community's strengths. *Plan can build on strengths to address areas of weakness.*[2]
- Identify and prioritize goals to facilitate accomplishment. *Helps to bring the community together to meet a common concern/threat, maintain focus, and facilitate accomplishment.*[5]
- Identify and interact with available resources (e.g., persons, groups, financial, governmental, as well as other communities). *Promotes cooperation. Major catastrophes, such as earthquakes, floods, and terrorist activity, affect more than the local community, and communities need to work together to deal with and accomplish reconstruction and future growth.*[6]
- Make a joint plan with the community and the larger community to deal with adaptation and problem-solving. *Promotes management of problems/stressors to enable most effective solution for identified concern.*[3]
- Seek out and involve underserved/at-risk groups within the community, including the homeless. *Supports communication and commitment of community as a whole.*[3]

Cultural   Collaborative   Community/Home Care   Diagnostic Studies   Pediatric/Geriatric/Lifespan   Medications

NURSING PRIORITY NO. 3 To promote optimal well-being of community:

🏠 • Assist the community to form partnerships within the community and between the community and the larger society. *Promotes long-term developmental growth of the community.*[5]

🏠 • Support development of plans for maintaining these interactions.

🏠 • Establish mechanism for self-monitoring of community needs and evaluation of efforts. *Facilitates proactive—rather than reactive—responses by the community.*

🏠 • Use multiple formats to disseminate information, such as TV, radio, print media, billboards, as well as computer bulletin boards, speakers' bureau, and reports to community leaders/groups on file and accessible to the public. *Keeps community informed regarding plans, needs, outcomes to encourage continued understanding and participation.*[6]

DOCUMENTATION FOCUS

Assessment/Reassessment

• Assessment findings and community's perception of situation.
• Identified areas of concern, community strengths/weaknesses.

Planning

• Plan and who is involved and responsible for each action.
• Teaching plan.

Implementation/Evaluation

• Response of community entities to the actions performed.
• Attainment/progress toward desired outcomes.
• Modifications to plan.

Discharge Planning

• Short-range and long-range plans to deal with current, anticipated, and potential problems and who is responsible for follow-through.
• Specific referrals made, coalitions formed.

References

1. Higgs, Z. R., Gustafson, D. (1985). *Community as a Client: Assessment and Diagnosis.* Philadelphia: F. A. Davis.
2. Hunt, R. (1998). Community-based nursing. *AJN,* 98(10), 44.
3. Schaeder, C. et al. (1997). Community nursing organizations: A new frontier. *AJN,* 97(1), 63.
4. Lai, S. C., Cohen, M. N. (1999). Promoting lifestyle changes. *AJN,* 99(4), 63.
5. Doenges, M., Moorhouse, M., Geissler-Murr, A. (2002). *Nursing Care Plans Guidelines for Individualizing Patient Care.* 6th ed. Philadelphia: F. A. Davis.
6. Stanhope, M., Lancaster, J. (2000). *Community and Public Health Nursing.* 5th ed. St. Louis, MO: Mosby.

readiness for enhanced family Coping

Definition: Effective managing of adaptive tasks by family member involved with the patient's health challenge, who now exhibits desire and readiness for enhanced health and growth in regard to self and in relation to the patient

RELATED FACTORS
Needs are sufficiently gratified to enable goals of self-actualization to surface

Adaptive tasks effectively addressed to enable goals of self-actualization to surface [Developmental stage, situational crises/supports]

DEFINING CHARACTERISTICS

Subjective
Family member attempts to describe growth impact of crisis [on his or her own values, priorities, goals, or relationships]
Individual expresses interest in making contact with others who have experienced a similar situation

Objective
Family member moves in direction of health-promotion/enriching lifestyle
Chooses experiences that optimize wellness

Sample Clinical Applications: Genetic disorders (e.g., Down syndrome, cystic fibrosis, neural tube defects), traumatic injury (e.g., amputation, spinal cord), chronic conditions (e.g., asthma, AIDS, Alzheimer's disease)

DESIRED OUTCOMES/EVALUATION CRITERIA
Sample NOC linkages:
Family Participation in Professional Care: Family involvement in decision making, delivery, and evaluation of care provided by healthcare personnel
Family Coping: Family actions to manage stressors that tax family resources
Family Functioning: Capacity of the family system to meet the needs of its members during developmental transitions

Family Will (Include Specific Time Frame)

- Express willingness to look at own role in the family's growth.
- Verbalize desire to undertake tasks leading to change.
- Report feelings of self-confidence and satisfaction with progress being made.

ACTIONS/INTERVENTIONS

Sample NIC linkages:
Normalization Promotion: Assisting parents and other family members of children with chronic diseases or disabilities in providing normal life experiences for their children and families
Family Support: Promotion of family values, interests, and goals
Family Involvement Promotion: Facilitating family participation in the emotional and physical care of the patient

NURSING PRIORITY NO. I To assess situation and adaptive skills being used by the family members:

🏠 • Determine individual situation and stage of growth family is experiencing/demonstrating. *Essential elements needed to identify family needs and develop plan of care for improving communication and interactions. Changes that are occurring may help family adapt and grow and thrive when faced with these transitional events.*[1,7]

🌐 Cultural 🅰 Collaborative 🏠 Community/Home Care ⚗ Diagnostic Studies ∞ Pediatric/Geriatric/Lifespan 💊 Medications

- Ascertain motivation/expectations for change. *Motivation to improve and high expectations can encourage individuals to make changes that will improve their lives; however, presence of external locus of control or unrealistic expectations may hamper efforts.*
- Observe communication patterns of family. Listen to family's expressions of hope, planning, effect on relationships/life. *Provides clues to difficulties that individuals may have in expressing themselves effectively to others. Beginning to plan for the future with hope promotes changes in relationships that can enhance living for those involved.*[3]
- Note expressions such as "Life has more meaning for me since this has occurred." *Such statements identify change in values that may occur with the diagnosis/stress of a serious or potentially fatal illness.*[1]
- Identify cultural/religious health beliefs and expectations. *For example: Navajo parents may define family as nuclear, extended, or clan, and it is important to identify who are the primary child-rearing persons. Beliefs about causes of condition may affect how family interacts with client (e.g., African Americans may believe the condition is punishment for improper behavior and may react with anger and statements of condemnation).*[6]

NURSING PRIORITY NO. 2 To assist family to develop/strengthen potential for growth:

- Provide time to talk with family to discuss their view of the situation. *Provides an opportunity to hear family's understanding and determine how realistic their ideas are for planning how they are going to deal with situation in the most positive manner.*[3]
- Establish a relationship with family/client. *Therapeutic relationships foster growth and enable family to identify skills needed for coping with difficult situation/illness.*[3]
- Provide a role model with whom the family may identify. *Setting a positive example can be a powerful influence in changing behavior, and as family members learn more effective communication skills, consideration for others, warmth and understanding, family relationships will be enhanced.*[2]
- Discuss importance of open communication and of not having secrets. *Functional communication is clear, direct, open, and honest, with congruence between verbal and nonverbal. Dysfunctional communication is indirect, vague, controlled, with many double-bind messages. Awareness of this information can enhance relationships among family members.*[3]
- Demonstrate techniques such as Active-listening, I-messages, and problem-solving. *Learning these skills can facilitate effective communication and improve interactions within the family.*[2]
- Establish social goals of achieving and maintaining harmony with oneself, family, and community. *Enables client to interact with others in positive ways.*[3]

NURSING PRIORITY NO. 3 To promote optimum family well-being (Teaching/Discharge Considerations):

- Assist family to support the client in meeting own needs within ability or constraints of the illness/situation. *Family members may do too much for client or may not do enough, believing client "wants to be babied." With information and support, they can learn to allow client to take the lead in doing what he or she is able to do.*[3]
- Provide experiences for the family to help them learn ways of assisting/supporting client. *Learning is enhanced when individual participates in hands-on opportunities to try out new activities.*[4]
- Discuss cultural beliefs and practices that may impact family members' interaction with client and dealing with condition. *Preconceived biases may interfere with efforts toward positive growth.*[6]

- Identify other individuals/groups with similar conditions and assist client/family to make contact (groups such as Reach for Recovery, CanSurmount, Al-Anon, and so on). *Provides ongoing support for sharing common experiences, problem-solving, and learning new behaviors.*[5]
- Assist family members to learn new, more effective ways of dealing with feelings/reactions. *Growth process is essential to reach the goal of enhancing the family relationships.*[3]
- Encourage family members to persue personal interests/hobbies/leisure activities *to promote individual well-being and strengthen coping abilities.*[7]

DOCUMENTATION FOCUS

Assessment/Reassessment

- Adaptive skills being used, stage of growth.
- Family communication patterns.
- Motivation and expectations for change.

Planning

- Plan of care/interventions and who is involved in planning.
- Teaching plan.

Implementation/Evaluation

- Client's responses to interventions/teaching and actions performed.
- Attainment/progress toward desired outcome(s).
- Modifications to plan of care.

Discharge Planning

- Identified needs/referrals for follow-up care, support systems.
- Specific referral.

References

1. Doenges, M., Moorhouse, M., Murr, A. (2002). *Nursing Care Plans, Guidelines for Individualizing Patient Care.* 6th ed. Philadelphia: F. A. Davis.
2. Doenges, M., Townsend, M., Moorhouse, M. (1998). *Psychiatric Care Plans: Guidelines for Individualizing Care.* 3d ed. Philadelphia: F. A. Davis.
3. Townsend, M. (2003). *Psychiatric Mental Health Nursing: Concepts of Care.* 4th ed. Philadelphia: F. A. Davis.
4. Cox, H., Hinz, M., Lubno, M. A., Newfield, S., Ridenour, N., Slater, M., Sridaromont, K. (2002). *Clinical Applications of Nursing Diagnosis: Adult, Child, Women's Psychiatric, Gerontic and Home Health Considerations.* 4th ed. Philadelphia: F. A. Davis.
5. Sims, D. (1993). *If I Could Just See Hope.* Louisville, KY: Grief Inc. Available at www.griefinc.com.
6. Lipson, J. G., Dibble. S. L., Minarik, P. A. (1996). *Culture & Nursing Care: A Pocket Guide.* San Francisco: School of Nursing, UCSF Nursing Press.
7. Beckett, C. (2000). Family Theory as a Framework for Assessment. Available at http://jan.ucc.nau.edu/~nur350-c/class/2_family/theory/lesson2-1-3.html.

risk for sudden infant Death Syndrome

Definition: Presence of risk factors for sudden death of an infant under 1 year of age [Sudden Infant Death Syndrome (SIDS) is the sudden death of an infant under 1 year of age, which remains unexplained after a thorough case investigation, including performance of a complete autopsy, examination of the death scene, and review of the clinical history. SIDS

Cultural · Collaborative · Community/Home Care · Diagnostic Studies · Pediatric/Geriatric/Lifespan · Medications

is a subset of Sudden Unexpected Death in Infancy (SUDI) that is the sudden and unexpected death of an infant due to natural or unnatural causes.]

RISK FACTORS

Modifiable
Delayed/lack of prenatal care
Infants placed to sleep in the prone/side-lying position
Soft underlayment (loose articles in the sleep environment)
Infant overheating/overwrapping
Prenatal/postnatal smoke exposure

Potentially Modifiable
Young maternal age
Low birth weight; prematurity

Nonmodifiable
Male gender
Ethnicity (e.g., African American, Native American)
Seasonality of SIDS deaths (higher in winter and fall months)
Infant age of 2 to 4 months
NOTE: A risk diagnosis is not evidenced by signs and symptoms, as the problem has not occurred; rather, nursing interventions are directed at prevention.

Sample Clinical Applications: Any child during first year of life

DESIRED OUTCOMES/EVALUATION CRITERIA
Sample NOC linkages:
Risk Detection: Activities taken to identify personal health threats
Risk Control: Actions to eliminate or reduce actual, personal, and modifiable health threats
Knowledge: Infant Care: Extent of understanding conveyed about caring for a baby up to 12 months

Parent Will (Include Specific Time Frame)
- Verbalize knowledge of modifiable factors.
- Make changes in environment to prevent death occurring from other factors.
- Follow medically recommended regimen for prenatal and postnatal care.

ACTIONS/INTERVENTIONS

Sample NIC linkages:
Risk Identification: Analysis of potential risk factors, determination of health risks, and prioritization of risk-reduction strategies for an individual or group
Parent Education: Infant: Instruction on nurturing and physical care during the first year of life
Teaching: Infant Safety: Instruction on safety during first year of life

NURSING PRIORITY NO. 1 To assess causative/contributing factors:

- Identify individual risk factors pertaining to situation. *Determines modifiable or potentially modifiable factors that can be addressed and treated. SIDS is the most common cause of unexplained death between 2 weeks and 1 year of age, with peak incidence occurring between the second and fourth month.*[1,7]

- Determine ethnicity, cultural background of family. *Although the overall rate of SIDS in the United States has declined by more than 50% since 1990, rates have declined less among non-Hispanic black and American Indian/Alaska Native infants.*[7,8,9]

- Note whether mother smoked during pregnancy or is currently smoking. *Many risk factors for SIDS also apply to non-SIDS deaths as well, and smoking is known to negatively affect the fetus prenatally as well as after birth.*[1,2] *Some reports indicate an increased risk of SIDS in babies of smoking mothers.*[3]

- Assess extent of prenatal care, how early begun, extent to which mother followed recommended care measures. *Prenatal care is important for all pregnancies to afford the optimal opportunity for all infants to have a healthy start to life.*[4]

- Provide information about signs of premature labor and actions to be taken in the event they occur. *Prompt action can prevent early delivery and the complications of prematurity.*[4]

- Note use of alcohol/other drugs (including prescribed medications) during and after pregnancy. *While these are not known to affect the occurrence of SIDS, a healthy baby will be less apt to have problems.* **Note:** *Studies have shown that Native American infants whose mothers drank any amount of alcohol 3 months before conception through the first trimester had six times the risk of SIDS as those whose mothers did not drink. Mothers who consumed five or more drinks at one sitting during the first trimester had eight times the risk as those whose mothers did not binge drink.*[5]

NURSING PRIORITY NO. 2 To promote use of activities to minimize risk of SIDS:

- Stress importance of placing infant on his or her back to sleep, both at nighttime and naptime. *Research confirms that fewer babies die of SIDS when they sleep on their backs and that side-lying position is not to be used.*[6,8]

- Advise all formal child care providers as well as grandparents, babysitters, neighbors, or anyone who will have responsibility for the care of the child during sleep to maintain correct sleeping position. *The recommendation is to always place the child on his or her back until they roll over on their own; then repositioning is not required.*[1,7]

- Encourage parents to schedule "tummy time" only while infant is awake. *This activity promotes strengthening of back and neck muscles while parents are close and baby is not sleeping.*[1]

- Encourage early and medically recommended prenatal care and continue with well-baby checkups and immunizations after birth. *Prematurity presents many problems for the newborn, and keeping babies healthy prevents problems that could put the infant at risk for SIDS. Immunizing infants prevents many illnesses that can be life-threatening.*[1,4]

- Encourage breastfeeding, if possible. *Breastfeeding has many advantages (immunological, nutritional, and psychosocial), promoting a healthy infant. While this does not preclude the occurrence of SIDS, healthy babies are less prone to many illnesses/problems.*[1,4]

- Discuss issues of bedsharing/co-sleeping and the concerns regarding sudden unexpected infant deaths from accidental entrapment under a sleeping adult or suffocation by becoming wedged in a couch or cushioned chair. *While co-sleeping is controversial, there are concerns about problems of accidental death from suffocation. Bedsharing or putting infant to sleep on an unsafe surface results in dangerous sleep environments that place infants at substantial risk for sudden unexpected death in infancy (SUDI).*[6]

- Note cultural beliefs about bedsharing. *Bedsharing is more common among breastfed infants, young, unmarried, low income, or those from a minority group. Additional study is needed to better understand bedsharing practices and its associated risks and benefits.*[6]

Cultural Collaborative Community/Home Care Diagnostic Studies Pediatric/Geriatric/Lifespan Medications

NURSING PRIORITY NO. 3 To promote wellness (Teaching/Discharge Considerations):

🏠 • Discuss known facts about SIDS with parents. *SIDS is not preventable, although research indicates that SIDS deaths have reduced since back-sleeping position policy was implemented. It is not contagious or hereditary and is not an unusual disease. The cause, while not known, is not suffocation, aspiration, or regurgitation.*[.7]

🏠 • Recommend attention to factors below that may help in reducing risk:

Avoid overdressing or overheating infants during sleep. *Babies should be kept warm, but not too warm. Too many layers of clothing or blankets can overheat the infant. Room temperature that is comfortable for an adult will be comfortable for the baby. Infants who were dressed in two or more layers of clothes as they slept had six times the risk of SIDS as those dressed in fewer layers.*[1,4]

Place infant on a firm mattress in an approved crib. *Avoiding soft mattresses, sofas, cushions, waterbeds, other soft surfaces, while not known to prevent SIDS, will minimize chance of suffocation.*[1]

Remove fluffy and loose bedding from sleep area, making sure baby's head and face are not covered during sleep. *Using only sleep clothing without a blanket, or if a blanket is used, making sure it is below baby's face and tucked in at the foot of the bed minimizes possibility of suffocation.*[1]

Verify that day care center/provider(s) are trained in observation and modifying risk factors (e.g., sleeping position) *to reduce risk of death while infant in their care.*

Discourage excessive checking of the infant. *Since there is nothing that can currently be done (beyond proper sleep positioning) to reduce the occurrence of SIDS, excessive checking only tires the parents and creates an atmosphere of tension and anxiety.*[1,2]

• Discuss the use of apnea monitors. *Apnea monitors are not recommended to prevent SIDS but may be used to monitor other medical problems. Only a small percentage of infants who died of SIDS were known to have prolonged apnea episodes, and monitors are also not medically recommended for subsequent siblings.*[1,2]

• Recommend contacting public health nurse for visit to new mother at least once or twice following discharge. *Researchers found that Native American infants whose mothers received such visits were 80% less likely to die from SIDS than those who were never visited.*[4]

• Refer parents to local SIDS programs/resources for learning (e.g., National SIDS/Infant Death Resouce Center and simliar Web sites). *Provides reassurance and information for self-paced learning.*[1]

• Encourage consultation with primary care provider if baby shows any signs of illness or behaviors that concern parent. *Promotes timely evaluation and intervention for treatable problems.*[1]

DOCUMENTATION FOCUS

Assessment/Reassessment

• Baseline findings, degree of parental anxiety/concern.
• History of infant deaths within family.

Planning

• Plan of care/interventions and who is involved in planning.
• Teaching plan.

Implementation/Evaluation

• Parent's responses to interventions/teaching and actions performed.

- Attainment/progress toward desired outcome(s)
- Modifications to plan of care.

Discharge Planning

- Long-term needs and actions to be taken.
- Support systems available, specific referrals made, and who is responsible for actions to be taken.

References

1. The Colorado SIDS Program, Inc., 6825 East Tennessee Ave, Suite 300, Denver, CO 80224–1631.
2. Beers, M. H., Berkow, R. (1999). *The Merck Manual of Diagnosis and Therapy.* 17th ed. Whitehouse Station, NJ: Merck Research Laboratories.
3. Phillips, C. R. (1996). *Family-Centered Maternity and Newborn Care.* 4th ed. St. Louis, MO: Mosby.
4. London, M., Ladewig, P., Ball, J., Bindler, R. (2003). *Maternal-Newborn & Child Nursing; Family-Centered Care.* Upper Saddle River, NJ: Prentice Hall.
5. Iyasu, S., Randall, L. L., et al. (2002). Risk factors for sudden infant death syndrome among Northern Plains Indians. *JAMA,* 288(21), 2717.
6. American Academy of Pediatrics, Task Force on Sleep Position and SIDS. (2000). Changing concepts of sudden infant death syndrome: Implications for infant sleep environment and position. *Pediatrics,* 105, 650–656.
7. No author or publication date listed. What is SIDS? Public information of the National SIDS/Infant Death Resource Center. Health Resources and Services Administration (HRSA) Maternal and Child Health Bureau Web site. Retrieved February 2007 at www.sidscenter.org/WhatIsSIDS.aspx?fromparent=parent&heading=WhatIsSIDS?
8. No author listed. (2005). The changing concept of sudden infant death syndrome: Diagnostic coding shifts, controversies regarding the sleeping environment, and new variations to consider in reducing risk. *Pediatr,* 116(5), 1245–1255. Available at http://aappolicy.aappublications.org/cgi/content/full/pediatrics;116/5/1245.
9. CDC Office of Minority Health and Health Disparities (OMHD). (2006). Eliminate disparities in infant mortality. Available at www.cdc.gov/omhd/AMH/factsheets/infant.htm.

readiness for enhanced Decision Making

Definition: A pattern of choosing courses of action that are sufficient for meeting short- and long-term health-related goals and can be strengthened

RELATED FACTORS
To be developed by nurse researchers and submitted to NANDA

DEFINING CHARACTERISTICS

Subjective
Expresses desire to enhance:
Decision making
Congruency of decisions with personal sociocultural values and goals
Risk benefit analysis of decisions
Understanding of choices for decision making
Understanding of the meaning of choices
Use of reliable evidence for decisions

Sample Clinical Applications: Any acute or chronic condition, or healthy individual looking to improve well-being

DESIRED OUTCOMES/EVALUATION CRITERIA
Sample NOC linkages:

Cultural Collaborative Community/Home Care Diagnostic Studies Pediatric/Geriatric/Lifespan Medications

Decision Making: Ability to choose between two or more alternatives

Personal Autonomy: Personal actions of a competent individual to exercise governance in life decisions

Health-Promoting Behavior: Personal actions to sustain or increase wellness

Client Will (Include Specific Time Frame)

- Identify risks and benefit of decisions.
- Express beliefs about the meaning of choices.
- Make decisions that are congruent with personal and sociocultural values and goals.
- Use reliable evidence for decisions.

ACTION/INTERVENTIONS

Sample NIC linkages:

Decision-Making Support: Providing information and support for a person who is making a decision regarding healthcare

Values Clarification: Assisting another to clarify her or his own values in order to facilitate effective decision making

Self-Awareness Enhancement: Assisting a patient to explore and understand his or her thoughts, feelings, motivations, and behaviors

NURSING PRIORITY NO. 1 To assess causative/contributing factors:

- Determine usual ability to manage own affairs. Provides baseline for understanding client's decision-making process. *There may be variations in attitudes toward risk in different areas of the country that will affect this individual's decision-making preferences.*[8]
- Note expressions of decision, dependability, availability of support persons. *Having support for decision making and having good information regarding pros and cons of choices helps client to feel comfortable with the decisions made.*[8]
- Active-listen/identify reason(s) client would like to improve decision-making abilities and expectations for change. *As client articulates reasons for improvement, they are clarified and direction is provided.*[2] *Motivation to improve and high expectations can encourage client to make changes that will improve his or her life. However, presence of external locus of control or unrealistic expectations may hamper efforts.*
- Note presence of physical signs of anxiety. *Client may be excited about the quest for improvement, and excitement may be interpreted as anxiety. It is important to clarify meaning of physical signs.*[2]
- Identify cultural values/beliefs or moral obligations/principles that guide or affect decision-making process. *Preconceived biases may color decisions and need to be recognized in order to enhance efforts toward growth.*[5]
- Discuss meaning of life/reasons for living, belief in God or higher power, and how these relate to current desire for improvement or growth. *Helps client to clarify beliefs and how they relate to decision-making process.*[6] (Refer to ND readiness for enhanced Spiritual Well-Being.)

NURSING PRIORITY NO. 2 To assist client to improve/effectively use problem-solving skills:

- Promote safe and hopeful environment and help client identify own inner control. *Will help client understand the control he or she has over decisions made.*[1]

- Encourage verbalization of ideas, concerns, particular decisions that need to be made.
- Correct misperceptions client may have and provide factual information as needed. *Promotes understanding and enables client to make better decisions for own situation.*[1,8]
- Clarify and prioritize individual's goals, noting possible conflicts or "stumbling" blocks that may be encountered. *As client weighs pros and cons of decision making, taking into account negative aspects of situation, decisions will be more realistic and acceptable to client.*[3]
- Discuss dependence on others, involvement of support persons, and possibility for conflicting advice/goals. *While it is appropriate to consider the opinions of others when making choices, one needs to be aware of the potential for conflicting views when seeking advice and make own decisions free of pressure from others.*[8]
- Identify positive aspects of this experience and assist client to view it as a learning opportunity. *As client reframes experience as an opportunity, he or she will be able to use this learning for future situations.*[3]
- Assist client in learning how to find factual information (e.g., use of the library, Internet). *Individual who takes advantage of these resources will benefit from the knowledge gained. Client will need to be cautious in evaluating information to verify accuracy.*[8]
- Discuss the process of performing risk-benefit analysis to aid in making decisions. *The individual who learns this skill will be able to use it in many areas of life to enhance relationships, both personal and business.*[2]
- Have client list some alternatives to present decisions, using a brainstorming process. Include SO/family in this activity if appropriate. *Looking at different options can strengthen decision-making process.*[7]
- ∞ Encourage children to make age-appropriate decisions. *Learning problem-solving at an early age will enhance sense of self-worth and ability to exercise coping skills.*
- ⊕ Discuss/clarify spiritual beliefs, accepting client's values in a nonjudgmental manner. *Client may be able to decide what is really acceptable or unacceptable in the choice situation related to beliefs/values that have been expressed.*[8]

NURSING PRIORITY NO. 3 To promote optimum well-being (Teaching/Discharge Considerations):

- 🏠 Identify opportunities for using conflict-resolution skills. *Emphasizing each step as they are used will help with learning these skills.*[6]
- 🏠 Provide positive feedback for efforts, growth in use of skills, and learning efforts. As *individual is moving forward in learning new skills, hearing positive feedback provides reinforcement for individuals to continue efforts.*
- 🏠 Encourage involvement of family/SOs as desired/appropriate. *Helps all family members to improve conflict-resolution skills. When family works together, relationships are enhanced and family members can live fuller lives.*[4]
- 🏠 Recommend attending stress reduction, assertiveness classes as desired. *Individual can learn additional skills to enhance decision making, improving ability to make life better.*[2]
- ⊛ Refer to other resources as necessary (e.g., clergy, psychiatrist, clinical psychiatric nurse specialist, family/marital therapist). *May need additional counseling to help with specific concerns.*[4]

DOCUMENTATION FOCUS

Assessment/Reassessment

- Assessment findings/behavioral responses.
- Individuals involved in improving conflict skills.
- Personal values/beliefs, motivation for change.

Planning

- Plan of care/interventions and who is involved in the planning process.
- Teaching plan.

Implementation/Evaluation

- Client's and involved individual's responses to interventions/teaching and actions performed.
- Ability to express feelings, identify options, use resources.
- Attainment/progress toward desired outcomes(s).
- Modifications to plan of care.

Discharge Planning

- Long-term needs/referrals, action to be taken and who is responsible for doing.
- Specific referrals made.

References

1. Doenges, M., Moorhouse, M., Murr, A. (2002). *Nursing Care Plans, Guidelines for Individualizing Patient Care.* 6th ed. Philadelphia: F. A. Davis.
2. Doenges, M., Townsend, M., Moorhouse, M. (1998). *Psychiatric Care Plans: Guidelines for Individualizing Care.* 3d ed. Philadelphia: F. A. Davis.
3. Townsend, M. (2003). *Psychiatric Mental Health Nursing: Concepts of Care.* 4th ed. Philadelphia: F. A. Davis.
4. Cox, H., Hinz, M., Lubno, M. A., Newfield, S., Scott-Tilley, D., Slater, M., Sridaromont, K. (2002). *Clinical Applications of Nursing Diagnosis: Adult, Child, Women's Psychiatric, Gerontic and Home Health Considerations.* 4th ed. Philadelphia: F. A. Davis.
5. Lipson, J. G., Dibble, S. L., Minarik, P. A. (1996). *Culture & Nursing Care: A Pocket Guide.* San Francisco: School of Nursing, UCSF Nursing Press.
6. Hareven, T. K., Adams, K. J. (eds). (1982). *Aging and Life Course Transitions: An Interdisciplinary Perspective.* New York: Guilford.
7. Liken, M. A. (2001). Caregivers in crisis: Moving a relative with Alzheimer's to assisted living. *Clin Nurs Res,* 10(1), 53–69.
8. Llewellyn-Thomas, H. (2004). Helping Patients Make Health Care Decisions. Evaluative Clinical Sciences Dartmouth Medical School. Retrieved July 2007 at www.dartmouthatlas.org/atlas/DecisionSupport.pdf.

ineffective Denial

Definition: Conscious or unconscious attempt to disavow the knowledge or meaning of an event to reduce anxiety/fear, but leading to the detriment of health

RELATED FACTORS

Anxiety; threat of inadequacy in dealing with strong emotions
Lack of control of life situation; fear of loss of autonomy
Overwhelming stress; lack of competency in using effective coping mechanisms
Threat of unpleasant reality
Fear of separation/death, loss of autonomy
Lack of emotional support from others

DEFINING CHARACTERISTICS

Subjective

Minimizes symptoms; displaces source of symptoms to other organs
Unable to admit impact of disease on life pattern

Displaces fear of impact of the condition
Does not admit fear of death/invalidism

Objective

Delays seeking healthcare attention to the detriment of health
Does not perceive personal relevance of symptoms or danger
Unable to admit impact of disease on life pattern; does not perceive personal relevance of danger
Makes dismissive gestures/comments when speaking of distressing events
Displays inappropriate affect
Uses self-treatment

Sample Clinical Applications: Chronic illnesses, eating disorders, substance abuse, Alzheimer's disease, terminal conditions, bipolar disorder, body dysmorphic disorder

DESIRED OUTCOMES/EVALUATION CRITERIA

Sample NOC linkages:

Acceptance: Health Status: Reconciliation to significant change in health circumstances

Health Beliefs: Perceived Threat: Personal conviction that a threatening health problem is serious and has potential negative consequences for lifestyle

Psychosocial Adjustment: Life Change: Adaptive psychosocial response of an individual to a significant life change

Client Will (Include Specific Time Frame)

- Acknowledge reality of situation/illness.
- Express realistic concern/feelings about symptoms/illness.
- Seek appropriate assistance for presenting problem.
- Display appropriate affect.

ACTIONS/INTERVENTIONS

Sample NIC linkages:

Anxiety Reduction: Minimizing apprehension, dread, foreboding, or uneasiness related to an unidentified source or anticipated danger

Counseling: Use of an interactive helping process focusing on the needs, problems, or feelings of the patient and significant others to enhance or support coping, problem solving, and interpersonal relationships

Coping Enhancement: Assisting a patient adapt to perceived stressors, changes, or threats that interfere with meeting life demands and roles

NURSING PRIORITY NO. I To assess causative/contributing factors:

- Identify situational crisis/problem and client's perception of the situation. *Identification of both reality and client's perception, which may not be the same as the reality, are necessary for planning care accurately.*[1]
- Ascertain cultural values/religious beliefs affecting perception of situation, sense of personal responsibility for crisis. *Knowing that lifestyle/choices may have caused or contributed to current situation may limit client's ability to accept outcome or view event realistically, and make choices regarding therapeutic regimen or lifestyle changes.*[5]

Cultural Collaborative Community/Home Care Diagnostic Studies Pediatric/Geriatric/Lifespan Medications

- Determine stage and degree of denial. *These factors will help identify whether the client is in early stages of denial and may be more amenable to intervention than those who are well entrenched in their beliefs. Treatment needs to begin where the client is and progress from there.*[1,6]
- Compare client's description of symptoms/conditions to reality of clinical picture and impact of illness/problem on lifestyle. *Identifies extent of discrepancy between the two and where treatment needs to start to help client accept reality.*[1]

NURSING PRIORITY NO. 2 To assist client to deal appropriately with situation:

- Develop nurse-client relationship using therapeutic communication skills of Active-listening and I-messages. *Promotes trust in which client can begin to look at reality of situation and deal with it in a positive manner.*[2]
- Provide safe, nonthreatening environment. Allows client to feel comfortable enough to talk freely without fear of judgment and to deal with issues realistically.[2]
- Encourage expressions of feelings, accepting client's view of the situation without confrontation. Set limits on maladaptive behavior *to promote safety. Helps client to work through and understand feelings. Unacceptable behavior is counterproductive to making progress, as client will view self negatively.*[2]
- Present accurate information as appropriate, without insisting that the client accept what has been presented. *Avoids confrontation, which may further entrench client in denial. Open manner permits client to begin to accept reality.*[2]
- Discuss client's behaviors in relation to illness (e.g., diabetes mellitus, alcoholism, terminal cancer) and point out the results of these behaviors. *Information can help client accept reality and opt to change behaviors.*[3]
- Encourage client to talk with SO(s)/friends. *May clarify concerns and reduce isolation and withdrawal. Constructive feedback from others facilitates understanding.*[4]
- Involve in group sessions. *Promotes discussion and feedback to enhance learning. Client can hear other views of reality and test own perceptions.*[4]
- Avoid agreeing with inaccurate statements/perceptions. *Prevents perpetuating false reality.*[2]
- Provide positive feedback for constructive moves toward independence. *Promotes repetition of desired behavior.*[4]

NURSING PRIORITY NO. 3 To promote wellness (Teaching/Discharge Considerations):

- Provide written information about illness/situation for client and family. *Can refer to resource for reminders as they consider options.*[1]
- Involve family members/SO(s) in long-range planning. *Provides support, helps to identify and meet individual needs for the future.*[4]
- Refer to appropriate community resources (e.g., Diabetes Association, Multiple Sclerosis Society, Alcoholics Anonymous). *May be needed to help client with long-term adjustment.*[2]
- Refer to ND ineffective Coping.

DOCUMENTATION FOCUS

Assessment/Reassessment

- Assessment findings, degree of personal vulnerability/denial.
- Impact of illness/problem on lifestyle.

Planning

- Plan of care and who is involved in the planning.
- Teaching plan.

Implementation/Evaluation

- Client's response to interventions/teaching and actions performed.
- Use of resources.
- Attainment/progress toward desired outcome(s).
- Modifications to plan of care.

Discharge Planning

- Long-term needs and who is responsible for actions taken.
- Specific referrals made.

References

1. Doenges, M. E., Moorhouse, M. F., Geissler-Murr, A. (2002). *Nursing Care Plans Guidelines for Individualizing Patient Care.* 6th ed. Philadelphia: F. A. Davis.
2. Doenges, M. E., Townsend, M. C., Moorhouse, M. F. (1998). *Psychiatric Care Plans.* 3d ed. Philadelphia: F. A. Davis.
3. Burgess, E. (1994). Denial and terminal illness. *Am J Hospice Palliative Care*, 11(2), 46–48.
4. Robinson, A. W. (1999). Getting to the heart of denial. *AJN*, 99(5), 38–42.
5. Lipson, J. G., Dibble, S. L., Minarik, P. A. (1996). *Culture & Nursing Care: A Pocket Guide.* San Francisco: School of Nursing, UCSF Nursing Press.
6. Roberto, D. (2003) Man in Denial. Available at www.insmkt.com/myhome.htm.

impaired Dentition

Definition: Disruption in tooth development/eruption patterns or structural integrity of individual teeth

RELATED FACTORS

Dietary habits; nutritional deficits

Selected prescription medications; chronic use of tobacco/coffee /tea/red wine

Ineffective oral hygiene; sensitivity to heat/cold; chronic vomiting

Deficient knowledge regarding dental health; excessive intake of fluorides/use of abrasive cleaning agents

Barriers to self-care; lack of access/economic barriers to professional care

Genetic predisposition; bruxism

[Traumatic injury/surgical intervention]

DEFINING CHARACTERISTICS

Subjective
Toothache

Objective
Halitosis

Tooth enamel discoloration; erosion of enamel; excessive plaque

Worn down/abraded teeth; crown/root caries; tooth fracture(s); loose teeth; missing teeth; absence of teeth

Premature loss of primary teeth; incomplete eruption for age (may be primary or permanent teeth)

Excessive calculus

Malocclusion/tooth misalignment; asymmetrical facial expression

Sample Clinical Applications: Facial trauma/surgery, malnutrition, eating disorders, head/neck cancer, seizure disorder

DESIRED OUTCOMES/EVALUATION CRITERIA
Sample NOC linkages:
Oral Hygiene: Condition of the mouth, teeth, gums, and tongue
Self-Care: Oral Hygiene: Ability to care for own mouth and teeth independently with or without assistive device
Knowledge: Health Behavior: Extent of understanding conveyed about the promotion and protection of health

Client/SO Will (Include Specific Time Frame)

- Display healthy gums and mucous membranes, and teeth in good repair.
- Report adequate nutritional/fluid intake.
- Verbalize understanding of appropriate oral hygiene regimen.
- Demonstrate effective dental hygiene skills.
- Follow through on referrals for appropriate dental care.

ACTION/INTERVENTIONS

Sample NIC linkages:
Oral Health Maintenance: Maintenance and promotion of oral hygiene and dental health for the patient at risk for developing oral or dental lesions
Oral Health Restoration: Promotion of healing for a patient who has an oral mucosa or dental lesion
Referral: Arrangement for services by another care provider or agency

NURSING PRIORITY NO. 1 To assess causative/contributing factors:

- Inspect oral cavity. Note presence/absence and intactness of teeth or dentures and appearance of gums. *Provides baseline for planning and interventions in terms of safety, nutritional needs, and aesthetics.*[1]
- Evaluate current status of dental hygiene and oral health *to determine need for instruction/coaching, assistive devices, and/or referral to dental care providers.*[1]
- Note presence of halitosis. *Bad breath may be result of numerous local or systemic conditions, including smoking, periodontal disease, dehydration, malnutrition, ketoacidosis, infections, or some antiseizure medications. Management can include simple mouth care or treatment of underlying conditions.*[2]
- Document age/developmental and cognitive status; manual dexterity. Evaluate nutritional and health state, noting presence of conditions such as bulimia/chronic vomiting; musculoskeletal impairments; or problems with mouth (e.g., bleeding disorders, cancer lesions/abscesses, facial trauma). *Factors affecting client's dental health and ability to provide own dental care.*[1]
- Note current situation that will affect dental health (e.g., presence of airway/ET intubation, facial fractures, jaw surgery, new braces, and use of anticoagulants or chemotherapy) that require special mouth care activities.[1,7]
- Document (photograph) facial injuries before treatment *to provide "pictorial baseline" for future comparison/evaluation.*

NURSING PRIORITY NO. 2 To treat/manage dental care needs:

- Ascertain client's usual method of oral care *to provide continuity of care or to build on client's existing knowledge base and current practices in developing plan of care.*[1]
- Assist with/provide oral care, as indicated:[1,8,9]
  Offer/provide tap water or saline rinses, diluted alcohol-free mouthwashes.
  Provide gentle gum massage and tongue brushing with soft toothbrush, using fluoride toothpaste *to manage tartar buildup, if appropriate.*
  Use foam sticks *to swab gums and oral cavity.*
  Assist with/encourage brushing and flossing when client is unable to do self-care.
  Provide/assist with electric or battery-powered mouth care devices (e.g., toothbrush, plaque remover, etc.) as indicated.
  Assist with/provide denture care when indicated (e.g., remove and clean after meals and at bedtime).
  Remind client to brush teeth as indicated. *Cues may be needed if client is young, elderly, or cognitively or emotionally impaired.*
- Reposition endotracheal tubes and airway adjuncts routinely, carefully padding/protecting teeth/prosthetics.[7]
- Suction as needed (if client is unable to manage secretions).
- Maintain good jaw/facial alignment when fractures are present.
- Provide appropriate diet for optimal nutrition, considering client's ability to chew (e.g., liquids or soft foods), and offering low-sugar, low-starch foods and snacks *to minimize tooth decay.*
- Avoid thermal stimuli when teeth are sensitive. Recommend use of specific designed toothpastes *to reduce sensitivity of teeth.*
- Administer antibiotics as needed t*o treat oral/gum infections that may be present and to prevent nosocomial infection in critically ill client whose teeth may be colonized by significant bacteria.*[3]
- Recommend use of analgesics and topical analgesics as needed *when dental pain is present.*
- Administer prophylactic antibiotic therapy prior to some dental procedures in susceptible individuals (e.g., presence of prosthetic heart valve, prior infective endocarditis, certain congential heart defects, cardiac transplant with subsequent valvulopathy) *to reduce risk of infective endocarditis resulting from manipulation of gingival tissue or the periapical region of teeth, or procedures that will perforate the oral mucosa.*[10]
- Direct client to notify dental care provider when bleeding disorder present/anticoagulant therapy (including aspirin) being used. *May impact choice of procedure/technique in order to prevent excess bleeding.*
- Refer to appropriate care providers (e.g., dental hygienists, dentists, periodontist, oral surgeon).

NURSING PRIORITY NO. 3 To promote wellness (Teaching/Discharge Considerations):

- Instruct client/caregiver to inspect oral cavity and in home-care interventions *to provide good oral care, and prevent tooth decay and periodontal disease.*[4]
- Review/demonstrate proper toothbrushing techniques (i.e., brushing with bristles perpendicular to teeth surfaces) after meals and flossing daily. Suggest brushing with fluoride-containing toothpaste if client able to swallow/manage oral secretions. *This is the most effective way of reducing plaque formation and preventing periodontal disease.*[8]
- Discuss dental and oral health needs, both as client perceives needs and according to professional standards. *Client's perceptions are shaped by self-image, family, and cultural expectations or conditions created by disease or trauma. Current healthcare practices and education are geared toward practices that improve client's appearance and health, including reduced consumption of refined sugars, optimal fluoridation, access to preventative and restorative dental care, prevention of oral cancers and prevention of craniofacial injuries.*[4]

- Recommend that clients of all ages decrease sugary/high-carbohydrate foods in diet and snacks *to reduce buildup of plaque and risk of cavities caused by acids associated with the breakdown of sugar and starch.*[4]
- Instruct older client and caregiver(s) concerning their special needs and importance of regular dental care. *Elderly are prone to (1) experience decay around older fillings (also have more fillings in mouth); (2) receding gums, exposing root surfaces, which decay easily; (3) have reduced production of saliva and use multiple medications that can cause dry mouth with loss of tooth and gum protection; and (4) loosening of teeth or poorly fitting dentures associated with gum/bone loss. These factors (often compounded by disease conditions and lack of funds) affect nutrient intake, chewing, swallowing, and oral cavity health.*[5]
- Advise mother regarding age-appropriate concerns:[1,4–6]

  Instruct mother to refrain from allowing baby to fall asleep with bottle containing formula, milk, or sweetened beverages. Suggest use of water and pacifier during night *to prevent bottle tooth decay.*

  Determine pattern of tooth appearance and tooth loss and compare to norms for primary and secondary teeth.

  Discuss tooth discoloration and needed follow-up. *Brown or black spots on teeth usually indicates decay, gray tooth color may indicate nerve injury, multiple cavities in adolescent could be caused from vomiting/bulimia.*

  Discuss pit and fissure sealants. *Painted-on tooth surface sealants are becoming widely available to reduce number of cavities and sometimes are available through community dental programs.*

  Determine if school dental health programs available or recommend regular professional dental examinations as child grows.

  Discuss with children/parents problems associated with oral piercing, if individual is contemplating piercing, or needs to know what to watch for after piercing. *Common symptoms that occur with piercing of lips, gums, and tongue include pain, swelling, infection, increased flow of saliva and chipped or cracked teeth requiring diligent oral care or more frequent dental examination to prevent complications.*

  Discuss use of/need for safety devices (e.g., helmets, face mask, mouth guards) *to prevent/limit severity of sports-related facial injuries and tooth damage/loss.*
- Discuss with pregnant women special needs and regular dental care. *Pregnant women need additional calcium and phosphorus to maintain good dental health and provide for strong teeth and bones in fetal development. Many women avoid dental care during pregnancy whether because of concerns for fetal health or other reasons (including lack of financial resources). However, one research study of 400 women suggests that pregnant women who receive treatment for periodontal disease can reduce their risk of giving birth to low-birth-weight or preterm baby.*[4]
- Review resources that are needed/available for the client to perform adequate dental hygiene care (e.g., toothbrush/paste, clean water, referral to dental care providers, access to financial assistance, personal care assistant).
- Encourage cessation of tobacco (especially smokeless) and enrolling in smoking cessation classes *to reduce risk of oral cancers and other health problems.*
- Discuss advisability of dental checkup and care prior to instituting chemotherapy or radiation *to minimize oral/dental/tissue damage.*

DOCUMENTATION FOCUS

Assessment/Reassessment

- Individual findings, including individual factors influencing dentition problems.
- Baseline photos/description of oral cavity/structures.

Planning

- Plan of care and who is involved in planning.
- Teaching plan.

Implementation/Evaluation

- Responses to interventions/teaching and actions performed.
- Attainment/progress toward desired outcome(s).
- Modifications to plan of care.

Discharge Planning

- Individual long-term needs, noting who is responsible for actions to be taken.
- Specific referrals made.

References

1. Doenges, M. E., Moorhouse, M. F., Murr, A. C. (2004). *Nurse's Pocket Guide: Diagnoses, Interventions, and Rationales.* 9th ed. Philadelphia: F. A. Davis.
2. Ayers, K. M., Colquhoun, A. N. (1998). *NZ Dent J*, 94(418), 156–160.
3. Scannapieco, F. A., Stewart, E. M., Mylotte, J. M. (1992). Colonization of dental plaque by respiratory pathogens in medical intensive care patients. *Crit Care Med*, 20, 740.
4. Public education pamphlets from the American Dental Association: Your diet and dental health; Oral changes with age; Sealants; Oral piercing; National Academy of Sciences panel reaffirms effectiveness of fluoride; Periodontal treatment can reduce risk of some pregnancy complications: study. (Original study from the University of Chile was published in *J Periodontology*, August 2002.) Pamphlets published at various times on the ADA.org Web site and accessed July 2003. Available at www.ada.org/public/media.
5. Diagnosis and management of dental caries throughout life. (2001). Office of Medical Applications of Research (OMAR). Bethesda, MD, March 2001. Available at http://consensus.nih.gov/2001/2001DentalCaries115html.htm.
6. Engel, J. (2002). *Moby's Pocket Guide to Pediatric Assessment.* 4th ed. St Louis, MO: Mosby.
7. Truman, B. I., Gooch, B. F., Sulemana, I., et al. (July 2002). Recommendations on selected interventions to prevent dental caries, oral and pharyngeal cancers, and sports-related craniofacial injuries. *Am J Prev Med*, 23(1 suppl), 21–54.
8. Stiefel, K. A., et al. (2000). Improving oral hygiene for the seriously ill patient: Implementing research-based practice. *Medsurg Nurs*, 9(1), 40.
9. No author listed. (2005). Tooth Decay: Prevention. Article for WebMD health topics Web site. Retrieved February 2007 at www.webmd.com/hw/dental/hw/172611.asp.
10. Stiles, S., Vega, C. P. (April 24, 2007). AHA updates recommendations for antibiotic prophylaxis for dental procedures. Retrieved July 2007 at www.medscape.com/viewarticle/555596.

risk for delayed Development

Definition: At risk for delay of 25% or more in one or more of the areas of social or self-regulatory behavior, or cognitive, language, gross or fine motor skills

RISK FACTORS

Prenatal

Maternal age <15 years or >35 years
Unplanned/unwanted pregnancy; lack of/late/poor prenatal care
Inadequate nutrition; poverty; illiteracy
Genetic/endocrine disorders; infections; substance abuse

Cultural • Collaborative • Community/Home Care • Diagnostic Studies • Pediatric/Geriatric/Lifespan • Medications

Individual

Prematurity; congenital/genetic disorders
Vision/hearing impairment; frequent otitis media
Inadequate nutrition; failure to thrive
Chronic illness; chemotherapy; radiation therapy
Brain damage (e.g., hemorrhage in postnatal period, shaken baby, abuse, accident); seizures
Positive drug screening(s); substance abuse; lead poisoning
Foster/adopted child
Behavior disorders
Technology-dependent
Natural disaster

Environmental

Poverty
Violence

Caregiver

Mental retardation; severe learning disability
Abuse
Mental illness

NOTE: A risk diagnosis is not evidenced by signs and symptoms, as the problem has not occurred; rather, nursing interventions are directed at prevention.

Sample Clinical Applications: Congenital/genetic disorders, prematurity, infection, nutritional problems (malnutrition, anorexia, failure to thrive), toxic exposures (e.g., lead), substance abuse, endocrine disorders, abuse/neglect, developmental delay

DESIRED OUTCOMES/EVALUATION CRITERIA
Sample NOC linkage:

Child Development: [specify age]: Milestones of physical, cognitive, and psychosocial progression by [specify] months/years of age

Client Will (Include Specific Time Frame)

• Perform motor, social, self-regulatory behavior, cognitive and language skills appropriate for age or within scope of present capabilities.

Sample NOC linkages:

Knowledge: Infant Care: Extent of understanding conveyed about caring for a baby from birth to first birthday

Parenting Performance: Parental actions to provide a child a nurturing and constructive physical, emotional, and social environment

Parent/Caregiver Will (Include Specific Time Frame)

• Verbalize understanding of age-appropriate development/expectations
• Identify individual risk factors for developmental delay/deviation
• Formulate plan(s) for prevention of developmental deviation.
• Intiate interventions/lifestyle changes promoting appropriate development.

ACTIONS/INTERVENTIONS

Sample NIC linkages:

Developmental Enhancement: Child [or] Adolescent: Facilitating or teaching parents/caregivers to facilitate the optimal gross motor, fine motor, language, cognitive, social, and emotional growth of preschool and school-age children during the transition from childhood to adulthood

Risk Identification: Analysis of potential risk factors, determination of health risks, and prioritization of risk-reduction strategies for an individual or group

NURSING PRIORITY NO. 1   To assess causative/contributing factors:

- Identify condition(s) that could contribute to developmental deviations as listed in Risk Factors (e.g., extremes of maternal age; prenatal substance abuse/fetal alcohol syndrome; brain injury/damage, especially that occurring before or at time of birth; prematurity; family history of developmental disorders; chronic severe illness, brain infections; mental illness or retardation; shaken baby syndrome abuse; family violence; failure to thrive; poverty; inadequate nutrition). *Developmental delay occurs when a child fails to achieve one or more developmental milestones and may be the result of one or multiple factors.*[1]
- Participate in multidisciplinary evaluation to assess client's development, including neurological exams or assessment tools such as Draw-a-Person, Denver Developmental Screening Test, Bender's Visual Motor Gestalt Test, Early Language Milestone (ELM) Scale 2 and developmental language disorders (DLD). *Delays may affect speech and language, fine or gross motor skills, or personal and social skills requiring a coordinated treatment approach based on client's specific needs.*[1,8–10]
- Obtain information from variety of sources. *Parents are often the first ones to think that there is a problem with their baby's development and should be encouraged to have routine well-baby checkups and screening for developmental delays. Teachers, family members, physicians, and others interacting with a client (older than infant) may have valuable input regarding behaviors that may indicate problems/developmental issues.*[1,2]
- Identify cultural beliefs, norms, and values, as they may impact parent/caregiver view of situation. *What is considered normal or abnormal development may be based on cultural beliefs/expectations.*[3]
- Ascertain nature of required parent/caregiver activities and evaluate caregiver's abilities to perform needed activities.
- Note severity/pervasiveness of situation (e.g., potential for long-term stress leading to abuse/neglect, versus situational disruption during period of crisis or transition that may eventually level out). *Situations require different interventions in terms of the intensity and length of time that assistance and support may be critical to the parent/caregiver. A crisis can produce great change within a family, some of which can be detrimental to the individual or family unit.*[4–6]
- Evaluate environment in which long-standing care will be provided. *The physical, emotional, financial, and social needs of a family are impacted and intertwined with the needs of the client. Changes may be needed in the physical structure of the home or family roles, resulting in disruption and stress, placing everyone at risk.*[4,6]

NURSING PRIORITY NO. 2   To assist in preventing or limiting developmental delays:

- Note chronological age and review expectations for "normal development" *to help determine developmental expectations (e.g., when child should roll over, sit up alone, speak first words, attain a certain weight/height, etc.), and how the expectations may be altered by child's condition. Note: Pediatrition may screen with a motor quotient (MQ; which is child's age calculated*

   Cultural   Collaborative   Community/Home Care   Diagnostic Studies   Pediatric/Geriatric/Lifespan   Medications

by milestones met divided by chronological age and multiplied by 100). MQ between 50 and 70 requires further evaluation/intervention.[1,7]

- Review expected skills/activities, using authoritative text (e.g., Gesell, Musen/Congor), reports of neurological exams, or assessment tools. *Provides guide for evaluation of growth and development, and for comparative measurement of individual's progress.*[2,4]

- Describe realistic, age-appropriate patterns of development to parent/caregiver and promote activities and interactions that support developmental tasks where client is at this time. *Important in planning interventions in keeping with the individual's current status and potential. Each child will have own unique strengths and challenges.*[1–3]

- Collaborate with related professional resources (e.g., physical/occupational/rehabilitation/speech therapists; home health agencies; social services, nutritionist; special-education teacher, family therapists; technological and adaptive equipment specialists; vocational counselor). *Multidisciplinary team care increases likelihood of developing a well-rounded plan of care that meets client/family's specialized and varied needs.*[4,10]

NURSING PRIORITY NO. 3 To promote wellness (Teaching/Discharge Considerations):

- Engage in/encourage prevention strategies (e.g., abstinence from drugs, alcohol and tobacco for pregnant women/child, referral for treatment programs, referral for violence prevention counseling, anticipatory guidance for potential handicaps [vision, hearing, failure to thrive]). *Promoting wellness starts with preventing complications and/or limiting severity of anticipated problems. Such strategies can often be initiated by nurses where the potential is first identified, in the community setting.*[1,4]

- Evaluate client's progress on continual basis. Identify target symptoms requiring intervention *to make referrals in a timely manner and/or to make adjustments in plan of care, as indicated.*[2]

- Provide/assist with follow-up appointments as indicated *to promote ongoing evaluation, support, or management of situation.*[2]

- Discuss proactive wellness actions to take (e.g., periodic laboratory studies to monitor nutritional status or getting immunizations on schedule to prevent serious infections) *to avoid preventable complications.*[2]

- Maintain positive, hopeful attitude. Encourage setting of short-term realistic goals for achieving developmental potential. *Small incremental steps are often easier to deal with, and successes enhance hopefulness and well-being.*[6]

- Provide information as appropriate, including pertinent reference materials, reliable Web sites. *Bibliotherapy provides opportunity to review data at own pace, enhancing likelihood of retention.*[1,2]

- Encourage attendance at educational programs (e.g., parenting classes, infant stimulation sessions, food buying/cooking/nutrition, home and family safety, anger management, seminars on life stresses, aging process) *to address specific learning need/desires and interact with others with similar life challenges.*[2]

- Identify available community and national resources as appropriate (e.g., early intervention programs, gifted and talented programs, sheltered workshop, crippled children's services, medical equipment/supplier, caregiver support and respite services). *Provides additional assistance to support family efforts and can help identify community responsibilities (e.g., services required to be provided to school-age child).*[1]

DOCUMENTATION FOCUS

Assessment/Reassessment

- Assessment findings/individual needs, including developmental level.
- Caregiver's understanding of situation and individual role.

Planning

- Plan of care and who is involved in the planning.
- Teaching plan.

Implementation/Evaluation

- Client's response to interventions/teaching and actions performed.
- Caregiver response to teaching.
- Attainment/progress toward desired outcome(s).
- Modifications to plan of care.

Discharge Planning

- Identified long-range needs and who is responsible for actions to be taken.
- Specific referrals made, sources for assistive devices, educational tools.

References

1. Developmental Delays: A Pediatrician's Guide to Your Children's Health and Safety. Accessed July 2003. Available at www.keepkidshealthy.com.
2. Practice parameters for the assessment and treatment of children, adolescents, and adults with autism and other pervasive developmental disorders. (1999). American Academy of Child and Adolescent Psychiatry Working Group on Quality Issues. *J Am Acad Child Adolesc Psychiatry*, 38 (12 Suppl), 55s–76s. Accessed July 2003 at www.guideline.gov.
3. Leininger, M. M. (1996). *Transcultural Nursing: Theories, Research and Practices*. 2d ed. Hilliard, OH: McGraw-Hill.
4. Doenges, M. E., Moorhouse, M. F., Geissler Murr, A. C. (2004). ND: Growth and Development, Delayed. In *Nurse's Pocket Guide: Diagnoses, Interventions, and Rationales*. 9th ed. Philadelphia: F. A. Davis.
5. Engel, J. (2002). *Mosby's Pocket Guide to Pediatric Assessment*. St Louis, MO: Mosby.
6. Cox, H. C., et al. (2002). *Clinical Applications of Nursing Diagnosis: Adult, Child, Women's Psychiatric, Gerontic, and Home Health Considerations*. 4th ed. Philadelphia: F. A. Davis.
7. Educating parents of extra-special children: Developmental delays. Available at www.epeconline.com/DeveolpmentalDelays.html.
8. Schiffman, R. F. (2004). Drug and subtance use in adolescents. *MCN, American J of Maternal/Child Nursing*, 29(1), 21–27.
9. Grenz, K., Bynum, G., Pine, D., et al (updated verson 2005). Preventive services for children and adolescents. Institute for Clinical Systems Improvement [ICSI]. Article for National Guideline Clearinghouse Web site. Retrieved February 2007 at www.guideline.gov.
10. Blann, L. E. (2005). Early intervention for children and families with special needs. *MCN, American J of Maternal/Child Nursing*, 30(4), 263–267.

Diarrhea

Definition: Passage of loose, unformed stools

RELATED FACTORS

Psychological
High stress levels; anxiety

Situational
Laxative/alcohol abuse; toxins; contaminants
Adverse effects of medications; radiation

Cultural Collaborative Community/Home Care Diagnostic Studies Pediatric/Geriatric/Lifespan Medications

Tube feedings
Travel

Physiological
Inflammation; irritation
Infectious processes; parasites
Malabsorption

DEFINING CHARACTERISTICS

Subjective
Abdominal pain
Urgency, cramping

Objective
Hyperactive bowel sounds
At least three loose liquid stools per day

Sample Clinical Applications: Inflammatory bowel disease, gastritis, enteral feedings, alcohol abuse, antibiotic use, food allergies/contamination, AIDS, radiation, parasites

DESIRED OUTCOMES/EVALUATION CRITERIA
Sample NOC linkages:
Bowel Elimination: Formation and evacuation of stool
Hydration: Adequate water in the intracellular and extracellular compartments of the body
Knowledge: Illness Care: Extent of understanding conveyed about illness-related information needed to achieve and maintain optimal health

Client Will (Include Specific Time Frame)

• Reestablish and maintain normal pattern of bowel functioning.
• Verbalize understanding of causative factors and rationale for treatment regimen.
• Demonstrate appropriate behavior to assist with resolution of causative factors (e.g., proper food preparation or avoidance of irritating foods).

ACTIONS/INTERVENTIONS

Sample NIC linkages:
Diarrhea Management: Management and alleviation of diarrhea
Fluid Monitoring: Collection and analysis of patient data to regulate fluid balance
Perineal Care: Maintenance of perineal skin integrity and relief of perineal discomfort

NURSING PRIORITY NO. 1   To assess causative factors/etiology:

∞ • Evaluate client/caregiver's perception of symptoms. *People perceive having diarrhea in many different ways, but generally if client is having loose watery stools occurring more than three times a day, the diagnosis of diarrhea can be made. The condition can affect people of all ages, although its effect is more dangerous for infants and frail elderly (due to risk of dehydration).*[1–3]
• Obtain comprehensive history of symptoms to help in identifying cause and treatment needs:[1,2,4–6,13,14]

Ascertain onset and pattern of diarrhea, noting whether acute or chronic. *Acute diarrhea caused by (1) viral/bacterial/parasitic infections (e.g., Norwalk, Rotavirus/salmonella, shigella/giardia, amebiasis, respectively); (2) bacterial food-borne toxins (e.g., staphylococcus aureus, E. coli); (3) medications (e.g., antibiotics, chemotherapy agents, colchicine, laxatives); and (4) enteral tube feedings lasting a few days up to a week.* **Chronic diarrhea** *caused by irritable bowel syndrome; infectious diseases; inflammatory bowel disease; colon cancer and treatments; severe constipation; malabsorption disorders; laxative abuse; certain endocrine disorders (e.g., hyperthyroidism, Addison's disease) almost always lasts more than 3 weeks.*

Review history/observe stools for **characteristics** (e.g., soft to watery stools, bloody, greasy), **frequency** (e.g., more than normal number of stools/day), **time of day** (e.g., after meals), **volume**, and **duration**.

Identify any **associated signs/symptoms** (e.g., fever/chills, abdominal cramping, emotional upset, weight loss), **aggravating factors** (e.g., stress, foods), or **mitigating factors** (e.g., changes in diet, use of prescription or OTC medications).

Note reports of abdominal or rectal pain. *Pain is often present with inflammatory bowel disease, irritable bowel syndrome, and mesenteric ischemia.*

- Note client's age. *Diarrhea in infant/young child and older or debilitated client can cause complications of dehydration and electrolyte imbalances.*
- Determine recent travel to developing countries/foreign environments; change in drinking water/food intake, consumption of unsafe food; swimming in untreated surface water, similar illness of family members/others close to client that *may help identify causative environmental factors.*[2,4-6]
- Review medications, noting side effects, possible interactions. *Many drugs (e.g., antibiotics, digitalis, ACE inhibitors, NSAIDS, hypoglycemia agents, cholesterol-lowering drugs) can cause/exacerbate diarrhea, particularly in the elderly. Beginning antibiotic therapy often causes changes in bowel habits.*[1,2,6-8]
- Evaluate diet history and note nutritional/fluid and electrolyte status *that may be causing/exacerbating diarrhea.*
- Auscultate abdomen for presence, location, and characteristics of bowel sounds. *High-pitched, rapidly occurring, loud or tinkling bowel sounds often accompany diarrhea.*[9]
- Determine if incontinence is present. *May indicate presence of fecal impaction, particularly in elderly, where impaction may be accompanied by diarrhea.*[3] (Refer to ND Bowel Incontinence.)
- Review results of laboratory testing on stool specimens. *Can reveal presence of bacterial/viral infection, parasites, fat, blood, offending drugs, metabolic disorder, malabsorption syndrome, gastroenteritis, colitis, etc.*[1,2,4-6]
- Assist with, prepare for additional evaluation as indicated. *Chronic diarrhea may require more invasive testing, including upper and/or lower GI radiographs, ultrasound, endoscopic evaluations, biopsy, etc.*[12]

NURSING PRIORITY NO. 2 To alleviate/limit condition:

- Assist with treatment of underlying conditions (e.g., infections, malabsorption syndrome, cancer) and complications of diarrhea. *Treatments are varied and may be as simple as allowing time for recovery from a self-limiting gastroenteritis, or may require complex treatments, including antimicrobials and rehydration, or community health interventions for contaminated food/water sources.*[14]
- Provide/encourage bedrest during acute episode. *Rest decreases intestinal motility and reduces metabolic rate when infection or hemorrhage is a complication.*[1-6,8,10]
- Restrict solid food intake, if indicated. *May help on short-term to allow for bowel rest/reduced intestinal workload, especially if cause of diarrhea is under investigation or vomiting is present.*

Note: Child's preferred/usual diet may be continued to prevent or limit dehydration, with the possible limitation of fruit, fruit juices, or milk, if these factors are exacerbating the diarrhea.[5,9]

- Limit caffeine and high-fat (e.g., butter, fried foods) or high-protein (e.g., meats) and foods known to cause/aggravate diarrhea (e.g., extremely hot/cold foods, chili), and milk and fruits/fruit juices as appropriate.[1-6,8,10]
- Adjust strength/rate of enteral tube feedings; change formula as indicated *when diarrhea is associated with tube feedings.*[1-6,8,10]
- Consider change in infant formula. *Diarrhea may be result of/aggravated by intolerance to specific formula.*[9,10]
- Change medications as appropriate (e.g., stopping magnesium-containing antacid or antibiotic causing diarrhea).[7,8]
- Promote the use of relaxation techniques (e.g., progressive relaxation exercise, visualization techniques) *to decrease stress/anxiety.*[1-6,8,10]
- Administer medications *to treat or limit diarrhea, as indicated, depending on cause. May include use of antidiarrheals, anti-infectives, antispasmodics, etc.*[1-6,8,10,14]
- Assist client to manage situation:[12]
  Respond to call for assistance promptly.
  Place bedpan in bed with client (if desired) or commode chair near bed *to provide quick access/reduce need to wait for assistance of others.*
  Provide privacy; remove stool promptly; use room deodorizers *to reduce noxious odors, limit embarrassment.*
  Use incontinence pads, depending on the severity of the problem.
  Provide emotional/psychological support. *Diarrhea can be source of great embarrassment and can lead to social isolation and feeling of powerlessness. Intimate relationship and sexual activity may be affected and need specific interventions to resolve.*
- Maintain skin integrity:[12]
  Assist as needed with pericare after each bowel movement *to prevent skin excoriation and breakdown.*
  Provide prompt diaper/incontinence pad change and gentle cleansing, *because skin breakdown can occur quickly with diarrhea.*
  Apply lotion/ointment skin barrier as needed.
  Provide dry linen as necessary.
  Expose perineum/buttocks to air/use heat lamp with caution if needed *to keep area dry.*
  Refer to ND impaired Skin Integrity.

NURSING PRIORITY NO. 3 To restore/maintain hydration/electrolyte balance:

- Note reports of thirst, less frequent or absent urination, dry mouth and skin, weakness, light-headedness, headache. *Signs/symptoms of dehydration and need for rehydration.*[1-3,5,6,10]
- Observe for/question parents about young child crying with no tears, fever, decreased urination, or no wet diapers for 6 to 8 hours, listlessness or irritability, sunken eyes, dry mouth and tongue, and suspected or documented weight loss. *Child needs emergency/inpatient treatment for dehydration if these signs are present and child is not taking fluids.*[1-3,5,6,10]
- Note presence of low blood pressure/postural hypotension, tachycardia, poor skin hydration/turgor. *Presence of these factors indicates severe dehydration and electrolyte imbalance. The frail elderly can progress quickly to this point, especially when vomiting is present or client's normal food and fluid intake is below requirements.*[1-3,5,6,10]
- Monitor total intake and output, including stool output as possible. *Provides estimation of fluid needs.*[1-3,5,6,10]
- Weigh infant's diapers to determine output.[1-3,5,6,10]

- Offer/encourage water, plus broth or soups that contain sodium, and fruit juices/soft fruits or vegetables that contain potassium *to replace water and electrolytes.*[1–3,5,6,10]
- Recommend oral intake of beverages such as Gatorade, Pedialyte, Infalyte, Smart Water. *Commercial rehydration solutions containing electrolytes may prevent/correct imbalances* .[1–3,5,6,10]
- Administer enteral/parenteral feedings and IV/electrolyte fluids as indicated. *Intravenous fluids may be needed either short-term to restore hydration status (e.g., acute gastroenteritis) or long-term (severe osmotic diarrhea). Enteral/parenteral nutrition is reserved for clients unable to maintain adequate nutritional status because of long-term diarrhea (e.g., wasting syndrome, malnutrition states).*[1–3,5,6,10]

NURSING PRIORITY NO. 4 To promote return to normal bowel functioning:

- Encourage intake of nonirritating liquids, increasing intake as tolerated and gradually returning to normal diet.[1,2,4-6,10,11]
- Recommend products such as natural fiber, plain natural yogurt, Lactinex *to restore normal bowel flora.*[1,2,4–6,10,11]
- Administer medications as ordered *to treat infectious process, decrease motility, and/or absorb water.*[1,2,4–6,10,11]

NURSING PRIORITY NO. 5 To promote wellness (Teaching/Discharge Considerations):

- Review individual's causative factors and appropriate interventions *to prevent recurrence.*
- Discuss medication regimen, including prescription and OTC drugs, *especially when client has multiple medications with potential for diarrhea as side effect or interaction.*[12]
- Instruct clients planning to travel outside the United States about traveler's diarrhea and ways to prevent/limit *(e.g., do not drink tap water, use tap water ice cubes, or brush your teeth with tap water; avoid raw fruits and vegetables, unless they can be peeled; avoid raw or rare meat or fish; discuss destination with local health department for particular recommendations, such as advisability of use of protective antibiotics).*[12]
- Assess home/living environment, if indicated. *Discussion with client/caregivers may be needed regarding (1) sanitation and hygiene (e.g., handwashing and laundry practices), (2) safe food storage and preparation (to reduce risk of food-borne infections), and (3) particular risks in select populations (e.g., persons with chronic liver disease should avoid shellfish; persons with impaired immune defenses are at increased risk for diarrhea associated with raw dairy products or unheated deli meats; pregnant women should avoid undercooked meats [infectious diarrhea]).*[12]
- Emphasize importance of handwashing *to prevent spread of infectious causes of diarrhea such as clostridium difficile (C.difficile), staph-A, etc.*[15]
- Instruct parent/caregiver in signs of dehydration and importance of fluid and electrolyte replacement, as well as simple food/fluids to provide rehydration.

DOCUMENTATION FOCUS

Assessment/Reassessment

- Assessment findings, including characteristics/pattern of elimination.

Planning

- Plan of care and who is involved in planning.
- Teaching plan.

⊕ Cultural Ⓐ Collaborative 🏠 Community/Home Care ⟋ Diagnostic Studies ∞ Pediatric/Geriatric/Lifespan ⬭ Medications

Implementation/Evaluation

- Client's response to treatment/teaching and actions performed.
- Attainment/progress toward desired outcome(s).
- Modifications to plan of care.

Discharge planning

- Recommendations for follow-up care.

References

1. Hogan, C. M. (1998). The nurse's role in diarrhea management. *Oncol Nurs Forum*, 25(5), 879–885.
2. Diarrhea. National Digestive Diseases Information Clearinghouse. (NDDIC). National Institutes of Health Publication No. 01–2749 January 2001.
3. Carnaveli, D. L., Patrick, M. (1993). *Nursing Management for the Elderly*. 3d ed. Philadelphia: JB Lippincott.
4. Evidence based clinical practice guideline for children with acute gastroenteritis (AGE). (2001). Cincinnati (OH) Children's Hospital Medical Center. Accessed July 2003.
5. American Gastroenterological Association medical position statement: Guidelines for the evaluation of chronic diarrhea. (1999). Accessed July 2003 at www.guideline.gov.
6. Guerrant, R. L., et al. (2001). Practice guidelines for the management of infectious diarrhea. *Clin Infect Dis*, 32(3), 331–351.
7. Ratnaike, R. N. (2000). Drug-induced diarrhea in older persons. *Clin Geriatr*, 8(1), 67–76.
8. Vogel, L. C. (1995). Antibiotic-induced diarrhea. *Orthop Nurs*, 14, 38–41.
9. Engel, J. (2002). *Mosby's Pocket Guide to Pediatric Assessment*. 4th ed. St Louis, MO: Mosby.
10. Larson, C. E. (2000). Evidence-based practice: Safety and efficacy of oral rehydration therapy for the treatment of diarrhea and gastroenteritis in pediatrics. *Pediatr Nurs*, 26(2), 177–179.
11. Peikin, S. R. (1999). *Diarrhea in Gastrointestinal Health*. New York: HarperCollins.
12. Doenges, M. E., Moorhouse, M. F., Geissler-Murr, A. C. (2002). ND Diarrhea, risk for in Gastrointestinal Disorders. In *Nursing Care Plans: Guidelines for Individualizing Patient Care*. 6th ed. Philadelphia: F. A. Davis.
13. Marks, J. W., Lee, D. (2004). Diarrhea. Article for MedicineNet Web site. Retrieved February 2007 at www.medicinenet.com.
14. Diskin, A. (2006). Gastroenteritis. Article for Emedicine Web site. Retrived February 2007 at www.emedicine.com/emerg/topic213.htm.
15. DeNoon, D. (2006). C.Diff: New threat from old bug: Epidemic gut infection causing rapid rise in life-threatening disease. Article for MedicineNet Web site. Retrieved February 2007 at www.medicinenet.com.

risk for compromised human Dignity

Definition: At risk for perceived loss of respect and honor

RISK FACTORS
Loss of control of body functions; exposure of the body
Perceived humiliation/invasion of privacy
Disclosure of confidential information; stigmatizing label; use of undefined medical terms
Perceived dehumanizing treatment/intrusion by clinicians
Inadequate participation in decision making
Cultural incongruity
NOTE: A risk diagnosis is not evidenced by signs and symptoms, as the problem has not occurred; rather, nursing interventions are directed at prevention.

Sample Clinical Applications: Chronic conditions, eg: multiple sclerosis, stroke, quadraplegia, ALS

DESIRED OUTCOMES/EVALUATION CRITERIA
Sample NOC linkages:

Patient Satisfaction: Protection of Rights: Extent of positive perception of protection of a patient's legal and moral rights provided by nursing staff

Patient Satisfaction: Cultural Needs Fulfillment: Extent of positive perception of integration of cultural beliefs, values, and social structures into nursing care

Client Will (Include Specific Time Frame)

- Verbalize awareness of specific problem.
- Identify positive ways to deal with situation.
- Demonstrate problem-solving skills.
- Express sense of dignity in situation.

ACTIONS/INTERVENTIONS

Sample NIC linkages:

Cultural Brokerage: The deliberate use of culturally competent strategies to bridge or medicate between the patient's culture and the biomedical healthcare system

Patient Rights Protection: Protection of healthcare rights of a patient, especially a minor, incapacitated, or incompetent patient unable to make decisions

Emotional Support: Provision of reassurance, acceptance, and encouragement during times of stress

NURSING PRIORITY NO. 1 To determine individual situation as perceived by client:

- Determine client's perception and specific factors that could lead to sense of loss of dignity. *Human dignity is a totality of the individual's uniqueness—mind, body, and spirit, and all components must be considered.*[4]
- Note labels/items used by staff, friends/family that stigmatize the client. *Human dignity is threatened by insensitive, as well as inadequate healthcare and lack of client participation in care decisions.*[4]
- Identify cultural beliefs/values and degree of importance to client. *Some individuals cling to their basic culture, especially during times of stress, which may result in conflict with current circumstances.*[7]
- Identify client's/SO's healthcare goals/expectations. *Clarifies client's (or SO/family's) vision, provides framework for planning care, identifies possible conflicts.*[2]
- Note availability of support systems. *Client will feel loved and valued and will be able to manage difficult circumstances better when the support of family and friends surrounds individual.*[2]
- Ascertain response of family/SOs to client's situation. *It is important that family supports and values client to enable him or her to manage situation. If they are not supportive or conflicts arise, client may need to separate self from family members who are negative.*[3]

NURSING PRIORITY NO. 2 To assist client to deal with situation in positive ways:

- Ask client by what name he or she would like to be addressed. *A person's name is important to their identity and recognizes their individuality. Many older people prefer to be addressed in a formal manner (e.g., Mr. or Mrs.).*[2,7]
- Active-listen feelings, encouraging client to verbalize concerns. Be available for support and assistance. *Helps client to discover underlying reasons for feelings and discuss solutions.*[5]
- Respect the client's needs and wishes for quiet, privacy, talking, or silence. *Conveys respect and concern for client's dignity.*[3]

Cultural · Collaborative · Community/Home Care · Diagnostic Studies · Pediatric/Geriatric/Lifespan · Medications

- Provide for privacy when discussing sensitive/personal issues. *Demonstrates respect for client and promotes sense of safe environment for free exchange of thoughts/feelings.*[3]
- Use understandable terms when talking to client/family about the medical condition procedures/treatments. *Most lay people do not understand medical terms and may be hesitant to ask what is meant.*[6]
- Encourage family/SO(s) to treat client with respect and understanding, especially when the client is older and may be irritable and difficult to deal with. *Everyone needs to be treated with respect and dignity, regardless of individual abilities/frailty.*[4]
- Include client and family in decision making, especially regarding end-of-life issues. *Helps the individual feel respected/valued and involved in the care process.*[2]
- Involve facility/local ethics committee as appropriate *to facilitate mediation/resolution of conflicts between client/family and staff, or client and family members.*
- Protect client's privacy when providing personal care/during procedures. Assure client is covered adequately when care is being given. *Prevents embarrassment over unnecessary exposure and conveys a message of caring.*[6]
- Clean client immediately when vomiting, bleeding, or incontinence occurs. Speak in a gentle voice. *Assures client that these things cannot be helped and that nurses are glad to take care of the problem.*

NURSING PRIORITY NO. 3 To promote wellness (Teaching/Discharge Considerations):

- Discuss client's rights as an individual. *While hospitals and other care settings have a Client's Bill of Rights, a broader view of human dignity is stated in America's Constitution.*[1,6]
- Assist with planning for the future, taking into account client's desires and rights. *As the client plans for the future, the needs of the self as a human who has dignity are considered and incorporated to preserve that dignity.*[4]
- Incorporate familial, religious, and cultural factors that have meaning for client in planning process. *When these issues are addressed and incorporated in plan of care, they add to the feelings of inclusion for the client.*[4,7]
- Refer to other resources (e.g., pastoral care, counseling, organized support groups, classes), as appropriate. *May need additional assistance to deal with illness/situation.*[6]

DOCUMENTATION FOCUS

Assessment/Reassessment

- Assessment findings, including individual risk factors, client's perceptions, and concerns about involvement in care.
- Individual cultural/religious beliefs/values, healthcare goals.
- Responses/involvement of family/SOs.

Planning

- Plan of care and who is involved in planning
- Teaching Plan

Implementation/Evaluation

- Client's response to interventions/teaching and actions performed
- Attainment/progress toward desired outcome(s)
- Modifications to plan of care

Discharge Planning

- Long-term needs and who is responsible for actions to be taken
- Specific referrals made

References

1. Champion Aspirations for Human Dignity. The White House. Available at www.whitehouse.gov/nsc/nss2.html.
2. Schulman, A. (2005). Staff Working Paper. The Presidents' Council on Bioethics. Bioethics and Human Dignity.
3. Cheshire, W. P., Jr. (2007). Grey matters-when eloquence is inarticulate. *Ethics & Medicine: An International Journal of Bioethics* 22(3). Retrieved March 2007 from the Center for Bioethics Human Dignity at www.cbhd.org/resources/neuroethics/cheshire_2007-01-26.htm.
4. The Center for Ethics and Advocacy in Healthcare. Retrieved March 2007 at www.healthcare-ethics.org/about/.
5. Gordon, T. (2000). *Parent Effectiveness Training.* New York: Three Rivers Press.
6. Doenges, M., Moorhouse, M., Murr, A. (2002). *Nursing Care Plans, Guidelines for Individualizing Patient Care.* 6th ed. Philadelphia: F. A. Davis.
7. Lipson, J. G., Dibble, S. L., Minarik, P. A. (1996). *Culture & Nursing Care: A Pocket Guide.* San Francisco: School of Nursing, UCSF Nursing Press.

moral Distress

Definition: Response to the inability to carry out one's chosen ethical/moral decision/action

RELATED FACTORS

Conflict among decision makers, [e.g., client/family, healthcare providers, insurance payers, regulatory agencies]

Conflicting information guiding moral/ethical decision making; cultural conflicts

Treatment decisions; end-of-life decisions; loss of autonomy

Time constraints for decision making; physical distance of decision maker

DEFINING CHARACTERISTICS

Subjective

Expresses anguish (e.g., powerlessness, guilt, frustration, anxiety, self-doubt, fear) over difficulty of acting on one's moral choice

DESIRED OUTCOMES/EVALUATION CRITERIA

Sample NOC linkages:

Decision Making: Ability to make judgments and choose between two or more alternatives

Patient Satisfaction: Protection of Rights: Extent of positive perception of a patient's legal and moral rights provided by nursing staff

Participation in Healthcare Decision: Personal involvement in selecting and evaluating healthcare options to achieve desired outcome

Client Will (Include Specific Time Frame)

- Verbalize understanding of causes for conflict in own situation.
- Be aware of own moral values conflicting with desired/required course of action.
- Identify positive ways/actions necessary to deal with own self and situation.
- Express sense of satisfaction with/acceptance of resolution.

⊕ Cultural   Ⓐ Collaborative   🏠 Community/Home Care   Diagnostic Studies   ∞ Pediatric/Geriatric/Lifespan   Medications

ACTIONS/INTERVENTIONS

Sample NIC linkages:

Values Clarification: Assisting another to clarify her or his own values in order to facilitate effective decision making

Decision-Making Support: Providing information and support for a patient who is making a decision regarding healthcare

Mutual Goal-Setting: Collaborating with a patient to identify and prioritize care goals, then developing a plan of care for achieving those goals

NURSING PRIORITY NO. 1 To identify cause/situation in which moral distress is occurring:

- Note situations/individuals at high risk for conflict. *For example, family members may not agree on proper course of action for comatose loved one, parents faced with expectation of taking ventilator-dependent child home and effect on family as a whole,[8] care providers discontinuing life-support measures for preterm infant are likely to encounter some degree of distress with decision making but may be silent about their discomfort. Recognizing potential for moral distress allows for timely intervention and support for involved parties.*
- Determine client's perceptions and specific factors resulting in a sense of distress, and all parties involved in situation. *Conflict may be personal or job related. Moral conflict centers around lessening the amount of harm suffered, with the involved individuals usually struggling with decisions such as what "can be done" to prevent, improve, or cure a medical condition or what "ought to be done" in a specific situation, often within financial constraints or scarcity of resources.[6]*
- Note use of sarcasm, avoidance, apathy, crying, reports of depression/loss of meaning. *Individuals may not understand their feelings of uneasiness/distress or know that the emotional basis for moral distress is anger.[4]*
- Ascertain response of family/SOs to client's situation/healthcare choices. *May provide clues to emotional/conflictual problems individual is experiencing.*
- Identify healthcare goals/expectations. *New treatment options/technology can prolong life or postpone death based on the individual's personal viewpoint, increasing the possibility of conflict with others, including healthcare providers.[2]*
- Ascertain cultural beliefs/values and degree of importance to client. *Cultural diversity may lead to disparate views/expectations between clients, SO/family members, and healthcare providers. When tensions between conflicting values cannot be resolved, persons experience moral distress.[2]*
- Note attitudes and expressions of dissatisfaction of caregivers/staff. *Client may feel pressure/disapproval if own views are not congruent with expectations of those perceived to be more knowledgeable or in "authority." Furthermore, healthcare providers may themselves feel moral distress in carrying out or refraining from performing requested interventions.[7]*
- Determine degree of emotional and physical distress (e.g., fatigue, headaches, forgetfulness, anger, guilt, resentment) individual(s) are experiencing and impact on ability to function. *Moral distress can be very destructive, affecting one's ability to carry out daily tasks/care for self or others, and may lead to a crisis of faith.[5]*
- Assess sleep habits of involved parties. *Evidence suggests that sleep-deprivation can harm a person's physical and emotional well-being, hindering the ability to integrate emotion and cognition to guide moral judgment.[5]*
- Perform/review results of moral distress test, such as the Moral Distress Assessment questionnaire (MDAQ), or Moral Distress Scale to help measure degree of involvement and identify possible actions to improve situation.[3,10]
- Note availability of family/friends/coworkers. *Provides support and encouragement for difficult situation.[4]*

NURSING PRIORITY NO. 2 To assist client/involved individuals to develop/effectively use problem-solving skills:

- Encourage involved individuals to recognize and name the experience, resulting in moral sensitivity. *Brings concerns out in the open so they can be dealt with.*[1]
- Provide time for nonjudgmental discussion of philosophical issues/questions about impact of conflict leading to moral questioning of current situation. *Moral issues have been discussed and studied for many years (e.g., philosophers, such as Piaget [1932] with his early work in developmental moral psychology, discussed what is the basis for moral reasoning). It is not possible to accurately read another's mind, and open discussion helps those involved in conflict to better understand the situation and begin to look at options.*[9]
- Use skills such as Active-listening, I-messages, and problem-solving *to clarify feelings of anxiety and conflict. Helps to understand what the ethical dilemmas are that lead to moral distress (e.g., family members ignoring advanced directives of loved one, providing lifesaving care to a death-row inmate, terminally ill individual requesting assistance to die, families living with the moral experience of caring for a ventilator-assisted child in the home).*[8]
- Provide privacy when discussing sensitive personal issues. *Shows regard and concern for individual's self-worth.*[2]
- Ascertain coping behaviors client has used successfully in the past that may be used in the current situation. *When encouraged, individuals can recall past situations where they had a positive experience and used successful coping skills.*[4]
- Identify role models (e.g., other individuals who have experienced similar problems in their lives). *Sharing of experiences, identifying options can be helpful to deal with current situation.*[1]
- Involve facility/local ethics committee or ethicist as appropriate *to educate, make recommendations, and facilitate mediation/resolution of issues.*[3]

NURSING PRIORITY NO. 3 To promote wellness (Teaching/Discharge Considerations):

- Engage all parties as appropriate in developing plan to address conflict. *Resolving one's moral distress requires making changes or compromises while preserving one's integrity and authenticity.*[4]
- Incorporate identified familial, religious, and cultural factors that have meaning for client. *Can provide comfort for the person.*[7]
- Refer to appropriate resources for support/guidance (e.g., pastoral care, counseling, organized support groups, classes) as indicated. *These resources can help client as they pursue the search for moral resolution.*[8]
- Assist individual to recognize that if she or he follows their moral decisions, they may clash with the legal system, and refer to appropriate resource for legal opinion/options.[3]
- Encourage the work organization to provide better support resources and structures. Discuss changes in the healthcare system that have resulted in more complex healthcare decisions. *The complexity of healthcare choices, expectations of clients/families, increasing costs/limitations in resources has resulted in increased pressures on healthcare providers and has led to ethics becoming a required component of clinical practice. Acknowledging reality of potential areas of conflict and providing proactive discussions for staff as well as support for involved individuals when making difficult decisions can decrease moral distress for staff and families.*[2,8]

DOCUMENTATION FOCUS

Assessment/Reassessment

- Individual findings, including nature of moral conflict, individuals involved in conflict.
- Physical/emotional responses to conflict.

Cultural Collaborative Community/Home Care Diagnostic Studies Pediatric/Geriatric/Lifespan Medications

- Individual cultural/religious beliefs and values, healthcare goals.
- Responses/involvement of family/SOs or coworkers.

Planning

- Plan of care and who is involved in planning.
- Teaching Plan.

Implementation/Evaluation

- Responses to interventions/teaching.
- Effects of participation in classes/mediation activities.
- Attainment/progress toward desired outcome(s).
- Modifications to plan of care.

Discharge Planning

- Long-term needs and who is responsible for actions to be taken.
- Available resources.
- Specific referrals made.

References

1. Elpern, E. H., Covert, B., Kleinpell, R. (2005). Moral distress of staff nurses in a medical intensive care unit. *Am J of Critical Care*, 14, 523–539.
2. Kalvemark, S., Hoglund, A. A. T., Hansson M. G., Westerholm, P., Arnetz, B. (2004). Living with conflicts—ethical dilemmas and moral distress in the health care system. *Soc Sci Med*, 58(6), 1075–1084. Dept. of Public Health and Caring Sciences, Uppsala University, Uppsala, Sweden.
3. Hanna, D. R. (2002). Moral distress redefined: The lived experience of moral distress of nurses who participated in legal, elective, surgically induced abortions. Retrieved July 2007 at http://escholarship.bc.edu/dissertations/AAI3053658/.
4. Cheshire, W. P. (2007). Grey Matters When Eloquence Is Inarticulate. The Center for BioEthics Human Dignity. Retrieved July 2007 at www.cbhd.org/resources/neuroethics/cheshire_2007-02-26.htm.
5. Preidt, R. (2007). Sleeplessness Clouds Moral Choices. American Academy of Sleep Medicine. Retrieved July 2007 at www.ktvotv3.com/Global/story.asp?S=6170132&nav=menu124_5.
6. Kopala, B., Burkhart, L. (2005). Ethical dilemma and moral distress: Proposed new NANDA diagnoses. *International Journal of Nursing Terminologies and Classifications*, 16(1).
7. Nichols, S. (2002). Mindreading and the Core Architecture of Moral Psychology, Department of Philosophy, College of Charleston, Charleston, SC. *Cognition* 84, 221–236. Retrieved July 2007 at http://ruccs.rutgers.edu/ArchiveFolder/Research%20Group/Publications/MCMP/MCAMP1b.htm.
8. Carnevale, F. A., Alexander, E., Renneck, J. (2006). Daily living with distress and enrichment: The moral experience of families with ventilator-assisted children at home. *Pediatrics*, 117(1), e48–e60 (doi:10.1542/peds. 2005-0789). Retrieved July 2007 at http://pediatrics.aappublications.org/cgi/content/abstract/117/1/e48.
9. Piaget, J. (1932). *The Psychology of Moral Development: The Nature and Validity of Moral Stages*. M. Gabain, trans. New York: Free Press. (Translation published 1965.)
10. Corley, M. (1993). Moral distress of critical care nurses. *Am J of Critical Care Nurses*, 4(4), 280–285.

risk for Disuse Syndrome

Definition: At risk for deterioration of body systems as the result of prescribed or unavoidable musculoskeletal inactivity

Note: Complications from immobility can include pressure ulcer, constipation, stasis of pulmonary secretions, thrombosis, urinary tract infection and/or retention, decreased strength or endurance, orthostatic hypotension, decreased range of joint motion, disorientation, body image disturbance, and powerlessness.

RISK FACTORS

Severe pain; [chronic pain]

Paralysis; [other neuromuscular impairment]

Mechanical/prescribed immobilization

Altered level of consciousness

[Chronic physical or mental illness]

NOTE: A risk diagnosis is not evidenced by signs and symptoms, as the problem has not occurred; rather, nursing interventions are directed at prevention.

Sample Clinical Applications: Multiple sclerosis, cerebral palsy, muscular dystrophy, post-polio syndrome, brain injury/stroke, spinal cord injury, arthritis, osteoporosis, fractures, amputation, dementia

DESIRED OUTCOMES/EVALUATION CRITERIA

Sample NOC linkages:

Immobility Consequences: Physiological: Severity of compromise in physiological functioning due to impaired physical mobility

Risk Control: Personal actions to prevent, eliminate, or reduce modifiable health threats

Immobility Consequences: Psycho-Cognitive: Severity of compromise in psychco-cognitive functioning due to impaired physical mobility

Client Will (Include Specific Time Frame)

- Display intact skin/tissues or achieve timely wound healing.
- Maintain/reestablish effective elimination patterns.
- Be free of signs/symptoms of infectious processes.
- Demonstrate absence of pulmonary congestion with breath sounds clear.
- Demonstrate adequate peripheral perfusion with stable vital signs, skin warm and dry, palpable peripheral pulses.
- Maintain usual reality orientation.
- Maintain/regain optimal level of cognitive, neurosensory, and musculoskeletal functioning.
- Express sense of control over the present situation and potential outcome.
- Recognize and incorporate change into self-concept in accurate manner without negative self-esteem.

ACTIONS/INTERVENTIONS

Sample NIC linkages:

Energy Management: Regulating energy use to treat or prevent fatigue and optimize function

Environmental Management: Manipulation of the patient's surroundings for therapeutic benefit

Exercise Promotion: Facilitation of regular physical exercise to maintain or advance to a higher level of fitness and health

NURSING PRIORITY NO. 1 To evaluate probability of developing complications:

- Identify underlying conditions/pathology (e.g., cancer, trauma; fractures with casting, immobilization devices; surgery, chronic disease conditions, malnutrition; neurological conditions [e.g., stroke/other brain/spinal cord injury, post-polio syndrome, multiple sclerosis]; chronic pain conditions; use of predisposing medications [e.g., steroids]) *that cause/exacerbate problems associated with inactivity and immobility.*

Cultural Collaborative Community/Home Care Diagnostic Studies Pediatric/Geriatric/Lifespan Medications

- Identify potential concerns, including cognition, mobility, and exercise status. *Disuse syndrome can be a complication of and cause for bedridden state. The syndrome can include muscle and bone atrophy, stiffening of joints, brittle bones, reduction of cardiopulmonary function, loss of red blood cells, decreased sex hormones, decreased resistance to infections, increased proportion of body fat in relation to muscle mass and chemical changes in the brain, which adversely impact client's activities of daily living, social life, and quality of life.*[1,2]
- Note client's age. *Age-related physiological changes accompanied by chronic illness predispose older adults to functional decline related to inactivity and immobility.*[3,8]
- Determine if client's condition is acute/short-term or whether it may be a long-term/permanent condition. *Relatively short-term conditions (e.g., simple fracture treated with cast) may respond quickly to rehabilitative efforts. Long-term conditions (e.g., stroke, aged person with dementia, cancers, demyelinating or degenerative diseases, spinal cord injury, and psychological problems such as depression or learned helplessness) have a higher risk of complications for the client and caregiver.*
- Assess/document (ongoing) client's functional status, including cognition, vision, and hearing, social support, psychological well-being, abilities in performance of ADLs *for comparative baseline, to evaluate response to treatment and to identify preventative interventions or necessary services.*[8]
- Evaluate client's risk for injury. *Risk is greater in client with cognitive problems, lack of safe or stimulating environment, inadequate mobility aids, and/or sensory-perception problems.*[3]
- Ascertain attitudes of individual/SO about condition (e.g., cultural values, stigma). Note misconceptions. *The client may be influenced (positively or negatively) by peer group and family role expectations.*
- Evaluate client's/family's understanding and ability to manage care for prolonged period. Ascertain availability and use of support systems. *Caregivers may be influenced by their own physical/emotional limitations, degree of commitment to assisting the client toward optimal independence, or available time.*[3]
- Review psychological assessment of client's emotional status. *Potential problems that may arise from presence of condition need to be identified and dealt with to avoid further debilitation.*[3]

NURSING PRIORITY NO. 2 To identify/provide individually appropriate preventive or corrective interventions:

Skin:[6,7]

- Inspect skin on a frequent basis, noting changes. Monitor skin over bony prominences.
- Reposition frequently as individually indicated *to relieve pressure.*
- Provide skin care daily and prn, drying well and using gentle massage and lotion *to stimulate circulation.*
- Keep skin, clothing, and area clean/dry *to prevent/limit skin irritation and breakdown.*
- Initiate use of padding devices (e.g., foam, egg-crate/gel/water/air mattress or cushions) *to reduce pressure on/enhance circulation to compromised tissues.*
- Review nutritional status and promote diet with adequate protein, calorie, and vitamin/mineral intake *to aid in healing and promote general good health of skin/tissues.*
- Refer to NDs impaired Skin Integrity, impaired Tissue Integrity for additional interventions.

Elimination:[6-8]

- Observe elimination pattern, noting changes and potential problems.
- Encourage balanced diet, including fruits and vegetables high in fiber and with adequate fluids *for optimal stool consistency and to facilitate passage through colon.*

Nursing Diagnoses in Alphabetical Order

- Provide/encourage adequate fluid intake, include water and cranberry juice *to reduce risk urinary infections.*
- Maximize mobility at earliest opportunity.
- Evaluate need for stool softeners, bulk-forming laxatives.
- Implement consistent bowel management/bladder training programs, as indicated.
- Monitor urinary output/characteristics *to identify changes associated with infection.*
- Refer to NDs Constipation, Diarrhea, Bowel Incontinence, impaired Urinary Elimination, Urinary Retention for additional interventions.

🏠 **Respiration:**[6,7]

- Monitor breath sounds and characteristics of secretions *for early detection of complications (e.g., atelectasis, pneumonia).*
- Encourage ambulation and upright position. Reposition, cough, deep-breathe on a regular schedule *to facilitate clearing of secretions/prevent atelectasis.*
- Encourage use of incentive spirometry. Suction as indicated *to clear airways.*
- Demonstrate techniques/assist with postural drainage when indicated for long-term airway clearance difficulties.
- Assist with/instruct family and caregivers in quad coughing techniques/diaphragmatic weight training *to maximize ventilation (in presence of SCI).*
- Ⓐ Discourage smoking. Refer for smoking cessation program as indicated.
- Refer to NDs ineffective Airway Clearance, ineffective Breathing Pattern, impaired Gas Exchange, impaired spontaneous Ventilation for additional interventions.

🏠 **Vascular (tissue perfusion):**[6–8]

- Assess cognition and mental status (ongoing). *Changes can reflect state of cardiac health, cerebral oxygenation impairment, or be indicative of a mental/emotional state that could adversely affect safety and self-care.*
- Determine core and skin temperature. Investigate development of cyanosis, changes in mentation *to identify changes in oxygenation status.*
- Routinely evaluate circulation/nerve function of affected body parts. *Changes in temperature, color, sensation, and movement can be the effect of immobility, disease, aging, or injury.*
- Encourage/provide adequate fluid *to prevent dehydration and circulatory stasis.*
- Monitor blood pressure before, during, and after activity—sitting, standing, and lying if possible *to ascertain response to/tolerance of activity.*
- Assist with position changes as needed. Raise head gradually. Institute use of tilt table/sitting upright on side of bed and arising slowly where appropriate *to reduce incidence of injury that may occur as a result of orthostatic hypotension.*
- Maintain proper body position; avoid use of constricting garments/restraints *to prevent vascular congestion.*
- Ⓐ Provide range-of-motion exercise. Refer for/assist with physical therapy *for strengthening, restoration of optimal range of motion, and prevention of circulatory problems related to disuse.*[4]
- Ambulate as quickly and often as possible, using mobility aids and frequent rest stops to assist client in continuing activity. *Upright position and weight bearing helps maintain bone strength, increases circulation, and prevents postural hypotension.*[8]
- Ⓐ Institute peripheral vascular support measures (e.g., elastic hose, Ace wraps, sequential compression devices) *to enhance venous return and reduce incidence of thrombophlebitis.*
- Refer to NDs risk for Activity Intolerance; decreased Cardiac Output; risk for Peripheral Neurovascular Dysfunction; ineffective Tissue Perfusion for additional interventions.

🌐 Cultural Ⓐ Collaborative 🏠 Community/Home Care Diagnostic Studies ∞ Pediatric/Geriatric/Lifespan Medications

Musculoskeletal (mobility/range of motion, strength/endurance):[5–8]

- Perform/assist with range-of-motion exercises and involve client in active exercises with physical/occupational therapy *to promote bone health, muscle strengthening, flexibility, optimal conditioning, and functional ability.*
- Have client do exercises in bed if not contraindicated. *In-bed exercises help maintain muscle strength and tone.*
- Maximize involvement in self-care *to restore/maintain strength and functional abilities.*
- Intersperse activity with rest periods. Pace activities as possible *to increase strength and endurance in a gradual manner and reduce failure of planned exercise because of exhaustion or overuse of weak muscles/injured area.*
- Identify needs/use supportive devices (e.g. cane/walker/functional positioning splints) as appropriate *to assist with safe mobility and functional independence.*
- Evaluate role of pain in mobility problem. Implement pain management program as individually indicated.
- Limit/monitor closely the use of restraints and immobilize client as little as possible *to reduce possibility of agitation and injury.*
- Refer to NDs Activity Intolerance; risk for Falls; impaired physical Mobility; acute Pain; chronic Pain; impaired Walking for additional interventions.

Sensory-perception:[6–8]

- Orient client as necessary to time, place, person, and situation. Provide cues for orientation (e.g., clock, calendar). *Disturbances of sensory interpretation and thought processes are associated with immobility as well as aging, being ill, disease processes/treatments, and medication effects.*
- Provide appropriate level of environmental stimulation (e.g., music, television/radio, personal possessions, and visitors). *Needs vary depending on the client, the nature of the current problem, and whether client is at home or in a healthcare facility. Having normal life cues can help with mental stimulation and restoration of health.*
- Encourage participation in recreational/diversional activities and regular exercise program (as tolerated) *to decrease the sensory deprivation associated with immobility and isolation.*
- Promote regular sleep hours, use of sleep aids, and usual presleep rituals *to promote normal sleep/rest cycle.*
- Refer to NDs chronic Confusion, deficient Diversional Activity, Insomnia, disturbed Sensory Perception for additional interventions.

Self-esteem, Powerlessness, Hopelessness, Social Isolation:[6,7]

- Determine factors that may contribute to impairment of client's self-esteem and social interactions. *Many factors can be involved, including the client's age, relationship status, usual health state; presence of disabilities, including pain; or financial, environmental, and physical problems; current situation causing immobility and client's state of mind concerning the importance of the current situation in regard to the rest of client's life and desired lifestyle.*
- Ascertain if changes in client's situation are likely to be short-term/temporary or long-term/permanent. *Can affect both the client and care provider's coping abilities and willingness to engage in activities that prevent/limit effects of immobility.*
- Assess living situation (e.g., lives with spouse, parents, alone, etc.) and determine factors that may positively or adversely affect client's progress, roles, and/or safety.
- Explain/review all care procedures and plans. *Improves knowledge and facilitates decision making. Involves client in own care, enhances sense of control, and promotes independence.*
- Encourage questions and verbalization of feelings. *Aids in reducing anxiety and promotes learning about condition/specific needs.*
- Acknowledge concerns; provide presence and encouragement.

- Refer for mental/psychological/spiritual services as indicated *to provide counseling, support, and medications.*
- Provide for/assist with mutual goal-setting, involving SO(s). *Promotes sense of control and enhances commitment to goals.*
- Ascertain that client can communicate needs adequately (e.g., call light, writing tablet, picture/letter board, interpreter).
- Refer to NDs impaired verbal Communication, Powerlessness, ineffective Role Performance, Self-Esteem [specify], impaired Social Interaction for additional interventions.

Body Image:[6,7]

- Evaluate for presence/potential for emotional, mental, and behavioral conditions that may contribute to isolation and degeneration. *Disuse syndrome often affects those individuals who are already isolated for one reason or another (e.g., serious illness/injury with disfigurement, frail elderly living alone, individual with severe depression, person with unacceptable behavior or without support system).*
- Orient to body changes through discussion and written information *to promote acceptance and understanding of needs.*
- Promote interactions with peers and normalization of activities within individual abilities.
- Refer to NDs disturbed Body Image, disturbed Personal Identity, situational low Self-Esteem, Social Isolation for additional interventions.

NURSING PRIORITY NO. 3 To promote wellness (Teaching/Discharge Considerations):

- Assist client/caregivers in development of individualized plan of care *to best meet the client's potential, enhance safety, and prevent/limit affects of disuse.*
- Provide information about individual needs/areas of concerns (e.g., client's mental status, living environment, nutritonal needs). *Information can help client and care providers to understand what long-term goals could be attained, what barriers may need to be overcome, and what constitutes progress or lack of progress requiring further evaluation/intervention.*[6]
- Review therapeutic regimen. *Treatment may be required for underlying condition(s), stress management, medications, therapies, and needed lifestyle changes.*
- Encourage involvement in regular exercise program, including isometric/isotonic activities, active or assistive range of motion *to limit consequences of disuse and maximize level of function.*[2]
- Promote self-care and SO-supported activities *to gain/maintain independence.*
- Encourage/recommend suitable balanced nutrition as well as use of supplements if needed *to provide energy for healing and maximal organ function.*
- Refer to appropriate community health providers and resources *to provide necessary assistance (e.g., help with meal preparation, financial help for groceries, dietitian/nutritionist, etc.).*[7]
- Review signs/symptoms requiring medical evaluation/follow-up *to promote timely interventions and limit adverse effects of situation.*[6]
- Identify community support services (e.g., financial, counseling, home maintenance, respite care, transportation).
- Refer to appropriate rehabilitation/home-care and support resources *to help client/care providers learn more about specific condition and acquire needed assistance, adaptive devices/necessary equipment.*

DOCUMENTATION FOCUS

Assessment/Reassessment

- Assessment findings, noting individual areas of concern, functional level, degree of independence, support systems/available resources.

Cultural Collaborative Community/Home Care Diagnostic Studies Pediatric/Geriatric/Lifespan Medications

Planning

- Plan of care and who is involved in planning.
- Teaching plan.

Implementation/Evaluation

- Client's response to interventions/teaching and actions performed.
- Changes in level of functioning.
- Attainment/progress toward desired outcome(s).
- Modifications to plan of care.

Discharge Planning

- Long-term needs and who is responsible for actions to be taken.
- Specific referrals made, resources for specific equipment needs.

References

1. Disuse Syndrome. (1999). Department for the Care of the Aged: Laboratory of Rehabilitation Research National Institute for Longevity Sciences Web site. Accessed August 2003. Available at www.nils.go.jp/organ/dca/lrr/reh-e.html.
2. Hanson, R. W. (2000). Physical Exercise, in Self-Management of Chronic Pain. Patient Handbook. Accessed July 2007. Available at www.long-beach.med.va.gov/Our_Services/Patient_Care/cpmpbook/cpmp-11.html.
3. Blair, K. A. (1999). Immobility and activity intolerance in older adults. In Stanley, M., Beare, P. G. (eds). *Gerontological Nursing: A Health Promotion/Protection Approach.* 2d ed. Philadelphia: F. A. Davis.
4. Jiricka, M. K. (1994). Alterations in activity intolerance. In Port, C. M. (ed). *Pathophysiology: Concepts of Altered Health States.* Philadelphia: JB Lippincott.
5. Metzlar, D. J., Harr, J. (1996). Positioning your patient properly. *Am J Nurs*, 96, 33–37.
6. Doenges, M. E., Moorhouse, M. F., Geissler-Murr, A. C. (2004). *Nurse's Pocket Guide: Diagnoses, Interventions, and Rationales.* 9th ed. Philadelphia: F. A. Davis.
7. Cox, H. C., et al. (2002). *Clinical Applications of Nursing Diagnosis: Adult, Child, Women's, Psychiatric, Gerontic, and Home Health Considerations.* 4th ed. Philadelphia: F. A. Davis.
8. Graf, C. (2006). Functional decline in hospitalized older adults. *AJN*, 106(1), 58–67.

deficient Diversional Activity

Definition: Decreased stimulation from (or interest or engagement in) recreational or leisure activities [Note: Internal/external factors may or may not be beyond the individual's control.]

RELATED FACTORS

Environmental lack of diversional activity [e.g., long-term hospitalization; frequent, lengthy treatments, homebound]

[Physical limitations, bedridden, fatigue, pain]

[Situational, developmental problem, lack of sources]

[Psychological condition such as depression]

DEFINING CHARACTERISTICS

Subjective

Client's statements regarding boredom (e.g., wish there were something to do, to read, etc.)

Usual hobbies cannot be undertaken in hospital [home or other care setting]

[Changes in abilities/physical limitations]

Objective
[Flat affect, disinterest, inattentiveness]
[Restlessness, crying]
[Lethargy, withdrawal]
[Hostility]
[Overeating or lack of interest in eating: weight loss or gain]

Sample Clinical Applications: Traumatic injuries, chronic pain, prolonged recovery (e.g., postoperative, complicated fractures), cancer therapy, chronic/debilitating conditions (e.g., congestive heart failure, COPD, renal failure, multiple sclerosis), awaiting organ transplantation

DESIRED OUTCOMES/EVALUATION CRITERIA
Sample NOC linkages:
Leisure Participation: Use of relaxing, interesting, and enjoyable activities to promote well-being
Social Involvement: Social interactions with persons, groups, or organizations
Health-Promoting Behavior: Personal actions to sustain or increase wellness

Client Will (Include Specific Time Frame)
• Recognize own psychological response (e.g., hopelessness and helplessness, anger, depression) and initiate appropriate coping actions.
• Engage in satisfying activities within personal limitations.

ACTIONS/INTERVENTIONS

Sample NIC linkages:
Recreation Therapy: Purposeful use of recreation to promote relaxation and enhancement of social skills
Activity Therapy: Prescription of and assistance with specific physical, cognitive, social, and spiritual activities to increase the range, frequency, or duration of an individual's (or group's) activity
Exercise Promotion: Facilitation of regular physical exercise to maintain or advance to a higher level of fitness and health

NURSING PRIORITY NO. 1 To assess precipitating/etiological factors:

• Assess/review client's physical, cognitive, emotional, and environmental status. *Validates reality of diversional deprivation when it exists, or identifies the potential for loss of desired diversional activity, in order to plan for prevention or early intervention where possible.*
• Observe for restlessness, flat facial expression, withdrawal, hostility, yawning, or statements of boredom as noted above, especially in individual likely to be confined either temporarily or long-term. *May be indicative of need for diversional interventions.*[1]
• Note potential impact of current disability/illness on lifestyle (e.g., young child with leukemia, elderly person with fractured hip, individual with severe depression). *Provides comparative baseline for assessments and interventions.*[9]
• Be aware of age/developmental level, gender, and cultural factors, and the importance of a given activity in client's life. *When illness interferes with individual's ability to engage in usual*

activities, such as a lifelong dancer with incapacitating osteoporosis, a Latino woman who is unable to take care of her family, the person may have difficulty engaging in meaningful substitute activities.

- Determine client's actual ability to participate in available activities, noting attention span, physical limitations and tolerance, level of interest/desire, and safety needs. *Presence of depression/disinterest in life, problems of immobility, protective isolation, and lack of stimulation, developmental delay, or sensory deprivation may interfere with desired activity. However, lack of involvement may not reflect client's actual abilities, but may rather be a matter of misperception about abilities.*[9]

NURSING PRIORITY NO. 2 To motivate and stimulate client involvement in solutions:

- Institute/continue appropriate actions to deal with concomitant conditions such as anxiety, depression, grief, dementia, physical injury isolation and immobility, malnutrition, acute or chronic pain, etc. *These conditions interfere with the individual's ability to engage in meaningful activities that will stimulate his or her interest.*
- Introduce activities at client's current level of functioning, progressing to more complex activities, as tolerated. *Provides opportunity for client to experience successes, reaffirming capabilities and enhancing self-esteem.*[8]
- Establish therapeutic relationship, acknowledging reality of situation and client's feelings. *May be feeling sense of loss when unable to participate in usual activities or to interact socially as desired.*[8]
- Accept hostile expressions while limiting aggressive acting-out behavior. *Permission to express feelings of anger, hopelessness allows for beginning resolution. However, destructive behavior is counterproductive to self-esteem and problem-solving.*[8]
- Involve client, and parent/SO/caregiver in determining client's needs, desires, and available resources. *Helps ensure that plan is attentive to client's interests and resources, increasing likelihood of client participation.*[2]
- Encourage parent/caregiver of young child to engage in play with confined child. *Reduces child's boredom, and play is essential to young child's development.*[3]
- Review history of lifelong activities and hobbies client has enjoyed. Discuss reasons client is not doing these activities now, and whether client can/would like to resume these activities. *Diversional activities can provide positive and productive avenues into which client can channel thoughts and time.*[4]
- Assist client/caregiver to set realistic goals for diversional activities, communicating hope and patience. *Can help client realize that this situation is not hopeless, that there are choices for improving the current situation, and that the future can hold the promise for improvement.*
- Encourage/instruct in relaxation techniques (e.g., meditation, sharing experiences, reminiscence, soft music, guided visualization) *to enhance coping skills.*[8]
- Participate in decisions about timing and spacing of visitors, leisure and care activities *to promote relaxation/reduce sense of boredom as well as prevent overstimulation and exhaustion.*[8]
- Encourage client to assist in scheduling required and optional activity choices. *For example, client may want to watch favorite television show at bath time; if bath can be rescheduled later, client's sense of control is enhanced.*[8]
- Encourage mix of desired activities/stimuli (e.g., music, news/educational presentations, movies, computer/Internet access, books/other reading materials, visitors, games, arts and crafts, sensory enrichment [e.g., massage, aromatherapy], grooming/beauty care, cooking, social outings, gardening, discussion groups, as appropriate). *Activities need to be personally meaningful and not physically/ emotionally overwhelming for client to derive the most benefit.*[4,10]

- Refrain from making changes in schedule without discussing with client. *It is important for staff to be sensitive and responsible in making and following through on commitments to client.*[8]

 • Provide change of scenery (indoors and out where possible). Provide for periodic changes in the personal environment when client is confined inside, eliciting the client's input for likes and desires. *Change (e.g., new pictures on the wall, seasonal colors/flowers, altering room furniture, or outdoor light and air) can provide positive sensory stimulation, reduce client's boredom, improve sense of normalcy and control.*[5]

- Suggest activities such as bird feeders/baths for bird-watching, a garden in a window box/terrarium, or a fishbowl/aquarium *to stimulate observation as well as involvement and participation in activity (e.g., bird identification, picking out feeders and seeds).*[8]

- Involve recreational/occupational/play/music/movement therapist as appropriate *to help identify enjoyable activities for client; to procure assistive devices or modify activities for individual situation. Assists client to express needs/feelings, share experiences, escape healthcare routines, and participate in self-healing.*[1,6,7]

NURSING PRIORITY NO. 3 To promote wellness (Teaching/Discharge Considerations):

- Explore options for useful activities using the person's strengths/abilities and interests to engage the client/SO.
- Make appropriate referrals to available resources (e.g., exercise groups, senior activities, hobby clubs, volunteering, companion and service organizations) *to introduce or continue diversional activities in community/home settings.*
- Refer to NDs ineffective Coping; Hopelessness; Powerlessness; Social Isolation for additional interventions.

DOCUMENTATION FOCUS

Assessment/Reassessment

- Specific assessment findings, including blocks to desired activities.
- Individual choices for activities.

Planning

- Plan of care/interventions and who is involved in planning.

Implementation/Evaluation

- Client's responses to interventions/teaching and actions performed.
- Attainment/progress toward desired outcome(s).
- Modifications to plan of care.

Discharge Planning

- Long-term needs and who is responsible for actions to be taken.
- Referrals/community resources.

References

1. Radziewicz, R. M. (1992). Using diversional activities to enhance coping. *Cancer Nurs*, 15(4), 293.
2. Cox, H. C., et al. (2002). *Adult, Child, Women's, Psychiatric, Gerontic, and Home Health Considerations.* 4th ed. Philadelphia: F. A. Davis, pp. 275–78.
3. Engel, J. (2002). *Mosby's Pocket Guide to Pediatric Assessment.* 4th ed. St. Louis, MO: Mosby.

Cultural Collaborative Community/Home Care Diagnostic Studies Pediatric/Geriatric/Lifespan Medications

4. Harley, K., et al. (2002). Making each moment count Developing a diversional therapies program for patients with hematologic malignancies. Abstract from Oncology Nursing Society Convention.
5. Dossey, B. M. (1998). Holistic modalities & healing moments. *AJN*, 98(6), 44.
6. Williams, M. A. (1988). The physical environment and patient care. *Am Rev Nurs Res*, 6, 61.
7. Coaten, R. (2002). Movement matters. *National Healthcare J*, (5), 53.
8. Psychosocial aspects of care. (2002). In Doenges, M. E., Moorhouse, M. F., Geissler-Murr, A. C. *Nursing Care Plans: Guidelines for Individualizing Patient Care.* 6th ed. Philadelphia: F. A. Davis.
9. Heriot, C. S. (1999). Developmental tasks and development in the later years of life. In Stanley, M., Bear, P. G. (eds). *Gerontological Nursing: A Health Promotion/Protection Approach.* 2d ed. Philadelphia: F. A. Davis.
10. Wheeler, S. L., Houston, K. (2005). The role of diversional activities in the general medical hospital setting. *Holistic Nursing Practice,* 19(2), 67–69.

disturbed Energy Field

Definition: Disruption of the flow of energy [aura] surrounding a person's being that results in a disharmony of the body, mind, or spirit

RELATED FACTORS

Slowing or blocking of energy flow secondary to:

Pathophysological factors—Illness, pregnancy, injury

Treatment-related factors—Immobility, labor and delivery, perioperative experience, chemotherapy

Situational factors—Pain, fear, anxiety, grieving

Maturational factors—Age-related developmental difficulties/crisis

DEFINING CHARACTERISTICS

Objective

Perception of changes in patterns of energy flow, such as:

Movement (wave, spike, tingling, dense, flowing)

Sounds (tone, words)

Temperature change (warmth, coolness)

Visual changes (image, color)

Disruption of the field (deficient, hole, spike, bulge, obstruction, congestion, diminished flow in energy field)

Sample Clinical Applications: Illness, trauma, cancer, pain, impaired immune system, fatigue, surgical procedures

DESIRED OUTCOMES/EVALUATION CRITERIA

Sample NOC linkages:

Personal Well-Being: Extent of positive perception of one's health status and life circumstances

Coping: Personal actions to manage stressors that tax an individual's resources

Symptom Severity: Severity of perceived adverse changes in physical, emotional, and social functioning

Client Will (Include Specific Time Frame)

- Acknowledge feelings of anxiety and distress.
- Verbalize sense of relaxation/well-being.
- Display reduction in severity/frequency of symptoms.

ACTIONS/INTERVENTIONS

Sample NIC linkages:

Therapeutic Touch: Attuning to the universal healing field, seeking to act as an instrument for healing influence, and using the natural sensitivity of the hands to gently focus and direct the intervention process

Meditation Facilitation: Facilitating a person to alter his or her level of awareness by focusing specifically on an image or thought

Pain Management: Alleviation of pain or a reduction in pain to a level of comfort that is acceptable to the patient

NURSING PRIORITY NO. 1 To determine causative/contributing factors:

- Review current situation/concerns of client. Encourage client to talk about condition, past history, emotional state, or other relevant information. Note body gestures, tone of voice, words chosen to express feelings/issues. *Recent studies reported that therapeutic touch (TT) produced positive outcomes by decreasing levels of anxiety and pain perception and improving sense of well-being/quality of life; TT may also be beneficial in reducing behavioral symptoms of dementia (e.g., manual manipulation/restlessness, vocalization, pacing).*[8,10–14]
- Determine client's motivation/desire for treatment. *Following explanation of TT process and expected results, client may have unrealistic expectations or may understand purpose and believe process will be helpful.*[2] *Although attitude can affect success of therapy, TT is often successful even when the client is skeptical.*[11]
- Note use of medications, other drug use (e.g., alcohol). *May affect client's ability to relax and take full advantage of the TT process.*[4] *However, TT may be helpful in reducing anxiety level in individuals undergoing alcohol withdrawal.*[9]
- Perform/review results of testing, as indicated, such as the State-Trait Anxiety Inventory (STAI) or the Affect Balance Scale. *Provides measure of the client's anxiety to evaluate need for treatment/intervention.*[3]

NURSING PRIORITY NO. 2 To evaluate energy field:

- Develop therapeutic nurse-client relationship, initially accepting role of healer/guide as client desires. *This relationship is one in which both participants recognize each other as unique and important human beings and in which mutual learning occurs. The role of the nurse and the use of self as a therapeutic tool is recognized.*[3]
- Place client in sitting or supine position with legs/arms uncrossed. Place pillows or other supports *to enhance comfort. Promotes relaxation and feelings of peace, calm, and security, preparing the client to derive the most benefit from the procedure.*[1]
- Center self physically and psychologically. *A quiet mind and focused attention turns to the healing intent.*[6]
- Move hands slowly over the client at level of 2 to 6 inches above skin. *Assesses state of energy field and flow of energy within the system. The feelings that may be noted are tingling, warmth, coolness, comfort, peace, calm, and security.*[5]
- Identify areas of imbalance or obstruction in the field. *Areas of asymmetry; feelings of heat/cold, tingling, congestion or pressure, decreased or disrupted energy flow, pulsation, congestion, heaviness, decreased flow may be identified.*[7]

Cultural   Collaborative   Community/Home Care   Diagnostic Studies   Pediatric/Geriatric/Lifespan   Medications

NURSING PRIORITY NO. 3 To provide therapeutic intervention:

- Explain the process of TT and answer questions as indicated *to prevent unrealistic expectation. TT is the knowledgeable and purposeful patterning of the client environmental energy field to relieve discomfort and anxiety. Providing information that the fundamental focus of TT is on healing and wholeness, not curing signs/symptoms of disease helps the client to understand the process.*[6]

- Discuss findings of evaluation with client. *Including the client in the process by sharing the findings of the nurse combined with sensations the client experienced provides the best opportunity to derive benefit from the procedure.*[2]

- Assist client with exercises to promote "centering." *Deep breathing, guided imagery, and the process of centering increases the potential to self-heal, enhance comfort, reduce anxiety.*[2]

- Perform unruffling process, keeping hands 2 to 6 inches from client's body and sweeping them downward and out of the field from head to toe, concentrating on areas of congestion. *Dissipates impediments to free flow of energy within the system and between nurse and client, promoting the reception of healing energy and allowing the client to use own resources for self-healing.*[6]

- Focus on areas of disturbance identified, holding hands over or on skin, or place one hand in back of body with other hand in front. At the same time, concentrate on the intent to help the client heal. *This move allows the client's body to pull/repattern energy as needed and corrects energy imbalances.*[1]

- Shorten duration of treatment 2 to 3 minutes as appropriate. *Children, elderly individuals, those with head injuries, and others who are severely debilitated are generally more sensitive to overloading energy fields.*[1,2]

- Make coaching suggestions in a soft voice. *Pleasant images/other visualizations, deep breathing enhance feelings of relaxation and help to relieve anxiety.*[1,2]

- Use hands-on massage/apply pressure to acupressure points as appropriate during process. *The addition of these methods can enhance the relaxation and benefit client receives from TT.*[6]

- Note changes in energy sensations as session progresses. Stop when the energy field is symmetrical and there is a change to feelings of peaceful calm. *Signifies energy is balanced, further intervention is not necessary, and client is ready to rest.*[1,2]

- Hold client's feet for a few minutes at end of session. *Assists in "grounding" the body energy, completing the session.*[1]

- Provide client time for a period of peaceful rest following procedure. *TT promotes feelings of peace and comfort, relieving anxiety and promoting self-healing.*[1]

NURSING PRIORITY NO. 4 To promote wellness (Teaching/Discharge Considerations):

- Allow period of client dependency, as appropriate. *Period of dependency permits clients to strengthen own inner resources at their own pace.*[1]

- Encourage ongoing practice of the therapeutic process. *Helping client and family members to learn skill of TT will promote feelings of control of illness and health. It can be used anytime, anywhere, and with friends and family.*[4]

- Instruct in use of stress-reduction activities (e.g., centering/meditation, relaxation exercises, guided imagery). *Continuous use of these activities can promote harmony between mind-body-spirit.*[2]

- Discuss importance of integrating techniques into daily activity plan, for sustaining/enhancing sense of well-being. *Helps client to understand that making these a way of life will help them in dealing with challenges of illness and promote a healthy lifestyle.*[1]

Nursing Diagnoses in Alphabetical Order

- Have client practice each step and demonstrate the complete TT process following the session. *Client displays readiness to assume responsibilities for self-healing as he or she learns the TT process.*[1,2]

- Promote attendance at a support group where members can help each other practice and learn the techniques of TT. *The support of others helps the client to become proficient in new skill.*[2]

- Reinforce that TT is a complementary intervention and stress importance of seeking timely evaluation/continuing other prescribed treatment modalities as appropriate. *Failure to follow prescribed therapeutic regimen may result in poor outcome/worsening of condition.*

- Refer to other resources as identified (e.g., psychotherapy, clergy, medical treatment of disease processes, hospice). *Encourages the individual to address total well-being/facilitate peaceful death.*[6]

DOCUMENTATION FOCUS

Assessment/Reassessment

- Assessment findings, including characteristics and differences in the energy field.
- Client's perception of problem/need for treatment.

Planning

- Plan of care and who is involved in planning.
- Teaching plan.

Implementation/Evaluation

- Changes in energy field.
- Client's response to interventions/teaching and actions performed.
- Attainment/progress toward desired outcomes.
- Modifications to plan of care.

Discharge Planning

- Long-term needs and who is responsible for actions to be taken.
- Specific referrals made.

References

1. Krieger, D. (1979). *The Therapeutic Touch: How to Use Your Hands to Heal.* Englewood Cliffs, NJ: Prentice Hall.
2. Buguslawski, M. (1980). Therapeutic touch: A facilitator of pain relief. *Top Clin Nurs*, 2(27).
3. Townsend, M. C. (2003). *Psychiatric Mental Health Nursing Concepts of Care.* 4th ed. Philadelphia: F. A. Davis.
4. Daglish, S. (1999). Therapeutic touch in an acute care community hospital. *Can Nurse*, 95(3), 57–58.
5. Hayes, J., Cox, C. (1999). The experience of therapeutic touch from a nusing perspective. *Br JNurs*, 8(18), 1249.
6. Meehan, T. (1998). Therapeutic touch as a nursing intervention. *J Adv Nurs*, 28(1), 117.
7. Marnhinweg, G. (1996). Energy field disturbance validation study. *Healing Touch Newsletter*, 6(11).
8. Woods, D. L., Craven, R. F., Whitney, J. (January–February 2005). The effect of therapeutic touch on behavioral symptoms of persons with dementia. *Altern-Ther-Health-Med*, 11(1), 66–74.
9. Larden, C. N., Palmer, M. L., Janssen, P. (December 2004). Efficacy of therapeutic touch in treating pregnant inpatients who have a chemical dependency. *J Holist-Nurs*, 22(4), 320–332.
10. Woods, D. L., Dimond, M. (October 2002). The effect of therapeutic touch on agitated behavior and cortisol in persons with Alzheimer's disease. *Biol Res Nurs*, 4(2), 104–114.
11. Denison, B. (May–June 2004). Touch the pain away: New research on therapeutic touch and persons with fibromyalgia syndrome. *Holist-Nurs-Pract*, 18(3), 142–151.

Cultural · Collaborative · Community/Home Care · Diagnostic Studies · Pediatric/Geriatric/Lifespan · Medications

12. Smith, D. W., Arnstein, P., Rosa, K. C., Wells-Federman, C. (December 2002). Effects of integrating therapeutic touch into a cognitive behavioral pain treatment program. Report of a pilot clinical trial. *J Holist Nurs*, 20(4), 367–387.
13. Samarel, N., Fawcett, J., Davis, M. M., Ryan, F. M. (September 1998). Effects of dialogue and therapeutic touch on preoperative and postoperative experiences of breast cancer surgery: An exploratory study. *Oncology Nursing Forum*, 25(8), 1369–1376.
14. Giasson, M., Bouchard L. (September 1998). Effect of therapeutic touch on the well-being of persons with terminal cancer. *J of Holistic Nursing*, 16(3), 383–398.

impaired Environmental Interpretation Syndrome

Definition: Consistent lack of orientation to person, place, time, or circumstances over more than 3 to 6 months, necessitating a protective environment

RELATED FACTORS
Dementia [Alzheimer's disease, multi-infarct, Pick's disease, AIDS dementia]
Huntington's disease
Depression

DEFINING CHARACTERISTICS

Objective
Consistent disorientation
Chronic confusional states
Inability to follow simple directions
Inability to reason/concentrate; slow in responding to questions
Loss of occupation/social functioning

Sample Clinical Applications: Dementia (e.g., Alzheimer's, AIDS, alcoholism), depression, brain injury, Huntington's disease

DESIRED OUTCOMES/EVALUATION CRITERIA
Sample NOC linkages:
Physical Injury Severity: Severity of injuries from accidents and trauma
Cognitive Orientation: Ability to identify person, place, and time accurately

Client Will (Include Specific Time Frame)

- Be free of harm.
- Sustain/demonstrate improvement in cognition.

Safe Home Environment: Physical arrangements to minimize environmental factors that might cause physical harm or injury in the home

Caregiver Will (Include Specific Time Frame)

- Identify individual client safety concerns/needs.
- Modify activities/environment to provide for safety.

ACTIONS/INTERVENTIONS

Sample NIC linkages:
Environment Management: Manipulation of the patient's surroundings for therapeutic benefit

Reality Orientation: Promotions of patient's awareness of personal identity, time, and environment

Surveillance: Purposeful and ongoing acquisition, interpretation, and synthesis of patient data for clinical decision making

(Refer to NDs acute Confusion, chronic Confusion; impaired Memory; disturbed Thought Processes, for additional relevant assessment and intervetions)

NURSING PRIORITY NO. 1 To assess causative/precipitating factors:

- Determine presence of conditions or behaviors leading to client's current problem. (Note: It is possible that there is no identifiable event.) *Can provide clues for likelihood for improvement, as well as helping to identify potentially useful interventions and therapies.*[1]
- Note presence/reports of client's misinterpretation of environmental information (e.g., sensory, cognitive, or social cues), history and progression of condition, length of time since onset, future expectations, and incidents of injury/accidents. *Identifies specific areas of concern, potential risks.*
- Review client's behavioral changes with client/SO(s) regarding baseline behaviors, length of time since onset/progression of problem, their perception of prognosis; as well as to identify additional impairments. *The client's SO/primary caregiver is an invaluable and essential source of information regarding past history and current situation, as both cognitive and behavioral symptoms tend to change over time and are often variable from day to day.*[1]
- Obtain information regarding recent changes or disruptions in client's health (e.g., decreased agility, loss of balance, decline in visual acuity, failure to eat, loss of interest in personal grooming, forgetfulness resulting in unsafe actions) or routine (e.g., hospitalization, change in medications, or moving to new home). *Decline in physical health or disruption in daily living situation can exacerbate symptoms, causing agitation or delirium.*[1]
- Test ability to receive and send effective communication. *Client may be nonverbal or require assistance with/interpretation of verbalizations.*
- Determine anxiety level in relation to situation. Note behavior that may be indicative of potential for violence. *Places both client and SO at risk and requires prompt intervention for safety of all.*
- Evaluate client's response to primary care providers as well as receptiveness to interventions. *Awareness of these dynamics is helpful for evaluation of ongoing needs for both client and caregiver, as client becomes increasingly dependent on caregivers or resistant to interventions.*[3]
- Identify potential environmental dangers and evaluate client's level of awareness (if any) of threat. *Highlights problems that may impact client care and safety, or add to client's difficulties in interpretation of sensory input.*
- Evaluate responses on diagnostic examinations (e.g., memory impairments, reality orientation, attention span, calculations). *A combination of tests, including (but not limited to) MRI/brain scan; Confusion Assessment Method (CAM); Mini-Mental State Examination (MMSE); Brief Dementia Severity Rating Scale (BDSRS); Alzheimer's Disease Assessment Scale, cognitive subsection (ADAS-cog); Functional Assessment Questionnaire (FAQ); Clinical Global Impression of Change (CGIC); Neuropsychiatric Inventory (NPI) is often needed to determine client's overall condition relating to chronic/irreversible condition.*[2,11]

NURSING PRIORITY NO. 2 To provide/promote safe environment:

- Collaborate in mangement of treatable conditions (e.g., infections, malnutrition, electrolye imbalances, and adverse medication reactions) *that may contribute to/exacerbate confusion.*

🌐 Cultural   Ⓐ Collaborative   🏠 Community/Home Care   ⬭ Diagnostic Studies   ∞ Pediatric/Geriatric/Lifespan   💊 Medications

- Include SO(s)/caregivers in planning process. Identify previous/usual patterns for activities, such as sleeping, eating, self-care, etc., *to incorporate into plan of care to the extent possible and lessen confusion.*
- Implement behavioral and environmental management interventions, *to promote orientation, provide opportunity for client interaction using current cognitive skills, preserve client's dignity and safety:*[1-6]

  Provide calm environment, eliminate extraneous noise/stimuli.

  Introduce yourself at each contact if needed. Call client by preferred name.

  Keep communication/questions simple. Use concrete terms. Use symbols instead of words when hearing/other impaired *to improve communication.*

  Avoid speaking in loud voice, crowding, restraining, shaming, demanding, or condescending actions toward client.

  Use touch judiciously. Tell client what is being done before touching.

  Simplify client's tasks and routines, limit number of decisions/choices client needs to make at one time, offer guided choices between two options.

  Promote and structure activities and rest periods, allow adequate rest between stimulating events.

  Recommend limiting number of visitors client interacts with at one time.

  Avoid challenging illogical thinking *because defensive reactions may result.*

  Distract/redirect client's attention when behavior is agitated or dangerous. Set limits on acting-out behavior.

  Remove from stressors and agitation triggers or danger; move client to quieter place; offer privacy.

  Use lighting and visual aides *to reduce confusion about surroundings.*

  Maintain continuity of caregivers, care routines, and surroundings as much as possible.

  Provide simple orientation measures, such as one-number calendar, personal items, seasonal decorations, etc.

  Be supportive and sensitive to fears, misperceived threats, and frustration with expressing what is wanted.
- Be open and honest when discussing client's disease, abilities, and prognosis. Use positive statements. *Promotes trust without diminishing hope in ability to deal with situation.*
- Provide safety measures (e.g., close supervision, alarms on exits, lock doors to unprotected areas/stairwells, toxic substances and medication lockup, supervision of outdoor activities and wandering, removal of car/car keys; lowered temperature on hot water tank); discourage/supervise smoking, monitor ADLs (e.g., use of stove/sharp knives, choice of clothing in relation to environment/season). *Impaired judgment and inattention to detail place client at increased risk for injury to self and others.*
- Place identity tags in clothes/belongings, provide bracelet/necklace to facilitate identification and safe return if client wanders away/gets lost.
- Avoid use of restraints. Use vest (instead of wrist) restraints if restraints required. *Although restraints can prevent falls, they can increase client's agitation and distress, and possibly cause intrapment/death.*[12]
- Administer medications *to manage symptoms and maximize abilities.* Use lowest possible therapeutic dose and monitor for expected or adverse responses, side effects, and interactions.
- Implement complementary therapies as indicated/desired, such as music therapy, hand massage, Therapeutic Touch (if touch is tolerated), aromatherapy, bright-light treatment. *May help client relax, refocus attention, stimulate memories.*[7]
- Refer to NDs impared verbal Communication; acute Confusion; chronic Confusion; impaired Memory; disturbed Sensory Perception; disturbed Thought Processes; risk for Trauma; Wandering for additional interventions.

NURSING PRIORITY NO. 3 To assist caregiver to deal with situation:

🏠 • Determine family dynamics, cultural values, resources, availability, and willingness to participate in meeting client's needs.

• Evaluate SO's attention to own needs, including health status, grieving process, and respite. Discuss caregiver burden, if appropriate. *Primary caregiver and other members of family will suffer from the stress that accompanies caregiving and require information and support.*[2–6,9,10] (Refer to ND risk for Caregiver Role Strain for additional interventions.)

🏠 • Involve SO(s) in care and discharge planning. Maintain frequent interactions with SOs *to relay information, to change care strategies, try different responses, or implement other problem-solving solutions.*

🏠 • Provide educational materials reflecting SO/family needs and learning styles and lists of available resources, such as newsletters, books, reliable Web sites, telephone help lines, etc. *Reduces sense of overload, allows individuals to review/refer to resources as needed on their own time frame.*

🏠 • Review safety measures regarding client's environmental impairments. *Client can not only lose items, but also can get lost in familiar places, requiring special attention to client's possessions, as well as to physical safety in the home and community. The client may believe that caregivers are stealing the "lost" items; or the client may leave home and be unable to get back.*[8]

🏠 • Avoid leaving client alone in home. Suggest instillation of home security system/motion detectors. Register client with Safe Return program of Alzheimer's Association. Talk with neighbors and police if client is prone to wander. *If the general public is on alert for a person with dementia who may need help, the chances of finding that person are greatly enhanced.*[8]

🅐 • Identify appropriate community resources (e.g., Alzheimer's Disease and Related Disorders Association [ADRDA]; stroke or other brain injury support groups; senior support groups; respite care, clergy, social services, therapists, attorney services for advance directives and durable power of attorney) *to provide support for client and SOs, and assist with problem-solving, decision making.*

NURSING PRIORITY NO. 4 To promote wellness (Teaching/Discharge Considerations):

🏠 • Provide specific information about disease process/prognosis and client's particular needs. *Client usually requires more social and behavioral support than medical management, although intermittent medical evaluations are needed to determine client's general health, any deterioration in cognitive function, requiring adjustment in medication regimen, etc.*[13]

🏠 • Develop plan of care with family to meet client's and SO('s) specific needs. *Success of the individual plan is dependent on cultural and belief patterns, as well as family (personal, emotional, and financial) resources.*

🏠 • Perform home assessment *to identify specific safety issues and approriate solutions, including using keyed locks for exterior doors to prevent client from wandering off while SO engaged in other household activities, locking up matches/smoking material, removing knobs from the stove so client does not turn on burner and leave it unattended, securing sharp knives/firearms.*

💊 • Instruct SO/caregivers to share information about client's condition, functional status, and medications whenever encountering new providers. *Clients often have multiple doctors, each of whom may prescribe medications, with potential for adverse effects and overmedication.*[3,7]

🅐 • Investigate local resources; provide appropriate referrals (e.g., case managers, counselors, support groups, financial services, Meals on Wheels, adult day care, adult foster care, respite care for family, home-care agency, nursing home placement). *Individuals are generally not capable of carrying alone the heavy burdens of caring for a relative with this problem.*

Caregivers need help and support (whether or not they are trying to provide total care) to deal with exhaustion and unresolved feelings.[9,10]

• Discuss need for/appropriateness of genetic testing/counseling for family members. *Diagnosis of dementias such as early onset Alzheimer's or Huntington's disease necessitate additional support for family members who may be at risk themselves.*

DOCUMENTATION FOCUS

Assessment/Reassessment

• Assessment findings, including degree of impairment.
• Involvement/availability of family members to provide care.

Planning

• Plan of care and who is involved in planning.
• Teaching plan.

Implementation/Evaluation

• Response to treatment plan/interventions and actions performed.
• Attainment/progress toward desired outcomes.
• Modifications to plan of care.

Discharge Planning

• Long-range needs, who is responsible for actions to be taken.
• Specific referrals made

References

1. Bostwick, J. M. (2000). The many faces of confusion: Timing and collateral history often holds the key to diagnosis. *Postgrad Med*, 108(6), 60–72.
2. About Alzheimer's. (2003). Physicians and Care Professionals, Various Educational Materials. Alzheimer's Disease and Related Disorders Association (ADRDA). Available at www.alz.org. Accessed 2003.
3. Doenges, M. E., Moorhouse, M. F., Geissler-Murr, A. C. (2002). *Nurse's Pocket Guide: Diagnoses, Interventions, and Rationales.* 8th ed. Philadelphia: F. A. Davis, pp. 145–147.
4. Expert Consensus Guideline Series: Agitation in older persons with dementia: A guide for families and caregivers. (1998). Expert Knowledge Systems, LLC. Ross Editorial Services. Available at www.psychguides.com. Accessed 2003.
5. Sommers, M. S., Johnson, S. A. (1997). Alzheimer's disease and delirium/dementia. In *Davis' Manual of Nursing Therapeutics for Diseases and Disorders.* Philadelphia: F. A. Davis.
6. Kovach, C. R., Wilson, S. A. (1999). Dementia in older adults. In Stanley, M., Beare P. G. *Gerontologic Nursing: A Health Promotion/Protection Approach.* 2d ed. Philadelphia: F. A. Davis.
7. Burns, A., Byrne, J., Ballard, C. (2002). Sensory stimulation in dementia: An effective option for managing behavioral problems. *BMJ*, 325, 1312–1313. Summarized on Dementia Center Health and Age Web site. Available at www.healthandage.com.
8. Rowe, M. A. (2003). People with dementia who become lost. *AJN*, 103(7), 32.
9. Brynes, G. (2000). Dealing with dementia: Help for relatives, friends and caregivers. Information brochure. Baltimore: Northern County Psychiatric Associates.
10. The mid stage of Alzheimer's disease: Tips for dealing with dementia sufferers. Available at www.dementia.com. Accessed August 13, 2003.
11. Naylor, M. D., Stephens, C., Bowles, K. H., et al. (2005). Cognitively impaired older adults. *AJN*, 105(2), 52–61.
12. Jacobs, D. H. (2006). Confusional states and acute memory disorders. Article for Emedicine Web site. Retrieved January 2007 at www.emedicine.com/neuro/topic435.htm.
13. Beatty, G. E. (2006). Shedding light on Alzheimer's. The nurse practitioner. *American J of Primary Health Care*, 31(9), 32–43.

adult Failure to Thrive

Definition: Progressive functional deterioration of a physical and cognitive nature; individual's ability to live with multisystem diseases, cope with ensuing problems, and manage his or her care are remarkably diminished

RELATED FACTORS
Depression
[Major disease/degenerative condition]
[Aging process]

DEFINING CHARACTERISTICS

Subjective
Expresses loss of interest in pleasurable outlets
Altered mood state
Verbalizes desire for death

Objective
Inadequate nutritional intake; consumption of minimal to no food at most meals (i.e., consumes less than 75% of normal requirements); anorexia
Unintentional weight loss (e.g., 5% in 1 month, 10% in 6 months)
Physical decline (e.g., fatigue, dehydration, incontinence of bowel and bladder)
Cognitive decline (e.g., problems with responding to environmental stimuli; demonstrated difficulty in reasoning, decision making, judgment, memory, concentration; decreased perception)
Apathy
Decreased participation in activities of daily living; self-care deficit; neglect of home environment/financial responsibilities
Decreased social skills/social withdrawal
Frequent exacerbations of chronic health problems

Sample Clinical Applications: Chronic debilitating conditions (e.g., AIDS, Alzheimer's disease, multiple sclerosis), cancer/terminal illnesses, major depression

DESIRED OUTCOMES/EVALUATION CRITERIA
Sample NOC linkages:
Will to Live: Desire, determination, and effort to survive

Client Will (Include Specific Time Frame)

• Express sense of optimism for future.

Sample NOC linkages:
Psychosocial Adjustment: Life Change: Adaptive psychosocial response of an individual to a significant life change
Physical Aging: Normal physical changes that occur with the natural aging process

Client/Caregiver Will (Include Specific Time Frame)

• Acknowledge presence of factors affecting well-being.
• Identify corrective/adaptive measures for individual situation.
• Demonstrate behaviors/lifestyle changes necessary to enhance functional status.

🌐 Cultural   Ⓐ Collaborative   🏠 Community/Home Care   🔬 Diagnostic Studies   ∞ Pediatric/Geriatric/Lifespan   💊 Medications

ACTIONS/INTERVENTIONS

Sample NIC linkages:

Mood Management: Providing for safety, stabilization, recovery, and maintenance of a patient who is dysfunctionally depressed or elevated mood

Hope Instillation: Facilitation of the development of a positive outlook in a given situation

Self-Care Assistance: Assisting another to perform activities of daily living

Refer to NDs Activity Intolerance; risk prone health Behaviors; chonic Confusion; ineffective Coping; impaired Dentition; risk for Falls complicated Grieving; risk for Loneliness; imbalanced Nutrition, less than body requirements; Relocation Stress Syndrome; Self-Care Deficit (specify); chronic low Self-Esteem risk for Spiritual Distress; impaired Swallowing, as appropriate, for additional relevant interventions.

NURSING PRIORITY NO. 1 To identify causative/contributing factors:

- Assess client's/SO's perception of factors leading to present condition, noting onset, duration of decline. *Adult failure to thrive (FTT) is characterized by malnutrition associated with consistent weight loss; loss of physical, cognitive, and social functioning; impaired immune function; and depression.[1] The condition may be diagnosed when client is hospitalized for such problems as urinary tract infection, decubitus ulcers, falls, and mental confusion. Although it can occur as a result of an acute health problem or elder abuse, FTT is most often associated with chronic health conditions, social isolation, and budgetary constraints.[2,10]*

- Note presence/absence of physical complaints (e.g., fatigue, weight loss, others as noted in Defining Characteristics) and presence of conditions (e.g., heart disease, undetected diabetes mellitus, dementia, stroke, renal failure, terminal conditions). *These contributing factors may/may not be recognized by the client or SOs.*

- Assist with/review results of testing, as indicated (e.g., endocrine/metabolic testing, gastrointestinal endoscopy, psychiatric evaluation). *Aversion to eating and decline in mental function could reflect physical problem (e.g., gastric infection with Helicobacter pylori) or be the result of an emotional/psychological condition (e.g., depression).[9,11]*

- Identify cultural beliefs, norms, and values that are influencing client/caregiver understanding of dietary needs. *Although many cultures have their own distinct theories of nutritional practices for health promotion and disease prevention, the need for nutritional balance of a diet is almost universally recognized as essential for healing, general health, and sustaining a quality life.[3]*

- Review with client/SO previous and current life situations, including role changes, multiple losses (e.g., death of loved ones, change in living arrangements, finances, independance), social isolation, and grieving *to identify stressors that may be affecting current situation.*

- Determine nutritional status. *Malnutrition (e.g., weight loss and laboratory abnormalities) and factors contributing to failure to eat (e.g., chronic nausea, loss of appetite, no access to food or cooking, poorly fitting dentures, no one with which to share meals, depression, financial problems) greatly impact health status and quality of life—especially for the elderly individual.[4–6,10,11]*

- Evaluate client's level of adaptive behavior and client/caregiver knowledge and skills about health maintenance, environment, and safety *in order to instruct, intervene, and refer appropriately.*

- Ascertain safety of home environment and persons providing care *to identify potential for/presence of neglectful or abusive situations and/or need for referrals.*

NURSING PRIORITY NO. 2 To assess degree of impairment:

- Collaborate with multidisciplinary team to determine severity of client's nutritional and functional limitations. *Various scales may be used to determine the extent of problem, to implement treatment, and to make appropriate referrals. Note: FTT is a recognized diagnosis for admission to hospice care.*[7]
- Obtain current weight *to provide comparative baseline and evaluate response to interventions.*
- Active-listen client's/caregiver's perception of problem. *Conveys sense of confidence in client's ability to identify and solve current problems.*[8]
- Discuss individual concerns about feelings of loss/loneliness and relationship between these feelings and current decline in well-being. Note desire/willingness to change situation. *Motivation/lack thereof can impede—or facilitate—achieving desired outcomes.*[10]

NURSING PRIORITY NO. 3 To assist client to achieve/maintain general well-being:

- Assist with treatment of underlying medical/psychiatric conditions *that could positively influence current situation (e.g., resolution of infection, addressing depression).*
- Develop plan of action with client/caregiver *to meet immediate needs for nutrition, safety, and self-care and facilitate implementation of actions.*
- Refer to dietitian/nutritionist to assist in planning meals to meet client's specific needs, taste, and abilities. *Plans could include offering client's favorite food(s), attending social events (e.g., ice cream social, happy hour), or participating in family style meals. In additon, interventions may be geared toward treatment of depression/grief/loss and cutural or environmental adaptation measures.*[11,12] (Refer to ND imbalanced Nutrition: less than body requirements for additional interventions.)
- Monitor caloric intake and weigh regularly, as indicated. Maintain food diary, as appropriate. *Provides data to evaluate effectiveness of interventions.*
- Explore strengths/successful coping skills the individual has previously used and apply to current situation. Refine/develop new strategies, as appropriate. *Incorporating these into problem-solving builds on past successes.*[8]
- Assist client to develop goals for dealing with life/illness situation. Involve SO in long-range planning. *Promotes commitment to goals and plan, thereby maximizing outcomes.*

NURSING PRIORITY NO. 4 To promote wellness (Teaching/Discharge Considerations):

- Assist client/SO(s) to identify useful community resources (e.g., support groups, Meals on Wheels, social worker, home care/assistive care, placement services). *Enhances coping, assists with problem-solving, and may reduce risks to client and caregiver.*
- Encourge client to talk about positive aspects of life and to keep as physically active as possible *to reduce effects of dispiritedness (e.g., "feeling low," sense of being unimportant, disconnected).*[12]
- Introduce concept of mindfulness (living in the moment). *Promotes feeling of capability and belief that this moment can be dealt with.*
- Promote socialization within individual limitations *to provide additional stimulation, reduce sense of isolation.*
- Help client explore reasons for living or begin to deal with end-of-life issues and provide support for grieving. *Enhances hope and sense of control, providing opportunity for client to take charge of own future.*[8,12]
- Offer opportunities to discuss life goals and support client/SO in setting/attaining new goals for this time in their lives *to enhance hope for the future.*

 Cultural   Collaborative   Community/Home Care   Diagnostic Studies   Pediatric/Geriatric/Lifespan   Medications

- Assist client/SO/family to understand that FTT commonly occurs near the end of life and cannot always be reversed.[10]
- Refer to pastoral care, counseling/psychotherapy *for grief work.*
- Discuss appropriateness of/refer to palliative services or hospice care, as indicated.

DOCUMENTATION FOCUS

Assessment/Reassessment

- Individual findings, including current weight, dietary pattern, perceptions of self, food and eating, motivation for loss, support/feedback from SOs.
- Perception of losses/life changes.
- Ability to perform ADLs/participate in care, meet own needs.
- Motivation for change, support/feedback from SO(s).

Planning

- Plan of care/interventions and who is involved in planning.
- Teaching plan.

Implementation/Evaluation

- Responses to interventions and actions performed, general well-being, weekly weight.
- Attainment/progress toward desired outcome(s).
- Modifications to plan of care.

Discharge Planning

- Long-term needs and who is responsible for actions to be taken.
- Community resources/support groups.
- Specific referrals made.

References

1. Groom, D. D. (1993). Elder care: A diagnostic model for failure to thrive. *J Gerontol Nurs,* 19, 6.
2. Stanley, M. (1999). The aging gastrointestinal system, with nutritional considerations. In Stanley, M., Beare, P. G. (eds). *Gerontological Nursing: A Health Promotion/Protection Approach.* 2d ed. Philadelphia: F. A. Davis.
3. Purnell's Model for Cultural Competence. (1998). In Purnell, L. D., Paulanka, B. J. (eds). *Transcultural Health care: A Culturally Competent Approach.* Philadelphia: F. A. Davis, p. 34.
4. Wallace, J. I., Schwartz, R. S. (1997). Involuntary weight loss in elderly outpatients. *Clin Geriatr Med,* 13, 717.
5. Scott, D. D., Chase, M. (2003). Nutritional management in the rehabilitation setting. Accessed July 2007. Available at www.emedicine.com/pmr/topic159.htm.
6. Karnofsky Performance Status Scale Rating Criteria. (1993). *Oxford Textbook of Palliative Medicine.* Oxford University Press.
7. Adult Failure to Thrive/Debility, Unspecified. (1993). Medicare worksheet for determining prognosis. Hospice of Southern Illinois, Inc.
8. Townsend, M. C. (2003). Psychiatric Mental Health Nursing Concepts of Care. 4th ed. Philadelphia: F. A. Davis.
9. Portnoi, V. A. (1997). Helicobacter pylori infection and anorexia of aging. *Arch Intern Med,* 157, 269.
10. Robertson, R. G., Montagnini, M. (2004). Geriatric failure to thrive. *Am Fam Physician* 70(2), 343–350.
11. diMaria-Ghalili, R. A., Amelia, E. (2005). Nutrition in older adults: Interventions and assessment can help curb the growing threat of malnutrition. *AJN,* 105(3), 4050.
12. Butcher, H. K., McGonigal-Kenney. (2005). Depression & dispiritedness in later life. *AJN,* 105(12), 52–61.

risk for Falls

Definition: Increased susceptibility to falling that may cause physical harm

RISK FACTORS

Adults
History of falls
Wheelchair use; use of assistive devices (e.g., walker, cane)
Age 65 or over; lives alone
Lower-limb prosthesis

Physiological
Presence of acute illness; postoperative conditions
Visual/hearing difficulties
Arthritis
Orthostatic hypotension; faintness when turning/extending neck
Sleeplessness
Anemias; vascular disease
Neoplasms (i.e., fatigue/limited mobility)
Urgency; incontinence; diarrhea
Postprandial blood sugar changes/[hypoglycemia]
Impaired physical mobility; foot problems; decreased lower extremity strength
Impaired balance; difficulty with gait; proprioceptive deficits [e.g., unilateral neglect]
Neuropathy

Cognitive
Diminished mental status [e.g., confusion, delirium, dementia, impaired reality testing]

Medications
Antihypertensive agents; ACE inhibitors; diuretics; tricyclic antidepressants; antianxiety agents; hypnotics; tranquilizers; narcotics
Alcohol use

Environment
Restraints
Weather conditions (e.g., wet floors/ice)
Cluttered environment; throw/scatter rugs; no antislip material in bath/shower
Unfamiliar/dimly lit room

Children
<2 years of age; male gender when >1 year of age
Lack of gate on stairs, window guards, auto restraints
Unattended infant on elevated surface (e.g., bed/changing table); bed located near window
Lack of parental supervision
NOTE: A risk diagnosis is not evidenced by signs and symptoms, as the problem has not occurred; rather, nursing interventions are directed at prevention.

Sample Clinical Applications: Osteoporosis, seizure disorder, cerebrovascular disease, cataracts, dementia, paralysis, hypotension, cardiac dysrhythmias, amputation, inner ear infection, alcohol abuse/intoxication

Cultural Collaborative Community/Home Care Diagnostic Studies Pediatric/Geriatric/Lifespan Medications

DESIRED OUTCOMES/EVALUATION CRITERIA
Sample NOC linkages:
Physical Injury severity: Severity of injuries from accidents and trauma

---

Client Will (Include Specific Time Frame)

- Be free of injury.

Knowledge: Fall Prevention: Extent of understanding conveyed about prevention of falls
Fall Prevention Behavior: Personal or family caregiver actions to minimize risk factors that might precipitate falls in the personal environment

---

Client/Caregivers Will (Include Specific Time Frame)

- Verbalize understanding of individual risk factors that contribute to possibility of falls.
- Demonstrate behaviors, lifestyle changes to reduce risk factors and protect self from injury.
- Modify environment as indicated to enhance safety.

ACTIONS/INTERVENTIONS

Sample NIC linkages:
Fall Prevention: Instituting special precautions with patient at risk for injury from falling
Environment Management: Safety: Manipulation of the patient's surroundings for therapeutic benefit
Risk Identification: Analysis of potential risk factors, determination of health risks, and prioritization of risk-reduction strategies for an individual or group

NURSING PRIORITY NO. 1 To evaluate source/degree of risk:

- Review client's general health status *noting factors that may affect safety such as chronic/debilitating conditions, polypharmacy, recent trauma, prolonged bedrest/immobility, sedentary lifestyle.*
- Assess and document client's fall risk using a fall scale (e.g., Morse Fall Scale [MFS], Functional Ambulation Profile [FAP], Tinetti Balance and Gait Assessment, etc.) upon admission, change in status, transfer, and discharge. *Fall risk scales are widely used in acute care and long-term settings and include numbered rating scales for (1) history of falls, (2) secondary diagnosis, (3) use of ambulatory aid, (4) presence of IV, (5) gait/transfer abilities, and (6) mental status. An MFS score of >51 indicates the client is at high risk for falls and requires high fall-prevention interventions.*[1,2,7,8]
- Note client's age/developmental level, gender, and decision-making ability, level of competence. *Infants, young children (e.g. climbing on objects, stairs); young adults (e.g., sports activities), and elderly (e.g., significant vision, cognitive, or mobility impairments; osteoporosis; or loss of muscle, fat, and subcutaneous tissue) are at greatest risk because of developmental issues or impaired/lack of ability to self-protect.*[2]
- Assess client's cognitive status (e.g., presence of brain injury, dementia, neurological disorders of multiple kinds). *Affects ability to perceive own limitations or recognize danger. If client is unable to protect self, responsibility falls upon primary care provider(s).*
- Evaluate client's muscle strength, balance, gross and fine motor coordination. Review history of past or current physical injuries (e.g., musculoskeletal injures; orthopedic surgery) *that may be altering coordination, gait, and balance.*

- Assess mood, coping abilities, personality styles. *Individual's temperament, typical behavior, stressors, and level of self-esteem can affect attitude toward safety issues, resulting in carelessness or increased risk-taking without consideration of consequences.*[7,8]
- Determine client's/SO('s) level of knowledge about/attendance to safety needs. *May reveal lack of knowlege needed/required to provide for safety or chooses to make a different decision for some reason (e.g., "We can't hire a home assistant; I can't watch him every minute; it's not manly . . .") or may not have resources to attend to safety issues in all settings.*[3]
- Evaluate client's use/misuse or failure to use assistive aids when indicated. *Client may have assistive device but is at high risk for falls while adjusting to altered body state and use of unfamiliar device. Client might refuse to use devices for various reasons (e.g., waiting for help; just doesn't like it for whatever reason).*[7,8]
- Identify environmental hazards in the care setting or home/other environment. *Determining needs/deficits provides opportunities for intervention and instruction (e.g., concerning clearing of hazards, intensifying client supervison; obtaining safety equipment; referring for vision evaluation, etc.).*[7,8]
- 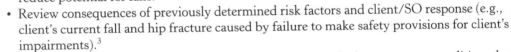 Ascertain caregiver's expectations of client (whether child, cognitively impaired and/or elderly family member) and compare with actual abilities. *Reality of client's abilities and needs may be different than perception or desires of caregivers.*
- Note socioeconomic status/availability and use of resources in other circumstances. *Can affect current coping abilities.*

NURSING PRIORITY NO. 2 To assist client/caregiver to reduce or correct individual risk factors:

- Collaborate in treatment of disease/condition(s) (e.g., acute illness, dementia, incontinence, neurological or musculoskeletal conditions) to improve client's overall health and thereby reduce potential for falls.
- Review consequences of previously determined risk factors and client/SO response (e.g., client's current fall and hip fracture caused by failure to make safety provisions for client's impairments).[3]
- Recommend/implement needed interventions and safety devices *to manage conditions that could contribute to falling and to promote safe environment for individual and others:*[1–6]
  Situate bed to enable client to exit toward his or her stronger side whenever possible.
  Place bed in lowest possible position, use raised-edge mattress, pad floor at side of bed, or place mattress on floor as appropriate.
  Use half side rail instead of full side rails or upright pole to assist individual in arising from bed.
  Provide chairs with firm, high seats and lifting mechanisms when indicated.
  Provide adequate day/night lighting; evaluate vision/encourage use of prescription eyewear.
  Assist with transfers and ambulation; show client/SO ways to move safely.
  Provide/instruct in use of mobility devices and safety devices, like grab bars and call light/personal assistance systems.
  Clear environment of hazards (e.g., obstructing furniture, small items on the floor, electrical cords, throw rugs).
  Lock wheels on movable equipment (e.g., wheelchairs, beds).
  Encourage use of treaded slippers, socks, and shoes, and maintain nonskid floors and floor mats.
  Provide foot and nail care.
- Provide/encourage use of analgesics before activity if pain is interfering with desired activities. *Balance and movement can be impaired by pain associated with multiple conditions such as trauma or arthritis.*[1,2]

🌐 Cultural   Ⓐ Collaborative   🏠 Community/Home Care   🧪 Diagnostic Studies   ∞ Pediatric/Geriatric/Lifespan   💊 Medications

- Follow up with physician to review client's usual medication regimen (e.g., narcotics/opiates; psychotropics, antihypertensives, diuretics), *which can contribute to weakness, confusion, balance and gait disturbances. May benefit from dose adjustment, change in choice of medication prescribed, or time of administration.*[6-8]

- Refer to physical medicine specialist, physical or occupational therapist, recreation therapist as appropriate. *May require evaluation (e.g., balance, muscle strength) and exercises to improve client's balance, strength, or mobility, to improve/relearn ambulation, to identify and obtain appropriate assistive devices for mobility, environmental safety, or home modification.*

- Perform home visit when appropriate. *Useful in determining client's specific needs and available resources, or verifying that home safety issues are addressed, including supervision, access to emergency assistance, and client's ability to manage self-care in the home.*

NURSING PRIORITY NO. 3 To promote wellness (Teaching/Discharge Considerations):[1-6]

- Educate client/SO/caregivers in fall prevention, address the need for exercise balanced with need for client/care provider safety. *While fall prevention is necessary, the need to protect the client from harm must be balanced with preserving client's independence. If the client is overly afraid of falling, the lack of activity will result in deconditioning and even greater risk of falling.*[3]

- Discuss importance of monitoring client/intervening in conditions (e.g., client fatigue; acute illness; depression, etc.; objects that block traffic patterns in home; insufficient lighting; unfamiliar surroundings; client attempting tasks that are too difficult for present level of functioning, inability to contact someone when help is needed, etc.) *that have been shown to contribute to occurrence of falls.*[7,8]

- Address individual environmental factors associated with falling and create/instruct in safe physical environment such as bed height, room lighting, removal of loose carpet or throw rugs, repair of uneven flooring, installing grab bars in bathrooms.

- Refer to community resources as indicated. Provide written material for review/reinforcement of learning. *Client/caregivers may need/desire information (now or later) about financial assistance, home modifications, referrals for counseling, home care, sources for safety equipment, or placement in extended care facility.*

- Connect client/family with sources of assistance (e.g., neighbors, friends, support groups) *to check on client on regular basis, to assist elderly/handicapped individuals in providing such things as structural maintenance, clearing of snow, gravel, or ice from walks and steps, etc.*

- Promote community awareness about the problems of design of buildings, equipment, transportation, and workplace accidents that contribute to falls.

DOCUMENTATION FOCUS

Assessment/Reassessment

- Individual risk factors noting current physical findings (e.g., bruises, cuts, anemia, and use of alcohol, drugs, and prescription medications).
- Client's/caregiver's understanding of individual risks/safety concerns.
- Caregiver's expectations of client's abilities.

Planning

- Plan of care and who is involved in planning.
- Teaching plan.

Implementation/Evaluation

- Individual responses to interventions/teaching and actions performed.
- Specific actions and changes that are made.
- Attainment/progress toward desired outcomes.
- Modifications to plan of care.

Discharge Planning

- Long-range plans for discharge needs, lifestyle, home setting and community changes, and who is responsible for actions to be taken.
- Specific referrals made.

References

1. Falls and fall risk. (1999). Clinical practice guideline. American Medical Directors Association (AMDA). Columbia MD. Accessed July 2007. Available at www.amda.com/tools/cpg/falls.cfm.
2. VA National Center for Patient Safety (NCPS) Fall Prevention and Management (updated 2002). Includes articles on Morse Fall Scale, standard and high risk fall prevention measures and safety education. Accessed July 2007. Available at www.va.gov/ncps/CogAids/FallPrevention/index.html.
3. Henkel, G. (2002). Beyond the MDS. Team approach to falls assessment, prevention & management. *Caring for the Aged*, 3(4), 15–20.
4. Nursing Care Plan: Extended care, falls, risk for. (2002). In Doenges, M. E., Moorhouse, M. F., Geissler-Murr, A. C. (eds). *Nursing Care Plans: Guidelines for Individualizing Patient Care*. 6th ed. (CD-ROM). Philadelphia: F. A. Davis.
5. Daus, C. (1999). Maintaining mobility: Assistive equipment helps the geriatric population stay active and independent. *Rehab Management*, 12(5), 58–61.
6. Horn, L. B. (2000). Reducing the risk of falls in the elderly. *Rehab Management*, 13(3), 36–38.
7. Bright, L. (2005). Strategies to improve the patient safety outcome indicator: Preventing or reducing falls. *Home Healthcare Nurse*, 23(1), 29–36.
8. Poe, S. S., Cvach, M. M., Gartrell, D. G., et al. (2005). An evidence-based approach to fall risk assessment, prevention, and management: Lessons learned. *Journal of Nursing Care Quality*, 20(2), 107–116.

dysfunctional Family Processes: alcoholism [/substance abuse]

Definition: Psychosocial, spiritual, and physiological functions of the family unit are chronically disorganized, which leads to conflict, denial of problems, resistance to change, ineffective problem-solving, and a series of self-perpetuating crises

RELATED FACTORS

Abuse of alcohol [/addictive substances]
Family history of alcoholism/resistance to treatment
Inadequate coping skills; addictive personality; lack of problem-solving skills
Biochemical influences; genetic predisposition

DEFINING CHARACTERISTICS

Subjective

Feelings
Anxiety/tension/distress; decreased self-esteem/worthlessness; lingering resentment
Anger/suppressed rage; frustration; shame/embarrassment; hurt; unhappiness; guilt
Emotional isolation/loneliness; powerlessness; insecurity; hopelessness; rejection
Responsibility for alcoholic's behavior; vulnerability; mistrust

Cultural Collaborative Community/Home Care Diagnostic Studies Pediatric/Geriatric/Lifespan Medications

Depression; hostility; fear; confusion; dissatisfaction; loss

Being different from other people; misunderstood

Emotional control by others; being unloved; lack of identity

Abandonment; confused love and pity; moodiness; failure

Roles and Relationships

Family denial; deterioration in family relationships/disturbed family dynamics; ineffective spouse communication; marital problems; intimacy dysfunction

Altered role function; disrupted family roles/rituals; inconsistent parenting; low perception of parental support; chronic family problems

Lack of skills necessary for relationships; lack of cohesiveness

Pattern of rejection; economic problems; neglected obligations

---

Objective

Feelings

Repressed emotions

Roles and Relationships

Closed communication systems

Triangulating family relationships; reduced ability of family members to relate to each other for mutual growth and maturation

Family does not demonstrate respect for individuality/autonomy of its members

Behavioral

Alcohol abuse; substance abuse other than alcohol; nicotine addiction

Enabling to maintain drinking [/substance use]; inadequate understanding/deficient knowledge about alcoholism [/substance abuse]

Family special occasions are alcohol-centered

Rationalization/denial of problems; refusal to get help; inability to accept/receive help appropriately

Inappropriate expression of anger; blaming; criticizing; verbal abuse of children/spouse/parent

Lying; broken promises; lack of reliability; manipulation; dependency

Inability to express/accept wide range of feelings; difficulty with intimate relationships; diminished physical contact

Harsh self-judgment; difficulty having fun; self-blaming; isolation; unresolved grief; seeking approval/affirmation

Impaired communication; contradictory/paradoxical communication; controlling communication; power struggles

Ineffective problem-solving skills; lack of dealing with conflict; orientation toward tension relief rather than achievement of goals; agitation; escalating conflict; chaos

Disturbances in concentration; disturbances in academic performance in children; failure to accomplish developmental tasks; difficulty with life-cycle transitions

Inability to meet emotional/security/spiritual needs of its members

Inability to adapt to change; immaturity; stress-related physical illnesses; inability to accept health; inability to deal constructively with traumatic experiences

Sample Clinical Applications: Alcohol abuse/withdrawal, prescription/illicit drug abuse

DESIRED OUTCOMES/EVALUATION CRITERIA

Sample NOC linkages:

Family Functioning: Capacity of the family system to meet the needs of its members during developmental transitions

---

Family Social Climate: Supportive milieu as characterized by family member relationships and goals

Substance Addiction Consequences: Severity of change in health status and social functioning due to substance addiction

Family Will (Include Specific Time Frame)

- Verbalize understanding of dynamics of codependence.
- Participate in individual/family treatment programs.
- Identify ineffective coping behaviors/consequences of choices/actions.
- Demonstrate/plan for necessary lifestyle changes.
- Take action to change self-destructive behaviors/alter behaviors that contribute to client's drinking/substance use.
- Demonstrate improvement in parenting skills.

ACTIONS/INTERVENTIONS

Sample NIC linkages:

Substance Use Treatment: Supportive care of patient/family members with physical and psychosocial problems associated with the use of alcohol or drugs

Family Process Maintenance: Minimization of family process disruption effects

Counseling: Use of an interactive helping process focusing on the needs, problems, or feelings of the patient and SOs to enhance or support coping, problem-solving, and interpersonal relationships

NURSING PRIORITY NO. I To assess contributing factors/underlying problem(s):

- Assess current level of functioning of family members. *Information necessary for planning care determines areas for focus, potential for change.*[2]
- Ascertain family's understanding of current situation; note results of previous involvement in treatment. *Family with a member who is addicted to alcohol has often had frequent hospitalizations in the past. Knowing what has brought about the current situation will determine a starting place for this treatment plan.*[2]
- Review family history, explore roles of family members and circumstances involving substance use. *Although one member may be identified as the client, all of the family members are participants in the problem and need to be involved in the solution.*[5]
- Determine history of accidents/violent behaviors within family and current safety issues. *Identifies families at risk and degree of concern/or disregard of individual members to determine course of action to prevent further violence.*[2,4]
- Discuss current/past methods of coping. *Family members have developed coping skills to deal with behaviors of client, which may or may not be useful to changing the situation. Skills identified as useful can help to change the present situation. Those identified as not helpful (enabling behaviors) can be targeted for intervention to bring about desired changes and improve family functioning.*[1,2,5]
- Determine extent and understanding of enabling behaviors being evidenced by family members. *Family members may have developed behaviors that support the client continuing the pattern of addiction. Awareness, identification, and knowledge of these behaviors provide opportunity for individuals to begin the process of change.*[2,5]
- Identify sabotage behaviors of family members. *Issues of secondary gain (conscious or unconscious) may impede recovery. Even though family member(s) may verbalize a desire for the*

Cultural Collaborative Community/Home Care Diagnostic Studies Pediatric/Geriatric/Lifespan Medications

individual to become substance-free, the reality of interactive dynamics is that they may unconsciously not want the individual to recover because this would affect the family member(s) own role in the relationship.[2]

- Note presence/extent of behaviors of family, client, and self that might be "too helpful," such as frequent requests for assistance, excuses for not following through on agreed-on behaviors, feelings of anger/irritation with others. *Identification of specific behaviors (enabling) can help family members see what they do that complicates acceptance of situation by substance abuser and that need to be changed to facilitate resolution of problem.*[5]

NURSING PRIORITY NO. 2 To assist family to change destructive behaviors:

- Mutually agree on behaviors/responsibilities for nurse and client/family members. *Maximizes understanding of what is expected of each person and minimizes opportunity for manipulation of each individual.*[5]
- Confront and examine denial and sabotage behaviors used by family members. *Identifies specific behaviors that individuals can be aware of and begin to change so they can recognize and move beyond what can be blocks to recovery.*[6]
- Discuss use of anger, rationalization, or projection and ways in which these interfere with problem resolution. *Awareness of own feelings can lead to a decision to change, client then has to face the consequences of his or her own actions and may choose to get well.*[6]
- Encourage family to identify and deal with anger. Solve concerns and develop solutions. *Understanding what leads to anger and violence can lead to new behaviors and changes in the family for healthier relationships.*[3]
- Determine family strengths, areas for growth, individual/family successes. *Family members may not have realized they have strengths, and as they identify these areas, they can choose to learn and develop new strategies for a more effective family structure.*[2]
- Remain nonjudgmental in approach to family members and to member who uses alcohol/drugs. *Individual already sees self as unworthy, and judgment on the part of caregivers to family will interfere with ability to be a change agent.*[5]
- Provide information regarding effects of addiction on mood/personality of the involved person. *Family members have been dealing with client's behavior for a time, and information can help them to understand and cope with negative behaviors without being judgmental or reacting angrily.*[2]
- Distinguish between destructive aspects of enabling behavior and genuine motivation to aid the user. *Family members often want to help but need to identify behavior that is helpful and that which is not, to begin to solve problems of addiction.*[6]
- Identify use of manipulative behaviors and discuss ways to avoid/prevent these situations. *The client often manipulates the people around him or her to maintain the status quo. When family begins to interact in a straightforward, honest manner, manipulation is not possible and healing can begin.*[2]

NURSING PRIORITY NO. 3 To promote wellness (Teaching/Discharge Considerations):

- Provide factual information to client/family about the effects of addictive behaviors on the family and what to expect after discharge from program. *Family may have unrealistic expectations about changes that have occurred in therapy, and having information will help them deal more effectively with the difficulties of continuing the changes as they return to their new life without alcohol/substance.*[5]
- Provide information about enabling behavior, addictive disease characteristics for both user and nonuser who is codependent. *Education is a prime ingredient in treatment of addiction and can assist family members to deal realistically with these issues.*[6]

🏠 • Discuss importance of restructuring life activities, work/leisure relationships. *Previous lifestyle/relationships supported substance use requiring change to prevent relapse.*[7]

🏠 • Encourage family to refocus celebrations to exclude alcohol use. *Because celebrations often include the use of alcohol, this is one area where change can be made that can reduce the risk of relapse.*[7]

🏠 • Provide support for family members; encourage participation in group work. *Support is essential to changing client and family behaviors. Participating in group provides an opportunity to practice new skills of communication and behavior.*[5]

Ⓐ • Encourage involvement with/refer to self-help groups, Al-Anon, AlaTeen, Narcotics Anonymous, family therapy groups. *Regular attendance at a group can provide support; help client see how others are dealing with similar problems; and learn new skills, such as problem solving, for handling family disagreements.*[7]

🏠 • Provide bibliotherapy/reliable Web sites, as appropriate. *Reading provides helpful information for making desired changes, especially when client/family members are dedicated to making change and willing to learn new ways of interacting within the family.*[7]

• Refer to NDs compromised/disabled family Coping, interrupted Family Processes as appropriate, for additional interventions.

DOCUMENTATION FOCUS

Assessment/Reassessment

• Assessment findings, including history of substance(s) that have been used, and family risk factors/safety concerns.
• Family composition and involvement.
• Results of previous treatment involvement.
• Cultural/religious beliefs and values.

Planning

• Plan of care and who is involved in planning.
• Teaching plan.

Implementation/Evaluation

• Responses of family members to treatment/teaching and actions performed.
• Attainment/progress toward desired outcome(s).
• Modifications to plan of care.

Discharge Planning

• Long-term needs, who is responsible for actions to be taken.
• Specific referrals made.

References

1. Messina, J., Messina, C. (2007). Tools for Handling Control: Eliminating Manipulation. Retrieved July 2007 at www.coping.org/control/manipul.htm.
2. Townsend, M. C. (2003). *Psychiatric Mental Health Nursing Concepts of Care.* 4th ed. Philadelphia: F. A. Davis.
3. Gordon, T. (2000). *Parent Effectiveness Training* (updated edition). NY: Three Rivers Press.
4. No author listed. Screening for family violence. Retrieved Aug 2007, at ahrq.gov/clinic/2ndcps/famviol.pdf
5. American Nurses Association (1987). Task Force on Substance Abuse Nursing Practice: The care of clients with addictions; dimensions of nursing practice. Kansas City, MO. American Nurses Association.

6. Nye, C. L., Zucker, R. A., Fitzgerald H. E. (1999). Early family-based intervention in the path to alcohol problems, rationale and relationship between treatment process characteristics and child and parenting outcomes. *J Stud Alcohol Suppl*, 13, 10–21.
7. Sielhamer, R. A., Jacob, T., Dunn N. J. (1993). The impact of alcohol consumption on parent-child relationships in families of alcoholics. *J Stud Alcohol*, 54, 189.

interrupted Family Processes

Definition: Change in family relationships and/or functioning

RELATED FACTORS
Situational transition/crises
Developmental transition/crises
Shift in health status of a family member
Family roles shift; power shift of family members
Modification in family finances/family social status
Interaction with community

DEFINING CHARACTERISTICS

Subjective
Changes in power alliances; satisfaction with family, expressions of conflict within family, effectiveness in completing assigned tasks, stress-reduction behaviors, expressions of conflict with/isolation from community resources, somatic complaints
[Family expresses confusion about what to do, verbalizes they are having difficulty responding to change]

Objective
Changes in assigned tasks, participation in problem-solving/decision making, communication patterns, mutual support, availability for emotional support/affective responsiveness, intimacy, patterns/rituals

Sample Clinical Applications: Chronic illness, cancer, surgical procedures, traumatic injury, substance abuse, Alzheimer's, pregnancy, adolescent rebellion/conduct disorder

DESIRED OUTCOMES/EVALUATION CRITERIA
Sample NOC linkages:
Family Functioning: Capacity of the family system to meet the needs of its members during developmental transitions
Family Normalization: Capacity of the family system to maintain routines and develop strategies for optimal functioning when a member has a chronic illness or disability
Family Social Climate: Supportive milieu as characterized by family member relationships and goals

Family Will (Include Specific Time Frame)

- Express feelings freely and appropriately.
- Demonstrate individual involvement in problem-solving processes directed at appropriate solutions for the situation/crisis.
- Direct energies in a purposeful manner to plan for resolution of the crisis.
- Verbalize understanding of illness/trauma, treatment regimen, and prognosis.

- Encourage and allow member who is ill to handle situation in own way, progressing toward independence.

ACTIONS/INTERVENTIONS

Sample NIC linkages:

Family Process Maintenance: Minimization of family process disruption effects

Family Integrity Promotion: Facilitating family participation in the emotional and physical care of the patient

Normalization Promotion: Assisting parents and other family members of children with chronic diseases or disabilities in providing normal life experiences for their children and families

NURSING PRIORITY NO. 1 To assess individual situation for causative/contributing factors:

- Determine pathophysiology, illness/trauma, developmental crisis present. *Identifies areas of need for planning care for this family.*[2]
- Identify family developmental stage (e.g., marriage, birth of a child, children leaving home, death of a spouse). *Developmental stage will affect family functioning; for instance, a couple who are newly married will be dealing with issues of learning how to live with each other; children leaving home may result in problems of "empty-nest syndrome"; or death of a spouse radically changes life for the survivor.*[2,8]
- Note components of family: parent(s), children, male/female, extended family available. *Affects how individuals deal with current stressors. Relationships among members may be supportive or strained.*[6]
- Observe patterns of communication in this family. Are feelings expressed? Freely? Who talks to whom? Who makes decisions? For whom? Who visits? When? What is the interaction between family members? *Not only identifies weakness/areas of concern to be addressed, but also strengths that can be used for resolution of problem(s).*[6,9]
- Assess boundaries of family members. Do members share family identity and have little sense of individuality? Do they seem emotionally distant, not connected with one another? *These factors are critical to understanding individual family dynamics and developing strategies for change. Boundaries need to be clear so individual family members are free to be responsible for themselves.*[6]
- Ascertain role expectations of family members. Who is the ill member (e.g., nurturer, provider)? How does the illness affect the roles of others? *Each person may see the situation in own individual manner, and clear identification and sharing of these expectations promotes understanding. Family members may expect client to continue to perform usual role or may not allow them to do anything. Either action can create problems for the ill member, and realistic planning can provide positive sense of self for the client.*[2,8]
- Determine "family rules." For example, adult concerns (finances, illness, and so on) are kept from the children. *Rules may be imposed by adults rather than through a democratic process involving all family members, leading to conflict and angry confrontations. Setting positive family rules with all family members participating can promote a functional family.*[2,3]
- Identify parenting skills and expectations. *Ineffective parenting and unrealistic expectations may contribute to abuse. Understanding normal responses, progression of developmental milestones may help parent cope with changes necessitated by current crisis.*[2,3]

Cultural · Collaborative · Community/Home Care · Diagnostic Studies · Pediatric/Geriatric/Lifespan · Medications

- Note energy direction. Are efforts at resolution/problem-solving purposeful or scattered? *Provides clues about interventions that may be appropriate to assist client and family in directing energies in a more effective manner.*[2,9]

- Listen for expressions of despair/helplessness (e.g., "I don't know what to do") to note degree of distress. *Such feelings may contribute to difficulty adjusting to situation (e.g., teenage independence, change in health status of household breadwinner, dependence of aging parent on grown child) and ability to cooperate with plan of care/treatment regimen required.*[4]

- Note cultural and/or religious beliefs and values affecting perceptions/expectations of family members. *These factors affect client/SO reactions and adjustment to situation, and may limit choice of interventions/potential for successful resolution. For example, Arab-American family relationships often include nuclear and extended family, make collective decisions, men are expected to be responsible for carrying out decisions, women are usually delegated care for daily needs of the family, children may have little independence, and birth control may not be allowed for teenagers.*[7]

- Assess support systems available outside of the family. *Having these resources can help the family begin to pull together and deal with current situation and problems they are facing.*[2]

NURSING PRIORITY NO. 2 To assist family to deal with situation/crisis:

- Deal with family members in warm, caring, respectful way. *Provides feelings of empathy and promotes individual's sense of worth and competence in ability to handle current situation.*[2]
- Acknowledge difficulties and realities of the situation. *Communicates message of understanding and reinforces that some degree of conflict is to be expected and can be used to promote growth.*[3]
- Encourage expressions of anger. Avoid taking them personally. *Feelings of anger are to be expected when individuals are dealing with difficult situation. Appropriate expression enables progress toward resolution of the stages of the grieving process when indicated. Not taking their anger personally maintains boundaries between nurse and family.*[2,5]
- Stress importance of continuous, open dialogue between family members to facilitate ongoing problem-solving. *Promotes understanding and assists family members to maintain clear communication and resolve problems effectively.*[6,10]
- Provide information, verbal and written, and reinforce as necessary. *Promotes understanding and opportunity to review as needed.*[2]
- Assist family to identify and encourage their use of previously successful coping behaviors. *Most people have developed effective coping skills that when identified can be useful in current situation.*[6,10]
- Recommend contact by family members on a regular, frequent basis. *Promotes feelings of warmth and caring and brings family closer to one another, enabling them to manage current difficult situation.*[2]
- Arrange for/encourage family participation in multidisciplinary team conference/group therapy as appropriate. *Participation in family and group therapy for an extended period increases likelihood of success as interactional issues (e.g., marital conflict, scapegoating of children) can be addressed and dealt with. Involvement with others can help family members to experience new ways of interacting and gain insight into their behavior, providing opportunity for change.*[2,5]
- Involve family in social support and community activities of their interest and choice. *Involvement with others outside of family constellation provides opportunity to observe how others handle problems and deal with conflict.*[2,8]

NURSING PRIORITY NO. 3 To promote wellness (Teaching/Discharge Considerations):

- Encourage use of stress-management techniques (e.g., appropriate expression of feelings, relaxation exercises). *The relaxation response helps members think more clearly, deal more*

effectively with conflict, and promote more effective relationships to enhance family interactions.[4]

🏠 • Provide educational materials and information. *Learning about the problems they are facing can assist family members in resolution of current crisis.*[2]

ⓐ • Refer to classes (e.g., Parent Effectiveness, specific disease/disability support groups, self-help groups, clergy, psychological counseling/family therapy as indicated). *Can assist family to effect positive change/enhance conflict-resolution skills. Presence of substance abuse problems requires all family members to seek support/assistance in dealing with situation to promote a healthy outcome.*[2,3] (Refer to dysfunctional Family Processes: alcoholism for additional interventions as appropriate.)

🏠 • Assist family to identify situations that may lead to fear/anxiety (e.g., diagnosis of chronic debilitating condition, decline in mental functioning of aging spouse/parent, sexually active teenager). (Refer to NDs Anxiety; Fear.) *Promotes opportunity to provide anticipatory guidance.*[1,5]

🏠 • Involve family in mutual goal-setting to plan for the future. *When all members of the family are involved, commitment to goals/continuation of plan are more likely to be maintained.*[3]

ⓐ • Identify community agencies (e.g., Meals on Wheels, visiting nurse, trauma support group, American Cancer Society, Veterans Administration). *Provides both immediate and long-term support.*[6]

DOCUMENTATION FOCUS

Assessment/Reassessment

- Assessment findings, including family composition, developmental stage of family, and role expectations.
- Family communication patterns.
- Cultural/religious beliefs and values.

Planning

- Plan of care/interventions and who is involved in planning.
- Teaching plan.

Implementation/Evaluation

- Each individual's response to interventions/teaching and actions performed.
- Attainment/progress toward desired outcome(s).
- Modifications to plan of care.

Discharge Planning

- Long-range needs, noting who is responsible for actions to be taken.
- Specific referrals made.

References

1. Doenges, M. E., Moorhouse, M. F., Geissler-Murr, A. C. (2004). *Nurse's Pocket Guide: Diagnoses, Interventions, and Rationales.* 9th ed. Philadelphia: F. A. Davis.
2. Townsend, M. C. (2003). Psychiatric Mental Health Nursing Concepts of Care. 4th ed. Philadelphia: F. A. Davis.
3. Gordon, T. (2000). *Parent Effectiveness Training* (updated edition). New York: Three Rivers Press.
4. Cox, H. C., et al. (2002). *Clinical Applications of Nursing Diagnosis: Adult, Child, Women's, Psychiatric, Gerontic, and Home Health Considerations.* 4th ed. Philadelphia: F. A. Davis.

5. Amato, P. R., Booth, A. (2000). *A Generation at Risk: Growing up in an Era of Family Upheaval.* First Harvard University Press.
6. Wright, L., Leahey, M. (2000). *Nurses and Families: A Guide to Assessment and Intervention.* 3d ed. Philadelphia: F. A. Davis.
7. Lipson, J. G., Dibble, S. L., Minarik, P. A. (1995). *Culture & Nursing Care: A Pocket Guide.* San Francisco: UCSF Nursing Press.
8. Kreal's Guide to the Sociology of the Family. Available at www.trinity.edu/~mkearl/family.html.
9. Family Relations: Interdisciplinary Journal of Applied Family Studies and Journal of Marriage and Family. From the National Council on Family Relations.
10. Popenoe, D., DaFo Whitehead, B. The State of Our Unions: The Social Health of Marriage in America 2004. From Rutger's National Marriage Project.

readiness for enhanced Family Processes

Definition: A pattern of family functioning that is sufficient to support the well-being of family members and can be strengthened

RELATED FACTORS

To be developed by nurse researchers and submitted to NANDA

DEFINING CHARACTERISTICS

Subjective

Expresses willingness to enhance family dynamics

Communication is adequate

Relationships are generally positive; interdependent with community; family tasks are accomplished

Energy level of family supports activities of daily living

Family adapts to change

Objective

Family functioning meets needs of family members

Activities support the safety/growth of family members

Family roles are appropriate/flexible for developmental stages

Respect for family members is evident; boundaries of family members are maintained

Family resilience is evident

Balance exists between autonomy and cohesiveness

Sample Clinical Applications: Chronic health conditions (e.g., asthma, diabetes mellitus, arthritis, systemic lupus, multiple sclerosis, AIDS), mental health concerns (e.g., seasonal affective disorder, attention deficit disorder, Down syndrome)

DESIRED OUTCOMES/EVALUATION CRITERIA

Sample NOC linkages:

Family Social Climate: Supportive milieu as characterized by family member relationships and goals

Family Health Status: Overall health and social competence of family unit

Family Resiliency: Capacity of the family system to successfully adapt and function competently following significant adversity or crises

Client Will (Include Specific Time Frame)

• Express feelings freely and appropriately.

- Verbalizes understanding of desire for enhanced family dynamics.
- Demonstrate individual involvement in problem-solving to improve family communications.
- Acknowledges awareness of and respect for boundaries of family members.

ACTIONS/INTERVENTIONS

Sample NIC linkages:

Family Support: Promotion of family values, interests, and goals

Parent Education: Childrearing Family: Assisting parents to understand and promote the physical, psychological, and social growth and development of their toddler, preschool, or school-age child/children

Normalization Promotion: Assisting parents and other family members of children with chronic illnesses or disabilities in providing normal life experiences for their children and families

NURSING PRIORITY NO. 1 To determine current status of family:

- Determine family composition: parent(s), children, male/female, extended family involved. *Many family forms exist in society today, such as biological, nuclear, single-parent, stepfamily, communal, and homosexual couple or family. A better way to determine a family may be to determine the attribute of affection, strong emotional ties, a sense of belonging, and durability of membership.*[1,6]
- Identify participating members of family: parent(s), children, male/female, extended family. *Identifies members of family who need to be involved and taken into consideration in developing plan of care to improve family functioning.*[1]
- Note stage of family development. *While the North American middle-class family stages may be described as single, young adult, newly married, family with young children, family with adolescents, grown children, later life, these developmental tasks may vary greatly among cultural groups. This information provides a framework for developing a plan to enhance family processes.*[1]
- Ascertain motivation/expectations for change. *Motivation to improve and high expectations can encourage family to make changes that will improve their life. However, unrealistic expectations may hamper efforts.*[7]
- Observe patterns of communication in the family. Are feelings expressed: Freely? Who talks to whom? Who makes decisions? For whom? Who visits? When? What is the interaction between family members? *Not only identifies possible weakness/areas of concern to be addressed, but also strengths that can be used for planning improvement in family communication. Effective communication is that in which verbal and nonverbal messages are clear, direct, and congruent.*[1,2]
- Assess boundaries of family members. Do members share family identity and have little sense of individuality? Do they seem emotionally connected with one another? *Individuals need to respect one another, and boundaries need to be clear so family members are free to be responsible for themselves.*[1,3]
- Identify "family rules" that are accepted in the family. *Families interact in certain ways over time and develop patterns of behavior that are accepted as the way "we behave" in this family. "Functional families'" rules are constructive and promote the needs of all family members.*[1]
- Note energy direction. *Efforts at problem-solving, resolution of different opinions, growth may be purposeful or may be scattered and ineffective.*[3]

- Determine cultural and/or religious factors influencing family interactions. *Expectations related to socioeconomic beliefs may be different in various cultures; for instance, traditional views of marriage and family life may be strongly influenced by Roman Catholicism in Italian-American and Latino-American families. In some cultures, the father is considered the authority figure and the mother is the homemaker. These beliefs may be functional or dysfunctional in any given family and may change with stressors/circumstances (e.g., financial, loss/gain of a family member, personal growth).*[1,3,7]
- Note health of married individuals. *Recent reports have determined that marriage inceases life expectancy by as much as 5 years.*[5]

NURSING PRIORITY NO. 2 To assist the family to improve family interactions:

- Establish nurse-family relationship. *Promotes a warm, caring atmosphere in which family members can share thoughts, ideas, and feelings openly and nonjudgmentally.*[3]
- Acknowledge difficulties and realities of individual situation. *Reinforces that some degree of conflict is to be expected in family interactions that can be used to promote growth.*[1,3]
- Stress importance of continuous, open dialogue between family members. *Facilitates ongoing expression of open, honest feelings and opinions and effective problem-solving.*[1,4]
- Assist family to identify and encourage use of previously successful coping behaviors. *Promotes recognition of previous successes and confidence in own abilities to learn and improve family interactions.*[2,4]
- Acknowledge differences among family members with open dialogue about how these differences have occurred. *Conveys an acceptance of these differences among individuals and helps to look at how they can be used to strengthen the family process.*[3]
- Identify effective parenting skills already being used and additional ways of handling difficult behaviors that may develop. *Allows the individual family members to realize that some of what has been done already has been helpful and helps them to learn new skills to manage family interactions in a more effective manner.*[3]

NURSING PRIORITY NO. 3 To promote optimum well-being (Teaching/Discharge Considerations):

- Discuss and encourage use and participation in stress-management techniques. *Relaxation exercises, visualization, and similar skills can be useful for promoting reduction of anxiety and ability to manage stress that occurs in their lives.*[1]
- Encourage participation in learning role-reversal activities. *Helps individuals to gain insight and understanding of other person's feelings and point of view.*[3]
- Provide educational materials and information. *Enhances learning to assist in developing positive relationships among family members.*[4]
- Assist family members to identify situations that may create problems and lead to stress/anxiety. *Thinking ahead can help individuals anticipate helpful actions to handle/prevent conflict and untoward consequences.*[4]
- Refer to classes/community resources as appropriate. *Family Effectiveness, self-help, psychotherapy, religious affiliations can provide new information to assist family members to learn and apply to enhancing family interactions.*[4]
- Involve family members in setting goals and planning for the future. *When individuals are involved in the decision making, they are more committed to carrying through on plan to enhance family interactions as life goes on.*[2]

DOCUMENTATION FOCUS

Assessment/Reassessment

- Assessment findings, including family composition, developmental stage of family, and role expectations.
- Cultural/religious values and beliefs regarding family and family functioning.
- Family communication patterns.
- Motivation and expectations for change.

Planning

- Plan of care/interventions and who is involved in planning.
- Educational plan.

Implementation/Evaluation

- Each individual's response to interventions/teaching and actions performed.
- Attainment/progress toward desired outcome(s).
- Modifications to lifestyle/treatment plan.

Discharge Planning

- Long-range needs, noting who is responsible for actions to be taken.
- Specific referrals made.

References

1. Townsend, M. (2003). *Psychiatric Mental Health Nursing Concepts of Care.* 4th ed. Philadelphia: F. A. Davis.
2. Gordon, T. (2000). *Parent Effectiveness Training.* New York: Three Rivers Press.
3. Doenges, M. E., Townsend, M. C., Moorhouse, M. F. (1998). *Psychiatric Care Plans Guidelines for Individualizing Care.* 3d ed. Philadelphia: F. A. Davis.
4. Doenges, M. E., Moorhouse, M. F., Geissler-Murr, A. C. (2004). *Nurse's Pocket Guide Diagnoses, Interventions, and Rationales.* 9th ed. Philadelphia: F. A. Davis.
5. Schoenborn, C. Marital Status and Health: United States, 1999–2002. Advance Data from Vital and Health Statistics, no 351. Retrieved March 2007 at www.cdc.gov/nchs/data/ad/ad351.pdf.
6. Marriage and Family Processes, Kearl's Guide to the Sociology of the Family. Retrieved July 2007 at www.trinity.edu/~mkearl/family.html.
7. Lipson, J. G., Dibble, S. L., Minarik, P. A. (1996). *Culture & Nursing Care: A Pocket Guide.* San Francisco: School of Nursing, UCSF Nursing Press.

Fatigue

Definition: An overwhelming sustained sense of exhaustion and decreased capacity for physical and mental work at usual level

RELATED FACTORS

Psychological
Stress; anxiety; boring lifestyle; depression

Environmental
Noise; lights; humidity; temperature

🌐 Cultural 🔗 Collaborative 🏠 Community/Home Care 🧪 Diagnostic Studies ∞ Pediatric/Geriatric/Lifespan 💊 Medications

Situational
Occupation; negative life events

Physiological
Increased physical exertion; sleep deprivation
Pregnancy; disease states; malnutrition; anemia
Poor physical condition
[Altered body chemistry (e.g., medications, drug withdrawal, chemotherapy)]

DEFINING CHARACTERISTICS

Subjective
Verbalization of an unremitting/overwhelming lack of energy; inability to maintain usual routines/level of physical activity
Perceived need for additional energy to accomplish routine tasks; increase in rest requirements
Tired; inability to restore energy even after sleep
Feelings of guilt for not keeping up with responsibilities
Compromised libido
Increase in physical complaints

Objective
Lethargic; listless; drowsy; lack of energy
Compromised concentration
Disinterest in surroundings; introspection
Decreased performance, [accident-prone]

Sample Clinical Applications: Anemia, hypothyroidism, cancer, multiple sclerosis, Lyme disease, post-polio syndrome, AIDS, chronic renal failure, chronic fatigue syndrome, depression

DESIRED OUTCOMES/EVALUATION CRITERIA
Sample NOC linkages:
Endurance: Capacity to sustain activity
Energy Conservation: Personal actions to manage energy for initiating and sustaining activity
Activity Tolerance: Physiological response to energy-consuming movements with daily activities

Client Will (Include Specific Time Frame)
- Report improved sense of energy.
- Identify basis of fatigue and individual areas of control.
- Perform ADLs and participate in desired activities at level of ability.
- Participate in recommended treatment program.

ACTIONS/INTERVENTIONS

Sample NIC linkages:
Energy Management: Regulating energy use to treat or prevent fatigue and optimize function

Exercise Promotion: Facilitation of regular physical exercise to maintain or advance to a higher level of fitness and health

Nutrition Management: Assisting with or providing a balanced dietary intake of foods and fluids

NURSING PRIORITY NO. 1 To assess causative/contributing factors:

- Identify presence of physical and/or psychological conditions (e.g., pregnancy, infectious processes, blood loss/anemia, autoimmune disorders [e.g., multiple sclerosis, lupus, rheumatoid arthritis], trauma/chronic pain syndomes [e.g., arthritis], cardiopulmonary disorders, cancer/cancer treatments, hepatitis, AIDS, major depressive disorder, anxiety states, substance use/abuse). *Important information can be obtained from knowing if fatigue is a result of an underlying condition or disease process (acute or chronic); whether an exacerbating/remitting condition is in exacerbation; and/or whether fatigue has been present over a long time without any identifiable cause.*
- Note diagnosis of chronic fatigue syndrome (CFS). *This condition has been defined as a distinct disorder (affecting children and adults) characterized by chronic (often relapsing but always debilitating) fatigue, lasting for at least 6 months (often for much longer), causing impairments in overall physical and mental functioning and without an apparent etiology.*[1]
- Note client's age, gender, and developmental stage. *Some studies show a prevalence of fatigue in adolescent girls.*[11]
- Assess general well-being—cardiovascular and respiratory status, musculoskeletal strength, emotional health, and nutritional/fluid status. *Treatment of underlying conditions may resolve fatigue.*
- Note changes in life (e.g., relationship problems, family illness/injury/death, expanded responsibilities/demands of others, job-related conflicts) that can be causing or exacerbating level of fatigue. *Stress may be the result of dealing with disease or situational crises, dealing with the "unknowns" or trying to meet expectations of others.*[2] *Also, grief and depression can sap energy and cause avoidance of social and/or physical interactions that could stimulate the mind and body. Persons with AIDS and the elderly are especially prone to this fatigue because they experience significant losses, often on a regular/recurring basis.*[3,4]
- Assess sleep pattern—hours/quality of sleep. *Sleep disturbance is both a contributor to and a manifestation of fatigue (e.g., a client with chronic pain or depression may be sleeping long periods but not experience refreshing sleep, or may not be able to fall/stay asleep).*
- Test for/determine ability to participate in activities/level of mobility. *While many illness conditions negatively affect client's energy and activity tolerance, if the client is not engaged in light to moderate exercise, he or she may simply adjust to more sedentary activities, which can in turn exacerbate deconditioning and debilitation (chronic fatigue syndrome, cancer). However, there are certain conditions (e.g., multiple sclerosis [MS] and post-polio syndrome) where the client's ability to do things reduces as he or she does them (e.g., at the beginning of a walk the client feels okay, but fatigue sets in [out of proportion to the activity] and the client is exhausted as if running a marathon).*[5,6]
- Review medication regimen/use. *Many medications have the potential side effect of causing/exacerbating fatigue (e.g., beta-blockers, chemotherapy agents, narcotics, sedatives, muscle relaxants, antiemetics, antidepressants, antiepileptics, diuretics, cholesterol-lowering drugs, HIV treatment agents, and combinations of drugs and/or substances).*
- Assess psychological and personality factors that may affect reports of fatigue level. *Client with severe/chronic fatigue may have issues affecting desire to be active (or work), resulting in secondary gain from exaggerating fatigue reports.*
- Evaluate aspect of "learned helplessness" that may be manifested by giving up. *Can perpetuate a cycle of fatigue, impaired functioning, increased anxiety and fatigue.*

Cultural   Collaborative   Community/Home Care   Diagnostic Studies   Pediatric/Geriatric/Lifespan   Medications

NURSING PRIORITY NO. 2 To determine degree of fatigue/impact on life:

- Ask client to describe fatigue, noting particular phrases (e.g., drained, exhausted, lousy, weak, lazy, worn out, whole-body tiredness, etc.). *Helpful in clarifying client's expressions for symptoms, pattern/timing of fatigue, which varies over time and may also vary in duration, unpleasantness, and intensity from person to person.*[7]
- Have client rate fatigue (1 to 10 scale) and describe its effects on ability to participate in desired activities. *Fatigue is often accompanied by irritability, lack of concentration, difficulty making decisions, problems with leisure, relationship difficulties that can add to stress level and aggravate sleep problems.*[12]
- Assess severity of fatigue using a recognized scale (e.g., the Multidimensional Assessment of Fatigue [MAF], Piper Fatigue Self-Report Scale, Global Fatigue Index, etc.), as appropriate. *In initial evaluations, these scales can help determine manifestation, intensity, duration, and emotional meaning of fatigue. The scales can be used in ongoing evaluations to determine current status and estimate response to treatment strategies.*[2,7–9,13,14]
- Measure blood pressure and heart/respiratory rate before and after activity as indicated. *Physiological response to activity (e.g., changes in blood pressure or heart/respiratory rate) may indicate need for interventions to improve cardiovascular health, pulmonary status and conditioning.* (Refer to risk for Activity Intolerance for additional interventions.)
- Review availability and current use of assistance with daily activities, support systems, and resources.
- Evaluate need for individual assistance/assistive devices. *Certain conditions causing fatigue (e.g., post-polio syndrome) worsen with overuse of weakened muscles. Client benefits from protection provided by braces, canes, power chairs, etc.*[6,7]

NURSING PRIORITY NO. 3 To assist client to cope with fatigue and manage with individual limitations:

- Accept reality of client's fatigue and avoid underestimating effect on quality of life the client experiences. *Fatigue is subjective and often debilitating (e.g., clients with cancer, AIDS, or MS are prone to more frequent episodes of severe fatigue following minimal energy expenditure and require longer recovery period; post-polio clients often display a cumulative effect if they fail to pace themselves and rest when early signs of fatigue are encountered).*[5,7,10]
- Active-listen concerns, encourage expression of feelings. *Provides support to help client deal with very frustrating and taxing situation.*
- Treat underlying conditions where possible (e.g., manage pain, depression, or anemia; treat infections, reduce numbers of interacting medications, etc.), *to reduce fatigue caused by treatable conditions.*
- Involve client/SO/caregivers(s) in planning care *to incorporate their input, choices, and assistance.*
- Encourage client to do whatever activity possible (e.g., self-care, sit up in chair, walk for 5 minutes), pacing self, increasing activity level gradually. Schedule activities for periods when client has the most energy, *to maximize participation.*
- Structure daily routines and establish realistic activity goals with client, especially when depression is a factor in fatigue. *May enhance client's commitment to efforts and promote sense of self-esteem in accomplishing goals.*
- Instruct client/caregivers in alternate ways of doing familiar activities and methods to conserve energy, such as the following:[2,3,7–10,13]
  Sit instead of standing during daily care/other activities.
  Adjust the level/height of work surface for ergonomic benefit/to prevent bending over.

Carry several small loads instead of one large load.

Use assistive devices (e.g., wheeled walkers/chairs, electrically raised chairs, stair-climbers).

Plan steps of activity before beginning so that all needed materials are at hand.

Take frequent short rest breaks and return to activity.

Delegate tasks/duties whenever possible.

Combine and simplify activities.

Ask for/accept assistance.

Say "no" or "later."

- Provide environment conducive to relief of fatigue, avoid temperature and humidity extremes. *Temperature and level of humidity are known to affect exhaustion (especially in clients with MS).*[5]

- Encourage nutritional foods/refer to dietitian as indicated. *Nutritionally balanced diet with proteins, complex carbohydrates, vitamins, and minerals may boost energy. Frequent, small meals and simple-to-digest foods are beneficial when combating fatigue. Reduced amounts of caffeine and sugar can improve sleep and energy.*[3,7,10]

- Provide supplemental oxygen as needed. *If fatigue is related to oxygenation/perfusion problems, oxygen may improve energy level and ability to be active.* (Refer to ND Activity Intolerance for additional interventions.)

- Provide diversional activities (e.g., visiting with friends/family, TV/music, doing hobbies or schoolwork). *Participating in pleasurable activities can refocus energy and diminish feelings of unhappiness, sluggishness, worthlessness, which can accompany fatigue.* (Refer to deficient Diversional Activity for additional interventions.)

- Avoid over/understimulation (cognitive and sensory). *Impaired concentration can limit ability to block competing stimuli/distractions.*

- Recommend/implement routines that promote restful sleep, such as the following:
Regular sleep hours at night with beneficial nighttime rituals
Short naps during day hours
Mild exercise, yoga, tai chi
Quiet activities in the evening
Meditation, visualization
Warm baths
Refer to NDs Insomnia, Sleep Deprivation for additional interventions.

- Instruct in/refer for stress-management skills of visualization, deep breathing, relaxation, and biofeedback *to deal with situation, aid in relaxation, and to reduce boredom, pain, and sense of fatigue.*

- Participate in comprehensive rehabilitation program with physical or occupational therapist, exercise or rehabilitation physiologist. *Collaborative program with short-term achievable goals enhances likelihood of success and may motivate client to adopt a lifestyle for enhancement of health.*[2,7,8]

- Discuss appropriateness of other therapies (e.g., massage, acupuncture, osteopathic/chiropractic manipulations). *Complementary therapies may be helpful in reducing muscle tension/pain to promote relaxation and rest.*

NURSING PRIORITY NO. 4 To promote wellness (Teaching/Discharge Considerations):

- Discuss therapy regimen relating to individual causative factors (e.g., physical and/or psychological illnesses) and help client/SO(s) to understand relationship of fatigue to illness. Promotes acceptance of situation, allowing client to focus attention on finding ways to live with fatigue.

⊕ Cultural   Ⓐ Collaborative   🏠 Community/Home Care   Diagnostic Studies   ∞ Pediatric/Geriatric/Lifespan   Medications

- 🏠 • Assist client/SO(s) to develop plan for activity and exercise within individual ability. *Enhances sense of control and commitment to attaining goals.*
- 🏠 • Stress necessity of allowing sufficient time to finish activities. *Client is more likely to succeed when he or she does not feel rushed and is allowed to proceed at a measured pace.*
- 🏠 • Instruct client in ways to monitor response to activity and significant signs/symptoms to heed. *Changes in pulse/respiratory rate, or development of worsened/unrelenting fatigue is a signal to stop, rest, and to modify activity level.*
- 🏠 • Promote overall health measures (e.g., good nutrition, adequate fluid intake, appropriate vitamin/iron supplementation).
- 🏠 • Encourage client to develop assertiveness skills and prioritizing of goals/activities.
- 🏠 • Discuss burnout syndrome when appropriate and actions client can take to change individual situation.
- 🏠 • Assist client to identify appropriate coping behaviors. *Promotes sense of control and improves self-esteem.*
- 🏠 • Identify support groups/resources (e.g., condition-specific groups, reliable Web sites) *to provide information, share experiences, enhance problem-solving.*
- 🏠 • Refer to community resources for assistance with routine needs (e.g., Meals on Wheels, homemaker/housekeeper services, yard care, transportation options).
- 🏠 • Refer to counseling/psychotherapy as indicated *to deal with stressors and effects of condition.*

DOCUMENTATION FOCUS

Assessment/Reassessment

- Manifestations of fatigue and other assessment findings.
- Degree of impairment/effect on lifestyle.
- Expectations of client/SO relative to individual abilities/specific condition.

Planning

- Plan of care/interventions and who is involved in the planning.
- Teaching plan.

Implementation/Evaluation

- Client's response to interventions/teaching and actions performed.
- Attainment/progress toward desired outcome(s).
- Modifications to plan of care.

Discharge Planning

- Discharge needs/plan, actions to be taken, and who is responsible.
- Specific referrals made.

References

1. Fukuda, K., Straus, S. D., Hickie, I., et al. (1994). The chronic fatigue syndrome: A comprehensive approach to its definition and study. International Chronic Fatigue Syndrome Study Group. *Ann Intern Med*, 121(12), 953–959 [Medline].
2. Vogin, G. (2001). Colorectal Cancer: Coping with Fatigue. The Cleveland Clinic Condition Center. Accessed July 2007. Available at www.webmd.com/colorectalcancer/colorectal_cancer_coping_with_fatigue?page=1
3. Zimmerman, J. (2002). Nutrition for health and healing in HIV. ACRIA Update, 11(2). Accessed July 2007 at www.thebody.com/content/art14418.html.

4. Ackley, B. J. (2002). Fatigue. In Ackley, B. J., Ladwig, G. B. (eds). *Nursing Diagnosis Handbook: A Guide to Planning Care*. 5th ed. St. Louis, MO: Mosby.
5. Understanding the unique role of fatigue in multiple sclerosis. (Updated 9/7/02). Multiple Sclerosis Encyclopedia Web site. Accessed July 2007 at www.mult-sclerosis.org/fatigue.html.
6. Perlman, S. (1999). Coping with fatigue of post-polio syndrome. Rancho Los Amigos Post Polio Support Group Newsletter.
7. Wells, J. N., Fedric, T. (2001). Helping patients manage cancer-related fatigue. *Home Healthcare Nurse*, 19(8), 486.
8. VHA/DoD. (2001). Clinical practice guidelines for the management of medically unexplained symptoms: Chronic pain and fatigue. Veterans Health Administration, Department of Defense. Washington, DC. Accessed July 2007 at www.oqp.med.va.gov/cpg/cpgn/mus/D/CFS_Summary.pdf.
9. Tolan, R. W., Stewart, J. M. (2001). Chronic Fatigue Syndrome. Accessed July 2007 at www.emedicine.com/ped/topic2795.htm.
10. American Health Consultants. (1996). Common sense about AIDS: Fighting fatigue requires battle on many fronts.
11. terWolbeek, M., vanDoormen, L. J., Kavelaars, A., et al. (2006). Severe fatigue in adolescents: A common phenomenon? *Pediatrics*, 117(6), e1078–e1086. Accessed February 2007 at www.medscape.com/medline/abstract.
12. Barton-Burke, M. (2006). Cancer-related fatigue and sleep disturbances: Further research on the prevalence of these two symptoms in long-term cancer survivors can inform education, policy, and clinical practice. *AJN*, 106(3), Suppl:72–7.13.
13. Belza, B. (1994). The impact of fatigue on exercise performance. *Arthritis Care and Research*, 7(4), 176–180.
14. Trendall, J. (2005). Concept analysis: Chronic fatigue. *J of Advanced Nursing*, 32(5), 1126–1131.

Fear [specify focus]

Definition: Response to perceived threat [real or imagined] that is consciously recognized as a danger

RELATED FACTORS

Innate origin (e.g., sudden noise, height, pain, loss of physical support); innate releasers (neurotransmitters); phobic stimulus

Learned response (e.g., conditioning, modeling from or identification with others)

Unfamiliarity with environmental experience(s)

Separation from support system in potentially stressful situation (e.g., hospitalization, hospital procedures [/treatments])

Language barrier, sensory impairment

DEFINING CHARACTERISTICS

Subjective

Report of apprehension; excitement; being scared; alarm; panic; terror; dread; decreased self-assurance; increased tension; jitteriness

Cognitive: Identifies object of fear; stimulus believed to be a threat

Physiological: Anorexia, nausea, fatigue, dry mouth, [palpitations]

Objective

Cognitive: Diminished productivity/learning ability/problem-solving

Behaviors: Increased alertness; avoidance[/flight]; attack behaviors; impulsiveness; narrowed focus on the source of the fear

Physiological: Increased pulse; vomiting; diarrhea; muscle tightness; increased respiratory rate; dyspnea; increased systolic blood pressure; pallor; increased perspiration; pupil dilation

Sample Clinical Applications: Phobias, hospitalization/diagnostic procedures, diagnosis of chronic/life-threatening condition

Cultural   Collaborative   Community/Home Care   Diagnostic Studies   Pediatric/Geriatric/Lifespan   Medications

DESIRED OUTCOMES/EVALUATION CRITERIA

Sample NOC linkages:

Fear Self-Control: Personal actions to eliminate or reduce disabling feelings of apprehension, tension, or uneasiness from an identifiable source

Coping: Personal actions to manage stressors that tax an individual's resources

Fear Level: Severity of manifested apprehension, tension, or uneasiness arising from an identifiable source

---

Client Will (Include Specific Time Frame)

- Acknowledge and discuss fears, recognizing healthy versus unhealthy fears.
- Verbalize accurate knowledge of/sense of safety related to current situation.
- Demonstrate understanding through use of effective coping behaviors (e.g., problem-solving) and resources.
- Display lessened fear as evidenced by appropriate range of feelings and relief of signs/symptoms (specific to client).

ACTIONS/INTERVENTIONS

Sample NIC linkages:

Anxiety Reduction: Minimizing apprehension, dread, foreboding, or uneasiness related to an unidentified source or anticipated danger

Security Enhancement: Intensifying a patient's sense of physical and psychological safety

Coping Enhancement: Assisting a patient to adapt to perceived stressors, changes, or threats that interfere with meeting life demands and roles

NURSING PRIORITY NO. 1 To assess degree of fear and reality of threat perceived by the client:

- Ascertain client/SO(s) perception of what is occurring and how this affects life. *Fear is a natural reaction to frightening events and how client views the event will determine how he or she will react.*[1]
- Determine client's age/developmental level. *Helps in understanding usual/typical fears experienced by individuals (e.g., toddler has entirely different fears than adolescent or older person with dementia).*[3]
- Note ability to concentrate, level of attention, degree of incapacitation (e.g., "frozen with fear," inability to engage in necessary activities). *Indicative of extent of anxiety/fear related to what is happening and need for specific interventions to reduce physiological reactions. Presence of severe reaction (phobia), requires more intensive intervention.*[1,4]
- Compare verbal/nonverbal responses. *Noting congruencies or incongruencies can help to identify client's misperceptions of situation and what actions may be helpful.*[1]
- Be alert to signs of denial/depression. *Client may deny existance of problem until overwhelmed and unable to deal with situation. Depression may be associated with fear that interferes with productive life/daily activities.*[2]
- Identify sensory deficits that may be present, such as vision/hearing impairment. *Affects reception and interpretation and inabilty to correctly sense and perceive stimuli leads to misundertanding, increasing fear.*[4]
- Measure vital signs/physiological responses to situation. *Provides baseline information of extent of response for comparison as needed at a later date. Stabilization can indicate effectiveness of interventions by lessening of response to identified fear.*[6]

- Investigate client's reports of subjective experiences (may reflect delusions/hallucinations). *It is important to understand how the client views the situation and identify need for reality orientation and further evaluation.*[4]
- Be alert to and evaluate potential for violence. *Client who is fearful may feel need to protect himself or herself and strike out at closest person. Proactive planning can avert or manage violent behaviors.*[5]
- 🏠 Assess family dynamics. *Actions and responses of family members may exacerbate or soothe fears of client.*[1] (Refer to NDs Anxiety, readiness for enhanced family Coping, compromised/disabled family Coping, interrupted Family Processes for additional interventions.)

NURSING PRIORITY NO. 2 To assist client/SOs in dealing with fear/situation:

- Stay with the client or make arrangements to have someone else be there. *Provides non-threatening environment in which the presence of a calm, caring person can provide reassurance that individual will be safe. Sense of abandonment can exacerbate fear.*[6]
- Active-listen client concerns. *Conveys message of belief in competence and ability of client. Promotes understanding of issues when client feels listened to, so problem-solving can begin.*[2]
- Acknowledge normalcy of fear, pain, despair, and give "permission" to express feelings appropriately/freely. *Feelings are real, and it is helpful to bring them out in the open so they can be discussed and dealt with.*[6]
- Present objective information when available and allow client to use it freely. Avoid arguing about client's perceptions of the situation. *Limits conflicts when fear response may impair rational thinking.*[6]
- 🏠 Speak in simple sentences and concrete terms, include written materials as appropriate. *Intense state of fear interferes with reception and interpretation of verbal information; supplementing it with written information facilitates understanding and retention of information.*[4]
- Provide opportunity for questions, answering honestly. *Enhances sense of trust and promotes positive nurse-client relationship in which individual can verbalize fears and begin to problem-solve.*[1]
- ∞ Manage environmental factors, such as loud noises, harsh lighting, changing person's location without knowledge of family/SO; strangers in care area/unfamiliar people, high traffic flow, *which can cause/exacerbate stress, especially to very young or to older individuals.*
- ∞ Be truthful with client when painful procedures anticipated; be present, provide physical contact (e.g., hugging, refocusing attention, rocking a child) as appropriate, *to soothe fears and provide assurance.*[9]
- Modify procedures as possible (e.g., substitute oral for intramuscular medications, combine blood draws/use fingerstick method) *to limit degree of stress, avoid overwhelming a fearful individual.*[3]
- Promote client control where possible and help client identify and accept those things over which control is not possible. *Life changes and stressful events are viewed differently by each individual. Providing opportunity to make own decision when possible strengthens internal locus of control. Individual with external locus of control may attribute feelings of anxiety and fear to an external source and may perceive it as beyond his or her control.*[1]
- 🅐 Provide touch, Therapeutic Touch, massage, and other adjunctive therapies as indicated. *Aids in meeting basic human need, decreasing sense of isolation, and assisting client to feel less anxious. Note: Therapeutic Touch requires the nurse to have specific knowledge and experience to use the hands to correct energy field disturbances by redirecting human energies to help or heal.* (Refer to ND disturbed Energy Field.)[2,7]
- 🏠 Encourage contact with a peer who has successfully dealt with a similarly fearful situation. *Provides a role model, which can enhance sense of optimism. Client is more likely to believe others who have had similar experience(s).*[1]

NURSING PRIORITY NO. 3 To assist client in learning to use own responses for problem-solving:

- Acknowledge usefulness of fear for taking care of self. *Provides new idea that can be a motivator to focus on dealing appropriately with situation.*[1]
- Explain relationship between disease and symptoms if appropriate. *Providing accurate information promotes understanding of why the symptoms occur, allaying anxiety about them.*[1]
- Identify client's responsibility for the solutions while reinforcing that the nurse will be available for help if desired/needed. *Enhances sense of control, self-worth, and confidence in own ability, diminishing fear.*[8]
- Determine internal/external resources for assistance (e.g., awareness/use of effective coping skills in the past; SOs who are available for support). *Provides opportunity to recognize and build on resources client/SO may have used successfully in the past.*[1]
- Explain actions/procedures within level of client's ability to understand and handle being aware of how much information client wants *to prevent confusion/overload. Complex and/or anxiety-producing information can be given in manageable amounts over an extended period as opportunities arise and facts are given; individual will accept what he or she is ready for.*[8]
- Discuss use of antianxiety medications and reinforce use as prescribed. *Antianxiety agents may be useful for brief periods to assist client to reduce anxiety to managable levels, providing opportunity for initation of client's own coping skills.*[1]

NURSING PRIORITY NO. 4 To promote wellness (Teaching/Discharge Considerations):

- Support planning for dealing with reality. *Assists in identifying areas in which control can be exercised and those in which control is not possible, enabling client to handle fearful situation/feelings.*[1]
- Assist client to learn relaxation/visualization and guided imagery skills (e.g., imagining a pleasant place, use of music/tapes, deep-breathing, meditation, and mindfulness.) *Promotes release of endorphins and aids in developing internal locus of control, reducing fear/anxiety. May enhance coping skills, allowing body to go about its work of healing. Note: Mindfulness is a method of being in the here and now, concentrating on what is happening in the moment.*[7,8]
- Encourage regular physical activity. Assist client/refer to physical therapist to develop exercise program within limits of ability. *Provides a healthy outlet for energy generated by feelings and promotes relaxation. Has been shown to raise endorphin levels to enhance sense of well-being.*[2]
- Provide for/deal with sensory deficits in appropriate manner (e.g., speak clearly and distinctly, use touch carefully as indicated by situation). *Hearing or visual impairments, other deficits can contribute to feelings of fear. Recognizing and providing for appropriate contact can enhance communication, promoting understanding.*[4]
- Refer to support groups, community agencies/organizations as indicated. *Provides information, ongoing assistance to meet individual needs, and opportunity for discussing concerns.*[2]

DOCUMENTATION FOCUS

Assessment/Reassessment

- Assessment findings, noting individual factors contributing to current situation, source of fear.
- Manifestations of fear.

Planning

- Plan of care and who is involved in the planning.
- Teaching plan.

Implementation/Evaluation

• Client's responses to treatment plan/interventions and actions performed.
• Attainment/progress toward desired outcome(s).
• Modifications to plan of care.

Discharge Planning

• Long-term needs and who is responsible for actions to be taken.
• Specific referrals made.

References

1. Townsend, M. C. (2003). *Psychiatric Mental Health Nursing Concepts of Care*. 4th ed. Philadelphia: F. A. Davis.
2. Doenges, M. E., Moorhouse, M. F., Geissler-Murr, A. C. (2004). *Nurse's Pocket Guide: Diagnoses, Interventions, and Rationales*. 9th ed. Philadelphia: F. A. Davis.
3. Lawrence, S. (2005). When health fears are overblown. Article for WebMD Health and Balance Feature Stories. Retrieved February 2007 at www.webmd.com/balance/features.
4. Cox, H. C., et al. (2002). *Clinical Applications of Nursing Diagnosis: Adult, Child, Women's, Psychiatric, Gerontic, and Home Health Considerations*. 4th ed. Philadelphia: F. A. Davis.
5. Lewis, M. I., Dehn, D. S. (1999). Violence against nurses in outpatient mental health settings. *J Psychosoc Nurs*, 37(6), 28.
6. Bay, E. J., Algase, D. L. (1999). Fear and anxiety. A simultaneous concept analysis, *Nurs Diagn*, 10, 103.
7. Olson, M., Sneed N. (1995). Anxiety and therapeutic touch. *Issues Ment Health Nurs*, 16(2), 97.
8. Kabat-Zinn, J. (1994). *Wherever You Go There You Are, Mindfulness Meditation in Everyday Life*. New York: Hyperion.

readiness for enhanced Fluid Balance

Definition: A pattern of equilibrium between fluid volume and chemical composition of body fluids that is sufficient for meeting physical needs and can be strengthened

RELATED FACTORS
To be developed by nurse researchers and submitted to NANDA

DEFINING CHARACTERISTICS

Subjective
Expresses willingness to enhance fluid balance
No excessive thirst

Objective
Stable weight; no evidence of edema
Moist mucous membranes
Intake adequate for daily needs
Straw-colored urine; specific gravity within normal limits; urine output appropriate for intake
Good tissue turgor; [no signs of] dehydration

Sample Clinical Applications: Heart failure, irritable bowel syndrome, Addison's disease, enteral/parenteral feeding

Cultural Collaborative Community/Home Care Diagnostic Studies Pediatric/Geriatric/Lifespan Medications

DESIRED OUTCOME/EVALUATION CRITERIA
Sample NOC Linkages:
Hydration: Adequate water in the intracellular and extracellular compartments of the body
Fluid Balance: Water balance in the intracellular compartments of the body
Risk Control: Personal actions to prevent, eliminate, or reduce actual, modifiable health threats

Client Will (Include Specific Time Frame)

- Maintain fluid volume at a functional level as indicated by adequate urinary output, stable vital signs, moist mucous membranes, good skin turgor.
- Demonstrate behaviors to monitor fluid balance.
- Be free of thirst.
- Be free of evidence of fluid deficit or fluid overload.

ACTIONS/INTERVENTIONS

Sample NIC Linkages:
Fluid Management: Promotion of fluid balance and prevention of complications resulting from abnormal or undesired fluid levels
Fluid Monitoring: Collection and analysis of patient data to regulate fluid balance
Surveillance: Purposeful and ongoing acquisition, interpretation, and synthesis of patient data for clinical decision making

NURSING PRIORITY NO. 1   To assess potential for fluid imbalance, ways that client is managing:

- Note presence of factors with potential for fluid imbalance: (1) diagnoses/disease processes (e.g., hyperglycemia, ulcerative colitis, COPD, burns, cirrhosis of the liver, vomiting, diarrhea, hemorrhage) or situations (e.g., diuretic therapy, hot/humid climate, prolonged exercise; getting overheated/fever; diuretic effect of caffeine/alcohol) that may lead to deficits; or (2) conditions/situations potentiating fluid excess (e.g., renal failure, cardiac failure, stroke, cerebral lesions, renal/adrenal insufficiency, psychogenic polydipsia, acute stress, surgical/anesthetic procedures, excessive or rapid infusion of IV fluids). *Body fluid balance is regulated by intake (food and fluid), output (kidney, gastrointestinal tract, skin, and lungs), and regulatory hormonal mechanisms. Balance is maintained within a relatively narrow margin and can be easily disrupted by multiple factors.*[4]
- Determine potential effects of age and developmental stage. *Elderly individuals have less body water than younger adults, decreased thirst response, and reduced effectiveness of compensatory mechanisms (e.g., kidneys are less efficient in conserving sodium and water). Infants and children have a relatively higher percentage of total body water and metabolic rate, and are often less able than adults to control their fluid intake.*[1,2,5]
- Evaluate environmental factors that could impact fluid balance. *Persons with impaired mobility, diminished vision or confined to bed cannot as easily meet their own needs and may be reluctant to ask for assistance. Persons whose work environment is restrictive or outside may also have greater challenges in meeting fluid needs.*[3]
- Assess vital signs (e.g., temperature, blood pressure, heart rate), skin/mucous membrane moisture, and urine output. Weigh as indicated. *Predictors of fluid balance that should be in client's usual range in a healthy state.*[4]

- Ascertain motivation/expectations for change. *Motivation to improve and high expectations can encourage client to make changes that will improve his or her life. However, unrealistic expectations may hamper efforts.*

NURSING PRIORITY NO. 2 To prevent occurrence of imbalance:

- Monitor intake and output (e.g., frequency of voids/diaper changes) as appropriate, being aware of insensible losses (e.g., diaphoresis in hot environment, use of oxygen/permanent tracheostomy) and "hidden sources" of intake (e.g., foods high in water content) *to ensure accurate picture of fluid status.*[4]
- Weigh client regularly and compare with recent weight history. *Useful in early recognition of water retention/unexplained losses.*[1,4]
- Establish/review individual fluid needs and replacement schedule with client. Distribute fluids over 24-hour period. *Enhances likelihood of cooperation with meeting therapeutic goals while avoiding periods of thirst if fluids are restricted.*[1]
- Encourage regular oral intake of fluids (e.g., between meals, additional fluids during hot weather or when exercising) interspersed with high-fluid-content foods of client's choice. *Adds variety to maximize intake while maintaining fluid balance.*[1]
- Provide adequate free water with enteral feedings.
- Administer/discuss judicious use of medications as indicated (e.g., antiemetics, antidiarrheals, antipyretics, and diuretics). *Medications may be indicated to prevent fluid imbalance if individual becomes ill.*[1]

NURSING PRIORITY NO. 3 To promote optimum wellness (Teaching/Discharge Considerations):

- Discuss client's individual conditions/factors that could cause occurrence of fluid imbalance as appropriate, paying special attention to environmental factors such as hot/humid climate, lack of air conditioning, outdoor work setting *so that client/SO can take corrective action/modify risks.*[1,3,6]
- Identify and instruct in ways to meet specific fluid needs (e.g., keep fluids near at hand/carry water bottle when leaving home, or measure specific 24-hour fluid portions if restrictions apply) *to manage fluid intake over time.*[1,3]
- Instruct client/SO(s) in how to measure and record I/O, including weighing diapers/continence pads when used, *if data needed for home management.*
- Establish regular schedule for weighing. *To help monitor changes in fluid status.*
- Identify actions (if any) client may take to correct imbalance (e.g., limiting salt or caffeine intake, as needed use of diuretics, tight control of blood sugar).
- Review/instruct in medication regimen and administration and discuss potential for interactions/side effects that could disrupt fluid balance.[1,4,5]
- Instruct in signs and symptoms indicating need for immediate/further evaluation and follow-up to prevent complications and/or allow for timely intervention.[1,4,5]

DOCUMENTATION FOCUS

Assessment/Reassessment

- Individual findings, including factors affecting ability to manage (regulate) body fluids.
- I/O, fluid balance, changes in weight, and vital signs.
- Results of diagnostic testing/laboratory studies.
- Motivation/expectations for change.

Cultural   Collaborative   Community/Home Care   Diagnostic Studies   Pediatric/Geriatric/Lifespan   Medications

Planning

- Plan of care and who is involved in the planning.
- Teaching plan.

Implementation/Evaluation

- Client's responses to treatment/teaching and actions performed.
- Attainment/progress toward desired outcome(s).
- Modifications to plan of care.

Discharge Planning

- Long-term needs, noting who is responsible for actions to be taken.
- Specific referrals made.

References

1. Cox, H. C., et al. (2002). *Clinical Applications of Nursing Diagnosis: Adult, Child, Women's Psychiatric, Gerontic, and Home Health Considerations.* 4th ed. Philadelphia: F. A. Davis.
2. Miller-Huey, R. Hydration in Elders: More than just a glass of water. Caregiver.com. Today's Caregiver Magazine. Accessed July 2007 at www.caregiver.com/articles/general/hydration_in_elders.htm.
3. Curtis, R. (1997). Guide to Heat Related Illnesses & Fluid Balance. Outdoor Action. Princeton University.
4. Metheny, N. (2000). *Fluid and Electrolyte Balance: Nursing Considerations.* 4th ed. Philadelphia: J. B. Lippincott.
5. Engle, J. (2002). *Pocket Guide to Pediatric Assessment.* 4th ed. St. Louis, MO: Mosby.
6. Bennett, J. A. (2000). Dehydration: hazards and benefits. *Geriatr Nurs,* 21(2), 84–88.

[deficient Fluid Volume: hyper/hypotonic]

[**NOTE:** NANDA has restricted deficient Fluid Volume to address only isotonic dehydration. For client needs related to dehydration associated with alterations in sodium, the authors have provided this second diagnostic category.]

Definition: [Decreased intravascular, interstitial, and/or intracellular fluid. This refers to dehydration with changes in sodium.]

RELATED FACTORS

[Hypertonic dehydration: uncontrolled diabetes mellitus/insipidus, HHNC, increased intake of hypertonic fluids/IV therapy, inability to respond to thirst reflex/inadequate free water supplementation (high-osmolarity enteral feeding formulas), renal insufficiency/failure]

[Hypotonic dehydration: chronic illness/malnutrition, excessive use of hypotonic IV solutions (e.g., D5W), renal insufficiency]

DEFINING CHARACTERISTICS

Subjective
[Reports of fatigue, nervousness, exhaustion]
[Thirst]

Objective
[Increased urine output, dilute urine (initially), or decreased output/oliguria]
[Weight loss]
[Decreased venous filling; hypotension (postural)]

[deficient FLUID VOLUME: hyper/hypotonic]

[Increased pulse rate; decreased pulse volume and pressure]
[Decreased skin turgor; dry skin/mucous membranes]
[Increased body temperature]
[Change in mental status (e.g., confusion)]
[Hemoconcentration; altered serum sodium]

Sample Clinical Applications: Diabetes mellitus, diabetic ketoacidosis, renal failure, conditions requiring IV therapy or enteral feeding, heat exhaustion/stroke, presence of draining wounds/fistulas

DESIRED OUTCOMES/EVALUATION CRITERIA
Sample NOC linkages:
Fluid Balance: Water balance in the intracellular and extracellular compartments of the body
Hydration: Adequate water in the intracellular and extracellular compartments of the body
Electrolyte and Acid/Base Balance: Balance of electrolytes and non-electrolytes in the intracellular and extracellular compartments of the body

Client Will (Include Specific Time Frame)

- Maintain fluid volume at a functional level as evidenced by individually adequate urinary output, stable vital signs, moist mucous membranes, good skin turgor.
- Verbalize understanding of causative factors and purpose of individual therapeutic interventions and medications.
- Demonstrate behaviors to monitor and correct deficit as indicated when condition is chronic.

ACTIONS/INTERVENTIONS

Sample NIC linkages:
Fluid/Electrolyte Management: Regulation and prevention of complications from altered fluid and/or electrolyte levels
Hypovolemia Management: Expansion of intracellular fluid volume in a patient who is volume depleted
Shock Management: Volume: Promotion of adequate tissue perfusion for a patient with severely compromised intravascular volume.

NURSING PRIORITY NO. 1   To assess causative/precipitating factors:

- Note possible medical diagnoses/disease processes that may lead to fluid deficits: (1) fluid loss (e.g., diarrhea/vomiting; fever; excessive sweating; heat stroke; diabetic ketoacidosis; burns, other draining wounds; gastrointestinal obstruction; salt-wasting diuretics; rapid breathing/mechanical ventilation, surgical drains); (2) limited intake (e.g., sore throat or mouth; client dependent on others for eating and drinking; vomiting); (3) fluid shifts (e.g., ascites, effusions, burns, sepsis); and (4) environmental factors (e.g., isolation, restraints, malfunctioning air conditioning, exposure to extreme heat).
- ∞ Determine effects of age, gender. Obtain weight and measure subcutaneous fat/muscle mass (influences total body water [TBW], which is approximately 60% of an adult's weight and 75% of an infant's weight).[1] *In general, men have higher TBW than women, and the elderly's TBW is less than that of a youth. Elderly individuals are often at risk because of decreased thirst reflex, repeated infections, chronic conditions, and polypharmacy.*[2,9]

Cultural   Collaborative   Community/Home Care   Diagnostic Studies   ∞ Pediatric/Geriatric/Lifespan   Medications

Infants/young children and other nonverbal persons cannot describe thirst. Worldwide, dehydration (secondary to diarrheal illness) is the leading cause of infant and child mortality.[3,9]

- Evaluate nutritional status, noting current intake, weight changes, problems with oral intake, use of supplements/tube feedings.
- Collaborate with physician to identify/characterize the nature of fluid/electrolyte imbalance(s). *Dehydration is often categorized according to serum sodium concentration. Isonatremic (i.e., isotonic) dehydration is the most common type of dehydration. However, hypernatremic (also called "hypertonic dehydration" when relatively less sodium than water is lost) and hyponatremic (or hypotonic dehydration when relatively less water than sodium is lost) can both cause neurological complications, and thus may be more dangerous.*[3] *More than one cause may exist at a given time (e.g., increased loss of salt and water caused by diuretics that leads to decreased fluid intake as a result of lethargy and confusion).*[5 10,11]

NURSING PRIORITY NO. 2 To evaluate degree of fluid deficit:

- Obtain history of usual pattern of fluid intake and recent alterations. *Intake may be reduced because of current physical or environmental issues (e.g., swallowing problems, vomiting; severe heat wave with inadequate fluid replacement); or a behavior pattern (e.g., elderly person refuses to drink water trying to control incontinence).*[8]
- Assess vital signs, including temperature (often elevated), pulse (elevated), respirations, and blood pressure (may be low). Measure blood pressure (lying/sitting/standing *to evaluate orthostatic blood pressure*), and monitor invasive hemodynamic parameters as indicated (e.g., central venous pressure [CVP]) *to determine degree of intravascular deficit and replacement needs.*[7–9]
- Note presence of dry mucous membranes, poor skin turgor, delayed capillary refill, flat neck veins, reports of thirst or weakness, child crying without tears, sunken eyeballs, fever, weight loss, little or no urine output. *Assessment signs of dehydration that client/SO may notice.*[8,9]
- Note change in usual mentation/behavior/functional abilities (e.g., confusion, falling, loss of ability to carry out usual activities, lethargy, dizziness). *These signs indicate sufficient dehydration to cause poor cerebral perfusion and/or electrolyte imbalance.*[10,11]
- Observe/measure urinary output hourly or for 24 hours as indicated. Note color *(may be dark because of concentration)* and specific gravity *(high number associated with dehydration with usual range being 1.010 to 1.025).*[4]
- Estimate or measure other fluid losses, (e.g., gastric, respiratory, and wound losses) *to more accurately determine fluid replacement needs.*[8]
- Review laboratory data (e.g., Hb/Hct, electrolytes [sodium, potassium, chloride, bicarbonate]; blood urea nitrogen [BUN], creatinine) *to evaluate body's response to fluid loss and to determine replacement needs.*[4]

NURSING PRIORITY NO. 3 To correct/replace fluid losses to reverse pathophysiological mechanisms:

- Assist with treatment of underlying conditions causing or contributing to dehydration and electrolyte imbalances (e.g., change antibiotics causing diarrhea, treat fever/infection, malnutrition or severe depression; discontinue medications contributing to dehydration).
- Administer fluids and electrolytes as indicated. *Fluid used for replacement depends on the(1) type of dehydration present (e.g., hypertonic/hypotonic), and (2) degree of deficit determined by age, weight, and type of trauma/condition causing the fluid deficit. Multiple fluid resuscitation formulas (e.g., Parkland, Evans, Brooke burn formulas) exist with variations in both the*

volumes per weight suggested and the type or types of crystalloid or crystalloid-colloid combinations. Regardless of the formula or strategy used, the first 24 to 48 hours of fluid resuscitation require constant evaluation of the client's response, as well as frequent adjustments in fluid rates/solutions, to prevent complications (e.g., under/overhydration).[2,6,10]

- Establish 24-hour replacement schedule and routes to be used (e.g., IV/PO/tube feeding). *Entire fluid replacement may be done by IV or tube feeding if client is NPO, acutely ill, or severely dehydrated. However, if client is be rehydrated orally, fluid replacement may be calculated to replace certain amount with meals (e.g., 75% to 80%) with the remainder offered during nonmeal times. Steady rehydration rate reduces thirst, helps to balance electrolytes, and prevents peaks/valleys in fluid level. Managing oral rehydration in this manner can replace fluids, without resorting to IV therapy. These interventions should also be in place to prevent dehydration.*[2,3,5,6,9]

- Spread fluid intake throughout the day *to prevent periods of uncomfortable thirst.*[8]

- Encourage increased intake of water and other fluids based on individual needs (up to 2.5 L/day or amount determined by physician for client's age, weight, and condition).

- Provide a variety of fluids in small frequent offerings, attempting to incorporate client's preferred beverage and temperature (e.g., iced or hot) *to enhance cooperation with regimen.*[8]

- Suggest intake of high-water content foods (e.g., popsicles, gelatin, soup, eggnog, watermelon) and/or electrolyte replacement drinks (e.g., Gatorade, Pedialyte) as appropriate. *Variety may stimulate intake.*

- Limit intake of alcohol/caffeinated beverages that tend to exert a diuretic effect.

- Engage client, family, and all caregivers in fluid management plan. *Everyone is responsible for the prevention or treatment of dehydration and should be involved in the planning and provision of adequate fluid on a daily basis.*

- Review diet orders to remove any nonessential fluid and salt restrictions.

- Provide nutritionally balanced diet and/or enteral feedings (avoiding use of hyperosmolar or excessively high-protein formulas) and provide adequate amount of free water with feedings.

- Maintain accurate intake and output (I/O), calculate 24-hour fluid balance, and weigh regularly (daily, in unstable client) *in order to monitor/document trends. Note: A 1-pound weight loss reflects fluid loss of about 500 mL in an adult.*[7]

NURSING PRIORITY NO. 4 To promote comfort and safety:

- Change position frequently. Bathe infrequently, using mild cleanser/soap and provide optimal skin care with suitable emollients *to maintain skin integrity and prevent excessive dryness caused by dehydration.*

- Provide frequent oral care and eye protection *to prevent injury from dryness.*

- Provide for safety measures when client is confused. (Refer to NDs acute Confusion, chronic Confusion for additional interventions.)

- Adjust or discontinue medications (e.g., diuretics, laxatives, steroids, psychotropics, ACE inhibitors, etc.) *that may be contributing to dehydration.*[2,5]

- Observe for sudden/marked elevation of blood pressure, restlessness, moist cough, dyspnea, basilar crackles, and frothy sputum. *Too rapid a correction of fluid deficit may compromise the cardiopulmonary system, causing fluid overload and edema, especially if colloids are used in initial fluid resuscitation.*[8]

NURSING PRIORITY NO. 5 To promote wellness (Teaching/Discharge Considerations):

- Discuss factors related to occurrence of deficit as individually appropriate. *Early identification of risk factors can decrease occurrence and severity of complications associated with hypovolemia.*[7]

🌐 Cultural Ⓐ Collaborative 🏠 Community/Home Care ✏ Diagnostic Studies ∞ Pediatric/Geriatric/Lifespan   Medications

- Recommend drinking more water when exercising/engaged in physical exertion, or during hot weather. Suggest carrying water bottle when away from home as appropriate.
- Identify and instruct in ways to meet specific fluid and nutritional needs.
- Offer fluids on a regular basis to infants, young children, and the elderly, *who may not sense/or be able to report thirst.*
- Instruct client/SO(s) in how to monitor color of urine (dark urine equates with concentration/dehydration) and/or how to measure and record I/O (may include weighing or counting diapers in infant/toddler).
- Review/instruct in medication regimen and administration. Stress interactions/side effects to be reported to healthcare provider. *Facilitates timely intervention to prevent/lessen complications.*[8]
- Instruct in signs and symptoms indicating need for immediate/further evaluation and follow-up.

DOCUMENTATION FOCUS

Assessment/Reassessment

- Individual findings, including factors affecting ability to manage (regulate) body fluids and degree of deficit.
- I/O, fluid balance, changes in weight, urine-specific gravity, and vital signs.
- Results of diagnostic testing/laboratory studies.

Planning

- Plan of care and who is involved in the planning.
- Teaching plan.

Implementation/Evaluation

- Client's responses to treatment/teaching and actions performed.
- Attainment/progress toward desired outcome(s).
- Modifications to plan of care.

Discharge Planning

- Long-term needs, noting who is responsible for actions to be taken.
- Specific referrals made.

References

1. Cox, H. C., et al. (2002). *Clinical Applications of Nursing Diagnosis: Adult, Child, Women's, Psychiatric, Gerontic, and Home Health Considerations.* 4th ed. Philadelphia: F. A. Davis, p. 88.
2. Mentes, J. C. (1998). Hydration management. The Iowa Veterans Affairs Nursing Research Consortium. Iowa City, IA: University Iowa Gerontological Nursing Interventions Research Center, Research Dissemination Core.
3. Ellsbury, D. L., George, C. S. (2006 update). Dehydration. Accessed July 2007 at www.emedicine.com/ped/topic556.htm.
4. Cavanaugh, B. M. (1999). *Nurse's Manual of Laboratory and Diagnostic Tests.* 3d ed. Philadelphia: F. A. Davis.
5. Dehydration and fluid maintenance. (2001). American Medical Directors Association (AMDA). Columbia, MD. Accessed July 2007 at www.guideline.gov/summary/.
6. Oliver, R. I., Spain, D. (2006 update). Burns, resuscitation and early management. Accessed July 2007 at www.emedicine.com/plastic/topic159.htm.
7. Matheny, N. (2000). *Fluid and Electrolyte Balance: Nursing Considerations.* 4th ed. Philadelphia: J. B. Lippincott.
8. Fluid and Electrolyte Imbalances. In Doenges, M. E., Moorhouse, M. F., Geissler-Murr, A. C. (2002). *Nursing Care Plans: Guidelines for Individualizing Patient Care.* 6th ed. CD ROM. Philadelphia: F. A. Davis.

9. Mayo Clinic Staff. (2007). Dehydration. Article for MayoClinic.com Web site. Retrieved February 2007 at www.mayoclinic.com/health/dehydration/DS00561/DSECTION=1.
10. Astle, S. M. (2005). Restoring electrolyte balance. Article for RNWeb. Retrieved February 2007 at www.rnweb.com/content/printContentPopup.jsp?id=158212.
11. Viele, C. S., Quin, A. M., Daly, C. F. (2006). Dehydration and electrolyte requirements in oncology care. Retrieved July 2007 at www.cmknowledge.com/Downloads/215393_enewsletter.pdf.

deficient Fluid Volume: [isotonic]

[**NOTE:** This diagnosis has been structured to address isotonic dehydration (hypovolemia) when fluids and electrolytes are lost in even amounts and excluding states in which changes in sodium occur. For client needs related to dehydration associated with alterations in sodium, refer to [deficient Fluid Volume: hyper/hypotonic]

Definition: Decreased intravascular, interstitial, and/or intracellular fluid; refers to dehydration, water loss alone without change in sodium

RELATED FACTORS

Active fluid volume loss [e.g., hemorrhage, gastric intubation, acute/prolonged diarrhea; wounds; abdominal cancer; burns, fistulas, ascites (third spacing); use of hyperosmotic radiopaque contrast agents]

Failure of regulatory mechanisms [e.g., fever/thermoregulatory response, renal tubule damage]

DEFINING CHARACTERISTICS

Subjective
Thirst
Weakness

Objective
Decreased urine output; increased urine concentration
Decreased venous filling; decreased pulse volume/pressure
Sudden weight loss (except in third spacing)
Decreased BP; increased pulse rate/body temperature
Decreased skin/tongue turgor; dry skin/mucous membranes
Change in mental state
Elevated hematocrit

Sample Clinical Applications: Hemorrhage, severe burns, gastroenteritis (with vomiting and diarrhea), malnutrition, uncontrolled diabetes mellitus

DESIRED OUTCOMES/EVALUATION CRITERIA
Sample NOC linkages:
Hydration: Adequate water in the intracellular and extracellular compartments of the body
Fluid Balance: Water balance in the intracellular and extracellular compartments of the body
Blood Loss Severity: Severity of internal or external bleeding/hemorrhage

Client Will (Include Specific Time Frames)

• Maintain fluid volume at a functional level as evidenced by individually adequate urinary output with normal specific gravity, stable vital signs, moist mucous membranes, good skin turgor, and prompt capillary refill, resolution of edema.

Cultural Collaborative Community/Home Care Diagnostic Studies Pediatric/Geriatric/Lifespan Medications

- Verbalize understanding of causative factors and purpose of individual therapeutic interventions and medications.
- Demonstrate behaviors to monitor and correct deficit, as indicated.

ACTIONS/INTERVENTIONS

Sample NIC linkages:

Hypovolemia Management: Reduction in extracellular or intracellular fluid volume and prevention of complications in a patient who is fluid overloaded

Shock Management: Volume: Promotion of adequate tissue perfusion for a patient with severely compromised intravascular volume

Bleeding Precautions: Reduction of stimuli that may induce bleeding or hemorrhage in at-risk patients

NURSING PRIORITY NO. 1 To assess causative/precipitating factors:

- Identify relevant diagnoses *that may create a fluid volume depletion (decreased intravascular plasma volume, such as might occur with rapid blood loss/hemorrhage from trauma; or vascular, pregnancy-related, or GI bleeding disorders; significant fluid (other than blood) loss such as might occur with severe gastroenteritis with vomiting and diarrhea, or extensive burns.*[1]
- Note presence of other factors (e.g., laryngectomy/tracheostomy tubes, drainage from wounds/fistulas or suction devices; water deprivation/fluid restrictions; decreased level of consciousness; dialysis; hot/humid climate, prolonged exercise; increased metabolic rate secondary to fever; increased caffeine/alcohol) *that may contribute to lack of fluid intake or loss of fluid by various routes.*
- Prepare for/assist with diagnostic evaluations (e.g., imaging studies, x-rays, etc.) *to locate source of bleeding/cause for hypovolemia.*
- Determine effects of age, gender. Obtain weight and measure subcutaneous fat/muscle mass (influences total body water [TBW], which is approximately 60% of an adult's weight and 75% of an infant's weight).[1] *In general, men have higher TBW than women, and the elderly's TBW is less than that of a youth. Elderly individuals are often at risk because of decreased thirst reflex, decreased effectiveness of compensatory mechanisms, repeated infections, chronic conditions, and polypharmacy.*[2,3,9] *Infants/young children and other nonverbal persons cannot describe thirst. Worldwide, dehydration (secondary to diarrheal illness) is the leading cause of infant and child mortality.*[4,9]

NURSING PRIORITY NO. 2 To evaluate degree of fluid deficit:

- Estimate/measure traumatic or procedural fluid losses. Note possible routes of insensible fluid losses. Determine customary and current weight. *These factors are used to determine degree of dehydration and method of fluid replacement. The body surface area (BSA) method states that dehydration is related to deficit of TBW and assumes that loss of weight is loss of water. The caloric method states that the degree of dehydration is related to body weight (e.g., loss of 10% of usual body weight is considered "10% dry").*[5]
- Assess vital signs, including temperature (often elevated), pulse and respirations (elevated), and blood pressure (may be low). Measure blood pressure (lying/sitting/standing to evaluate orthostatic blood pressure), and monitor invasive hemodynamic parameters as indicated (e.g., central venous pressure [CVP]) *to determine degree of intravascular deficit and replacement needs.*[8-10]
- Note presence of dry mucous membranes, poor skin turgor, delayed capillary refill, flat neck veins, and reports of thirst or weakness, child crying without tears, sunken eyeballs (or

fontanels in infant), fever, weight loss, little or no urine output. *Assessment signs of dehydration that client/SO may notice. In an acute, life-threatening hemorrhage state, cold, pale, moist skin may be noted reflecting body compensatory mechanisms to profound hypovolemia.*[1,9,10]

- Note change in usual mentation/behavior/functional abilities (e.g., confusion, falling, loss of ability to carry out usual activities, lethargy, and dizziness). *These signs indicate sufficient dehydration to cause poor cerebral perfusion or electrolyte imbalance. In hypovolemic shock state, mentation changes rapidly and client may present in coma.*
- *Observe/measure urinary output (hourly/24-hour totals). Note color* (may be dark because of concentration) *and specific gravity* (high number associated with dehydration with usual range being 1.010 to 1.025).[6]
- Review laboratory data (e.g., Hb/Hct, electrolytes [sodium, potassium, chloride, bicarbonate]; blood urea nitrogen [BUN], creatinine) *to evaluate body's response to fluid loss and to determine replacement needs.*[6] *In isotonic dehydration, electrolyte levels may be lower, but concentrations remain near normal.*[5]

NURSING PRIORITY NO. 3 To correct/replace losses to reverse pathophysiological mechanisms:

- Stop blood loss (e.g., gastric lavage with room temperature or cool saline solution, drug administration, prepare for surgical intervention).
- Stop fluid loss (e.g., administer medication to stop vomiting/diarrhea, fever).[8]
- Administer fluids and electrolytes (e.g., blood, isotonic sodium chloride solution, lactated Ringer solution, fresh frozen plasma, dextran, hetastarch).[8,10]
- Establish/continually reevaluate 24-hour fluid replacement needs and routes to be used *to prevent peaks/valleys in fluid level and to prevent fluid overload.*[8,9]
- Control humidity and ambient air temperature as appropriate, especially when major burns are present, or in presence of fever *to reduce insensible losses.*
- Reduce bedding/clothes, provide tepid sponge bath.
- Assist with hypothermia therapy as indicated *to decrease severe fever and elevated metabolic rate.* (Refer to ND Hyperthermia for additional interventions.)
- Maintain accurate I/O and weigh daily. Measure urine specific gravity. Monitor blood pressure and invasive hemodynamic parameters as indicated (e.g., CVP, PAP/PCWP) *to evaluate effectiveness of resuscitation measures.*[8]

NURSING PRIORITY NO. 4 To promote comfort and safety:

- Change position frequently. Bathe infrequently, using mild cleanser/soap, and provide optimal skin care with emollients *to maintain skin integrity and prevent excessive dryness caused by dehydration.*
- Provide frequent oral care and eye care *to prevent injury from dryness.*
- Change dressings as needed/use adjunct appliances as indicated for draining wounds *to protect skin and to monitor/replace losses.*
- Administer medications (e.g., antiemetics, antidiarrheals *to limit gastric/intestinal losses;* antipyretics *to reduce fever*). (Refer to NDs Diarrhea, Hyperthermia for additional interventions.)
- Observe for sudden/marked elevation of blood pressure, restlessness, moist cough, dyspnea, basilar crackles, and frothy sputum. *Too rapid a correction of fluid deficit may compromise the cardiopulmonary system, causing fluid overload and edema, especially if colloids are used in initial fluid resuscitation.*[8]

⊕ Cultural Ⓐ Collaborative 🏠 Community/Home Care ⬭ Diagnostic Studies ∞ Pediatric/Geriatric/Lifespan Medications

NURSING PRIORITY NO. 5 To promote wellness (Teaching/Discharge Considerations):

- Discuss factors related to occurrence of fluid deficit as individually appropriate (e.g., reason for hemorrhage, potential for dehydration in children with fever/diarrhea, inadequate fluid replacement when performing strenuous work/exercise, living in hot climate, improper use of diuretics) *to reduce risk of recurrence.*[7]

- Identify actions (if any) client may take to prevent/correct deficiencies. *Carrying water bottle when away from home aids in maintaining fluid volume. Dressing in weather-appropriate clothing, staying in shade during heat of day, engaging in exercise during early morning or evening hours, and installation of room cooler or electric fan for hot climates helps reduce risk of heat stress/hyperthermia. In cases of mild-to-moderate dehydration, use of oral solutions (e.g., Gatorade, Rehydralyte), soft drinks, breast milk, or formula can provide adequate rehydration.*[7]

- Instruct client/SO(s) in how to monitor color of urine (dark urine equates with concentration/dehydration) or how to measure and record I/O (may include weighing or counting diapers in infant/toddler).

- Review medications and interactions/side effects, especially medications that can cause or exacerbate fluid loss (e.g., diuretics, laxatives), and those indicated to prevent fluid loss (e.g., antidiarrheals or anticoagulants).[9]

- Discuss signs/symptoms indicating need for emergent/further evaluation and follow-up. *Promotes timely intervention.*

DOCUMENTATION FOCUS

Assessment/Reassessment

- Assessment findings, including degree of deficit and current sources of fluid intake.
- I/O, fluid balance, changes in weight/edema, urine-specific gravity, and vital signs.
- Results of diagnostic studies.

Planning

- Plan of care and who is involved in planning.
- Teaching plan.

Implementation/Evaluation

- Client's responses to interventions/teaching and actions performed.
- Attainment/progress toward desired outcome(s).
- Modifications to plan of care.

Discharge Planning

- Long-term needs, plan for correction, and who is responsible for actions to be taken.
- Specific referrals made.

References

1. Kolecki, P., Meckhoff, C. R. (2001). Shock, hypovolemic. Article from Emedicine.com. Available at www.emedicine.com. Accessed August 2003.
2. Cox, H. C., et al. (2002). *Clinical Applications of Nursing Diagnosis: Adult, Child, Women's, Psychiatric, Gerontic, and Home Health Considerations.* 4th ed. Philadelphia: F. A. Davis, p. 88.
3. Mentes, J. C. (1998). Hydration management. The Iowa Veterans Affairs Nursing Research Consortium. Iowa City, IA: University Iowa Gerontological Nursing Interventions Research Center, Research Dissemination Core.

4. Ellsbury, D. L., George, C. S. (2006 update). Dehydration. Accessed July 2007 at www.emedicine.com/ped/topic556.htm.
5. Welch, J. (1998). Isotonic dehydration. Accessed August 2003. Available at http://gucfm.georgetown.edu/welchjj/netscut/fen/isotonic_dehydration.html.
6. Cavanaugh, B. M. (1999). *Nurse's Manual of Laboratory and Diagnostic Tests*. 3d ed. Philadelphia: F. A. Davis.
7. Koch, H., Graber, M. A. *Pediatrics: Vomiting, Diarrhea, and Dehydration. University of Iowa Family Practice Handbook*. 4th ed. Available at www.vh.org. Accessed August 2003.
8. Fluid and Electrolyte Imbalances. In Doenges, M. E., Moorhouse, M. F., Geissler-Murr, A. C. (2002). *Nursing Care Plans: Guidelines for Individualizing Patient Care*. 6th ed. CD ROM. Philadelphia: F. A. Davis.
9. Mayo Clinic Staff. (2007). Dehydration. Article for MayoClinic.com Web site. Retrieved February 2007 at www.mayoclinic.com/health/dehydration/DS00561/DSECTION=1.
10. Diel-Oplinger, L., Kaminski, M. F. (2004). Choosing the right fluid to counter hypovolemic shock. *Nursing 2004*, 34(3), 52–54.

excess Fluid Volume

Definition: Increased isotonic fluid retention

RELATED FACTORS
Compromised regulatory mechanism [e.g., syndrome of inappropriate antidiuretic hormone (SIADH), or decreased plasma proteins as found in conditions such as malnutrition, draining fistulas, burns, organ failure]
Excess fluid intake
Excess sodium intake
[Drug therapies such as chlorpropamide, tolbutamide, vincristine, triptylines, carbamazepine]

DEFINING CHARACTERISTICS

Subjective
Anxiety
[Difficulty breathing]

Objective
Edema; anasarca; weight gain over short period of time
Intake exceeds output; oliguria; specific gravity changes
Adventitious breath sounds [rales or crackles]; changes in respiratory pattern; dyspnea; orthopnea
Pulmonary congestion; pleural effusion; pulmonary artery pressure changes; blood pressure changes
Increased central venous pressure; jugular vein distention; positive hepatojugular reflex
S_3 heart sound
Change in mental status; restlessness
Decreased Hb/Hct, azotemia, altered electrolytes

Sample Clinical Applications: Congestive heart failure, renal failure, cirrhosis of liver, cancer, toxemia of pregnancy, conditions associated with SIADH (e.g., meningitis, encephalitis, Guillain-Barré syndrome), schizophrenia (where polydipsia is a prominent feature)

DESIRED OUTCOMES/EVALUATION CRITERIA
Sample NOC linkages:
Fluid Balance: Water balance in the intracellular and extracellular compartments of the body

Electrolyte and Acid/Base Balance: Balance of electrolytes and non-electrolytes in the intracellular and extracellular compartments of the body

Cardiac Pump Effectiveness: Adequacy of blood volume ejected from the left ventricle to support systemic perfusion pressure

Client Will (Include Specific Time Frame)

- Stabilize fluid volume as evidenced by balanced I/O, vital signs within client's normal limits, stable weight, and free of signs of edema.
- Verbalize understanding of individual dietary/fluid restrictions.
- Demonstrate behaviors to monitor fluid status and reduce recurrence of fluid excess.
- List signs that require further evaluation.

ACTIONS/INTERVENTIONS

Sample NIC linkages:

Hypervolemia Management: Reduction in extracellular or intracellular fluid volume and prevention of complications in a patient who is fluid overloaded

Electrolyte Management: Promotion of electrolyte balance and prevention of complications resulting from abnormal or undesired serum electrolyte levels

Peritoneal Dialysis/Hemodialysis Therapy: Administration and monitoring of dialysis solution into and out of the peritoneal cavity/or management of extracorporeal passage of the patient's blood through a dialyzer

NURSING PRIORITY NO. 1 To assess causative/precipitating factors:

- Note presence of medical conditions or situations (e.g., heart failure, chronic kidney disease, renal/adrenal insufficiency, excessive or rapid infusion of IV fluids, cerebral lesions, psychogenic polydipsia, acute stress, surgical/anesthetic procedures, decreased/loss of serum proteins) *that can contribute to excess fluid intake or retention.*[1]
- Determine/estimate amount of fluid intake from all sources: oral, intravenous, enteral feedings, ventilator, etc.
- Review nutritional issues (e.g., intake of sodium, potassium, and protein). *Imbalances in these areas are associated with fluid imbalances.*

NURSING PRIORITY NO. 2 To evaluate degree of excess:

- Compare current weight with admission or previously stated weight. Weigh daily or on a regular schedule, as indicated. *Provides a comparative baseline and evaluates the effectiveness of diruetic therapy when used (i.e., if I/O is 1 liter negative, weight loss of 2.2 pounds should be noted).*[8] *Note: Volume overload can occur over weeks to months in clients with unrecognized renal failure where lean muscle mass is lost and fluid overload occurs with relatively little change in weight.*[4]
- Measure vital signs and invasive hemodynamic parameters (e.g., CVP, PAP/PCWP) if available. *Blood pressures may be high because of excess fluid volume, or be low if cardiac failure is occurring.*
- Note presence of tachycardia, irregular rhythms. Auscultate heart tones for S_3, ventricular gallop. *Signs suggestive of heart failure, which results in decreased cardiac output and tissue hypoxia.*[7]

- Auscultate breath sounds for presence of crackles/congestion. Record occurrence of exertional breathlessness, dyspnea at rest, or paroxysmal nocturnal dyspnea. *Indication of pulmonary congestion and potential of developing pulmonary edema that can interfere with oxygen—carbon dioxide exchange at the capillary level.*[3]
- Note presence and location of edema (e.g., puffy eyelids, dependent swelling ankles/feet if ambulatory or up in chair; sacrum and posterior thighs when recumbent). Determine whether lower extremity edema is new or increasing. *Heart failure and renal failure are associated with dependent edema because of hydrostatic pressures, with dependent edema being a defining characteristic for excess fluid. Generalized edema (e.g., upper extremities and eyelids) is associated with nephrotic syndrome.*[2]
- Assess for presence of neck vein distention/hepatojugular reflux with head of bed elevated 30 to 45 degrees. *Signs of increased intravascular volume.*[6]
- Measure abdominal girth *to evaluate changes that may indicate increasing fluid retention/edema.*[7]
- Measure/record intake and output accurately. Include "hidden" fluids (e.g., IV antibiotic additives, liquid medications, ice chips). Calculate 24-hour fluid balance (plus/minus). Note patterns, times, and amount of urination (e.g., nocturia, oliguria).[6]
- Evaluate mentation for restlessness, anxiety, confusion, and personality changes. *Signs of decreased cerebral oxygenation (e.g., cerebral edema) or electrolyte imbalance (e.g., hyponatremia).*[1,9]
- Assess appetite; note presence of nausea/vomiting. Assess neuromuscular reflexes *to determine presence of problems associated with imbalance of electrolytes (e.g., glucose, sodium, potassium, calcium).*[9]
- Observe skin and mucous membranes. *Edematous tissues are prone to ischemia and breakdown/ulceration.*[5]
- Review laboratory data (e.g., BUN/Cr, Hb/Hct, serum albumin, proteins, and electrolytes; urine specific gravity/osmolality/sodium excretion) and chest radiograph. *These tests may be repeated to ascertain baseline imbalances and to monitor response to therapy.*

NURSING PRIORITY NO. 3 To promote mobilization/elimination of excess fluid:

- Restrict fluid intake as indicated (especially when sodium retention is less than water retention or when fluid retention is related to renal failure).[6]
- Provide for sodium restrictions if needed (as might occur in sodium retention in excess of water retention). *Restricting sodium favors renal excretion of excess fluid and may be more useful than fluid restriction.*[1]
- Set an appropriate rate of fluid intake/infusion throughout 24-hour period. Maintain steady rate of all IV infusions *to prevent exacerbation of excess fluid volume and to prevent peaks/valleys in fluid level.*[6]
- Administer medications (e.g., diuretics, cardiotonics, plasma or albumin volume expanders) in order to improve cardiac output and kidney function, thereby *reducing congestion and edema.*
- Evaluate edematous extremities *to enhance venous return/prevent further edema formation.*[7]
- Encourage bedrest when ascites is present and place in semi-Fowler's position as appropriate. *May promote recumbency-induced diuresis and facilitate respiratory effort when movement of the diaphragm is limited/breathing is impaired because of lung congestion.*
- Prepare for/assist with procedures as indicated (e.g., peritoneal or hemodialysis, mechanical ventilation). *May be done to correct volume overload, electrolyte and acid-base imbalances, or to support individual during shock state.*[7]

Cultural Collaborative Community/Home Care Diagnostic Studies Pediatric/Geriatric/Lifespan Medications

NURSING PRIORITY NO. 4 To maintain integrity of skin and tissues:

- Promote early ambulation *to mobilize fluids and prevent/limit damage from venous stasis complications.*
- Change position frequently *to reduce tissue pressure and risk of skin breakdown.*[7]
- Offer frequent mouth care when fluids are restricted using nondrying mouthwash and hard candies, etc., *to promote comfort of dry mucous membranes and prevent oral complications.*[7]
- Avoid use of restraints/use safety precautions if client is confused/debilitated as may occur with cerebral edema, electrolyte imbalance, heart failure, etc. *There is an increased risk of skin/tissue trauma with the use of restraints as well as increased agitation that may lead to more serious injury/death.*[7]
- Refer to NDs impaired Oral Mucous Membrane, impaired/risk for impaired Skin [or] Tissue Integrity for additional interventions.

NURSING PRIORITY NO. 5 To promote wellness (Teaching/Discharge Considerations):

- Consult dietitian as needed *to develop dietary plan/identify foods to be limited or omitted:* Review dietary restrictions and safe substitutes for salt (e.g., lemon juice or spices such as oregano).
  Discuss fluid restrictions and "hidden sources" of fluids (e.g., foods high in water content such as fruits, ice cream, sauces, custard, etc.). Use small drinking cup or glass.
  Avoid salty or spicy foods, as they increase thirst or fluid retention. Suck ice chips, hard candy, or slices of lemon *to help allay thirst.*[7]
- Suggest chewing gum, use of lip balm *to reduce discomforts of fluid restrictions.*[7]
- Instruct client/family in ways to keep track of intake. For example, use a marked water bottle/container; refill as needed.[6]
- Measure output, encourage use of voiding record when it is appropriate, or weigh daily and report gain of more than 2 pounds/day (or as indicated by individual physician order). *If weight is higher than target weight, fluid is likely being retained.*[6,7]
- Review drug regimen/side effects of agents used to increase urine output or manage hypertension, kidney disease, or heart failure. *Many drugs have an impact on kidney function and fluid balance, especially in the elderly or those with cardiac and kidney impairments.*
- Stress need for mobility or frequent position changes *to prevent stasis and reduce risk of tissue injury.*[7]
- Identify "danger" signs requiring notification of healthcare provider *to ensure timely evaluation/intervention.*[6]

DOCUMENTATION FOCUS

Assessment/Reassessment

- Assessment findings, noting existing conditions contributing to and degree of fluid retention (vital signs; amount, presence and location of edema; and weight changes).
- I/O, fluid balance.
- Results of laboratory tests/diagnostic studies.

Planning

- Plan of care and who is involved in the planning.
- Teaching plan.

Implementation/Evaluation

- Response to interventions and teaching and actions performed.
- Attainment/progress toward desired outcome(s).
- Modifications to plan of care.

Discharge Planning

- Long-range needs, noting who is responsible for actions to be taken.

References

1. Fauci, A. S., et al. (eds). (1998). *Harrison's Principles of Internal Medicine.* 14th ed. New York: McGraw-Hill, pp. 268–269, 1292–1293.
2. Rios, H., et al. (1991). Validation of defining characteristics of four nursing diagnoses using a computerized database. *J Prof Nurs, 7,* 293–299.
3. Matheny, N. (2000). *Fluid and Electrolyte Balance: Nursing Considerations.* 4th ed. Philadelphia: J. B. Lippincott.
4. Veterans Health Administration, Department of Defense. VHA/DoD clinical practice guideline for the management of chronic kidney disease and pre-ERSD in the primary care setting. Department of Veterans Affairs (U.S.), Veterans Health Administration (2001), various pages. Available at www.guideline.gov. Accessed August 2003.
5. Cullen, L. (1992). Interventions related to fluid and electrolyte imbalance. *Nurs Clin North Am, 27,* 569–597.
6. Hydration management. (2004 update). American Medical Directors Association (AMDA). Columbia, MD: National Guideline Clearinghouse. Accessed July 2007. Available at www.guideline.gov/summary/summary.aspx?doc_id=4832.
7. Fluid and Electrolyte Imbalances. In Doenges, M. E., Moorhouse, M. F., Geissler-Murr, A. C. (2002). *Nursing Care Plans: Guidelines for Individualizing Patient Care.* 6th ed. CD ROM. Philadelphia: F. A. Davis.
8. Riggs, J. M. (2006). Manage heart failure. *Nursing2006 Critical Care, 1*(4), 18–28.
9. Astle, S. M. (2005). Restoring electrolyte balance. *RN, 68*(5), 31–34.

risk for deficient Fluid Volume

Definition: At risk for experiencing vascular, cellular, or intracellular dehydration

RISK FACTORS
Extremes of age/weight
Loss of fluid through abnormal routes (e.g., indwelling tubes)
Knowledge deficiency
Factors influencing fluid needs (e.g., hypermetabolic states)
Medications (e.g., diuretics)
Excessive losses through normal routes (e.g., diarrhea)
Deviations affecting access, intake, or absorption of fluids (e.g., physical immobility)
NOTE: A risk diagnosis is not evidenced by signs and symptoms, as the problem has not occurred; rather, nursing interventions are directed at prevention.

Sample Clinical Applications: Conditions with fever, diarrhea, nausea/vomiting; irritable bowel syndrome, draining wounds, dementia, depression, eating disorders

DESIRED OUTCOMES/EVALUATION CRITERIA
Sample NOC linkages:
Fluid Balance: Water balance in the intracellular and extracellular compartments of the body

Cultural   Collaborative   Community/Home Care   Diagnostic Studies   Pediatric/Geriatric/Lifespan   Medications

Client Will (Include Specific Time Frame)

- Maintain fluid volume at a functional level as evidenced by individually adequate urinary output with normal specific gravity, stable vital signs, moist mucous membranes, good skin turgor, and prompt capillary refill.

Risk Control: Personal actions to prevent, eliminate, or reduce modifiable health threats
Knowledge: Disease Process: Extent of understanding conveyed about a specific disease process

Client/Caregiver Will (Include Specific Time Frame)

- Identify individual risk factors and appropriate interventions.
- Demonstrate behaviors or lifestyle changes to prevent development of fluid volume deficit.

ACTIONS/INTERVENTIONS

Sample NIC linkages:
Fluid Monitoring: Collection and analysis of patient data to regulate fluid balance
Hemodynamic Regulation: Optimization of heart rate, preload, afterload, and contractility
Bleeding Precautions: Reduction of stimuli that may indicate bleeding or hemorrhage in at-risk patients

NURSING PRIORITY NO. 1   To assess causative/contributing factors:

- Note possible conditions/processes *that may lead to fluid deficits*: (1) fluid loss (e.g., indwelling tubes, diarrhea/vomiting, fever, excessive sweating, diabetic ketoacidosis; burns, other draining wounds; gastrointestinal obstruction; use of diuretics); (2) limited intake (e.g., extremes of age, immobility, client dependent on others for eating and drinking; lack of knowledge related to fluid intake; heat exhaustion/stroke); (3) fluid shifts (e.g., ascites, effusions, burns, sepsis); or (4) environmental factors (e.g., isolation, restraints, very high ambient temperatures, malfunctioning air conditioning).[4,8]
- ∞ Determine effects of age, gender. Obtain weight and measure subcutaneous fat/muscle mass. These factors affect ratio of lean body mass to body fat, influencing total body water (TBW). *In general, men have higher TBW than women, and the elderly's TBW is less than that of a youth. Elderly individuals are often at risk for underhydration because of a decreased thirst reflex, repeated infections, and chronic conditions. They may not be aware of water or nutritional needs, may be depressed or cognitively impaired, incontinent, and taking many medications.[2] Infants, children, and developmentally delayed individual cannot verbalize or self-manage thirst. Worldwide, dehydration (secondary to diarrheal illness) is the leading cause of infant and child mortality.[3]*
- ♠ Evaluate nutritional status, noting current food intake, type of diet (e.g., client is NPO or is on a restricted/pureed diet). Note problems *that can negatively affect fluid intake* (e.g., impaired mentation, nausea, wired jaws, immobility, insufficient time for meals, lack of finances restricting availability of food).
- Refer to NDs [deficient Fluid Volume: hyper/hypotonic] or [isotonic] for additional interventions.

NURSING PRIORITY NO. 2   To prevent occurrence of deficit:

- Monitor I/O balance being aware of altered intake or output, as well as insensible losses *to ensure accurate picture of fluid status.*[4]

- Weigh client and compare with recent weight history. Perform serial weights *to determine trends.*[5]
- Monitor vital signs for changes (e.g., orthostatic hypotension, tachycardia, fever) *that may cause dehydration.*[4]
- Assess skin turgor/oral mucous membranes for signs of dehydration.

- Review laboratory data (e.g., Hb/Hct, electrolytes, BUN/Cr) as indicated *to evaluate fluid and electrolyte status.*[4]

- Administer medications as appropriate (e.g., antiemetics, antidiarrheals, antipyretics) *to stop/limit fluid losses.*[4,5]
- Determine individual fluid needs and establish replacement schedule. Distribute fluids over 24 hours *to prevent periods of thirst.*[5]
- Provide supplemental fluids (tube feed, IV) as indicated. *Fluids may be given in this manner if client is unable to take oral fluid or is NPO for procedures.*
- Encourage oral intake:[4–6]

    Provide water and other fluids to a minimum amount daily (up to 2.5 L/day or amount determined by healthcare provider for client's age, weight, and condition).

    Offer fluids between meals and regularly throughout the day.

    Allow adequate time for eating and drinking at meals.

    Provide fluids in manageable cup, bottle, or with drinking straw.

    Ensure that immobile/restrained client is assisted.

    Encourage a variety of fluids in small frequent offerings, attempting to incorporate client's preferred beverage and temperature (e.g., iced or hot).

    Limit fluids that tend to exert a diuretic effect (e.g., caffeine, alcohol).

    Promote intake of high-water content foods (e.g., popsicles, gelatin, soup, eggnog, watermelon) or electrolyte replacement drinks (e.g., Smartwater, Gatorade, Pedialyte), as appropriate.

    Encourage client to increase fluids when exercising/physical exertion, or during hot weather.

    Review diet orders to remove any nonessential fluid and salt restrictions.
- Provide nutritionally balanced diet and/or enteral feedings, when indicated (avoiding use of hyperosmolar or excessively high-protein formulas) and provide adequate amount of free water with feedings.

NURSING PRIORITY NO. 3 To promote wellness (Teaching/Discharge Considerations):

- Discuss individual risk factors/potential problems and specific interventions *to reduce risk of heat injury and dehydration* (e.g., proper clothing/bedding for infants and elderly during hot weather, use of room cooler/fan for comfortable ambient environment).[7]
- Review appropriate use of medications and inform client of side effects of medications *that have potential for causing/exacerbating dehydration.*
- Encourage client/caregiver to maintain diary of food/fluid intake, number and amount of voidings, and estimate of other fluid losses (e.g., wounds, liquid stools) as necessary *to determine replacement needs.*
- Engage client, family, and all caregivers in fluid management plan. *Enhances cooperation with regimen and achievement of goals.*[5]

DOCUMENTATION FOCUS

Assessment/Reassessment

- Individual findings, including individual factors influencing fluid needs/requirements.
- Baseline weight, vital signs.

- Results of laboratory tests.
- Specific client preferences for fluids.

Planning

- Plan of care and who is involved in planning.
- Teaching plan.

Implementation/Evaluation

- Responses to interventions/teaching and actions performed.
- Attainment/progress toward desired outcome(s).
- Modifications to plan of care.

Discharge Planning

- Individual long-term needs, noting who is responsible for actions to be taken.
- Specific referrals made.

References

1. Cox, H. C., et al. (2002). *Clinical Applications of Nursing Diagnosis: Adult, Child, Women's, Psychiatric, Gerontic, and Home Health Considerations*. 4th ed. Philadelphia: F. A. Davis, p. 88.
2. Mentes, J. C. (1998). Hydration management. The Iowa Veterans Affairs Nursing Research Consortium. Iowa City, IA: University Iowa Gerontological Nursing Interventions Research Center, Research Dissemination Core.
3. Ellsbury, D. L., George, C. S. (2006 update). Dehydration. Accessed July 2007 at www.emedicine.com/ped/topic556.htm.
4. No author listed. (2001). Dehydration and fluid maintenance. American Medical Directors Association (AMDA). Columbia, MD. Accessed July 2007 at www.guideline.gov/summary/.
5. Fluid and Electrolyte Imbalances. In Doenges, M. E., Moorhouse, M. F., Geissler-Murr, A. C. (2002). *Nursing Care Plans: Guidelines for Individualizing Patient Care*. 6th ed. CD-ROM. Philadelphia: F. A. Davis.
6. Matheny, N. (2000). *Fluid and Electrolyte Balance: Nursing Considerations*. 4th ed. Philadelphia: J. B. Lippincott.
7. Curtis, R. (1997). OA guide to heat related illnesses & fluid balance. Article for Princeton University Outdoor Action Web site. Accessed July 2007 at www.princeton.edu/~oa/safety/heatill.html.
8. Laskowski-Jones, L. (2006). Responding to trauma: Your priorities in the first hour. *Nursing2006*, 36(9), 52–58.

risk for imbalanced Fluid Volume

Definition: At risk for a decrease, an increase, or a rapid shift from one to the other of intravascular, interstitial, or intracellular fluid; refers to body fluid loss, gain, or both

RISK FACTORS
Scheduled for major invasive procedures
[Rapid/sustained loss, e.g., hemorrhage, burns, fistulas]
[Rapid fluid replacement]
Other risk factors to be determined
NOTE: A risk diagnosis is not evidenced by signs and symptoms, as the problem has not occurred; rather, nursing interventions are directed at prevention.

Sample Clinical Application: Major surgical procedures, renal dialysis, conditions requiring IV therapy or parenteral/enteral nutrition, heart failure with use of diuretic therapy

DESIRED OUTCOMES/EVALUATION CRITERIA

Sample NOC linkages:

Fluid Balance: Water balance in the intracellular and extracellular compartments of the body

Risk Control: Personal actions to prevent, eliminate, or reduce modifiable health threats

Cardiac Pump Effectiveness: Adequacy of blood volume ejected from the left ventricle to support systemic perfusion pressure

Client Will (Include Specific Time Frame)

- Demonstrate adequate fluid balance as evidenced by stable vital signs, palpable pulses/good quality, normal skin turgor, moist mucous membranes, individual appropriate urinary output, lack of excessive weight fluctuation (loss/gain), and no edema present.
- Identify individual risk factors and appropriate interventions.
- Demonstrate behaviors or lifestyle changes to prevent development of fluid imbalance.

ACTIONS/INTERVENTIONS

Sample NIC linkages:

Fluid Monitoring: Collection and analysis of patient data to regulate fluid balance

Intravenous [IV] Therapy: Administration and monitoring of intravenous fluids and medication

Bleeding Precautions: Reduction of stimuli that may induce bleeding or hemorrhage in at-risk patients

NURSING PRIORITY NO. 1   To determine risk/contributing factors:

- Note potential sources of fluid imbalances (e.g., presence of conditions such as diabetes insipidus, hyperosmolar nonketotic syndrome, bowel obstruction, heart/kidney/liver failure), major invasive procedures (e.g., surgery), use of anesthesia, preoperative vomiting and dehydration, draining wounds, use/overuse of certain medications (e.g., anticoagulants, diuretics, laxatives), use of IV fluids and delivery device, administration of total parenteral nutrition (TPN).
- Note client's age, current level of hydration, and mentation. *Provides information regarding ability to tolerate fluctuations in fluid level and risk for creating or failing to respond to a problem (e.g., confused client may have inadequate intake, disconnect tubings, or readjust IV flow rate; infant or child unable to self-monitor or manage).*[1]

NURSING PRIORITY NO. 2   To prevent fluctuations/imbalances in fluid levels:

- Measure and record intake:
  Include all sources (e.g., oral, intravenous, antibiotic additives, liquids with medications).
- Measure and record output:
  Monitor urine output (hourly, or as often as needed). Report urine output <30. mL/hr or 0.5 mL/kg/hr *because it may indicate deficient fluid volume or cardiac or kidney failure.*
  Observe color of all excretions *to evaluate for bleeding.*
  Estimate volume/measure emesis when vomiting.
  Measure/estimate amount of liquid stool; weigh diapers/continence pads when indicated.
  Inspect dressing(s), weigh dressings, estimate blood loss in surgical sponges, count dressings/pads saturated per hour. *Note: Small losses can be life-threatening to pediatric clients.*[2]
  Measure output from drainage devices (e.g., gastric, wound, chest).

Estimate/calculate insensible fluid losses *to include losses in replacement calculations. Note: Losses from diffusion through skin and via respiratory tract, are estimated at about 700 mL/24 hours in adult at ambient temperature,*[3] *while a diaphoretic episode requiring a full linen change may represent a fluid loss of as much as 1 L.*[5]

Calculate 24-hour fluid balance (noting intake > output, or output > intake).

- Weigh daily or as indicated, using same scale and clothing and evaluate changes as they relate to fluid status. *Provides for early detection and prompt intervention as needed.*[5]
- Monitor vital signs:

Evaluate vital signs at rest and with activities. *Blood pressure, heart and respiratory rate often increase initially when either volume deficit or fluid excess is present.*[5]

Calculate pulse pressure. *Pulse pressure often widens before systolic BP drops in response to fluid loss.*

Evaluate hemodynamic pressures when available. *Central venous pressure (CVP) and pulmonary artery wedge pressures (PAWP) may be used in critically ill to determine fluid balance and guide administration of vasoactive medications.*[2]

- Maintain IVs on volumetric infusion pumps, rapid infusion devices, as appropriate *to deliver fluids accurately at desired rates to prevent either under- or overinfusion.*[5] Tape tubing connections longitudinally *to reduce risk of disconnection and loss of fluids.*
- Assess for dry skin/mucous membranes, delayed capillary refill, soft eyeballs, sunken fotanels (in infant). *Clinical signs of dehydration.*[4,5]
- Assess for peripheral/dependent edema, adventitious breath sounds, and distended neck veins. *Clinical signs of fluid excess. Note: Intravascular volume depletion can be present at the same time as extravascular fluid excess (seen as edema) is present, so hypertension or hypotension could be found.*[4,5]
- Note increased lethargy or reports of dizziness, weakness, muscle cramping. *Electrolyte imbalances (e.g., sodium, potassium, magnesium, calcium) may be present.*[5,6]
- Review laboratory data (e.g., electrolytes, Hgb/Hct), chest radiograph *to determine changes indicative of electrolyte and/or fluid imbalance and fluid needs.*[5,6]
- If fluid volume deficit is possible:

Anticipate fluid replacement needs (e.g., need for blood/plasma transfusion in client with major trauma, planned surgery where blood and fluid loss can be expected, major burn injury, person with heat stroke, or vomiting/diarrhea/inability to take fluids).[5]

Establish/promote oral intake, incorporating beverage preferences when possible. Administer IV fluids (e.g., crystalloids, colloids, blood/blood components) *to support fluid management.*[4,5]

Administer medications (e.g., antidiarrheals, antiemetics, agents to reduce blood loss/promote clotting) as indicated *to reduce fluid loss.*[4,5]

Refer to NDs deficient Fluid Volume: [hypertonic/hypotonic], deficient Fluid Volume: [isotonic], and risk for deficient Fluid Volume for additional interventions.

- If fluid volume excess is possible:

Maintain fluid/sodium restrictions when needed. Offer small amounts of fluid over 24 hours.

Administer medications (e.g., diuretics, cardiotonics) *to assist in management of fluid excess/edema.*[4,5]

Assist with/prepare for rotating tourniquets, phlebotomy, dialysis, or ultrafiltration *to correct fluid overload situation.*[5]

Refer to ND excess Fluid Volume for additional interventions.

NURSING PRIORITY NO. 3 To promote wellness (Teaching/Discharge Considerations):

- Engage client, family, and all caregivers in fluid management plan. *Enhances cooperation with regimen and achievement of goals.*[5]

- Discuss individual risk factors/potential problems and specific interventions *to prevent or limit fluid imbalance/complications.*
- Instruct client/SO in how to measure and record I/O as appropriate.
- Review/instruct in medications or nutritional regimen (e.g., enteral/parenteral) *to alert to potential complications and ways to manage.*
- Identify signs and symptoms indicating need for prompt evaluation/follow-up by primary healthcare provider *for timely intervention/correction.*[5]

DOCUMENTATION FOCUS

Assessment/Reassessment

- Individual findings, including individual factors influencing fluid needs/requirements.
- Baseline weight, vital signs.
- Specific client preferences for fluids.

Planning

- Plan of care and who is involved in planning.
- Teaching plan.

Implementation/Evaluation

- Responses to interventions/teaching and actions performed.
- Attainment/progress toward desired outcome(s).
- Modifications to plan of care.

Discharge Planning

- Individual long-term needs, noting who is responsible for actions to be taken.
- Specific referrals made.

References

1. Cox, H. C., et al. (2002). *Clinical Applications of Nursing Diagnosis: Adult, Child, Women's, Psychiatric, Gerontic, and Home Health Considerations.* 4th ed. Philadelphia: F. A. Davis, p. 136.
2. Ackley, B. J., Ladwig, G. B. (2002). *Nursing Diagnosis Handbook: A Guide to Planning Care.* 5th ed. St. Louis, MO: Mosby, pp. 359–360.
3. Guyton, A. C., Hall, J. E. (1996). *Textbook of Medical Physiology.* 9th ed. Philadelphia: W. B. Saunders.
4. Matheny, N. (2000). *Fluid and Electrolyte Balance: Nursing Considerations.* 4th ed. Philadelphia: J. B. Lippincott.
5. Fluid and Electrolyte Imbalances, and Surgical Interventions. In Doenges, M. E., Moorhouse, M. F., Geissler-Murr, A. C. (2002). *Nursing Care Plans: Guidelines for Individualizing Patient Care.* 6th ed. CD-ROM. Philadelphia: F. A. Davis.
6. Astle, S. M. (2005). Restoring electrolyte balance. *RN*, 68(5), 31–34.

impaired Gas Exchange

Definition: Excess or deficit in oxygenation and/or carbon dioxide elimination at the alveoli-capillary membrane [this may be an entity of its own but also may be an end result of other pathology with an interrelatedness between airway clearance and/or breathing pattern problems]

Cultural   Collaborative   Community/Home Care   Diagnostic Studies   Pediatric/Geriatric/Lifespan   Medications

RELATED FACTORS

Ventilation perfusion imbalance [as in the following: altered blood flow (e.g., pulmonary embolus, increased vascular resistance), vasospasm, heart failure, hypovolemic shock]

Alveolar-capillary membrane changes [e.g., acute respiratory distress syndrome; chronic conditions such as restrictive/obstructive lung disease, pneumoconiosis, asbestosis/silicosis]

[Altered oxygen supply (e.g., altitude sickness)]

[Altered oxygen-carrying capacity of blood (e.g., sickle cell/other anemia, carbon monoxide poisoning)]

DEFINING CHARACTERISTICS

Subjective

Dyspnea

Visual disturbances

Headache upon awakening

[Sense of impending doom]

Objective

Confusion [decreased mental acuity]

Restlessness; irritability; [agitation]

Somnolence; [lethargy]

Abnormal ABGs/arterial pH, hypoxia/hypoxemia, hypercapnia, hypercarbia, decreased carbon dioxide

Cyanosis (in neonates only), abnormal skin color (e.g., pale, dusky)

Abnormal breathing (e.g., rate, rhythm, depth); nasal flaring

Tachycardia; [dysrhythmias]

Diaphoresis

[Polycythemia]

Sample Clinical Applications: COPD, asthma, pneumonia, tuberculosis, heart failure, respiratory distress syndrome, high-altitude pulmonary edema, carbon monoxide poisoning

DESIRED OUTCOMES/EVALUATION CRITERIA

Sample NOC linkages:

Respiratory Status: Gas Exchange: Alveolar exchange of carbon dioxide and oxygen to maintain arterial blood gas concentrations

Tissue Perfusion: Pulmonary: Adequacy of blood flow through pulmonary vasculature to perfuse alveoli/capillary unit

Respiratory Status: Ventilation: Movement of air in and out of the lungs

Client Will (Include Specific Time Frame)

• Demonstrate improved ventilation and adequate oxygenation of tissues by ABGs within client's normal limits and absence of symptoms of respiratory distress (as noted in Defining Characteristics).

• Verbalize understanding of causative factors and appropriate interventions.

• Participate in treatment regimen (e.g., breathing exercises, effective coughing, and use of oxygen) within level of ability/situation.

ACTIONS/INTERVENTIONS

Sample NIC linkages:

Respiratory Monitoring: Collection and analysis of patient data to ensure airway patency and adequate gas exchange

Oxygen Therapy: Administration of oxygen and monitoring of its effectiveness

Airway Management: Facilitation of patency of air passages

NURSING PRIORITY NO. 1 To assess causative/contributing factors:

• Note presence of factors listed in Related Factors. *Gas exchange problems can be related to multiple factors, including anemias, anesthesia/surgical procedures, high altitude, allergic response, altered level of consciousness, anxiety/fear, aspiration, decreased lung compliance, excessive or thick secretions, immobility, infection, medication and drug toxicity/overdose, neuromuscular impairment of breathing pattern, pain, smoking.*

• Refer to NDs ineffective Airway Clearance, ineffective Breathing Pattern for additional nursing interventions and rationale as appropriate.

NURSING PRIORITY NO. 2 To evaluate degree of compromise:

• Evaluate respirations:

Observe respiratory rate, depth. *Increasing both rate and depth of respirations increases alveolar ventilation and occurs normally in response to exercise and stressors. Tachypnea is usually present to some degree and can progress to hyperventilation with shallow respirations, dyspnea, and respiratory depression.*[1]

Note client's reports/perceptions of breathing ease. *Client may report a range of symptoms (e.g., air hunger; shortness of breath with speaking, activity, or at rest).*

Observe for dyspnea on exertion, gasping; changing positions frequently to ease breathing; tendency to assume three-point position (bending forward while supporting self by placing one hand on each knee) *to maximize respiratory effort.*

Note use of accessory muscles (e.g., scalene muscles, pectoralis minor, sternocleidomastoids, and external intercostal muscles) *to assist diaphragm in increasing volume of thoracic cavity, which aids in inspiration.*[2]

∞ Observe infants/young children for nasal flaring and sternal retractions *indicating increased work of breathing/progressing respiratory distress.*

Note use of abdominal muscles during expiration (normally a passive process) *to reduce thoracic dimensions and overcome airway resistance to expiration.*[2]

• Evaluate lungs:

Auscultate and percuss chest, describing presence/absence of breath sounds, note adventitious breath sounds. *Although air may be heard moving through the lung fields, breath sounds may be faint because of decreased airflow or areas of consolidation. In this nursing diagnosis, ventilatory effort is insufficient to deliver enough oxygen, or to get rid of sufficient amounts of carbon dioxide. Abnormal breath sounds are indicative of numerous problems (e.g., hypoventilation such as might occur with atelectasis or presence of secretions, improper endotracheal tube placement, collapsed lung) and must be evaluated for further intervention.*[3,4]

• Note character and effectiveness of cough mechanism. *Affects ability to clear airways of secretions.*

• Evaluate skin/mucous membrane color noting areas of pallor/cyanosis, for example, peripheral (nailbeds) versus central (around lips or earlobes) or general duskiness. *Duskiness and central cyanosis are indicative of advanced hypoxemia.*[4]

Cultural Collaborative Community/Home Care Diagnostic Studies Pediatric/Geriatric/Lifespan Medications

- Evaluate behavior:
  Assess level of consciousness and mentation changes. *Decreased level of consciousness impairs one's ability to protect the airway, potentially adversely affecting oxygenation that in turn further impairs mentation.*
  Note somnolence, restlessness, reports of headache on arising.
  Assess energy level and activity tolerance, noting reports/evidence of fatigue, weakness, problems with sleep *that are associated with decreased oxygenation.*
- Monitor vital signs:
  Measure temperature. *High fever greatly increases metabolic demands and oxygen consumption.*
  Monitor heart rate/rhythm. *Tachycardia and dysrhythmias may be noted as heart reacts to ischemia, especially during activity.*
  Monitor blood pressure. *BP can be variable, depending on underlying condition and cardiopulmonary response.*
  Note increased pulmonary artery/right ventricular wedge pressures in critically ill client with central lines. *Indicative of increased pulmonary vascular resistance.*
- Review pertinent diagnostic data (e.g., ABGs, Hgb, red blood cells, electrolytes); chest radiography. Evaluate pulse oximetry (can be typical measurement along with vital signs in many facilities) and pulmonary function studies (e.g., lung volumes and capacities) *to determine presence/degree of lung function, and/or respiratory insufficiency and acid-base status; also used to monitor response to therapies. Client in respiratory failure typically shows hypoxemia and metabolic acidosis and is high risk for developing respiratory acidosis.*[5,8]

NURSING PRIORITY NO. 3 To correct/improve existing deficiencies:

- Elevate head of bed/position client appropriately. *Elevation/upright position facilitates respiratory function by gravity; however, client in severe distress will seek position of comfort. In ventilated client, prone position may be indicated to improve pulmonary perfusion and increase oxygen diffusion.*[4]
- Provide airway adjuncts and suction as indicated *to clear/maintain airway and improve gas diffusion when client is unable to clear secretions or is showing desaturation of oxygen by oximetry or ABGs.*[4,6,7]
- Encourage frequent position changes, deep-breathing/directed coughing exercises, use of incentive spirometer, chest physiotherapy as indicated. *Promotes optimal chest expansion, mobilization of secretions, and oxygen diffusion.*[4]
- Provide supplemental oxygen (via cannula, mask) using lowest concentration possible *dictated by pulse oximetry, ABGs, and client symptoms/underlying condition.*
- Ensure availability of proper emergency equipment, including ET/trach set and suction catheters appropriate for age and size of infant/child/adult. Avoid use of face mask in elderly emaciated client.
- Prepare for/assist with intubation and mechanical ventilation. *The decision to intubate and ventilate is made on a clinical diagnosis of increased work of breathing, hypoventilation, impaired mental status, or presence of a moribund state.*[5]
- Monitor/adjust ventilator settings (e.g., FIo_2, tidal volume, inspiratory/expiratory ratio, sigh, positive end–expiratory pressure—PEEP) as indicated when mechanical support is being used.
- Monitor for carbon dioxide narcosis (e.g., change in level of consciousness, changes in O_2 and CO_2 blood gas levels, flushing, decreased respiratory rate and headaches), *which may occur in clients receiving long-term oxygen therapy.*[8]
- Maintain adequate intake *for mobilization of secretions*, but avoid fluid overload *that may increase pulmonary congestion.*

- Provide psychological support, Active-listen questions/concerns. Address client's/SO's fears/anxiety that may be present. Maintain calm attitude while working with client/SOs. *Anxiety is contagious, and associated agitation can increase oxygen consumption/dyspnea.*
- Encourage adequate rest and limit activities to within client tolerance. Promote calm/restful environment. *Facilitates relaxation and helps limit oxygen needs/consumption.*[4]
- Administer medications as indicated (e.g., inhaled and systemic glucocorticosteroids, antibiotics, bronchodilators, methylxanthines, expectorants, heparin) *to treat underlying conditions. Medications may be aerosolized/nebulized for enhanced response and limitation of side effects.*[4]
- Monitor therapeutic and adverse effects/interactions of drug therapy *to determine efficacy and need for change.*
- Use sedation judiciously *to avoid depressant effects on respiratory functioning.*[4]
- Minimize blood loss from procedures (e.g., blood draws—especially in neonates/infants, hemodialysis) *to limit effects of anemia and related gas diffusion impairment.*
- Assist with procedures as individually indicated (e.g., transfusion, phlebotomy, bronchoscopy) *to improve respiratory function/oxygen-carrying capacity.*
- Keep environment allergen/pollutant-free *to reduce irritant effect of dust and chemicals on airways.*

NURSING PRIORITY NO. 4 To promote wellness (Teaching/Discharge Considerations):

- Review risk factors, particularly genetic/environmental/employment-related conditions (e.g., sickle-cell anemia, altitude sickness, exposure to toxins) *to help client/SO prevent complications or manage risk factors.*
- Discuss implications of smoking related to the illness/condition. Encourage client and SO(s) to stop smoking, attend cessation programs as necessary *to reduce health risks and or prevent further decline in lung function.*[9]
- Review oxygen-conserving techniques (e.g., organizing tasks before beginning, sitting instead of standing to perform tasks, eating small meals, performing slower-purposeful movements) *to reduce oxygen demands.*[4]
- Reinforce need for adequate rest, while encouraging activity and exercise (e.g., upper and lower extremity endurance/strength training and flexibility) *to decrease dyspnea and improve quality of life.*[10]
- Emphasize the importance of good general nutrition *for improving stamina and reducing the work of breathing.*[4,10]
- Refer to dietician *for nutritional assessment/individual dietary plan as indicated.*[10]
- Instruct in the use of relaxation, stress-reduction techniques as appropriate.
- Review job description/work activities *to identify need for job modifications/vocational rehabilitation.*[4]
- Discuss home oxygen therapy use and instruct in safety concerns as indicated *to ensure client's safety, especially when used in the very young, fragile elderly, or when cognitive or neuromuscular impairment is present.*[4]
- Identify specific supplier for supplemental oxygen/necessary respiratory devices, as well as other individually appropriate resources, such as home-care agencies, Meals on Wheels, etc., *to facilitate independence.*[4]

DOCUMENTATION FOCUS

Assessment/Reassessment

- Assessment findings, including respiratory rate, character of breath sounds; frequency, amount, and appearance of secretions; presence of cyanosis; laboratory findings; and mentation level.

Cultural Collaborative Community/Home Care Diagnostic Studies Pediatric/Geriatric/Lifespan Medications

- Conditions that may interfere with oxygen delivery/exchange.

Planning

- Plan of care/interventions and who is involved in the planning.
- Ventilator settings, liters of supplemental oxygen.
- Teaching plan.

Implementation/Evaluation

- Client's responses to treatment/teaching and actions performed.
- Attainment/progress toward desired outcome(s).
- Modifications to plan of care.

Discharge Planning

- Long-range needs, identifying who is responsible for actions to be taken.
- Community resources for equipment/supplies postdischarge.
- Specific referrals made.

References

1. Seay, S. J., Gay, S. L., Strauss, M. (2002). Tracheostomy emergencies. *AJN*, 102(3), 59.
2. Waldorf, A. (2003). Online course: Physiology of Exercise and Health. Pulmonary structure and function and gas exchange and transport. Cal State San Marcus. iLearn (Internet Learning Environments and Resource Network). Available at http://courses.csusm.edu/resources/biol325aw/chapter12_13.
3. Cox, H. C., et al. (2002). *Clinical Applications of Nursing Diagnosis: Adult, Child, Women's Gerontic, and Home Health Considerations.* 4th ed. Philadelphia: F. A. Davis, pp. 256–261.
4. Doenges, M. E., Moorhouse, M. F., Geissler, Murr, A. C. (2002). *Nursing Care Plans: Guidelines for Individualizing Patient Care.* 6th ed. Philadelphia: F. A. Davis, pp. 112, 118–120, 130–131, 167.
5. Carcillo, J. A., Fields A. I. (2002). Clinical practice parameters for hemodynamic support of pediatric and neonatal patients in septic shock. *Crit Care Med*, 30(6). 1365–1378.
6. Fink, J. B., Hess, D. R. (2002). Secretion clearance techniques. In Hess, D. R., et al. (eds). *Respiratory Care: Principles and Practices.* Philadelphia: W. B. Saunders.
7. Blair, K. A. (1999). The aging pulmonary system. In Stanley, M., Beare, P. G. (eds). *Gerontological Nursing: A Health Promotion/Protection Approach.* 2d ed. Philadelphia: F. A. Davis.
8. Argyle, B. (1996). Blood Gases Computer Program. Retrieved from Mad Scientist Software's Blood Gas tutorial. Accessed July 2007 at www.madsci.com/manu/indexgas.htm.
9. Anderson, N. R. (2006). The role of the home healthcare nurse in smoking cessation: Guidelines for successful intervention. *Home Healthcare Nurse,* 24(7), 424–431.
10. McAllister, M. (2005). Promoting physiologic-physical adaptation in chronic obstructive pulmonary disease: Pharmacotherapeutic evidence-based research and guidelines. *Home Healthcare Nurse,* 23(8), 523–531.

risk for unstable blood Glucose

Definition: Risk for variation of blood glucose/sugar levels from the normal range

RISK FACTORS
Lack of acceptance of diagnosis; deficient knowledge of diabetes management (e.g., action plan)
Lack of diabetes management/adherence to diabetes management (e.g., action plan); inadequate blood glucose monitoring; medication management
Dietary intake; weight gain/loss; rapid growth periods; pregnancy
Physical health status/activity level

Stress; mental health status

Developmental level

NOTE: A risk diagnosis is not evidenced by signs amd symptoms, as the problem has not occurred; rather, nursing interventions are directed at prevention.

Sample Clinical Applications: Diabetes mellitus, diabetic ketoacidosis, hypoglycemia, gestational diabetes, coticosteroid use, total parenteral nutrition

DESIRED OUTCOMES/EVALUATION CRITERIA

Sample NOC linkages:

Knowledge: Diabetes Management: Extent of understanding conveyed about diabetes mellitus and the prevention of complications

Diabetes Self-Management: Personal actions to manage diabetes mellitus and prevent disease progression

Blood Glucose Level: Extent to which glucose levels in plasma and urine are maintained in normal range

Client Will (Include Specific Time Frame)

- Acknowledge factors that may lead to unstable glucose.
- Verbalize understanding of body and energy needs.
- Verbalize plan for modifying factors to prevent/minimize shifts in glucose level.
- Maintain glucose in satisfactory range.

ACTIONS/INTERVENTIONS

Sample NIC linkages:

Hyperglycemia Management: Preventing and treating above-normal blood glucose levels

Teaching: Disease Process: Assisting the patient to understand information related to a specific disease process

Teaching: Prescribed Medication: Preparing a patient to safely take prescribed medications and monitor for their effects

NURSING PRIORITY NO. 1   To assess risk/contributing factors:

- Determine individual factors as listed in Risk Factors. *Client or family history of diabetes; known diabetic with poor glucose control; eating disorders (e.g., morbid obesity); poor exercise habits; failure to recognize changes in glucose needs/control due to adolescent growth spurts/pregnancy can result in problems with glucose stability.*
- Ascertain client's/SO's knowledge/understanding of condition and treatment needs.
- Identify individual perceptions and expectations of treatment regimen.
- Note influence of cultural/religious factors impacting dietary practices, taking responsibility for own care, expectations of outcomes. *These factors will influence client's ability to manage condition and must be considered when planning care.*
- Determine client's awareness/ability to be responsible for dealing with situation. *Age, developmental level, and current health status affect client's ability to provide for own safety.*
- Assess client family/SO(s) support of client. *Client may need assistance with lifestyle changes (e.g., food preparation/consumption, timing of intake and/or exercise, administration of medications).*
- Note availability/use of resources.

Cultural   Collaborative   Community/Home Care   Diagnostic Studies   Pediatric/Geriatric/Lifespan   Medications

NURSING PRIORITY NO. 2 To assist client to develop preventative strategies to avoid glucose instability:

- Ascertain whether client/SOs are adept at operating client's home glucose-monitoring device. *All available machines will provide satisfactory readings if properly used, maintained, and routinely calibrated.*[1]
- Provide information on balancing food intake, antidiabetic agents, and energy expenditure.
- Review medical necessity for regularly scheduled lab screening tests for diabetes. *Tests including fasting and daily glucose levels, HgbA1c help identify acute and long-term glucose control.*[2,3]
- Discuss home glucose-monitoring according to individual parameters (e.g., 6x/day for normal day and more frequently during times of stress) *to identify and manage glucose fluctuations.*[2]
- Identify common situations that contribute to client's glucose instability on daily, occasional, or crisis basis. *Multiple factors can be in play at any time, such as missing meals, an adolescent growth spurt, infection/other illness.*
- Review client's diet, especially carbohydrate intake. *Glucose balance is determined by the amount of carbohydrates consumed, which should be determined in needed grams/day.*[4]
- Encourage client to read labels and choose foods described as having a low glycemic index (GI), higher fiber, and low-fat content. *These foods produce a slower rise in blood glucose and more stable release of insulin.*[5]
- Discuss how client's antidiabetic medication(s) work. *Drugs and combinations of drugs work in varying ways with different blood glucose control and side effects. Understanding drug actions can help client avoid/reduce risk of potential for hypoglycemic reactions.*[6]

For client receiving insulin:

- Emphasize importance of checking expiration dates of medication, inspecting insulin for cloudiness if it is normally clear, and monitoring proper storage and preparation (when mixing required). *Affects insulin absorbability/effectiveness.*[1]
- Review type(s) of insulin used (e.g., rapid, short, intermediate, long-acting, premixed) and delivery method (e.g., subcutaneous, intramuscular injection; inhaled; pump). Note time when short-acting and long-acting insulins are administered. Remind client that only short-acting insulin is used in pump. *Affects timing of effects and provides clues to potential timing of glucose instability.*[1,7]
- Check injection sites periodically. *Insulin absorption can vary from day to day in healthy sites and is less absorbable in lumpy sites.*[7]
- Ascertain that all injections are being given. *Children, teenagers, and elderly client may forget injections or be unable to self-inject, may need reminders and supervision.*[7]

NURSING PRIORITY NO. 3 To promote wellness (Teaching/Discharge Considerations):

- Review individual risk factors and provide information *to assist client in efforts to avoid complications, such as caused by chronic hyperglycemia and acute hypoglycemia. Note: Hyperglycemia is most commonly caused by alterations in nutrition needs, inactivity, or inadequate use of antidiabetic medications. Hypoglycemia is the most common complication of antidiabetic therapy, stress, and exercise.*[1,8–10]
- Emphasize consequences of actions/choices—both immediate and long-term. *Close control of glucose levels over time has been shown to delay onset/reduce severity of complications enhancing quality of life.*
- Engage client/family/caregiver in formulating plan *to manage blood glucose level incorporating lifestyle, age/developmental level, physical/psychological ability to manage condition.*

Nursing Diagnoses in Alphabetical Order

- Consult with dietitian about specific dietary needs based on individual situation (e.g., growth spurt, pregnancy, change in activity level following injury).
- Encourage client to develop a system for self-monitoring *to provide a sense of control and enable client to follow own progress and assist with making choices.*
- Refer to appropriate community resources, diabetic educator, and/or support groups as needed *for lifestyle modification, medical management, referral for insulin pump or glucose monitor, financial assistance for supplies, etc.*

DOCUMENTATION FOCUS

Assessment/Reassessment

- Findings related to individual situation, risk factors, current caloric intake/dietary pattern; prescription medication use; monitoring of condition.
- Client's/caregiver's understanding of individual risks/potential complications.
- Results of laboratory tests/fingerstick testing.

Planning

- Plan of care and who is involved in planning.
- Teaching plan.

Implementation/Evaluation

- Individual responses to interventions/teaching and actions performed.
- Specific actions and changes that are made.
- Attainment/progress toward desired outcomes.
- Modifications to plan of care.

Discharge Planning

- Long-range plans for ongoing needs, monitoring, and management of condition, and who is responsible for actions to be taken.
- Sources for equipment/supplies.
- Specific referrals made.

References

1. No author listed. Monitoring Diabetes Control. Diabetes Manual. Royal Children's Hospital. Retrieved January 2007 at www.rch.org.au/diabetesmanual.cfm.
2. Gardner, B. M. (2002). Current Approaches to Type 2 Diabetes Mellitus. Article for Medscape CME. American Academy of Family Physicians (AAFP) 2002 Annual Scientific Assembly Common Clinical Problem Update and Family Medicine research. Retrieved December 2006 at www.medscape.com/viewarticle/444348.
3. Buse, J. B. (2003). Normal A1C but Unstable Blood Glucose. Article for Medscape Diabetes asnd Endocrinology site. Retrieved January 2007 at www.medscape.com/viewarticle/46302.
4. Moshang, J. (2005). The growing problem of type 2 diabetes. *LPN2005*,1(3), 26–34.
5. No author listed. Diabetes and Healthy Eating. Better Health Channel Fact Sheet. (2000-2004). Victoria, Australia. Retrieved January 2007 at www.betterhealth.vic.gov.au.
6. Davis, J. L. (2006). New Type 2 Diabetes Treatment Options. Article for WebMD. Retrieved January 2007 at www.webmd.com/content/Article/129/117304.htm.
7. Haines, C. (2006). Diabetes: Treating Diabetes with Insulin. Article for WebMD. Retrieved January 2007 at www.webmd.com/content/Article/46/1667_50931.htm.
8. Iscoe, K. E., Campbell, J. E., Jamnik, V., et al. (2006). Efficacy of continuous real-time blood glucose monitoring during and after prolonged high-intensity cycling exercise: Spinning with a continuous glucose monitoring system. *Diabetes Technology and Therapeutic*, 8(6), 627–635. Mary Ann Liebert, Inc.

Cultural   Collaborative   Community/Home Care   Diagnostic Studies   Pediatric/Geriatric/Lifespan   Medications

9. McLeod, M. E. (2006). Interventions for clients with diabetes mellitus. In Ignativicius, D. D., Workman, M. L. (eds). *Medical-Surgical Nursing: Critical Thinking for Collaborative Care*. 5th ed. Elsevier Saunders, Philadelphia.
10. Asp, A. A. (2005). Diabetes mellitus. In Copstead, L. C., Banasik, J. L. (eds.). *Pathophysiology*. 3rd ed. Elsevier Saunders, Philadelphia.

Grieving

Definition: A normal complex process that includes emotional, physical, spiritual, social, and intellectual responses and behaviors by which individuals, families, and communities incorporate an actual, anticipated, or perceived loss into their daily lives

RELATED FACTORS

Anticipatory loss/loss of significant object (e.g., possessions, job, status, home, parts and processes of body)
Anticipatory loss/death of a significant other

DEFINING CHARACTERISTICS

Subjective
Anger; pain; suffering; despair; blame
Alteration in activity level; sleep/dream patterns
Making meaning of the loss; personal growth
Experiencing relief

Objective
Detachment; disorganization; psychological distress; panic behavior
Maintaining the connection to the deceased
Alterations in immune/neuroendocrine function

Sample Clinical Applications: Cancer, traumatic injuries (e.g., brain/spinal cord), amputation, chronic/debilitating conditions (e.g., renal failure, COPD, MS, ALS), genetic/birth defects, community disaster

DESIRED OUTCOMES/EVALUATION CRITERIA
Sample NOC linkages:
Grief Resolution: Adjustment to actual or impending loss
Caregiver Emotional Health: Emotional well-being of a family care provider while caring for a family member

Client Will (Include Specific Time Frame)

- Identify and express feelings (e.g., sadness, guilt, fear) freely/effectively.
- Acknowledge impact/effect of the grieving process (e.g., physical problems of eating, sleeping) and seek appropriate help.
- Look toward/plan for future, one day at a time.

Sample NOC linkages:
Community Competence: Capacity of a community to collectively problem-solve to achieve community goals

Community Will (Include Specific Time Frame)

- Recognize needs of citizens, including underserved population.
- Activate/develop plan to address identified needs.

ACTIONS/INTERVENTIONS

Sample NIC linkages:
Grief Work Facilitation: Assistance with the resolution of a significant loss
Grief Work Facilitation: Perinatal Death: Assistance with the resolution of a perinatal loss
Dying Care: Promotion of physical comfort and psychological peace in the final phase of life

NURSING PRIORITY NO. 1 To assess causative/contributing factors:

- Determine circumstances of current situation (e.g., sudden death, prolonged fatal illness, loved one kept alive by extreme medical interventions). *Grief can be anticipatory (mourning the loss of loved one's former self before actual death) or actual. Both types of grief can provoke a wide range of intense and often conflicting feelings. Grief also follows losses other than death (e.g., traumatic loss of a limb, or loss of home by a tornado, loss of known self due to brain injury).*[11,12]
- Determine significance of loss to community (e.g., school bus accident with loss of life, major storm with damage to community infrastructure, financial failure of major employer).
- Determine client's perception of anticipated/actual loss and meaning to him or her. "What are your concerns?" "What are your fears? Your greatest fear?" "How do you see this affecting you/your lifestyle?" *Identifying the needs to be addressed and acknowledging the client's responses are integral to planning care.*[9] *Some individuals may use anticipatory grieving as a defense against the inevitable loss. While some people may find this helpful when the loss occurs, many people find that intense feelings occur regardless of the period of anticipation.*[2]
- Ascertain response of family/SO(s) to client's situation/concerns. *Family concerns affect client and need to be listened to and appropriate interventions taken. Problems may arise if family completes grieving prematurely and disengages from the dying member, who then feels abandoned at a time when the support is needed.*[2]

NURSING PRIORITY NO. 2 To determine current response:

- Note emotional responses, such as withdrawal, angry behavior, crying. Provide information about normal stages of grieving. *Awareness allows for appropriate choice of interventions because individuals handle grief in different ways. Knowledge promotes understanding of emotional responses.*[4]
- Observe client's body language and check out meaning with the client. Note congruency of body language with verbalizations. *Body language is open to interpretation and needs to be validated so misinterpretation does not occur. Client may be saying one thing, but often body language is saying something else; identifying incongruencies can provide opportunity for individual to understand self in relation to grieving process.*[2]
- Note cultural and religious factors/expectations that may impact client's responses to situation. *Beliefs vary with the individual/community and will affect respones to the situation (e.g., Arab Americans may want to pray in silence or private; African Americans may use faith and root healers in conjunction with biomedical resources; groups may congregate at site of disaster or at church to grieve together).*[5,8]

⊕ Cultural ⊛ Collaborative 🏠 Community/Home Care ⬥ Diagnostic Studies ∞ Pediatric/Geriatric/Lifespan ❙ Medications

- Determine impact on general well-being (e.g., increased frequency of minor illnesses, exacerbation of chronic condition, problems with eating, activity level, sexual desire, role performance [e.g., work, parenting]). *Indicators of severity of feelings client is experiencing and need for specific interventions to resolve these issues.*[5]

- Note family communication/interaction patterns. *Dysfunctional patterns of communication such as avoidance, preaching, giving advice can block effective communication and isolate family members.*[3]

- Discuss with client and family/SOs, and others as appropriate, plans that need to be made as well as anticipated adjustments/role changes related to the situation. Encourage/answer questions as needed. *This type of discussion will bring concerns out in the open and help with adaptation to the loss.*[5,11]

- Determine use/availability of community resources/support groups. *Appropriate use of support can help the individual feel less isolated and can promote feelings of inclusion and comfort.*[6]

- Note community plans in place to deal with major loss (e.g., team of crisis counselors stationed at a school to address the loss of classmates, vocational counselors/retraining programs, outreach of services from neighboring communities).

NURSING PRIORITY NO. 3 To assist client/community to deal with situation:

- Provide open environment and trusting relationship. *Promotes a free discussion of feelings and concerns in a safe enviroment where client can reveal innermost fears and beliefs about anticipated loss.*[2]

- Use therapeutic communication skills of Active-listening, silence, acknowledgment. Respect client desire/request not to talk. *These skills convey belief in ability of client to deal with situation and develop a sense of competence. Client may not be ready to discuss feelings and situation, and respecting client's own timeline conveys confidence.*[2,3]

- Inform children about the anticipated or actual death/loss in age-appropriate language. *Providing accurate information about loss or change in life situation will help the child begin the mourning process.*[10]

- Give permission to child to express feelings about situation and ask questions, being careful to provide honest answers within child's understanding. *Adults may be uncomfortable or upset talking about death/loss and children may be excluded from adult conversation about what is happening.*[10]

- Provide puppets or play therapy for toddlers/young children. *Young children do not have the capacity to express their feelings, and the use of play may help them express grief and help deal with loss in ways that are appropriate to the age.*[2]

- Permit appropriate expressions of anger, fear. Note hostility toward/feelings of abandonment by spiritual power. *Anger is a normal part of the grieving process, and talking about these feelings allows individual to think about them and move on, coming to some resolution regarding the anticipated loss.*[6] (Refer to ND Spiritual Distress for additional interventions.)

- Provide information about normalcy of individual grief reaction. *Many people are not familiar with grief and are concerned that what they are experiencing is not normal. Letting them know that grief takes many forms and what they are feeling is all right helps them deal with what is happening.*[9]

- Be honest when answering questions, providing information. *Enhances nurse-client relationship, promoting trust and confidence.*[2]

- Provide assurance to child that cause for situation is not his or her own doing, bearing in mind age and developmental level. *May lessen sense of guilt and affirm there is no need to assign blame to self or any family member.*[2]

🏠 • Provide hope within parameters of individual situation. *Assisting client to find the positives will help with management of current situation.* Do not give false reassurance. *Comments such as "Everything will be all right" or "Don't worry" are not helpful and convey lack of understanding to the client.*[2]

🏠 • Review past life experiences/previous loss(es), role changes, and coping skills used, noting strengths/successes. *Useful in dealing with current situation and problem-solving existing needs.*[4]

🏠 • Discuss control issues, such as what is in the power of the individual to change and what is beyond control. *Recognition of these factors helps client focus energy for maximal benefit/outcome on what can be done.*[4]

🏠 • Incorporate family/SO(s) in problem-solving. *Encourages family to support/assist client to deal with situation while meeting needs of family members.*[6]

🏠 • Determine client's status and role in family (e.g., parent, sibling, child), and address loss of family member role. *Client's illness affects usual activities in the role he or she has in the family, and inevitably affects all the other family members as responsibilities are taken over by them.*[6]

🏠 • Instruct in use of visualization and relaxation techniques. *These skills can be helpful to reduce anxiety and stress and help client and family members manage grief more effectively.*[7]

💊 • Use sedatives/tranquilizers with caution. *While the use of these medications may be helpful in the short term, too much dependence on them may retard passage through the grief process.*[2]

🏠 • Mobilize resources when client is the community. *When anticipated loss affects community as a whole, such as closing of manufacturing plant, impending disaster (e.g., wildfire, terrorist concerns), multiple supports will be required to deal with size and complexity of situation. Indeed, when more people are directly or indirectly involved in the anticipated/actual loss, emotions/anxiety tend to be amplified and transmitted, thus complicating the situation.*[1]

🏠 • Encourage community members/groups to engage in talking about event/loss and verbalizing feelings. Seek out underserved populations to include in process. *Increases likelihood that the needs of the entire community are identified/addressed.*

🏠 • Encourage individuals to participate in activities to deal with loss/rebuild community. *Exercising control in a productive manner empowers individuals and promotes rebuilding of life/community.*

NURSING PRIORITY NO. 4 To promote wellness (Teaching/Discharge Considerations):

🏠 • Provide information that feelings are okay and are to be expressed appropriately. Set limits regarding destructive behavior. *Talking about feelings can facilitate the grieving process, but destructive behavior can be damaging to the self-esteem.*[2]

🏠 • Discuss recurring nature of grief reactions. *On birthdays, major holidays, at times of significant personal events, or anniversary of loss, intense grief reactions may occur for a long time after the loss. If these reactions start to disrupt day-to-day functioning, client may need to seek help.*[1] (Refer to NDs such as ineffective community Coping, complicated Grieving.)

🏠 • Encourage continuation of usual activities/schedule and involvement in appropriate exercise program, as appropriate and able. *Promotes sense of control and self-worth, enabling client to feel more positive about ability to handle situation.*[6]

🏠 • Identify/promote involvement of family and social support systems. *A supportive environment enhances the effectiveness of interventions and promotes a successful grieving process.*[4]

🏠 • Discuss and assist with planning for future/funeral, as appropriate. *Involving family members in this discussion assures that everyone knows what is desired and what is planned, thus avoiding unexpected disagreements.*[4]

🌐 Cultural   ⚛ Collaborative   🏠 Community/Home Care   ✎ Diagnostic Studies   ∞ Pediatric/Geriatric/Lifespan   💊 Medications

- Refer to additional resources, such as pastoral care, counseling/psychotherapy, community/organized support groups, as indicated, for both client and family/SO. *Useful for ongoing needs and facilitation of grieving process.*[6,8]
- Identify resources/develop community plan to address anticipated large-scale losses. *Preparation for complex challenges facilitates prompt response as needs occur.*
- Support community efforts to strengthen support/develop plan *to foster recovery and growth.*

DOCUMENTATION FOCUS

Assessment/reassessment

- Assessment findings, including client's perception of anticipated loss and signs/symptoms that are being exhibited.
- Responses of family/SO(s) or community members, as indicated.
- Availability/use of resources.

Planning

- Plan of care and who is involved in planning.
- Teaching plan.

Implementation/Evaluation

- Client's response to interventions/teaching and actions performed.
- Attainment/progress toward desired outcome(s).
- Modifications to plan of care.

Discharge planning

- Long-range needs and who is responsible for actions to be taken.
- Specific referrals made.

References

1. Sharma, V. P. (1996). Normal mourning and "complicated grief." Article for Mind Publications Web site. Retrieved March 2007 at www.Mindpub.com/art045.htm.
2. Townsend, M. C. (2003). *Psychiatric Mental Health Nursing Concepts of Care.* 4th ed. Philadelphia: F. A. Davis.
3. Gordon, T. (2000). *Parent Effectiveness Training* (updated edition). New York: Three Rivers Press.
4. Cox, H. C., et al. (2002). *Clinical Applications of Nursing Diagnosis: Adult, Child, Women's, Psychiatric, Gerontic, and Home Health Considerations.* 4th ed. Philadelphia: F. A. Davis.
5. Lipson, J. G., Dibble, S. L., Minarik, P. A. (1996). *Culture & Nursing Care: A Pocket Guide.* San Francisco: UCSF Nursing Press.
6. Doenges, M. E., Townsend, M. C., Moorhouse, M. F. (1998). Psychiatric Care Plans Guidelines for Individualizing Care. 3d ed. Philadelphia: F. A. Davis.
7. Pearce, J. C. (2002). *The Biology of Trancendence a Blueprint of the Human Spirit.* Rochester, VT: Park St Press.
8. Matzo, M., et al. (2002). Teaching cultural consideration at the end of life. End of Life Nursing Education Consortium program recommendations. *J Contin Edu Nurs,* 33(6), 270–278.
9. Neeld, E. H. (2003). *Seven Choices.* 4th ed. Austin, TX: Centerpoint Press.
10. Riely, M. (2003). Facilitating Children's Grief. *J School Nurs,* 19(4), 212–218.
11. No author or pub date listed. Anticipatory Grief. Featured Columns under Life Topics/Grief & Loss for Psychologist 4therapy Web site. Retrieved March 2007 at www.4therapy.com.

complicated Grieving

Definition: A disorder that occurs after the death of a significant other, in which the experience of distress accompanying bereavement fails to follow normative expectations and manifests in functional impairment

RELATED FACTORS

Death/sudden death of a significant other
Emotional instability
Lack of social support
[Loss of significant object (e.g., possessions, job, status, home, parts and processes of body)]

DEFINING CHARACTERISTICS

Subjective
Verbalizes anxiety; lack of acceptance of the death; persistant painful memories; distressful feelings about the deceased; self-blame
Verbalizes feelings of anger; disbelief; detachment from others
Verbalizes feeling dazed; empty; stunned; in shock
Decreased sense of well-being; fatigue; low levels of intimacy; depression
Yearning

Objective
Decreased functioning in life roles
Persistant emotional distress; separation/traumatic distress
Preoccupation with thoughts of the deceased; longing for the deceased; searching for the deceased; self-blame
Experiencing somatic symptoms of the deceased
Rumination
Grief avoidance

Sample Clinical Applications: Death of significant other, traumatic loss, depression, attempted suicide

DESIRED OUTCOMES/EVALUATION CRITERIA
Sample NOC linkages:
Grief Resolution: Adjustment to actual or impending loss
Family Coping: Family actions to manage stressors that tax family resources
Psychosocial Adjustment: Life Change: Adaptive psychosocial responses of an individual to a significant life change

Client Will (Include Specific Time Frame)

- Acknowledge presence/impact of dysfunctional situation.
- Demonstrate progress in dealing with stages of grief at own pace.
- Participate in work and self-care/ADLs, as able.
- Verbalize a sense of progress toward resolution of the grief and hope for the future.

Cultural   Collaborative   Community/Home Care   Diagnostic Studies   Pediatric/Geriatric/Lifespan   Medications

ACTIONS/INTERVENTIONS

Sample NIC linkages:

Grief Work Facilitation: Assistance with the resolution of a significant loss

Grief Work Facilitation: Perinatal Death: Assistance with the resolution of a perinatal loss

Coping Enhancement: Assisting a patient to adapt to perceived stressors, changes, or threats that interfere with meeting life demands and roles

NURSING PRIORITY NO. 1 To determine causative/contributing factors:

- Identify loss that is present. Note circumstances of death such as sudden or traumatic (e.g., fatal accident, homicide), related to socially sensitive issue (e.g., AIDS, suicide), or associated with unfinished business (e.g., spouse died during time of crisis in marriage, son has not spoken to parent for years). *These situations can sometimes cause individual to become stuck in grief and unable to move forward with life.*[11–13]
- Determine significance of the loss to client (e.g., presence of chronic condition leading to divorce/disruption of family unit and change in lifestyle/financial security). *The more complicated or devastating the loss is to the individual, the more likely she or he will have difficulty reaching resolution.*
- Identify cultural/religious beliefs and expectations *that may impact or dictate client's response to loss.*
- Ascertain response of family/SO(s) to situation (e.g., sympathetic or urging client to "just get over it"). Assess needs of SO(s). *Response of family members will affect how client is dealing with situation—this information is important for planning care to enable all members to effectively cope with events.*[9]

NURSING PRIORITY NO. 2 To determine degree of impairment/dysfunction:

- Observe for cues of sadness (e.g., sighing, faraway look, unkempt appearance, inattention to conversation, somatic complaints such as exhaustion, headaches). *Indicators of the extent of grief and how individual is dealing with situation.*[6]
- Identify stage of grief being expressed: denial, isolation, anger, bargaining, depression, acceptance. *Helps to establish how client is dealing with grieving and degree of difficulty client is having adjusting to the death/loss.*[10]
- Listen to words/communications indicative of renewed/intense grief (e.g., constantly bringing up death/loss even in casual conversation long after event; outbursts of anger at relatively minor events; expressing desire to die), *indicating person is possibly unable to adjust/move on from feelings of intense grief.*[12]
- Determine level of functioning, ability to care for self, and use of support systems and community resources. *Individual may be incapacitated by depth of loss and be unable to manage day-to-day activities adequately, necessitating intervention/assistance.*[6]
- Be aware of avoidance behaviors (e.g., anger, withdrawal, long periods of sleeping or refusing to interact with family, sudden or radical changes in lifestyle, inability to handle everyday responsiblities at home/work/school, conflict). *Additional indicators of depth of grieving being experienced and need for more intensive support/monitoring to help client deal effectively with death/loss.*[10,11]
- Determine if client is engaging in reckless/self-destructive behaviors (e.g., substance abuse, heavy drinking, promiscuity, or aggression) *to identify safety issues.*[1]

- ⊕ • Identify cultural factors and ways individual(s) has dealt with previous loss(es). *Way of expressing self may reflect cultural background and religious beliefs. Understanding cultural expectations will help put current behavior/responses in context and determine the nature/degree of dysfunction.*[8]
- ⊘ • Perform/refer for psychological testing, as indicated (e.g., Beck's Depression Scale). *Determines degree of depression and indication of need for medication.*[2]

NURSING PRIORITY NO. 3 To assist client/others to deal appropriately with loss:

- 🏠 • Encourage verbalization without confrontation about realities. *It is helpful to listen without correcting misperceptions in the beginning, allowing free flow of expression. Provides opportunity for reflection aiding resolution and acceptance.*[6]
- 🏠 • Encourage client to choose topics of conversation and refrain from forcing client to "face the facts." *Talking freely about concerns can help client identify what is important to deal with and how to cope with situation.*[9]
- 🏠 • Active-listen to feelings and be available for support/assistance. Speak in soft, caring voice. *Communicates acceptance and caring, enabling client to seek own answers to current situation.*[3]
- 🏠 • Encourage expression of anger/fear and anxiety. (Refer to appropriate NDs.) *These feelings are part of the grieving process, and to accomplish the work of grieving, they need to be expressed and accepted.*[9]
- 🏠 • Permit verbalization of anger with acknowledgment of feelings and setting of limits regarding destructive behavior. *Enhances client safety, promotes resolution of grief process by encouraging expression of feelings that are not usually accepted, and supports self-esteem.*[2]
- 🏠 • Acknowledge reality of feelings of guilt/blame, including hostility toward spiritual power. Do not minimize loss; avoid clichés and easy answers. (Refer to ND Spiritual Distress.) *Reinforces that feelings are acceptable and allows client to become aware of own thoughts and begin to deal with feelings.*[1,7]
- 🏠 • Respect the client's needs and wishes for quiet, privacy, talking, or silence. *Individual may not be be ready to talk about or share grief and needs to be allowed to make own timeline.*[6]
- 🏠 • Give "permission" to be at this point when the client is depressed. *Assures client that feelings are normal and can be a starting point to deal in a positive manner with loss/death that has occurred.*[9]
- 🏠 • Provide comfort and availability as well as caring for physical needs. *Client needs to know he or she will be supported and helped when not able to care for self.*[6]
- 🏠 • Reinforce use of previously effective coping skills. Instruct in/encourage use of visualization and relaxation techniques. *Identifying and discussing how client has dealt with loss in the past can provide opportunities in the current situation. Use of these techniques helps client to learn to relax and consider options for dealing with loss.*[2]
- 🏠 • Assist SOs to cope with client's response. Include age-specific interventions. *Family/SO(s) may not understand/be intolerant of client's distress and inadvertantly hamper client's progress. Family members, including children, may express their feelings in anger, resulting in punishment for behavior that is deemed unacceptable, rather than recognizing the basis in grief.*[10]
- 🏠 • Include family/SO(s) in setting realistic goals for meeting needs of client and family members. *Involving all members enhances the probability that each member will express their needs and hear what the needs of others are, ensuring a more effective outcome.*[2]
- 💊 • Use sedatives/tranquilizers with caution. *While the use of these medications may be helpful in the short term, too much dependence on them may retard passage through the grief process.*[2]
- ⊛ • Refer to mental health provider for specific diagnostic studies and intervention in issues associated with complicated grief.[13]
- • Refer to ND Grieving for additional interventions as appropriate.

NURSING PRIORITY NO. 4 To promote wellness (Teaching/Discharge Considerations):

* Discuss with client/SO healthy ways of dealing with difficult situations. *Identifying ways individual(s) has dealt with losses in the past will help identify strengths/successes and what might be useful in the current situation.*[2]

* Have individual(s) identify familial, religious, and cultural factors that have meaning. *One's family of origin has a major impact on what the individuals learn about these issues and how to deal with losses. Identifying and discussing how they affect the current situation may help bring loss into perspective and facilitate grief resolution.*[8]

* Encourage involvement in usual activities, exercise, and socialization within limits of physical ability and psychological state. *Keeping life to a somewhat normal routine can provide individual(s) with some sense of control over events that are not controllable.*[8]

* Suggest client keep a journal of experiences and feelings. *As client writes about what is happening, new insights may occur. Reading over what has been written can help individual see progress that has been made and begin to have hope for the future.*[9]

* Advocate planning for the future as appropriate to individual situation (e.g., staying in own home after death of spouse, returning to sporting activities following traumatic amputation, choice to have another child or to adopt, rebuilding home following a disaster). *Provides a sense of control and purpose and ensures that individual's wishes will be heard and respected.*[10]

* Identify volunteer opportunities (e.g., working with children at risk, raising funds for favorite charity, investigating new employment/relocation opportunities, participating in community reorganization/cleanup). *Exercising control in a productive manner empowers individuals and promotes rebuilding of life/community.*

* Refer to other resources (e.g., pastoral care, family counseling, psychotherapy, organized support groups—widow's group) as indicated. *Provides additional support to resolve situation, continue grief work.*[8]

DOCUMENTATION FOCUS

Assessment/Reassessment

* Assessment findings, including meaning of loss to the client, current stage of the grieving process, and responses of family/SOs.
* Cultural/religious beliefs and expectations.
* Availability/use of resources.

Planning

* Plan of care and who is involved in the planning.
* Teaching plan.

Implementation/Evaluation

* Client's response to interventions/teaching and actions performed.
* Attainment/progress toward desired outcome(s).
* Modifications to plan of care.

Discharge Planning

* Long-term needs and who is responsible for actions to be taken.
* Specific referrals made.

References

1. Lubit, R. (2005). Acute treatment of disaster survivors. Article for Emedicine Web site. Retrieved March 2007 at www.emedicine.com/med/topic3540.htm.
2. Townsend, M. C. (2003). *Psychiatric Mental Health Nursing Concepts of Care.* 4th ed. Philadelphia: F. A. Davis.
3. Gordon, T. (2000). *Parent Effectiveness Training* (updated edition). New York: Three Rivers Press.
4. Cox, H. C., et al. (2002). *Clinical Applications of Nursing Diagnosis: Adult, Child, Women's, Psychiatric, Gerontic, and Home Health Considerations.* 4th ed. Philadelphia: F. A. Davis.
5. Lipson, J. G., Dibble, S. L., Minarik, P. A. (1996). *Culture & Nursing Care: A Pocket Guide.* San Francisco: UCSF Nursing Press.
6. Doenges, M. E., Townsend, M. C., Moorhouse, M. F. (1998). *Psychiatric Care Plans Guidelines for Individualizing Care.* 3rd ed. Philadelphia: F. A. Davis.
7. Pearce, J. C. (2002). *The Biology of Trancendence, a Blueprint of the Human Spirit.* Rochester, VT: Park St Press.
8. Matzo M., et al. (2002). Teaching cultural consideration at the end of life. End of Life Nursing Education Consortium program recommendations. *J Contin Edu Nurs,* 33(6), 270–278.
9. Neeld, E. H. (2003). *Seven Choices.* 4th ed. Austin, TX: Centerpoint Press.
10. Riely, M. (2003). Facilitating children's grief. *J School Nurs,* 19(4), 212–218.
11. Sharma, V. P. (1996). Normal Mourning and "Complicated Grief." Article for Mind Publications Web site. Retrieved March 2007 at www.Mindpub.com/art045.htm.
12. No author or pub date listed. Sometimes grief becomes complicated, unresolved or stuck. Featured Columns under Life Topics/Grief & Loss for Psychologist 4therapy Web site. Retrieved March 2007 at www.4therapy.com.
13. Kersting, K. (2004). A new approach to complicated grief. *Monitor on Psychology,* 35(10), 51.

risk for complicated Grieving

Definition: At risk for a disorder that occurs after the death of a significant other, in which the experience of distress accompanying bereavement fails to follow normative expectations and manifests in functional impairment

RISK FACTORS

Death of a significant other

Emotional instability

Lack of social support

[Loss of significant object (e.g., possessions, job, status, home, parts and processes of body)]

NOTE: A risk diagnosis is not evidenced by signs and symptoms, as the problem has not occurred; rather, nursing interventions are directed at prevention.

Sample Clinical Applications: Death of significant other, depression

DESIRED OUTCOMES/EVALUATION CRITERIA

Sample NOC linkages:

Grief Resolution: Adjustment to actual or impending loss

Family Coping: Family actions to manage stressors that tax family resources

Psychosocial Adjustment: Life Change: Psychosocial adaptation of an individual to a life change

Client Will (Include Specific Time Frame)

- Acknowledge awareness of individual factors affecting client in this situation. (See Risk Factors)
- Identify emotional responses and behaviors occurring after the death or loss.
- Participate in therapy to learn new ways of dealing with anxiety and feelings of inadequacy.
- Discuss meaning of loss to individual/family.
- Verbalize a sense of beginning to deal with grief process.

🌐 Cultural   🅐 Collaborative   🏠 Community/Home Care   🧪 Diagnostic Studies   ∞ Pediatric/Geriatric/Lifespan   💊 Medications

ACTIONS/INTERVENTIONS

Sample NIC linkages:

Grief Work Facilitation: Assistance with the resolution of a significant loss
Grief Work Facilitation: Perinatal Death: Assistance with the resolution of a perinatal loss
Coping Enhancement: Assisting a patient to adapt to perceived stressors, changes, or threats that interfere with meeting life demands and roles

NURSING PRIORITY NO. 1 To identify risk/contributing factors:

- Determine loss that has occurred and meaning to client. Note if death was sudden or traumatic (e.g., fatal accident, homicide), related to socially sensitive issue (e.g., AIDS, suicide), or associated with unfinished business (e.g., spouse died during time of crisis in marriage, son has not spoken to parent for years). *These situations can sometimes cause individual to become stuck in grief and unable to move forward with life.*[1]

- Ascertain circumstances surrounding loss of fetus/infant/child (e.g., gestational age of fetus; multiple miscarriages; death due to violence or fatal illness, etc.). *Repeated losses and/or violent death can increase client's/SO's sense of futility and compromise resolution of grieving process.*[2]

- Meet with both parents following loss of child *to determine how they are dealing with the loss together and individually. Death of child is often more difficult for parents/family, based on individual values and sense of life unlived.*[2]

- Note stage of grief client is experiencing (e.g., denial, anger, bargaining, depression, etc.). *Stages of grief may progress in a predictable manner or stages may be random/revisited.*[3]

- Assess client's ability to manage activities of daily living and period of time since loss has occurred. *Periods of crying, feelings of overwhelming sadness, loss of appetite, and insomnia can occur with grieving; however, when they persist and interfere with normal activities, client may need additional assistance.*[3]

- Note availability/use of support systems, community resources.

- Listen to words/communications indicative of renewed/intense grief (e.g., constantly bringing up death/loss even in casual conversation long after event; outbursts of anger at relatively minor events; expressing desire to die), *indicating person is possibly unable to adjust/move on from feelings of intense grief.*[4]

- Identify cultural/religious beliefs and expectations that may impact or dictate client's response to loss. *These factors affect current situation and may help bring loss into perspective and promote grief resolution.*[5]

- Assess status of relationships/marital difficulties and adjustments to loss. *Responses of family/SOs affect how client deals with situation.*[6]

NURSING PRIORITY NO. 2 To assist client to deal appropriately with loss:

- Discuss meaning of loss to client, Active-listen to responses without judgment. *The more complicated or devastating the loss is to the individual, the more likely she or he will have difficulty reaching resolution.*

- Respect client's desire for quiet, privacy, talking, or silence. *Individual may not be ready to talk about or share grief and needs to be allowed to make own timeline.*[3]

- Encourage expression of feelings, including anger/fear and anxiety. Let client know that all feelings are okay, while setting limits on destructive behavior. *These feelings are part of the grieving process, and to accomplish the work of grieving, they need to be expressed and accepted.*[3,6]

- Acknowledge client's sense of relief when death follows a long and debilitating course. *Sadness and loss are still there, but the death may be a release, or client may feel guilty about having a sense of relief.*
- Assist SOs/family to understand and be tolerant of client's feelings and behavior. *Family/SO(s) may not understand/be intolerant of client's distress and inadvertantly hamper client's progress. Family members, including children, may express their feelings in anger, resulting in punishment for behavior that is deemed unacceptable, rather than recognizing the basis in grief.*[8]

NURSING PRIORITY NO. 3 To promote wellness (Teaching/Discharge Considerations):

- Assist client/SOs to identify successful coping skills they have used in the past. *These can be used in current situation to facilitate dealing with grief.*[3]
- Support client and family in setting goals for meeting needs of members for moving on beyond the grieving process.
- Encourage resuming involvement in usual activities, exercise, and socialization within physical and psychological abilities. *Keeping life to a somewhat normal routine can provide individual with some sense of control over events that are not controllable.*[5]
- Advocate planning for the future as appropriate to individual situation (e.g., staying in own home after death of spouse, returning to sporting activities following traumatic amputation, choice to have another child or to adopt, rebuilding home following a disaster). *Provides a sense of control and purpose and ensures that individual's wishes will be heard and respected.*[8]
- Refer to other resources, as needed, such as psychotherapy, family counseling, religious references/pastor, grief support group. *Depending upon meaning of the loss, individual may require ongoing support to work through grief.* [5]

DOCUMENTATION FOCUS

Assessment/Reassessment
- Assessment findings, including meaning of loss to the client, current stage of the grieving process, psychological status, and responses of family/SOs.
- Cultural/religious beliefs, expectations, and rituals.
- Availability/use of resources.

Planning
- Plan of care and who is involved in the planning.
- Teaching plan.

Implementation/Evaluation
- Client's response to interventions/teaching and actions performed.
- Attainment/progress toward desired outcome(s)
- Modifications to plan of care.

Discharge Planning
- Long-term needs and who is responsible for actions to be taken.
- Specific referrals made.

References

1. Sharma, V. P. (1996). Normal Mourning and "Complicated Grief." Article for Mind Publications Web site. Retrieved March 2007 at www.Mindpub.com/art045.htm.

🌐 Cultural   Ⓐ Collaborative   🏠 Community/Home Care   Diagnostic Studies   ∞ Pediatric/Geriatric/Lifespan   Medications

2. Doenges, M. E., Moorhouse, M. F., Murr, A. C. (2006). Risk for dysfunctional Grieving. In *Nurse's Pocket Guide: Diagnoses, Prioritized Interventions, and Rationales*. 10th ed. Philadelphia: F. A. Davis.
3. Doenges, M. E., Townsend, M. C., Moorhouse, M. F. (1998). *Psychiatric Care Plans: Guidelines for Individualizing Care*. 3d ed. Philadelphia: F. A. Davis.
4. No author or pub date listed. Sometimes grief becomes complicated, unresolved or stuck. Featured Columns under Life Topics/Grief & Loss for Psychologist 4therapy Web site. Retrieved March 2007 at www.4therapy.com.
5. Matzo, M., et al. (2002). Teaching cultural considerations at the end of life. End of Life Nursing Education Consortium program recommendations. *J Contin Edu Nurs*, 33(6), 212–218.
6. Neeld, E. H. (2003). *Seven Choices*. 4th ed. Austin, TX: Centerpoint Press.
7. Kersting, K. (2004). A new approach to complicated grief. *Monitor on Psychology*, 35(10), 51.
8. Riely, M. (2003). Facilitating children's grief. *J School Nurs*, 19(4), 212–218.

risk for disproportionate Growth

Definition: At risk for growth above the 97th percentile or below the third percentile for age, crossing two percentile channels; disproportionate growth

RISK FACTORS

Prenatal
Maternal nutrition/infection; multiple gestation
Substance use/abuse; teratogen exposure
Congenital/genetic disorders [e.g., dysfunction of endocrine gland, tumors]

Individual
Prematurity
Malnutrition; caregiver/individual maladaptive feeding behaviors; insatiable appetite; anorexia; [impaired metabolism, greater-than-normal energy requirements]
Infection; chronic illness [e.g., chronic inflammatory diseases]
Substance [use]/abuse [including anabolic steroids]

Environmental
Deprivation, poverty
Violence, natural disasters
Teratogen, lead poisoning

Caregiver
Abuse
Mental illness/retardation, severe learning disability
NOTE: A risk diagnosis is not evidenced by signs and symptoms, as the problem has not occurred and nursing interventions are directed at prevention.

Sample Clinical Applications: Congenital/genetic disorders, prematurity, infection, nutritional problems (malnutrition, anorexia, failure to thrive, excessive intake), toxic exposures (e.g., lead), abuse/neglect, endocrine disorders, pituitary tumor

DESIRED OUTCOMES/EVALUATION CRITERIA
Sample NOC linkages:
Growth: Normal increase in bone size and body weight during growth years
Weight: Body Mass: Extent to which body weight, muscle, and fat are congruent to height, frame, gender, and age

Client Will (Include Specific Time Frame)

- Receive appropriate nutrition as dictated by individual needs.
- Demonstrate weight/growth stabilizing or progress toward age-appropriate size.
- Participate in plan of care as appropriate for age/ability.

Sample NOC linkages:

Child Development: [specify age group]: Milestones of physical, cognitive, and psychosocial progression by [specify] months/years of age

Client/Caregiver Will (Include Specific Time Frame)

- Verbalize understanding of potential for growth delay/deviation and plans for prevention

ACTIONS/INTERVENTIONS

Sample NIC linkages:

Nutritional Monitoring: Collection and analysis of patient data to prevent or minimize malnourishment

Teaching: Infant/Toddler Nutrition: Instruction on nutrition and feeding practices during the first, second, and third years of life

Weight Management: Facilitating maintenance of optimal body weight and percent body fat

NURSING PRIORITY NO. 1   To assess causative/contributing factors:

- Determine factors/condition(s) existing that could contribute to growth deviation as listed in Risk Factors, including familial history (e.g., pituitary tumors, Marfan's syndrome, genetic anomalies); prematurity with complications; use of certain drugs/substances during pregnancy; maternal diabetes/other chronic illness; poverty/inability to attend to nutritional issues; eating disorders; etc. *Information essential to developing plan of care.*[1]
- Identify nature and effectiveness of parenting/caregiving activities. *Inadequate, inconsistent caregiving, unrealistic/insufficient expectations, lack of stimulation, inadequate limit-setting; lack of responsiveness indicates problems in parent-child relationship.*[4]
- Note severity/pervasiveness of situation (e.g., individual/SO showing effects of long-term physical/emotional abuse/neglect versus individual experiencing recent-onset situational disruption or inadequate resources during period of crisis or transition).
- Evaluate nutritional status. *Overfeeding or malnutrition (protein and other basic nutrients) on a constant basis prevents individual from reaching healthy growth potential, even if no disorder/ disease exists.*
- Review results of x-rays/bone scans/MRI *to determine bone age/extent of bone and soft-tissue overgrowth; presence of tumors*; note laboratory studies (e.g, growth hormone levels/other endocrine studies) *to identify pathology.*
- Determine cultural/familial/societal values that may impact situation/parental expectations (e.g., some cultures equate a "plump" baby with a healthy baby, childhood obesity now a risk for American children; parental concern for amount of food intake; expectations for "normal growth").
- Assess significant stressful events, losses, separation, and environmental changes (e.g., abandonment, divorce, death of parent/sibling, aging, move).

Cultural   Collaborative   Community/Home Care   Diagnostic Studies   Pediatric/Geriatric/Lifespan   Medications

- Assess cognition, awareness, orientation, behavior of the client/caregiver. *Actions such as withdrawal/aggression, reactions to environment and stimuli provide information for identifying needs and planning care.*[1]
- Active-listen concerns about body size, ability to perform competitively (e.g., sports, body building) *to ascertain the potential for inappropriate use of anabolic steroids/other drugs.*

NURSING PRIORITY NO. 2 To prevent/limit deviation from growth norms:

- Determine chronological age, familial factors (body build/stature) to clarify growth expectations. Note reported losses/alterations in functional level. *Provides comparative baseline.*
- Identify present growth age/stage. *Measurements are compared to "standard" or normal range for children of same gender and age.*
- Review expectations for current height/weight percentiles and degree of deviation. Plan for periodic evaluations. *Growth rates are measured in terms of how much a child grows within a specified time. These rates vary dramatically as a child grows (normal growth is a discontinuous process) and must be evaluated periodically over time to ascertain that child has definite growth disturbance. Accelerated or slowed growth rates are rarely normal and warrant further evaluation.*[1]
- Investigate deviations in height/weight/head size. *Deviations may include weight only (increased or decreased) or height (increased or decreased) and head size (disproportionate to rest of body). These deviations may be seen alone or in combination, all requiring additional testing over time to determine cause and effect on child's growth and development. Some are more urgent than others (e.g., small head size is evaluated further/treated as soon as identified, whereas short stature may require a longer evaluation period to determine if developmental problem exists).*[1]
- Determine if child's growth is above 97th percentile (very tall and large) for age. *Child should be further evaluated for endocrine disorders/pituitary tumor (could result in gigantism). Other disorders may be characterized by excessive weight for height (e.g., hypothyroidism, Cushing syndrome), abnormal sexual maturation or abnormal body/limb proportions.*[2,8]
- Determine if child's growth is below third percentile (very short and small) for age. *Child should have further evaluations for failure to thrive related to intrauterine growth retardation, prematurity/very low birth weight, small parents, poor nutrition, stress/trauma, or medical condition (e.g., intestinal disorders with malabsorption, diseases of heart, kidneys, diabetes mellitus). Treatment of underlying condition may alter/improve child's growth pattern.*[3,9,10]
- Assist with therapies *to treat/correct underlying conditions (e.g., Crohn's disease, cardiac problems, or renal disease); endocrine problems (e.g., hyperpituitarism, hypothyroidism, type 1 diabetes mellitus, growth hormone abnormalities); genetic/intrauterine growth retardation; infant feeding problems, nutritional deficits.*
- Include nutritionist and other specialists as indicated (e.g., physical/occupational therapist) in developing plan of care. *Helpful in determining specific dietary needs for growth/weight issues, assistive devices, or appropriate exercise/rehabilitation programs.*[6]
- Note reports of changes in facial features, joint pain, lethargy, sexual dysfunction, or progressive increase in hat/glove/ring/shoe size in adults, especially after age 40. *Individual should be referred for further evaluation for hyperpituitarism/growth hormone imbalance/acromegaly.*

NURSING PRIORITY NO. 3 To promote wellness (Teaching/Discharge Considerations):

- Provide information regarding growth issues, as appropriate, including pertinent reference materials, including books, audiovisual materials, credible Web sites, etc. *Provides opportunity to review data at own pace, enhancing likelihood of retention, and opportunity to make informed decisions.*

Nursing Diagnoses in Alphabetical Order

- Discuss with pregnant women and adolescents consequences of substance use/abuse. *Prevention of growth disturbances depends on many factors but includes the cessation of smoking, alcohol, and many drugs that have the potential for causing CNS or orthopedic disorders in the fetus.*[5,7]
- Refer for genetic screening as appropriate. *There are many reasons for referral, including (and not limited to) positive family history of a genetic disorder (e.g., fragile X syndrome, muscular dystrophy), woman with exposure to toxins/potential teratogenic agents, women older than 35 years at delivery, previous child born with congenital anomalies, history of intrauterine growth retardation, etc.*
- Address parent/caregiver issues (e.g., parental abuse, learning deficiencies, environment of poverty) *where they could impact client's ability to thrive.*
- Promote client lifestyle that prevents/limits complications (e.g., management of obesity, hypertension, sensory/perceptial impairments); regular medical follow-up; nutritionally balanced meals, socialization for age/development, etc., *to enhance functional independence and quality of life.*
- Recommend involvement in regular monitored exercise/sports program *to enhance muscle tone/strength and appropriate body building.*
- Review medications being considered (e.g., appetite stimulant, growth hormone, thyroid replacement, antidepressant) noting potential side effects/adverse reactions *to promote adherence to regimen and reduce risk of untoward responses.*
- Identify available community resources as appropriate (e.g., public health programs such as WIC, medical equipment suppliers, nutritionist, substance abuse programs, specialists in endocrine problems/genetics).
- Stress importance of regular follow-up with healthcare provider *to monitor progress of growth/weight changes.*

DOCUMENTATION FOCUS

Assessment/Reassessment
- Assessment findings/individual needs, including current growth status and trends.
- Caregiver's understanding of situation and individual role.
- Cultural/familial values and expectations.

Planning
- Plan of care and who is involved in the planning.
- Teaching plan.

Implementation/Evaluation
- Client's responses to interventions/teaching and actions performed.
- Caregiver response to teaching.
- Attainment/progress toward desired outcome(s).
- Modifications to plan of care.

Discharge Planning
- Identified long-range needs and who is responsible for actions to be taken.
- Specific referrals made, sources for assistive devices, educational tools.

References

1. Leglar, J. D., Rose, L. C. (1998). Assessment of abnormal growth curves. Article for "Problem-Oriented Diagnoses" series for Department of Family Practice, University of Texas Health Science Center, San Antonio,

🌐 Cultural   Collaborative   🏠 Community/Home Care   Diagnostic Studies   ∞ Pediatric/Geriatric/Lifespan   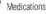 Medications

TX: American Academy of Family Physicians Web site. Accessed July 2007 at www.aafp.org/afp/980700ap/legler.html.

2. Gigantism. (2003). Fact sheet: University of Pennsylvania Health System Web site. Accessed July 2007 at http://pennhealth.com/ency/article/001174.htm.

3. Endocrinology and short stature. (2001). Patient Fact Sheets. The Endocrine Society Web site. Available at www.endo society.org.

4. Gordon, T. (2000). *Parent Effectiveness Training* (updated edition). New York: Three Rivers Press.

5. Maloni J. A., et al. (2003). Implementing evidence-based practice: Reducing risk for low birth weight through pregnancy smoking cessation. *J Obstet Gynecol Neonatal Nurs*, 32(5), 676–682.

6. American Dietetic Association. (1997). Nutrition in comprehensive program planning for persons with developmental disabilities. *J Am Diet Assoc*, 97(2), 189–193.

7. Schiffman, R. F. (2004). Drug and subtance use in adolescents. *MCN, American J of Maternal/Child Nursing*, 29(1), 21–27.

8. Ferry, R. J., Shim, M. (2006). Gigantism and acromegaly. Article for Emedicine Web site. Retrieved March 2007 at www.emedicine.com/ped/topic2634.htm.

9. Kemp, S., Gungor, N. (2005). Growth failure. Article for Emedicine Web site. Retrieved March 2007 at www.emedicine.com/ped/topic902.htm.

10. Owens, T. A. (2005). Medical Encyclopedia: Delayed Growth. Article for MedlinePlus Web site. Retrieved March 2007 at http://nim.nih.gov/medlineplus/ency/aritcle/003021.htm.

delayed Growth and Development

Definition: Deviations from age-group norms

RELATED FACTORS

Inadequate caretaking, [physical/emotional neglect or abuse]
Indifference, inconsistent responsiveness, multiple caretakers
Separation from significant others
Environmental and stimulation deficiencies
Effects of physical disability [handicapping condition]
Prescribed dependence [insufficient expectations for self-care]
[Physical/emotional illness (chronic, traumatic), such as chronic inflammatory disease, pituitary tumors, impaired nutrition/metabolism, greater-than-normal energy requirements, prolonged/painful treatments, prolonged/repeated hospitalizations]
[Sexual abuse]
[Substance use/abuse]

DEFINING CHARACTERISTICS

Subjective
Inability to perform self-care/self-control activities appropriate for age

Objective
Delay/difficulty in performing skills typical of age group; [loss of previously acquired skills, precocious or accelerated skill attainment]
Altered physical growth
Flat affect, listlessness, decreased responses
[Sleep disturbances, negative mood/response]

Sample Clinical Applications: Congenital/genetic disorders, prematurity, infection, nutritional problems (malnutrition, anorexia, failure to thrive), toxic exposures (e.g., lead), substance abuse, endocrine disorders, abuse/neglect, Down syndrome/developmental delay delayed GROWTH AND DEVELOPMENT

DESIRED OUTCOMES/EVALUATION CRITERIA

Sample NOC linkages:

Child Development: [specify age group]: Milestones of physical, cognitive, and psychosocial progression by [specify] months/years of age

Physical Maturation: Female/Male: Normal physical changes in the female/male that occur with the transition from childhood to adulthood

Growth: Normal increase in bone size and body weight during growth years

---

Client Will (Include Specific Time Frame)

- Perform motor, social, and expressive skills typical of age group within scope of present capabilities.
- Perform self-care and self-control activities appropriate for age.
- Demonstrate weight/growth stabilization or progress toward age-appropriate size.

Sample NOC linkages:

Knowledge: Parenting: Extent of understanding conveyed about provision of a nurturing and constructive environment for a child from 1 to 17 years of age

---

Parents/Caregivers Will (Include Specific Time Frame)

- Verbalize understanding of growth/developmental delay/deviation and plan(s) for intervention.

ACTIONS/INTERVENTIONS

Sample NIC linkages:

Developmental Enhancement: Child/Adolescent [specify]: Facilitating or teaching parents/caregivers to facilitate the optimal gross motor, fine motor, language, cognitive, social, and emotional growth of preschool and school-age children/of individuals during the transition from childhood to adulthood

Nutritional Monitoring: Collection and analysis of patient data to prevent or minimize malnourishment

Developmental Care: Structuring the environment and providing care in response to the behavioral cues and states of the preterm infant

NURSING PRIORITY NO. 1   To assess causative/contributing factors:

- Determine existing condition(s) (e.g., limited intellectual capacity, physical disabilities, accelerated physical growth, early or delayed puberty, chronic illness, tumors, genetic anomalies, substance use/abuse, violence, poverty, multiple birth [twins]/minimal length of time between pregnancies). *These conditions contribute to growth/developmental deviation, necessitating specific evaluation and interventions depending on the situation.*[6]
- Determine developmental delays using standard screening tests assessing cognitive abilities, communication, and social interactions. *Developmental surveillance is a flexible, ongoing process that involves the use of both skilled observation of the child and concerns of parents, health professionals, teachers, and others to identify children with variations in normal growth and development.*[1,10,11]
- Review results of lab tests (e.g., pituitary hormones)/diagnostic studies (e.g., radiographs/bone scans assessing bone growth plates/age) *to evaluate problems with growth and assist in determining interventions/treatment needs.*

Cultural   Collaborative   Community/Home Care   Diagnostic Studies   Pediatric/Geriatric/Lifespan   Medications

- Active-listen to client's/parents' concerns about body size and actual/perceived limitations, ability to perform competitively (e.g., ability to participate in desired activities and lifestyle, perform in sports, body building). *Helps in identifying actual needs and provides emotional support in situation that is often difficult to manage over time.*
- Ascertain cultural beliefs, norms, and values. *What is considered normal and abnormal growth/development may be influenced by familial and cultural perceptions.*[5]
- Determine nature of parenting/caretaking activities. *Presence of conflict and negative interaction between parent/caregiver and child (e.g., inadequate, inconsistent parenting, unrealistic/insufficient expectations; lack of stimulation, limit-setting, and responsiveness) interferes with the development of age-appropriate skills and maturation.*[1,3,12]
- Assess occurrence/frequency of significant stressful events, losses, separation, and environmental changes (e.g., loss, separation, abandonment, divorce; death of parent/sibling; aging; unemployment, new job; moves; new baby/sibling, marriage, new stepparent). *Lack of resolution or repetition of stressor can have a cumulative effect over time and result in regression in/or deterioration of functional level.*
- Determine presence of environmental risk factors (e.g., exposure to toxins; active substance abusers in home; or child of parent(s) who are abusive, neglectful, or mentally disabled).[13,14]
- Note severity/pervasiveness of situation (e.g., long-term physical/emotional abuse versus situational disruption or inadequate assistance during period of crisis or transition). *Problems existing over a long period may have more severe effects and require longer course of treatment to reverse.*
- Evaluate home/day care/hospital/institutional environment *to determine adequacy of care provided, including nourishing meals, healthy sleep/rest time, stimulation, diversional or play activities.*

NURSING PRIORITY NO. 2 To determine degree of deviation from growth/developmental norms:

- Measure present growth age/stage. Record height/weight over time. *Provides baseline for identification of needs and determines trends/effectiveness of therapy.*[2]
- Determine expectations for current height/weight percentiles. *Measurements are compared to "standard" or normal range for children of same gender and age to determine degree of deviation.*[2]
- Note chronological age, familial factors (e.g., body build/stature) *to help determine individual developmental expectations (e.g., when child should roll over, sit up alone, speak first words, attain a certain weight/height, etc.), and how the expectations may be altered by child's condition. Pediatrician may screen with a motor quotient (MQ), which is child's age calculated by milestones met divided by chronological age and multiplied by 100). MQ between 50 and 70 requires further evaluation.*[3,9]
- Identify present developmental age/stage. Note reported deficits in functional level/evidence of precocious development. *Provides comparative baseline.*
- Review expected skills/activities, using authoritative text (e.g., Gesell, Musen/Congor), reports of neurological examinations, or assessment tools (e.g., Draw-a-Person, Denver Developmental Screening Test, Bender's Visual Motor Gestalt test. Early Language Milestone [ELM] Scale 2 and developmental language disorders [DLD]). *Provides guide for evaluation of growth and development, and for comparative measurement of individual's progress.*[4]
- Note degree of individual deviation, multiple skills affected (e.g., speech, motor activity, socialization versus one area of difficulty such as toileting) and whether difficulty is

temporary or permanent (e.g., setback or delay versus irreversible condition, such as brain damage, stroke).

- Note signs of sexual maturation in child (e.g., development of pubic/axillary hair, breast enlargement, presence of body odor, acne, rapid linear growth, and adolescent-type behavior, with or without maturation of gonads). *Precocious puberty in females before age 8 or males before age 10 may occur because of lesions of hypothalamus/intracranial tumors.*
- Evaluate sexual behavior, as indicated. Investigate sexual acting-out behaviors inappropriate for age. *May indicate sexual abuse.*
- Note findings of psychological evaluation of client and family *to determine factors that may impact growth or development of client, or impair the psychological health of the family.*

NURSING PRIORITY NO. 3 To correct/minimize growth deviations and associated complications:

- Assist in therapies to treat/correct underlying medical/psychological conditions (e.g., intestinal malabsorption/malnourishment; infant feeding problems; kidney failure, congenital heart disease; cystic fibrosis, inflammatory bowel disease; bone/cartilage conditions; endocrine disorders [e.g., hypothyroidism, diabetes, growth hormone abnormalities]; adverse side effects of medications; mental illness, substance abuse) as appropriate.[10] *May result in restoration of more normal developmental levels or growth patterns.*
- Collaborate with physician, nutritionist, and other specialists (e.g., physical/occupational therapists) in developing plan of care. *Multidisciplinary team care increases likelihood of developing a well-rounded plan of care that meets client's/family's specialized and varied needs.*
- Recommend involvement in regular exercise/sports program *to enhance muscle tone/strength and appropriate body building.*
- Administer/monitor responses to medications. *May be given to stimulate growth as appropriate, or possibly to shrink tumor when present.* Stress necessity of not stopping medications without approval of healthcare provider *in order to maximize benefit and limit adverse side effects.*
- Discuss appropriateness and potential complications of surgical interventions/radiation therapy when indicated (e.g., *to treat pituitary tumor, bone-lengthening procedures*).
- Plan for/stress importance of periodic evaluations. *Growth rates are measured in terms of how much a child grows within a specified time. These rates vary dramatically as a child grows (normal growth is a discontinuous process) and must be evaluated periodically over time to ascertain that child has definite growth disturbance. Accelerated or slowed growth rates are rarely normal and warrant further evaluation.*[2]

NURSING PRIORITY NO. 4 To assist clients (and/or caregivers) to prevent, minimize, or overcome delay/regressed or precocious development:

- Asssist with treatment of underlying condition (e.g., inborn errors of metabolism-galactosemia, phenylketonuria; attention deficit disorder, autism), correct environmental factors (e.g., removal of lead paint) as appropriate.
- Provide anticipatory guidance for parents/care providers regarding expectations for client's development *to clarify misconceptions and assist them in dealing with reality of situation. May help in providing nurturing care.*[7]
- Describe realistic, age-appropriate patterns of development to parent/caregiver, whether child's deviation is likely to be temporary or permanent (setback or delay versus permanent brain injury); and promote activities and interactions that support developmental tasks

Cultural   Collaborative   Community/Home Care   Diagnostic Studies   Pediatric/Geriatric/Lifespan   Medications

where client is at this time. *Increases likelihood of commitment to interventions in keeping with the child's current status and potential. Each child will have own unique strengths and difficulties. Some children will catch up with other children in early childhood; some will have problems into adulthood.*[1,5,6]

🏠 • Encourage recognition that certain deviations/behaviors are appropriate for a specific developmental age level (e.g., 14-year-old child functioning at level of 6-year-old child is not able to anticipate the consequences of his or her actions) or chronological age (e.g., 9-year-old is displaying pubertal changes). *Promotes acceptance of client as presented and helps shape expectations reflecting actual situation.*

🏠 • Encourage participation in "early intervention services" for child birth to 3 years of age with developmental delays. *Federally funded entitlement program for qualified child (e.g., Down syndrome or cerebral palsy; prematurity; deprived physical/social environment) aimed at maximizing child's development. Services include nursing, occupational/physical/speech thereapy, service coordination, social work and assistive technologies.*[12]

🏠 • Communicate with client at appropriate cognitive level of development. Give client tasks and responsibilities appropriate to age or functional level *to model age and cognitively appropriate caregiver skills.*[8]

🏠 • Encourage client to perform activities of daily living (ADLs) as able. Discuss appropriateness of appearance, grooming, touching, language, play, safety, and other associated developmental issues. *Promotes independence and helps client develop sense of what is appropriate for age.*

🏠 • Involve client in opportunities to practice progress in activities of life or to try new behaviors (e.g., role play, group activities). *Facilitates learning process/retention of new skills.*

🏠 • Encourage setting of short-term, realistic goals for achieving developmental potential. Evaluate progress on continual basis *to increase complexity of tasks/goals as indicated.*

• Collaborate with additional professional resources (e.g., occupational/rehabilitation/speech therapists, special education teacher, job counselor) *to address specific individual needs.*

🏠 • Maintain positive, hopeful attitude. Support self-actualizing nature of the client and attempts to achieve or return to optimal level of self-control or self-care activities.

🏠 • Provide positive feedback for efforts/successes and adaptation while minimizing failures. *Encourages continuation of efforts, improving outcome.*

🏠 • Identify equipment needs/refer to suppliers (e.g., adaptive/growth-stimulating computer programs, communication devices) *to provide client/caregivers access to assistive devices that could improve involvement in/quality of life.*

🏠 • Assist client/caregivers to accept and adjust to irreversible developmental deviations (e.g., Down syndrome is not currently correctable). *Helps refocus attention and energy to areas that can be changed/improved.*

🏠 • Assist client/family to identify lifestyle changes that may be required (e.g., care for handicaps [blindness, musculoskeletal or cognitive deficits], proper use of assistive devices, learning new skills, development of routines and support systems).

🏠 • Provide support for caregiver during transitional crises (e.g., residential schooling, institutionalization).

• Refer family/client for counseling/psychotherapy to deal with issues of grief and loss, time and stress management, lifestyle changes, abuse/neglect and other needs as indicated.

NURSING PRIORITY NO. 5 To promote wellness (Teaching/Discharge Considerations):

🏠 • Provide information regarding normal growth and development process as appropriate. *Individuals need to know about normal process so deviations can be recognized when necessary.*

- Avoid blame when discussing contributing factors. *Parent/caregivers usually feel inadequate and blame themselves for being "a poor parent/care provider." Adding blame further diverts the individual's focus from learning new/changing behaviors to achieve the desired outcomes.*
- Review reasonable expectations for individual without restricting potential (i.e., set realistic goals that, if met, can be advanced). *Provides hope for achievement and promotes continued personal growth.*
- Recommend involvement in regular exercise/sport medicine program *to enhance muscle tone/strength and appropriate body building.*
- Review use of medications (e.g., steroids, growth hormones), *which can affect body growth and development. Potential for good and for harm exists in the use of these agents.*
- Recommend wearing medical alert bracelet when taking replacement hormones. *Provides information in case of an emergency.*
- Discuss consequences of substance use/abuse. *May be involved in the problems of growth/development that individual is experiencing.*[14]
- Suggest genetic testing/counseling for family/client dependent on causative factors. *May be necessary for planning for future pregnancies.*
- Stress importance of periodic reassessment of growth/development (e.g., periodic laboratory studies *to monitor hormone levels/nutritional status). Aids in evaluating effectiveness of interventions over time, and promotes early identification of need for additional actions, avoid preventable complications.*
- Encourage attendance at appropriate educational programs (e.g., parenting and expectant parent classes, infant stimulation sessions, seminars on life stresses, aging process). *Can provide information for client/family to learn to manage current situation and adapt to future changes.*
- Provide pertinent reference materials/reliable Web sites regarding normal growth/development as appropriate. *Bibliotherapy provides opportunity to review data at own pace, enhancing likelihood of retention.*
- Discuss community responsibilities (e.g., services required to be provided to school-age child). Include social worker/special education team in planning process *to meet educational, physical, psychological, and monitoring needs of child.*
- Identify community resources: public health programs such as Women, Infants, and Children (WIC), well-baby care provider; nutritionist, substance abuse programs; early intervention programs, seniors' activity/support groups, gifted and talented programs, Sheltered Workshop, crippled children's services, medical equipment/supplier. *Provides additional assistance to support family efforts in treatment program.*
- Evaluate/refer to social services as indicated *to determine/monitor safety of client and consideration of placement in foster care.*
- Refer to the NDs interrupted Family Processes, impaired Parenting for additional interventions.

DOCUMENTATION FOCUS

Assessment/Reassessment

- Assessment findings/individual needs, including current growth status/trends and developmental level/evidence of regression.
- Caregiver's understanding of situation and individual role.
- Cultural beliefs/values and expectations.
- Drug use/substance abuse.
- Safety of individual/need for placement.

Cultural   Collaborative   Community/Home Care   Diagnostic Studies   Pediatric/Geriatric/Lifespan   Medications

Planning

- Plan of care and who is involved in the planning.
- Teaching plan.

Implementation/Evaluation

- Client's responses to interventions/teaching and actions performed.
- Caregiver response to teaching.
- Attainment/progress toward desired outcome(s).
- Modifications to plan of care.

Discharge Planning

- Identified long-range needs and who is responsible for actions to be taken.
- Specific referrals made; sources for assistive devices, educational tools.

References

1. Curry, D. M., Duby, J. C. (1994). Developmental surveillance by pediatric nurses. *Pediatr Nurs,* 20, 40–44.
2. Leglar, J. D., Rose, L. C. (1998). Assessment of abnormal growth curves. Article for "Problem-Oriented Diagnoses" series for Department of Family Practice, San Antonio, TX: University of Texas Health Science Center. Accessed July 2007 at www.aafp.org/afp/980700ap/legler.html.
3. Developmental Delays: A Pediatrician's Guide to Your Children's Health and Safety. Accessed July 2007 at www.keepkidshealthy.com/welcome/conditions/developmentaldelays.html.
4. American Academy of Child and Adolescent Psychiatry Working Group on Quality Issues. (1999). *J Am Acad Child Adolesc Psychiatry,* 38 (12 Suppl), 55S–76S. Accessed July 2003 at www.guideline.gov.
5. Leininger, M. M. (1996). *Transcultural Nursing: Theories, Research and Practices.* 2d ed. Hilliard, OH: McGraw-Hill.
6. Engel, J. (2002). *Mosby's Pocket Guide to Pediatric Assessment.* St. Louis, MO: Mosby.
7. Denehy, J. A. (1990). Anticipatory guidance. In Craft, M. J., Denehy, J. A. (eds). *Nursing Interventions for Infants and Children.* Philadelphia: WB Saunders.
8. McCloskey, J. C., Bulechek, G. M. (eds). (1992). *Nursing Interventions Classification (NIC).* St. Louis, MO: Mosby.
9. Educating parents of extra-special children: Developmental delays. Accessed January 2004 at www.epeconline.com/DevelopmentalDelays.html.
10. Kemp, S., Gungor, N. (2005). Growth failure. Article for Emedicine Web site. Retrieved March 2007 at www.emedicine.com/ped/topic902.htm.
11. Owens, T. A. (2005). Medical Encyclopedia: Delayed Growth. Article for MedlinePlus Web site. Retrieved March 2007 at http://nim.nih.gov/medlineplus/ency/aritcle/003021.htm.
12. Blann, L. E. (2005). Early intervention for children and families with special needs. *MCN, American J of Maternal/Child Nursing,* 30(4), 263–267.
13. Grenz, K., Bynum, G., Pine, D., et al. (updated verson 2005). Preventive services for children and adolescents. Institute for Clinical Systems Improvement [ICSI]. Article for National Guideline Clearinghouse. Web site. Retrieved February 2007 at www.guideline.gov.
14. Schiffman, R. F. (2004). Drug and subtance use in Adolescents. *MCN, American J of Maternal/Child Nursing,* 29(1), 21–27.

ineffective Health Maintenance

Definition: Inability to identify, manage, and/or seek out help to maintain health
[This diagnosis contains components of other NDs. We recommend subsuming health maintenance interventions under the "basic" nursing diagnosis when a single causative factor is identified (e.g., deficient Knowledge [specify], ineffective Therapeutic Regimen Management, chronic Confusion, impaired verbal Communication, disturbed Thought Process, ineffective Coping, compromised family Coping, delayed Growth and Development).]

RELATED FACTORS

Deficient communication skills [written, verbal, or gestural]
Unachieved developmental tasks
Inability to make appropriate judgments
Perceptual/cognitive impairment
Diminished/lack of gross motor skills; diminished/lack of fine motor skills
Ineffective individual/family coping; complicated grieving; spiritual distress
Insufficient resources (e.g., equipment, finances); [lack of psychosocial supports]

DEFINING CHARACTERISTICS

Subjective

Lack of expressed interest in improving health behaviors
[Reported compulsive behaviors]

Objective

Demonstrated lack of knowledge regarding basic health practices
Inability to take the responsibility for meeting basic health practices; history of lack of health-seeking behavior
Demonstrated lack of adaptive behaviors to environmental changes
Impairment of personal support system
[Observed compulsive behaviors]

Sample Clinical Applications: Chronic conditions (e.g., MS, rheumatoid arthritis, chronic pain), brain injury/stroke, spinal cord injury/paralysis, laryngectomy, dementia/Alzheimer's disease, developmental delay

DESIRED OUTCOMES/EVALUATION CRITERIA
Sample NOC linkages:
Health Promoting Behaviors: Personal actions to sustain or increase wellness
Knowledge: Health Behaviors: Extent of understanding conveyed about the promotion and protection of health
Participation in Healthcare Decisions: Personal involvement in selecting and evaluating healthcare options to achieve desired outcome

Client Will (Include Specific Time Frame)

- Identify necessary health maintenance activities.
- Verbalize understanding of factors contributing to current situation.
- Assume responsibility for own healthcare needs within level of ability.
- Adopt lifestyle changes supporting individual healthcare goals.

Sample NOC linkages:
Risk Detection: Personal actions to identify personal health threats
Social Support: Perceived availability and actual provision of reliable assistance from others

SO/Caregiver Will (Include Specific Time Frame)

- Verbalize ability to cope adequately with existing situation, provide support/monitoring as indicated.

Cultural   Collaborative   Community/Home Care   Diagnostic Studies   Pediatric/Geriatric/Lifespan   Medications

ACTIONS/INTERVENTIONS

Sample NIC linkages:

Health System Guidance: Facilitating a patient's location and use of appropriate health services

Support System Enhancement: Facilitation of support to patient by family, friends, and community

Health Education: Developing and providing instruction and learning experiences to facilitate voluntary adaptation of behavior conducive to health in individuals, families, groups, or communities

NURSING PRIORITY NO. 1 To assess causative/contributing factors:

- Identify risk factors in client's personal and family history, including health values/religious/cultural beliefs and expectations regarding healthcare. *May not view current situation as a problem or be unaware of routine health maintenance practices/needs.*[11]
- Note client's age (e.g., very young or elderly age); cognitive, emotional, physical, and developmental status, and level of dependence/independence. *Client's status may range from complete dependence (dysfunctional) to partial or relative independence and determines type of interventions/support needed.*[1]
- Note whether impairment is related to an acute/sudden onset situation, or a progressive illness/long-term health problem. *Determines type/intensity and length of time support may be required.*[4]
- Ascertain client's ability and desire to learn. Determine barriers to learning (e.g., can't read, speaks/understands different language, is overcome with stress or grief). *May not be physically, emotionally, or mentally capable at present because of current situation or may need information in small, manageable increments.*[1]
- Assess communication skills/ability/need for interpreter. Identify support person requiring/willing to accept information. *Ability to understand is essential to identification of needs and planning care. May need to provide the information to another individual if client is unable to comprehend.*[9]
- Evaluate for substance use/abuse (e.g., alcohol/other drugs). *Affects client's desire/ability to accept responsibility for self.*[6]
- Note client's desire/level of ability to meet health maintenance needs, as well as self-care ADLs. *Care may begin with helping client make a decision to improve situation, as well as identifying factors that are currently interfering with meeting needs.*[3]
- Note setting where client lives (e.g., long-term care facility, homebound, or homeless). *May contribute to inability/desire to meet healthcare needs.*[10]
- Ascertain recent changes in lifestyle. *For instance, a man whose spouse dies and who has no skills for taking care of his own/family's health needs may need assistance to learn how to manage new situation, or newly unemployed individual without healthcare benefits may require referral to public assistance agencies.*[8]
- Determine level of adaptive behavior, knowledge, and skills about health maintenance, environment, and safety. *Will determine beginning point for planning and intervening to help client learn necessary skills to maintain health in a positive manner.*[7]
- Evaluate environment *to note individual adaptation needs (e.g., supplemental humidity, air purifier, change in heating system).*[1]
- Note client's use of professional services and resources (i.e., appropriate or inappropriate/nonexistent).[9]

NURSING PRIORITY NO. 2 To assist client/caregiver(s) to maintain and manage desired health practices:

🏠 • Discuss with client/SO beliefs about health and reasons for not following prescribed plan of care. *Determines client's view about current situation and potential for change.*

🏠 • Identify realistic health goals and develop plan with client/SO(s) for self-care. *Allows for incorporating existing disabilities with client's/SO's desires, adapting and organizing care as necessary.*[1]

⊛ • Involve comprehensive specialty health teams when available/indicated (e.g., pulmonary, psychiatric, enterostomal, IV therapy, nutritional support, substance abuse counselors).[9]

🏠 • Provide time to Active-listen concerns of client/SO(s). *Provides opportunity to clarify expectations/misconceptions.*

🏠 • Provide anticipatory guidance *to maintain and manage effective health practices during periods of wellness and to identify ways client can adapt when progressive illness/long-term health problems occur.*[9,11]

🏠 • Encourage socialization, "buddy system," and personal involvement *to enhance support system, provide pleasant stimuli, and limit permanent regression.*[2]

⊛ • Provide for communication and coordination between healthcare facility teams and community healthcare providers *to promote continuation of care/maximize outcomes.*[2]

💊 • Monitor adherence to prescribed medical regimen *to problem-solve difficulties in adherence and alter the plan of care as needed.*[1]

NURSING PRIORITY NO. 3 To promote wellness (Teaching/Discharge Considerations):

🏠 • Provide information about individual healthcare needs, using client's preferred learning style (e.g., pictures, words, video, Internet). *Can help client to understand own situation and enhance cooperation with the plan of care.*[8]

🏠 • Limit amount of information presented at one time, especially when dealing with elderly or cognitively impaired client. Present new material through self-paced instruction when possible. *Allows client time to process and store new information.*[8]

🏠 • Help client/SO(s) prioritize healthcare goals. Provide a written copy to those involved in planning process *for future reference/revision as appropriate. Promotes planning to enable the client to maintain a healthy/productive lifestyle.*[10]

🏠 • Assist client/SO(s) to develop stress-management skills. *Knowing ways to manage stress helps individual to develop and maintain a healthy lifestyle.*[3]

🏠 • Identify ways to make adaptions in exercise program *to meet client's changing needs/abilities and environmental concerns.*[5]

⊛ • Identify signs and symptoms requiring further screening, evaluation, and follow-up. *Essential to identify developing problems that could interfere with maintaining well-being.*[10,11]

⊛ • Make referral as needed for community support services (e.g., homemaker/home attendant, Meals on Wheels, skilled nursing care, community/free clinic, Well-Baby Clinic, senior citizen healthcare activities). *May need additional assistance to maintain self-sufficiency.*[9]

⊛ • Refer to social services as indicated. *May need assistance with financial, housing, or legal concerns (e.g., conservatorship).*[2]

⊛ • Refer to support groups as appropriate (e.g., senior citizens, Red Cross, Salvation Army, Alcoholics or Narcotics Anonymous). Provides information and help for specific needs/at times of crisis.[9]

⊛ • Arrange for hospice service for client with terminal illness. *Will help client and family deal with end-of-life issues in a positive manner.*[3,4]

DOCUMENTATION FOCUS

Assessment/Reassessment

- Assessment findings, including individual abilities, family involvement, and support factors/availability of resources.
- Cultural/religious beliefs and healthcare values.

Planning

- Plan of care and who is involved in planning.
- Teaching plan.

Implementation/Evaluation

- Responses of client/SO(s) to plan/interventions/teaching and actions performed.
- Attainment/progress toward desired outcome(s).
- Modifications to plan of care.

Discharge Planning

- Long-range needs and who is responsible for actions to be taken.
- Specific referrals made.

References

1. Bohny, B. (1997). A time for self-care: Role of the home healthcare nurse. *Home Healthcare Nurs,* 15(4), 281–286.
2. Callaghan, P., Morrissey, G. (1993). Social support and health: A review. *J Adv Nurs,* 203, 18.
3. Dossey, B. M., Dossey, L. (1998). Body-mind-spirit: Attending to holistic care. *AJN,* 998(6), 44.
4. Gregory, C. M. (1997). Caring for caregivers: Proactive planning eases burden on caregivers. *Lifelines,* 1(2), 51.
5. Lai, S. C., Cohen, M. N. (1999). Promoting lifestyle changes. *AJN,* 99(4), 63.
6. Larsen, L. S. (1998). Effectiveness of counseling intervention to assist family caregivers of chronically ill relatives. *J Psychosoc Nurs,* 36(8), 26.
7. MacNeill, D., Weis, T. (1998). Case study: Coordinating care. *Continuing Care,* 17(4), 78.
8. Pocinki, K. (1990). Writing for an older audience: Ways to maximize understanding and acceptance. *AMWA,* 3(5), 6.
9. Stuifbergen, A. (1997). Health promotion: An essential component of rehabilitation for persons with chronic disabling conditions. *Adv Nurs Sci,* 19(4), 138–147.
10. Healthy People 2010 Toolkit: A Field Guide for Health Planning. Washington, DC: Public Health Foundation. Accessed July 2007 at www.phf.org/HPtools/state.htm.
11. No author or pub date listed. Health maintenance evaluation: Replacing the "annual physical." Fact sheet for Palo Alto Medical Foundation Web site. Retrieved March 2007 at www.pamf.org/children/maintenance/healtheval.html.

Health-Seeking Behaviors (specify)

Definition: Active seeking (by a person in stable health) of ways to alter personal health habits and/or the environment in order to move toward a higher level of health (Note: Stable health is defined as achievement of age-appropriate illness-prevention measures; client reports good or excellent health, and signs and symptoms of disease, if present, are controlled.)

RELATED FACTORS
To be developed by nurse researchers and submitted to NANDA
[Situational/maturational occurrence precipitating concern about current health status]

HEALTH-SEEKING BEHAVIORS (specify)

DEFINING CHARACTERISTICS

Subjective
Expressed desire to seek a higher level of wellness
Expressed desire for increased control of health practice
Expressed concern about current environmental conditions on health status
Stated unfamiliarity with wellness community resources
[Expressed desire to modify codependent behaviors]

Objective
Demonstrated lack of knowledge in health-promotion behaviors
Observed unfamiliarity with wellness community resources

Sample Clinical Applications: Seasonal allergies/episodic asthma, familial risk factors for major disease conditions (e.g., myocardial infarction, breast cancer, hypertension), well-controlled chronic diseases (e.g., diabetes, MS, Crohn's)

DESIRED OUTCOMES/EVALUATION CRITERIA
Sample NOC linkages:
Health-Seeking Behavior: Personal actions to promote optimal wellness, recovery, and rehabilitation
Health Promoting Behavior: Personal actions to sustain or increase wellness
Knowledge: Health Promotion: Extent of understanding conveyed about information needed to obtain and maintain optimal health

Client Will (Include Specific Time Frame)
- Express desire to change specific habit/lifestyle patterns to achieve/maintain optimal health.
- Participate in planning for change.
- Seek community resources to assist with desired change.

ACTIONS/INTERVENTIONS

Sample NIC linkages:
Self-Modification Assistance: Reinforcement of self-directed change initiated by the patient to achieve personally important goals
Health Education: Developing and providing instruction and learning experiences to facilitate voluntary adaptation of behavior conducive to health in individuals, families, groups, or communities
Health System Guidance: Facilitating a patient's location and use of appropriate health services

NURSING PRIORITY NO. 1 To assess specific concerns/habits/issues client desires to change:
- Determine client's current health status and perception of possible threats to health.
- Ascertain client's beliefs about health and his or her ability to maintain health. *Belief in ability to accomplish desired action is predictive of performance.*[7]
- Active-listen to concerns to identify underlying issues (e.g., physical or emotional stressors; or external factors such as environmental pollutants or other hazards) that could impact

Cultural Collaborative Community/Home Care Diagnostic Studies Pediatric/Geriatric/Lifespan Medications

client's ability to control own health. *Helps to determine client's level of satisfaction with current health issues and readiness for change.*

- Review knowledge base and note coping skills that have been used previously to change behavior/promote health. *Brings these to client's awareness and provides useful tools for current situation.*[1]

- Determine familial/cultural perspectives, values, concerns, and behaviors about health, well-being, and illness. *Influences client/SO and healthcare provider's perception of health and needs, which are not necessarily congruent. Also affects healthcare delivery systems and client's desire for/access to services.*[8]

- Perform testing such as Myers-Briggs or other psychological tests, as indicated, and review results with client/SO(s). *Can identify client strengths and help with development of plan of action. May also help client make decisions for the future.*[1]

- Identify risk-prone behaviors associated with health habits/poor health practices and propagation of chronic health problems (i.e., tobacco use; not wearing seat belts, helmets, water-flotation device when appropriate; alcohol and substance use; lack of exercise/sedentary lifestyle; sexual behavior that causes unintended pregnancy and disease). *Identifies areas client may choose to change for a healthier future.*[3,9,10]

NURSING PRIORITY NO. 2 To assist client to develop plan for improving health:

- Explore with client/SO(s) areas of health over which each individual has control and discuss barriers to healthy practices (e.g., chooses fast food instead of cooking for one; lack of time, access to convenient facilities or safe environment in which to exercise). *Identifies actions individual can take to plan for improving health practices.*[5]

- Address barriers to healthcare (e.g., finding a primary healthcare provider, transportation services, lack of insurance, costs of services, unavailability of child/elder care, communication barriers, fear of/actual criticism from peers, etc.). *Nurse/other professionals can help reduce some of these barriers by advocating for the client and encouraging client's efforts in self-management of health.*[6]

- Provide information about conditions/health risk factors or concerns in desired format (e.g., pictures, TV programs, articles, handouts, audio/visual materials; classes, group discussions, Web sites, and other databases) as appropriate. *Use of multiple modalities enhances acquisition/retention of information and gives client choices for accessing and applying information.*

- Problem-solve options for change. *Helps identify actions to be taken to achieve desired improvement.*[6]

- Discuss assertive behaviors and provide opportunity for client to practice new behaviors. *Promotes positive change to improve lifetime healthcare practices for the individual.*[6]

- Use therapeutic communication skills. *Promotes effective interactions within the family and with helping resources to provide support for desired changes.*[1]

NURSING PRIORITY NO. 3 To promote wellness (Teaching/Discharge Considerations):

- Acknowledge client's strengths in present health management and build on in planning for future. *Promotes feelings of self-esteem and recognition of current positive actions can help client progress in own care.*[5]

- Encourage use of exercise, relaxation skills, yoga, meditation, visualization, and guided imagery *to assist in management of stress and promote general health/well-being.*[2]

- Instruct in individually appropriate wellness behaviors. *Regular scheduling of breast self-examination/mammogram, testicular self-examination/prostate examination; flu shots, immunizations, smoking cessation, regular medical and dental examinations, healthy diet/ exercise program; screening and early treatment of risk factors (e.g., family history of diabetes/heart disease/hypertension, obesity, etc.) helps client comprehensively manage healthcare practices.*[6]

 • Identify and refer child/family member to health resources for immunizations, basic health services, and to learn health-promotion/monitoring skills (e.g., monitoring hydration, measuring fever). *May facilitate long-term attention to health issues and recognition of developing problems to facilitate timely intervention.*

 • Refer to community resources (e.g., nutritionist/weight-control program; exercise training; smoking-cessation program; driving safety, violence prevention; Alcoholics Anonymous, codependency support groups, assertiveness training/Parent Effectiveness classes, etc.) *to address specific concerns and apply health-promotion skills.*[6]

• Refer to other wellness NDs such as Knowledge, Nutrition, Parenting, or readiness for enhanced Therapeutic Regimen Management for additional interventions as appropriate.

DOCUMENTATION FOCUS

Assessment/Reassessment

• Assessment findings, including individual concerns/risk factors.
• Pertinent cultural/religious beliefs and values.
• Client's request/expectation for change.

Planning

• Plan of care and who is involved in planning.
• Teaching plan.

Implementation/Evaluation

• Responses to wellness plan, interventions/teaching and actions performed.
• Attainment/progress toward desired outcome(s).
• Modifications to plan of care.

Discharge Planning

• Long-range needs and who is responsible for actions to be taken.
• Specific referrals.

References

1. Townsend, M. C. (2003). *Psychiatric Mental Health Nursing Concepts of Care.* 4th ed. Philadelphia: F. A. Davis.
2. Herrick, C. M., Ainsworth, A. F. (2000). Invest in yourself: Yoga as a self-care strategy. *Nurs Forum,* 35(2), 32–36.
3. Patel, A. M. (2001). Using the Internet in the management of asthma. *Curr Opin Pulm Med,* 7(1), 39–42.
5. U.S. Department of Health and Human Services: Healthy People 2000 national health promotion and disease prevention objectives. DHHS No (PHS) 91–50212, Washington, DC, 1991, U.S. Government Printing Office.
6. Healthy People 2010 Toolkit: A Field Guide to Health Planning. Accessed July 2007 at www.phf.org/HPtools/state.htm.
7. Fenn, M. (1998). Health promotion: Theoretical perspectives and clinical applications. *Holis Nurs Pract,* 19(2), 1–7.
8. Purnell, L. D., Paulanka, B. J. (1998). *Transcultural Health Care: A Culturally Competent Approach.* Philadelphia: F. A. Davis.

  Cultural   Collaborative   Community/Home Care   Diagnostic Studies   Pediatric/Geriatric/Lifespan   Medications

9. No author listed. (2002). World Health Report. Reducing risks, promoting healthy life. Report of the World Health Organization (WHO). Retrieved March 2007 at www.who.int/whr/2002/en/whr02_en.pdf.

10. No author listed. (2007). Preventing leading causes of premature death, disease and disability. Fact sheet of the World Health Organization (WHO). Retrieved March 2007 at www.who.int/school_youth_health/en/.

impaired Home Maintenance

Definition: Inability to independently maintain a safe growth-promoting immediate environment

RELATED FACTORS

Disease; injury
Insufficient family organization/planning
Insufficient finances
Impaired functioning
Lack of role modeling
Unfamiliarity with neighborhood resources
Deficient knowledge
Inadequate support systems

DEFINING CHARACTERISTICS

Subjective

Household members express difficulty in maintaining their home in a comfortable [safe] fashion
Household members request assistance with home maintenance
Household members describe outstanding debts/financial crises

Objective

Disorderly/unclean surroundings; offensive odors
Inappropriate household temperature
Presence of vermin
Repeated unhygienic disorders/infections
Lack of necessary equipment; unavailable cooking equipment
Insufficient/lack of clothes/linen
Overtaxed family members

Sample Clinical Applications: Chronic conditions (e.g., AIDS, MS, rheumatoid arthritis), depression, dementia, developmental delay

DESIRED OUTCOMES/EVALUATION CRITERIA

Sample NOC linkages:

Self-Care: Instrumental Activities of Daily Living [IADL]: Ability to perform activities needed to function in the home or community independently with or without assistive device

Family Functioning: Capacity of the family system to meet the needs of its members during developmental transitions

Family Physical Environment: Physical arrangements in the home that provide safety and stimulation to family members

Client/Caregiver Will (Include Specific Time Frame)

- Identify individual factors related to difficulty in maintaining a safe environment.
- Verbalize plan to eliminate health and safety hazards.
- Adopt behaviors reflecting lifestyle changes to create and sustain a healthy/growth-promoting environment.
- Demonstrate appropriate, effective use of resources.

ACTIONS/INTERVENTIONS

Sample NIC linkages:

Home Maintenance Assistance: Helping the patient/family to maintain the home as a clean, pleasant place to live

Environmental Management: Manipulation of the patient's surroundings for therapeutic benefit

Support System Enhancement: Facilitation of support to patient by family, friends, and community

NURSING PRIORITY NO. 1   To assess causative/contributing factors:

- Identify presence of/potential for conditions such as diabetes, fractures/spinal cord injury, amputation, multiple sclerosis, arthritis, stroke, Parkinson's disease, mental illness (schizophrenia) *that can compromise client's/SO's functional abilities in taking care of home.*[3]
- Note personal or environmental factors (e.g., family member with multiple care tasks, substance abuse, absence of family/support systems, lifestyle of self-neglect, client comfortable with home environment/has no desire for change) *that can contribute to neglect of home.*[2,5]
- Determine problems in the household and degree of discomfort/unsafe conditions noted by client/SO. *Some safety problems may be immediately obvious (e.g., lack of heat, water), while other problems may be more subtle and difficult to manage (e.g., lack of sufficient finances for home repairs, or lack of knowledge about food storage or rodent control). Client and/or SO may need assistance or teaching regarding safety of their environment, especially if it is negatively impacting their health.*[2]
- Assess client's/SO's level of cognitive/emotional/physical functioning *to ascertain client's needs and caregiver's capabilities when developing plan of care for preventive, supportive, and therapeutic care.*[1]
- Identify lack of knowledge/misinformation *to determine need for health education/home safety program.*
- Identify support systems available to client/SO(s) *to determine needs and initiate referrals (e.g., companionship, daily care, respite care, homemaking, running errands, meal preparation or meal-service program, financial assistance, etc.).*[1]
- Determine financial resources to meet needs of individual situation. *May need referral to social services for funds, necessary equipment, home repairs, transportation, etc.*[2]

NURSING PRIORITY NO. 2   To help client/SO(s) to create/maintain a safe, growth-promoting environment:

- Coordinate planning with multidisciplinary team and client/SO as appropriate. *Coordination and cooperation of team improves motivation and maximizes outcomes.*

Cultural   Collaborative   Community/Home Care   Diagnostic Studies   Pediatric/Geriatric/Lifespan   Medications

- Assist client/SO(s) to develop plan for maintaining a clean, healthful environment. *Activities such as sharing of household tasks/repairs between family members, contract services, exterminators, trash removal can promote ongoing maintenance.*
- Discuss home environment/perform home visit as indicated to *determine client's ability to care for self, to identify potential health and safety hazards, and to determine adaptations that may be needed (e.g., wheelchair-accessible doors/hallways, safety bars in bathroom, safe place for child play, clean water available, working cook stove/microwave, screens on windows).*[2]
- Assist client/SO(s) to identify and acquire necessary equipment and services (e.g., chair/stair lifts, commode chair, safety grab bar, structural adaptations, service animals, aids for hearing/seeing, mobility; trash removal, cleaning supplies) *to meet individual needs.*[3]
- Identify resources available for appropriate assistance (e.g., visiting nurse, budget counseling, homemaker, Meals on Wheels, physical/occupational therapy, social services).[2]
- Discuss options for financial assistance with housing needs. *Client may be able to stay in home with minimal assistance or may need significant assistance over a wide range of possibilities, including removal from the home.*[2]

NURSING PRIORITY NO. 3 To promote wellness (Teaching/Discharge Considerations):

- Evaluate client at each community contact or before facility discharge *to determine if home maintenance needs are ongoing in order to initiate appropriate referrals.*[3]
- Discuss environmental hazards *that may negatively affect health or ability to perform desired activities.*
- Discuss long-term plan *for taking care of environmental needs (e.g., assistive personnel, specialized controls for electrical equipment, trash removal and pest control services, etc.).*[4]
- Provide information necessary for the individual situation. *Helps client/family decide what can be done to improve situation.*[3]
- Identify ways to access/use community resources and support systems (e.g., extended family, neighbors, church group, seniors program).
- Refer to NDs Caregiver Role Strain, compromised family Coping, ineffective Coping, risk for Injury, deficient Knowledge [specify], Self-Care Deficit [specify] for additional interventions as appropriate.

DOCUMENTATION FOCUS

Assessment/Reassessment

- Assessment findings include individual/environmental factors, presence and use of support systems.

Planning

- Plan of care and who is involved in planning; support systems and community resources identified.
- Teaching plan.

Implementation/Evaluation

- Client's/SO's responses to interventions/teaching and actions performed.
- Attainment/progress toward desired outcome(s).
- Modifications to plan of care.

Discharge Planning

- Long-term needs and who is responsible for actions to be taken.
- Specific referrals made, equipment needs/resources.

References

1. Townsend, M. C. (2003). *Psychiatric Mental Health Nursing Concepts of Care.* 4th ed. Philadelphia: F. A. Davis.
2. MSU Extension. (2003). Home Maintenance and Repair. Accessed July 2007 at http://web1.msue.msu.edu/msue/imp/mod02/master02.html.
3. Fenn, M. (1998). Health promotion: Theoretical perspectives and clinical application. *Holis Nurs Pract,* 19(2), 1–7.
4. Schmelling, S. (2005). Home, adapted home. *Rehab Management,* 18(6), 12–19.
5. Gibbons, S., Lauder, W., Ludwick, R. (2006). Self-neglect: A proposed new NANDA diagnosis. *International J Nursing Terminologies and Classifications,* 17(1), 10–18.

readiness for enhanced Hope

Definition: A pattern of expectations and desires that is sufficient for mobilizing energy on one's own behalf and can be strengthened

RELATED FACTORS
To be developed by nurse researchers and submitted to NANDA

DEFINING CHARACTERISTICS

Subjective
Expresses desire to enhance: hope; belief in possibilities; congruency of expectations with desires; ability to set achievable goals; problem-solving to meet goals
Expresses desire to enhance: sense of meaning to life; interconnectedness with others; spirituality

Sample Clinical Applications: Any acute or chronic condition, or healthy individual looking to improve well-being

DESIRED OUTCOMES/EVALUATION CRITERIA
Sample NOC linkages:
Hope: Optimism that is personally satisfying and life supporting
Quality of Life: Extent of positive perception of current life circumstances
Personal Well-Being: Extent of positive perception of one's health status and life circumstances

Client Will (Include Specific Time Frame)

- Identify and verbalize feelings related to expectations and desires.
- Verbalize belief in possibilities for the future.
- Discuss current situation and desire to enhance hope.
- Set short-term goals that will lead to behavioral changes to meet desire for enhanced hope.

Cultural · Collaborative · Community/Home Care · Diagnostic Studies · Pediatric/Geriatric/Lifespan · Medications

ACTIONS/INTERVENTIONS

Sample NIC linkages:

Hope Instillation: Facilitation of the development of a positive outlook in a given situation

Self-awareness Enhancement: Assisting a patient to explore and understand his or her thoughts, feelings, motivations, and behaviors

Spiritual Growth Facilitation: Facilitation of growth in patient's capacity to identify, connect with, and call upon the source of meaning, purpose, comfort, strength, and hope in his or her life

NURSING PRIORITY NO. 1 To determine needs and desire for improvement:

- Review familial/social history to identify past situations (e.g., illness, emotional conflicts, alcoholism) that have led to decision to improve life. *When trials of life have been resolved, individuals may look toward making life better.*[1]
- Determine current physical condition of client/SO. *Treatment regimen and indicators of healing can influence ability to promote positive feelings of hope.*[2]
- Ascertain client's perception of current state and expectations/goals for the future (e.g., general well-being, prosperity, independence). *Perception is more important than reality in individual's mind and can help to pursue realistic goals for self.*[3]
- Identify spiritual beliefs/cultural values that guide or influence client's spirituality and view of self. *Influences sense of hope and connectedness.*[4]
- Determine meaning of life/reasons for living, belief in God or higher power. *Helps client to clarify beliefs and how they relate to desire for improvement in life.*[6]
- Ascertain motivation/expectations for change. Note congruency of expectations with desires for change. *Motivation to improve and high expectations can encourage client to make changes that will improve his or her life. However, presence of unrealistic expectations may hamper efforts.*[3,4]
- Note degree of involvement in activities/relationships with others. *Interactions with others can promote a sense of connectedness and enjoyment of relationships.*[3]

NURSING PRIORITY NO. 2 To assist client to achieve goals and strengthen sense of hope:

- Establish a therapeutic relationship showing positive regard and hopefulness for the client. *Enhances feelings of worth and comfort, inspiring client to continue pursuit of goals.*[3]
- Help client recognize areas that are in his or her control versus those that are not. *To be most effective, client needs to expend energy in those areas where he or she has control and let the others go.*[2]
- Assist client to develop manageable short-term goals. *Success at short-term goals that are manageable will lead to attainment of long-term goals too.*[2]
- Identify activities to achieve goals, and facilitate contingency planning. *Promotes dealing with situation in manageable steps, enhancing chances for success and sense of control.*[5]
- Explore interrelatedness of relationship between unresolved emotions, anxieties, fears, and guilt. *Provides opportunity to address issues that may be limiting individual's ability to improve life situation.*[5]
- Assist client to acknowledge current coping behaviors and defense mechanisms that may hamper moving toward goals. *Allows client to focus on coping mechanisms that are more successful in problem-solving.*[3]

🏠 • Encourage client to concentrate on progress not perfection. *If client can accept that perfection is difficult/not always the desirable outcome, he or she may be able to view own accomplishments with pride.*[3]

🏠 • Involve client in care and explain all procedures thoroughly, answering questions truthfully. *Enhances trust and relationship, promoting hope for a positive outcome.*[2]

🏠 • Express hope to client and encourage SO(s) and other heath team members to do so. *Enhances client's sense of hope and belief in possibilities of a positive outcome.*[1]

🏠 • Identify ways to strengthen sense of interconnectedness or harmony with others *to support sense of belonging and connection that promotes feelings of wholeness and hopefulness.*[1]

NURSING PRIORITY NO. 3 To promote optimum wellness:

🏠 • Demonstrate and encourage use of relaxation techniques, guided imagery, and meditation activities. *Learning to relax can help client decrease tension resulting in refreshment of body and mind, enabling individual to perform and think more successfully.*[3]

🏠 • Provide positive feedback for efforts taken to improve situation, growth in use of skills, and learning efforts. *Acknowledges client's efforts as individual is moving forward in learning new skills, and reinforces gains.*[3]

🏠 • Explore ways that beliefs give meaning and value to daily living. *As client's understanding of these issues improves, hope for the future is strengthened.*[1]

🏠 • Encourage life-review by client. *Acknowledges own successes, identifies opportunity for change, and clarifies meaning in life.*[5]

🏠 • Identify ways for spiritual expression, strengthening spirituality. *There are many options for enhancing spirituality through connectedness with self/others (e.g., volunteering, mentoring, involvement in religious activities).* (Refer to ND: readiness for enhanced Spiritual Well-being.)[5]

🏠 • Encourage client to join groups with similar or new interests. *Expanding knowledge and making friendships with new people will widen horizons for the individual.*

Ⓐ • Refer to community resources/support groups, spiritual advisor as indicated.

DOCUMENTATION FOCUS

Assessment/Reassessment

• Assessment findings, including client's perceptions of current situation, relationships, sense of desire for enhancing life.
• Cultural/spiritual values and beliefs.
• Motivation and expectations for improvement.

Planning

• Plan of care and who is involved in planning.
• Teaching plan

Implementation/Evaluation

• Responses to interventions/teaching and actions performed
• Attainment/progress toward desired outcome(s)
• Modifications to plan of care

 🌐 Cultural   Ⓐ Collaborative   🏠 Community/Home Care   ✏ Diagnostic Studies   ∞ Pediatric/Geriatric/Lifespan   💊 Medications

Discharge Planning

- Identifies long-range needs/goals for change and who is responsible for actions to be taken
- Specific referrals made

References

1. Hope for Today Al-Anon Group. Retrieved March 2007 at http://health.groups.yahoo.com/group/HopeForTodayGroup/.
2. Doenges, M., Moorhouse, M., Murr, A. *Nursing Care Plans, Guidelines for Individualizing Patient Care.* 6th ed. Philadelphia: F. A. Davis.
3. Townsend, M. (2006). Psychiatric Mental Health Nursing Concepts of Care in Evidenced-Based Practice. 5th ed. Philadelphia: F. A. Davis.
4. Lipson, J. G., Dibble, S., Minarik, P. (eds). (1999). *Culture and Nursing Care: A Pocket Guide.* UCSF Nursing Press.
5. Cox, H. C., et al. (2002). *Clinical Applications of Nursing Diagnosis: Adult, Child, Women's, Psychiatric, Gerontic, and Home Health Considerations.* 4th ed. Philadelphia: F. A. Davis.
6. Hareven, T. K., Adams, K. J. (eds). (1982). *Aging and Life Course Transitions: An Interdisciplinary Perspective.* New York: Guilford.

Hopelessness

Definition: Subjective state in which an individual sees limited or no alternatives or personal choices available and is unable to mobilize energy on own behalf

RELATED FACTORS
Prolonged activity restriction creating isolation
Deteriorating physiological condition
Long-term stress; abandonment
Lost belief in spiritual power/transcendent values[/God]

DEFINING CHARACTERISTICS

Subjective
Verbal cues (despondent content, "I can't," sighing); [believes things will not change/problems will always be there]

Objective
Passivity; decreased verbalization
Decreased affect/appetite/response to stimuli
[Depressed cognitive functions, problems with decisions, thought processes; regression]
Lack of initiative/involvement in care
Sleep pattern disturbance, [increased/decreased sleep]
Turning away from speaker; shrugging in response to speaker; [withdrawal from environs; closing eyes]
[Lack of involvement/interest in SOs (children, spouse)]
[Angry outbursts]
[Substance abuse]

Sample Clinical Applications: Chronic conditions, terminal diagnoses, infertility

DESIRED OUTCOMES/EVALUATION CRITERIA

Sample NOC linkages:

Depression Self-Control: Personal actions to minimize melancholy and maintain interest in life events

Hope: Optimism that is personally satisfying and life supporting

Quality of Life: Extent of positive perception of current life circumstances

Client Will (Include Specific Time Frame)

- Recognize and verbalize feelings.
- Identify and use coping mechanisms to counteract feelings of hopelessness.
- Involve self in, and control (within limits of the individual situation), own self-care and ADLs.
- Set progressive short-term goals that develop/foster/sustain behavioral changes and positive outlook.
- Participate in diversional activities of own choice.

ACTIONS/INTERVENTIONS

Sample NIC linkages:

Hope Instillation: Facilitation of the development of a positive outlook in a given situation

Emotional Support: Provision of reassurance, acceptance, and encouragement during times of stress

Mood Management: Providing for safety, stabilization, recovery, and maintenance of a patient who is experiencing dysfunctionally depressed or elevated mood

NURSING PRIORITY NO. 1   To identify causative/contributing factors:

- Review familial/social history and physiological history contributing to current problems. *History of poor coping abilities, disorder of familial relating patterns, emotional problems, language/cultural barriers (leading to feelings of isolation), recent or long-term illness of client or family member, multiple social and/or physiological traumas to individual or family members can all affect client's feelings of hopelessness.*[2]

- Identify current familial/social/physical factors contributing to sense of hopelessness. *Issues such as a newly diagnosed chronic/terminal disease, lack of support system, recent job loss, loss of spiritual/religious faith, recent multiple traumas can result in an individual giving up. Identification of the issues involved in each person's situation is necessary to appropriately plan for care.*[2,5]

- Determine client's locus of control (internal/external) and associated cultural factors influencing self-view. Note expressions of responsibility for self versus expressions of lack of control over self and environment. *Individuals views life change and stressful events differently. Those with internal locus of control tend to be more optimistic about their ability to deal with adversity even in the face of current difficulties. Individual with external locus of control may attribute feelings of hopelessness to an external source perceiving it as beyond his or her control and will look to others to solve problems and take care of them.*[2,5]

- Identify coping behaviors and defense mechanisms displayed previously and in current situation as well as client's perception of effectiveness then and now. *It is important to identify client's strengths and encourage their use as client begins to deal with what is currently happening.*[2]

• Have client describe events that lead to feeling inadequate or having no control. *Identifies sources of frustration and defines problem areas so action can be taken to learn how to deal with them in more positive ways.*[6]

• Determine presence of suicidal ideation, availability of plan, and means to follow through with plan. (Refer to ND risk for Suicide.) *Hopelessness is identified as a central underlying factor in the predisposition to suicide, and the client sees no other way out of a hopeless situation.*[7]

• Perform physical examination, review results of lab tests/diagnostic studies. *Current situation may be the result of a decline in physical well-being/progression of a chronic condition, or physical symptoms may be associated with effects of depression (e.g., loss of appetite, lack of sleep).*

NURSING PRIORITY NO. 2 To assess level of hopelessness:

• Note behaviors indicative of hopelessness as listed in Defining Characteristics. *Identifies problem areas to be addressed in developing an effective plan of care and suggests possible resources needed.*[6]

• Evaluate/discuss use of defense mechanisms (useful or not). *Identifying behaviors such as increased sleeping, dependence on medications, illness behaviors, eating disorders, denial, forgetfulness, daydreaming, ineffectual organizational efforts, exploiting own goal-setting, and regression can provide accurate information for client to begin changing behavior/inaccurate beliefs.*[6]

• Discuss problem/duration of alcohol/drug abuse. Behavior may be an effort to provide psychological numbing in an attempt to lessen pain of situation, or may have preceded and contributed to sense of hopelessness. *Client may feel hopeless about stopping behavior and believe that it is impossible.*[2]

• Evaluate degree of hopelessness using psychological testing such as Beck's Depression Scale. Note client's feelings about life not being worth living and other signs of hopelessness and worthlessness. *Identifying the degree of hopelessness and possible suicidal thoughts is crucial to instituting appropriate treatment to protect client.*[10]

NURSING PRIORITY NO. 3 To assist client to identify feelings and to begin to cope with problems as perceived by the client:

• Establish a therapeutic/facilitative relationship showing positive regard for the client. Answer questions truthfully. *Enhances trust so that client may feel safe to disclose feelings, talk openly about concerns and feel understood and listened to.*[2,3,10]

• Encourage client to verbalize and explore feelings and perceptions of what is happening. *Talking about feelings of anger, helplessness, powerlessness, confusion, despondency, isolation, and grief (which can lead to a sense of hopelessness and the belief that nothing can be done) provides opportunity for reflection and enables client to begin to understand self and that there are actions that can be helpful.*[3]

• Provide opportunity for children to "play out" feelings (e.g., puppets or art for preschooler, peer discussions for adolescents). *Provides insight into perceptions and can give direction for developing coping strategies.*[2]

• Engage teens and parents in discussions and arrange to do activities with them. *Parents can make a difference in their children's lives by being with them, discussing sensitive topics, and going different places with them.*[3,4]

• Express hope to client and encourage SOs and other health-team members to do so as well. Avoid expressions of false hope. *Client may not identify positives in own situation and may find it difficult to accept them from others, but will hear them. False reassurances will undermine sense of security.*[2]

- Help client recognize areas in which he or she has control versus those that are not within his or her control. *Often the individual who is feeling hopeless is focusing on issues that cannot be changed. When the client begins to focus energy in those areas where he or she has control, a sense of hope can be nurtured.*[6]
- Use client's locus of control to develop individual plan of care. *Tailoring care to the individual's ability will maximize effectiveness. For instance, client with internal control can take control of own destiny, and those with external control may need to begin with small tasks and add as tolerated, moving toward learning to take more control of personal choices.*[13]
- Encourage client to identify short-term goals. Promote activities to achieve goals, and facilitate contingency planning. *Dealing with situation in manageable steps, enhances chances for success, promotes sense of control, and encourages belief that there is hope for resolution of situation/moving forward.*[6]
- Discuss current options with client and list actions that can be taken. Correct misconceptions expressed by the client. *Encourages use of own actions, validates reality, and promotes sense of control of the situation.*[2]
- Endeavor to prevent situations that might lead to feelings of isolation or lack of control in client's perception. *Client will interpret these occurrences as further proof that there is no hope.*[6]
- Promote client control in establishing time, place, and frequency of treatment/therapy sessions. Involve family members in the appointments as appropriate. *Allows individual to assume control over own situation, engendering positive feelings of ability to manage what is happening. Involvement of family members provides source of support and encouragement for client.*[2]
- Encourage risk-taking in situations in which the client can succeed. *Succeeding in new ventures can improve self-esteem and hope for more successful actions.*[2]
- Help client begin to develop new coping mechanisms. *New skills need to be learned and used effectively to counteract hopelessness.*[3]
- Encourage structured/controlled increase in physical activity as tolerated. *Promotes the release of endorphins, enhancing sense of well-being.*[2]
- Demonstrate and encourage use of relaxation exercises, guided imagery. *Anxious feelings create tension, and learning to relax can help client begin to look at possibilities of feeling more hopeful.*[9]
- Discuss safe use of prescribed antidepressants. *May require short-term use to elevate mood while client pursues other therapeutic measures to regain sense of hope.*[2]

NURSING PRIORITY NO. 4 To promote wellness (Teaching/Discharge Considerations):

- Provide positive feedback for actions taken to deal with and overcome feelings of hopelessness. *Encourages changes in thinking patterns and continuation of desired behaviors.*[10,12]
- Assist client/family to become aware of factors/situations leading to feelings of hopelessness. *Helps individuals to identify precipitating events and provides opportunities to avoid/modify situation, promoting sense of control over life.*[8]
- Discuss initial signs of hopelessness. *Helps client to identify behaviors such as procrastination, increased need for sleep, decreased physical activity, and withdrawal from social/familial activities and how they have affected thinking and ability to deal with current situation. Awareness provides the opportunity to begin to change.*[9]
- Facilitate client's incorporation of personal loss. *Often losses in individual's life result in feelings of hopelessness and lack of control in current events that are happening. Hopelessness*

means a loss of hope rather than just an absence of hope. Enhancing grief work and promoting resolution of feelings helps client to begin to feel hope again and look forward to life.[9]

- Encourage client/family to develop support systems in the immediate community. *Having support nearby provides individuals with assistance, advocacy for moving forward, enabling them to look toward future with hope.*[4,6]

- Help client to become aware of, nurture, and expand spiritual self. (Refer to ND Spiritual Distress.) *Spiritual needs are an integral part of being human. Acknowledging and learning about spiritual aspect of self can help client look toward the future with hope for improved sense of well-being.*[11]

- Encourage/facilitate interaction with religious representative/spiritual counselor as indicated. *Client's sense of hopelessness may include the loss of spiritual connectedness or client may view spiritual being as responsible for current situation.*[1]

- Introduce the client into a support group before the individual therapy is terminated for continuation of therapeutic process. *Provides for a smooth transition so client feels accepted and comfortable in the presence of others.*[6]

- Stress need for continued monitoring of medication regimen by healthcare provider. *Necessary to evaluate effectiveness and prevent/minimize possible side effects. Antidepressant agents are not be discontinued abruptly without consulting healthcare provider.*[2]

- Refer to other resources for assistance as indicated (e.g., clinical nurse specialist, psychiatrist, social services, Alcoholics/Narcotics Anonymous. Anon/Alateen). *May need additional help to develop hope for the future, sustain efforts for change.*[2]

DOCUMENTATION FOCUS

Assessment/Reassessment

- Assessment findings, including what has been lost in hopelessness, degree of impairment, locus of control, use of coping skills and support systems.
- Cultural/religious beliefs and expectations.
- Spiritual concerns.

Planning

- Plan of care and who is involved in planning.
- Teaching plan.

Implementation/Evaluation

- Responses to interventions/teaching and actions performed.
- Attainment/progress toward desired outcome(s).
- Modifications to plan of care.

Discharge Planning

- Identified long-range needs/client's goals for change and who is responsible for actions to be taken.
- Specific referrals made.

References

1. Geiter, H. (2002). The spiritual side of nursing. *RN*, 65(5), 43–44.
2. Townsend, M. C. (2006). *Psychiatric Mental Health Nursing Concepts of Care*. 5th ed. Philadelphia: F. A. Davis.
3. Gordon, T. (2000). *Parent Effectiveness Training* (updated edition). New York: Three Rivers Press.

4. Cox, H. C., et al. (2002). *Clinical Applications of Nursing Diagnosis: Adult, Child, Women's, Psychiatric, Gerontic, and Home Health Considerations*. 4th ed. Philadelphia: F. A. Davis.
5. Lipson, J. G., Dibble, S. L., Minarik, P. A. (1999). *Culture & Nursing Care: A Pocket Guide*. San Francisco: UCSF Nursing Press.
6. Doenges, M. E., Townsend, M. C., Moorhouse, M. (1998). *Psychiatric Care Plans Guidelines for Individualizing Care*. 3d ed. Philadelphia: F. A. Davis.
7. Ghosh, T. B., Victor, B. S. (1994). Suicide. In Hales, R. R., Yudofsky, S. C., Talbott, J. A. (eds). *The American Psychiatric Press Textbook of Psychiatry*. 2d ed. Washington, DC: American Psychiatric Press.
8. Drew, B. (1990). Differentiation of hopelessness, helplessness, and powerlessness using Erik Erikson's "Roots of Virtue." *Arch Psychiatr Nurs*, 4, 332.
9. Miller, J. F. (2000). *Coping with Chronic Illness: Overcoming Powerlessness*. Philadelphia: F. A. Davis.
10. Beck, A. T., Brown, G., Berchick, R. J. (1990). Relationship between hopelessness and ultimate suicide: A replication with psychiatric out-patients. *Am J Psychiatry*, 147, 190–195.
11. Pearce, J. C. (2000). *The Biology of Trancendence, a Blueprint of the Human Spirit*. Rochester, VT: Park St Press.
12. Seligman, M. E. P. (1998). *Learned Optimism: How to Change Your Mind & Your Life*. New York Pocket Books/Simon & Schuster.
13. Kunert, P. K. (2002). Stress and adaptation. In Porth, C. M. (ed). *Pathophysiology: Concepts of Altered Health States*. Philadelphia: J. B. Lippincott.

Hyperthermia

Definition: Body temperature elevated above normal range

RELATED FACTORS
Exposure to hot environment; inappropriate clothing
Vigorous activity; dehydration
Decreased perspiration
Medications; anesthesia
Increased metabolic rate; illness; trauma

DEFINING CHARACTERISTICS

Subjective
[Headache]
[Weakness, dizziness, nausea]

Objective
Increase in body temperature above normal range
Flushed skin; warm to touch
Increased respiratory rate, tachycardia; [unstable BP]
Seizures; convulsions; [muscle rigidity/fasciculations]
[Confusion]

Sample Clinical Applications: Infectious diseases, head trauma, hyperthyroidism, heat exhaustion/heatstroke, surgical procedure/anesthesia

DESIRED OUTCOMES/EVALUATION CRITERIA
Sample NOC linkages:
Thermoregulation: Balance among heat production, heat gain, and heat loss
Thermoregulation: Newborn: Balance among heat production, heat gain, and heat loss during the first 28 days of life
Personal Safety Behavior: Personal actions of an adult to control behaviors that can cause physical injury

Cultural   Collaborative   Community/Home Care   Diagnostic Studies   Pediatric/Geriatric/Lifespan   Medications

Client Will (Include Specific Time Frame)
- Maintain core temperature within normal range.
- Be free of complications such as irreversible brain/neurological damage, and acute renal failure.
- Identify underlying cause/contributing factors and importance of treatment, as well as signs/symptoms requiring further evaluation or intervention.
- Demonstrate behaviors to monitor and promote normothermia.
- Be free of seizure activity.

ACTIONS/INTERVENTIONS

Sample NIC linkages:

Temperature Regulation: Attaining or maintaining body temperature within a normal range

Fever Treatment: Management of a patient with hyperpyrexia caused by nonenvironmental factors

Malignant Hyperthermia Precautions: Prevention or reduction of hypermetabolic response to pharmacological agents used during surgery

NURSING PRIORITY NO. 1 To assess causative/contributing factors:

- Identify underlying cause (e.g., *excessive heat production such as occurs with strenuous exercise, fever, shivering, tremors, convulsions, hyperthyroid state, infection/sepsis; malignant hyperpyrexia/heatstroke, sympathomimetic drugs; impaired heat dissipation such as occurs with heatstroke, dermatological diseases, burns, inability to perspire such as occurs with spinal cord injury and certain medications [e.g., diuretics, sedatives, certain heart and blood pressure medications]; loss of thermoregulation such as may occur in infections, brain lesions, drug overdose).*[1,10,11]
- Note chronological and developmental age of client. *Infants, young children, and elderly persons are most susceptible to damaging hyperthermia. Environmental factors and relatively minor infections can produce a much higher temperature in infants and young children than in older children and adults. Infants, children, or impaired individuals are not able to protect themselves and cannot recognize and/or act on symptoms of hyperthermia. Elderly persons have age-related risk factors (e.g., poor circulation, inefficient sweat glands, skin changes caused by normal aging, chronic diseases).*[1-4,11]

NURSING PRIORITY NO. 2 To evaluate effects/degree of hyperthermia:

- Monitor core temperature by appropriate route (e.g., tympanic, rectal). Note presence of temperature elevation (>98.6°F [37°C]) or fever (100.4°F [38°C]). *Rectal and tympanic temperatures most closely approximate core temperature; however, shell temperatures (oral, axillary, touch) are often measured at home and are predictive of fever. Rectal temperature measurement may be the most accurate but is not always expedient (e.g., client declines, is agitated, has rectal lesions or surgery, etc.). Abdominal temperature monitoring may be done in the premature neonate.*[1-3,5,6]
- Assess whether body temperature reflects heatstroke. *Defined as body temperature higher than 106°F (41.1°C) that is associated with neurological dysfunction and is potentially life-threatening.*[1]

- Assess neurological response, noting level of consciousness and orientation, reaction to stimuli, reaction of pupils, presence of posturing or seizures. *High fever accompanied by changes in mentation may indicate septic state or heatstroke.*[1–3,5,6]
- Monitor blood pressure and invasive hemodynamic parameters if available (e.g., cardiac output, arterial pressures). *Hypodynamic state can occur, especially in person with preexisting cardiovascular disease if heat-related illness (e.g., heatstroke or malignant hyperthermia reaction to anesthesia) has rendered the client critically ill.*[1–3,5,6]
- Monitor heart rate and rhythm. *Tachycardia, dysrhythmias, and ECG changes are common due to electrolyte and acid-base imbalance, dehydration, specific action of catecholamines, and direct effects of hyperthermia on blood and cardiac tissue.*[1-3,5,6]
- *Monitor respirations. Hyperventilation may initially be present, but ventilatory effort may eventually be impaired by seizures, hypermetabolic state (shock and acidosis).*
- Auscultate breath sounds *to note presence/progression of adventitious sounds such as crackles (rales), especially when heart failure or pneumonia is present.*[1–3,5,6]
- Monitor/record all sources of fluid loss such as urine (*oliguria or renal failure may occur due to hypotension, dehydration, shock, and tissue necrosis*), vomiting and diarrhea, wounds/fistulas, and insensible losses (*potentiates fluid and electrolyte losses*).[1–3,5,6]
- Note presence/absence of sweating. *The body attempts to increase heat loss by evaporation, conduction, and diffusion. Evaporation is decreased by environmental factors of high humidity and high ambient temperature as well as body factors producing loss of ability to sweat or sweat gland dysfunction (e.g., spinal cord transection, cystic fibrosis, dehydration, and vasoconstriction).*[10,11]

- Monitor laboratory studies such as ABGs, electrolytes, cardiac and liver enzymes (*may reveal tissue degeneration*); glucose (*hypoglycemia*); BUN/Cr (*acute renal failure*); urinalysis (*myoglobinuria, proteinuria, and hemoglobinuria can occur as products of tissue necrosis*).[1]

NURSING PRIORITY NO. 3 To assist with measures to reduce body temperature/restore normal body/organ function[1–3,5,6,10,11]

- Administer antipyretics, orally/rectally (e.g., acetaminophen, aspirin), as ordered.
  Avoid use of aspirin products in children (*may cause Reye's syndrome*) or in individuals with a clotting disorder or receiving anticoagulant therapy.
- Promote cooling by means of:
  Limiting clothing/dress in lightweight, loose-fitting clothes. *Encourages heat loss by radiation and conduction.*
  Cool the environment with air-conditioning or fans. *Promotes heat loss by convection.*
  Provide cool/tepid sponge baths or immersion if temperature is >104°F (*heat loss by evaporation and conduction*), or local ice packs, especially in groin and axillae (*areas of high blood flow*). Note: In pediatric clients, tepid water is preferred. Alcohol sponge baths are contraindicated *because they increase peripheral vascular constriction and CNS depression; cold-water sponges/immersion can increase shivering, producing heat.*
  Keep clothing and linens dry *to reduce shivering.*
  Monitor use of hypothermia blanket and wrap extremities with bath towels *to minimize shivering.* Turn off hypothermia blanket when core temperature is within 1° to 3° of desired temperature *to allow for downward drift.*
  Administer medications (e.g., dantrolene, chlorpromazine, or diazepam) as ordered, *to manage hyperthermia, control shivering and seizures.*
  Assist with internal cooling methods in presence of malignant hyperthermia *to promote rapid core cooling.*

- Provide hydration:
  Offer/force plenty of fluids, by appropriate route even if client is not thirsty *to replace fluids lost through perspiration and respiration.*
  Avoid alcohol and caffeinated beverages *(increases fluid loss by diuresis).*
   Administer replacement IV fluids and electrolytes *to support circulating volume and tissue perfusion and treat acid-base imbalance.*
- Promote client safety (e.g., maintain patent airway, padded side rails, quiet environment, mouth care for dry mucous membranes, skin protection from cold when hypothermia blanket is used, observation of equipment safety measures).
- Maintain bedrest *to reduce metabolic demands/oxygen consumption.*
- Provide supplemental oxygen *to offset increased oxygen demands and consumption.*
- Administer medications as indicated to treat underlying cause, such as antibiotics *(for infection)*, dantrolene *(for malignant hyperthermia)*, ß-blockers *(for thyroid storm).*
- Provide high-calorie diet, enteral/parenteral nutrition *to meet increased metabolic demands.*

NURSING PRIORITY NO. 4 To promote wellness (Teaching/Discharge Considerations):

- Teach parents how to measure child's temperature, at what body temperature to give antipyretic medications, and what symptoms to report to physician. *Low-grade fever enhances immune system functioning in presence of infection and is not harmful as long as individual is not dehydrated or susceptible to febrile seizures.*[3,7] *Fever may be treated at home to relieve the general discomfort and lethargy associated with fever. Fever is reportable, however, especially if it is unresponsive to antipyretics and fluids, because it often accompanies a treatable infection (viral or bacterial).*[5]
- Review with client/SO specific cause of hyperthermia. Helps to identify those factors that client can control (if any), such as *correction of underlying disease process (e.g., thyroid suppression medication); ways to protect oneself from excessive exposure to environmental heat (e.g., proper clothing, restriction of activity, scheduling outings during cooler part of day); and understanding of family traits (e.g., malignant hyperthermia reaction to anesthesia is often familial).*[9,11]
- Discuss importance of adequate fluid intake at all times and ways to improve hydration status when ill or when under stress (e.g., exercise, hot environment).
- Instruct families/caregivers (of young children, persons who are outdoors in very hot climate, elderly living alone) in dangers of heat exhaustion and heatstroke and ways to manage hot environments. Instruct parents to avoid leaving young children in unattended car. *Heat injuries can be immediately life-threatening. Being aware of environmental hazards and hydration levels can save one's life.*[8,12]
- Recommend avoidance of hot tubs/saunas as appropriate (e.g., client with cardiac conditions compromised by decreased cardiac output associated with peripheral vasodilation; pregnancy that may affect fetal development or increase maternal cardiac workload).
- Review signs/symptoms of hyperthermia (e.g., flushed skin, increased body temperature, increased respiratory/heart rate; fainting, loss of consciousness, seizures). *Indicates need for prompt intervention.*
- Identify community resources, especially for elderly clients, to address specific needs *(e.g., provision of fans for individual use, location of cooling rooms—usually in a community center—during heatwaves, daily telephone contact to assess wellness).*

Assessment/Reassessment

- Temperature and other assessment findings, including vital signs and state of mentation.

Planning

- Plan of care/interventions and who is involved in the planning.
- Teaching plan.

Implementation/Evaluation

- Responses to interventions/teaching and actions performed.
- Attainment/progress toward desired outcome(s).
- Modifications to plan of care.

Discharge Planning

- Referrals that are made, those responsible for actions to be taken.

References

1. Helman, R. S. (2002, update 2005). Heatstroke. Emedicine article. Accessed July 2007 at www.emedicine.com/med/topic956.htm.
2. Evidence-based clinical practice guideline of fever of uncertain source: Outpatient evaluation and management for children 2 months to 36 months of age. (2002). Cincinnati, OH: Cincinnati Children's Hospital Medical Center. Accessed July 2007 at www.guideline.gov/summary/summary.aspx?doc_id=5613.
3. Engel, J. (2002). *Mosby's Pocket Guide to Pediatric Assessment*. 4th ed. St. Louis, MO: Mosby.
4. Brody, G. M. (1994). Hyperthermia and hypothermia in the elderly. *Clin Geriatr Med,* 10, 213.
5. Doenges, M. E., Moorhouse, M. F., Geissler-Murr, A. C. (2004). *Nurse's Pocket Guide: Diagnoses, Interventions, and Rationales.* 9th ed. Philadelphia: F. A. Davis.
6. Sepsis/Septicemia. (2002). In Doenges, M. E., Moorhouse, M. F., Geissler-Murr, A. C. *Nursing Care Plans: Guidelines for Individualizing Patient Care.* 6th ed. Philadelphia: F. A. Davis, pp. 676–677.
7. Roberts, N. J. (1991). The immunological consequences of fever. In Mackowiak, P. A. (ed). *Fever: Basic Mechanisms and Management.* New York: Raven.
8. Curtis, R. (1997). Outdoor Action guide to heat related illnesses & fluid balance. Article for Princeton University Outdoor Action Web site. Accessed July 2007 at www.princeton.edu/~oa/safety/heatill.html.
9. Malignant Hyperthermia. (1989). Dantrolene-Medstudents-Anesthesiology. Fact Sheet. National Institute on Aging. U.S. Dept Health and Human Services.
10. Hoppe, J., Sinert, R. (2006). Heat exhaustion and heatstroke. Article for Emedicine Web site. Retrieved March 2007 at www.emedicine.com/emert/topic236.htm.
11. No author listed. (2005). Hyperthermia: Too hot for your health. Article for National Institute on Aging Web site. Retrieved March 2007 at www.niapublications/org/agepages/hyperther.asp.
12. Null, J. (2007). Hyperthermia deaths of children in vehicles. Fact sheet for San Fransisco State University department of Geosiences Web site. Retrieved March 2007 at http://ggweather.com/heat/.

Hypothermia

Definition: Body temperature below normal range

RELATED FACTORS

Exposure to cool environment [prolonged exposure (e.g., homeless, immersion in cold water/near-drowning; induced hypothermia/cardiopulmonary bypass)]

Inadequate clothing

Evaporation from skin in cool environment

Decreased ability to shiver
Aging [or very young]
[Debilitating] illness; trauma; damage to hypothalamus
Malnutrition; decreased metabolic rate; inactivity
Consumption of alcohol; medications [/drug overdose]

DEFINING CHARACTERISTICS

Objective
Body temperature below normal range
Shivering; piloerection
Cool skin
Pallor; slow capillary refill; cyanotic nailbeds
Hypertension; tachycardia
[Core temperature 95°F/35°C: increased respirations, poor judgment, shivering]
[Core temperature 95°F to 93.2°F/35° to 34°C: bradycardia or tachycardia, myocardial irritability/dysrhythmias, muscle rigidity, shivering, lethargic/confused, decreased coordination]
[Core temperature 93.2°F to 86°F/34°C to 30°C: hypoventilation, bradycardia, generalized rigidity, metabolic acidosis, coma]
[Core temperature below 86°F/30°C: no apparent vital signs, heart rate unresponsive to drug therapy, comatose, cyanotic, dilated pupils, apneic, areflexic, no shivering (appears dead)]

Sample Clinical Applications: Dementia, malnutrition/anorexia nervosa, brain trauma/stroke, endocrine disorders, some surgical procedures (e.g., craniotomy), alcohol intoxication, abuse/neglect, prematurity, near-drowning/cold water immersion

DESIRED OUTCOMES/EVALUATION CRITERIA
Sample NOC linkages:
Thermoregulation: Balance among heat production, heat gain, and heat loss
Thermoregulation: Newborn: Balance among heat production, heat gain, and heat loss during the first 28 days of life
Personal Safety Behavior: Personal actions of an adult to control behaviors that can cause physical injury

Client Will (Include Specific Time Frame)

- Display core temperature within normal range.
- Be free of complications such as cardiac failure, respiratory infection/failure, thromboembolic phenomena.
- Identify underlying cause/contributing factors that are within client control.
- Verbalize understanding of specific interventions to prevent hypothermia.
- Demonstrate behaviors to monitor and promote normothermia.

ACTIONS/INTERVENTIONS

Sample NIC linkages:
Hypothermia Treatment: Rewarming and surveillance of a patient whose core body temperature is below 35°C

Temperature Regulation: Attaining or maintaining body temperature within a normal range

Temperature Regulation: Intraoperative: Attaining or maintaining desired intraoperative body temperature

NURSING PRIORITY NO. 1 To assess causative/contributing factors:

• Note underlying cause, e.g., (1) *decreased heat production such as occurs with hypopituitary, hypoadrenal and hypothyroid conditions, hypoglycemia and neuromuscular inefficiencies seen in extremes of age;* (2) *increased heat loss (e.g., exposure to cold weather/winter outdoor activities; cold-water drenching or immersion, improper clothing/shelter/food for conditions; vasodilation from medications, drugs, or poisons; skin-surface problems such as burns or psoriasis; fluid losses/dehydration; surgery, open wounds/exposed skin/viscera; multiple rapid infusions of cold solutions or transfusions of banked blood; overtreatment of hyperthermia);* (3) *impaired thermoregulation (e.g., hypothalamus failure such as might occur with CNS trauma or tumor; intracranial bleeding/stroke; toxicological and metabolic disorders; Parkinson's disease, multiple sclerosis).*[1,2,5,6]

 • Note contributing factors: age of client (e.g., premature neonate, child, elderly person); concurrent/coexisting medical problems (e.g., brainstem injury, CNS trauma; near-drowning, sepsis, hypothyroidism); other factors (e.g., alcohol/other drug use/abuse; homelessness); nutrition status (e.g., thin tall person loses heat easier than short stature, fat person); living condition/relationship status (e.g., aged/cognitive impaired client living alone).[1,2,5]

NURSING PRIORITY NO. 2 To prevent further decrease in body temperature:

Mild-to-moderate hypothermia:[1–6]

Remove wet clothing/bedding.

Add layers of clothing, wrap in warm blankets.

Increase physical activity if possible.

Provide warm liquids after shivering stops if client is alert and can swallow.

Provide warm nutrient-dense food (carbohydrates, proteins, and fats) and fluids (hot sweet liquids are easily digestible and absorbable).

Avoid alcohol, caffeine, and tobacco (*to prevent vasodilation, diuresis, or vasoconstriction, respectively*).

Place in warm ambient temperature environment, protect from drafts; provide external heat sources.

Prevent pooling of antiseptic/irrigating solutions under client in operating room; cover skin areas outside of operative field; wrap in warmed blankets.

Provide stocking hat for newborn; place under open radiant warmer/in isolette, or use heating blanket—monitoring temperature closely.

Severe hypothermia:[1–6]

Remove client from causative/contributing factors.

Dry the skin, cover with blankets, provide shelter with warm ambient temperature; use radiant lights.

Provide heat to trunk, not to extremities, initially. Avoid use of heat lamps or hot water bottles. *Surface rewarming can result in rewarming shock due to surface vasodilation.*

Keep individual lying down. Avoid jarring (*can trigger an abnormal heart rhythm*).

NURSING PRIORITY NO. 3 To evaluate effects of hypothermia:

- Measure core temperature with low register thermometer (measuring below 94°F/34°C).
- Assess respiratory effort (*rate and tidal volume are reduced when metabolic rate decreases and respiratory acidosis occurs*).
- Auscultate lungs, noting adventitious sounds. *Pulmonary edema, respiratory infection, and pulmonary embolus are potential complications of hypothermia.*
- Monitor heart rate and rhythm. *Cold stress reduces pacemaker function, and bradycardia (unresponsive to atropine), atrial fibrillation, atrioventricular blocks, and ventricular tachycardia can occur. Ventricular fibrillation occurs most frequently when core temperature is 82°F/28°C or below.*[1,2,4,5]
- Monitor blood pressure, noting hypotension. *Can occur due to vasoconstriction, and shunting of fluids as a result of cold injury effect on capillary permeability.*
- Measure urine output. *Oliguria/renal failure can occur due to low flow state and/or following hypothermic osmotic diuresis.*
- Note CNS effects (e.g., mood changes, sluggish thinking, amnesia, complete obtundation); and peripheral CNS effects (e.g., paralysis—87.7°F/31°C; dilated pupils—below 86°F/30°C; flat EEG—68°F/20°C).[1,2,4,5]
- Monitor laboratory studies such as ABGs (*respiratory and metabolic acidosis*); electrolytes; CBC (*increased hematocrit, decreased white blood cell count*); cardiac enzymes (*myocardial infarct may occur owing to electrolyte imbalance, cold stress catecholamine release, hypoxia, or acidosis*); coagulation profile; glucose; pharmacological profile (*for possible cumulative drug effects*).

NURSING PRIORITY NO. 4 To restore normal body temperature/organ function:

- Assist with surface warming. Cover head/neck and thorax, leaving extremities uncovered as appropriate *to maintain peripheral vasoconstriction*. Note: Do not institute surface rewarming prior to core rewarming in severe hypothermia (*causes afterdrop of temperature by shunting cold blood back to heart in addition to rewarming shock as a result of surface vasodilation*).[1–4]
- Assist with core rewarming measures, such as warmed IV solutions and warm-solution lavage of body cavities (gastric, peritoneal, bladder) or cardiopulmonary bypass if indicated to normalize core temperature. Rewarm no faster than 1°F to 2°F per hour *to avoid sudden vasodilation, increased metabolic demands on heart, and hypotension (rewarming shock).*[5,6]
- Protect skin/tissues by repositioning, applying lotion/lubricants, and avoiding direct contact with heating appliance/blanket. *Impaired circulation can result in severe tissue damage.*
- Keep client quiet; handle gently *to reduce potential for fibrillation in cold heart.*
- Provide CPR as necessary, with compressions initially at one-half normal heart rate. *Severe hypothermia causes slowed conduction, and cold heart may be unresponsive to medications, pacing, and defibrillation.*[4,6,7]
- Maintain patent airway. Assist with intubation if indicated. Provide heated, humidified oxygen when used.
- Turn off warming blanket when temperature is within 1°F to 3°F of desired temperature *to accommodate drift/avoid hyperthermia situation.*
- Administer IV fluids with caution *to prevent overload as the vascular bed expands. Cold heart is slow to compensate for increased volume.*
- Avoid vigorous use of pharmacological therapy. *As rewarming occurs, organ function returns, correcting endocrine abnormalities, and tissues become more receptive to the effects of drugs previously administered, creating risk for overdose.*

- Perform range-of-motion exercises, provide support hose/sequential compression device (SCDs), reposition, encourage coughing/deep-breathing exercises, avoid restrictive clothing/restraints *to reduce effects of circulatory stasis.*
- Provide well-balanced, high-calorie diet/feedings *to replenish glycogen stores and nutritional balance.*

NURSING PRIORITY NO. 5 To promote wellness (Teaching/Discharge Considerations):

- Review specific risk factors/causes of hypothermia. Note that hypothermia can be accidental (see Related Factors) or intentional (*such as occurs when induced-hypothermia therapy is used after cardiac arrest or brain injury*) requiring interventions to protect client from adverse affects.[6,7]
- Identify factors that client can control (if any), such as protection from environment/adequate heat in home; layering clothing and blankets; minimize heat loss from head with hat/scarf; appropriate cold-weather clothing; avoidance of alcohol/other drugs if anticipating exposure to cold; potential risk for future hypersensitivity to cold, etc.
- Discuss signs/symptoms of early hypothermia (e.g., changes in mentation, somnolence, impaired coordination, slurred speech) *to facilitate recognition of problem and timely intervention. Information may be especially important if client works or plays outdoors (e.g., camping, skiing, hiking).*[1,2,5]
- Identify assistive community resources, as indicated (social services, emergency shelters, clothing suppliers, food bank, public service company, financial resources, etc.). *Individual/SO may be in need of numerous resources if hypothermia was associated with inadequate housing, homelessness, malnutrition.*

DOCUMENTATION FOCUS

Assessment/Reassessment

- Findings, noting degree of system involvement, respiratory rate, ECG pattern, capillary refill, and level of mentation.
- Graph temperature.

Planning

- Plan of care and who is involved in planning.
- Teaching plan.

Implementation/Evaluation

- Responses to interventions/teaching, actions performed.
- Attainment/progress toward desired outcome(s).
- Modifications to plan of care.

Discharge Planning

- Long-term needs, identifying who is responsible for each action.

References

1. Curtis, R. (2002). Outdoor Action guide to hypothermia and cold weather injuries. Princeton University Outdoor Action Web site. Accessed July 2007 at www.princeton.edu/~oa/safety/hypocold.html.

Cultural Collaborative Community/Home Care Diagnostic Studies Pediatric/Geriatric/Lifespan Medications

2. Decker, W., et al. (2001, updated 2005). Hypothermia. Article for Emedicine Web site. Accessed July 2007 at www.emedicine.com/emerg/topic279.htm.
3. Surgical Intervention. (2002). In Doenges, M. E., Moorhouse, M. F., Geissler-Murr, A. C. *Nursing Care Plans: Guidelines for Individualizing Patient Care*. 6th ed. Philadelphia: F. A. Davis, pp. 771–772.
4. State of Alaska cold injuries and cold water near drowning guidelines. (Revised 2003). Accessed July 2007 at www.chems.alaska.gov/EMS/documents/AKColdInj2005.pdf.
5. Li, J., Decker, W. (2005). Hypothermia. Article for Emedicine Web site. Retrieved March 2007 at www.emedicine.com/emerg/topic279.htm.
6. Good, K. K., Verble, J. A., Secrest, J. et al. (2006) Postoperative hypothermia—the chilling consequences. *AORN*, 83(5), 1055–1066.
7. Calver, P., Braungardt, T., Kupchik, N., et al. (2005). The big chill: Improving the odds after cardiac arrest. CE Home Study Program for RNweb. Retrieved March 2007 at www.rnweb.com.

disturbed personal Identity

Definition: Inability to distinguish between self and nonself

RELATED FACTORS

To be developed by nurse researchers and submitted to NANDA
[Organic brain syndrome; traumatic brain injury]
[Poor ego differentiation, as in schizophrenia]
[Panic/dissociative states]
[Biochemical body change, e.g., eating disorders]
[Illness/trauma affecting body image, e.g., multiple sclerosis, amputation]

DEFINING CHARACTERISTICS

To be developed by nurse researchers and submitted to NANDA

Subjective
[Confusion about sense of self, purpose or direction in life, sexual identification/preference]
[Questioning "Who am I?"; what does it take to be a person as opposed to a nonperson]

Objective
[Difficulty in making decisions]
[Poorly differentiated ego boundaries]
[Problems with physical ability to move as desired]
[See ND Anxiety for additional characteristics]

Sample Clinical Applications: Schizophrenia, dissociative disorders, borderline personality disorder, developmental delay, autism, gender identity conflict, dementia, traumatic injury (e.g., amputation, spinal cord injury, brain injury)

DESIRED OUTCOMES/EVALUATION CRITERIA

Sample NOC linkages:
Identity: Distinguish between self and nonself and characterize one's essence
Distorted Thought Self-Control: Self-restraint of disruption in perception, thought processes, and thought content
Anxiety Self-Control: Personal actions to eliminate or reduce feelings of apprehension, tension, or uneasiness from an unidentifiable source

Client Will (Include Specific Time Frame)

- Acknowledge threat to personal identity.
- Integrate threat in a healthy, positive manner (e.g., state anxiety is reduced, make plans for the future).
- Verbalize acceptance of changes that have occurred.
- State ability to identify and accept self (long-term outcome).

ACTIONS/INTERVENTIONS

Sample NIC linkages:

Self-Esteem Enhancement: Assisting a patient to increase his or her personal judgment of self-worth

Self-Awareness Enhancement: Assisting a patient to explore and understand his or her thoughts, feelings, motivations, and behaviors

Decision-Making Support: Providing information and support for a person who is making a decision regarding healthcare

NURSING PRIORITY NO. 1 To assess causative/contributing factors:

- Ascertain client's perception of the extent of the threat to self and how client is handling the situation. *Many factors can affect an individual's self-image: illness (chronic or terminal), injuries, changes in body structure (amputation, spinal cord damage, burns), and client's view of what has happened will affect development of plan of care and interventions to be used.*[1,6]

- Determine speed of occurrence of threat. *An event, such as an accident or sudden diagnosis of diabetes, cancer, that has happened quickly may be more threatening.*[7]

- Have client define own body image. *Body image is the basis of personal identity, and changes that prevent individual from achieving ideals and expectancies can have a negative impact. Erickson's stages of psychosocial development describe an identity crisis during the teenage years as a struggle between feelings of identity versus role confusion.*[1]

- Note age of client. *An adolescent may struggle with the developmental task of personal/sexual identity, whereas an older person may have more difficulty accepting/dealing with a threat to identity, such as progressive loss of memory, or aging body changes.*[3]

- Assess availability and use of support systems. Note response of family/SO(s). *During stressful situations, support is essential for client to cope with changes that are occurring. Engaging family in choosing supportive interventions will help client and family members deal with situation/illness.*[3]

- Note withdrawn/automatic behavior, regression to earlier developmental stage, general behavioral disorganization, or display of self-mutilation behaviors in adolescent or adult; delayed development, preference for solitary play, display of self-stimulation in child. *Indicators of poor coping skills and need for specific interventions to help client develop sense of self and identity. Inability to identify self interferes with interactions with others.*[3]

- Be aware of physical signs of panic state. *Presence of severe anxiety state may progress to panic when concerns seem overwhelming to client.* (Refer to ND Anxiety.)

- Determine presence of hallucinations/delusions, distortions of reality. *Indicators of presence of psychosis and need for immediate interventions to deal with inability to distinguish between self and nonself.*[1,3]

⊕ Cultural ⒶCollaborative 🏠 Community/Home Care ✏ Diagnostic Studies ∞ Pediatric/Geriatric/Lifespan ⚕ Medications

NURSING PRIORITY NO. 2 To assist client to manage/deal with threat:

- Make time to listen/Active-listen to client, encouraging appropriate expression of feelings, including anger and hostility. *Conveys a sense of confidence in client's ability to identify extent of threat, how it is affecting sense of identity, and how to deal with feelings in acceptable ways.*[7,8]
- Note use of alcohol/other drugs. *Individual may turn to these substances to relieve painful feelings, especially in the presence of fearful diagnoses (e.g., cancer, multiple sclerosis).*[8]
- Provide calm environment. *Feelings of anxiety are contagious, and calm surroundings can help client to relax/maintain control and be able to think more clearly about how illness/situation can be managed effectively.*[9]
- Use crisis-intervention principles when indicated. *May be necessary to help client restore equilibrium when situation escalates.*[1]
- Discuss client's commitment to an identity. *Those who have made a strong commitment to an identity tend to be more comfortable with self and happier than those who have not.*[3]
- Assist client to develop strategies to cope with threat to identity. *Reduces anxiety, promotes self-awareness, and enhances self-esteem, enabling client to deal with threat more realistically.*[10]
- Engage client in activities appropriate to individual situation. *Using activities such as a mirror for visual feedback, tactile stimulation to reconnect with parts of the body (amputation, unilateral neglect), can help to identify self as an individual.*[2]
- Provide for simple decisions, concrete tasks, calming activities. *Promotes sense of control and positive expectations to enable client to regain sense of self.*[3]
- Allow client to deal with situation in small steps. *May have difficulty coping with larger picture when in stress overload. Taking small steps promotes feelings of success and ability to manage illness/situation.*[9]
- Encourage client to develop/participate in an individualized exercise program. *While walking is an excellent beginning program, it is helpful to choose activities that client enjoys. Exercise releases endorphins, thereby reducing stress and anxiety, promoting a sense of well-being.*[1]
- Provide concrete assistance as needed. *Until basic-level needs, such as ADLs and food, are met, individual is unable to deal with higher-level needs. Once these needs are met, client can begin to deal with threat to identity.*[1]
- Take advantage of opportunities to promote growth. Realize that client will have difficulty learning while in a dissociative state. *Alterations in mental status can interfere with ability to process information, and new information can increase confusion and disorientation.*[3]
- Maintain reality orientation without confronting client's irrational beliefs. *Client may become defensive, blocking opportunity to look at other possibilities. Arguing does not change the perceptions and can interfere with/damage nurse-client relationship.*[1]
- Use humor judiciously when appropriate. *While humor can lift spirits and provide a moment of levity, it is important to note the mood/receptiveness of the client before using it.*[3]
- Discuss options for dealing with issues of gender identity. *Identification of client's concerns about role dysfunction/conflicting feelings about sexual identity will indicate need for therapy, possible gender-change surgery when client is a transsexual, or other available choices.*[2]
- Refer to NDs disturbed Body Image, Self-Esteem [specify], Spiritual Distress.

NURSING PRIORITY NO. 3 To promote wellness (Teaching/Discharge Considerations):

- Provide accurate information about threat to and potential consequences for individual in current situation. *Fear and anxiety regarding the threat represented by the illness/situation can be potentiated by lack of knowledge, unknown consequences, and inaccurate beliefs. Accurate information can help client incorporate new knowledge into changed self-concept.*[7]

• Assist client and SO(s) to acknowledge and integrate threat into future planning. *A diagnosis, accident, etc., can require major life changes, such as wearing identification bracelet when prone to mental confusion; a new lifestyle to accommodate change of gender for transsexual client; diet and medication routine with the diagnosis of diabetes mellitus. Planning can help the client to make the changes required to move forward with new life.*[4,5]

• Refer to appropriate support groups. *May need additional assistance, such as day-care program, counseling/psychotherapy, gender identity, family/marriage counseling, parenting classes.*[2]

DOCUMENTATION FOCUS

Assessment/Reassessment

• Findings, noting degree of impairment.
• Nature of and client's perception of the threat.

Planning

• Plan of care and who is involved in the planning.
• Teaching plan.

IMPLEMENTATION/EVALUATION

• Client's response to interventions/teaching and actions performed.
• Attainment/progress toward desired outcome(s).
• Modifications to plan of care.

Discharge Planning

• Long-term needs and who is responsible for actions to be taken.
• Specific referrals made.

References

1. Townsend, M. (2006). *Psychiatric Mental Health Nursing: Concepts of Care.* 5th ed. Philadelphia: F. A. Davis.
2. Doenges, M., Moorhouse, M., Murr, A. (2006). *Nursing Care Plans, Guidelines for Individualizing Patient Care.* 7th ed. Philadelphia: F. A. Davis.
3. Doenges, M., Townsend, M., Moorhouse, M. (1998). *Psychiatric Care Plans: Guidelines for Individualizing Care.* 3d ed. Philadelphia: F. A. Davis.
4. Pinhas-Hamiel, O., Dolan, L. M., et al. (1996). Increased incidence of non-insulin-dependent diabetes mellitus among adolescents. *J Pediatr,* 128(8), 608.
5. Deckelbaum, R. J., Williams, C. L. (2001). Childhood obesity: The health issue. *Obesity Res,* 9(5), 239s.
6. Badger, J. M. (2001). Burns: The psychological aspect. *AJN,* 101(11), 38–41.
7. Bartol, T. (2002). Putting a patient with diabetes in the driver's seat. *Nursing,* 32(2), 53–55.
8. Bruera, E., et al. (1995). The frequency of alcoholism among patients with pain due to terminal cancer. *J Pain Symptom Management,* 10(8), 599–603.
9. Paice, J. (2002). Managing psychological conditions in palliative care. *AJN,* 102(11), 36–43.
10. Cox, H., Hinz, M., Lubno, M. A., Newfield, S., Ridenour, N., Slater, M., Sridaromont, K. (2002). *Clinical Applications of Nursing Diagnosis: Adult, Child, Women's Psychiatric, Gerontic and Home Health Considerations.* 4th ed. Philadelphia: F. A. Davis.

readiness for enhanced Immunization Status

Definition: A pattern of conforming to local, national, or international standards of immunization to prevent infectious disease(s) that is sufficient to protect a person, family, or community and can be strengthened

🌐 Cultural 🔗 Collaborative 🏠 Community/Home Care 🧪 Diagnostic Studies ∞ Pediatric/Geriatric/Lifespan 💊 Medications

RELATED FACTORS
To be developed by nurse researchers and submitted to NANDA

DEFINING CHARACTERISTICS

Subjective
Expresses desire to enhance:
Knowledge of immunization standards
Immunization status
Identification of providers of immunizations
Record-keeping of immunizations
Identification of possible problems associated with immunizations
Behavior to prevent infectious diseases

Sample Clinical Applications: Traumatic brain injury (TBI), cerebral edema, cranial tumors/hematomas, hydrocephalus

DESIRED OUTCOMES/EVALUATION CRITERIA
Sample NOC linkages:
Immunization Behavior: Personal actions to obtain immunization to prevent a communicable disease

Client Will (Include Specific Time Frame)

- Express understanding of immunization recommendations.
- Develop plan to obtain appropriate immunizations.
- Identify/adopt behaviors to reduce risk of infectious disease.
- Maintain and update immunization records.

Community Health Status: Immunity: Resistance of community members to the invasion and spread of an infectious agent that could threaten public health

Community Will (Include Specific Time Frame)

- Provide information to community regarding immunization requirements/recommendations.
- Identify underserved populations requiring immunization support and ways to meet their needs.
- Develop a plan to provide mass immunizations in time of major threat/disease outbreak.

ACTIONS/INTERVENTIONS

Sample NIC linkages:
Immunization/Vaccination Management: Monitoring immunization status, facilitating access to immunizations, and providing immunizations to prevent communicable disease

NURSING PRIORITY NO. 1 To determine current immunization status:

- Assess client's history of immunizations. *Response may vary widely, depending on client's age (infant to adult), cultural influences, travel history, family beliefs about immunization, and medical conditions (e.g., some vaccines should not be given to children with certain cancers or persons taking immunosuppressant drugs or with serious allergies to eggs).*[1]

- Ascertain motivation/expectations for change. *Motivation to improve and high expectations can encourage client to make changes that will improve his or her life. However, unrealistic expectations may hamper efforts.*
- Determine if adult client works in/frequents high-risk areas (e.g., doctor's office, home care, homeless or immigrant shelters or clinics, correctional facility, international travel) *to review potential exposures and determine new vaccines or boosters client may need.*
- Address client/SO concerns (e.g., client may wonder if annual flu shots are truly beneficial or whether adult boosters may be needed for particular immunizations received in childhood; parent is concerned about safety of vaccine supply). *Helps to clarify plans and deal with misconceptions or myths.*[2]
- Ascertain/discuss conditions that may preclude client receiving specific immunizations *(e.g., history of prior adverse reaction, current fever/illness, pregnancy, undergoing cancer/other immunosuppressant treatments).*
- Review community plan for dealing with imunnizations/disease outbreak. *Identifies strengths to build on and limitations to be addressed.*

NURSING PRIORITY NO. 2 To assist client/SO/community to develop/strengthen plan to meet identified needs:

- Review parents' knowledge/information regarding immunizations recommended/required to enter school: (1) prior to kindergarten (e.g., hepatitis B, rotavirus, H influenza, mumps/measles/rubella, varicella, and hepatitis A; (2) by junior high/middle school age: tetanus/diphtheria/pertussis; human papillomavirus; (3) for college freshmen planning to live in dorm: meningitis *to document status, plan for boosters, and/or discuss appropriate intervals for follow-up.*[1-4]
- Examine/discuss protective benefit of each vaccine, route of administration, expected side effects, and potential adverse reactions. *Information necessary for client/SO to make informed decisions.*
- Discuss appropriate time intervals for all recommended immunizations, as well as catch-up and booster options for children birth to 18 years.[4]
- Review travel requirements for client preparing for international travel *to ascertain potential for contracting vaccine-preventable disease in geographic area of client's travel so that vaccines can be provided if needed.*[3]
- Inform of exemptions when client/SO desires. *Some states permit medical, religious, personal, and philosophical exemptions when parent does not want child to participate in immunization programs.*[5] Refer to appropriate care providers for further discussion/intervention.
- Define and discuss current needs and anticipated or projected concerns of community health-promotion programs. *Agreement on scope/parameters of needs is essential for effective planning.*
- Prioritize goals *to facilitate accomplishment.*
- Identify available community resources (e.g., persons, groups, financial, governmental, as well as other communities). *Inclusion of all stakeholders enhances support for plan and increases likelihood of success.*
- Seek out and involve underserved/at-risk groups within the community. *Supports communication and commitment of community as a whole.*

NURSING PRIORITY NO. 3 To promote optimum wellness:

- Review reasons to continue immunization programs. *Viruses and bacteria that cause vaccine-preventable disease and death still exist and can be passed on to people who are not protected, increasing medical, social, and economic costs.*[6]

⊕ Cultural ⊛ Collaborative 🏠 Community/Home Care ⟋ Diagnostic Studies ∞ Pediatric/Geriatric/Lifespan ✎ Medications

- Provide reliable vaccine information in written form or Web sites (e.g., brochures/facts sheets form CDC, American Academy of Pediatrics, National Network for Immunization Information, etc.). *Allows client/SO to review at own pace in order to make informed decisions.*[1-4]
- Identify community resources for obtaining immunizations such as Public Health Department/community clinic, family physician.
- Discuss management of common side effect symptoms (e.g., muscle pain, rash, fever, site swelling).
- Support development of community plans for maintaining/enhancing efforts *to increase immunization level of population.*
- Establish mechanism for self-monitoring of community needs and evaluation of efforts.
- Use multiple formats for client instruction (e.g., TV, radio, print media, billboards, and computer bulletin boards, speakers' bureau, reports to community leaders/groups on file and accessible to the public), *to keep community informed regarding immunization needs, disease prevention.*

DOCUMENTATION FOCUS

Assessment/Reassessment

- Assessment findings of immunization status, potential risks/disease exposure.
- Identified areas of concern, strengths/limitations.
- Understanding of immunization needs/safety, and disease prevention.
- Motivation and expectations for change.

Planning

- Action plan and who is involved in planning.
- Teaching plan.

Implementation/Evaluation

- Individual/family responses to interventions/teaching and actions performed.
- Response of community entities to the actions performed.
- Attainment/progress toward desired outcome(s).
- Modifications to plan.

Discharge Planning

- Identified needs/referrals for follow-up care, support systems.
- Short-range and long-range plans to deal with current, anticipated, and potential community needs and who is responsible for follow-through.
- Specific referrals made, coalitions formed.

References

1. Mosocco, D. (2007). Clipboard: Childhood vaccines. *Home Healthcare Nurse,* 25(1), 7–8.
2. Engle, J. (2002). *Mosby's Pocket Guide to Pediatric Assessment.* 4th ed. St. Louis, MO: Mosby.
3. Center for Disease Control and Prevention. (2007). Adult immunization schedule. Fact sheet for National Immunization Program. Retrieved March 2007 at www.cdc.gov/nip.
4. Center for Disease Control and Prevention. (2006). Recommended immunization schedules for persons aged 0–18 years—United States. *MMWR,* 55, (51–52), Q1–Q4.

5. Salmon, D. A., Moulton, L.H., Omer, S. B., et al. (2005). Factors associated with refusal of childhood vaccines among parents of school-aged children: A case-control. *Arch Pediatr Adolesc Med,* 159(5), 470–476.
6. Center for Disease Control and Prevention. (2003). What would happen if we stopped vaccinations? Fact sheet for National Immunization Program. Retrieved March 2007 at www.cdc.gov/nip.

disorganized Infant Behavior

Definition: Disintegrated physiological and neurobehavioral responses of infant to the environment

RELATED FACTORS

Prenatal
Congenital/genetic disorders; teratogenic exposure; [exposure to drugs]

Postnatal
Prematurity; oral/motor problems; feeding intolerance; malnutrition
Invasive procedures; pain

Individual
Gestational/postconceptual age; immature neurological system
Illness; [infection]; [hypoxia/birth asphyxia]

Environmental
Physical environment inappropriateness
Sensory inappropriateness/overstimulation/deprivation
Lack of containment within environment

Caregiver
Cue misreading; cue knowledge deficit
Environmental stimulation contribution

DEFINING CHARACTERISTICS

Objective
Regulatory Problems
Inability to inhibit startle; irritability
State-Organization System
Active-awake (fussy, worried gaze); quiet-awake (staring, gaze aversion)
Diffuse sleep; state-oscillation
Irritable crying
Attention-Interaction System
Abnormal response to sensory stimuli (e.g., difficult to soothe, inability to sustain alert status)
Motor System
Finger splay; fisting; hands to face; hyperextension of extremities
Tremors; startles; twitches; jittery; uncoordinated movement
Changes to motor tone; altered primitive reflexes
Physiological
Bradycardia; tachycardia; arrhythmias

Cultural   Collaborative   Community/Home Care   Diagnostic Studies   Pediatric/Geriatric/Lifespan   Medications

Skin color changes

"Time-out signals" (e.g., gaze, grasp, hiccough, cough, sneeze, sigh, slack jaw, open mouth, tongue thrust)

Feeding intolerances

Sample Clinical Applications: Prematurity, congenital/genetic disorders, meconium aspiration, respiratory distress syndrome, small for gestational age

DESIRED OUTCOMES/EVALUATION CRITERIA

Sample NOC linkage:

Neurological Status: Ability of the peripheral and central nervous system to receive, process, and respond to internal and external stimuli

Infant Will (Include Specific Time Frame)

- Exhibit organized behaviors that allow the achievement of optimal potential for growth and development as evidenced by modulation of physiological, motor, state, and attentional-interactive functioning.

Sample NOC linkages:

Child Development: [specify age group]: Milestones of physical, cognitive, and psychosocial progression by [specify] months of age

Growth: Normal increase in bone size and body weight during growth years

Parent/Caregiver Will (Include Specific Time Frame)

- Recognize individual infant cues.
- Identify appropriate responses (including environmental modifications) to infant's cues.
- Verbalize readiness to assume caregiving independently.

ACTIONS/INTERVENTIONS

Sample NIC linkages:

Environmental Management: Manipulation of the patient's surroundings for therapeutic benefit

Developmental Care: Structuring the environment and providing care in response to the behavioral cues and states of the preterm infant

Newborn Care: Management of neonate during the transition to extrauterine life and subsequent period of stabilization

NURSING PRIORITY NO. 1 To assess causative/contributing factors:

- Determine infant's chronological and developmental age; note length of gestation. *These factors (prematurity, infant maturity, and stages of development) help to determine plan of care.*[1,2,5]
- Observe for cues suggesting presence of situations that may result in pain/discomfort. *Some behavior that appears to be disorganized may be caused by a pain source that once identified may be alleviated.*[1]
- Determine adequacy of physiological support. *Identifies areas of additional need.*[1]

- Evaluate level/appropriateness of environmental stimuli. *Infant behavior is affected by a wide range of stimuli. Careful assessment narrows focus of concerns.*[2]
- Ascertain parents' understanding of infant's needs/abilities. *Identifies knowledge base and areas of learning needed.*[2–4]
- Listen to parents' concerns about their capabilities to meet infant's needs. *Active-listening can reassure parents, pinpoint areas to be addressed, as well as provide opportunity to correct misconceptions.*[2,3]

NURSING PRIORITY NO. 2 To assist parents in providing co-regulation to the infant:

- Provide a calm, nurturant physical and emotional environment. *Provides optimal infant comfort. Models behavior for parent(s) and optimizes learning.*[2,3]
- Encourage parents to hold infant, including skin-to-skin contact as appropriate. *Touch enhances parent-infant bonding, as well as provides means of calming.*[3] *Research suggests skin-to-skin contact/Kangaroo Care (KC) may have a positive effect on infant development by enhancing neurophysiological organization as well as an indirect effect by improving parental mood, perceptions, and interactive behavior.*[6]
- Model gentle handling of baby and appropriate responses to infant behavior. *Provides cues to parent.*[3]
- Support and encourage parents to be with infant and participate actively in all aspects of care. *Situation may seem overwhelming to new parents. Emotional and physical support enhances coping. Parents who are able to help in the care of their infant express lower levels of helplessness and powerlessness.*[1,2]
- Provide positive feedback for progressive parental involvement in caregiving process. *Transfer of care from staff to parents progresses along a continuum as parents' confidence level increases, and they are able to take on more complex care activities.*[7]
- Discuss infant growth/development, pointing out current status and progressive expectations as appropriate. *Augments parent knowledge of co-regulation.*[2]
- Incorporate the parents' observations and suggestions into plan of care. *Demonstrates valuing of parents' input and encourages continued involvement.*[2,4]

NURSING PRIORITY NO. 3 To deliver care within the infant's stress threshold:

- Provide a consistent caregiver. *Facilitates recognition of infant cues/changes in behavior. Communication is optimized if family is familiar with caregiver.*[2]
- Identify infant's individual self-regulatory behaviors (e.g., sucking, mouthing; grasp, hand-to-mouth, face behaviors; foot clasp, brace; limb flexion, trunk tuck; boundary seeking).
- Support hands to mouth and face; offer pacifier or nonnutritive sucking at the breast with gavage feedings. *Provides opportunities for infant to self-regulate.*[2]
- Avoid aversive oral stimulation, such as routine oral suctioning; suction ET tube only when clinically indicated. *Maximizes infant comfort, preventing undue/noxious stimulation.*[1,2]
- Use oxy-hood large enough to cover the infant's chest so arms will be inside the hood. *Allows for hand-to-mouth self-calming activities during this therapy.*[2]
- Provide opportunities for infant to grasp. *Helps with development of motor function skills.*[2]
- Provide boundaries or containment during all activities. Use swaddling, nesting, bunting, caregiver's hands as indicated. *Enhances infant's feelings of security and safeness. Avoids startle reflex and accompanying distress.*[2,3]
- Allow adequate time/opportunities to hold infant. Handle infant very gently, move infant smoothly, slowly, and contained, avoiding sudden/abrupt movements. *Provides comfort to infant and models behavior to parent(s).*[3]

🌐 Cultural ⓐ Collaborative 🏠 Community/Home Care 🧪 Diagnostic Studies ∞ Pediatric/Geriatric/Lifespan 💊 Medications

- Maintain normal alignment, position infant with limbs softly flexed, shoulders and hips adducted slightly. Use appropriate-sized diapers. *Avoids unnecessary discomfort.*[2]
- Evaluate chest for adequate expansion, placing rolls under trunk if prone position indicated. *Provides for ease of respirations.*[2]
- Avoid restraints, including at IV sites. If IV board is necessary, secure to limb positioned in normal alignment. *Optimizes comfort and movement.*[1,2]
- Provide a sheepskin, egg-crate mattress, waterbed, or gel pillow/mattress for infant who does not tolerate frequent position changes. *Minimizes tissue pressure and risk of tissue injury.*[2]
- Visually assess color, respirations, activity, invasive lines without disturbing infant. Assess with "hands on" every 4 hours as indicated and PRN. *Allows for undisturbed rest/quiet periods.*[2,3]
- Schedule daily activities, time for rest, and organization of sleep/wake states to maximize tolerance of infant. Defer routine care when infant in quiet sleep. *Gives infant a sense of routine and also provides for undisturbed rest/quiet periods.*[2,3]
- Provide care with baby in side-lying position. Begin by talking softly to the baby, then placing hands in containing hold on baby, allow baby to prepare. Proceed with least invasive manipulations first. *Gradual build from comforting touch, to nursing care, to invasive interventions decreases overall stress of infant. Shortens perception of "being bothered" time and facilitates more rapid calming phase.*[3]
- Respond promptly to infant's agitation or restlessness. Provide "time-out" when infant shows early cues of overstimulation. Comfort and support the infant after stressful interventions. *Decreases stress for both infant and family. Facilitates calming phase.*[3]
- Remain at infant's bedside for several minutes after procedures/caregiving to monitor infant's response and provide necessary support. *Allows for more rapid intervention(s) if infant becomes overstressed.*[3]
- Administer analgesics as individually appropriate. *Maintains optimal comfort.*[1–4]

NURSING PRIORITY NO. 4   To modify the environment to provide appropriate stimulation:

- Introduce stimulation as a single mode and assess individual tolerance.
Light/Vision
- Reduce lighting perceived by infant, introduce diurnal lighting (and activity) when infant achieves physiological stability. (Daylight levels of 20 to 30 candles and nightlight levels of less than 10 candles are suggested.) Change light levels gradually to allow infant time to adjust. *Lowering light levels reduces visual stimulation, provides comforting environment. Diurnal lighting allows the stable infant to begin perception of day and night cycles and to establish circadian rhythms.*[1]
- Protect the infant's eyes from bright illumination during examinations/procedures, as well as from indirect sources such as neighboring phototherapy treatments. *Prevents retinal damage and reduces visual stressors.*[2]
- Deliver phototherapy (when required) with Biliblanket devices if available. *Alleviates need for eye patches to protect vision.*[2]
- Provide caregiver face (preferably parent's) as visual stimulus when infant shows readiness (awake, attentive). *Begins process of visual recognition.*[1]

Sound

- Identify sources of noise in environment and eliminate/reduce *to minimize auditory stimulus, reduces startle response in infant, provides comforting environment:*[2]
Speak in a low voice.
Reduce volume on alarms/telephones to safe but not excessive volume.

Nursing Diagnoses in Alphabetical Order

Pad metal trash can lids.

Open paper packages such as IV tubing and suction catheters slowly and at a distance from bedside.

Conduct rounds/report away from bedside.

Place soft/thick fabric such as blanket rolls and toys near infant's head *to absorb sound.*

Keep all incubator portholes closed, closing with two hands *to avoid loud snap with closure and associated startle response.*

- Refrain from playing musical toys or tape players inside incubator. *Even very soft sounds echo in an enclosed space. What an adult may find soothing is likely to overstimulate an infant.*[2,3]
- Avoid placing items on top of incubator; if necessary to do so, pad surface well. *Contact with the external parts of the incubator causes reverberation inside the chamber.*
- Conduct regular decibel checks of interior noise level in incubator (recommended not to exceed 60 dB). *Verifies that decibel levels are within acceptable range.*[2]
- Provide auditory stimulation to console, support infant before and through handling or to reinforce restfulness. *Provides modeling of behavior for family and increased comfort for infant.*[3]

Olfactory

- Be cautious in exposing infant to strong odors (such as alcohol, Betadine, perfumes). *Olfactory capability of the infant is very sensitive.*[1]
- Place a cloth or gauze pad scented with milk near the infant's face during gavage feeding. *Enhances association of milk with act of feeding/gastric fullness.*[2]
- Invite parents to leave a handkerchief that they have scented by wearing close to their body near infant. *Strengthens infant recognition of parents.*[2]

Vestibular

- Move and handle the infant slowly and gently. Do not restrict spontaneous movement. *Maintains comfort while at the same time encouraging motor function skill.*[2]
- Provide vestibular stimulation *to console, stabilize breathing/heart rate, or enhance growth.* Use a waterbed (with or without oscillation), a motorized/moving bed or cradle, or rocking in the arms of a caregiver.

Gustatory

- Dip pacifier in milk and offer to infant for sucking and tasting during gavage feeding. *Further enhances feeding recognition with touch and taste cues.*[2]

Tactile

- Maintain skin integrity and monitor closely. Limit frequency of invasive procedures. *Decreases chance of infections. Decreases infant discomfort.*[1]
- Minimize use of chemicals on skin (e.g., alcohol, povidone-iodine, solvents) and remove afterward with warm water. *Chemical compounds remove the natural protective mechanisms of skin, and infants are often very sensitive to integumentary injury.*[1]
- Limit use of tape and adhesives directly on skin. Use DuoDerm under tape. *Helps prevent dermal injury/allergic reactions.*[1]
- Touch infant with a firm containing touch, avoid light stroking. Provide a sheepskin, soft linen. Note: Tactile experience is the primary sensory mode of the infant. *Light stroking can cause tickle sensations that are irritating rather than pleasurable. Firm touch is reassuring.*[2]
- Encourage frequent parental holding of infant (including skin-to-skin). Supplement activity with extended family, staff, volunteers. *For family members, touch enhances bonding. If family is not readily available, infant needs regular skin-to-skin contact from caregivers for comfort and reassurance.*[3]

🌐 Cultural   Ⓐ Collaborative   🏠 Community/Home Care   Diagnostic Studies   ∞ Pediatric/Geriatric/Lifespan   Medications

NURSING PRIORITY NO. 5 To promote wellness (Teaching/Discharge Considerations):

- Evaluate home environment to identify appropriate modifications. *Helps the family identify needs and begin to mentally prepare for infant homecoming.*[3]
- Identify community resources (e.g., early stimulation program, qualified child-care facilities/respite care, visiting nurse, home-care support, specialty organizations). *Begins process of resource utilization.*[2–4]
- Determine sources for equipment/therapy needs. *Facilitates transition to at-home care.*[3]
- Refer to support/therapy groups as indicated. *Provides role models, facilitates adjustment to new roles/responsibilities, and enhances coping.*[2,3]
- Provide contact number, as appropriate (e.g., primary nurse). *Supports adjustment to home setting, enhances problem-solving.*[3]
- Refer to additional NDs such as risk for impaired parent/infant/child Attachment, risk for Caregiver Role Strain, compromised/disabled/readiness for enhanced family Coping, delayed Growth and Development.

DOCUMENTATION FOCUS

Assessment/Reassessment

- Findings, including infant's cues of stress, self-regulation, and readiness for stimulation; chronological/developmental age.
- Parent's concerns, level of knowledge.

Planning

- Plan of care and who is involved in the planning.
- Teaching plan.

Implementation/Evaluation

- Infant's responses to interventions/actions performed.
- Parents' participation and response to interactions/teaching.
- Attainment/progress toward desired outcome(s).
- Modifications of plan of care.

Discharge Planning

- Long-term needs and who is responsible for actions to be taken.
- Specific referrals made.

References

1. Creasy, R., Resnik, R. (1999). *Maternal-Fetal Medicine.* 4th ed. Philadelphia: W. B. Saunders.
2. London, M., Ladewig, P., Ball, J., Bindler, R. (2003) *Maternal-Newborn & Child Nursing; Family-Centered Care.* Upper Saddle River, NJ: Prentice Hall.
3. Ladewig, P., London, M., Moberly, S., Olds, S. (2002). *Contemporary Maternal-Newborn Nursing Care.* 5th ed. Upper Saddle River, NJ: Prentice Hall.
4. Lowdermilk, D., Perry, S., Bobak, I. (2001). *Maternity & Women's Health Care.* 6th ed. St. Louis, MO: Mosby.
5. Mandeville, L., Troiano, N. (1999). *High-Risk & Critical Care; Intrapartum Nursing.* 2d ed. Philadelphia: Lippincott.
6. Feldman, R., Eidelman, A. I., Sirota, L., Weller, A. (2002). Comparison of skin-to-skin (kangaroo) and traditional care: Parenting outcomes and preterm infant development. *Pediatrics,* 110(1), 16–26.
7. Scharer, K., Brooks, G. (1994). Mothers of chronically ill neonates and primary nurses in the NICU: Transfer of care. *Neonatal Network,* 13(5), 37–46.

risk for disorganized Infant Behavior

Definition: Risk for alteration in integration and modulation of the physiological and behavioral systems of functioning (i.e., autonomic, motor, state, organizational, self-regulatory, and attentional-interactional systems)

RISK FACTORS

Pain

Oral/motor problems

Environmental overstimulation

Lack of containment within environment

Invasive/painful procedures

Prematurity; [immaturity of the CNS; genetic problems that alter neurological and/or physiological functioning, conditions resulting in hypoxia and/or birth asphyxia]

[Malnutrition; infection; drug addiction]

[Environmental events or conditions such as separation from parents, exposure to loud noise, excessive handling, bright lights]

NOTE: A risk diagnosis is not evidenced by signs and symptoms, as the problem has not occurred; rather, nursing interventions are directed at prevention.

Sample Clinical Applications: Prematurity, congenital/genetic disorders, meconium aspiration, respiratory distress syndrome, small for gestational age

DESIRED OUTCOMES/EVALUATION CRITERIA

Sample NOC linkages:

Preterm Infant Behavior: Extrauterine integration of physiological and behavioral function by the infant born 24 to 37 weeks gestation

Neurological Status: Ability of the peripheral and central nervous system to receive, process, and respond to internal and external stimuli

Infant Will (Include Specific Time Frame)

• Exhibit organized behaviors that allow the achievement of optimal potential for growth and development as evidenced by modulation of physiological, motor, state, and attentional-interactive functioning.

Sample NOC linkages:

Child Development: [specify age group 2/4/6/12 months]: Milestones of physical, cognitive, and psychosocial progression by [specify] months of age

Knowledge: Infant Care: Extent of understanding conveyed about caring for a baby from birth to 1 year

Parent/Caregiver Will (Include Specific Time Frame)

• Identify cues reflecting infant's stress threshold and current status.
• Develop/modify responses (including environment) to promote infant adaptation and development.

ACTIONS/INTERVENTIONS AND DOCUMENTATION FOCUS

Refer to ND disorganized Infant Behavior for Actions/Interventions and Documentation Focus.

Cultural   Collaborative   Community/Home Care   Diagnostic Studies   Pediatric/Geriatric/Lifespan   Medications

readiness for enhanced organized Infant Behavior

Definition: A pattern of modulation of the physiological and behavioral systems of functioning (i.e., autonomic, motor, state-organizational, self-regulators, and attentional-interactional systems) in an infant that is satisfactory but that can be improved

RELATED FACTORS
Prematurity
Pain

DEFINING CHARACTERISTICS

Objective
Stable physiological measures
Definite sleep-wake states
Use of some self-regulatory behaviors
Response to stimuli (e.g., visual, auditory)

Sample Clinical Applications: Prematurity, congenital/genetic disorders, meconium aspiration, respiratory distress syndrome, small for gestational age

DESIRED OUTCOMES/EVALUATION CRITERIA
Sample NOC linkage:
Neurological Status: Ability of the peripheral and central nervous system to receive, process, and respond to internal and external stimuli

Infant Will (Include Specific Time Frame)

• Continue to modulate physiological and behavioral systems of functioning.
• Achieve higher levels of integration in response to environmental stimuli.

Sample NOC linkages:
Child Development: [specify age group 2/4/6/12 months]: Milestones of physical, cognitive, and psychosocial progression by [specify] months of age
Knowledge: Infant Care: Extent of understanding conveyed about caring for a baby from birth to first birthday

Parent/Caregiver Will (Include Specific Time Frame)

• Identify cues reflecting infant's stress threshold and current status.
• Develop/modify responses (including environment) to promote infant adaptation and development.

ACTIONS/INTERVENTIONS

Sample NIC linkages:
Developmental Care: Structuring the environment and providing care in response to the behavioral cues and states of the preterm infant
Environmental Management: Manipulation of the patient's surroundings for therapeutic benefit

Nursing Diagnoses in Alphabetical Order

NURSING PRIORITY NO. 1 To assess infant status and parental skill level:

- Determine infant's chronological and developmental age; note length of gestation. *These factors (prematurity, infant maturity, and stages of development) help to determine plan of care.*[1,2,5]
- Identify infant's individual self-regulatory behaviors: suck, mouth; grasp, hand-to-mouth, face behaviors; foot clasp, brace; limb flexion, trunk tuck; boundary seeking. *Assessing the infant's own regulatory coping tools alerts family and caregiver when infant is entering a stress cycle and helps determine if the infant needs assistance coping. This knowledge also helps development of a care plan if situation warrants.*[1,2,4]
- Observe for cues suggesting presence of situations that may result in pain/discomfort. *Some behavior that appears to be disorganized may be caused by a pain source that once identified may be alleviated.*[1]
- Evaluate level/appropriateness of environmental stimuli. *Infant behavior is affected by a wide range of stimuli. Careful assessment narrows focus of concerns.*[2]
- 🏠 Ascertain parents' understanding of infant's needs/abilities. *Identifies knowledge base and areas of additional learning need.*[2–4]
- 🏠 Listen/Active-listen to parents' perceptions of their capabilities to promote infant's development. *When parents feel their thoughts/concerns are heard, they will feel reassured that they will be able to handle situation.*[2,3]

NURSING PRIORITY NO. 2 To assist parents to enhance infant's integration:

- Provide positive feedback for parental involvement in caregiving process. Transfer of care from staff to parents progresses along a continuum as parents' confidence level increases, and they are able to take on more responsibility.[7]
- Discuss use of skin-to-skin contact (kangaroo care) as appropriate. Research suggests KC may have a positive effect on infant development by enhancing neurophysiological organization as well as an indirect effect by improving parental mood, perceptions, and interactive behavior.[6]
- 🏠 Review infant growth/development, pointing out current status and progressive expectations. *Increases parental knowledge base and level of confidence.*[2–4]
- 🏠 Identify cues reflecting infant stress. *Attention to cues allow for early intervention in case of problem development.*[2–4]
- 🏠 Discuss parents' perceptions of needs/provide recommendations for modifications of environmental stimuli/activity schedule, sleep and pain control needs. *While care provided is satisfactory, some modifications may enhance infant's integration/development.*[1,4]
- 🏠 Incorporate parents' observations and suggestions into plan of care. *Demonstrates value of and regard for parents' input and enhances sense of ability to deal with situation.*[2,4]

NURSING PRIORITY NO. 3 To promote wellness (Teaching/Learning Considerations):

- Ⓐ Identify community resources (e.g., visiting nurse, home-care support, childcare). *Begins process of resource utilization.*[2–4]
- Ⓐ Refer to support group/individual role model *to facilitate ongoing adjustment to new roles/responsibilities and problem-solving.*[2,3]
- Refer to additional NDs, for example, readiness for enhanced family Coping.

🌐 Cultural Ⓐ Collaborative 🏠 Community/Home Care Diagnostic Studies ∞ Pediatric/Geriatric/Lifespan Medications

DOCUMENTATION FOCUS

Assessment/Reassessment

- Findings, including infant's self-regulation and readiness for stimulation; chronological/developmental age.
- Parents' concerns, level of knowledge.

Planning

- Plan of care and who is involved in the planning.
- Teaching plan.

Implementation/Evaluation

- Infant's responses to interventions/actions performed.
- Parents' participation and response to interactions/teaching.
- Attainment/progress toward desired outcome(s).
- Modifications of plan of care.

Discharge Planning

- Long-term needs and who is responsible for actions to be taken.
- Specific referrals made.

References

1. Creasy, R., Resnik, R. (1999). *Maternal-Fetal Medicine.* 4th ed. Philadelphia: W. B. Saunders.
2. London, M., Ladewig, P., Ball, J., Bindler, R. (2003). *Maternal-Newborn & Child Nursing: Family-Centered Care.* Upper Saddle River, NJ: Prentice Hall.
3. Ladewig, P., London, M., Moberly, S., Olds, S. (2002). *Contemporary Maternal-Newborn Nursing Care.* 5th ed. Upper Saddle River, NJ: Prentice Hall.
4. Lowdermilk, D., Perry, S., Bobak, I. (2001). *Maternity & Women's Health Care.* 6th ed. St. Louis, MO: Mosby.
5. Mandeville, L., Troiano, N. (1999). *High-Risk & Critical Care; Intrapartum Nursing.* 2d ed. Philadelphia: Lippincott.
6. Feldman, R., Eidelman, A. I., Sirota, L., Weller, A. (2002). Comparison of skin-to-skin (kangaroo) and traditional care: Parenting outcomes and preterm infant development. *Pediatrics,* 110(1), 16–26.
7. Scharer, K., Brooks, G. (1994). Mothers of chronically ill neonates and primary nurses in the NICU: Transfer of care. *Neonatal Network,* 13(5), 37–46.

ineffective Infant Feeding Pattern

Definition: Impaired ability of an infant to suck or coordinate the suck/swallow response resulting in inadequate oral nutrition for metabolic needs

RELATED FACTORS
Prematurity
Neurological impairment/delay
Oral hypersensitivity
Prolonged NPO
Anatomic abnormality

DEFINING CHARACTERISTICS

Subjective
[Caregiver reports infant is unable to initiate or sustain an effective suck]

Objective
Inability to initiate/sustain an effective suck
Inability to coordinate sucking, swallowing, and breathing

Sample Clinical Applications: Prematurity, cleft lip/palate, thrush, hydrocephalus, cerebral palsy, fetal alcohol syndrome, respiratory distress, severe developmental delay

DESIRED OUTCOMES/EVALUATION CRITERIA
Sample NOC linkages:
Swallowing Status: Oral Phase: Preparation, containment, and posterior movement of fluids and/or solids in the mouth
Breastfeeding Establishment: Infant: Infant attachment to and sucking from the mother's breast for nourishment during the first 3 weeks of breastfeeding
Hydration: Adequate water in the intracellular and extracellular compartments of the body

Infant Will (Include Specific Time Frame)

• Display adequate output as measured by sufficient number of wet diapers daily.
• Demonstrate appropriate weight gain.
• Be free of aspiration.

ACTIONS/INTERVENTIONS

Sample NIC linkages:
Lactation Counseling: Use of an interactive helping process to assist in maintenance of successful breastfeeding
Swallowing Therapy: Facilitating swallowing and preventing complications of impaired swallowing
Nutrition Monitoring: Collection and analysis of patient data to prevent or minimize malnourishment

NURSING PRIORITY NO. I To identify contributing factors/degree of impaired function:

• Assess infant's suck, swallow, and gag reflexes. *Provides comparitive baseline and useful in determining appropriate feeding method.*
• Note developmental age, structural abnormalities (e.g., cleft lip/palate), mechanical barriers (e.g., ET tube, ventilator). *These factors (infant maturity and structural/mechanical barriers to infant feeding) help to determine plan of care.*[1,2,4]
• Determine level of consciousness, neurological impairment, seizure activity, presence of pain. *Provides baseline information and identifies areas of special need.*[1,2]
• Observe parent/infant interactions *to determine level of bonding/comfort that could impact stress level during feeding activity.*
• Note type/scheduling of medications. *May cause sedative effect/impair feeding activity.*[2]

Cultural Collaborative Community/Home Care Diagnostic Studies Pediatric/Geriatric/Lifespan Medications

- Compare birth and current weight/length measurements. *Monitors effectiveness of infant feeding technique.*[1,2,4]
- Assess signs of stress when feeding (e.g., tachypnea, cyanosis, fatigue/lethargy). *Detects areas of increased need for alternate feeding methods and/or rest periods.*[1]
- Note presence of behaviors indicating continued hunger after feeding. *Determines if infant is receiving adequate amount during feeding.*[2,4]

NURSING PRIORITY NO. 2 To promote adequate infant intake:

- Determine appropriate method for feeding (e.g., special nipple/feeding device, gavage/enteral tube feeding) and choice of breast milk/formula to meet infant needs. *Individualizes care and maintains infant health status.*[1]
- Review early infant feeding cues (e.g., rooting, lip smacking, sucking fingers/hand) versus late cue of crying. *Early recognition of infant hunger promotes timely/more rewarding feeding experience for infant and mother.*[5]
- Demonstrate techniques/procedures for feeding. Note proper positioning of infant, "latching-on" techniques, rate of delivery of feeding, frequency of burping. (Refer to ND ineffective Breastfeeding as appropriate.) *Models appropriate feeding methods, increases parental knowledge base and confidence.*[2–4]
- Limit duration of feeding to maximum of 30 minutes based on infant's response (e.g., signs of fatigue) *to balance energy expenditure with nutrient intake.*
- Monitor caregiver's efforts. Provide feedback and assistance as indicated. *Enhances learning, encourages continuation of efforts.*[2,3]
- Refer mother to lactation specialist for assistance and support in dealing with unresolved issues (e.g., teaching infant to suck). *Provides resource for future needs and problem-solving. Begins pattern of resource utilization.*[2–4]
- Emphasize importance of calm/relaxed environment during feeding *to reduce detrimental stimuli and enhance mother/infant's focus on feeding activity.*
- Adjust frequency and amount of feeding according to infant's response. *Prevents infant's frustration associated with under/overfeeding.*
- Advance diet, adding solids or thickening agent as appropriate for age and infant needs. *Provides for infant's nutrition and health needs.*[2,4]
- Alternate feeding techniques (e.g., nipple and gavage) according to infant's ability and level of fatigue. *Individualizes plan of care to enhance successful feeding.*[1]
- Alter medication/feeding schedules as indicated to minimize sedative effects. *Altered states of function and consciousness interfere with feeding and may lead to choking or aspirating.*[1]

NURSING PRIORITY NO. 3 To promote wellness (Teaching/Discharge Considerations):

- Instruct caregiver in techniques to prevent/alleviate aspiration. *Helps parent/caregiver feel more confident, promotes infant safety.*[1,4]
- Discuss anticipated growth and development goals for infant, corresponding caloric needs. *Accommodating infant maturity and development help to individualize and update plan of care.*[1,2,5]
- Suggest recording infant's weight and nutrient intake periodically. *Monitors effectiveness of infant feeding technique by providing measurable data. Provides positive reinforcement to implementation of care plan.*[1,2,4]
- Recommend participation in classes as indicated (e.g., first aid, infant cardiopulmonary resuscitation). *Increases knowledge base for infant safety and caregiver confidence.*[2–4]

- Refer to support groups (e.g., La Leche League, parenting support groups, stress reduction, or other community resources as indicated).
- Provide bibliotherapy/appropriate Web sites for further information.

DOCUMENTATION FOCUS

Assessment/Reassessment

- Type and route of feeding, interferences to feeding and reactions.
- Infant's measurements.

Planning

- Plan of care/interventions and who is involved in planning.
- Teaching plan.

Implementation/Evaluation

- Infant's response to interventions (e.g., amount of intake, weight gain, response to feeding) and actions performed.
- Caregiver's involvement in infant care, participation in activities, response to teaching.
- Attainment of/progress toward desired outcome(s).
- Modifications to plan of care.

Discharge Planning

- Long-term needs/referrals and who is responsible for follow-up actions.

References

1. Creasy, R., Resnik, R. (1999). *Maternal-Fetal Medicine.* 4th ed. Philadelphia: W. B. Saunders.
2. London, M., Ladewig, P., Ball, J., Bindler, R. (2003). *Maternal-Newborn & Child Nursing; Family-Centered Care.* Upper Saddle River, NJ: Prentice Hall.
3. Ladewig, P., London, M., Moberly, S., Olds, S. (2002). *Contemporary Maternal-Newborn Nursing Care.* 5th ed. Upper Saddle River, NJ: Prentice Hall.
4. Lowdermilk, D., Perry, S., Bobak, I. (2001). *Maternity & Women's Health Care.* 6th ed. St. Louis, MO: Mosby.
5. American Academy of Family Physicians: Breastfeeding (Position paper). Accessed February 2007 at www.aafp.org/online/en/home/policy/policies/b/breastfeedingpositionpaper.html.

risk for Infection

Definition: At increased risk for being invaded by pathogenic organisms

RISK FACTORS

Inadequate primary defenses (broken skin, traumatized tissue, decrease in ciliary action, stasis of body fluids, change in pH secretions, altered peristalsis)

Inadequate secondary defenses (e.g., decreased hemoglobin, leukopenia, suppressed inflammatory response)

Inadequate acquired immunity; immunosuppression

Tissue destruction; increased environmental exposure to pathogens; invasive procedures

Chronic disease, malnutrition, trauma

Pharmaceutical agents (e.g.,immunosuppressants, [antibiotic therapy])

Cultural   Collaborative   Community/Home Care   Diagnostic Studies   Pediatric/Geriatric/Lifespan   Medications

Rupture of amniotic membranes

Insufficient knowledge to avoid exposure to pathogens

NOTE: A risk diagnosis is not evidenced by signs and symptoms, as the problem has not occurred; rather, nursing interventions are directed at prevention.

Sample Clinical Applications: Immune suppressed conditions (e.g., HIV positive/AIDS, cancer), COPD, long-term use of steroids (e.g., asthma, rheumatoid arthritis, SLE), diabetes mellitus, malnutrition, surgical/invasive procedures, substance abuse, burns, premature rupture of membranes

DESIRED OUTCOMES/EVALUATION CRITERIA

Sample NOC linkages:

Immune Status: Natural and acquired appropriately targeted resistance to internal and external antigens

Knowledge: Infection Control: Extent of understanding conveyed about prevention and control of infection

Risk Control: Personal actions to prevent, eliminate, or reduce modifiable health threats

Client Will (Include Specific Time Frame)

- Verbalize understanding of individual causative/risk factor(s).
- Identify interventions to prevent/reduce risk of infection.
- Demonstrate techniques, lifestyle changes to promote safe environment.
- Achieve timely wound healing; be free of purulent drainage or erythema; be afebrile.

ACTIONS/INTERVENTIONS

Sample NIC linkages:

Infection Protection: Prevention and early detection of infection in a patient at risk

Infection Control: Minimizing the acquisition and transmission of infectious agents

Surveillance: Purposeful and ongoing acquisition, interpretation, and synthesis of patient data for clinical decision making

NURSING PRIORITY NO. 1 To determine risk/contributing factors:

- Assess for presence of host-specific factors that affect immunity:[1,12–14]
  ∞ **Extremes of age:** *Newborns and the elderly are more susceptible to disease/infection than general population.*
  Presence of underlying disease: *Client may have disease that directly impacts immune system (e.g., cancer, AIDS, autoimmune disorder) or may be weakened by prolonged disease condition/treatment.*
  Lifestyle: *Personal habits or living situations such as persons sharing close quarters and/or equipment (e.g., college dorm, group home/long-term care facility, day care, correctional facility); IV drug use/shared needles, unprotected sex can increase susceptibility to infections.*
  Nutritional status: *Malnutrition weakens the immune system; elevated serum glucose levels (e.g., administration of total parenteral nutrition [TPN] or poorly controlled diabetes mellitus) provides growth media for pathogens.*

Trauma: Loss of skin or mucous membrane integrity, or invasive procedures (e.g., surgery/invasive procedures: urinary catheterizations, oral intubation, parenteral injection, sharps/needle sticks) *are common paths of pathogen entry.*

Certain medications: *Steroids, chemotherapeutic agents directly affect immune system. Long-term or improper antibiotic treatment can disrupt body's normal flora and result in increased susceptibility to antibiotic-resistant organisms.*

Presence or absence of immunity: *Natural immunity may be acquired as a result of development of antibodies to a specific agent following infection, preventing recurrence of specific disease (e.g., chickenpox). Active immunization (via vaccination, e.g., measles, polio) and passive immunization (e.g., antitoxin or immune globulin administration) can prevent certain communicable diseases.*

Environmental exposure: *May be accidental or intentional (e.g., act of terrorism).*

- Observe skin/tissues surrounding injuries (e.g., knife cuts, toe injuries, insect/animal bites); also inspect insertion sites of invasive lines, sutures, surgical incisions/wounds. *Redness, warmth, swelling, pain, red streaks are signs of developing localized infection that may have systemic implications if treatment is delayed.*[9,10,14,17]
- Assess and document skin conditions around insertions of orthopedic pins, wires, and tongs. *Direct connection to bone increases the risk of infections in bone sites that can lead to osteomyelitis and long-term delays of healing, or bone loss.*[9,10,14,17]
- Review laboratory values (e.g., white blood cell count and differential, blood/urine/wound cultures) *to identify presence of pathogens/treatment options.*
- Note onset of fever, chills, diaphoresis, altered level of consciousness. *Signs and symptoms of sepsis (systemic infection), requiring intensive medical treatment and evaluation for source of infection and specific pathogen.*

NURSING PRIORITY NO. 2 To reduce/correct existing risk factors:

Healthcare environment:

- Stress proper handwashing techniques (using antibacterial soap and running water) before and after all care contacts, and after contact with items likely to be contaminated. Wash hands after glove removal. Instruct client/SO/visitors to wash hands, as indicated. *A first-line defense against healthcare-associated infections (HAI).*[1,3,15]
- Provide clean, well-ventilated environment (may require turning off central air-conditioning and opening window for good ventilation; room with negative air pressure, etc.).[6]
- Postvisual alerts in healthcare settings instructing clients/SO to inform healthcare providers if they have symptoms of respiratory infections/influenza-like symptoms. *Can limit/prevent transmission to and from client and may reveal additional cases.*[1,8,11,12,15]
- Monitor client's visitors/caregivers for respiratory illnesses. Offer masks and tissues to client/visitors who are coughing/sneezing *to limit exposures, reduce cross-contamination.*
- Encourage parents of sick children to keep them away from child care settings and school until afebrile for 24 hours.
- Provide for isolation as indicated (e.g., wound/skin, resipatory, reverse). Educate staff in infection-control procedures. *Reduces risk of cross-contamination.*[18]
- Stress proper use of personal protective equipment (PPE) by staff/visitors as dictated by agency policy *for particular exposure risk (e.g., airborne, droplet, splash risk), including mask/respiratory filter of appropriate particulate regulator, gowns, aprons, head covers, face shields, protective eyewear.*[1,4,6,8,11]
- Include information in preoperative teaching about ways *to reduce potential for postoperative infection (e.g., respiratory measures to prevent pneumonia, wound/dressing care, avoidance of others with infection).*[5,9]

Cultural Collaborative Community/Home Care Diagnostic Studies Pediatric/Geriatric/Lifespan Medications

- Encourage early ambulation, deep breathing, coughing, position changes, and early removal of endotracheal and/or nasal/oral feeding tubes *for mobilization of respiratory secretions and prevention of aspiration/respiratory infections.*[15,16]
- Monitor/assist with use of adjuncts (e.g., respiratory aids such as incentive spirometry) *to prevent pneumonia.*[15,16]
- Maintain adequate hydration and electrolyte balance *to prevent imbalances that would predispose to infection.*
- Provide/encourage balanced diet, emphasizing proteins to feed the immune system. *Immune function is affected by protein intake, the balance between omega-6 and omega-3 fatty acid intake, and adequate amounts of vitamins A, C, and E and the minerals zinc and iron. A deficiency of these nutrients puts the client at an increased risk of infection.*[2]
- Handle and properly package tissue/fluid specimens.[1,7]
- Administer prophylactic antibiotics and immunizations as indicated.
- Assist with medical procedures (e.g., wound/joint aspiration, incision and drainage of abscess, bronchoscopy) as indicated.
- Administer/monitor medication regimen (e.g., antimicrobials, drip infusion into osteomyelitis, subeschar clysis, topical antibiotics) and note client's response *to determine effectiveness of therapy/presence of side effects.*

Medical Devices:

- Maintain sterile technique for invasive procedures (e.g., IV, urinary catheter, tracheostomy care, pulmonary suctioning).[1]
- Use disposable equipment whenever possible. Sterilize reusable equipment and surfaces according to manufacturer recommendations.[1,8]
- Dispose of needles and sharps in approved containers *to reduce risk of needle stick/sharps injury.*[1,8]
- Choose proper vascular access device based on anticipated treatment duration and solution/medication to be infused and best available aseptic insertion techniques; cleanse incisions/insertion sites daily/per facility protocol with appropriate solution *to reduce potential for catheter-related bloodstream infections.*[17]
- Maintain appropriate hang times for parenteral solutions (IVs, additives, nutritional solutions) *to reduce opportunity for contamination/bacterial growth.*[2]
- Assist with weaning from mechanical ventilator as soon as possible *to reduce risk of venitalor-associated pneumonia (VAP).*[18]
- Fill bubbling humidifiers/nubulizers with *sterile* water—not distilled or tap water. Use heat and moisture exchangers (HME) instead of heated humidifier with mechanical ventilator.[16,18]

Skin/tissues:

- Change surgical/other wound dressings as needed/indicated, using proper technique for changing/disposing of contaminated materials.[8,9,19]
- Cleanse incisions/insertion sites daily and as needed with povidone-iodine or other appropriate solution *to prevent growth of bacteria.*[9]
- Separate touching surfaces of excoriated skin (e.g., in herpes zoster, burns, weeping dermatitis) and apply appropriate skin barriers. Use gloves when caring for open lesions *to minimize autoinoculation/transmission of viral diseases.*[9]
- Perform/instruct in daily mouth care. Include use of antiseptic mouthwash for individuals in acute/long-term care settings *at high-risk for nosocomial/healthcare associated infections.*[18]
- Provide regular urinary catheter/perineal care. *Reduces risk of ascending urinary tract infection.*

- Cover perineal/pelvic region dressings/casts with plastic when using bedpan *to prevent contamination when wound is in perineal/pelvic region.*
- Discuss routine or preoperative body shower/scrubs when indicated (e.g., orthopedic, plastic surgery) *to reduce bacterial colonization.*[15]

Community:

- Recommend individuals/staff isolate self at home when ill *to prevent spread of infection to others, including coworkers.*[11]
- Alert infection control officer/proper authorities to presence of specific infectious agents and number of cases as required. *Provides for case finding and helps curtail outbreak.*[11,21]
- Group/cohort individuals with same diagnosis/exposure as resources require. *Limited resources (as may occur with an outbreak/epidemic) may dictate a wardlike environment but need for regular precautions to control spread of infection still exists.*[11]
- Encourage contacting healthcare provider for prophylactic therapy as indicated following exposure to individuals with infectious disease (e.g., tuburcluosis, hepatitis, influenza).

NURSING PRIORITY NO. 3 To promote wellness (Teaching/Discharge Considerations):

- Review individual nutritional needs, appropriate exercise program, and need for rest *to enhance immune system function and healing.*[2,10,11]
- Instruct client/SO(s) in techniques to protect the integrity of skin, care for lesions, temperature measurement, and prevention of spread of infection in the home setting. *Provides basic knowledge for self-help and self-protection.*[7,10]
- Emphasize necessity of taking antivirals/antibiotics as directed (e.g., dosage and length of therapy). *Premature discontinuation of treatment when client begins to feel well may result in return of infection and potentiate drug-resistant strains.*[20]
- Discuss importance of not taking antibiotics/using "leftover" drugs unless specifically instructed by healthcare provider. *Inappropriate use can lead to development of drug-resistant strains/secondary infections.*[10]
- Discuss the role of smoking and secondhand smoke in respiratory infections. Refer to smoking cessation programs as indicated.
- Promote safer-sex practices and reporting sexual contacts of infected individuals *to prevent the spread of HIV/other sexually transmitted diseases.*[1,10,20]
- Encourage high-risk persons, including healthcare workers, to have influenza and pneumonia vaccinations *to reduce individual risk as well as help prevent spread of flu and viral pneumonias to others.*[1,11,21]
- Promote childhood immunization program. Encourage adults to update immunizations as appropriate.[12]
- Discuss precautions with client engaged in international travel, and refer for immunizations *to reduce incidence/transmission of global infections.*[13]
- Review use of prophylactic antibiotics if appropriate *(e.g., before dental work for clients with history of rheumatic fever, heart valve replacements, etc.).*[10]
- Identify resources available to the individual (e.g., substance abuse/rehabilitation or needle-exchange program as appropriate; available/free condoms, and so on).
- Provide information/involve in appropriate community and national education programs *to increase awareness of and prevention of communicable diseases.*[1,10,11]
- Refer to NDs risk for Disuse Syndrome; ineffective Health Maintenance; impaired Home Maintenance; readiness for enhanced Immunization Status for additional interventions as appropraite.

DOCUMENTATION FOCUS

Assessment/Reassessment

- Individual risk factors that are present, including recent/current antibiotic therapy.
- Wound and/or insertion sites, character of drainage/body secretions.
- Signs/symptoms of infectious process

Planning

- Plan of care/interventions and who is involved in planning.
- Teaching plan.

Implementation/Evaluation

- Responses to interventions/teaching and actions performed.
- Attainment/progress toward desired outcome(s).
- Modifications to plan of care.

Discharge Planning

- Discharge needs/referrals and who is responsible for actions to be taken.
- Specific referrals made.

References

1. Mechanisms of transmission and pathogenic organisms in the health care setting and strategies for prevention and control. (2001). Elements One and Two of online course of Infection Control Learning Institute. Available at www.proceo.com. Accessed September 2003.
2. Lehmann, S. (1991). Immune function and nutrition: The clinical role of the intravenous nurse. *J Intraven Nurs*, 14, 406.
3. Garner, J., Favero, M. (1986). CDC Guideline for handwashing and hospital environmental control. *Am J Infection Control*, 16, 28–40.
4. Borton, D. (1997). Isolation precautions: Clearing up the confusion. *Nursing 97*, 21(1), 49.
5. Emori, L., Culver, D., Horan, T. (1995). National Nosocomial Infections Surveillance System (NNIS): Description of surveillance methods. *Am J Infection Control*, 19, 259–257.
6. Garner, J. S. (1996). Guideline for isolation precautions in hospitals. *Infection Control and Hospital Epidemiology*, 17(1), 53–80.
7. Friedman, M. M. (2002). Improving infection control in home care: From ritual to science-based practice. *Home Healthcare Nurse*, 18(2), 99.
8. Hospital infection control guidance: Communicable disease surveillance & response (CSR). World Health Organization (WHO) Web site. Available at www.who.int/csr/en.
9. Thompson, J. (2000). A practical guide to wound care. *RN*, 63(1), 48–52.
10. Androwich, I., Burkhart, L., Gettrust, K. V. (1995). *Community and Home Health Nursing*. Albany, NY: Delmar.
11. Care Plan: Disaster Considerations; and ND Infection, Risk for, in Numerous Care Plans. In Doenges, M. E., Moorhouse, M. F., Geissler-Murr, A. C. (2002). *Nursing Care Plans: Guidelines for Individualizing Patient Care*. 6th ed. Philadelphia: F. A. Davis.
12. Goldrick, B. A., Goetz, A. M. (2006). 'Tis the season for influenza. *Nurse Practitioner*, 31(12), 24–33.
13. Hunter, A., Denman-Vitale, S., Garzon, L. (2007). Global infections: Recognition, management, and prevention. *Nurse Practitioner*, 32(2), 34–41.
14. Romero, D. V., Treston, J., O'Sullivan, A. L. (2006). Hand-to-hand combat: Preventing MRSA infection. *Advances in Skin & Wound care: J for Prevention and Healing*, 19(6), 328–333.
15. Houghton, D. (2006). HAI prevention: The power is in your hands. *Nursing Management*, 37(5), Supl, 1–7.
16. Lorente, L., Lecuona, M., Jimenez, A., Mora, M. L., Sierra, A. (2006). Ventilator-associated pneumonia using a heated humidifier or a heat and moisture exchanger: A randomized controlled trial. *Crit Care*, 10, 4.
17. Rosenthal, K. (2006). Guarding against vascular site infection. *Nursing Management*, 37(4), 54–66.

18. Tablan, O. C., Anderson, L. J., Besser, R., Bridges, C., Hajjeh, R. (2004). Guidelines for preventing health-care associated pneumonia, 2003—Recommendations of CDC and Healthcare Infection Control Practices Advisory Committee. *MMWR*, 53(RRO3), 1–36.
19. Odom-Forren, J. (2006). Preventing surgical site infections. *Nursing2006*, 36(6), 59–63.
20. Kirton, C. (2005). The HIV/AIDS epidemic: A case of good news/bad news. *Nursing Made Incredibly Easy!*, 3(2), 28–40.
21. Lashley, F. R. (2006). Emerging infectious dieases at the beginning of the 21st century. *Online Journal of Issues in Nursing*, 11(1). Retrieved March 2007 at www.nursingworld.org.ojin/topic29_1.htm.

risk for Injury

Definition: At risk of injury as a result of environmental conditions interacting with the individual's adaptive and defensive resources

RISK FACTORS

Internal

Physical (e.g., broken skin, altered mobility); tissue hypoxia; malnutrition

Abnormal blood profile (e.g., leukocytosis/leukopenia, altered clotting factors, thrombocytopenia, sickle cell, thalassemia, decreased hemoglobin)

Biochemical dysfunction; sensory dysfunction

Integrative/effector dysfunction; immune-autoimmune dysfunction

Psychological (affective, orientation); developmental age (physiological, psychosocial)

External

Biological (e.g., immunization level of community, microorganism)

Chemical (e.g., pollutants, poisons, drugs, pharmaceutical agents, alcohol, nicotine, preservatives, cosmetics, dyes); nutritional (e.g., vitamins, food types)

Physical (e.g., design, structure, and arrangement of community, building, and/or equipment), mode of transport

Human (e.g., nosocomial agents, staffing patterns; cognitive, affective, psychomotor factors)

NOTE: A risk diagnosis is not evidenced by signs and symptoms, as the problem has not occurred; rather, nursing interventions are directed at prevention.

Sample Clinical Applications: Seizure disorder, dementia/AIDS, cataracts, glaucoma, Parkinson's, substance abuse, malnutrition, developmental delay/mental retardation

In reviewing this ND, it is apparent there is much overlap with other diagnoses. We have chosen to present generalized interventions. Although there are commonalities to injury situations, we suggest that the reader refer to other primary diagnoses as indicated, such as risk for acute/chronic Confusion; risk for Contamination; impaired Evinromental Intepretation Syndrome; risk for Falls; ineffective Health Maintenance; impaired Home Maintenance; risk for Infection; impaired physical Mobility; impaired/risk for impaired Parenting; risk for Poisoning; impaired/risk for impaired Skin Integrity; disturbed Thought Processes; risk for Trauma; risk for other-directed Violence; Wandering for additional interventions.

DESIRED OUTCOMES/EVALUATION CRITERIA

Sample NOC linkage:

Physical Injury Severity: Severity of injuries from accidents and trauma

Cultural ⓐCollaborative Community/Home Care Diagnostic Studies ∞ Pediatric/Geriatric/Lifespan Medications

Client Will (Include Specific Time Frame)

• Be free of injury.

Sample NOC linkages:

Personal Safety Behavior: Personal actions of an adult to control behaviors that might cause physical injury

Risk Control [specify]: Personal actions to prevent, eliminate, or reduce modifiable health threats [such as alcohol/drug use, altered visual function]

Client/Caregivers Will (Include Specific Time Frame)

• Verbalize understanding of individual factors that contribute to possibility of injury.
• Demonstrate behaviors, lifestyle changes to reduce risk factors and protect self from injury.
• Modify environment as indicated to enhance safety.

ACTIONS/INTERVENTIONS

Sample NIC linkages:

Surveillance: Safety: Purposeful and ongoing collection and analysis of information about the patient and the environment for use in promoting and maintaining client safety

Risk Identification: Analysis of potential risk factors, determination of health risks, and prioritization of risk-reduction strategies for an individual or group

Environmental Management: Safety: Manipulation of the patient's surroundings for therapeutic benefit

NURSING PRIORITY NO. 1 To evaluate degree/source of risk inherent in the individual situation:

• Identify client at risk (e.g., acute illness/surgery/trauma; chronic illness conditions with weakness, immunosuppression, or prolonged immobility; acute/chronic confusion/dementia/head injury; use of multiple medications; use of alcohol/other drugs; mental/emotional illness; cultural, familial, and socioeconomic factors adversely affecting lifestyle and home; exposure to environmental chemicals/other hazards).

∞ • Note age and gender (*children, young adults, elderly persons, and men are at greater risk*). *Affects client's ability to protect self and others and influences choice of interventions or teaching.*[15]

• Evaluate developmental level, decision-making ability, level of cognition, competence, and independence. *Determines client's/SO's ability to attend to safety issues.*

• Assess mood, coping abilities, personality styles (i.e., temperament, aggression, impulsive behavior, level of self-esteem). *May result in careless/increased risk-taking without consideration of consequences.*[1,2]

🏠 • Evaluate individual's emotional and behavioral response to violence in surroundings (e.g., neighborhood, television, peer group). *May affect client's view of/and regard for own/others' safety.*[1,2,15]

• Assess muscle strength, gross and fine motor coordination *to identify risk for falls.*

🏠 • Observe client for signs of injury and age (e.g., old/new bruises, history of fractures, frequent absences from school/work). Determine potential for abusive behavior by family members/SO(s)/peers. *Client or care providers may require further evaluation/investigation for abuse.*[5]

- Perform thorough assessments regarding safety issues when planning for client care/discharge. *Failure to accurately assess and intervene or refer regarding these issues can place the client at needless risk and creates negligence issues for the healthcare practitioner.*[14]
- Ascertain knowledge of safety needs/injury prevention and motivation to prevent injury in home, community, and work setting. *Information may reveal areas of misinformation, lack of knowledge, need for teaching.*[4]
- Note socioeconomic status/availability and use of resources.

NURSING PRIORITY NO. 2 To assist client/caregiver to reduce or correct individual risk factors:

- Provide healthcare within a culture of safety (e.g., adherence to nursing standards of care and facility safe-care policies) *to prevent errors resulting in client injury, promote client safety, and model safety behaviors for client/SO):*[14]
  Maintain bed/chair in lowest position with wheels locked.
  Provide seat raisers for chairs, use stand-assist/repositioning/lifting devices.
  Ensure that pathway to bathroom is unobstructed and properly lighted.
  Place assistive devices (e.g., walker, cane, glasses, hearing aid) within reach.
  Instruct client/SO to request assistance, as needed; make sure call light is within reach and client knows how to operate.
  Monitor environment for potentially unsafe conditions/hazards, modify as needed.
  Place confused client/young child near nurses' station *to provide for frequent observation.*[6]
  Orient/reorient client to environment, as needed.
  Safety lock exit/stairwell doors *when client can wander away.*
  Avoid use of restraints (*can increase client's agitation and risk of entrapment/death*).
  Administer medications and infusions using "5 rights" system (right client, right medication, right route, right dose, right time).[8]
  Inform and educate client/SO regarding all treatments and medications.
- Provide client/SO information regarding client's specific disease/condition and consequences of continuing unhealthy behaviors (e.g., increase in oral cancer among teenagers using smokeless tobacco; fetal alcohol syndrome/neonatal addiction in prenatal women using tobacco/alcohol/other drugs) *to enhance decision making, clarify expectations and individual needs.*
- Determine if risk-prone behavior is occurring/likely to occur *to initiate appropriate wellness counseling/referrals.*
- Review client's level of physical activity in his or her lifestyle *to determine changes/adaptations that may be required by current situation.*
- Refer to physical or occupational therapist as appropriate *to identify high-risk tasks, conduct site visits; select, create, modify equipment/assistive devices; and provide education about body mechanics and musculoskeletal injuries, in addition to providing therapies as indicated.*[6]
- Perform home assessment/identify safety issues such as[1–13]
  locking up medications/poisonous substances;
  using window grates/locks *to prevent young children from falls;*
  properly installing of handrails, ramps, bathtub safety tapes;
  using electrical outlet covers/lockouts;
  locking exterior doors *to prevent confused individual from wandering off while SO is engaged in other household activities;*
  removing matches/smoking material and knobs from the stove *so young children/confused individual do not turn on burner and leave it unattended;*
  properly placing alarms/fire extinguishers;

Cultural · Collaborative · Community/Home Care · Diagnostic Studies · Pediatric/Geriatric/Lifespan · Medications

discussing safe use of oxygen;
obtaining medical alert device/home monitoring service.

- Review specific employment concerns/worksite issues and needs (e.g., ergonomic chairs/workstations; proper fitting safety equipment, footwear; regular use of safety glasses/goggles and ear protectors; safe storage of hazardous substances; number of hours worked per shift/week).
- Demonstrate/encourage use of techniques to reduce/manage stress and vent emotions such as anger, hostility. *Identifying and dealing with emotions appropriately enables individual to maintain control of behavior and avoid possibility of violent outbursts.*[2,5,7]
- Discuss importance of self-monitoring of factors that can contribute to occurrence of injury (e.g., fatigue, anger, irritability). *Client/SO may be able to modify risk through monitoring of actions, or postponement of certain actions, especially during times when client is likely to be highly stressed.*
- Encourage participation in self-help programs, such as assertiveness training, anger management, positive self-image *to enhance self-esteem.*
- Review expectations caregivers have of children, cognitively impaired, and/or elderly family members. Discuss concerns about discipline practices.[13]
- Discuss need for and sources of supervision (e.g., before- and after-school programs, elderly day care).

NURSING PRIORITY NO. 3 To promote wellness (Teaching/Discharge Considerations):

- Identify individual needs/resources for safety education (e.g., home hazard information; fall prevention; firearm safety; CPR/first aid, etc.).[3,10,11]
- Stress importance of correct use of child safety seats, car seat belt restraints, bicycle/other helmets; regular use of sports safety equipment; etc.
- Provide instruction/refer to classes for back safety and proper use of injury-prevention devices. Recommend use of ergonomic bed/chair as appropriate.
- Provide telephone numbers and other contact numbers as individually indicated (e.g., doctor, 911, poison control, police, elder advocate).
- Provide bibliotherapy/written resource lists/reliable Web sites *for later review and self-paced learning.*
- Refer to other resources as indicated (e.g., counseling/psychotherapy, budget counseling, and parenting classes).
- Refer to/assist with community education programs *to increase awareness of safety measures and resources available to the individual.*[4]
- Promote community awareness about the problems of design of buildings, equipment, transportation, and workplace practices that contribute to accidents.[4]
- Identify community resources/neighbors/friends to assist elderly/handicapped individuals in providing such things as structural maintenance, snow and ice removal from walks and steps, etc.
- Identify emergency escape plans/routes for home and community *to be prepared in the event of natural or man-made disaster (e.g., fire, hurricane, earthquake, toxic chemical release).*[4]

DOCUMENTATION FOCUS

Assessment/Reassessment

- Individual risk factors, noting current physical findings (e.g., bruises, cuts).
- Client's/caregiver's understanding of individual risks/safety concerns.

Planning

- Plan of care and who is involved in planning.
- Teaching plan.

Implementation/Evaluation

- Individual responses to interventions/teaching and actions performed.
- Specific actions and changes that are made.
- Attainment/progress toward desired outcome(s).
- Modifications to plan of care.

Discharge Planning

- Long-range plans for discharge needs, lifestyle and community changes, and who is responsible for actions to be taken.
- Specific referrals made.

References

1. Gorman-Smith, D., Tolan, P. (1998). The role of exposure to community violence and developmental problems among inner city youth. *Dev Psychopathol,* 10(1), 101.
2. Youth Violence in the United States. National Center for Injury Prevention and Control. Accessed July 2007 at www.cdc.gov/ncipc/factsheets/yvfacts.htm.
3. Gun Safety. ENA Fact sheet. Accessed July 2007 at www.ena.org/ipinstitute/fact/ENAIPFactSheet-GunSafety.pdf.
4. Care Plan: Disaster Considerations; and ND Infection, risk for, in numerous care plans. In Doenges, M. E., Moorhouse, M. F., Geissler-Murr, A. C. (2002). *Nursing Care Plans: Guidelines for Individualizing Patient Care.* 6th ed. Philadelphia: F. A. Davis.
5. Intimate Partner Violence. National Center for Injury Prevention and Control. Accessed July 2007 at www.cdc.gov/ncipc/factsheets/ipvfacts.htm.
6. Nelson, A., et al. (2003). Safe patient handling & movement. *AJN,* 103(3), 32–43.
7. Sexual Violence. National Center for Injury Prevention and Control. Accessed July 2007 at www.cdc.gov/ncipc/factsheets/svfacts.htm.
8. Cohen, M. (2000). *Medication Errors: Causes, Prevention and Risk Management.* Boston: Jones and Bartlett.
9. Bicycle/Helmet Safety. Available at www.ena.org. Accessed January 2004.
10. Water Safety. Emergency Nurses Association. Available at www.ena.org. Accessed January 2004.
11. Drowning Prevention. National Center for Injury Prevention and Control. Accessed July 2007 at www.cdc.gov/ncipc/factsheets/drown.htm.
12. Suicide in the United States. National Center for Injury Prevention and Control. Accessed July 2007 at www.cdc.gov/ncipc/factsheets/suifacts.
13. Safety for older consumers' home safety checklist. Consumer Product Safety Commission (CPSC) document no. 701. Accessed July 2007 at www.gardencitymi.org/departments/fire/seniorsafetychecklist.pdf.
14. Keepnews, D., Mitchell, P. H. (2003). Health Systems' Accountability for patient safety. *Online J of Issues in Nursing,* 8(2). Manuscript 2. Retrieved March 2007 at http://nursingworld.org/ojin/topic22/tpc22_2.htm.
15. Schwebel, D. C., Barton, B. K. (2005). Contributions of multiple risk factors to child injury. *J of Pediatr Psychol,* 30(7), 553–61.

risk for perioperative positioning Injury

Definition: At risk for injury as a result of the environmental conditions found in the perioperative setting

RISK FACTORS
Disorientation; sensory/perceptual disturbances due to anesthesia
Immobilization; muscle weakness; [preexisting musculoskeletal conditions]

Cultural Collaborative Community/Home Care Diagnostic Studies Pediatric/Geriatric/Lifespan Medications

Obesity; emaciation; edema

[Elderly]

NOTE: A risk diagnosis is not evidenced by signs and symptoms, as the problem has not occurred; rather, nursing interventions are directed at prevention.

Sample Clinical Applications: Operative procedures, arthritis, obesity, malnutrition, peripheral vascular disease

DESIRED OUTCOMES/EVALUATION CRITERIA

Sample NOC linkages:

Risk Detection: Personal actions to identify personal health threats

Risk Control: Personal actions to prevent, eliminate, or reduce modifiable health threats

Circulation Status: Unobstructed, unidirectional blood flow at an appropriate pressure through large vessels of the systemic and pulmonary circuits

Client Will (Include Specific Time Frame)

- Be free of injury related to perioperative disorientation.
- Be free of untoward skin and tissue injury or changes lasting beyond 24 to 48 hours post-procedure.
- Report resolution of localized numbness, tingling, or changes in sensation related to positioning within 24 to 48 hours as appropriate.

ACTIONS/INTERVENTIONS

Sample NIC linkages:

Positioning: Intraoperative: Moving the patient body part to promote surgical exposure while reducing the risk of discomfort and complications

Skin Surveillance: Collection and analysis of patient data to maintain skin and mucous membrane integrity

Circulatory Precautions: Protection of a localized area with limited perfusion

NURSING PRIORITY NO. 1 To identify individual risk factors/needs:

- Consider anticipated type and length of procedure, type of anesthesia to be used, and customary required position (e.g., supine, lithotomy, prone, lateral, sitting) *to increase awareness of potential postoperative complications (e.g., supine position may cause low back pain and skin pressure at heels/elbows/sacrum; lateral chest position can cause shoulder and neck pain, or eye and ear injury on the client's downside. Also normal defense mechanisms are altered due to anesthetic agents and medications as well as forced prolonged immobility during the procedure).*[1,2,8]
- Review client's history, noting age, weight, height, nutritional status, physical limitations (e.g., prostheses, implants, range-of-motion restrictions) and preexisting conditions (vascular, respiratory, circulatory, neurological, immunocompromise). *These factors affect choice of position for the procedure (e.g., elderly person with no subcutaneous padding or severe arthritis). Presence of certain conditions can cause the risk of skin/tissue integrity problems during surgery (e.g., diabetes mellitus, obesity, presence of peripheral vascular disease, level of hydration, temperature of extremities).*[1,2,10,11]
- Evaluate/document client's preoperative reports of neurological, sensory or motor deficits *for comparative baseline of perioperative/postoperative sensations.*

- Assess the individual's responses to preoperative sedation/medication, noting level of sedation or adverse effects (e.g., drop in blood pressure) and report to surgeon as indicated. *Hypotension is a common factor associated with nerve ischemia.*[3]
- Evaluate environmental conditions/safety issues surrounding the sedated client (e.g., client alone in holding area, siderails up on bed/cart, use of tourniquets/armloads, need for local injections, etc.) *that predispose client to potential tissue injury.*[1,3,9,11]

NURSING PRIORITY NO. 2 To position client to provide protection for anatomic structures and to prevent injury:

- Stabilize/lock transport cart/bed when transferring client to and from operating room table. Provide body and limb support for client during transfers, using adequate numbers of personnel *to prevent client fall, shear and friction injuries, as well as to prevent injury to personnel.*[4,11]
- Position client, using appropriate positioning equipment/devices, *to provide protection for anatomic structures and to prevent injury:*[1,2]

  Keep head in neutral position (when client in supine position) and arm boards at less than 90-degree angle and level with floor *to prevent neural injuries.*

  Maintain cervical neck alignment and provide protection/padding for forehead, eyes, nose, chin, breasts, genitalia, knees, and feet *when client in prone position.*

  Protect bony prominences and pressure points on dependent side (e.g., axillary roll for dependent axilla, lower leg flexed at hip, upper leg straight padding between knees, ankles, and feet) *when client in lateral position.*

  Place legs in stirrups simultaneously, adjusting stirrup height to client's legs, maintaining symmetrical position, pad popliteal space as indicated *to reduce risk of peroneal and tibial nerve damage, prevent muscle strain, and reduce risk of hip dislocation when lithotomy position used.*
- Check that positioning equipment is correct size for client, is firm and stable, and is adjusted accordingly.[2,4]
- Use gel pads or similar devices over the operating room bed. *Decreases pressure at any given point by redistributing overall pressures across a larger surface area.*[2,8]
- Limit use of pillows, blankets, molded foam devices, towels, and sheet rolls, *which may produce only a minimum of pressure reduction or contribute to friction injuries.*[2]
- Place safety straps strategically *to secure client for specific procedure.* Avoid pressure on extremities when securing straps *to limit possibility of compromising circulation/pressure injuries.*[4]
- Realign/maintain body alignment during procedure as needed. *Changes in position may expose or damage otherwise protected body tissue. The position change may be planned, or imperceptible, and may result from adding or deleting positioning devices, adjusting the procedure bed in some manner, or moving the client on the procedure bed.*[2]
- Apply and periodically reposition padding of pressure points/bony prominences (e.g., arms, shoulders, ankles) and neurovascular pressure points (e.g., breasts, knees, ears) *to maintain position of safety and prevent injury from prolonged pressure.*
- Protect body from contact with metal parts of the operating table, *which could produce electrical injury/burns.*[1,5]
- Position extremities to facilitate periodic evaluation of hands, fingers, and toes. *Prevents accidental trauma from moving table attachments, allows for repositioning of extremities to prevent neurovascular injuries from prolonged pressure. Extremities should not extend beyond the end of operating table to reduce risk of compression or stretch injury.*[6,10]
- Check peripheral pulses and skin color/temperature periodically *to monitor circulation.*

Cultural   Collaborative   Community/Home Care   Diagnostic Studies   Pediatric/Geriatric/Lifespan   Medications

- Ascertain that eyelids are closed and secured *to prevent corneal abrasions.*[6]
- Prevent pooling of prep and irrigating solutions, and body fluids. *Pooling of liquids in areas of high pressure under client increases risk of pressure ulcer development and presents electrical hazard.*[7,8]
- Reposition slowly at transfer and in bed (especially halothane-anesthetized client) *to prevent severe drop in blood pressure, dizziness, or unsafe transfer.*
- Position client following extubation *to protect airway and facilitate respiratory effort.*
- Determine specific postoperative positioning guidelines (e.g., head of bed slightly elevated following spinal anesthesia *to prevent headache;* turn to unoperated side following pneumonectomy *to facilitate maximal respiratory effort).*[1]

NURSING PRIORITY NO. 3 To promote wellness (Teaching/Discharge Considerations):

- Maintain equipment in good working order *to identify potential hazards in the surgical suite and implement corrections as appropriate.*[8]
- Provide perioperative teaching relative to client safety issues (including not crossing legs during procedures performed under local or light anesthesia, postoperative needs/limitations, and signs/symptoms requiring medical evaluation) *to reduce incidence of preventable complications.*
- Inform client and postoperative caregivers of expected/transient reactions (such as low backache, localized numbness, and reddening or skin indentations, which should quickly resolve), *to help them identify problems/concerns that require follow-up.*
- Assist with therapies/nursing actions, including skin care measures, application of elastic stockings, early mobilization *to enhance circulation and venous return, and promote skin and tissue integrity.*
- Encourage/assist with frequent range-of-motion exercises *to prevent/reduce joint stiffness.*
- Refer to appropriate resources, as needed.

DOCUMENTATION FOCUS

Assessment/Reassessment

- Findings, including individual risk factors for problems in the perioperative setting/need to modify routine activities or positions.
- Periodic evaluation of monitoring activities.

Planning

- Plan of care and who is involved in planning.
- Teaching plan.

Implementation/Evaluation

- Response to interventions and actions performed.
- Attainment/progress toward desired outcome(s).
- Modifications to plan of care.

Discharge Planning

- Long-term needs and who is responsible for actions to be taken.

References

1. Surgical Intervention. (2002). In Doenges, M. E., Moorhouse, M. F., Geissler-Murr, A. C. *Nursing Care Plans: Guidelines for Individualizing Patient Care.* 6th ed. Philadelphia: F. A. Davis, pp. 766–767.
2. AORN Standards and Recommended Practices for Perioperative Nursing (2001). Denver, CO: Association of Perioperative Registered Nurses (AORN).
3. No author listed. (1997–2004). Prevention of injuries in the anaesthetised patient. Accessed July 2007 at www.surgical-tutor.org.uk/default-home.htm?principles/perioperative/perioperative_injuries.htm~right.
4. Gruendemann, B. J., Fernsebner, B. (1995). *Comprehensive Perioperative Nursing,* vol. 1. Boston: Jones & Bartlett.
5. Rothrock, J. (1996). *Perioperative Nursing Care Planning.* St. Louis, MO: Mosby.
6. Spry, C. (1997). *Essentials of Perioperative Nursing.* Gaithersburg, MD: Aspen.
7. Meeker, M., Rothrock, J. (1999). *Alexander's Care of the Patient in Surgery.* 11th ed. St. Louis, MO: Mosby.
8. Lafreniere, R., Berguer, R., Seifert, P. C., et al. (2005). Preparation of the operating room. Article for Medscape. Retrieved March 2007 at www.medscape.com/viewarticle/503004.
9. Dunn, D. (2005). Preventing perioperative complicatons in special populations. *Nursing2005,* 35(11), 36–43.
10. Renter, T. A. (No pub date listed). Upper extremity positioning injuries during operative/other invasive procedures. Article for Anesthesia Consulting Web site. Retrieved March 2007 at www.anesthesia-consulting.com.
11. Dunn, D. (2006). Age-smart care: Preventing perioperative complications in older adults. *Nursing2006,* 4(3), 30–39.

Insomnia

Definition: A sustained disruption in amount and quality of sleep that impairs functioning

RELATED FACTORS
Intake of stimulants/alcohol; medications; gender-related hormonal shifts

Stress (e.g., ruminative presleep pattern); depression, fear, anxiety, grief

Impairment of normal sleep pattern (e.g., travel, shift work, parental responsibilities, interruptions for interventions); inadequate sleep hygiene (current)

Activity pattern (e.g., timing, amount)

Physical discomfort (e.g., body temperature, pain, shortness of breath, cough, gastroesophageal reflux, nausea, incontinence/urgency)

Environmental factors (e.g., ambient noise, daylight/darkness exposure, ambient temperature/humidity, unfamiliar setting

DEFINING CHARACTERISTICS

Subjective
Client Reports
Difficulty falling/staying asleep
Waking up too early
Dissatisfaction with sleep (current); nonrestorative sleep
Sleep disturbances that produce next-day consequences; lack of energy; difficulty concentrating; changes in mood
Decreased health status/quality of life
Increased accidents

Objective
Observed lack of energy
Observed changes in affect
Increased work/school absenteeism

Sample Clinical Applications: Chronic pain, substance use/abuse, hyperthyroidism, pulmonary diseases (e.g., COPD, asthma), sleep apnea, restless leg syndrome, depression,

Alzheimer's/senile dementia, anxiety disorders, bipolar disorders, pregnancy—prenatal/ postnatal period

DESIRED OUTCOMES/EVALUATION CRITERIA

Sample NOC linkages:

Sleep: Natural periodic suspension of consciousness during which the body is restored

Rest: Quality and pattern of diminished activity for mental and physical rejuvenation

Client Will (Include Specific Time Frame)

- Verbalize understanding of sleep impairment.
- Identify individually appropriate interventions to promote sleep.
- Adjust lifestyle to accommodate chronobiological rhythms.
- Report improvement in sleep/rest pattern.
- Report increased sense of well-being and feeling rested.

ACTIONS/INTERVENTIONS

Sample NIC linkages:

Sleep Enhancement: Facilitation of regular sleep/wake cycle

Simple Relaxation Therapy: Use of techniques to encourage and elicit relaxation for the purpose of decreasing undesirable signs and symptoms such as pain, muscle tension, or anxiety

Environmental Management: Comfort: Manipulation of the patient's surroundings for promotion of optimal comfort

NURSING PRIORITY NO. 1   To identify causative/contributing factors:

- Identify presence of Related Factors that can contribute to insomnia (e.g., chronic pain, arthritis, dyspnea; movement disorders; dementia; obseity; pregnancy, menopause; psychiatric disorders); metabolic diseases (such as hyperthyroidism and diabetes); prescribed/ OTC drugs; alcohol, stimulant/other recreational drug use; circadian rhythm disorders (e.g., shift work, jet lag); environmental factors (e.g., noise, no control over thermostat, uncomfortable bed); major life stressors (e.g., grief, loss, finances).[1–6,12,13]
- Note age. *Increased sleep latency (time required to fall asleep), decreased sleep efficiency, and increased awakenings are common in the elderly.*[2]
- Observe parent-infant interactions/provision of emotional support. Note mother's sleep-wake pattern. *Lack of knowledge of infant cues/problem relationships may create tension interfering with sleep. Structured sleep routines based on adult schedules may not meet child's needs.*[7]
- Ascertain presence/frequency of enuresis, incontinence, or need for frequent nighttime voidings, interrupting sleep.[2]
- Assist with/review psychological assessment, noting individual and personality characteristics *if anxiety disorders or depression could be affecting sleep.*
- Determine recent traumatic events in client's life (e.g., a death in family, loss of job).[2,3]
- Review client's medication regimen, including prescription (e.g., beta-blockers, steroids, antihypertensives, bronchodilators, weight-loss drugs, thyroid preparations, sedatives, etc.); OTC products (e.g., decongestants); herbals. *Use or timing may be interfering with falling alseep or staying asleep requiring adjustments such as change in dose or time medication is taken, or choice of drug prescribed.*[8,13]

- Note caffeine and alcohol intake. *May interfere with falling asleep/quality of sleep.*
- Assist with diagnostic testing (e.g., EEG, full-night sleep studies) *to determine cause/type of sleep disturbance.*

NURSING PRIORITY NO. 2 To evaluate sleep pattern and dysfunction(s):

- Observe or obtain feedback from client/SO(s) regarding client's sleep problems, usual bedtime, rituals/routines, number of hours of sleep, time of arising, and environmental needs *to determine usual sleep pattern and provide comparative baseline.*
- Listen to subjective reports of sleep quality (e.g., client never feels rested or feels sleepy during day). *Provides opportunity to address misconceptions/unrealistic expectations and plan for interventions.*[9]
- Determine type of insomnia (e.g., transient, short-term, chronic). *Transient episodes are occasional restless nights caused by such factors as jet lag, first night in a new bed, etc. Short-term lasts a few weeks and arises from temporary stressful experience, such as pressures at work, loss of job, death in family, and usually resolves over time as client adapts to stressor. Chronic insomnia lasts for more than 3 weeks and can be caused by many physical and psychological factors as well as use/misuse of medications and drugs.*[5]
- Investigate whether client snores and in what position(s) this occurs. Also determine if obese individual experiences loud periodic snoring, along with unusual nighttime activities (e.g., sitting upright, sleepwalking); morning headaches, sleepiness, depression. *Sleep studies may need to be done to rule out obstructive sleep disorder.*[2,4]
- Note alteration of habitual sleep time such as change of work pattern/rotating shifts, change in normal bedtime (hospitalization). *Helps identify circumstances that are known to interrupt sleep patterns resulting in mental and physical fatigue, affecting concentration, interest, energy, and appetite.*[6]
- Observe physical signs of fatigue (e.g., restlessness, hand tremors, thick speech).
- Graph "circadian" rhythms of individual's biological internal chemistry per protocol as indicated. *Note: Studies have shown sleep cycles are affected by body temperature at onset of sleep.*
- Assist with diagnostic testing (e.g., electroencephalogram [EEG], electrooculogram [EOG], and electromyogram [EMG]; psychological assessment/testing, chronological chart). *Polysmnography (the three electrical tests noted above) are performed in a sleep laboratory to measure several parameters of sleep, including brain wave activity, eye movement, and leg muscle tone. These tests may be performed after initial clinical evaluation or symptom management fails to discover or resolve a particular sleep disturbance or point to appropriate interventions and treatments.*[1,2,4]

NURSING PRIORITY NO. 3 To assist client to establish optimal sleep/rest patterns:

- Collaborate in treatment of underlying medical problem (e.g., obstructive sleep apnea, pain, GERD, lower UTI/prostatic hypertropy; depression, complicated grief).
- Arrange care to provide for uninterrupted periods for rest. *Allows for longer periods of sleep, especially during night.*[9]
- Limit fluid intake in evening if nocturia is a problem *to reduce need for nighttime elimination.*[10]
- Provide quiet environment and comfort measures (e.g., back rub, washing hands/face, cleaning and straightening sheets). *Promotes relaxation and readiness for sleep.*[9]
- Administer pain medications (if required) 1 hour before sleep *to relieve discomfort and take maximum advantage of analgesic and sedative effect.*[5]

∞ • Discuss/implement effective age-appropriate bedtime rituals (e.g., going to bed at same time each night, drinking warm milk, rocking, story reading, cuddling, favorite blanket/toy) *to enhance client's ability to fall asleep, reinforce that bed is a place to sleep, and promote sense of security for child or confused elder.*[7]

🏠 • Recommend limiting intake of chocolate and caffeine/alcoholic beverages, especially prior to bedtime. *Substances known to impair falling asleep or staying asleep. Alcohol may help individual fall asleep, but ensuing sleep is fragmented.*[7]

🏠 • Explore other sleep aids (e.g., warm bath/milk, light protein snack before bedtime, soothing music, favorite TV show). *Nonpharmaceutical aids may enhance falling asleep free of concern of medication side effects such as morning hangover or drug dependence.*[5]

🏠 • Develop behavioral program for insomnia, such as [1–6,13]
establishing routine at bedtime and arising;
thinking relaxing thoughts when in bed;
not napping in the daytime;
not reading or watching TV in bed;
getting out of bed if not asleep in 15 minutes;
limiting sleep to 7 hours a night;
geting up the same time each day—even on weekends/days off;
geting adequate exposure to bright light during day;
individually tailoring stress-reduction program, music therapy, relaxation routine.

🏠 • Recommend/assist with implementing/facilitating program to "reset" sleep clock (chronotherapy when client has delayed sleep-onset insomnia). *These sleep-wake problems are commom among shift workers and airplane travelers. Shift workers can benefit by adhereing to a set routine and ensuring that noises and interruptions are kept to a minimum. Those who travel across time zones can benefit by adjusting their sleep time to match the time zone of their arrival and avoiding caffiene and alcohol.*[11]

💊 • Use barbiturates or other sleeping medications sparingly. *Research indicates long-term use of these medications can actually induce sleep disturbances.*

⊘ • Encourage routine use of continuous positive airway pressure (CPAP) therapy when indicated *to obtain optimal benefit of treatment for sleep apnea.*

💊 • Monitor effects of therapeutic use of amphetamines or stimulants (such as may be used for attention deficit disorder or narcolepsy). *Use of these medications can induce or potentiate sleep disturbances.*[8]

⊘ • Refer to sleep specialist as indicated/desired. *Follow-up evaluation/intervention may be needed when insomnia is having a serious impact on client's quality of life, productivity, and safety (e.g., on the job, at home, on the road).*[2,15]

NURSING PRIORITY NO. 4 To promote wellness (Teaching/Discharge Considerations):

🏠 • Assure client that occasional sleeplessness should not threaten health. *Knowledge that occasional insomnia is universal and usually not harmful may promote relaxation and relief from worry, which can perpetuate the problem.*[4]

🏠 • Assist client to develop individual program of relaxation. Demonstrate techniques (e.g., biofeedback, self-hypnosis, visualization, progressive muscle relaxation). *Methods that reduce sympathetic response and decrease stress can help induce sleep, particulary in persons suffering frrom chronic and long-term sleep disturbances.*[3]

🏠 • Encourage participation in regular exercise program during day *to aid in stress control/release of energy. Note: Exercise at bedtime may stimulate rather than relax client and actually interfere with sleep.*[2]

- Investigate use of aids (e.g., sleep mask, darkening shades/curtains, earplugs, monotonous sounds [white noise]) *to block out ambient light/noise.*
- Assist individuals with insomnia associated with shift work to develop individual schedule *to take advantage of peak performance times as identified in chronobiological chart.*
- Recommend midmorning nap if one is required. *Napping, especially in the afternoon, can disrupt normal sleep patterns.*
- Assist client to deal with grieving process if grief is causing/excacerbating insomina. (Refer to ND Grieving.)

DOCUMENTATION FOCUS

Assessment/Reassessment

- Assessment findings, including specifics of sleep pattern (current and past) and effects on lifestyle/level of functioning.
- Medications/interventions, previous therapies.
- Results of testing.

Planning

- Plan of care and who is involved in planning.
- Teaching plan.

Implementation/Evaluation

- Client's response to interventions/teaching and actions performed.
- Attainment/progress toward desired outcome(s).
- Modifications to plan of care.

Discharge Planning

- Long-term needs and who is responsible for actions to be taken.
- Specific referrals made.

References

1. National Sleep Foundation. When you can't sleep: ABCs of ZZZs. Accessed July 2007 at www.sleepfoundation.org.
2. Grandjean, C. K., Gibbons, S. W. (2000). Assessing geriatric sleep complaints. *Nurse Pract: Am J Prim Health Care*, 25(9), 25.
3. Sleep Pattern, disturbed. In Cox, H. C., Hinz, M. D., Lubano, M. A., et al. (2002). *Clinical Applications of Nursing Diagnosis: Child, Women's, Psychiatric, Gerontic, and Home Health Considerations*. 4th ed. Philadelphia: FA Davis, pp. 375–380.
4. Brain basics. Understanding sleep. National Institute of Neurological Disorders and Stroke (NINDS). Accessed July 2007 at www.ninds.nih.gov/disorders/brain_basics/understanding_sleep.htm.
5. Bahr, R. T. (1999). Sleep disturbances. In Stanley, M., Beare, P. G. *Gerontological Nursing: A Health Promotion/Protection Approach*. 2d ed. Philadelphia: FA Davis, pp. 335–341.
6. Pronitis-Ruotolo, D. (2001). Surviving the night shift: Making Zeitgerber work for you. *AJN*, 101(7), 63.
7. Olds, S., London, M., Ladwig, P. (1999). *Maternal-Newborn Nursing: A Family and Community-Based Approach*. 6th ed. Upper Saddle River, NJ: Prentice Hall.
8. Deglin, J. H., Vallerand, A. H. (2003). *Davis's Drug Guide for Nurses*. 8th ed. Philadelphia: F. A. Davis.
9. Doenges, M. E., Moorhouse, M. F., Geissler-Murr, A. C. (2004). *Nurse's Pocket Guide: Diagnoses, Interventions and Rationales*. 9th ed. Philadelphia: F. A. Davis.
10. Townsend, M. C. (2000). Psychiatric Mental Health Nursing Concepts of Care. 4th ed. Philadelphia: F. A. Davis.

Cultural   Collaborative   Community/Home Care   Diagnostic Studies   Pediatric/Geriatric/Lifespan   Medications

11. Somer, E., Snyderman, N. L. (1999). *Food & Mood: The Complete Guide to Eating Well and Feeling Your Best.* 2nd ed. New York: Owl Books.
12. Vij, S., Gentili, A. (2005). Sleep disorder, geriatric. Article for Emedicine Web site. Retrieved December 2006 at www.emedicine.com/med/topic3179.htm.
13. Hertz, G., Cataletto, M. E. (2006). Sleep dysfunction in women. Article for Emedicine Web site. Retrieved December 2006 at www.emedicine.com/med/topic656.htm.
14. Turkowski, B. B. (2006). Managing insomnia. *Orthopaedic Nursing*, 25(5), 339–345.
15. Nadolski, M. (2005). Getting a good night's sleep: Diagnosing and treating insomnia. *Plastic Surgical Nursing*, 25(4), 167–173.

decreased Intracranial Adaptive Capacity

Definition: Intracranial fluid dynamic mechanisms that normally compensate for increases in intracranial volume are compromised, resulting in repeated disproportionate increases in intracranial pressure (ICP) in response to a variety of noxious and non-noxious stimuli

RELATED FACTORS

Brain injuries
Sustained increase in ICP = 10 to 15 mm Hg
Decreased cerebral perfusion pressure <50 to 60 mm Hg
Systemic hypotension with intracranial hypertension

DEFINING CHARACTERISTICS

Objective

Repeated increases in ICP of >10 mm Hg for more than 5 minutes following a variety of external stimuli
Disproportionate increase in ICP following stimulus
Elevated P_2 ICP waveform
Volume pressure response test variation (volume-pressure ratio 2, pressure-volume index <10)
Baseline ICP <10 mm Hg
Wide amplitude ICP waveform
[Altered level of consciousness—coma]
[Changes in vital signs, cardiac rhythm]

Sample Clinical Applications: Traumatic brain injury (TBI), cerebral edema, stroke, cranial tumors/hematomas, hydrocephalus

DESIRED OUTCOMES/EVALUATION CRITERIA

Sample NOC linkages:

Tissue Perfusion: Cerebeal: Adequacy of blood flow through the cerebral vasculature to maintain brain function

Neurological Status: Ability of the peripheral and central nervous system to receive, process, and respond to internal and external stimuli

Client Will (Include Specific Time Frame)

- Demonstrate stable ICP as evidenced by normalization of pressure waveforms/response to stimuli.
- Display improved neurological signs.

ACTIONS/INTERVENTIONS

Sample NIC linkages:

Cerebral Edema Management: Limitation of secondary cerebral injury resulting from swelling of brain tissue

Cerebral Perfusion Promotion: Promotion of adequate perfusion and limitation of complications for a patient experiencing or at risk for inadequate cerebral perfusion

Intracranial Pressure (ICP) Monitoring: Measurement and interpretation of patient data to regulate intracranial pressure

NURSING PRIORITY NO. 1 To assess causative/contributing factors:

- Determine factors related to individual situation (e.g., traumatic brain injury, infection such as meningitis/encephalitis; brain tumor) and potential for increased intracranial pressure [ICP]). *Deterioration in neurological signs/symptoms or failure to improve after initial insult may reflect decreased adaptive capacity.*[1]

- Review results of diagnostic imaging (e.g., cerebral CT scans) *to note location, type, and severity of tissue injury.*
- Monitor for change in intracranial pressure (e.g., worsening neurological signs or variations in ICP monitor waveform/pressure) and corresponding event (e.g., coughing, suctioning, position change, noise such as monitor alarms, family visit, etc.). *Elevated pressure can be caused by the injury, environmental stimuli, or treatment modalities.*[1,2]

NURSING PRIORITY NO. 2 To note degree of impairment:

- Evaluate level of consciousness using Glasgow Coma Scale (GCS). *GCS assesses eye opening (e.g., awake, opens only to painful movement, keeps eyes closed); position/movement (e.g., spontaneous, purposeful, posturing); pupils (size, shape, equality, light reactivity), and consciousness/mental status (e.g., comatose, responds to pain, awake/confused, etc.). Low numbers (e.g., <9) are typically seen in clients with severe head injury and impaired cerebral perfusion requiring critical care interventions.*[1–3,7]
- Note purposeful and nonpurposeful motor response (e.g., posturing), comparing right/left sides. *Posturing and abnormal flexion of extremities usually indicates diffuse cortical damage. Absence of spontaneous movement on one side indicates damage to the motor tracts in the opposite cerebral hemisphere.*[1]
- Test for presence/absence of reflexes (e.g., blink, cough, gag, Babinski's reflex), nuchal rigidity. *Helps identify location of injury (e.g., loss of blink reflex suggests damage to the pons and medulla, absence of cough and gag reflexes reflects damage to medulla, and presence of Babinski's reflex indicates injury along pyramidal pathways in the brain).*[1]
- Monitor vital signs and cardiac rhythm before/during/after activity. *Helps determine parameters for "safe" activity. Mean arterial blood pressure should be maintained above 90 mm Hg to maintain cerebral perfusion pressure (CCP) greater than 70 mm Hg, which reflects adequate blood supply to the brain. Fever in brain injury can be associated with injury to the hypothalamus or bleeding, systemic infection (e.g., pneumonia), or drugs. Hyperthermia exacerbates cerebral ischemia. Irregular respiration patterns can suggest location of cerebral insult. Cardiac dysrhythmias can be due to brainstem injury and stimulation of the sympathetic nervous system. Bradycardia may occur with high ICP.*[1,3]
- Monitor pulse oximetry/arterial blood gases (ABGs), particularly pH, CO_2, and Pao_2. *$Paco_2$ level of 28 to 30 mm Hg decreases cerebral blood flow while maintaining adequate*

🌐 Cultural   🅐 Collaborative   🏠 Community/Home Care   ⟋ Diagnostic Studies   ∞ Pediatric/Geriatric/Lifespan   💊 Medications

cerebral oxygenation, while a PaO₂ of less than 65 mm Hg may cause cerebral vascular dilation.[1-3]

- Monitor urine output and serum sodium (Na). *Posttraumatic neuroendocrine dysfunction can result in a hyponatremic or hypernatremic state. When hyponatremia exists, cerebral edema or syndrome of inappropriate antidiuretic hormone (SIADH) can occur requiring correction with fluid restriction and hypertonic IV solution. Hypernatremia can occur because of injury to the hypothalamus or pituitary stalk, causing diabetes insipidus (DI), resulting in huge urine losses; or be the result of excessive diuresis due to use of mannitol or furosemide administered to reduce cerebral edema.*[3]

NURSING PRIORITY NO. 3 To minimize/correct causative factors/maximize perfusion:

- Elevate head of bed as individually appropriate. *Optimal head of bed position is determined by both ICP and CPP measurements—that is, which degree of elevation lowers ICP while maintaining adequate cerebral blood flow.*[4] *Studies show that in most cases, 30 degrees elevation significantly decreases ICP while maintaining cerebral blood flow.*[1,7,8]
- Maintain head/neck in neutral position, supporting with small towel rolls or pillows *to maximize venous return. Note: Lateral and rotational neck flexion has been shown to be the most consistent trigger of sustained increases in ICP.*[5]
- Avoid causing hip flexion of 90 degrees or more. *Hip flexion may trap venous blood in the intra-abdominal space, increasing abdominal and intrathoracic pressure, and reducing venous outflow from the head, increasing cerebral pressure.*[6]
- Limit/prevent activities *that increase intrathoracic/abdominal pressures (e.g., coughing, vomiting, straining at stool). Avoid/limit use of restraints (often increases agitation and markedly increasing ICP).*[1]
- Suction with caution and only when needed, limiting to two passes of 10 seconds each with negative pressure no more than 120 mm Hg. Pass catheter just beyond end of endo/tracheal tube without touching tracheal wall or carina. Administer lidocaine intratracheally if indicated, *to reduce cough reflex.*[3]
- Hyperoxygenate before suctioning as appropriate *to minimize hypoxia. Note: Routine hyperventilation is to be avoided; however, therapeutic hyperventilation (PaCO₂ of 30 to 35 mm) may be used for a short period of time in acute neurological deterioration to reduce intracranial hypertension, while other methods of ICP control are initated.*[3,8,9]
- Investigate increased restlessness *to determine causative factors and initiate corrective measures as indicated:*

  Decrease extraneous stimuli/provide comfort measures (e.g., quiet environment, soft voice, tapes of familiar voices played through earphones, back massage, gentle touch as tolerated) *to reduce CNS stimulation and promote relaxation.*[1,5]

  Limit painful procedures (e.g., venipunctures, redundant neurological evaluations) to those that are absolutely necessary *in order to minimize preventable elevations in ICP.*[1,3]

  Provide rest periods between care activities and limit duration of procedures. Lower lighting/noise level, schedule and limit activities *to provide restful environment and limit spikes in ICP associated with noxious stimuli.*[1]

  Encourage family/SOs to talk to client. *Familiar voices appear to have a relaxing effect on many comatose individuals (thereby reducing ICP).*[1]

- Administer/restrict fluid intake as necessary, administer IV fluids via pump/control device *to maintain intravascular volume sufficient to maintain cerebral perfusion while preventing inadvertent vascular overload, cerebral edema, and increased ICP.*[1]

- Weigh as indicated. Calculate fluid balance every shift/daily *to determine fluid needs/maintain hydration and prevent fluid overload.*[1]
- Monitor and manage body temperature. Regulate environmental temperature/bed linens, use cooling blanket as indicated *to decrease metabolic and oxygen needs when fever present or when therapeutic hypothermia therapy is used. Lowering the body temperature has been shown to lower ICP and improve outcomes for recovery.*[3]
- Provide appropriate safety measures/initiate treatment for seizures *to prevent injury/increase of ICP/hypoxia.*
- Administer medications (e.g., antihypertensives, diuretics, analgesics/sedatives, antipyretics, vasopressors, antiseizure drugs, neuromuscular blocking agents, and corticosteroids) as appropriate *to maintain cerebral homeostasis and manage symptoms associated with neuological injury.*
- Administer enteral/parenteral nutrition *to achieve positive nitrogen balance, reducing effects of post-brain injury metabolic and catabolic states, which can lead to complications such as immunosuppression, infection, poor wound healing, loss of body mass, and multiple organ dysfunction.*[3]
- Prepare client for surgery as indicated (e.g., evacuation of hematoma/space-occupying lesion) *to reduce ICP/enhance circulation.*

NURSING PRIORITY NO. 4 To promote wellness (Teaching/Discharge Considerations):

- Identify signs/symptoms suggesting increased ICP (in client at risk without an ICP monitor), for example, restlessness, deterioration in neurological responses. Review appropriate interventions.

DOCUMENTATION FOCUS

Assessment/Reassessment

- Neurological findings noting right/left sides separately (such as pupils, motor response, reflexes, restlessness, nuchal rigidity); Glasgow Coma Scale.
- Response to activities/events (e.g., changes in pressure waveforms/vital signs).
- Presence/characteristics of seizure activity.

Planning

- Plan of care and who is involved in planning.
- Teaching plan.

Implementation/Evaluation

- Response to interventions and actions performed.
- Attainment/progress toward desired outcome(s).
- Modifications to plan of care.

Discharge Planning

- Future needs, plan for meeting them, and determining who is responsible for actions.
- Referrals as identified.

References

1. Craniocerebral trauma (acute rehabilitative phase). In Doenges, M. E., Moorhouse, M. F., Geissler-Murr, A. C. (2002): *Nursing Care Plans: Guidelines for Individualizing Patient Care.* 6th ed. Philadelphia: F. A. Davis.

🌐 Cultural   Collaborative   🏠 Community/Home Care   Diagnostic Studies   ∞ Pediatric/Geriatric/Lifespan   Medications

2. Part 1: Guidelines for the management of severe traumatic brain injury. (2000). Brain Trauma Foundation, Inc. New York: American Association of Neurological Surgeons. Accessed July 2007 at www.guideline.gov/summary/summary.aspx?doc_id=3794.
3. Acute care management of severe traumatic brain injuries. (2001). *Crit Care Nurse Q*, 23(4), 1.
4. Simmons, B. J. (1997). Management of intracranial hemodynamics in the adult: A research analysis of head positioning and recommendations for clinical practice and future research. *J Neurosci Nurs*, 29, 44.
5. Mitchell, P. H., Habermann, B. (1999). Rethinking physiological stability: Touch and intracranial pressure. *Biol Res Nurs*, 1(1), 12–19.
6. Vos, H. R. (1993). Making headway with intracranial hypertension. *Am J Nurs*, 93, 28.
7. Salinas, P., Hanbali, F. (2006). Closed Head Trauma. Article for Emedicine Web site. Retrieved March 2007 at www.emedicine.com/med/topic3403.htm.
8. Reddy, L. (2006) Heads up on cerebral bleeds. *Nursing 2006*, 3(5), Suppl, ED Insider, pp. 4–9.
9. Zink, E. K., McQuillan, K. (2005). Managing traumatic brain injury. *Nursing2005*, 35(9), 36–43.

deficient Knowledge [Learning Need] (specify)

Definition: Absence or deficiency of cognitive information related to specific topic [Lack of specific information necessary for clients/SO(s) to make informed choices regarding condition/treatment/lifestyle changes]

RELATED FACTORS
Lack of exposure/recall
Information misinterpretation; [inaccurate/incomplete information presented]
Unfamiliarity with information resources
Cognitive limitation
Lack of interest in learning; [request for no information]

DEFINING CHARACTERISTICS

Subjective
Verbalization of the problem
[Request for information]
[Statements reflecting misconceptions]

Objective
Inaccurate follow-through of instruction/performance of test
Inappropriate or exaggerated behaviors (e.g., hysterical, hostile, agitated, apathetic)
[Development of preventable complication]

Sample Clinical Applications: Any newly diagnosed disease or traumatic injury, progression of/deterioration in a chronic condition

DESIRED OUTCOMES/EVALUATION CRITERIA
Sample NOC linkages:
Knowledge: [specify—25 choices]: Extent of understanding conveyed about a specific disease process, the promotion and protection of health, maintaining optimal health, etc.
Information Processing: Ability to acquire, organize, and use information

Client Will (Include Specific Time Frame)
• Participate in learning process.
• Identify interferences to learning and specific action(s) to deal with them.

deficient KNOWLEDGE [Learning Need] (specify)

- Exhibit increased interest/assume responsibility for own learning by beginning to look for information and ask questions.
- Verbalize understanding of condition/disease process and treatment.
- Identify relationship of signs/symptoms to the disease process and correlate symptoms with causative factors.
- Perform necessary procedures correctly and explain reasons for the actions.
- Initiate necessary lifestyle changes and participate in treatment regimen.

ACTIONS/INTERVENTIONS

Sample NIC linkages:

Teaching: Individual [or 13 other choices]: Planning, implementation, and evaluation of a teaching program designed to address a patient's particular needs

Learning Facilitation: Promoting the ability to process and comprehend information

Learning Readiness Enhancement: Improving the ability and willingness to receive information

NURSING PRIORITY NO. 1 To assess readiness to learn and individual learning needs:

- Ascertain level of knowledge, including anticipatory needs. *Learning needs can include many things (e.g., disease cause and process, factors contributing to symptoms, procedures for symptom control, needed alterations in lifestyle, ways to prevent complications). Client may or may not ask for information or may express inaccurate perceptions of health status and needed behaviors to manage self-care.*[1]
- Engage in Active-listening. *Conveys expectation of confidence in client's ability to determine learning needs and best ways of meeting them.*[5]
- Determine client's ability/readiness and barriers to learning. *Client may not be physically, emotionally, or mentally capable at this time and may need time to work through and express emotions before learning.*[1]
- Be alert to signs of avoidance. *May need to allow client to suffer the consequences of lack of knowledge before client is ready to accept information.*[1]
- Identify SO(s)/family members requiring information. *Providing appropriate information to others can provide reinforcement for learning, as everyone will understand what is to be expected.*[4]

NURSING PRIORITY NO. 2 To determine other factors pertinent to the learning process:

- Note personal factors (e.g., age/developmental level, gender, social/cultural influences, religion, life experiences, level of education, emotional stability) *that affect ability and desire to learn/assimilate new information, take control of situation, accept responsibility for change.*[2,11]
- Determine blocks to learning, including (1) language barriers (e.g., can't read or write, speaks/understands a different language than that spoken by teacher); (2) physical factors (e.g., cognitive impairment, sensory deficits [e.g., aphasia, dyslexia, hearing or vision impairment]); (3) physical constraints (e.g., acute illness, activity intolerance, impaired thought processes); (4) complexity of material to be learned (e.g., caring for colostomy, giving own insulin injections); (5) forced change in lifestyle (e.g., stopping smoking); or (6) have stated no need/desire to learn. *Many factors affect the client's ability and desire to learn, and his or her expectations of the learning process must be addressed if learning is to be successful.*[1,11]

Cultural · Collaborative · Community/Home Care · Diagnostic Studies · Pediatric/Geriatric/Lifespan · Medications

- Assess the level of the client's capabilities and the possibilities of the situation. *May need to assist SO(s) or caregivers to learn by introducing one new idea, by building on previous information, or by finding pictures to demonstrate an idea, etc., to adapt teaching to client's specific needs.*[6]

NURSING PRIORITY NO. 3 To assess the client's/SO('s) motivation:

- Identify motivating factors for the individual (e.g., client needs to stop smoking because of advanced lung cancer, or client wants to lose weight because family member died of complications of obesity). *Motivation may be negative (e.g., smoking caused lung cancer) or positive (e.g., client wants to promote health/prevent disease). Provides information that can guide content specific to client's situation and motivations.*[3,12]
- Provide information relevant only to the situation. *Reducing the amount of information at any one given time helps to keep the client focused and prevents client from feeling overwhelmed.*[4]
- Provide positive reinforcement rather than negative reinforcers (e.g., criticism and threats). *Enhances cooperation and encourages continuation of efforts.*[5]

NURSING PRIORITY NO. 4 To establish priorities in conjunction with client:

- Determine client's most urgent need from both client's and nurse's viewpoint. *Identifies whether client and nurse are together in their thinking and provides a starting point for teaching and outcome planning for optimal success.*[6]
- Discuss client's perception of need. *Takes into account the client's personal desires/needs and values/beliefs, providing a basis for planning appropriate care.*[6]
- Differentiate "critical" content from "desirable" content. *Identifies information that must be learned now as well as content that could be addressed at a later time. Client's emotional state may preclude hearing much of what is presented, and by only providing what is essential, client may hear it.*[3]

NURSING PRIORITY NO. 5 To determine the content to be included:

- Identify information that needs to be remembered (cognitive) at client's level of development and education. *Enhances possibility that information will be heard and understood.*[6]
- Identify information having to do with emotions, attitudes, and values (affective). *The affective learning domain addresses a learner's emotions toward learning experiences, and attitudes, interest, attention, awareness, and values are demonstrated by affective behaviors. Knowing the client's affective state enhances learning possibilities.*[7,12]
- Identify psychomotor skills that are necessary for learning. *Psychomotor learning involves both cognitive learning and muscular movement. The phases for learning these skills are cognitive (what), associative (how), and autonomous (practice to automaticity). Learners need to know what, why, and how they will learn. For instance, papers need to be typed, so the psychomotor skill will be touch typing. The individual will learn touch typing finger placement and how to type smoothly and rhythmically.*[8]

NURSING PRIORITY NO. 6 To develop learner's objectives:

- State objectives clearly in learner's terms *to meet learner's (not instructor's) needs. Understanding why the material is important to the learner provides motivation to learn.*[8]
- Identify outcomes (results) to be achieved. *Understanding what the outcomes will be helps the client realize the importance of learning the material, providing the motivation necessary to learning.*[8]

deficient KNOWLEDGE [Learning Need] (specify)

- Recognize level of achievement, time factors, and short-term and long-term goals. *Learning progresses in stages. Stage 1: unconsciously unskilled where we don't know we don't know. Stage 2: consciously unskilled, we know we don't know and start to learn. Stage 3: consciously skilled, we know how to do it but need to think and work hard to do it. And stage 4: we become unconsciously skilled, where the new skills are easier and even seem natural.*[9]
- Include the affective goals (e.g., reduction of stress). *The learner's emotional behaviors affect the learning experience and need to be actively addressed for maximum effectiveness.*[7]

NURSING PRIORITY NO. 7 To identify teaching methods to be used:

- Determine client's/SO's method of accessing information and preferred learning mode (e.g., auditory/visual, kinesthetic; group classes, one-to-one instruction, online) and include in teaching plan. *Using multiple modes of instruction facilitates learning/enhances retention, especially when faced with a stressful situation, illness/new treatment regimen.*[3,10]
- Involve the client/SO(s) by using age-appropriate materials tailored to client's interest and literacy skills (e.g., interactive programmed books, questions/dialogue, and audio/visual materials). *Accesses familiar mental images at client's developmental level to help individual learn more effectively.*[3,12,13]
- Involve with others who have same problems/needs/concerns. *Group presentations, support groups provide role models and opportunity for sharing of information to enhance learning.*
- Use team and group teaching as appropriate.

NURSING PRIORITY NO. 8 To facilitate learning:

- Provide mutual goal-setting and learning contracts. *Clarifies expectations of teacher and learner.*
- Provide written information/guidelines and self-learning modules for client to refer to as necessary. *Reinforces learning process.*
- Pace and time learning sessions and learning activities to individual's needs. Involve and evaluate effectiveness of leaning activities with client. *Client statements, questions, comments provide feedback about ability to grasp information being presented.*
- Provide an environment that is conducive to learning *to limit distractions and allow client to focus on the material presented.*
- Be aware of factors related to teacher in the situation (e.g., vocabulary, dress, style, knowledge of the subject, and ability to impart information effectively) *that may affect client's reaction to teacher/ability to learn from this individual.*
- Begin with information the client already knows and move to what the client does not know, progressing from simple to complex. *Can arouse interest/limit sense of being overwhelmed.*[12]
- Deal with the client's anxiety/other strong emotions. Present information out of sequence, if necessary, dealing first with material that is most anxiety-producing *when the anxiety is interfering with the client's learning process.*
- Provide active role for client in learning process, including questions and discussion. *Promotes sense of control over situation.*
- Have client paraphrase content in own words, perform return demonstration, and explain how learning can be applied in own situation *to enhance internalization of material and to evaluate learning.*[3]
- Provide for feedback (positive reinforcement) and evaluation of learning/acquisition of skills. *Validates current level of understanding and identifies areas requiring follow-up.*[5]
- Be aware of informal teaching and role modeling that takes place on an ongoing basis. *Answering specific questions/reinforcing previous teaching during routine contacts/care enhances learning on a regular basis.*[1]

🌐 Cultural Ⓐ Collaborative 🏠 Community/Home Care Diagnostic Studies ∞ Pediatric/Geriatric/Lifespan Medications

🏠 • Assist client to use information in all applicable areas (e.g., situational, environmental, personal). *Enhances learning to promote better understanding of situation/illness.*[1]

NURSING PRIORITY NO. 9 To promote wellness (Teaching/Discharge Considerations):

🏠 • Provide access information for contact person *to answer questions/validate information after discharge.*[1]

🏠 • Identify available community resources/support groups *to assist with problem-solving, provide role models, and support personal growth/change.*[4]

🏠 • Provide additional learning resources (e.g., bibliography, reliable Web sites, audio/visual media), as appropriate. *May assist with further learning/promote learning at own pace.*[7]

DOCUMENTATION FOCUS

Assessment/Reassessment

• Individual findings/learning style and identified needs, presence of learning blocks (e.g., hostility, inappropriate behavior).

Planning

• Plan for learning, methods to be used, and who is involved in the planning.
• Teaching plan.

Implementation/Evaluation

• Responses of the client/SO(s) to the learning plan and actions performed. How the learning is demonstrated.
• Attainment/progress toward desired outcome(s).
• Modifications to plan of care.

Discharge Planning

• Additional learning/referral needs.

References

1. Bohny, B. A. (1997). A time for self-care: Role of the home healthcare nurse. *Home Health Nurse*, 15(4), 281–286.
2. Purnell, L. D., Paulanka, B. J. (1998). Purnell's model for cultural competence. In Purnell, L. D., Paulanka, B. J. (eds): *Transcultural Health Care: A Culturally Competent Approach.* Philadelphia: F. A. Davis.
3. Duffy, B. (1997). Using a creative teaching process with adult patients. *Home Health Nurse,* 15(2), 102–108.
4. Bartholomew L. K., et al. (2000). Watch, discover, think, and act: A model for patient education program development. *Patient Educ Couns*, 39(2–3), 269–280.
5. Gordon, T. (2000). *Parent Effectiveness Training.* New York: Three Rivers Press.
6. Townsend, M. C. (2003). *Psychiatric Mental Health Nursing Concepts of Care.* 4th ed. Philadelphia: F. A. Davis.
7. Bloom B. Bloom's Learning Domains. From Encyclopedia of Educational Technology. Available at: http://coe.sdsu.edu/eet/Articles/BloomsLD. Accessed March 2004.
8. Cook, S. L. Strategies for Psychomotor Skills. From Instructional Strategies. Available at www. signaleader.com/IDTPortfolio/IT800/psychomotor.html. Accessed March 2004.
9. Adams, L. (March 2004). Learning a New Skill Is Easier Said Than Done. Working Together (electronic newsletter). Gordon Training International.
10. Kolb, D. A. (1984). *Experiential Learning: Experience as the Source of Learning and Development.* Englewood Cliffs, NJ: Prentice Hall.
11. No author listed. (2005). Understanding transcultural nursing. *Nursing2005*, 35(1), Suppl: Career Directory, pp. 14–23.

12. Anderson, N. R. (2006). The role of the home healthcare nurse in smoking cessation: Guidelines for successful intervention. *Home Healthcare Nurse, 24*(7), 424–431.
13. Pieper, B., Sieggreen, M., Freeland, B., et al. (2006). Discharge information needs of clients after surgery. *J of Wound, Ostomy and Continence Nursing, 33*(3), 281–290.

readiness for enhanced Knowledge (specify)

Definition: The presence or acquisition of cognitive information related to a specific topic that is sufficient for meeting health-related goals and can be strengthened

RELATED FACTORS
To be developed by nurse researchers and submitted to NANDA

DEFINING CHARACTERISTICS

Subjective
Expresses an interest in learning
Explains knowledge of the topic; describes previous experiences pertaining to the topic

Objective
Behaviors congruent with expressed knowledge

Sample Clinical Applications: As a health-seeking behavior, the patient may be healthy or this diagnosis can occur in any clinical condition

DESIRED OUTCOMES/EVALUATION CRITERIA
Sample NOC linkages:
Knowledge: [specify—25 choices]: Extent of understanding conveyed about a specific disease process, the promotion and protection of health, maintaining optimal health, etc.
Information Processing: Ability to acquire, organize, and use information

Client Will (Include Specific Time Frame)

- Exhibit responsibility for own learning by seeking answers to questions.
- Verify accuracy of informational resources.
- Verbalize understanding of information gained.
- Use information to develop individual plan to meet healthcare needs/goals.

ACTIONS/INTERVENTIONS

Sample NIC linkages:
Teaching: Individual: Planning, implementation, and evaluation of a teaching program designed to address a patient's particular needs
Learning Facilitation: Promoting the ability to process and comprehend information
Learning Readiness Enhancement: Improving the ability and willingness to receive information

NURSING PRIORITY NO. 1 To develop plan for learning:

- Verify client's level of knowledge about specific topic. *Provides opportunity to assure accuracy and completeness of knowledge base for future learning.*[4]

Cultural   Collaborative   Community/Home Care   Diagnostic Studies   Pediatric/Geriatric/Lifespan   Medications

- Determine motivation/expectation for learning. *Provides insight useful in developing goals and identifying information needs.*[4]
- Assist client to identify learning goals/outcomes. *Helps to frame or focus content to be learned. Provides motivation for learning and a measure to evaluate learning process.*[5,8]
- Ascertain preferred methods of learning (e.g., auditory, visual, interactive, or "hands-on"). *Identifies best approaches for the individual to facilitate learning process.*[5]
- Note personal factors (e.g., age/developmental level, gender, social/cultural influences, religion, life experiences, level of education) *that may impact learning style, choice of informational resources, willingness to take control of situation, accept responsibility for change.*[2]
- Determine challenges to learning: language barriers (e.g., client cannot read, speaks/understands language other than that of care provider, dyslexia), physical factors (e.g., sensory deficits such as vision/hearing impairments, aphasia), physical stability (e.g., acute illness, activity intolerance), difficulty of material to be learned. *Identifies special needs to be addressed if learning is to be successful.*[6]

NURSING PRIORITY NO. 2 To facilitate learning:

- Identify/provide information in varied formats appropriate to client's learning style (e.g., audiotapes, print materials, videos, classes/seminars, online). *Use of multiple formats increases learning and retention of material.*[3]
- Provide information about additional/outside learning resources (e.g., bibliography, pertinent Web sites). *Promotes ongoing learning at own pace.*[7]
- Discuss ways to verify accuracy of informational resources. *Encourages independent search for learning opportunities while reducing likelihood of acting on erroneous or unproven data that could be detrimental to client's well-being.*[4]
- Identify available community resources/support groups. *Provides additional opportunities for role modeling, skill training, anticipatory problem-solving, and so forth.*[1]
- Be aware of/discuss informal teaching and role modeling that takes place on an ongoing basis. *Incongruencies in community/peer role models, support group feedback, print advertisements, popular music/videos may exist, creating questions/potentially undermining learning process.*[4]

NURSING PRIORITY NO. 3 To enhance optimum wellness:

- Assist client to identify ways to integrate and use information in all applicable areas (e.g., situational, environmental, personal). *Ability to apply/use information increases desire to learn and retention of information.*[5]
- Encourage client to journal, keep a log, or graph as appropriate. *Provides opportunity for self-evaluation of effects of learning, such as better management of chronic condition, reduction of risk factors, acquisition of new skills.*[6,9]

DOCUMENTATION FOCUS

Assessment/Reassessment

- Individual findings/learning style and identified needs, presence of challenges to learning.
- Motivation/expectations for learning.

Planning

- Plan for learning, methods to be used, and who is involved in the planning.
- Educational plan.

Implementation/Evaluation

- Responses of the client/SO(s) to the educational plan and actions performed.
- How the learning is demonstrated.
- Attainment/progress toward desired outcome(s).
- Modifications to lifestyle/treatment plan.

Discharge Planning

- Additional learning/referral needs.

References

1. Bohny, B. A. (1997). A time for self-care: Role of the home healthcare nurse. *Home Health Nurse,* 15(4), 281–286.
2. Purnell, L. D., Paulanka, B. J. (1998). Purnell's model for cultural competence. In Purnell, L. D., Paulanka, B. J. (eds). *Transcultural Health Care: A Culturally Competent Approach.* Philadelphia: F. A. Davis.
3. Duffy, B. (1997). Using a creative teaching process with adult patients. *Home Health Nurse,* 15(2), 102–108.
4. Bartholomew, L. K., et al. (2000). Watch, discover, think, and act: A model for patient education program development. *Patient Educ Couns,* 39(2–3), 269–280.
5. Clark, D. (1999). Learning Styles, or How We Go from the Unknown to the Known. Accessed July 2007 at www.nwlink.com/~donclark/hrd/learning/styles.html.
6. Townsend, M. C. (2003). *Psychiatric Mental Health Nursing Concepts of Care.* 4th ed. Philadelphia: F. A. Davis.
7. Bloom, B. Bloom's Learning Domains. From Encyclopedia of Educational Technology. Accessed July 2007 at http://coe.sdsu.edu/eet/articles/BloomsLD/.
8. Cook, S. L. Strategies for Psychomotor Skills. From Instructional Strategies. Available at www.signaleader.com/IDTPortfolio/IT800/psychomotor.html. Accessed March 2004.
9. Adams, L. Learning a New Skill Is Easier Said Than Done. From Gordon Training International. Accessed July 2007 at www.gordontraining.com/article-learning-a-new-skill-is-easier-said-than-done.html.

sedentary Lifestyle

Definition: Reports a habit of life that is characterized by a low physical activity level

RELATED FACTORS
Lack of interest/motivation/resources (time, money, companionship, facilities)
Lack of training for accomplishment of physical exercise
Deficient knowledge of health benefits of physical exercise

DEFINING CHARACTERISTICS

Subjective
Verbalizes preference for activities low in physical activity

Objective
Chooses a daily routine lacking in physical exercise
Demonstrates physical deconditioning

Sample Clinical Applications: Chronic/debilitating conditions (e.g., arthritis, MS, COPD, heart failure, paralysis), chronic pain, obesity, depression

DESIRED OUTCOMES/EVALUATION CRITERIA
Sample NOC linkages:
Knowledge: Prescribed Activity: Extent of understanding conveyed about prescribed
activity and exercise
Endurance: Capacity to sustain activity

Client Will (Include Specific Time Frame)

- Verbalize understanding of importance of regular exercise to general well-being.
- Identify necessary precautions/safety concerns and self-monitoring techniques.
- Formulate/implement realistic exercise program with gradual increase in activity.

ACTIONS/INTERVENTIONS

Sample NIC linkages:
Exercise Promotion: Facilitation of regular physical activity to maintain or advance to a
higher level of fitness and health
Teaching: Prescribed Activity/Exercise: Preparing a patient to achieve or maintain a prescribed level of activity

NURSING PRIORITY NO. 1 To assess precipitating/etiological factors:

- Identify client's specific condition(s) (e.g., obesity, depression, MS, arthritis, Parkinson's,
surgery, hemiplegia/paraplegia, chronic pain, brain injury) *that may contribute to immobility
or the onset and continuation of inactivity/sedentary lifestyle.*
- Assess client's age/developmental level, motor skills, ease and capability of movement, posture and gait. *Determines type and intensity of needed interventions related to activity.*[1]
- Determine client's current weight and body mass index (BMI); note dietary habits. *If client
is overweight and BMI is not in healthy range, weight-loss program will be required.*[8]
- Assess physical capabilities to participate in exercise/activities, noting attention span, physical limitations/tolerance, level of interest/desire, and safety needs. *Identifies barriers that
need to be addressed.*[1,6]
- Review usual activities, work requirements/environment. *Absence of regular exercise, stressful
job with little physical exercise increases likelihood of deconditioning and affects choice of interventions and need for involvement of primary healthcare provider in determining safe program.*[8]
- Note emotional/behavioral responses to problems associated with self- or condition-imposed
sedentary lifestyle. *Feelings of frustration and powerlessness may impede attainment of goals.*[2]
- Determine family dynamics and support provided by family/friends. *Major lifestyle change
will require support of others to achieve and maintain goals or client is at increased risk of slipping back into "old" ways.*[8]
- Discuss availability of resources (e.g., financial for gym membership, transportation, exercise
facility/gym at work site, proximity of bike path, safety of neighborhood for outdoor activity).

NURSING PRIORITY NO. 2 To motivate and stimulate client involvement:

- Establish therapeutic relationship, acknowledging reality of situation and client's feelings.
*Changing a lifelong habit can be difficult, and client may feel discouraged with body and hope-
less to turn situation around into a positive experience.*[2]

- Ascertain client's perception of current activity/exercise patterns, impact on life, and cultural expectations of client/others. *Helps to determine whether or not client perceives need for change, and potential limitations in choices for activities.*[8]
- Discuss client's stated motivation for change. *Concerns of client/SOs regarding threats to personal health/longevity, or acceptance by teen peers may be sufficient to cause client to initiate change; however, client must want to change for himself or herself in order to sustain change.*[4,8]
- Review necessity for/benefits of regular exercise. *Research confirms that exercise has benefits for the whole body (e.g., can boost energy, enhance coordination, reduce muscle deterioration, improve circulation, lower blood pressure, produce healthier skin and a toned body, prolong youthful appearance). Regular exercise has also been found to boost cardiac fitness in both conditioned and out-of-shape individuals.*[4]
- Counsel client regarding individual health risks. *Focuses attention on own situation and helps prioritize needs, making change more manageable.*[8]
- Involve client, SO/parent, or caregiver in developing exercise plan and goals *to meet individual needs, desires, and available resources. Also increases commitment to program and successful attainment of goals.*
- Introduce activities at client's current level of functioning, progressing to more complex activities, as tolerated. *Reduces likelihood of overwhelming client at the beginning and maintains interest over time.*
- Recommend mix of age/gender-appropriate activities/stimuli (e.g., movement classes, walking/hiking, jazzercise, swimming, biking, skating, bowling, golf, weight training). *Activities need to be personally meaningful for client to derive the most enjoyment and to sustain motivation to continue with program.*[2,6]
- Encourage change of scenery (indoors and outdoors where possible) and periodic changes in the personal environment when client is confined inside.

NURSING PRIORITY NO. 3 To promote optimal level of function and prevent exercise failure:

- Assist with treatment of underlying condition impacting participation in activities *to maximize function within limitations of situation.* Refer to dietician *for weight-loss program, as indicated.*
- Collaborate with physical medicine specialist or occupational/physical therapist in providing active or passive range-of-motion exercise, isotonic muscle contractions. *Techniques such as gait training, strength training, and exercise to improve balance and coordination can be helpful in rehabilitating client.*[1]
- Schedule ample time to perform exercise activities balanced with adequate rest periods.[1]
- Provide for safety measures as indicated by individual situation, including environmental management/fall prevention. (Refer to ND risk for Falls.)
- Reevaluate ability/commitment periodically. *Changes in strength/endurance signal readiness for progression of activities or possibly to decrease exercise if overly fatigued. Wavering commitment may require change in types of activities, addition of a workout buddy to reenergize involvement.*[2,5]
- Discuss discrepancies in planned and performed activities with client aware and unaware of observation. Suggest methods for dealing with identified problems. *May be necessary when client is using avoidance or controlling behavior or is not aware of own abilities due to anxiety/fear.*[2,5]

NURSING PRIORITY NO. 4 To promote wellness (Teaching/Discharge Considerations):

- Review components of physical fitness: (1) muscle strength and endurance, (2) flexibility, (3) body composition (muscle mass, percentage of body fat), and (4) cardiovascular health. *Fitness routines need to include all elements to attain maximized benefits/prevent deconditioning.*[4,5,7]

- Instruct in safety measures, as individually indicated (e.g., warm-up and cooldown activities; taking pulse before/during/after activity; adequate intake of fluids, especially during hot weather/strenuous activity; wearing reflective clothing when jogging/reflectors on bicycle; locking wheelchair before transfers; judicious use of medications; supervision, as indicated).[1]

- Recommend keeping an activity/exercise log, including physical/psychological responses, changes in weight, endurance, body mass. *Provides visual evidence of progress/goal attainment and encouragement to continue with program.*[2,6]

- Encourage client to involve self in exercise *as part of wellness management for the whole person.*[3,6]

- Encourage parents to set a positive example for children *by participating in exercise and engaging in an active lifestyle.*[3,6]

- Identify community resources, charity activities, support groups. *Community walking/hiking trails, sports leagues, etc.; provide free/low-cost options. Activities such as 5k walks for charity, participation in Special Olympics, or age-related competitive games provide goals to work toward. Note: Some individuals may prefer solitary activities; however, most individuals enjoy supportive companionship when exercising.*[3,4]

- Discuss alternatives for exercise program in changing circumstances (e.g., walking the mall during inclement weather, using exercise facilities at hotel when traveling, water aerobics at local swimming pool, joining a gym).

- Promote individual participation in community awareness of problem and discussion of solutions. *Physical inactivity (and associated diseases) is a major public health problem that affects large numbers of people in all regions of the world. Recognizing the problem and future consequences may empower the global community to develop effective measures to promote physical activity and improve public health.*[7]

- Promote community goals for increasing physical activity, such as school-based physical education; Sports, Play, and Active Recreation for Kids (SPARK); "buddy" system or contracting for specific physical activities; and Physician-Based Assessment and Counseling for Exercise (PACE) *to address national concerns about obesity and major barriers to physical activity, such as time constraints, lack of training in physical activity, or behavioral change methods, and lack of standard protocols.*[3,6,7,9]

DOCUMENTATION FOCUS

Assessment/Reassessment

- Individual findings, including level of function/ability to participate in specific/desired activities, motivation for change.

Planning

- Plan of care and who is involved in the planning.
- Teaching plan.

Implementation/Evaluation

- Responses to interventions/teaching and actions performed.
- Attainment/progress toward desired outcome(s).
- Modifications to plan of care.

Discharge Planning

- Discharge/long-range needs, noting who is responsible for each action to be taken.
- Specific referrals made.
- Sources of/maintenance for assistive devices.

References

1. Boesch, C., Meyers, J., Habersaat, A., et al. (2005). Maintenance of exercise capacity and physical activitity patterns after cardiac rehabilitation. *Cardiopulm Rehab*, 25(1), 14–21.
2. Sallis, J. F. (1996). The role of behavioral science in improving health through physical activity. Summary of presentation. Science Writers Briefing. Sponsored by OBSSR and the American Psychological Association. December 1996.
3. Wehling-Weepie, A. K., McCarthy, A. (2002). A healthy lifestyle program: Promoting child health in schools. *J School Nursing*, 18(6), 322.
4. McCormack, B. N., Yorkey, M. (2005). *Ten Great Things Exercise Can Do for You.* New York: Wiley Pub Inx. American Media, Inc.
5. Lai, S. C., Cohen, M. N. (1999). Promoting lifestyle changes. *AJN*, 99(4), 63.
6. Editorial staff. (2006). Fitness at any age. Article for MedicineNet Web site. Retrieved March 2007 at www.medicinenet.com.
7. World Health Organization (WHO). (2007). Sedentary lifestyle: A global public health problem. "Move for health" information sheet. Retrieved from WHO Web site March 2007 at www.who.int.
8. Morantz, C. (2004). Obesity and sedentary lifestyle guidelines. American Academy of Family Physicians. Retrieved July 2007 at http://findarticles.com/p/articles/mi_m3225/is_10_69/ai_n6048509.
9. Task Force on Community Preventive Services—Indpendent Expert Panel. (May 2002). Recommendations to increase physical activities in communities. *Am J Prev Med*, 22(2Suppl), 67–72.

risk for impaired Liver Function

Definition: At risk for liver dysfunction

RISK FACTORS
Viral infection (e.g., hepatitis A, hepatitis B, hepatitis C, Esptein-Barr)
HIV co-infection
Hepatotoxic medications (e.g., acetaminophen, statins)
Substance abuse (e.g., alcohol, cocaine)
NOTE: A risk diagnosis is not evidenced by signs and symptoms, as the problem has not occurred; rather, nursing interventions are directed at prevention.

Sample Clinical Applications: Hepatitis, HIV, substance abuse, drug overdose (acetaminophen), Epstein-Barr infection

DESIRED OUTCOMES/EVALUATION CRITERIA
Sample NOC linkages:
Knowledge: Disease Process: Extent of understanding conveyed about a specific disease process
Treatment Behavior: Illness or Injury: Personal actions to palliate or eliminate pathology

Client Will (Include Specific Time Frame)

- Verbalize understanding of individual risk factors that contribute to possibility of liver damage/failure.
- Demonstrate behaviors, lifestyle changes to reduce risk factors and protect self from injury.
- Be free of signs of liver failure as evidenced by liver function studies within normal range, and absence of jaundice, hepatic enlargement, or altered mental status.

Cultural   Collaborative   Community/Home Care   Diagnostic Studies   Pediatric/Geriatric/Lifespan   Medications

ACTIONS/INTERVENTIONS

Sample NIC linkages:

Risk Identification: Analysis of potential risk factors, determination of health risk, and prioritization of risk-reduction strategies for an individual or group

Infection Protection: Prevention and early detection of infection in a patient at risk

Substance Use Treatment: Supportive care of patient/family members with physical and psychosocial problems with the use of alcohol or drugs

NURSING PRIORITY NO. 1   To identify individual risk factors/needs:

- Determine presence of condition(s) as listed in Risk Factors, noting whether problem is acute (e.g., viral hepatitis, acetaminophen overdose) or chronic (e.g., alcoholic cirrhosis). *Influences choice of interventions.*[1]
- Note client history of known/possible exposure to virus, bacteria, or toxins *that can damage liver:*[2-8]

  Works in high-risk occupation [e.g., performs tasks that involve contact with blood, blood-contaminated body fluids, other body fluids, or sharps].

  Injects drugs, especially if client shared a needle; received tattoo or piercing with an unsterile needle.

  Received blood/blood products prior to 1992.

  Ingested contaminated food or water or experienced poor sanitation practices by food-service workers.

  Close contact (e.g., lives with or has sex with infected person/carriers).

  Regular exposure to toxic chemicals (e.g., carbon tetrachloride cleaning agents, bug spray, paint fumes, and tobacco smoke).

  Uses prescription drugs (e.g., sulfonamides, phenothiazines, isoniazid).

  Ingests certain herbal remedies or mega doses of vitamins.

  Uses alcohol with medications (including OTC medications).

  Consumes alcohol heavily and/or over long period of time.

  Ingested acetaminophen (accidentally, as may occur when client takes too large a dose, or has several medications containing acetaminophen over time; or intentionally, as may occur with suicide attempt).

  Travels internationally to/immigrates from countries such as China, Africa, southeast Asia, Middle East *(where hepatitis is endemic).*

- Review results of laboratory tests (e.g., liver function studies, such as alanine aminotransferase [ALT], alkaline phosphatase [ALP], bilirubin, gamma-glutamyl transferase [GGT], lactic acid dehydrogenase [LDH], albumin, total protein and prothrombin time [PT], drug levels, hepatitis titers)/diagnostic studies *that indicate presence of hepatotoxic condition and need for medical treatment.*[9]

NURSING PRIORITY NO. 2   To assist client to reduce or correct individual risk factors:

- Assist with medical treatment of underlying condition (e.g., hepatits, alcoholism, drug overdose) *to support organ function and minimize liver damage.*
- Educate client/SO on way(s) to prevent exposure to/incidence of hepatitis infections/limit damage to liver:[7]

  Practice safer sex (e.g., avoid multiple-partner sex, wear condoms, avoid sex with partners known to be infected).

Avoid injecting drugs or sharing needles.

Use proper protective equipment when working in high-risk occupations, such as health-care, emergency services, chemical manufacturing.

Avoid tap water and practice good hygiene and sanitation when traveling internationally.

Use harsh cleansers and aerosol products in well-ventilated room; wear mask and gloves, cover skin, and wash well afterward. *Insecticides and other chemicals can reach the liver through skin and destroy liver cells.*

- Discuss safe use/concerns about client's medication regimen (e.g., acetaminophen, NSAIDs, herbal/vitamin supplements, phenobarbitol, cholesterol-lowering drugs such as statins, certain antibiotics [e.g., sulfonamides, INH]; certain cardiovascular drugs [e.g., amiodarone, hydralazine]; certain antidepressants [e.g., tricyclics]) *known to cause hepatotoxicity, either alone or in combination, or in overdose situation. Note: Many OTC and prescription medicines, even "natural" or herbal remedies, contain chemicals that can harm the liver over time. Very high doses of certain pain relievers (such as acetaminophen) can cause liver failure.*[9–12]

- Encourage client who is routinely taking acetaminophen for pain management to read labels, determine strength of medication, note safe number of doses over 24 hours, become familiar with "hidden" sources of acetaminophen (e.g., Nyquil, Vicodin), and limit alcohol intake *to avoid/limit risk of liver damage.*[8]

- Stress importance of responsible drinking (e.g., men should limit alcohol to no more than two drinks a day, and women one drink/day); or avoid alcohol altogether when indicated (if client has any kind of liver disease) *to reduce incidence of cirrhosis/severity of liver damage/failure.*[7]

- Encourage smoking cessation. *The additives in cigarettes pose a challenge to the liver by reducing the liver's ability to eliminate toxins.*[7]

- Encourage client with liver dysfunction to avoid fatty foods. *Fat interferes with normal function of liver cells and can cause additional damage/permanent scarring to liver cells when they can no longer regenerate.*[11]

- Refer to nutritionist, as indicated, for dietary needs, including proteins, vitamins, *to promote healing.*

- Discuss signs/symptoms (e.g., increased abdominal girth; rapid weight loss/gain; increased peripheral edema; dyspnea, fever; blood in stool or urine; excess bleeding of any kind; jaundice) *that warrant prompt notification of healthcare provider for evaluation/treatment of severe liver dysfunction, possible organ failure.*[12]

- Refer to specialist/liver treatment center, as indicated. *May be beneficial for client with chronic liver disease when decompensating, for client with hepatitis and other coexisting disease condition (e.g., HIV), or for client with intolerance to treatment due to side effects.*

NURSING PRIORITY NO. 3 To promote wellness (Teaching/Discharge Considerations):

- Emphasize importance of hand hygiene, use of bottled water, and avoidance of fresh produce/raw meat/seafood *if client is traveling to area where hepatitis A is endemic or food/waterborne illness is a risk.*[13]

- Instruct in measures including protection from blood/other body fluids, sharps safety; safer sex practices; avoiding needle sharing; body tattoos/piercing *to prevent occupational and nonoccupational exposures to hepatitis.*

- Discuss need/refer for vaccination, as indicated (e.g., healthcare and public safety worker, children under 18, international traveler, recreational drug user, men who have sex with other men, client with clotting disorders or liver disease, anyone sharing household with an infected person) *to prevent exposure/transmission of blood/body fluid hepatitis/limit risk of liver injury.*[13]

⊕ Cultural   Collaborative   🏠 Community/Home Care   Diagnostic Studies   ∞ Pediatric/Geriatric/Lifespan   Medications

- Discuss appropriateness of prophylaxis immunizations. *Although the best way to protect against hepatitis B and C infections is to prevent exposure to viruses, post-exposure prophylaxis (PEP) should be initiated promptly to prevent/limit severity of infection, especially in persons with close contact with infected individual or in client with compromised immune system.*[14]
- Provide information regarding availability of gamma globulin, ISG, H-BIG, HB vaccine (Recombivax HB, Engerix-B), through health department or family physician.
- Stress necessity of follow-up care (in client with chronic liver disease) *to monitor liver function/effectiveness of interventions* and importance of adherence to therapeutic regimen *to prevent/minimize permanent liver damage.*
- Refer to community resources for immunizations/drug/alcohol treatment program, as indicated.

DOCUMENTATION FOCUS

Assessment/Reassessment

- Assessment findings, including individual risk factors.
- Results of laboratory tests/diagnostic studies.

Planning

- Plan of care and who is involved in planning.
- Teaching plan.

Implementation/Evaluation

- Response to interventions/teaching and actions performed.
- Attainment/progress toward desired outcome(s).
- Modifications to plan of care.

Discharge Planning

- Long-term needs, plan for follow-up and who is responsible for actions to be taken.
- Specific referrals made.

References

1. Smith, D. H. (2007). Managing acute acetaminophen toxicity. *Nursing2007*, 37(1), 58–63.
2. Bockhold, K. M. (2000). Who's afraid of hepatitis C? *AJN*, 100(5), 26.
3. Lambright, J. A. (1999). Preventing hepatitis. *Nursing99*, 29(8), 66.
4. Shovein, J. T., Camozo, R. J., Hyams, I. (2000). Hepatits A: How benign is it? *AJN*, 100(3), 43.
5. Klainberg, M. (1999). Primary biliary cirrhosis. *AJN*, 99(12), 38.
6. American Liver Society and National Institutes for Health. (2003). Viral Hepatitis: A through E and beyond. NIH Publication No. 03-4762 Retrieved July 2007 at http://digestive.niddk.nih.gov/ddiseases/pubs/viralhepatitis/index.htm.
7. American Liver Society and National Institutes for Health. (2006). You are at risk for liver damage or disease if . . . NIH Fact Sheet. Retrieved July 2007 at http://digestive.niddk.nih.gov/ddiseases/pubs/viralhepatitis/index.htm.
8. Fong, T. (2002). Acetaminopen (Tylenol) liver damage. Article for MedicineNet Web site. Retrieved December 2006 at www.medicinenet.com.
9. American Association for Clinical Chemistry. (2005). Liver Panel. Lab Tests Online Web site. Retrieved July 2007 at http://labtestsonline.org/understanding/analytes/liver_panel/glance.html.
10. No author listed. (2005). Liver blood enzymes. Article for MedicineNet Web site. Retrieved December 2006 at www.medicinenet.com.
11. Cormier, M. (2005). The role of hepatitis C support groups. *Gastroenterology Nursing*, 28(3,Suppl), S4–S9.
12. Whiteman, K., McCormick, C. (2005). When your patient is in liver failure. *Nursing2005*, 35(4), 58–63.

13. Durston, S. (2005). What you need to know about viral hepatitis. *Nursing2005*, 35(8), 36–41.
14. Kania, D. S., Scott, C. M. (2007). Postexposure prophylaxis considerations for occupational and nonoccupational exposures. *Advanced Emergency Nursing Journal*, 29(1), 20–32.

risk for Loneliness

Definition: At risk for experiencing discomfort associated with a desire or need for more contact with others

RISK FACTORS
Affectional deprivation
Physical/social isolation
Cathectic deprivation
[Problems of attachment for infants or adolescents]
[Chaotic family relationships]
NOTE: A risk diagnosis is not evidenced by signs and symptoms, as the problem has not occurred; rather, nursing interventions are directed at prevention.

Sample Clinical Applications: Debilitating conditions (e.g., MS, COPD, renal failure), cancer, AIDS, major depression

DESIRED OUTCOMES/EVALUATION CRITERIA
Sample NOC linkages:
Loneliness Severity: Severity of emotional, social, or existential isolation response
Social Involvement: Social interactions with persons, groups, or organizations

Client Will (Include Specific Time Frame)

• Identify individual difficulties and ways to address them.
• Engage in desired social activities.
• Report involvement in interactions/relationship client views as meaningful.

Sample NOC linkages:
Knowledge: Parenting: Extent of understanding conveyed about provision of a nurturing and constructive environment for a child from 1 year through 17 years of age

Parent Will (Include Specific Time Frame)

• Provide infant with consistent and loving caregiving.
• Participate in programs for adolescents and families.

ACTIONS/INTERVENTIONS

Sample NIC linkages:
Socialization Enhancement: Facilitation of another person's ability to interact with others
Hope Instillation: Facilitation of the development of a positive outlook in a given situation
Emotional Support: Provision of reassurance, acceptance, and encouragement during times of stress

Cultural　Collaborative　Community/Home Care　Diagnostic Studies　Pediatric/Geriatric/Lifespan　Medications

NURSING PRIORITY NO. 1 To identify causative/precipitating factors:

- Differentiate between ordinary loneliness and a state of constant sense of dysphoria. *Being alone is a different state than loneliness.*[3]

- Note client's age and duration of problem—that is, situational (such as leaving home for college) or chronic. *Adolescents may experience lonely feelings related to the changes that are happening as they become adults. Elderly individuals incur multiple losses associated with aging, loss of spouse, decline in physical health, and changes in roles, thus intensifying feelings of loneliness.*[3,12]

- Determine degree of distress, tension, anxiety, restlessness present. Note history of frequent illnesses, accidents, crises. *Identifies somatic complaints that can result from loneliness. Individuals under stress tend to have more illnesses and accidents related to inattention and anxiety.*[6]

- Note presence/proximity of family/SO(s). *Loneliness may not be related to being alone, but knowing that family is available can help with planning care. Client may be estranged from other family members or they may not be willing to be involved with client.*[6]

- Discuss with client whether there is a/are person(s) in his or her life who can be trustworthy and who will listen with empathy to the feelings that are expressed.

- Determine how individual perceives/deals with solitude. *Client may see being alone as positive, allowing time to pursue own interests, or may view solitude as sad and long for lost objects, such as spouse.*[6,13]

- Review issues of separation from parents as a child, loss of SO(s)/spouse. *Early separation from parents often affects the individual as other losses occur throughout life, leading to feelings of inadequacy and inability to deal with current situation.*[6,13]

- Assess sleep/appetite disturbances, ability to concentrate. *Feelings of loneliness often accompany depression, and identifying whether client is adequately taking care of self is important to planning care.*[7]

- Note expressions of "yearning" for an emotional partnership. *Widows and widowers are particularly prone to feelings of loneliness. Going from being a "couple" to being alone is a difficult transition, and these feelings are indicative of a desire to return to the "couple" state.*[7]

- Assess feelings of loneliness in client who is receiving palliative care. *These individuals often feel alienated and lonely as they face the end of their life and may need additional socialization to help them feel valued.*[5]

NURSING PRIORITY NO. 2 To assist client to identify feelings and situations in which he or she experiences loneliness:

- Establish therapeutic nurse-client relationship. *Provides a sense of connection with someone, thereby enabling client to feel free to talk about feelings of loneliness and current situation that is related to these feelings.*[1,10]

- Discuss individual concerns about feelings of loneliness and relationship between loneliness and lack of SOs. Note desire/willingness to change situation. *Motivation/lack thereof can facilitate/impede achieving desired outcomes. Often feelings of loneliness arise from underlying depression related to loss, thus affecting individual's coping abilities.*[7]

- Support expression of negative perceptions of others and whether client believes they are true. *Provides opportunity for client to clarify reality of situation, recognize own denial. Individual's view of the world is colored by feelings of loneliness/depression.*[1]

- Accept client's expressions of loneliness as a primary condition and not necessarily as a symptom of some underlying condition. *Provides a beginning point, which will allow the client to look at what loneliness means in life without having to search for deeper meaning.*[1,2]

Nursing Diagnoses in Alphabetical Order

NURSING PRIORITY NO. 3 To assist client to become involved:

🏠 • Discuss reality versus perception of situation. Have client identify people who he or she interacts with on a regular basis. *Provides opportunity for reality check and beginning to understand own feelings of loneliness related to what is happening in own life.*[2,13]

∞ • Discuss importance of emotional bonding (attachment) between infants/young children, parents/caregivers, as appropriate. *Understanding the importance of attachment provides parents with information that will help them take measures to ensure that this bonding occurs.*[2]

Ⓐ • Involve in classes such as assertiveness, language/communication, social skills. *Addressing individual needs will enhance socialization and provide client with the skills to become involved in social activities, thus promoting self-confidence and alleviating feelings of loneliness.*[3,8,11]

🏠 • Role-play situations that are new or are anxiety-provoking for client. *Practicing new situations helps develop self-confidence and provides client with information about what to expect and how to deal with the unexpected in a positive manner.*[2]

🏠 • Discuss positive health habits, including personal hygiene, exercise activity of client's choosing. *Improves feelings of self-esteem, thus enabling client to feel more confident in social situations.*[7]

🏠 • Identify individual strengths/areas of interest that client identifies and is willing to pursue. *Provides opportunities for involvement with others to develop new social skills.*[7,11]

Ⓐ • Encourage attendance at support groups (e.g., therapy, separation/grief, religious). *Participating in these activities can meet individual needs and help client begin to deal with feelings of loneliness.*[7]

🏠 • Help client establish plan for progressive involvement, beginning with a simple activity, such as calling an old friend, speaking to a neighbor, and then leading to more complicated interactions/activities. *Taking small steps promotes success, and confidence is gained as each step is taken, thus helping the client to be more involved and to resolve feelings of loneliness.*[7]

🏠 • Provide opportunities for interactions in a supportive environment (e.g., have client accompanied as in a "buddy system") during initial attempts to socialize. *Helps reduce stress, provides positive reinforcement, and facilitates successful outcome.*[7]

NURSING PRIORITY NO. 4 To promote wellness (Teaching/Discharge Considerations):

🏠 • Let client know that loneliness can be overcome. *It is up to the individual to build self-esteem and learn to feel good about self.*[4,13]

🏠 • Encourage involvement in special-interest groups (e.g., computers, bird watchers) or charitable services (e.g., serving in a soup kitchen, youth groups, animal shelter). *Becoming involved with others takes focus off of self and own concerns, promotes feelings of self-worth, and encourages client to again be an active part of society.*[7]

🏠 • Suggest volunteering for church committee or choir; attending community events with friends and family; becoming involved in political issues/campaigns; or enrolling in classes at local college/continuing education programs, as able. *When client is willing to become involved in these kinds of activities, perception of loneliness fades into the background, and even though individual may still be lonely, the sense of loneliness is not so pervasive.*[7]

Ⓐ • Refer to appropriate counselors for help with relationships, social skills, or other identified needs. *May provide additional assistance to help client deal with feelings of loneliness and isolation.*[9,10]

• Refer to NDs Anxiety, Hopelessness, and Social Isolation, for additional interventions, as appropriate.

🌐 Cultural Ⓐ Collaborative 🏠 Community/Home Care 🧪 Diagnostic Studies ∞ Pediatric/Geriatric/Lifespan   Medications

DOCUMENTATION FOCUS

Assessment/Reassessment

- Assessment findings, including client's perception of problem, availability of resources/support systems.
- Client's desire/commitment to change.

Planning

- Plan of care and who is involved in planning.
- Teaching plan.

Implementation/Evaluation

- Response to interventions/teaching and actions performed.
- Attainment/progress toward desired outcome(s).
- Modifications to plan of care.

Discharge Planning

- Long-term needs, plan for follow-up, and who is responsible for actions to be taken.
- Specific referrals made.

References

1. Doenges, M. E., Townsend, M., Moorhouse, M. F. (1998). *Psychiatric Care Plans: Guidelines for Individualizing Care.* 3d ed. Philadelphia: F. A. Davis.
2. Townsend, M. (2006). *Psychiatric Mental Health Nursing: Concepts of Care.* 5th ed. Philadelphia: F. A. Davis.
3. Lipson, J. G., Dibble, S. L., Minarik, P. A. (1999). *Culture & Nursing Care: A Pocket Guide.* San Francisco: School of Nursing, UCSF Nursing Press.
4. Doenges, M. E., Moorhouse, M. F., Geissler-Murr, A. C. (2006). *Nurse's Pocket Guide: Diagnoses, Interventions, and Rationales.* 11th ed. Philadelphia: F. A. Davis.
5. Paice, J. (2002). Managing psychological conditions in palliative care. *AJN,* 102(11), 36–43.
6. Killeen, C. (1998). Loneliness, an epidemic in modern society. *J Adv Nurs,* 28(4), 762–770.
7. McAuley, E., et al. (2000). Social relations, physical activity, and well-being in older adults. *Prev Med,* 31, 608–617.
8. Acorn, S., Bampton, E. (1992). Patient's loneliness: A challenge for rehabilitation nurses. *Rehabil Nurs,* 17, 22.
9. Davidson, L., Stayner, D. (1997). Loss, loneliness, and the desire for love: Perspectives on the social lives of people with schizophrenia. *Psychiatr Rehab J,* 20, 3–12.
10. Robinson, K. (2007). Loneliness. University of New York at Buffalo. Retrieved March 2007 at http://ub-counseling.buffalo.edu/loneliness.shtml .
11. Finch, A. (2007). Fed up with feeling alone? Retrieved February 2007 at www.selfesteem4women.com/_lib/eZine/articles/cc_0408.php.
12. Evans, M. Loneliness. Self-Help Information Counseling and Testing Center. Retrieved March 2007 at http://darkwing.uoregon.edu/~counsel/loneliness.htm.
13. Seepersad, S. (2007). Loneliness in Attachment and Family. Retrieved March 2007 at www.webofloneliness.com/publications/critical/pubintro.htm.

impaired Memory

Definition: Inability to remember or recall bits of information or behavioral skills [Impaired memory may be attributed to physiopathological or situational causes that are either temporary or permanent]

RELATED FACTORS

Hypoxia; anemia

Fluid and electrolyte imbalance; decreased cardiac output

Neurological disturbances [e.g., brain injury/concussion]

Excessive environmental disturbances; [manic state, fugue, traumatic event]

[Substance use/abuse; effects of medications]

[Age]

DEFINING CHARACTERISTICS

Subjective

[Reported] experiences of forgetting

Inability to recall recent or past events/factual information, [or familiar persons, places, items]

Objective

[Observed] experiences of forgetting

Inability to determine if a behavior was performed

Inability to learn/retain new skills/information

Inability to perform a previously learned skill

Forgets to perform a behavior at a scheduled time

Sample Clinical Applications: Brain injury/stroke, dementia/Alzheimer's disease, hypoxia (e.g., COPD, anemia, altitude sickness), alcohol intoxication/substance abuse

DESIRED OUTCOMES/EVALUATION CRITERIA

Sample NOC linkages:

Memory: Ability to cognitively retrieve and report previously stored information

Cognition: Ability to execute complex mental processes

Client Will (Include Specific Time Frame)

- Verbalize awareness of memory problems.
- Establish methods to help in remembering essential things when possible.
- Accept limitations of condition and use resources effectively.

ACTIONS/INTERVENTIONS

Sample NIC linkages:

Memory Training: Facilitation of memory

Surveillance: Safety: Purposeful and ongoing collection and analysis of information about the patient and the environment for use in promoting and maintaining patient safety

NURSING PRIORITY NO. 1 To assess causative factor(s)/degree of impairment:

- Determine physical/biochemical factors (e.g., recent surgery, infections, brain injury, use of multiple medications, exposure to toxic substances, use/abuse of alcohol/other drugs, pain, depression, etc.) *that may be related to changes in memory.*

Cultural Collaborative Community/Home Care Diagnostic Studies Pediatric/Geriatric/Lifespan Medications

- Note client's age and potential for depression symptoms in elderly. *Depressive disorders are particularly prevalent in older adults (approximately 15%) who report inability to concentrate and poor memory. Kuljis (2003) calls it a prevalent myth that substantial memory loss is a normal aspect of aging, barring effects of illness or injury. However, it is known that memory is somehow altered in the aging process and that generally, memory for past occurrences is superior to the retention and recall of more recent information.*[1,2,5,6]
- Note presence/degree of anxiety. *Can increase the client's confusion and disorganization and further interfere with attempts at recall.* (Refer to ND Anxiety for additional interventions as indicated.)
- Collaborate with medical and psychiatric providers *to evaluate extent of impairment to orientation, attention span, ability to follow directions, send/receive communication, and appropriateness of response.*
- Assist with/review results of cognitive testing (e.g., Blessed Information-Memory-Concentration [BIMC] test, Clinical Dementia Rating [CDR] Scale, Mini-Mental State Examination [MMSE]). *Although the etiology for some memory impairments may be obvious or established by client/SO/caregiver report, a combination of tests may be needed to complete picture of the client's overall condition and prognosis.*[3,6]
- Evaluate skill proficiency levels. *Evaluation may include many self-care activities (e.g., daily grooming, steps in preparing a meal, participating in a lifelong hobby, balancing a checkbook, and driving ability) to determine level of independence/needed assistance.*
- Ascertain how client/family view the problem (e.g., practical problems of forgetting to turn off the stove, client gets lost when driving, or role and responsibility impairments related to loss of memory and concentration) *to determine significance/impact of problem and suggest direction of interventions, especially as relates to basic safety issues.*[1]

NURSING PRIORITY NO. 2 To maximize level of function:

- Assist with treatment of underlying conditions (e.g., electrolyte imbalance, anemia, drug interactions/reaction to medications, alcohol/other drug intoxication, malnutrition, vitamin deficiencies, pain, etc.) *where treatment can improve memory processes.*
- Orient/reorient client, as needed, to environment. Introduce self with each client contact *to meet client's safety and comfort needs.* (Refer to NDs acute/chronic Confusion for additional interventions, as appropriate.)
- Implement appropriate memory-retraining techniques (e.g., keeping calendars, writing lists, memory cue games, mnemonic devices, using computers, etc.) *to provide restorative or compensatory training for cognitive function.*[4]
- Assist in/instruct client and family in associate-learning tasks (e.g., practice sessions recalling personal information, reminiscing, locating a geographic location [Stimulation Therapy]). *Practice may improve performance and integrate new behaviors into the client's coping strategies.*
- Support and reinforce client's efforts to remember information or behavioral skills. *Can decrease anxiety levels and perhaps help with further memory recovery*
- Encourage ventilation of feelings of frustration, helplessness, etc. Refocus attention to areas of control and progress *to diminsh feelings of powerlessness/hopelessness.*
- Provide for/emphasize importance of pacing learning activities and getting sufficient rest *to avoid fatigue that may further impair cognitive abilities.*
- Monitor client's behavior and assist in use of stress-management techniques (e.g., music therapy, reading, television, games, socialization) *to reduce frustration and enhance enjoyment of life.*
- Structure teaching methods and interventions *to client's level of functioning or potential for improvement.*[5]

• Determine client's response to/effects of medications prescribed to improve attention, concentration, memory processes, and to lift spirits/modify emotional responses. *Medications used for cognitive enhancement can be effective, but benefits need to be weighed against whether quality of life is improved when considering side effects/cost of drugs.*[3]

NURSING PRIORITY NO. 3 To promote wellness (Teaching/Discharge Considerations):

• Assist client/SO(s) to establish compensation strategies *to improve functional lifestyle and safety, such as menu planning with a shopping list; timely completion of tasks on a daily planner; and checklists at the front door to ascertain that lights and stove are off before leaving.*[6]

• Teach client and family/care providers memory involvement tasks, such as reminiscence and memory practice exercises *geared toward improving client's functional ability.*[6]

• Refer to/encourage follow-up with counselors, rehabilitation programs, job coaches, social/financial support systems *to help deal with persistent/difficult problems.*

• Refer to rehabilitation services *that are matched to the needs, strengths, and capacities of individual and modified as needs change over time.*[4]

• Discuss and encourage safety interventions, as indicated (e.g., assistance with meal preparation, evaluation of driving abilities, cessation of tobacco use or its use only under supervision, removal of guns and other weapons) *to prevent injury to client/others.*[1]

• Identify resources to meet individual needs (e.g., home-care assistant, companion, Meals on Wheels, etc.), *thereby maximizing independence and general well-being.*

DOCUMENTATION FOCUS

Assessment/Reassessment

• Individual findings, testing results, and perceptions of significance of problem.
• Actual impact on lifestyle and independence.

Planning

• Plan of care and who is involved in planning process.
• Teaching plan.

Implementation/Evaluation

• Responses to interventions/teaching and actions performed.
• Attainment/progress toward desired outcome(s).
• Modifications to plan of care.

Discharge Planning

• Long-term needs and who is responsible for actions to be taken.
• Specific referrals made.

References

1. Kuljis, R. O. (2003, update 2005). Minimal cognitive impairment. Available at www.emedicine.com./neuro/topic714.htm.
2. Roussel, L. A. (1999). The aging neurological system. In Stanley, M., Beare, P. G. (eds). *Gerontological Nursing: A Health Promotion/Protection Approach.* 2d ed. Philadelphia: F. A. Davis.
3. About Alzheimer's. (2003). Physicians and care professionals educational materials. Retrieved from Alzheimer's Disease and Related Disorders Association (AARDA) Web site. Available at www.alz.org.

Cultural   Collaborative   Community/Home Care   Diagnostic Studies   Pediatric/Geriatric/Lifespan   Medications

4. Rehabilitation of persons with traumatic brain injury. (1999). NIH Consensus Panel, *JAMA*, 8(10), 974–983.
5. Mayo Clinic. (2006). Mild cognitive impairment prevalent in elderly population; Risk increases as age goes up and education goes down. Ascribe Health News Service. Retrieved January 2007 at www.mayoclinic.org/news2006-rst/3306.html.
6. Jacobs, D. H. (2006). Confusional states and acute memory disorders. Article for Emedicine Web site. Retrieved Janury 2007 at www.emedicine.com/neuro/topic435.htm.

impaired bed Mobility

Definition: Limitation of independent movement from one bed position to another

RELATED FACTORS
Neuromuscular/musculoskeletal impairment
Insufficient muscle strength; deconditioning; obesity
Environmental contraints (i.e., bed size/type, treatment equipment, restraints)
Pain; sedating medications
Deficient knowledge
Cognitive impairment

DEFINING CHARACTERISTICS

Subjective
[Reported difficulty performing activities]

Objective
Impaired ability to turn side to side, move from supine to sitting or sitting to supine, "scoot," or reposition self in bed, move from supine to prone or prone to supine, from supine to long-sitting or long-sitting to supine

Sample Clinical Applications: Paralysis (e.g., spinal cord injury, stroke), traumatic brain injury, neuromuscular disorders (e.g., ALS), major chest/back surgery, severe depression, dementia, catatonic schizophrenia

DESIRED OUTCOMES/EVALUATION CRITERIA
Sample NOC linkages:
Body Positioning: Self-Initiated: Ability to change own body position independently with or without assistive device
Coordinated Movement: Adequacy of muscles to work together voluntarily for purposeful movement
Immobility Consequences: Physiological: Severity of compromise to physiological functioning due to impaired physical mobility

Client/Caregiver Will (Include Specific Time Frame)
• Verbalize willingness to/and participate in repositioning program.
• Verbalize understanding of situation/risk factors, individual therapeutic regimen, and safety measures.
• Demonstrate techniques/behaviors that enable safe repositioning.
• Maintain position of function and skin integrity as evidenced by absence of contractures, foot drop, decubitus, and other skin disorders.
• Maintain or increase strength and function of affected and/or compensatory body part.

ACTIONS/INTERVENTIONS

Sample NIC linkages:

Bedrest Care: Promotion of comfort and safety and prevention of complications for a patient unable to get out of bed

Positioning: Deliberative placement of the client or a body part to promote physiological and/or psychological well-being

Teaching: Prescribed Activity/Exercise: Preparing a patient to achieve or maintain a prescribed level of activity

NURSING PRIORITY NO. 1 To identify causative/contributing factors:

- Determine diagnoses that contribute to current immobility (e.g., MS, arthritis, Parkinson's, hemi/para/tetraplegia, fractures/multiple trauma, head injury, burns, etc.) *to identify interventions specific to client's mobility impairment and needs.*
- Note individual factors (e.g., surgery, casts, amputation, traction, pain, advanced age, general weakness/debilitation, severe depression, dementia) *that can contribute to problems related to bedrest and potential complications.*
- Determine degree of perceptual/cognitive impairment or ability to follow directions. *Impairments related to age, acute or chronic conditions (including severe depression, dementia), trauma, surgery, or medications require alternative interventions or changes in plan of care.*[1,3]

NURSING PRIORITY NO. 2 To assess functional ability:

- Determine functional level classification 1 to 4 *(level 1 requires use of equipment or device, level 2 requires help from another person for assistance, level 3 requires help from another person and equipment device, level 4 is totally dependent, does not participate in activity).*
- Note emotional/behavioral responses to problems of immobility. *Can negatively affect self-concept and self-esteem, autonomy, and independence. Feelings of frustration and powerlessness may impede attainment of goals. Social, occupational, and relationship roles can change, leading to isolation, depression, and economic consequences.*[4,5]
- Note presence of complications related to immobility. *Studies have shown that as much as 5.5% of muscle strength can be lost each day of rest and immobility.*[1] *Other complications include changes in circulation and impairments of organ function affecting the whole person (e.g., cognition, immune system function, emotional state, etc.).* (Refer to ND risk for Disuse Syndrome for additional interventions.)

NURSING PRIORITY NO. 3 To promote optimal level of function and prevent complications:

- Ascertain that dependent client is placed in best bed for situation (e.g., properly functioning equipment, correct size and support surface) *to promote environmental, client, and care provider safety.*[6]
- Instruct client/care providers in bed capabilities (e.g., mobility functions and set positions) encouraging client to participate as much as possible, even if only to move head or run bed controls. *Promotes independence and purposeful movement.*
- Change client's position frequently, moving individual parts of the body (e.g., legs, arms, head) using appropriate support and proper body alignment. Encourage periodic changes in head of bed (if not contraindicated by conditions such as acute spinal cord injury), with client in supine and prone positions at intervals *to improve circulation, reduce tightening of*

Cultural Collaborative Community/Home Care Diagnostic Studies Pediatric/Geriatric/Lifespan Medications

muscles and joints, normalizing body tone, and more closely simulating body positions individual would normally use.[2]

- Instruct caregivers in methods of moving client relative to specific situations (e.g., turning side to side, or prone or sitting) *to provide support for the client's body and to prevent injury to the lifter. Note: Positioning instructions and detailed sketches are available (e.g., Ossman)[7] on proper positions for certain conditions (e.g., paralyzed client) as well as the safe movement and positioning of body parts (e.g., rolling, bridging, scooting, sitting, etc.), which should become well known to caregivers in order to prevent injury to both the client and the caregivers.*

- Place client in upright position at intervals, or out of bed into upright chair, if condition allows. *Being vertical has been shown to reduce the work of heart, improve circulation and lung ventilation, and may improve cognition and awareness.*[3]

- Use egg-crate, alternating air-pressure, or water mattress; padding and positioning devices (e.g., foam wedge, pillows, hand rolls, etc., for bony prominences, feet, hands, elbows, head) *to prevent dermal injury/stress on tissues and reduce potential for disuse complications.*[3,6] (Refer to ND risk for Peripheral Neurovascular Dysfunction for additional interventions.)

- Perform/encourage regular skin examination for reddened or excoriated areas. Provide frequent skin care (e.g., cleansing, moisturizing, gentle massage) *to reduce pressure on sensitive areas and prevent development of problems with skin/tissue integrity.* (Refer to NDs impaired Skin Integrity; impaired Tissue Integrity.)

- Provide/assist with daily range-of-motion interventions (active and passive) *to maintain joint mobility, improve circulation, and prevent contractures.*

- Collaborate with rehabilitation team/physical/occupational therapists to create exercise and adaptive program designed specifically for client, identifying assistive devices (e.g., splints, braces, boots) and equipment (e.g., transfer board/sling, trapeze, hydraulic lift, specialty beds, etc.).

- Assist with activities of hygiene, feeding, and toileting, as indicated. Assist on/off bedpan and into sitting position (or use cardioposition bed or foot-egress bed) to facilitate elimination.

- Note change in strength to do more or less self-care (e.g., hygiene, feeding, toileting) *to promote psychological and physical benefits of self-care and to adjust level of assistance as indicated.*

- Administer medication before activity as needed for pain relief *to permit maximal effort/ involvement in activity.*

- Provide diversional activities (e.g., television, books, music, games, visiting) as appropriate *to decrease boredom and potential for depression.*

- Ensure telephone/call bell is within reach, client is able to activate surveillance alarm if provided. *Provides individually appropriate methods for client to communicate needs for assistance.*

- Refer to NDs, Activity Intolerance, impaired physical Mobility, impaired wheelchair Mobility, risk for Disuse Syndrome, impaired Transfer Ability, impaired Walking for additional interventions.

NURSING PRIORITY NO. 4 To promote wellness (Teaching/Discharge Considerations):

- Involve client/SO in determining activity schedule. *Promotes commitment to plan, maximizing outcomes.*

- Instruct all caregivers in safety concerns regarding body mechanics, as well as client's required positions and exercises *to prevent injury to both and to minimize potential for preventable complications.*

- Encourage continuation of regular exercise program *to maintain/enhance gains in strength/ muscle control.*

- Obtain/identify sources for assistive devices. Demonstrate safe use and proper maintenance. *Promotes independence and enhances safety.*

DOCUMENTATION FOCUS

Assessment/Reassessment

- Individual findings, including level of function/ability to participate in specific/desired activities.

Planning

- Plan of care and who is involved in the planning.

Implementation/Evaluation

- Responses to interventions/teaching and actions performed.
- Attainment/progress toward desired outcome(s).
- Modification to plan of care.

Discharge Planning

- Discharge/long-range needs, noting who is responsible for each action to be taken.
- Specific referrals made.
- Sources of/maintenance for assistive devices.

References

1. Pattillo, M. A., Stanley, M. (1999). The aging musculoskeletal system. In Stanley, M., Beare, P. G. (eds). *Gerontological Nursing: A Health Promotion/Protection Approach.* 2d ed. Philadelphia: F. A. Davis.
2. Kumagai, K. A. S. (1998). Physical management of the neurologically involved client: Techniques for bed mobility and transfers. In Chin, P. A., Finocchiaro, D., Rosebrough, A. (eds). *Rehabilitation Nursing Practice.* New York: McGraw-Hill.
3. Palmer, M., Wyness, M. A. (1988). Positioning and handling: Important considerations in the care of the severely head-injured patient. *J Neurosurg Nurs,* 20(1), 42–49.
4. Mass, M. L. (1989). Impaired physical mobility. Unpublished manuscript. Cited in research article for National Institutes for Health.
5. Hogue, C. C. (1984). Falls and mobility late in life: An ecological model. *J Am Geriatr Soc,* 32, 858–861.
6. Dionne, M. (2005). This bed is just right. *Rehab Management,* 18(1), 32–39.
7. Ossman, N. (1990). *Therapist Guide: Adult Positions, Transitions and Transfers.* Psychological Corporation.

impaired physical Mobility

Definition: Limitation in independent, purposeful physical movement of the body or of one or more extremities

RELATED FACTORS

Sedentary lifestyle; activity intolerance; disuse; deconditioning; decreased endurance; limited cardiovascular endurance

Decreased muscle strength/control mass; joint stiffness; contractures; loss of integrity of bone structures

Pain/discomfort

Neuromuscular/musculoskeletal impairment

Sensoriperceptual/cognitive impairment; developmental delay

Depressive mood state; anxiety

Cultural   Collaborative   Community/Home Care   Diagnostic Studies   Pediatric/Geriatric/Lifespan   Medications

Malnutrition; altered cellular metabolism; body mass index above 75th age-appropriate percentile

Deficient knowledge regarding value of physical activity; cultural beliefs regarding age-appropriate activity; lack of environmental supports (e.g., physical or social)

Prescribed movement restrictions; medications

Reluctance to initiate movement

DEFINING CHARACTERISTICS

Subjective
[Report of pain/discomfort on movement; unwillingness to move]

Objective
Limited range of motion; limited ability to perform gross fine/motor skills; difficulty turning

Slowed movement; uncoordinated/jerky movements, movement-induced tremor; decreased [slower] reaction time

Postural instability; gait changes

Engages in substitutions for movement (e.g., increased attention to other's activity, controlling behavior, focus on pre-illness disability/activity)

Sample Clinical Applications: Neuromuscular disorders (e.g., MS, ALS), Parkinson's disease, traumatic injuries (e.g., fractures, spinal cord/brain injuries), rheumatoid arthritis, severe depression

SUGGESTED FUNCTIONAL LEVEL CLASSIFICATION

0—Completely independent

1—Requires use of equipment or device

2—Requires help from another person for assistance, supervision, or teaching

3—Requires help from another person and equipment device

4—Dependent, does not participate in activity

DESIRED OUTCOMES/EVALUATION CRITERIA

Sample NOC linkages:

Mobility: Ability to move purposefully in own environment independently with or without assistive device

Immobility Consequences: Physiological: Severity of compromise in physiological functioning due to impaired physical mobility

Knowledge: Prescribed Activity: Extent of understanding conveyed about prescribed activity and exercise

Client Will (Include Specific Time Frame)

- Verbalize understanding of situation and individual treatment regimen and safety measures.
- Demonstrate techniques/behaviors that enable resumption of activities.
- Participate in ADLs and desired activities.
- Maintain position of function and skin integrity as evidenced by absence of contractures, footdrop, decubitus, and so forth.
- Maintain or increase strength and function of affected or compensatory body part.

ACTIONS/INTERVENTIONS

Sample NIC linkages:

Exercise Therapy: [specify]: Use of active or passive body movement to maintain or restore flexibility; use of specific activity or exercise protocols to enhance or restore controlled body movement, etc.

Pain Management: Alleviation of pain or a reduction in pain to a level of comfort acceptable to the patient

Traction/Immobilization Care: Management of a patient who has traction or a stabilizing device to immobilize and stabilize a body part

NURSING PRIORITY NO. 1   To identify causative/contributing factors:

- Determine diagnosis that contributes to immobility (e.g., MS, arthritis, Parkinson's, hemiplegia/paraplegia, depression, developmental delays, etc.). *These conditions can cause physiological and psychological problems that can seriously impact physical, social, and economic well-being.*[1]
- Note factors affecting current situation (e.g., surgery, fractures, amputation, tubings (chest tube, Foley catheter, IVs, pumps) and potential time involved (e.g., few hours in bed after surgery versus serious trauma requiring long-term bedrest/debilitating disease limiting movement). *Identifies potential impairments and determines type of interventions needed to provide for client's safety.*
- Assess client's developmental level, motor skills, ease and capability of movement, posture and gait to *determine presence of characteristics of client's unique impairment and to guide choice of interventions.*[8]
- Note older client's general health status. *Hogue (1984) identified mobility as the most important functional ability that determines the degree of independence and healthcare needs among older persons.*[2] *While aging per se does not cause impaired mobility, several predisposing factors in addition to age-related changes can lead to immobility (e.g., diminished body reserves of musculoskeletal system, chronic diseases, sedentary lifestyle, decreased ability to quickly and adequately correct movements affecting center of gravity). Thus, falls are a major source of morbidity and mortality for older persons.*[3,6,8]
- Evaluate for presence/degree of pain, listening to client's description about manner in which pain limits mobility *to determine needed interventions for pain management.*[4]
- Ascertain client's perception of activity/exercise needs and impact of current situation. Identify cultural beliefs and expectations affecting recovery/response to long-term limitations. *Helps to determine client's expectations/beliefs related to activity and potential long-term effect of current immobility. Also identifies barriers that may be addressed (e.g., lack of safe place to exercise, focus on pre-illness/disability activity, controlling behavior, depression, cultural expectations, distorted body image, etc.).*[5]
- Assess nutritional status and client's report of energy level. *Deficiencies in nutrients and water, electrolytes and minerals can negatively affect energy and activity tolerance.*
- Determine history of falls and relatedness to current situation. *Client may be restricting activity because of weakness/debilitation, actual injury during a fall, or from psychological distress (i.e., fear and anxiety) that can persist after a fall.*[6-8] (Refer to ND risk for Falls for additional interventions.)

NURSING PRIORITY NO. 2   To assess functional ability:

- Determine degree of immobility in relation to 0–4 scale, noting muscle strength and tone, joint mobility, cardiovascular status, balance, and endurance. *Identifies strengths and deficits*

Cultural   Collaborative   Community/Home Care   Diagnostic Studies   Pediatric/Geriatric/Lifespan   Medications

(e.g., ability to ambulate with/without assistive devices, or inability to transfer safely from bed to wheelchair) and may provide information regarding potential for recovery (e.g., client with severe brain injury may have permanent limitations because of impaired cognition affecting memory, judgment, problem-solving, and motor planning, requiring more intensive inpatient and long-term care).[1,6]

- Determine degree of perceptual/cognitive impairment and ability to follow directions. *Impairments related to age, chronic or acute disease condition, trauma, surgery, or medications require alternative interventions or changes in plan of care.*[3]
- Observe movement when client is unaware of observation *to note any incongruency with reports of abilities.*
- Note emotional/behavioral responses to problems of immobility. *Can negatively affect self-concept and self-esteem, autonomy, and independence. Feelings of frustration and powerlessness may impede attainment of goals. Social, occupational, and relationship roles can change, leading to isolation, depression, and economic consequences.*[1,2]
- Determine presence of complications related to immobility (e.g., pneumonia, elimination problems, contractures, decubitus, anxiety). *Studies have shown that as much as 5.5% of muscle strength can be lost each day of rest and immobility.*[5] *Other complications include changes in circulation and impairments of organ function affecting the whole person (e.g., cognition, bone demineralization, venous pooling, and thromboembolic pneumonia, weakened immune system function, muscle contractures, etc.).* (Refer to ND risk for Disuse Syndrome.)

NURSING PRIORITY NO. 3 To promote optimal level of function and prevent complications:

- Assist with treatment of underlying condition(s) *to maximize potential for mobility and optimal function.*
- Discuss discrepancies in movement with client aware and unaware of observation and methods for dealing with identified problems. *May be necessary when client is using avoidance or controlling behavior, or is not aware of own abilities due to anxiety/fear.*[7]
- Assist/have client reposition self on a regular schedule as dictated by individual situation (including frequent shifting of weight when client is wheelchair-bound) *to enhance circulation to tissues, reduce risk of tissue ischemia.*
- Review/encourage use of proper body mechanics *to prevent injury to client and caregiver.*
- Demonstrate/assist with use of side rails, overhead trapeze, roller pads, hydraulic lifts/chairs *for position changes/transfers.* Instruct in safe use of walker/cane *for ambulation.*
- Support affected body parts/joints using pillows/rolls, foot supports/shoes, gel pads, etc., *to maintain position of function and reduce risk of pressure ulcers.*
- Provide/recommend egg-crate, alternating air-pressure, or water mattress. *Reduces tissue pressure and aids in maximizing cellular perfusion to prevent dermal injury.*
- Use padding and positioning devices (e.g., foam wedge, pillows, hand rolls, etc., for bony prominences, feet, hands, elbows, head) *to prevent stress on tissues and reduce potential for disuse complications.*
- Collaborate with physical medicine specialist and occupational/physical therapists in providing range-of-motion exercise (active or passive), isotonic muscle contractions (e.g., flexion of ankles, push/pull exercises), assistive devices, and activities (e.g., early ambulation, transfers, stairs) *to limit/reduce effects and complications of immobility (e.g., contracture deformities, deep vein thromboses). Techniques such as gait training, strength training, and exercise to improve balance and coordination can be helpful in rehabilitating client.*[7]
- Encourage client's participation in self-care activities, physical/occupational therapies as well as diversional/recreational activities. *Reduces sensory deprivation, enhances self-concept and sense of independence, and improves body strength and function.*

- Provide client with ample time to perform mobility-related tasks. Schedule activities with adequate rest periods during the day *to reduce fatigue.*
- Avoid routinely assisting or doing for client those activities that client can do for self. *Caregivers can contribute to impaired mobility by being overprotective or helping too much.*
- Identify/encourage energy-conserving techniques for ADLs. *Limits fatigue, maximizing participation.*
- Provide for safety measures as indicated by individual situation, including environmental management/fall prevention. (Refer to ND risk for Falls.)
- Note change in strength to do more or less self-care (e.g., hygiene, feeding, toileting, therapies) *to promote psychological and physical benefits of self-care and to adjust level of assistance as indicated.*
- Administer medications before activity as needed for pain relief *to permit maximal effort/involvement in activity.*
- Perform/encourage regular skin examination and care *to reduce pressure on sensitive areas and to prevent development of problems with skin integrity.* (Refer to NDs risk for impaired Skin Integrity; risk for impaired Tissue Integrity for additional interventions.)
- Encourage adequate intake of fluids/nutritious foods. *Promotes well-being and maximizes energy production.*
- Refer to NDs Activity Intolerance, impaired bed Mobility, impaired wheelchair Mobility, impaired Transfer Ability, and impaired Walking for additional interventions.

NURSING PRIORITY NO. 4 To promote wellness (Teaching/Discharge Considerations):

- Encourage client's/SO's involvement in decision making as much as possible. *Enhances commitment to plan, optimizing outcomes.*
- Review importance and purpose of exercise (e.g., *increased cardiovascular and respiratory tolerance, improved flexibility, balance, and muscle strength/tone, enhanced sense of well-being).*
- Discuss safe ways that client can exercise. *Multiple options provide client choices and variety (e.g., walking around the block with companion or in a mall during bad air days, participating in a water aerobics class, attending regular rehab sessions).*
- Assist client/SO to learn safety measures as individually indicated. *May need instruction and to give return demonstration (e.g., use of heating pads, locking wheelchair before transfers, removal or securing of scatter/area rugs, judicious and accurate use of medications, supervised exercise).*[7]
- Involve client and SO(s) in care, assisting them to learn ways of managing problems of immobility, especially when impairment is expected to be long-term. *May need referral for support and community services to provide care, supervision, companionship, respite services, nutritional and ADL assistance, adaptive devices or changes to living environment, financial assistance, etc.*[7,8]
- Demonstrate use of standing aids and mobility devices (e.g., walkers, strollers, scooters, braces, prosthetics, etc.) and have client/careprovider demostrate knowledge about/safe use of device. Identify appropriate resources for obtaining and maintaining appliances/equipment. *Safe use of mobility aids promotes client's independence and enhances quality of life and safety for client and caregiver.*[9,10]

DOCUMENTATION FOCUS

Assessment/Reassessment

- Individual findings, including level of function/ability to participate in specific/desired activities.

　🌐 Cultural 　Ⓐ Collaborative 　🏠 Community/Home Care 　🧪 Diagnostic Studies 　∞ Pediatric/Geriatric/Lifespan 　💊 Medications

Planning

- Plan of care and who is involved in the planning.
- Teaching plan.

Implementation/Evaluation

- Responses to interventions/teaching and actions performed.
- Attainment/progress toward desired outcome(s).
- Modifications to plan of care.

Discharge Planning

- Discharge/long-range needs, noting who is responsible for each action to be taken.
- Specific referrals made.
- Sources of/maintenance for assistive devices.

References

1. Mass, M. L. (1989). Impaired physical mobility. Unpublished manuscript. Cited in research article for National Institutes for Health.
2. Hogue, C. C. (1984). Falls and mobility late in life: An ecological model. *J Am Geriatr Soc, 32,* 858–861.
3. Rowe, J. W., Kahn, R. L. (1987). Human aging: Usual and successful. *Science,* 237, 143–149.
4. McCaffrey, M., Pasero, C. (1999). Pain: *Clinical Manual.* 2d ed. St. Louis, MO: Mosby.
5. Pattillo, M. A., Stanley, M. (1999). The aging musculoskeletal system. In Stanley, M., Beare, P. G. *Gerontological Nursing: A Health Promotion/Protection Approach.* 2d ed. Philadelphia: F. A. Davis.
6. Tinetti, M. E., Williams, T. F., Mayewski, R. (1986). Fall risk index for elderly patients based on number of chronic disabilities. *Am J Med,* 80, 429–434.
7. Doenges, M. E., Moorhouse, M. F., Geissler-Murr, A. C. (2002). *Nursing Care Plans: Guidelines for Individualizing Patient Care.* 6th ed. Philadelphia: F. A. Davis.
8. Michael, K. M., Allen, J. K., Macko, R. F. (2006). Fatigue after stroke: Relationship to mobility, fitness, ambulatory activity, social support, and falls efficiency. *Rehabilitation Nursing,* 31(5), 210–217
9. Becker, B. (2005). To stand or not to stand. *Rehab Management,* 18(2), 28–34.
10. Dworak, P. A., Levy, A. (2005). Strolling along. *Rehab Management,* 18(9), 26–31.

impaired wheelchair Mobility

Definition: Limitation of independent operation of wheelchair within environment

RELATED FACTORS
Neuromuscular/musculoskeletal impairments (e.g., contractures)
Insufficient muscle strength; limited endurance; deconditioning; obesity
Impaired vision
Pain
Depressed mood; cognitive impairment
Deficient knowledge
Environmental constraints (e.g., stairs, inclines, uneven surfaces, unsafe obstacles, distances, lack of assistive devices or persons, wheelchair type)

DEFINING CHARACTERISTICS
Impaired ability to operate manual/power wheelchair on even/uneven surface; on an incline/decline; on curbs
NOTE: Specify level of independence using a standardized functional scale.

Sample Clinical Applications: Neuromuscular disorders (e.g., MS, ALS), paralysis (e.g., brain injury/stroke, spinal cord injury), muscular dystrophy, cerebral palsy, fractures

DESIRED OUTCOMES/EVALUATION CRITERIA
Sample NOC linkage:
Ambulation: Wheelchair: Ability to move from place to place in a wheelchair

Client Will (Include Specific Time Frame)

• Move safely within environment, maximizing independence.
• Identify and use resources appropriately.

Sample NOC linkages:
Fall Prevention Behavior: Personal or family caregiver actions to minimize risk factors that might precipitate falls in the personal environment

Caregiver Will (Include Specific Time Frame)

• Provide safe mobility within environment and community

ACTIONS/INTERVENTIONS

Sample NIC linkages:
Positioning: Wheelchair: Placement of a patient in a properly selected wheelchair to enhance comfort, promote skin integrity, and foster independence
Exercise Therapy: Muscle Control: Use of specific activity or exercise protocols to enhance or restore controlled body movement
Transport: Moving a patient from one location to another

NURSING PRIORITY NO. 1 To identify causative/contributing factors:

• Determine diagnosis that contributes to immobility (e.g., ALS, spinal cord injury, spastic cerebral palsy, brain injury) and client's functional level/individual abilities (e.g., 0–4 scale; see ND impaired physical Mobility).
• Identify factors in environments frequented by the client that contribute to inaccessibility (e.g., uneven floors/surfaces, lack of ramps, steep incline/decline, narrow doorways/spaces).
• Ascertain access to and appropriateness of public and/or private transportation.

NURSING PRIORITY NO. 2 To promote optimal level of function and prevent complications:

• Determine that client's underlying cognitive, emotional, and physical impairment(s) (e.g., brain injury, pain, depression, vision deficits, etc.) are treated/being managed *to maximize desire/motivation to participate in wheelchair activities.*[6]
• Collaborate with physical medicine, physical/occupational therapists in planning activities to improve client's ability to independently operate wheelchair within limits of tolerance and adjustment to various environments. *May require individual instruction and encouragement, strengthening exercises, assistance with various tasks and close supervision.*
• Ascertain that wheelchair provides the base mobility to maximize function. *Wheelchairs must be matched with client's age, size, developmental level, and unique functional needs (e.g.,*

proper seating and support for children in wheelchairs is critical to their ability to learn at school, to play and to interact with friends).[1] *Correct seating is essential for prevention, correction, and compensation for postural changes in order to maintain client's comfort and function. Chair should provide for maximum reach, maneuverability, function, and center of gravity positioning and propulsion; should recline to change back contours, hip angles, and pelvic restrictions; should have back adjustment for changing trunk stability requirements; and should tilt for reposition, pressure relief, and comfort.*[1,2,7,8]

- Perform periodic assessments of client and wheelchair to monitor chair usage and function as well as changes in client's postural, behavioral, and functional status. *Helps to identify problems (e.g., abnormal wear patterns on the chair requiring mechanical adjustments/repair; loss of client's strength where power add-ons to the chair would improve mobility; or alternate methods of mobility that might be needed).*[2]

- Provide for/instruct client in safety while in a wheelchair (e.g., cushions, supports for all body parts, repositioning and transfer assistive devices, position and pressure relief products, feet and leg support, armrest choices, and back and height adjustment).[7]

- Note evenness of surfaces client needs to negotiate and refer to appropriate sources for modifications (e.g., replacing carpet with tile, revising ramps that are too steep, narrow, or slippery). Clear pathways of obstructions.

- Recommend/arrange for modifications to home/work or school/recreational settings frequented by client. *Although most public buildings have certain adaptations in rooms and accesses, they are not always well constructed or in good working order. The client may need assistance in these settings and with requesting that appropriate alterations be carried out.*[9]

- Determine need for and capabilities of assistive persons. Provide training and support, as indicated. *Enhances safety for both client and caregiver.*

- Monitor client's use of joystick, sip and puff, sensitive mechanical switches, etc., *to provide necessary equipment if condition/capabilities change.*

- Monitor client for adverse effects of immobility (e.g., contractures, muscle atrophy, deep venous thrombosis, pressure ulcers). (Refer to NDs Disuse Syndrome; risk for Peripheral Neurovascular Dysfunction for additional interventions.)

NURSING PRIORITY NO. 3 To promote wellness (Teaching/Discharge Considerations):

- Identify/refer to medical equipment suppliers *to customize client's wheelchair for size, proper seating angle, positioning aids, incline/decline stability, accessories (e.g., side guards, headrests, heel loops, brake extenstions, tool packs, etc.) and electronics suited to client's ability (e.g., sip and puff, head movement, sensitive switches, etc.).*[6,8]

- Encourage client's/SO(s) involvement in decision making as much as possible. *Enhances sense of control and commitment to plan, thereby optimizing outcomes.*

- Involve client/SO in care, assisting them in managing immobility problems. *Promotes independence in self-evaluation and self-care, including managing the type of wheelchair/other assistive devices best for client, how the user's needs and abilities change over time, modifications that might be made (e.g., number and placement of ramps around the home, modifications to rooms, doors, and vehicles).*[3]

- Demonstrate/provide information regarding individually appropriate safety, including wheelchair preventative maintenance measures (e.g., for wheelchair locks, tires, axles, casters, metal parts, batteries). *Wheelchair safety involves the maintenance of the chair and provision for obtaining relief when chair malfunctions. Many states have enacted wheelchair lemon laws that "mandate warranties to maintain assistive technology in proper working condition, to assure availability of appropriate loaner replacement chairs during repair time, and to encourage manufacturers and dealers to cooperatively pool assistive technology resources for loaner purposes to assure availability without undue burden."*[4]

 • Refer to support groups relative to specific medical condition/disability and geared toward client's independence. Suggest involvement in political action group, as indicated. *Provides role modeling, assistance with problem-solving/social change.*

• Identify community resources to provide ongoing support. *The current societal view (that persons with disabilities have the right to be self-determining and to make their own choices about their lives and to achieve the quality of life each believes is personal best) places as much emphasis on community regarding integration as on physical rehabilitation and functional capabilities.*[5]

DOCUMENTATION FOCUS

Assessment/Reassessment

• Individual findings, including level of function/ability to participate in specific/desired activities.
• Type of wheelchair/equipment needs.
• Environmental factors/problems.

Planning

• Plan of care and who is involved in the planning.
• Teaching plan.

Implementation/Evaluation

• Responses to interventions/teaching and actions performed.

Discharge Planning

• Discharge/long-range needs, noting who is responsible for each action to be taken.
• Specific referrals made.
• Sources of/maintenance for assistive devices.

References

1. Taylor, S. J. (2000). Seating for children: What to consider. Article for Spin Tips Web site. Accessed July 2007 at www.spinlife.com/.
2. Buck, S. (2001). Mobility and the aged: The importance of adjustability and consistent reassessment when treating mobility-impaired elderly clients. Article retrieved from Rehab Management, Interdisciplinary Journal of Rehabilitation International Web site. Available at www.rehabinternationalpub.com/fall2001/7.asp.
3. Lathrop, D. (2000). Ramp the planet! Reprinted from New Mobility: Life on Wheels. Accessed July 2007 at www.spinlife.com/.
4. Colorado House Bill 97-1194, *Concerning Self-Sufficiency for Persons with Disabilities by Assuring Reliable Assistive Technology.* Bill signed into law April 30, 1997. Denver, CO.
5. Scherer, M. (2002). The importance of assistive technology outcomes. Article for Institute for Matching Person & Technology, Washington, DC.
6. Cohen, D. (2005). Optional but necessary. *Rehab Management,* 18(10), 26–29.
7. Rosen, L. (2005). Sit on it. *Rehab Management,* 18(2), 36–41.
8. Waugh, K. G. (2005). Measuring the right angle. *Rehab Management,* 18(1), 40–49.
9. McCullagh, M. C. (2006). Home modification. *AJN,* 106(10), 54–63.

Nausea

Definition: A subjective unpleasant, wavelike sensation in the back of the throat, epigastrium, or abdomen that may lead to the urge or need to vomit

RELATED FACTORS

Treatment
Gastric irritation [e.g., alcohol, blood]
Gastric distention
Pharmaceuticals [e.g., analgesics—aspirin/nonsteroidal anti-inflammatory drugs/opioids, anesthesia, antiviral for HIV, steroids, antibiotics, chemotherapeutic agents]
[Radiation therapy/exposure]

Biophysical
Biochemical disorders (e.g., uremia, diabetic ketoacidosis, pregnancy)
Localized tumors (e.g., acoustic neuroma, primary or secondary brain tumors, bone metastases at base of skull); intra-abdominal tumors
Toxins (e.g., tumor-produced peptides, abdominal metabolites due to cancer)
Esophageal/pancreatic disease; liver/splenetic capsule stretch
Gastric distention [e.g., delayed gastric emptying, pyloric intestinal obstruction, external compression of the stomach, other organ enlargement that slows stomach functioning (squashed stomach syndrome)]
Gastric irritation [e.g., pharyngeal and/or peritoneal inflammation]
Motion sickness; Meniere's disease; labyrinthitis
Increased intracranial pressure; meningitis

Situational
Noxious odors/taste; unpleasant visual stimulation
Pain
Psychological factors; anxiety; fear

DEFINING CHARACTERISTICS

Subjective
Report of nausea ["sick to my stomach"]

Objective
Aversion toward food
Increased salivation; sour taste in mouth
Increased swallowing; gagging sensation

Sample Clinical Applications: Surgery/anesthesia, cancer, pregnancy, AIDS, gastritis, peptic ulcer disease, renal failure, brain injury, meningitis, panic disorders/phobias

DESIRED OUTCOMES/EVALUATION CRITERIA
Sample NOC linkages:
Nausea & Vomiting Severity: Severity of nausea, retching, and vomiting symptoms
Nausea & Vomiting Control: Personal actions to control nausea, retching, and vomiting symptoms
Appetite: Desire to eat when ill or receiving treatment

Client Will (Include Specific Time Frame)

- Be free of nausea.
- Manage chronic nausea, as evidenced by acceptable level of dietary intake.
- Maintain/regain weight, as appropriate.

ACTIONS/INTERVENTIONS

Sample NIC linkages:

Nausea Management: Prevention and alleviation of nausea

Vomiting Management: Prevention and alleviation of vomiting

Fluid Management: Promotion of fluid balance and prevention of complications resulting from abnormal or undesired fluid levels

NURSING PRIORITY NO. 1 To determine causative/contributing factors:

- Assess for presence of conditions of the GI tract (e.g., peptic ulcer disease, cholecystitis, appendicitis, gastritis, intestinal blockage, ingestion of "problem" foods). *Dietary changes may be sufficient to decrease frequency of nausea in some situations.*
- Note systemic conditions that may result in nausea (e.g., pregnancy, cancer treatment, myocardial infarction, hepatitis, acid-base and metabolic disturbances, systemic infections, drug toxicity, migraine headache, presence of neurogenic causes—stimulation of the vestibular system, concussion, CNS trauma/tumor). *Helpful in determining appropriate interventions/need for treatment of underlying conditions.*[4]
- Identify situations that client perceives as anxiety-inducing, threatening, or distasteful (e.g., "this is nauseating") such as might occur if client is having multiple diagnostic studies, facing surgery. *May be able to limit/control exposure to situations or take medication prophylactically.*
- Note psychological factors, including those that are culturally determined (e.g., eating certain foods considered repulsive in one's culture).[4]
- Determine if nausea is potentially self-limiting and/or mild (e.g., first trimester of pregnancy, 24-hour GI tract viral infection) or is severe and prolonged (e.g., cancer treatment, hyperemesis gravidarum). *Indicates potential degree of effect on fluid/electrolyte balance and nutritional status.*[4]
- Record food intake and changes in symptoms *to help identify food intolerances when nausea is chronic.*
- Assess vital signs, especially for children and older clients, and note signs of dehydration. *Nausea may occur in the presence of postural hypotension/fluid volume deficit, or in severe hypertension.*
- Review medication regimen, especially in elderly client on multiple drugs. *Polypharmacy with drug interactions and side effects may cause/exacerbate nausea.*

NURSING PRIORITY NO. 2 To promote comfort and enhance intake:

- Collaborate with physician to treat underlying medical condition *when cause of nausea is known (e.g., infection, adverse side effect of medications, food allergies, gastrointestinal reflux).*
- Administer/monitor response to medications used to treat underlying cause of nausea (e.g., vestibular, bowel obstruction, dysmotility of upper gut, infection/inflammation, toxins).

 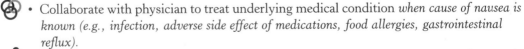 Cultural   Collaborative   Community/Home Care   Diagnostic Studies   Pediatric/Geriatric/Lifespan   Medications

Note: Older individuals are more prone to side effects of antiemitic and anti-anxiety/anti-psychotic medications (e.g., excessive sedation, extrapyramidal movements), and there is increased risk of aspiration in the sedated client.[5,8]

- Select route of medication administration best suited to client's needs (i.e., oral, sublingual, injectable, rectal, transdermal).[7]
- Administer antiemetic on regular schedule before/during and after administration of antineoplastic agents/radiation therapy as indicated. *Antiemetic agents may be administered prophylactically to prevent/limit severity of nausea and vomiting.*[1]
- Administer analgesics *when postoperative pain is a factor in nausea/vomiting.* Observe for nausea when opioids are used for pain management.[2]
- Review pain control regimen. *Converting to long-acting opioids or combination drugs may decrease stimulation of the chemotactic trigger zone (CTZ) reducing the occurrence of narcotic-related nausea.*[5,8]
- Manage food and fluids:

  Have client try dry foods such as toast, crackers, or dry cereal before arising *when nausea occurs in the morning or throughout the day,* as appropriate.[8]

  Encourage client to begin with ice chips or sips/small amounts of fluids—4 to 8 ounces for adult, 1 ounce or less for child.[6]

  Advise client to drink liquids 30 minutes before or after meals, instead of with meals.[8] Also advise client to sip fluids slowly and use cool, clear liquids (e.g., water, ginger ale/lemon-lime soda—if tolerated, and electrolyte drinks).

  Recommend avoiding milk/dairy products (especially during acute episodes), overly sweet, fried, or fatty foods, gas-forming vegetables (e.g., broccoli, cauliflower, cucumbers) *that may increase nausea/be more difficult to digest.*[4,6,8]

  Provide bland diet and snacks high in carbohydrates with substitutions of preferred foods (including bland/caffeine-free nondiet carbonated beverages, clear soup broth, non-acidic fruit juice, gelatin, sherbet/ices, skinless chicken) *to reduce gastric acidity and improve nutrient intake.*[4,6,8]

  Instruct client to eat small meals spaced throughout the day rather than large meals *so stomach does not feel too full.*[4,8]

  Instruct client to eat and drink slowly, chewing food well *for easier digestion.*[8]

  Advise client to suck on ice cubes or tart or hard candies and chew gum. *Keeps mucous membranes moist and can provide some fluid/nutrient intake.*

  Provide frequent oral care (especially after vomiting) *to cleanse mouth and minimize "bad tastes."*

  Time chemotherapy doses *for least interference with food intake.*

  Monitor infusion rate of tube feeding, if present, *to prevent rapid administration that can cause gastric distention/produce nausea.*

- Manage environment:

  Elevate head of bed or have client sit upright after meals *to promote digestion by gravity and eliminate feeling of fullness when that is causing nausea.*[8]

  Avoid sudden changes in position.

  Apply cool cloth to face and neck.

  Provide clean, pleasant-smelling, quiet environment and fresh air with fan/open window.

  Avoid offending odors (e.g., cooking smells, smoke, perfumes, mechanical emissions, etc.).[7,8]

- Discuss nonpharmacological measures:

  Encourage slow, deep breathing *to promote relaxation.*

  Use such distraction techniques as guided imagery, music therapy, chatting with family/friends, watching television *to refocus attention away from unpleasant sensations.*

  Provide frequent oral care *to cleanse mouth and minimize "bad tastes."*

• Investigate use of electrical nerve stimulation, or acupressure point therapy (e.g., elastic band worn around wrist with small, hard bump that presses against acupressure point). *Some individuals with chronic nausea/history of motion sickness report this to be helpful and without the sedative effect of medication.*[3]

NURSING PRIORITY NO. 3 To promote wellness (Teaching/Discharge Considerations):

• Review individual factors/triggers causing nausea and ways to avoid problem (e.g., identifying offending medications or foods). *Provides necessary information for client to manage own care. Note: Some individuals develop anticipatory nausea (a conditioned reflex) that recurs each time he or she encounters the situation that triggers the reflex.*[8]

• Instruct in proper use, side effects, and adverse reactions of antiemetic medications. *Enhances client safety and effective management of condition.*

• Discuss appropriate use of OTC medications/herbal products (e.g., Dramamine, antacids, antiflatulents, ginger) or in the use of THC (Marinol).[6,8]

• Encourage use of nonpharmacological interventions. *Activites such as self-hypnosis, progressive muscle relaxation, biofeedback, guided imagery, and systemic desensitization promote relaxation, refocus client's attention, increase sense of control, and decrease feelings of helplessness.*[7]

• Advise client/SO to prepare and freeze meals in advance, have someone else cook, or use microwave or oven instead of stovetop cooking for days when nausea is severe or cooking is impossible as with chemo/radiation therapy.[8]

• Suggest wearing loose-fitting clothing.[8]

• Recommend recording weight weekly, if appropriate, *to help monitor fluid/nutritional status.*

• Identify signs requiring immediate notification of healthcare provider (e.g., emesis appears bloody, black, or like coffee grounds; feeling faint) *to facilitate timely evaluation and intervention.*[8]

• Discuss potential complications and possible need for medical follow-up or alternative therapies. *Timely recognition and intervention may limit severity of complications (e.g., dehydration).*

• Review signs of dehydration and stress importance of replacing fluids and/or electrolytes (with products such as Gatorade for adults or Pedialyte for children) if vomiting occurs, especially in young children or frail elderly. *Increases likelihood of preventing potentially serious complications.*[6]

DOCUMENTATION FOCUS

Assessment/Reassessment

• Individual findings, including individual factors causing nausea.
• Baseline periodic weight, vital signs.
• Specific client preferences for nutritional intake.

Planning

• Plan of care and who is involved in planning.
• Teaching plan.

Implementation/Evaluation

• Response to interventions/teaching and actions performed.
• Response to medication.
• Attainment/progress toward desired outcome(s).
• Modifications to plan of care.

Discharge Planning

- Individual long-term needs, noting who is responsible for actions to be taken.
- Specific referrals made.

References

1. American Society of Health System Pharmacists (ASHP). (1999). Therapeutic guidelines on the pharmacologic management of nausea and vomiting in adult and pediatric patients receiving chemotherapy or radiation therapy or undergoing surgery. *Am J Health Syst Pharm,* 56(8), 729.
2. Thompson, H. J. (1999). The management of post-operative nausea and vomiting. *J Adv Nurs,* 29(5), 1130–1136.
3. Mann, E. (1999). Using acupuncture and acupressure to treat postoperative emesis. *Prof Nurs,* 14(10), 691–694.
4. The American Gastroenterological Association Medical Position Statement: Nausea and Vomiting. (2001). *Gastroenterology,* 120(1), 261–262. Available at www.guideline.gov. Accessed January 2004.
5. Hallenbeck, J., Weissman, D. (2007). Treatment of nausea and vomiting. Retrieved August 2007 at www.jasonprogram.org/nausea_treatment.htm.
6. Keim, S. M., Kent, M. (2005). Nausea and vomiting. Retrieved August 2007 at www.emedicinehealth.com/vomiting_and_nausea/article_em.htm.
7. National Comprehensive Cancer Network clinical practice guidelines: Nausea and vomiting: Treatment guidelines for patients with cancer. Vol 3, 2005. Retrieved August 2007 at www.cancer.org/downloads/CRI/NCCN_Nasuea.pdf.
8. Palliative Care & Symptom Management: Nausea & Vomiting. Retreived August 2007 at www.canceradvocacy.org/resources/essential/effects/nausea.aspx.

unilateral Neglect

Definition: Impairment in sensory and motor response, mental representation, and spatial attention to body and the corresponding environment characterized by inattention to one side and overattention to the opposite side; left-side neglect is more severe and persistent than right-side neglect

RELATED FACTORS
Brain injury from cerebrovascular problems; neurological illness; trauma; tumor
Left hemiplegia from CVA of the right hemisphere
Hemianopsia

DEFINING CHARACTERISTICS

Subjective
[Reports feeling that part does not belong to own self]

Objective
Marked deviation of the eyes/head/trunk (as if drawn magnetically) to the nonneglected side to stimuli and activities on that side
Failure to move eyes/head/limbs/trunk in the neglected hemisphere despite being aware of a stimulus in that space; failure to notice people approaching from the neglected side
Displacement of sounds to the nonneglected side
Appears unaware of positioning of neglected limb
Lack of safety precautions with regard to the neglected side
Failure to eat food from portion of the plate on the neglected side; dress/groom neglected side
Difficulty remembering details of internally represented familiar scenes that are on the neglected side

Use of only vertical half of page when writing; failure to cancel lines on the half of the page on the neglected side; substitution of letters to form alternative words that are similar to the original in length when reading

Distortion/omission of drawing on the half of the page on the neglected side

Perseveration of visual motor tasks on nonneglected side

Transfer of pain sensation to the nonneglected side

Sample Clinical Applications: Traumatic brain injury, cerebrovascular accident/ruptured cerebral aneurysm, brain tumor, glaucoma

DESIRED OUTCOMES/EVALUATION CRITERIA

Sample NOC linkages:

Adaption to Physical Disability: Adaptive response to a significant functional challenge due to a physical disability

Self-Care: Activities of Daily Living (ADL): Ability to perform the most basic physical tasks and personal care activities independently with or without assistive device

Personal Safety Behavior: Individual or caregiver efforts to control behaviors that might cause physical injury

Client/Caregiver Will (Include Specific Time Frame)

- Acknowledge presence of sensory-perceptual impairment.
- Identify adaptive/protective measures for individual situation.
- Demonstrate behaviors, lifestyle changes necessary to promote physical safety

Client Will (Include Specific Time Frame)

- Verbalize positive realistic perception of self, incorporating the current dysfunction.
- Perform self-care within level of ability.

ACTIONS/INTERVENTIONS

Sample NIC linkages:

Unilateral Neglect Management: Protecting and safely reintegrating the affected part of the body while helping the patient adapt to disturbed perceptual abilities

Positioning: Deliberative placement of the patient or a body part to promote physiological and/or psychological well-being

Environmental Management: Safety: Manipulation of the patient's surroundings for therapeutic benefit

NURSING PRIORTIY NO. 1 To assess the extent of altered perception and the related degree of disability:

- Identify underlying condition/reason for alterations in sensory/motor/behavioral perceptions as noted in Related Factors.
- Observe client's behaviors (as noted in Defining Characteristics) *to determine the extent of impairment (e.g., failure to respond to stimuli, objects, or people on the contralesional side).*
- Ascertain client's/SO's perception of problem/changes and impact on life/future, noting differences in perceptions. *Client may/may not be aware or able to express spatial perception problems or understand potential effect on future expectations.*

🌐 Cultural ⚛ Collaborative 🏠 Community/Home Care 🧪 Diagnostic Studies ∞ Pediatric/Geriatric/Lifespan 💊 Medications

- Measure visual acuity and field of vision *to determine presence/degree of interference if problem is due to actual loss of visual field as can occur with some types of stroke, causing (1) failure to recognize an object, or (2) define where an object is located. However, the client can have intact visual fields and still experience spatial neglect.*[1]
- Assess ability to distinguish between right and left. *Unilateral spatial neglect is observed in stroke, brain tumor, or accident victims with damage to the right parietal or parietal-occipital lobe, resulting in misperceptions of space opposite to brain damage. The individual with this condition has information from the left hemispace, but no conscious awareness of the information; thus they will pay no attention to the left space.*[1-4]
- Assess sensory awareness (e.g., response to stimulus of hot/cold, dull/sharp); note problems with awareness of motion and proprioception. *Disturbances in these areas may be result of spinal cord injury (where loss of sensation affects body awareness) or brain lesion (where sensation may be intact but awareness is impaired).*
- Note physical signs of neglect (e.g., disregard for position of affected limb[s], bumping into walls when ambulating, shaving only right side of face, skin irritation/injury, etc.).
- Observe ability to function within limits of impairment. Compare with client's perception of own abilities. *Client may or may not be able to learn from mistakes or from observing others, depending upon the location/severity of the brain lesion.*[5]
- Explore and encourage verbalization of feelings *to identify meaning of loss/dysfunction/change to the client and impact it may have on assuming ADLs.*
- Review results of testing done to determine cause or type of neglect syndrome (e.g., sensory, motor, representational, personal, spatial, behavioral inattention). *Aids in distinguishing neglect from visual field cuts, impaired attention, and planning or visuospatial abilities.*[6-8]

NURSING PRIORITY NO. 2 To promote optimal comfort and safety for the client in the environment:

- Collaborate in treatment strategies *focused on training of attention to the neglected hemispace:*[1-5,8,9]
  Encourage use of vision and hearing aids if condition requires/client usually wears them *to improve sensory input and interpretation.*
  Remove excess stimuli from the environment *to decrease confusion and reactive stress.*
  Orient/reorient to physical environment and persons interacting with client. *Client with unilateral neglect can also have numerous other cognitive defects affecting ability to think, remember, speak or understand language, and/or interpret environment.*[5]
  Approach client, and instruct others to approach client from the unaffected side (e.g., right side, or side where vision is not impaired) *to enhance client's awareness and potential for communication.*
  Encourage client to turn head and eyes in full rotation and "scan" the environment *to compensate for visual field loss or if neglect therapies include scanning.*
  Position bedside table and objects (such as telephone/call bell, tissues) *within functional field of vision or awareness to facilitate self-care.*
  Place nonessential items (e.g., television, pictures, hairbrush) on affected side during postacute phase once client begins to cross midline *to encourage continuation of retraining behaviors.*
  Discuss affected side while touching, manipulating, and stroking affected side *to focus client's attention on area* and provide objects of various weight, texture, and size for the client to handle *to provide tactile stimuli.*
  Describe where affected areas of body are *when moving/repositioning client.*
  Use descriptive terms to identify body parts rather than "left" and "right"; for example, "Lift this leg" (point to leg) or "Lift your affected leg."

Encourage client to accept affected limb/side as part of self even when it no longer feels like it belongs. Have client look at and handle affected side *to stimulate awareness* and bring the affected limb across the midline *for client to visualize during care.*

Provide visual cues/assist client to position the affected extremity carefully and teach to routinely visualize placement of the extremity.

Use a mirror to help client adjust position *by visualizing both sides of the body.*

- Provide assistance with ADLs (e.g., feeding, bathing, dressing, grooming, toileting, etc.), *which helps client tend to affected side or compensate for client's impairments.*
- Monitor neglected body part(s) for positioning/anatomic alignment, pressure points/skin irritation/injury, and dependent edema. *Increased risk of injury/ulcer formation necessitates close observation and timely intervention.* (Refer to NDs risk for Peripheral Vascular Dysfunction, impaired Tissue Integrity.)
- Assist with ambulation/movement, using appropriate mobility and assistive devices *to promote safety of client and caregiver.*
- Protect from falls and/or collision with objects:
  Position furniture and equipment *so travel path is unobstructed.*
  Remove articles that may create a safety hazard (e.g., footstool, throw rug).
  Ensure adequate lighting in the environment.
  Keep doors wide open or completely closed.
- Refer to NDs impaired Environmental Interpretation Syndrome, risk for Falls/Injury, and Self-Care Deficit (specify) for additional interventions regarding comfort and safety.

NURSING PRIORITY NO. 3 To promote wellness (Teaching/Discharge Considerations):

- Collaborate with rehabilitation team in strategies (e.g., sensory stimulation techniques such as tapping or stroking, active and passive range-of-motion exercises and temporary restraint of healthy limb while practicing motor skills) *to assist client to compensate for deficits.*[5]
- Refer to/participate in neuropsychological therapies, as indicated. *Rehabilitation may address (1) visual attention deficits (e.g., scanning, training) or (2) spatial representation deficits (e.g., mental imagery training, eye patching, stimulation therapy, etc.).*[3]
- Acknowledge and accept feelings of despondency, grief, and anger. *When feelings are openly expressed, client can deal with them and move forward.* (Refer to ND Grieving as appropriate.)
- Encourage family members/SO(s) to treat client normally, perform own care as able, and include in family activities/outings. *Promotes sense of self-worth and encourages participation in life activities to limit withdrawal/depression.*
- Reinforce to client the reality of the dysfunction and need to compensate. Avoid participating in the client's use of denial. *Delays dealing with reality of situation and limits progress toward goals.*
- Encourage client to continue rehabilitative services *to maximize recovery and enhance independence. Note: Research (Barrett, 2007) indicates that most clients with neglect show early recovery, particularly within the first month and marked improvement within 3 months. In approximately 10% of clients, classic (more severe) symptoms of spatial neglect persist after 6 months or longer. In these individuals, the deficit may be regarded as chronic neglect.*[9]
- Discuss/prepare for ongoing safety issues. *Client may continue to have some functional problems after apparent recovery of spatial neglect, including difficulty with navigating in familiar and unfamiliar environments and safe driving.*[9]
- Identify additional resources to meet individual needs (e.g., Meals on Wheels, home-care rehabilitation services) *to maximize independence, allow client to return to/succeed in community setting.*

Cultural Collaborative Community/Home Care Diagnostic Studies Pediatric/Geriatric/Lifespan Medications

DOCUMENTATION FOCUS

Assessment/Reassessment

• Individual findings, including extent of altered perception, degree of disability, effect on independence/participation in ADLs.

Planning

• Plan of care and who is involved in the planning.
• Teaching plan.

Implementation/Evaluation

• Responses to intervention/teaching and actions performed.
• Attainment/progress toward desired outcome(s).
• Modifications to plan of care.

Discharge Planning

• Long-term needs and who is responsible for actions to be taken.
• Available resources, specific referrals made.

References

1. Walker, R. (1994). Unilateral Neglect: Clinical and experimental studies edited by Ian H. Robertson and John C. Marshall. Review for Psyche: An Interdisciplinary Journal of Research on Consciousness. Accessed July 2007 at http://psyche.cs.monash.edu.au/v1/psyche-1-08-walker.html.
2. Mansoori, L. Hemispatial neglect syndrome. Student lecture for Brain, Thought and Action (MCDB 3650). University of Colorado, Boulder.
3. Ricci, R., Calhoun, J., Chatterjee, A. (2000). Orientation bias in unilateral neglect: Representational contributions. (Research article). Philadelphia: Department of Neurology and the Center for Cognitive Neuroscience, University of Pennsylvania.
4. Sinclair, C. (2001). Brain organization as seen in unilateral spatial neglect. Accessed July 2007 at http://serendip.brynmawr.edu/bb/neuro/neuro01/web2/Sinclair.html.
5. No author listed. Post-stroke rehabilitation fact sheet. Available at: National Institute for Neurological Disorders and Stroke (NINDS). Accessed July 2007 at www.ninds.nih.gov/disorders/stroke/poststrokerehab.htm.
6. Bates, B., Choi, J. Y., Duncan, P. W., et al. (2005). Veterans Affairs/Department of Defense clinical practice guidelines for the management of adult stroke rehabilitation care: An executive summary. *Stroke, 36*(9), 2049–2056.
7. Plummer, P., Morris, M. E., Dunai, J. (2003). Assessment of unilateral neglect. *Phys Ther, 83*(8), 732–740.
8. Swan, L. (2001). Unilateral spatial neglect. *Phys Ther, 81*(9), 1572–1580.
9. Barrett, A. M., John, S. T. (2007). Spatial neglect. Article for emedicine. Retrieved July 2007 at www.emedicine.com/neuro/topic719.htm.

Noncompliance [ineffective Adherence] (specify)

Definition: Behavior of person and/or caregiver that fails to coincide with a health-promoting or therapeutic plan agreed on by the person (or family or community) and healthcare professional; in the presence of an agreed-on health-promoting or therapeutic plan, person's or caregiver's behavior is fully or partially nonadherent and may lead to clinically ineffective or partially ineffective outcomes

[AUTHOR NOTE: When the plan of care is reviewed with client/SO, use of the term *noncompliance* may create a negative response and sense of conflict between healthcare providers and client. Labeling the client noncompliant may also lead to problems with third-party reimbursement. Where possible, use of the ND ineffective Therapeutic Regimen Management is recommended.]

RELATED FACTORS
Healthcare plan
Duration
Cost; intensity; complexity
Financial flexibility of plan
Individual factors
Personal/developmental abilities; knowledge/skill relevant to the regimen behavior; motivational forces
Individual's value system; health beliefs, cultural influences, spiritual values, significant others
[Altered thought processes such as depression, paranoia]
[Difficulty changing behavior, as in addictions]
[Denial; issues of secondary gain]
Health system
Individual health coverage
Credibility of provider; client-provider relationships; provider continuity/regular follow-up; provider reimbursement; communication/teaching skills of the provider
Access/convenience of care; satisfaction with care
Network
Involvement of members in health plan; social value regarding plan
Perceived beliefs of significant others

DEFINING CHARACTERISTICS

Subjective
Statements by client or SO(s) of failure to adhere; [does not perceive illness/risk to be serious, does not believe in efficacy of therapy, unwilling to follow treatment regimen or accept side effects/limitations]

Objective
Behavior indicative of failure to adhere
Objective tests (e.g., physiological measures, detection of physiological markers)
Failure to progress; evidence of development of complications/exacerbation of symptoms
Failure to keep appointments

Sample Clinical Applications: Any new diagnosis, chronic conditions, or situations requiring undesired/major lifestyle changes

DESIRED OUTCOMES/EVALUATION CRITERIA
Sample NOC linkages:
Compliance Behavior: Personal actions to promote wellness, recovery, and rehabilitation based on professional advice
Health Beliefs: [specify]: Personal convictions that influence health behaviors
Participation in Healthcare Decisions: Involvement in selecting and evaluating healthcare options to achieve desired outcomes

Client Will (Include Specific Time Frame)

- Verbalize accurate knowledge of condition and understanding of treatment regimen.
- Make choices at level of readiness based on accurate information.
- Verbalize commitment to mutually agreed-upon goals and treatment plan.
- Access resources appropriately.
- Demonstrate progress toward desired outcomes/goals.

ACTIONS/INTERVENTIONS

Sample NIC linkages:

Mutual Goal-Setting: Collaborating with patient to identify and prioritize care goals, then developing a plan for achieving those goals

Self-Modification Assistance: Reinforcement of self-directed change initiated by the patient to achieve personally important goals

Values Clarification: Assisting another to clarify her or his own values in order to facilitate effective decision making

NURSING PRIORITY NO. 1 To determine reason for alteration/disregard of therapeutic regimen/instructions:

- Determine client/SO(s) perception/understanding of the situation (illness/treatment). *Basic information needed to understand client's/SO(s) position and possible conflicts in order to develop plan of care.*[2]
- Listen to/Active-listen to client's complaints, comments. *Conveys confidence in individual's ability to understand and manage own care.*[1] *Helps to identify client's thinking about the treatment regimen (e.g., may be concerned about side effects of medications or success of procedures/transplantation).*[11]
- Note language spoken, read, and understood. *Lack of understanding of words that are used in explanations may result in client lack of cooperation with therapeutic regimen.*[2,10]
- Identify developmental level as well as chronological age of client. *Determines how to interact with client on appropriate level to enhance relationship and ability to discuss lack of cooperation with medical regimen.*[2]
- Assess level of anxiety, locus of control, sense of powerlessness, and so forth. *Presence of these factors will affect how client is managing illness/situation and therapeutic regimen.*[1,11]
- Note length of illness. *People tend to become passive and dependent in long-term, debilitating illnesses and find it difficult to expend energy to follow through with therapeutic regimen.*[6]
- Clarify value system: cultural/religious values, health/illness beliefs and practices of the client/SO(s). *These factors will influence individual's view of the therapeutic regimen and willingness to follow through on some interventions; for instance, Mexican Americans may believe the future is in God's hands; women may delay Pap smears and mammograms because of modesty.*[10]
- Determine social characteristics, demographic and educational factors, as well as personality of the client. *Educated individuals may be more oriented to health promotion and disease prevention, while lower-socioeconomic individuals may be focused on the basics of living and may not pay attention to/follow healthcare recommendations. Personality characteristics such as suspiciousness, obsessive features may affect how client views medical regimen.*[9]

- Verify psychological meaning of the behavior (e.g., may be denial). Note issues of secondary gain. *Family dynamics, school/workplace issues, involvement in legal system may unconsciously affect client's decision regarding care and necessary follow-through.*[3]
- Assess availability/use of support systems and resources. *Failure to follow through with recommended therapies may be due to lack of/incorrect usage of support that is available.*[9]
- Be aware of nurses'/healthcare providers' attitudes and behaviors toward the client. Do they have an investment in the client's compliance/recovery? What is the behavior of the client and healthcare provider when client is labeled "noncompliant"? *Some care providers may be enabling client whereas others' judgmental attitudes may impede treatment progress.*[1]
- Determine who (e.g., client, SO, other) manages the medication regime and whether individual knows what the medications are and why they are prescribed.
- Ascertain how client remembers to take medications and how many doses have been missed in the last 72 hours, last week, last 2 weeks, and last month. *While clients claiming to take their medication often do not, self-reported nonadherence is likely to be accurate and should be taken seriously.*[13]
- Identify factors that interfere with taking medications or lead to lack of adherence (e.g., depression, active alcohol/other drug use, low literacy, lack of support, lack of belief in treatment efficacy). *Forgetfulness is the most common reason given for not complying with the treatment plan.*[12]

NURSING PRIORITY NO. 2 To assist client/SO(s) to develop strategies for dealing effectively with the situation:

- Develop therapeutic nurse-client relationship. *Promotes trust, provides atmosphere in which client/SO(s) can freely express views/concerns and explore reasons for lack of compliance with therapeutic regimen. Adherence assessment is most successful when conducted in a positive, nonjudgmental atmosphere.*[1]
- Explore client involvement in or lack of mutual goal-setting. *Client will be more likely to follow through on goals he or she participated in developing.*[5,8]
- Review treatment strategies. Identify which interventions in the plan of care are most important in meeting therapeutic goals and which are least amenable to cooperation. *Sets priorities and encourages problem-solving areas of conflict, enabling client to make decisions related to choices of care.*[7]
- Contract with the client for participation in care. *Enhances commitment to follow-through.*[3]
- Encourage client to maintain self-care, providing for assistance when necessary. Accept client's evaluation of own strengths/limitations while working with client to improve abilities. *Promotes self-esteem, enabling client to have a sense of control over illness and treatment regimen.*[7]
- Provide for continuity of care in and out of the hospital/care setting, including long-range plans. *Supports trust, facilitates progress toward goals as client illness is dealt with over time.*[6,14]
- Provide information and help client to know where and how to find it on own. *Promotes independence and encourages informed decision making and control over illness, enhancing compliance with therapeutic regimen.*[4]
- Present information in manageable amounts, using verbal, written, and audiovisual modes at level of client's ability. *Individuals learn in many ways, and using different modes at client's own pace facilitates learning and enhances assimilation of the information.*[3]
- Have client/SO paraphrase instructions/information heard. *Validates understanding and reveals misconceptions so that corrections can be made and appropriate questions can be asked and answered.*[4]

🌐 Cultural   Ⓐ Collaborative   🏠 Community/Home Care   Diagnostic Studies   ∞ Pediatric/Geriatric/Lifespan   💊 Medications

- Accept the client's choice/point of view, even if it appears to be self-destructive. Avoid confrontation regarding beliefs. *Maintaining open communication is important to continuing to provide correct information and therapeutic relationship with the client/SO(s). If illness is terminal, accept client's wishes regarding continued care or treatments, providing what is accepted.*[1]
- Establish graduated goals or modified regimen as necessary. *Client with COPD who smokes a pack of cigarettes a day may be willing to reduce that amount but not give up smoking altogether. This choice may improve quality of life, and success with this goal may encourage progression to more advanced goals.*[3]

NURSING PRIORITY NO. 3 To promote wellness (Teaching/Discharge Considerations):

- Stress importance of the client's knowledge and understanding of the need for treatment/medication, as well as consequences of actions/choices. *Client who is not adhering to the treatment regimen may not have full information or may not understand the reasons for the recommendations. With full understanding, client can make a more informed decision about care.*[1,11,14]
- Develop a system for self-monitoring. *Provides a sense of control and enables the client to follow own progress, seek timely evaluation/intervention by healthcare provider, and assist with making choices.*[7]
- Suggest using a medication reminder system. *These have been shown to improve client adherence by a significant percentage.*
- Provide support systems to reinforce negotiated behaviors. Encourage client to continue positive behaviors, especially if client is beginning to see benefit. *Individuals who feel alone and do not hear any positive reinforcement for changes that have been made will have difficulty maintaining the changes. When clients do hear positive comments and see the results for themselves, they are more apt to be willing to continue treatment regimen.*[7,8]
- Refer to counseling/therapy or other appropriate resources. *May need additional assistance to resolve situation and enable client to progress as desired.*[1]
- Refer to NDs Anxiety; compromised family Coping; ineffective Coping; deficient Knowledge (specify); ineffective Therapeutic Regimen Management.

DOCUMENTATION FOCUS

Assessment/Reassessment

- Individual findings/deviation from prescribed treatment plan and client's reasons in own words.
- Cultural/religious values, beliefs, and expectations.
- Availability/use of resources.
- Involvement of SO/family.
- Consequences of actions to date.

Planning

- Plan of care and who is involved in planning.
- Teaching plan.

Implementation/Evaluation

- Response to interventions/teaching and actions performed.
- Attainment/progress toward desired outcome(s).
- Modifications to plan of care.

Discharge Planning

- Long-term needs and who is responsible for actions to be taken.
- Specific referrals made.

References

1. Doenges, M., Townsend, M., Moorhouse, M. (1998). *Psychiatric Care Plans: Guidelines for Individualizing Care.* 3d ed. Philadelphia: F. A. Davis.
2. Locher, J., et al. (2002). Effects of age and casual attribution to aging on health-related behaviors associated with urinary incontinence in older women. *Gerontologist,* 42(4), 525.
3. Cox, H., et al. (2002). *Clinical Applications of Nursing Diagnoses.* 4th ed. Philadelphia: F. A. Davis.
4. Pinhas-Hamiel, O., Dolan, L. M., et al. (1996). Increased incidence of non-insulin-dependent diabetes mellitus among adolescents. *J Pediatr,* 128(8), 608.
5. Deckelbaum, R. J., Williams, C. L. (2001). Childhood obesity: The health issue. *Obesity Research,* 9(5), 239s.
6. Badger, J. M. (2001). Burns: The psychological aspect. *AJN,* 101(11), 38–41.
7. Bartol, T. (2002). Putting a patient with diabetes in the driver's seat. *Nursing,* 32(2), 53–55.
8. Doughty, D. B. (2001). The state of ostomy care, tremendous progress, continued challenges. *J Wound Ostomy Continence Nurs,* 28(1), 1–2.
9. American Society of Pain Management Nurses. (2002). Position paper on pain management in patients with addictive disease. Pensacola, FL.
10. Lipson, J. G., Dibble, S. L., Minarik, P. A. (1999). *Culture & Nursing Care: A Pocket Guide.* San Francisco: UCSF Nursing Press.
11. Morrissey, P. (2005). Noncompliance after Transplantation. Retrieved August 2007 at www.lifespan.org/rih/services/transplant/news/02-07.htm.
12. Human Medication Noncompliance. Retrieved August 2007 at www.alrt.com/humnonc.html.
13. Zuger, A. (2001) Adherence By Any Measure Still Matters. Retrieved August 2007 at http://aids-clinical-care.jwatch.org/cgi/content/full/2001/701/1.
14. Clinical Manual for Management of the HIV-infected Adult, 2006 ed. Section 3: Antiretroviral Therapy Adherence, pp. 3–11. Retrieved April 2007 at www.aidsetc.org/aetc/pdf/AETC-CM_092206.pdf.

imbalanced Nutrition: less than body requirements

Definition: Intake of nutrients insufficient to meet metabolic needs

RELATED FACTORS
Inability to ingest/digest food; inability to absorb nutrients
Biological/psychological/economic factors
[Increased metabolic demands, such as with burns]
[Lack of information/misinformation/misconceptions]

DEFINING CHARACTERISTICS

Subjective
Reported food intake less than RDA (recommended daily allowances); lack of food
Lack of interest in food; aversion to eating; reported altered taste sensation; perceived inability to digest food
Satiety immediately after ingesting food
Abdominal pain/cramping
Lack of information/misinformation/misconceptions [NOTE: The authors view these as related factors rather than defining characteristics.]

Cultural Collaborative Community/Home Care Diagnostic Studies Pediatric/Geriatric/Lifespan Medications

Objective

Body weight 20% or more under ideal [for height and frame]; [decreased subcutaneous fat/muscle mass]

Loss of weight with adequate food intake

Hyperactive bowel sounds; diarrhea; steatorrhea

Weakness of muscles required for swallowing or mastication; poor muscle tone

Sore buccal cavity; pale mucous membranes; capillary fragility

Excessive loss of hair [or increased growth of hair on body (lanugo)]; [cessation of menses]

[Abnormal laboratory studies (e.g., decreased albumin, total proteins; iron deficiency; electrolyte imbalances)]

Sample Clinical Applications: Cancer, AIDS, anorexia/bulimia nervosa, burns, facial trauma, brain injury/coma, stroke, Parkinson's disease, cleft lip/palate, anemia, dementia/Alzheimer's disease, major depression, schizophrenia

DESIRED OUTCOMES/EVALUATION CRITERIA

Sample NOC linkages:

Nutritional Status: Extent to which nutrients are available to meet metabolic needs

Knowledge: Diet: Extent of understanding conveyed about recommended diet

Weight Control: Personal actions to achieve and maintain optimum body weight

Client Will (Include Specific Time Frame)

- Demonstrate progressive weight gain toward goal.
- Display normalization of laboratory values and be free of signs of malnutrition as reflected in Defining Characteristics.
- Verbalize understanding of causative factors when known and necessary interventions.
- Demonstrate behaviors, lifestyle changes to regain or maintain appropriate weight.

ACTIONS/INTERVENTIONS

Sample NIC linkages:

Nutrition Management: Assisting with or providing a balanced dietary intake of foods and fluids

Weight-Gain Assistance: Facilitating gain of body weight

Eating Disorders Management: Prevention and treatment of severe diet restrictions and overexercising or binging and purging of foods and fluids

NURSING PRIORITY NO. 1 To assess causative/contributing factors:

- ∞ • Identify client at risk for malnutrition (e.g., institutionalized elderly; client with chronic illness; child or adult living in poverty/low-income area; client with facial injuries/deformities; restrictive weight-loss program/surgical intervention; prolonged time of restricted intake, prior nutritional deficiencies; hypermetabolic states [e.g., hyperthyroidism]; malabsorption syndromes).[2,11,12]
- Obtain dietary history *to determine chronic problems/ongoing needs:*
  Increased caloric requirements with difficulty ingesting sufficient calories (e.g., cancer, burns, etc.)

∞   Maturational/developmental issues (e.g., premature baby with sucking difficulties, child with lack of emotional stimulation, frail elderly living alone)

Swallowing problems (e.g., stroke, Parkinson's disease, cerebral palsy/other neuromuscular disorders)[2]

Poor dentition: damaged or missing teeth, ill-fitting dentures, gum disease

Decreased absorption (e.g., lactose intolerance, Crohn's disease)

Diminished desire/refusal to eat (e.g., anorexia nervosa, cirrhosis, pancreatitis, alcoholism, bipolar disorder, chronic fatigue)[2,8]

Treatment-related issues (e.g., chemotherapy, radiation, stomatitis, facial surgery/wired jaw)

Personal/situational factors (e.g., inability to procure or prepare food, social isolation, grief/loss)[10]

∞ • Assess pediatric concerns (e.g., changes in nutritional needs related to growth phase; congenital anomalies, including tracheoesophageal fistula, cleft lip/palate; metabolic/malabsorption problems, such as diabetes, phenylketonuria, cerebral palsy; chronic infections).[5]

🏠 • Determine lifestyle factors that may affect weight. *Socioeconomic resources, amount of money available for purchasing food, proximity of grocery store, and available storage space for food are all factors that may impact food choices and intake.*

🌐 • Evaluate impact of cultural, ethnic, and religious influences. *The nutritional balance of a diet is recognized by most cultures, with distinct theories of nutritional practices for health promotion and disease prevention. Foods are used for prevention or treatment of disease (e.g., client may believe in use of "hot" or "cold" foods to treat certain conditions; or use low-fat, low-sodium foods to prevent heart disease). Certain foods may be thought to cause a disease condition (e.g., upset stomach caused from eating too many cold foods). Special diets or food preparation may be cultural or religious based (e.g., kosher preparation for Jewish client or eating no meat or meat by-products for vegetarian).*[1]

• Explore specific eating habits, the meaning of food to client (e.g., never eats breakfast, snacks throughout entire day, fasts for weight control, no time to eat properly), and individual food preferences and intolerances/aversions. *Identifies poor eating practices to be corrected and provides insight into dietary interventions that may appeal to client.*

• Obtain history or review diary of daily portion (or calorie) intake, patterns and times of eating *to reveal recent changes in client's weight or appetite; and identify strengths and weaknesses in client's dietary habits.*[2]

• Assess client's knowledge of nutritional needs and ways client is meeting these needs. *Identifies teaching needs and/or helps guide choice of interventions.*[2]

• Note availability/use of financial resources and support systems. *These factors affect/determine ability to acquire, prepare, and store food. Lack of support or socialization may impact client's desire to eat.*

💊 • Assess medication regimen, noting possible drug side effects/interactions, allergies, use of laxatives, diuretics. *These factors may be affecting appetite, food intake, or absorption.*[2,10]

• Note client's ability to feed self/presence of interfering factors. *Difficulties such as paralysis, tremor, or injury to hands/arms with inability to grasp or lift utensils to mouth; cognitive impairments affecting coordination or remembering to eat, age and/or developmental issues may require input of multiple providers/therapists to develop individualized plan of care.*[2]

• Auscultate for presence/character of bowel sounds *to determine ability/readiness of intestinal tract to handle digestive processes (e.g., hypermotility accompanies vomiting/diarrhea, while absence of bowel sounds may indicate bowel obstruction).*

🧪 • Determine psychological factors that may affect food choices. Perform psychological assessment as indicated, *to assess body image and congruency with reality, or to identify* factors (e.g., dementia, severe depression) that may be interfering with client's appetite and food intake.[2]

- Note occurrence of amenorrhea, tooth decay, swollen salivary glands, or report of constant sore throat. *May be signs of eating disorder, such as bulimia, affecting eating patterns and requiring additional evaluation.*[7,8]
- Review usual activities/exercise program noting repetitive activities (e.g., constant pacing) or inappropriate exercise (e.g., prolonged jogging). *Individuals with dementia may pace/be in contant motion increasing energy needs. Clients who have eating disorders, such as anorexia or bulimia, may use obsessive activities as weight-control measures.*[8]

NURSING PRIORITY NO. 2 To evaluate degree of deficit:

- Assess current weight, compared to usual weight, and norms for age and body size *to identify changes (e.g., sudden loss related to medical illness versus ongoing chronic depression with anorexia and weight loss; or toddler with failure to meet growth expectations) that affect choice of intervention and helps clarify expectations.*
- Obtain weights using same scale, same time of day, and same clothing, as much as possible *to provide for accurate comparison/evaluate effectiveness of therapeutic regimen.*[2]
- Calculate growth percentiles in infants/children using growth chart *to identify deviations from the norm.*[5]
- Measure/calculate body fat, body water, and muscle mass (via triceps skinfold/other anthropometric measurements), or calculate body mass index (BMI) *to establish baseline parameters and assist in determining therapeutic goals. Note: [BMI = weight (lb)/height (inches squared) x 704]. Desirable BMI is 23 to 25, with <19 being severely underweight.*[2,10]
- Observe for absence of subcutaneous fat/muscle wasting, loss of hair, fissuring of nails, delayed healing, gum bleeding, swollen abdomen, etc., that indicate protein-energy malnutrition.[11]
- Perform/review results of nutritional assessment using sreening tools such as Mini Nutritional Assessment (MNA).[8,13]
- Review laboratory studies (e.g., serum albumin/prealbumin, transferrin, aminoacid profile, iron, BUN, nitrogen balance studies, glucose, liver function, electrolytes, total lymphocyte count, indirect calorimetry *to determine degree of nutritional deficits and effect on body function dictating specific dietary needs. Note: Baseline screening may be done (e.g., albumin, cholesterol, and CBC) to determine whether more in-depth evaluation is needed.*[2,6]
- Assist with/review results of diagnostic procedures (e.g., Schilling's test, D-xylose test, 72-hour stool fat, gastrointestinal endoscopy, gastric reflux scanning, etc.).[2]

NURSING PRIORITY NO. 3 To establish a nutritional plan that meets individual needs:

- Collaborate with interdisicplinary *team* to set nutritional goals *when client has specific dietary needs, malnutrition is profound, or long-term feeding problems exist.*[2,9,11]
- Calculate basal energy expenditure (BEE) using Harris-Benedict (or similar) formula and estimate energy and protein requirements.
- Establish ongoing method of evaluating intake (e.g., calories/day, percent of food consumed at each feeding, etc.) *to assist in determining both amount of food taken and what food groups are consumed or left uneaten, to identify nutritional deficits.*[2]
- Discuss with client/SO aspects of diet that can remain unchanged *to preserve those that are valuable/meaningful.* Negotiate with client aspects of diet that need to be changed, especially if eating/psychiatric disorder is limiting food intake.

NURSING PRIORITY NO. 4 To address specific underlying condition/treatment needs:

- Assist in treatments to correct/control underlying causative factors *to improve intake and utilization of nutrients:*[2,9]

    Administer oral antifungal agent *to treat cutaneous lesions of the mouth (e.g., candidiasis) that limit client's ability or desire for food.*

    Medicate for pain or nausea, and manage drug side effects *to increase physical comfort and appetite.*

    Provide blenderized foods, formula tube feedings, or parenteral nutrition infusions when indicated by client's condition (e.g., wired jaws or paralysis following stroke) and degree of malnutrition. *Enteral route is preferred when oral feeding is not appropriate; however, parenteral nutrition is recommended if client is not able to tolerate at least 50% of the goal rate of enteral feedings.*[9]

    Consult occupational therapist *to identify appropriate assistive devices to facilitate independence in feeding and self-esteem.*

    Consult speech therapist *to develop specific exercises/activities to address swallowing difficulties related to neurological problems (e.g., stroke, ALS).* (Refer to ND impaired Swallowing for additional interventions.)

    Refer for dental care *to correct missing teeth/poorly fitting dentures that affect client's ability to chew food/enjoy process of eating.*

    Develop/refer client to structured (Behavioral Modification) program of nutrition therapy, which may include documenting time/length of eating period, putting food in a blender, and tube-feeding food not eaten. *These programs are used to change the maladaptive eating behaviors of clients with anorexia and bulimia and ensure adequate caloric intake. Because "control" is central to the etiology of these disorders, it is important to ensure that the client is perceived to be "in control."*[8]

    Recommend/support hospitalization for controlled environment, as indicated, in severe malnutrition/life-threatening situations.

NURSING PRIORITY NO. 5 To enhance dietary intake:

- Avoid/limit withholding of food (e.g., prolonged NPO for surgery) as much as possible and reinstitute oral feedings as early as possible *to reduce adverse effects of malnutrition.* Increase specific nutrients (e.g., protein, carbohydrates, fats, and calories), as needed, providing client with preferred food and seasoning choices where possible *to enhance intake.*[11]

- Determine when client prefers/tolerates largest meal of the day. Maintain flexibility in timing of food intake *to promote sense of control and give client opportunity to eat when feeling more rested, less pain or nausea, or family coming at mealtime, etc.*[2]

- Provide numerous small feedings, as indicated; supplement with easily digested snacks *to reduce feeling of fullness that can accompany larger meals, and to improve chances of increasing the amount of nutrients taken over 24-hour period.*[3]

- Promote adequate/timely fluid intake. *Fluid is essential to the digestive process and is often taken with meals. Fluids may need to be withheld before meals or with meals if interfering with food intake.*

- Encourage variety in food choices, varying textures and taste sensations (e.g., sweet, salty, fresh, methods of cooking) *to enhance food satisfaction and stimulate appetite.*[2]

- Offer/keep available to client finger foods and snacks *that are easy to self-feed.*

- Provide oral care before/after meals. *Reduces discomfort associated with nausea, vomiting, oral lesions, mucosal dryness and halitosis, making eating easier/food more palatable.*

- Encourage use of lozenges, gum, hard candy, beverages, etc., *to stimulate salivation when dryness is a factor.*

🌐 Cultural   Collaborative   🏠 Community/Home Care   Diagnostic Studies   ∞ Pediatric/Geriatric/Lifespan   Medications

- Use alternative flavoring agents (e.g., lemon and herbs) *to enhance taste of foods, especially if salt is restricted.*
- Add nonfat milk powder to foods with a high liquid content (e.g., gravy, puddings, cooked cereal) or sugar/honey in beverages if carbohydrates are tolerated *to increase caloric value.*[2]
- Avoid foods that cause intolerances/increase gastric motility (e.g., gas-forming foods, hot/cold, spicy, caffeinated beverages, milk products, and the like) *to reduce postprandial discomfort that may discourage client from eating.*[4]
- Limit high-fat foods or fiber/bulk if indicated, *because they may lead to early satiety.*
- Offer supplement drinks (or dispense in 2- to 4-oz portions several times/day). *Client may view this as a "medication" and thus will drink it, improving intake and energy level.*[2]
- Promote pleasant, relaxing environment, including socialization when possible. *Promotes focus on activity of eating, enhancing intake.*[2]
- Prevent/minimize unpleasant odors/sights, or cooking odors. *Often have a negative effect on appetite or activate gag reflex.*
- Administer pharmaceutical agents as indicated. *Appetite stimulants, dietary supplements; digestive drugs/enzymes, vitamins/minerals (e.g., iron), antacids, anticholinergics, antiemetics, or antidiarrheals, etc., may be used to enhance intake, improve digestion, and correct nutritional deficiencies.*[2]

NURSING PRIORITY NO. 6 To promote wellness (Teaching/Discharge Considerations):

- Discuss myths client/SO(s) may have about weight and weight gain *to address misconceptions and perhaps improve motivation for needed behavior changes.*
- Emphasize importance of well-balanced, nutritious intake. Provide nutritional information as indicated, taking into account client's age and developmental stage (e.g., toddler, teenager, pregnant woman, elderly person with chronic disease), physical health and activity tolerance, financial and socioeconomic factors, and client/SOs potential for management of underlying conditions. *For example, older adults need same nutrients as younger adults, but in smaller amounts and with attention to certain components, such as calcium, fiber, vitamins, protein, and water.*[4] *Infants/children require small meals and constant attention to needed nutrients for proper growth/development while dealing with child's food preferences and eating habits.*[5]
- Address financial issues/identify ways to meet dietary needs using nutrient-dense, low-budget foods.
- Involve SO(s) in treatment plan as much as possible *to provide ongoing support and increase likelihood of accomplishing dietary goals.*
- Consult with dietitian/nutritional support team as necessary *for long-term needs.*[2,9]
- Involve client in developing behavior modification program appropriate to specific needs based on consistent, realistic weight gain goal. *Enhances commitment to change and likelihood of accomplishing desired outcomes.*[8]
- Provide positive regard, love, and acknowledgment of "voice within" guiding client with eating disorder. *These efforts encourage the client to recognize maladaptive eating patterns as defense mechanisms to ease the emotional pain and begin to resolve underlying issues and develop more adaptive coping strategies for dealing with stressful situations.*[8]
- Weigh weekly and document results *to monitor effectiveness of dietary plan.*
- Develop regular exercise/stress-reduction program. *Enhances general well-being, improves organ function/muscle tone, and increases appetite.*[2]
- Review medical regimen and provide information/assistance as necessary. Discuss drug side effects and potential interactions with other medications/over-the-counter drugs.

- Assist client to identify/access community resources such as food stamps, budget counseling, Meals on Wheels, community food banks, or other appropriate assistance programs.
- Refer for dental hygiene/professional care, counseling/psychiatric care, family therapy as indicated.
- Provide/reinforce client teaching regarding preoperative/postoperative dietary needs when surgery is planned.
- Assist client/SO(s) to learn how to blenderize food or perform tube feeding when indicated. *Promotes independence/self-care and sense of some degree of control in a difficult situation.*
- Refer to home health resources *for initiation/supervision of home nutrition therapy when used.*

DOCUMENTATION FOCUS

Assessment/Reassessment

- Baseline and subsequent assessment findings to include signs/symptoms and laboratory diagnostic findings.
- Caloric/nutrient intake.
- Individual cultural/religious restrictions, personal preferences.
- Availability/use of resources.
- Personal understanding/perception of problem.

Planning

- Plan of care and who is involved in planning.
- Teaching plan.

Implementation/Evaluation

- Client's responses to interventions/teaching and actions performed.
- Results of periodic weigh-in.
- Attainment/progress toward desired outcome(s).
- Modifications to plan of care.

Discharge Planning

- Long-term needs/who is responsible for actions to be taken.
- Specific referrals made.

References

1. Purnell, L. D., Paulanka, B. J. (1998). *Transcultural Health Care: A Culturally Competent Approach*. Philadelphia: F. A. Davis, pp. 33–35.
2. Lawhorne, L. S. (2001). Altered nutritional status: Guideline. Columbia, MD: American Medical Directors Association (AMDA). Accessed July 2007 at www.guideline.gov.
3. Love, C. C., Seaton, H. (1991). Eating disorders: Highlights of nursing assessment and therapeutics. *Nurs Clin North Am, 26,* 667–697.
4. American Dietetic Association. (2005). Nutrition across the spectrum of aging. *J Am Diet Assoc,* 105(4), 616–633.
5. Engel, J. (2002). *Pocket Guide to Pediatric Assessment.* 4th ed. St. Louis, MO: Mosby.
6. Vogelzang, J. L. (2003). Making nutrition sense from OASIS. *Home Healthcare Nurse,* 21(9), 592–600.
7. Could You or Someone You Care about Have an Eating Disorder. Accessed July 2007 at www.eating-disorder.com.

8. Townsend, M. C. (2003). *Psychiatric Mental Health Nursing Concepts of Care*. 4th ed. Philadelphia: F. A. Davis.

9. Jacobs, D. G., Jacobs, D. O., Kudsk, K. A., et al. (2004). Practice management guidelines for nutritional support of the trauma patient. *J Trauma,* 57(3), 660–678.

10. Mealtime difficulties for older persons: Assessment and management. (2003). The John A. Hartford Foundation Institute for Geriatric Nursing. Accessed July 2007 at www.guideline.gov/.

11. Scheinfeld, N. S., Mokashi, A. (2007). Protein-energy malnutrition. Article for Emedicine Web site. Retrieved April 2007 at www.emedicine.com/derm/topic797.htm.

12. Sullivan, C. S., Logan, J., Kolasa, K. M. (2006). Medical nutrition therapy for the bariatric patient. *Nutrition Today,* 41(5), 207–212.

13. DiMaria, R. A., Amelia, E. (2005). Nutrition in older adults: Intervention and assessment can curb the growing threat of malnutrition. *AJN,* 105(3), 40-50.

imbalanced Nutrition: more than body requirements

Definition: Intake of nutrients that exceeds metabolic needs

RELATED FACTORS
Excessive intake in relationship to metabolic need

DEFINING CHARACTERISTICS

Subjective
Dysfunctional eating patterns (e.g., pairing food with other activities)
Eating in response to external cues (e.g., time of day, social situation)
Concentrating food intake at end of day
Eating in response to internal cues other than hunger (e.g., anxiety)
Sedentary activity level

Objective
Weight 20% over ideal for height and frame [obese]
Triceps skinfold >15 mm in men, >25 mm in women
[Percentage of body fat greater than 22% for trim women and 15% for trim men]

Sample Clinical Applications: Bulimia nervosa, morbid obesity, diseases requiring long-term steroid use (e.g., COPD), conditions associated with immobility (stroke/paralysis, MS, amputation), Alzheimer's disease, depression, developmental delay

DESIRED OUTCOMES/EVALUATION CRITERIA
Sample NOC linkages:
Weight Control: Personal actions to achieve and maintain optimum body weight
Knowledge: Diet: Extent of understanding conveyed about recommended diet
Nutritional Status: Extent to which nutrients are available to meet metabolic needs

Client Will (Include Specific Time Frame)

• Verbalize a more realistic self-concept/body image (congruent mental and physical picture of self).
• Demonstrate appropriate changes in lifestyle and behaviors, including eating patterns, food quantity/quality, and exercise program.
• Attain desirable body weight with optimal maintenance of health.

ACTIONS/INTERVENTIONS

Sample NIC linkages:
Weight-Reduction Assistance: Facilitating loss of weight or body fat
Nutrition Management: Assisting with or providing a balanced dietary intake of foods and
fluids
Eating Disorders Management: Prevention and treatment of severe diet restrictions and
overexercising or binging and purging of foods and fluids

NURSING PRIORITY NO. 1 To identify causative/contributing factors:

- Obtain weight history, noting if client has weight gain out of character for self or family, is/was obese child, or used to be much more physically active than is now *to identify trends.* *Note: Obesity is now the most prevalent nutritional disorder among children and adolescents in the United States.*[1]
- Assess risk/presence of factors/conditions associated with obesity (e.g., familial pattern of obeseity, decreased basal metabolic rate/hypothyroidism; type 2 diabetes; pregnancy; menopause; chronic disorders, such as heart, kidney disease, chronic pain; food/other substance addictions; stressful or sedentary lifestyle; depression; use of certain medications such as steroids, birth control pills; physical disabilities/limitations; lack of socioeconomic resources for obtaining or preparing healthy foods) *to determine treatments/interventions that may be indicated in addition to weight management.*[1,13]
- Assess client's knowledge of own body weight and nutritional needs, and determine cultural expectations regarding size. *Although nutritional needs are not always understood, being overweight or having large body size may not be viewed negatively by individual, since it is considered within relationship to family eating patterns, peer and cultural influences.*[1] *African American women's frame of reference for "normal body weight" is higher than standard indicators.*[2] *Some cultures place importance on large body size (e.g., Samoan people or Cuban children).*[3] *Life goals may dictate body size (e.g., wrestler/football lineman).*
- Identify familial and cultural influences regarding food. *People of many cultures place high importance on food and food-related events, while some cultures routinely observe fasting days (e.g., Arab, Greek, Irish, Jewish) that may be done for health or religious purposes.*[3]
- Ascertain how client perceives food and the act of eating. *Individual beliefs, values, and types of foods available influence what people eat, avoid, or alter. Client may be eating to satisfy an emotional need rather than physiological hunger, not only because food plays a significant role in socialization, but also because food can offer comfort, sense of security, and acceptance.*[3,4]
- Assess dietary practices by means of diary covering several days, asking for recall of foods/fluids ingested, times and patterns of eating, activities/place, whether alone or with other(s); and feelings before, during, and after eating. *Provides opportunity for individual to focus on/internalize realistic picture of the amount of food ingested and corresponding eating habits/feelings. Identifies patterns requiring change or a base on which to tailor dietary program.*[5]
- Calculate total calorie intake, using client's 24-hour recall or weekly food diary. Evaluate usual intake of different food groups. *Helps identify strengths and weaknesses. For example, client may report normal or excessive intake of food, but calories and intake of certain food groups (e.g., sweets and fats) are often underestimated.*[12-14]
- Ascertain previous dieting history. *Client may report experimentation with numerous types of diets, repeated dieting efforts ("yo-yo" dieting) with varying results, or may never have attempted a weight-management program.*

- Obtain comparative body drawing having client draw self on wall with chalk, then standing against it and having actual body outline drawn to note difference between the two. *Determines whether client's view of self-body image is congruent with reality.*[14]
- Ascertain occurrence of negative feedback from SO(s). *May reveal control issues, impact motivation for change.*
- Identify unhelpful eating behaviors (e.g., eating over sink, "gobbling, nibbling, or grazing") and address kinds of activities associated with eating (e.g., watching television or reading, being unmindful of eating or food) *that results in taking in too many calories as well as eliminating the joy of food because of failure to notice flavors or sensation of fullness/satiety.*[1,13,15]
- Review daily activity and exercise program *for comparative baseline and to identify areas for modification.*
- Review laboratory test results (e.g., total cholesterol/triglycerides, fasting glucose and insulin levels; thyroid/other hormones, etc.) *that may reveal medical conditions associated with obesity, and identify problems that may be treated with alterations in diet or medications.*[11,17]

NURSING PRIORITY NO. 2 To establish weight-reduction program:

- Determine client's motivation for weight loss (e.g., for own satisfaction/self-esteem, to improve health status, or to gain approval from another person). *Client is more likely to succeed and maintain desired weight when change is for self (e.g., acceptance of self "as is," general well-being) rather than to please others.*
- Discuss myths client/SO may have about weight and weight loss *to address misconceptions and possibly enhance motivation for needed behavior changes.*
- Obtain commitment/contract for weight loss. *Verbal agreement to goals or written contract formalizes the plan and may enhance efforts/maximize outcomes.*
- Involve SO(s) in treatment plan as much as possible *to provide ongoing support and increase likelihood of success.*
- Obtain anthropometric measurements *to determine presence/severity of obesity:*
  Evaluate body fat, body water, and muscle mass via scale skin caliper measurements and scale weight (*direct* measurement), bioelectric impedance analysis [BIA], dual-energy x-ray absorptiometry [DEXA], and hydrostatic weighing (*indirect* measurement).[13]
  Calculate body mass index (BMI) *to estimate percentage of body fat. Note: Desirable BMI is 23 to 25, with >30 being obese and >40 being morbidly obese.*[6] *Children who are 120% or more of ideal body weight for height and age are considered obese.*[7]
  Determine waist-to-hip ratio (WHR). *A WHR >8.2 in women and >1.0 in men (apple-shaped fat distribution in abdomen/around torso) is associated with increased risk of complications of obesity (e.g., diabetes and cardiovascular disease).*[8–10,16]
- Set realistic goals (short- and long-term) for weight loss. *Reasonable weight loss (1 to 2 lb/week) has been shown to have more lasting effects than rapid weight loss, although sustaining motivation for small losses often makes it difficult for client to stick with a program. Note: A loss of 5% to 20% of total body weight can reduce many of the health risks associated with obesity in adults.*[1,19]
- Collaborate with physician, nutritionist *to develop/implement comprehensive weight-loss program that includes food, activity, behavior alteration, and support.*
- Calculate calorie requirements based on physical factors and activity. *While many weight-reduction programs focus on portions size and food components (e.g., low-fat, high-protein, low-glycemic foods), reducing calorie intake is essential for weight loss.*[14] *Calories are usually counted according to three substances—carbohydrates = 4 calories/g, protein = 4 calories/g, fats = 9 calories/g. Note: Alcohol (a fourth separate group) = 7 calories/g. Decreasing calories by 500/day or expending 500 calories/day through exercise results in a weight loss of about 1 pound/week.*[9]

- Provide information regarding specific nutritional needs. *Individual may be deficient in needed nutrients (e.g., proteins, vitamins, or minerals) or may eat too much of one food group (e.g., fats or carbohydrates). Depending on client's desires and needs, many weight-management programs are available that focus on particular factors (e.g., low carbohydrates, low fat, low calories). Reducing portion size and following a balanced diet along with increasing exercise is often what is needed to improve health.*[12,18,19]

🏠 - Discuss modifications to achieve healthy body weight:[14,15,19,20]
   Eat from each food group (fruits, vegetables, whole grains, lean meats, low-fat dairy, and oils).
   Start with small changes, such as adding one more vegetable/day, introducing healthier versions of favorite foods.
   Choose "nutrient-dense" forms of foods that provide substantial amounts of fiber, vitamins, electrolytes, and minerals.
   Avoid saturated fats, trans fats, cholesterol, salt (sodium), and added sugars.
   Focus on portion sizes: calorie-dense foods (high in fat and/or sugar) should be eaten in smaller quantities, whereas high-fiber foods can be eaten in larger quantities.
   Discuss smart snacks (e.g., low-fat yogurt with fruit, nuts, apple slices with peanut butter, low-fat string cheese, etc.) *to assist client in finding healthy options.*

🏠 - Stress need for adequate fluid intake and taking fluids between meals rather than with meals to provide fluid while leaving more room for food intake at meals *to assist in digestive process and to quench thirst, which is often mistakenly identified as hunger.*

🏠 - Encourage involvement in planned activity program of client's choice and within physical abilities. Refer to formal exercise program, if desired. *Moderately increased physical activity for 30 to 45 minutes 5 days/week can expend an additional 1500 to 2000 calories/week, supporting both loss of pounds and maintenance of lower weight.*[13,20,21]

🏠 - Recommend weighing only once/week, same time/clothes, and graph on chart. Measure/monitor body fat when possible *to track progress while focusing more on the idea of being health-conscious and responsible than what scale may reveal.*[13]

- Provide positive reinforcement/encouragement for efforts as well as actual weight loss. *Enhances commitment to program and enhances person's sense of self-worth.*

🌐 - Refer to bariatric physician/surgeon when indicated. *Evaluation for special measures may be needed (e.g., supervised fasting or bariatric surgery) for morbidly obese persons with BMI >40.*[9,22]

NURSING PRIORITY NO. 3   To promote wellness (Teaching/Discharge Considerations):

🅐 - Assist in/encourage periodic evaluation of nutritional status and alteration of dietary plan. *May be desired/needed for addressing special needs (e.g., diabetes mellitus, age considerations, very low calorie/fasting) and monitoring health status.*[21]

🏠 - Emphasize importance of avoiding fad diets *that may be harmful to health and often do not produce long-term positive results.*

🏠 - Identify/encourage finding ways to reduce tension when eating. *Promotes relaxation to permit focus on act of eating and awareness of satiety.*

🏠 - Review and discuss strategies to deal appropriately with stressful events *to avoid overeating as a means of coping.*

🏠 - Discuss importance of an occasional treat by planning for inclusion in diet *to avoid feelings of deprivation arising from self-denial.*

🏠 - Advise planning for special occasions (birthday/holidays) by reducing intake before event and/or eating "smart" *to redistribute/reduce calories and allow for participation in food events.*

- Discuss normalcy of ups and downs of weight loss: plateau, set point (at which weight is not being lost), hormonal influences, etc. *Prevents discouragement when progress stalls.*
- Encourage buying personal items/clothing *as a reward for weight loss or other accomplishments.* Suggest disposing of "fat clothes" *to encourage positive attitude of permanent change and remove "safety valve" of having wardrobe available "just in case" weight is regained.*
- Review prescribed drug regimen (e.g., appetite suppressants, hormone therapy, vitamin/mineral supplements) *for benefits or adverse side effects/drug interactions.*
- Recommend reading labels of nonprescription diet aids if used. *Herbals containing diuretics or ma huang (product similar to ephedrine) may cause adverse side effects in vulnerable persons.*
- Encourage parents/school dieticians to model and offer good nutritional choices (e.g., offer vegetables, fruits, and lower-fat foods in daily meals and snacks) *to assist child in accepting healthy foodstyles.*[23]
- Refer to community support groups/psychotherapy, as indicated, *to provide role models, address issues of body image or self-worth.*
- Provide contact number for dietitian/nutritionist and/or audiovisual materials, bibliography, reliable Internet sites for resources *to address ongoing nutrition needs/dietary changes.*
- Refer to NDs disturbed Body Image and ineffective Coping for additional interventions, as appropriate.

DOCUMENTATION FOCUS

Assessment/Reassessment

- Individual findings, including current weight, dietary pattern; perceptions of self, food, and eating; motivation for loss, support/feedback from SO(s).
- Results of laboratory/diagnostic testing.
- Results of weekly weigh-in.

Planning

- Plan of care/interventions and who is involved in planning.
- Teaching plan.

Implementation/Evaluation

- Responses to interventions, weekly weight, and actions performed.
- Attainment/progress toward desired outcome(s).
- Modifications to plan of care.

Discharge Planning

- Long-term needs and who is responsible for actions to be taken.
- Specific referrals made.

References

1. Freemark, M. (2002, update 2006). Obesity. Accessed July 2007 at www.emedicine.com/ped/topic1699.htm.
2. Gore, S. V. (1999). African-American women's perceptions of weight: Paradigm shift for advanced practice. *Holist Nurs Pract,* 13(4), 71–79.
3. Purnell, L. D., Paulanka, B. J. (1998). *Transcultural Health Care: A Culturally Competent Approach.* Philadelphia: F. A. Davis, p. 22.
4. Leininger, M. E. (1988). Transcultural eating patterns and nutrition: Transcultural nursing and anthropological perspectives. *Holist Nurs Pract,* 3(1), 16–25.

5. Fleury, J. (1991). Empowering potential: A theory of wellness motivation. *Nurs Res*, 40, 288.
6. Lawhorne, L. S. (2001). Altered nutritional status: Guideline. Columbia, MD: American Medical Directors Association (AMDA). Accessed July 2007 at www.guideline.gov/.
7. Dimensions of Nutritional Assessment. In Engel, J. (2002). *Pocket Guide to Pediatric Assessment*. 4th ed. St. Louis, MO: Mosby, p. 58.
8. Stanley, M. (1999). The aging gastrointestinal system, with nutritional considerations. In Stanley, M., Beare, P. G. *Gerontological Nursing: A Health Promotion/Protection Approach*. 2d ed. Philadelphia: F. A. Davis.
9. Galletta, G. M. (2003). Obesity and weight control. Accessed November 2003 at www.emedicine.com.
10. Lutz, C. A., Przytulski, K. R. (2001). *Nutrition and Diet Therapy*. 3d ed. Philadelphia: F. A. Davis.
11. Woods, A. (2003). X marks the spot: Understanding metabolic syndrome. *Nursing Made Incredibly Easy!* 1(1), 19–26.
12. Nonas, C. A. (1998). A model for chronic obesity through dietary treatment. *J Am Diet Assoc* (suppl 2), S16.
13. Mathur, R. (2007). Obesity. Article for MedicineNet Web site. Retrieved April 2007 at www.medicinet.com.
14. Anne Collins Weight Management Program. (2000-2007). Article related to food portion size. Retrieved July 2007 at www.annecollins.com/food-portion-size-weight-management.htm.
15. U.S. Department of Health and Human Services, Department of Agriculture. The Dietary Guidelines for Americans, 2005. Retrieved July 2007 at www.heatlhierus.gov/dietaryguidelines.
16. U.S. Department of Health and Human Services, National Institutes of Heath. (2004). Weight and waist measurement. Fact sheet available on Weight-control Information Network (WIN). Retrieved July 2007 at http://win.niddk.nih.gov/statistics/index.htm.
17. Lab Test: Insulin. Retrieved July 2007 at www.labtestsonline.org/understanding/analytes/insulin/test.html.
18. Rippe, J. M., Hess, S. (1998). The role of physical activity in the prevention and management of obesity. *J Am Diet Assoc* (suppl 2), S9.
19. Miller, C. K., Ulbrecht, J. S., Lyons, J., et al. (2007). A reduced-carbohydrate diet improves outcomes in patients with metabolic syndrome: A transitional study. *Topics in Clinical Nutrition*, 22(1), 82–91.
20. Wing, R., Phelan, S. (2005). Long-term weight loss maintenance. *Am J Clin Nutr*, 82(Suppl), 222S–225S.
21. Meadows, M. (2006). Nutrition: Healthy eating. Article for MedicineNet Web site. Retrieved April 2007 at www.medicinet.com.
22. Beauchamp-Johnson, B. M. (2006). Scale down bariatric surgery risks. *Nursing Management*, 37(9), 27–32.
23. Doheny, K. (2006). Adults with children at home consume more fat, study shows. Article for WebMD Medical News. Retrieved January 2007 at www.webmd.com/content/Article/131/117923.htm.

imbalanced Nutrition: risk for more than body requirements

Definition: At risk for an intake of nutrients that exceeds metabolic needs

RISK FACTORS

Dysfunctional eating patterns; pairing food with other activities; eating in response to external cues other than hunger (e.g., time of day, social situation)/internal cues other than hunger (e.g., anxiety); concentrating food intake at end of day

Parental obesity

Rapid transition across growth percentiles in children; reported use of solid food as major food source before 5 months of age

Higher baseline weight at beginning of each pregnancy

Observed use of food as reward/comfort measure

[Frequent/repeated dieting]

[Alteration in usual activity patterns; sedentary lifestyle]

[Majority of foods consumed are concentrated, high-calorie/fat sources]

[Lower socioeconomic status]

NOTE: A risk diagnosis is not evidenced by signs and symptoms, as the problem has not occurred; rather, nursing interventions are directed at prevention.

Sample Clinical Applications: Bulimia nervosa, diseases requiring long-term steroid use (e.g., COPD), conditions associated with immobility (stroke/paralysis, MS, amputation), Alzheimer's disease, depression, developmental delay

🌐 Cultural Ⓐ Collaborative 🏠 Community/Home Care Diagnostic Studies ∞ Pediatric/Geriatric/Lifespan Medications

DESIRED OUTCOMES/EVALUATION CRITERIA
Sample NOC linkages:
Weight Control: Personal actions to achieve and maintenance of optimum body weight
Knowledge: Diet: Extent of understanding conveyed about recommended diet
Nutritional Status: Nutrient Intake: Adequacy of usual pattern of nutrient intake

Client/Caregiver Will (Include Specific Time Frame)

- Verbalize understanding of body and energy needs.
- Identify lifestyle/cultural factors that predispose to obesity.
- Demonstrate behaviors, lifestyle changes to reduce risk factors.
- Acknowledge responsibility for own actions and need to "act, not react" to stressful situations.

Sample NOC linkages:
Weight: Body Mass: Extent to which body weight, muscle, and fat are congruent to height, frame, gender, and age

Client Will (Include Specific Time Frame)

- Maintain weight at a satisfactory level for height, body build, age, and gender.

ACTIONS/INTERVENTIONS

Sample NIC linkages:
Weight Management: Facilitating maintenance of optimal body weight and percent body fat
Nutritional Counseling: Use of an interactive helping process focusing on the need for diet modification
Nutrition Management: Assisting with or providing a balanced dietary intake of foods and fluids

NURSING PRIORITY NO. 1 To assess potential factors for undesired weight gain:

- Note presence of factors/conditions that can contribute to weight gain/obesity (e.g., familial pattern of obesity; decreased basal metabolic rate/hypothyroidism; type 2 diabetes; pregnancy; menopause; chronic disorders such as heart, kidney disease, chronic pain; food/other substance addictions; stressful and/or sedentary lifestyle; depression; use of certain medications such as steroids, birth control pills; physical disabilities/limitations; lack of socioeconomic resources for obtaining or preparing healthy foods) *to determine treatment needs and possible behavioral changes for weight management.*[7]
- Note client's particular situation/number of risk factors *to help determine level of concern. For example, a high correlation exists between obesity in parents and children, which may reflect (in part) family patterns of food intake, exercise, selection of leisure activity (e.g., amount of television watching), family and cultural patterns of food selection. Also family studies (e.g., twin and adoption) suggest genetic factors.*[1,2]
- Evaluate familial and cultural influences *that often place high importance on food and food-related events, or groups that place importance on large body size (e.g., athletes such as football players or wrestlers; African American women [frame of reference for "normal body weight" is higher than standard indicators], Samoan people, or Cuban children).*[2]

∞ • Note client's age and activity level/exercise patterns *to identify areas where changes might be useful to prevent obesity/promote health. For example, older adults need same nutrients as younger adults but in smaller amounts and with attention to certain components, such as calcium, fiber, vitamins, protein, and water.*[4] *Infants/children require small meals and constant attention to needed nutrients for proper growth/development while dealing with child's food preferences and eating habits.*[5]

∞ • Calculate growth percentiles in infants/children using growth chart *to identify deviations from the norm.*

🧪 • Review laboratory data (e.g., growth hormones, thyroid, glucose and insulin levels, lipids, total protein) *to determine health status/presence of endocrine/metabolic disorders, thus dictating specific dietary needs.*[6]

🏠 • Assess eating patterns in relation to risk for obesity and disease conditions. *Food choices and amounts of certain food groups are known to impact health (in both children and adults) and cause/exacerbate disease conditions (e.g., heart disease, diabetes, hypertension, gallstones, colon cancer).*[3,8]

🏠 • Determine patterns of hunger and satiety. *Eating patterns often differ in those who are predisposed to weight gain and may include such factors as skipping meals (decreases the metabolic rate), fasting and binging (causes wide fluctuations in glucose and insulin), eating or overeating in response to emotions (e.g., loneliness, anger, happiness).*

🏠 • Note history of dieting/kinds of diets used. *Client may have tried multiple diets with varying degrees of success in the past, but often has history of regaining weight (yo-yo dieting) or finding that diets are not desirable.*

🏠 • Determine whether binging/purging (bulimia) is a factor *to identify potential for eating disorder requiring in-depth intervention.*

🏠 • Identify personality characteristics (e.g., rigid thinking patterns, external locus of control, negative body image/self-concept, negative monologues [self-talk], and dissatisfaction with life) *that are often associated with obesity.*

🏠 • Determine psychological significance of food to the client (e.g., derives love and comfort from food, uses food to escape deep unhappiness, eats when stressed/anxious).

🏠 • Listen to concerns and assess motivation to prevent weight gain. *If client's concern regarding weight control are motivated for reasons other than personal well-being (e.g., partner's expectations/demands), the likelihood of success is decreased.*

NURSING PRIORITY NO. 2 To assist client to develop preventive program to avoid weight gain:

🏠 • Assess client's knowledge of nutritional needs and ways client is meeting these needs. *Provides baseline for further teaching and/or interventions.*

∞ • Provide information, as indicated, on nutrition, taking into account client's age and developmental stage (e.g., toddler, teenager, pregnant woman, elderly person with chronic disease), physical health and activity tolerance, financial and socioeconomic factors, and client's/SO's potential for management of risk factors.

🏠 • Review guidelines for achieving/maintaining healthy body weight:[9,10]
   Eat from each food group (fruits, vegetables, whole grains, lean meats, low-fat dairy and oils).
   Start with small changes, such as adding one more vegetable/day, introducing healthier versions of favorite foods.
   Choose "nutrient-dense" forms of foods that provide substantial amounts of fiber, vitamins, electrolytes, and minerals.
   Avoid saturated fats, trans fats, cholesterol, salt (sodium), and added sugars.

Focus on portion sizes: calorie-dense foods (high in fat and/or sugar) should be eaten in smaller quantities, whereas high-fiber foods can be eaten in larger quantities.

Discuss smart snacks (e.g., low-fat yogurt with fruit, nuts, apple slices with peanut butter, low-fat string cheese, etc.) *to assist client in finding healthy options.*

- Review healthy eating patterns/habits (e.g., eating slowly and only when hungry; stopping when full; avoiding skipping meals; eating foods from every food group; using smaller plates; chewing food thoroughly; making healthy food choices even when eating fast food, etc.). *Most fast foods and packaged foods are highly processed or are high in sugar, fat, and calories.*
- Encourage involvement in planned exercises of client's choice and within physical abilities. Refer to formal exercise program, if desired. *Promotes incorporation of active lifestyle.*[11]
- Assist client to develop strategies for reducing stressful thinking/actions. *Promotes relaxation, reduces likelihood of stress/comfort eating.*

NURSING PRIORITY NO. 3 To promote wellness (Teaching/Discharge Considerations):

- Provide information about individual risk factors *to enhance decision making and support motivation.*
- Consult with nutritionist *to address client-specific issues (e.g., food groups, dietary restrictions that might be needed for certain chronic diseases such as kidney disease or diabetes).*
- Provide information to new mothers about nutrition for developing babies *to reduce potential for childhood obesity related to lack of knowledge.*
- Encourage parents/school dieticians to model and offer good nutritional choices (e.g., offer vegetables, fruits, and lower-fat foods in daily meals and snacks) *to assist child in accepting healthy foodstyles.*[2,3]
- Encourage the client to make a commitment to lead an active life, to manage food habits, and to develop a system for self-monitoring *to provide a sense of control and assist with making choices.*
- Provide bibliography/reliable Internet sites for resources *to reinforce learning, address ongoing nutrition needs, support informed decision making.*
- Refer to support groups and appropriate community resources for behavior modification, as indicated. *Provides role models and assistance for making lifestyle changes.*

DOCUMENTATION FOCUS

Assessment/Reassessment

- Findings related to individual situation, risk factors, current caloric intake/dietary pattern; activity level.
- Baseline height/weight, growth percentile.
- Results of laboratory tests.
- Motivation to reduce risks/prevent weight problems.

Planning

- Plan of care and who is involved in the planning.
- Teaching plan.

Implementation/Evaluation

- Response to interventions/teaching and actions performed.
- Attainment/progress toward desired outcome(s).
- Modifications to plan of care.

Discharge Planning

- Long-range needs, noting who is responsible for actions to be taken.
- Specific referrals made.

References

1. Freemark, M. (2002, update 2006). Obesity. Accessed July 2007 at www.emedicine.com/ped/topic1699.htm.
2. Purnell, L. D., Paulanka, B. J. (1998). *Transcultural Health Care: A Culturally Competent Approach*. Philadelphia: F. A. Davis.
3. Galletta, G. M. (2003). Obesity and weight control. Available at www.emedicine.com. Accessed November 2003.
4. American Dietetic Association. (2005). Nutrition across the spectrum of aging. *J Am Diet Assoc*, 105(4), 616s–633s
5. Engel, J. (2002). *Pocket Guide to Pediatric Assessment*. 4th ed. St. Louis, MO: Mosby.
6. Vogelzang, J. L. (2003). Making nutrition sense from OASIS. *Home Healthcare Nurse*, 21(9), 592–600.
7. Mathur, R. (2007). Obesity. Article for MedicineNet Web site. Retrieved April 2007 at www.medicinet.com.
8. Doheny, K. (2006). Adults with children at home consume more fat, study shows. Article for WebMD Medical News. Retrieved January 2007 at www.webmd.com/content/Article/131/117923.htm.
9. Anne Collins Weight Management Program. (2000–2007). Article related to food portion size. Retrieved July 2007 at www.annecollins.com/food-portion-size-weight-management.htm.
10. U.S. Department of Health and Human Services, Department of Agriculture. The Dietary Guidelines for Americans, 2005. Retrieved July 2007 at www.heatlhierus.gov/dietaryguidelines.
11. Rippe, J. M., Hess, S. (1998). The role of physical activity in the prevention and management of obesity. *J Am Diet Assoc* (suppl 2), S9.

readiness for enhanced Nutrition

Definition: A pattern of nutrient intake that is sufficient for meeting metabolic needs and can be strengthened

RELATED FACTORS

To be developed by nurse researchers and submitted to NANDA

DEFINING CHARACTERISTICS

Subjective

Expresses knowledge of healthy food and fluid choices/willingness to enhance nutrition
Eats regularly
Attitude toward eating/drinking is congruent with health goals

Objective

Consumes adequate food/fluid
Follows an appropriate standard for intake (e.g., the food pyramid or American Diabetic Association Guidelines)
Safe preparation/storage for food/fluids

Sample Clinical Applications: As a health-seeking behavior the client may be healthy or this diagnosis can occur in any clinical condition

DESIRED OUTCOMES/EVALUATION CRITERIA

Sample NOC linkages:

Nutritional Status: Extent to which nutrients are available to meet metabolic needs

Knowledge: Diet: Extent of understanding conveyed about recommended diet

Health-Promoting Behavior: Personal actions to sustain or increase wellness

Client Will (Include Specific Time Frame)

- Demonstrate behaviors to attain/maintain appropriate weight
- Be free of signs of malnutrition
- Be able to safely prepare and store foods

ACTIONS/INTERVENTIONS

Sample NIC linkages:

Nutrition Management: Assisting with or providing a balanced dietary intake of foods and fluids

Teaching: Prescribed Diet: Preparing a patient correctly follow a prescribed diet

Weight Management: Facilitating maintenance of optimal body weight and percent body fat

NURSING PRIORITY NO. 1 To determine current nutritional status and eating patterns:

- Assess client's knowledge of current nutritional needs and ways client is meeting these needs. *Provides baseline for further teaching or interventions.*
- Assess eating patterns and food/fluid choices in relation to any health-risk factors and health goals. *Helps to identify specific strengths and weaknesses that can be addressed.*
- Determine that age-related and developmental needs are met. *These factors are constantly present throughout the life span, although differing for each age group. For example, older adults need same nutrients as younger adults, but in smaller amounts and with attention to certain components, such as calcium, fiber, vitamins, protein, and water.[1] Infants/children require small meals and constant attention to needed nutrients for proper growth/development while dealing with child's food preferences and eating habits.[2]*
- Evaluate influence of cultural/religious factors *to determine what client considers to be normal dietary practice, as well as to identify food preferences/restrictions and eating patterns that can be strengthened or altered, if indicated.[3]*
- Assess how client perceives food, food preparation, and the act of eating *to determine client's feeling and emotions regarding food (including the use of food for celebrations or as a reward) and self-image.*
- Ascertain occurrence of/potential for negative feedback from SO(s). *May reveal control issues that could impact client's motivation for/commitment to change.*
- Determine patterns of hunger and satiety. *Helps identify strengths and weaknesses in eating patterns and potential for change (e.g., person predisposed to weight gain may need a different time for a big meal than evening or may need teaching as to what foods reinforce feelings of satisfaction).*
- Assess client's ability to shop for, safely store, and prepare foods *to determine if health information or financial resources might be needed.*

NURSING PRIORITY NO. 2 To assist client/SO(s) to develop plan to meet individual needs:

- Determine motivaton/expectation for change. *Motivation to improve and high expectations can encourage client to make changes that will improve his or her life. However, presence of unrealistic expectations may hamper efforts. Client may actually be satisfied with current nutritional state and eating behaviors or may be changing some aspect of food intake or preparation in response to new dietary information/change in health status.*

- Assist in obtaining/review results of individual testing, such as weight/height, body fat percent, lipids, glucose, complete blood count, total protein, etc., *to determine that client is healthy and/or identify dietary changes that may be helpful in attaining health goals.*[5]
- Encourage client's beneficial eating patterns/habits (e.g., controlling portion size, eating regular meals, reducing high-fat, high-sugar, or fast-food intake; following specific dietary program and drinking water and healthy beverages). *Provides reinforcement/ supports client's efforts to incorporate changes into lifestyle habits and continue with new behaviors.*[6,7]
- Provide instruction/reinforce information regarding special needs. *Client/SO may benefit from or desire assistance in learning new eating habits or following medically prescribed diets (e.g., very low-calorie diet, tube-feedings, diabetic or renal dialysis diet).*[4]
- Encourage the client to carefully read food labels, instructing in meaning of labeling, as indicated, *to assist client/SO in making healthful choices.*[7]
- Review safe preparation and storage of food *to maintain maximal nutrient value and avoid food-borne illnesses.*
- Consult/refer to nutritionist/physician, as indicated. *Client/SO may benefit from advice regarding specific nutrition/dietary issues or may require regular follow-up to determine that needs are being met when following a medically prescribed program.*
- Develop a system for self-monitoring *to provide a sense of control and enable the client to track own progress as well as to assist in making informed choices.*[6]

NURSING PRIORITY NO. 3 To promote optimum wellness (Teaching/Discharge Considerations):

- Review individual risk factors and provide additional information/response to concerns. *Assists the client with motivation and decision making.*
- Provide bibliotherapy and help client/SO(s) identify and evaluate resources they can access on their own. *Reinforces learning, allows client to progress at own pace, and encourages client to be responsible for own learning. When referencing the Internet or nontraditional/unproven resources, the individual must exercise some restraint and determine the reliability of the source/information before acting on it.*
- Encourage variety and moderation in dietary plan *to decrease boredom and encourage client in efforts to make healthy choices about eating and food.*
- Discuss use of nutritional supplements, OTC/herbal products. *Confusion may exist regarding the need for/use of these products in a balanced dietary regimen.*
- Assist client to identify/access community resources, when indicated. *May benefit from assistance, such as food stamps, budget counseling, Meals on Wheels, community food banks, and other assistance programs.*

DOCUMENTATION FOCUS

Assessment/Reassessment

- Baseline information, client's perception of need.
- Nutritional intake and metabolic needs.
- Motivation/expectations for change.

Planning

- Plan of care/interventions and who is involved in planning.
- Teaching plan.

⊕ Cultural   Ⓐ Collaborative   🏠 Community/Home Care   ⟋ Diagnostic Studies   ∞ Pediatric/Geriatric/Lifespan   ⚕ Medications

Implementation/Evaluation

- Client's responses to interventions/teaching and actions performed.
- Attainment/progress toward desired outcome(s).
- Modifications to plan of care.

Discharge Planning

- Long-term needs and actions to be taken
- Support systems available, specific referrals made, and who is responsible for actions to be taken.

References

1. American Dietetic Association. (2005). Nutrition across the spectrum of aging. *J Am Diet Assoc,* 105(4), 616–633.
2. Engel, J. (2002). *Pocket Guide to Pediatric Assessment.* 4th ed. St. Louis, MO: Mosby.
3. Purnell, L. D., Paulanka, B. J. (1998) *Transcultural Health Care: A Culturally Competent Approach.* Philadelphia: F. A. Davis.
4. Pignone, M. P., et al. (2003). Counseling to promote a healthy diet in adults: A summary of the evidence for the U. S. Preventive Services Task Force. *Am J Prev Med,* 24(1), 75–92.
5. Vogelzang, J. L. (2003). Making nutrition sense from CASIS. *Home Healthcare Nurse,* 21(9), 592–600.
6. Anne Collins Weight Management Program. (2000–2007). Article related to food portion size. Retrieved July 2007 at www.annecollins.com/food-portion-size-weight-management.htm.
7. U.S. Department of Health and Human Services, Department of Agriculture. The Dietary Guidelines for Americans, 2005. Retrieved July 2007 at www.heatlhierus.gov/dietaryguidelines.

impaired Oral Mucous Membrane

Definition: Disruption of the lips and/or soft tissue of the oral cavity

RELATED FACTORS

Dehydration; NPO for more than 24 hours; malnutrition

Decreased salivation; medication side effects; diminished hormone levels (women); mouth breathing

Deficient knowledge of appropriate oral hygiene

Ineffective oral hygiene; barriers to oral self-care/professional care

Mechanical factors (e.g., ill-fitting dentures; braces; tubes [endotracheal/nasogastric], surgery in oral cavity); loss of supportive structures; trauma; cleft lip/palate

Chemical irritants (e.g., alcohol, tobacco, acidic foods, regular use of inhalers or other noxious agents)

Chemotherapy; immunosuppression; immunocompromised; decreased platelets; infection; radiation therapy

Stress; depression

DEFINING CHARACTERISTICS

Subjective

Xerostomia [dry mouth]

Oral pain/discomfort

Reports bad taste in mouth; diminished taste; difficulty eating/swallowing

Objective

Coated tongue; smooth atrophic; geographic tongue

Gingival/mucosal pallor
Stomatitis; hyperemia; gingival hyperplasia; macroplasia; vesicles; nodules; papules
White patches/plaques, spongy patches; white curdlike exudate
Oral lesions/ulcers; fissures; bleeding; cheilitis; desquamation; mucosal denudation
Purulent drainage/exudates; presence of pathogens; enlarged tonsils
Edema
Halitosis
Gingival recession, pocketing deeper than 4 mm; [carious teeth]
Red or bluish masses (e.g., hemangiomas)
Difficult speech

Sample Clinical Applications: Oral trauma, cancer, chemo/radiation therapy, malnutrition, infection, oral surgery, cleft lip/palate, conditions requiring endotracheal intubation (e.g., brain or spinal cord injury/stroke, COPD, acute respiratory distress syndrome, ALS)

DESIRED OUTCOMES/EVALUATION CRITERIA
Sample NOC linkages:
Self-Care: Oral Hygiene: Ability to care for own mouth and teeth independently with or without assistive device
Tissue Integrity: Skin & Mucous Membranes: Structural intactness and normal physiological function of skin and mucous membranes

Client/Caregiver Will (Include Specific Time Frame)

• Verbalize understanding of causative factors.
• Identify specific interventions to promote healthy oral mucosa.
• Demonstrate techniques to restore/maintain integrity of oral mucosa.
Sample NOC linkages:
Oral Hygiene: Condition of the mouth, teeth, gums, and tongue

Client Will (Include Specific Time Frame)

• Report/demonstrate a decrease in symptoms/complaints as noted in Defining Characteristics.

ACTIONS/INTERVENTIONS

Sample NIC linkages:
Oral Health Restoration: Promotion of healing for a patient who has an oral mucosa or dental lesion
Oral Health Maintenance: Maintenance and promotion of oral hygiene and dental health for the patient at risk for developing oral or dental lesions
Oral Health Promotion: Promotion of oral hygiene and dental care for a patient with normal oral and dental health

NURSING PRIORITY NO. 1 To identify causative/contributing factors affecting oral health:

• Note presence of conditions (e.g., oral infections; facial fractures, head/neck cancer radiation; or systemic diseases such as Sjogren syndrome, systemic lupus erythematosus, rheumatoid arthritis, scleroderma, sarcoidosis, amyloidosis, hypothyroidism, diabetes) *that can affect health of oral tissues.*[10–12]

- Determine type of oral mucous membrane problem (e.g., severe/chronic dry mouth [xerostomia] associated with lack of saliva; abnormal tongue surfaces; gingivitis/periodontal disease; ulcerations/other lesions) that *may cause inflammation affecting ability to eat or more serious complications.*[1]
- Investigate reports of oral pain to determine possible source (e.g., oral lesion, gum disease, tooth abscess) *to identify needed interventions and reduce risk of complications such as systemic infection.*[1]
- Collaborate in evaluating abnormal lesions of mouth, tongue, and cheeks (e.g., white or red patches, ulcers, etc.). *White ulcerated spots may be canker sores, especially in children; white curd patches (thrush) are common in infants. Reddened, swollen bleeding gums may indicate infection, poor nutrition, or poor oral hygiene. A red tongue may be related to vitamin deficiencies.*[2] *Malignant lesions are more common in elderly than younger persons (especially if there is a history of smoking or alcohol use), and many elderly persons rarely visit a dentist.*[3]
- Note use of tobacco (including smokeless) and alcohol, *which may predispose mucosa to affects of nutritional deficiencies, infection, cell damage, and cancer.*[10,12]
- Observe for chipped or sharp-edged teeth. Note fit of dentures or other prosthetic devices when used. *Factors that increase the risk of injury to delicate tissues.*
- Review client's medications and evaluate possibility of side effects. *Many drugs (e.g., anticholinergics, antidepressants, anti-Parkinson's drugs, antihistamines/decongestants, urinary antispastics, antipsychotics, diuretics, hypnotics, systemic bronchodilators, muscle relaxants, reserpine, laxatives, beta-blockers, narcotics) can impair salivary function/promote xerostomia.*[8,10]
- Determine nutrition/fluid intake and reported changes (e.g., avoiding eating, reports change in taste, chews painstakingly, swallows numerous times for even small bites, unexplained weight loss). *Malnutrition and dehydration are associated with problems with oral mucous membranes.*[6,10]
- Determine allergies to food/drugs, other substances *that may result in irritation of oral mucosa.*
- Review oral hygiene practices, noting frequency and type (e.g., brushing/flossing/water appliances); inquire about client's professional dental care, regularity and date of last dental examination.
- Evaluate client's ability to provide self-care and availability of necessary equipment/assistance. *Client's age (very young or elderly) impacts ability to provide self-care, as well as current health issues (e.g., disease condition or treatment, weakness), and client's habits and lifestyle.*[4]

NURSING PRIORITY NO. 2 To correct identified/developing problems:

- Collaborate in treatment of underlying conditions (e.g., structural defects, infections, etc.) *that may correct/limit problem with oral tissues.*
- Routinely inspect oral cavity and recommend client establish regular schedule of self-inspection, such as when performing oral care activities. *Can help with early identification and management of mucous membrane concerns.*
- Adjust medication regimen *to reduce use of drugs with potential for causing/exacerbating painful dry mouth.*
- Administer medications, as ordered, (e.g., nonsteroidal anti-inflammatory drugs, antibiotics, antifungal agents, including antimicrobial mouth rinse or spray) *to treat oral infections or reduce potential for bacterial overgrowth.*[8–10]

- Provide anesthetic lozenges or analgesics such as Stanford solution, viscous lidocaine (Xylocaine), sulfacrate slurry, as indicated *to provide protection/reduce oral discomfort/pain.*[10]

- Disucss safe use of products used to treat xerostomia (e.g., artificial salivas mimic natural saliva to relieve soft tissue discomfort, are more effective and longer lasting than simple rinses but do not stimulate natural salivary gland production; cholinergic agonist preparations [e.g., pilocarpine, cevimeline] do stimulate saliva production).[13]

- Encourage use of tart, sour foods and drinks; chewing sugar-free gum or sucking hard candy to *stimulate saliva.*[11] Use citrus foods/liquids with caution *because may irritate mucosa/increase pain.*[13]

- Provide/encourage regular oral care (including after meals/at bedtime, and frequently to critically ill client):
    Use water, or rinses of normal saline or sodium bicarbonate solutions. *Note: Other rinses, including those containing chlorhexidine or sucralfate, available by prescription, and glutamine, an over-the-counter amino acid typically sold in powder form, can be costly, and studies have not demonstrated healing with their use.*[10]
    Avoid mouthwashes containing alcohol *(drying effect)* or hydrogen peroxide *(drying and foul tasting).*[5,13]
    Use soft-bristle brush or sponge/cotton-tip applicators to cleanse teeth and tongue. *Brushing the teeth is the most effective way of reducing plaque and manage periodontal disease.*[6]
    Floss gently/use WaterPik *to remove food particles that promote bacterial growth and gum disease.*
    Use foam sticks *to swab mouth, tongue, and gums when client has no teeth.*
    Use lemon/glycerin swabs with caution. *Glycerin absorbs water and actually dries the oral cavity; can result in decreased salivary amylase, as well as erosion of tooth enamel.*[6,13]
    Provide/assist with denture care, as needed. *Evidence-based protocol for denture care states that dentures are to be removed and scrubbed at least once daily, removed and rinsed after every meal, and kept in an appropriate solution at night.*[7]

- Change position of ET tube/airway every 8 hours and as needed when client is on ventilator *to minimize pressure on fragile tissues and improve access to all areas of oral cavity.*

- Suction oral cavity *if client cannot swallow secretions. Saliva contains digestive enzymes that may be erosive to exposed tissues (such as might occur because of heavy drooling following radical neck surgery).*

- Use gentle low-intensity suctioning *to reduce risk of aspiration in intubated clients or those with decreased gag/swallow reflexes.*[8]

- Lubricate lips and provide commercially prepared oral lubricant solution, when indicated. Encourage use of chewing gum, hard candy, etc., *to stimulate flow of saliva to neutralize acids and limit bacterial growth.*[10]

- Encourage adequate fluids *to prevent dehydration/oral dryness and limit bacterial overgrowth.*[8]

- Suggest use of vaporizer or room humidifier *to increase humidity if client is mouth breather or ambient humidity is low.*[13]

- Implement diet modifications, as indicated.[10]
    Offer foods with adequate nutritients and vitamins to promote healing *when deficits are impairing health of oral tissues.*
    Avoid sharp, hard, coarse, spicy, salty, and acidic foods *that can irritate or damage fragile mucosa and existing ulcers.*
    Include bland, low-acid, high-protein foods (e.g., milk shakes, bananas, applesauce, mashed potatoes, cooked cereals, soft-boiled or scrambled eggs, cottage cheese, macaroni and cheese, pudding, custard, and gelatin) *that are nutrient-dense and easy to eat.*

Provide moderate temperature foods/fluids, soft or pureed foods, popsicles; frozen yogurt or ice cream *that may be soothing to sensitive mucosa.*

Drink liquids with meals and use gravies and sauces *to make food easier to swallow.*[13]

Avoid dry foods, such as crackers, cookies, and toast, or soften them with liquids before eating.[13]

NURSING PRIORITY NO. 3 To promote wellness (Teaching/Discharge Considerations):

- Recommend regular dental checkups/care and episodic evaluation of oral health prior to certain medical treatments (e.g., chemotherapy/radiation) *to maintain oral health/reduce risks associated with impaired tissues.*[8]
- Review current oral hygiene concerns and provide informational resources/reliable Web sites about oral health *to reinforce learning, encourage proper care.*
- Promote general health/mental health habits *to prevent negative effects that altered immune response can exert on oral mucosa.*
- Provide nutritional information *to correct deficiencies, reduce mucosal inflammation/gum disease, and prevent dental caries.*
- Instruct parents in oral hygiene techniques and proper dental care for infants/children (e.g., safe use of pacifier, brushing of teeth and gums, avoidance of sweet drinks and candy, recognition and treatment of thrush). *Encourages early initiation of good oral health practices and timely intervention for treatable problems.*
- Stress importance of limiting nighttime regimen of bottle of milk for infant in bed. Suggest pacifier or use of water during night *to prevent bottle syndrome with decaying of teeth.*
- Discuss special mouth care required during and after illness/trauma, or following surgical repair (e.g., cleft lip/palate, facial fractures/jaw surgery, etc.) *to facilitate healing.*
- Recommend avoiding alcohol, smoking/chewing tobacco, *which can contribute to mucosal inflammation.*
- Identify need for/demonstrate use of special appliances (e.g., power toothbrushes, dental water jets, flossing instruments, applicators). *Enhances independence in self-care.*
- Identify community resources (e.g., low-cost dental clinics, smoking cessation resources, cancer information services/support group; Meals on Wheels/food stamps, home-care aide) *to meet individual needs.*

DOCUMENTATION FOCUS

Assessment/Reassessment

- Condition of oral mucous membranes, routine oral care habits and interferences.
- Availability of oral care equipment/products.
- Knowledge of proper oral hygiene/care.
- Availability/use of resources.

Planning

- Plan of care and who is involved in planning.
- Teaching plan.

Implementation/Evaluation

- Responses to interventions/teaching and actions performed.
- Attainment/progress toward desired outcome(s).
- Modifications to plan of care.

Discharge Planning

• Long-term needs and who is responsible for actions to be taken.
• Specific referrals made, resources for special appliances.

References

1. Carl, W., Havens, J. (2000). The cancer patient with severe mucositis. *Cur Rev Pain,* 4(3), 197–202.
2. Engel, J. (2002). *Pocket Guide to Pediatric Assessment.* 4th ed. St. Louis, MO: Mosby, pp. 155–156.
3. Aubertin, M. A. (1997). Oral cancer screening in the elderly: The home healthcare nurse's role. *Home Health Nurs,* 15(9), 594–604.
4. White, R. (2000). Nurse assessment of oral health: A review of practice and education. *Br J Nurs,* 9(5), 260–266.
5. Winslow, E. H. (1994). Don't use H_2O_2 for oral care. *Am J Nurse,* 94(3), 19.
6. Stiefel, K. A., et al. (2000). Improving oral hygiene for the seriously ill patient: Implementing research-based practice. *Medsurg Nurs,* 9(1), 40–43, 46.
7. Curzio, J., McCowan, M. (2000). Getting research into practice: Developing oral hygiene standards. *Br J Nurs,* 9(7), 434–438.
8. Trieger, N. (2004). Oral care in the intensive care unit. *Am J Crit Care,* 13(1), 24.
9. Munro, C., Grap, M. J. (2004). Oral health and care in the intensive care unit: Stat of science. *Am J Crit Care,* 13(1), 25–33.
10. Dahlin, C. (2004). Oral complications at the end of life. *AJN,* 104(7), 40–47.
11. Stegeman, C. A. (2005). Oral manifestations of diabetes. *Home Healthcare Nurse,* 23(4), 233–240.
12. No author listed. (2006). Oral cancer. Article for MedicineNet Web site. Retrieved April 2007 at www.medicinenet.com.
13. McKee, C. D. (1999). Xerostomia. Retrieved August 2007 at http://findarticles.com/p/articles/mi_m3374/is_7_21/ai_54563620/pg_1.

acute Pain

Definition: Unpleasant sensory and emotional experience arising from actual or potential tissue damage or described in terms of such damage (International Association for the Study of Pain); sudden or slow onset of any intensity from mild to severe with an anticipated or predictable end and a duration of less than 6 months

RELATED FACTORS
Injuring agents (biological, chemical, physical, psychological)

DEFINING CHARACTERISTICS

Subjective
Verbal report of pain; coded report [may be less from clients younger than age 40, men, and some cultural groups]
Changes in appetite

Objective
Observed evidence of pain
Guarding behavior; protective gestures; positioning to avoid pain
Facial mask; sleep disturbance (eyes lack luster, beaten look, fixed or scattered movement, grimace)
Expressive behavior (e.g., restlessness, moaning, crying, vigilance, irritability, sighing)
Distraction behavior (e.g., pacing, seeking out other people and/or activities, repetitive activities)
Change in muscle tone (may span from listless [flaccid] to rigid)

Cultural   Collaborative   Community/Home Care   Diagnostic Studies   Pediatric/Geriatric/Lifespan   Medications

Diaphoresis; change in blood pressure/heart rate/respiratory rate; pupillary dilation
Self-focusing; narrowed focus (altered time perception, impaired thought process, reduced interaction with people and environment)

Sample Clinical Applications: Traumatic injuries, surgical procedures, infections, cancer, burns, skin lesions, gangrene, thrombophlebitis/pulmonary embolus, neuralgia

DESIRED OUTCOMES/EVALUATION CRITERIA
Sample NOC linkages:
Pain Level: Severity of observed or reported pain
Pain Control: Personal actions to control pain
Pain: Adverse Psychological Response: Severity of observed or reported adverse cognitive and emotional responses to physical pain

Client Will (Include Specific Time Frame)

- Report pain is relieved/controlled.
- Follow prescribed pharmacological regimen.
- Verbalize methods that provide relief.
- Demonstrate use of relaxation skills and diversional activities as indicated for individual situation.

ACTIONS/INTERVENTIONS

Sample NIC linkages:
Pain Management: Alleviation of pain or a reduction in pain to a level of comfort that is acceptable to the patient
Analgesic Administration: Use of pharmacological agents to reduce or eliminate pain
Environmental Management: Comfort: Manipulation of the patient's surroundings for promotion of optimal comfort

NURSING PRIORITY NO. 1 To assess etiology/precipitating contributory factors:

- Note client's age/developmental level and current condition (e.g., infant/child, critically ill, ventilated/sedated, or cognitively impaired client) *affecting ability to report pain parameters.*[13,14]
- Obtain client's assessment of pain to include location, characteristics, onset/duration, frequency, quality, intensity. Identify precipitating/aggravating and relieving factors.
- Use pain rating scale appropriate for age/cognition (e.g., 0 to 10 scale, facial expression/Wong-Baker faces pain scale [pediatric, nonverbal], adolescent pediatric pain tool [APPT], pain assessment scale for seniors with limited ability to communicate [PACSLAC]; behavioral pain scale [BPS]).[1,2,17]
- Note possible pathophysiological/psychological causes of pain (e.g., inflammation, tissue trauma/burns, fractures, surgery; infections, heart attack/angina; abdominal conditions [e.g. appendicitis, cholecystitis] grief, fear/anxiety, depression, personality disorders, etc.). *Acute pain is that which follows an injury/trauma or procedure such as surgery, or occurs suddenly with the onset of a painful condition (e.g., herniated disk, migraine headache, pancreatitis).*[3,15]
- Note anatomical location of surgical incisions/procedures. *This can influence the amount of postoperative pain experienced; for example, vertical/diagonal incisions are more painful than*

transverse or S-shaped. Presence of known/unknown complication(s) may make the pain more severe than anticipated.[4,5,10]

- Determine history/presence of chronic conditions (e.g., multiple sclerosis, stroke, diabetes, depression, etc.) *that may also cause pain/be associated with an exacerbation of pain symptoms, or interfere with accurate assessment of acute pain.*[2]
- Assess client's perceptions of pain, along with behaviors and cultural expectations regarding pain. *Client's perception of pain is influenced by age and developmental stage, underlying problem causing pain, cognitive, behavioral and sociocultural factors.*[2]
- Note client's attitude toward pain and use of specific pain medications, including any history of substance abuse. *Client may have beliefs restricting use of medications, or may have a high tolerance for drugs because of recent/current use, or may not be able to take pain medications at all if participating in a substance abuse recovery program.*
- Note client's locus of control (internal/external). *Individuals with external locus of control may take little or no responsibility for pain management.*
- Determine medications (e.g., skeletal muscle relaxants, antibiotics, antidepressants, anticoagulants, etc.), alcohol/other drugs currently being used, and any medication allergies *that affect choice of analgesics.*[4,5]
- Collaborate with other medical providers in pain assessment, including neurological and psychological factors (pain inventory, psychological interview) as appropriate when pain persists.
- Refer for/review results of laboratory/diagnostic studies depending on results of history and physical examination.

NURSING PRIORITY NO. 2 To evaluate client's response to pain:

- Perform pain assessment each time pain occurs. Document and investigate changes from previous reports and evaluate results of pain interventions *to demonstrate improvement in status or to identify worsening of underlying condition/developing complications.*[6,16]
- Accept client's description of pain. Be aware of the terminology client uses for pain experience (e.g., young child may say "owie"; elderly may say "it aches so bad"). *Pain is a subjective experience and cannot be felt by others.*[2] Note: *Some elderly clients experience a reduction in perception of pain or have difficulty localizing/describing pain, and pain may be manifested as a change in behavior (e.g., restlessness, increased confusion/wandering, acting out).*
- Note cultural influences affecting pain response. *Verbal or behavioral cues may have no direct relationship to the degree of pain perceived (e.g., client may deny pain even when feeling uncomfortable, or reactions can be stoic or exaggerated, reflecting cultural/familial norms). These factors affect client's and caregiver's attitudes and beliefs regarding the pain experience, expressions of pain, and expectations regarding pain management.*[2,9,14]
- Observe nonverbal cues (e.g., how client walks, holds body, guarding behaviors; sleeplessness; grimacing facial expressions; distraction behaviors, narrowed focus; crying, poor feeding, lethargy in infants). Ask others who know client well (e.g., spouse, parent) to identify behaviors that may indicate pain in persons who cannot communicate verbally. *Helpful in recognizing presence of pain; however, cues not congruent with verbal reports indicate need for further evaluation.*[1-6,9]
- Assess for referred pain, as appropriate, *to help determine possibility of underlying condition or organ dysfunction causing pain to be perceived in area other than site of the problem.*
- Monitor vital signs during episodes of pain. *Blood pressure, respiratory and heart rate are usually altered in acute pain.*[1,2,4,5]
- Ascertain client's knowledge of and expectations about pain management. *Provides baseline for interventions and teaching, provides opportunity to allay common fears/misconceptions*

(e.g., fears about addiction to opiates, belief that complete pain relief is possible in every situation) or to address expected side effects of analgesics (e.g., constipation).[2]

- Review client's previous experiences with pain and methods found either helpful or unhelpful for pain control in the past. *Useful in determining appropriate interventions.*
- Be aware of client's "Right to Treatment" *that includes prevention of or adequate relief from pain*[7] *and that failure to meet the standard of assessing for pain can be considered negligence.*[8]

NURSING PRIORITY NO. 3 To assist client to explore methods for alleviation/control of pain:

- Determine client's acceptable level of pain/pain control goal. *Client may not be 100% pain-free but may feel that a "3" is a manageable level of discomfort, while another may require medication for pain at the same level, because the experience is subjective.*[1,2,4–6,9]
- Determine factors in client's lifestyle (e.g., alcohol/other drug use/abuse) that can affect responses to analgesics and/or choice of interventions for pain management.[14]
- Note when pain occurs (e.g., only with ambulation, every evening) *to medicate prophylactically as appropriate.*
- Collaborate in treatment of underlying condition/disease processes causing pain and proactive management of pain (e.g., epidural analgesia, nerve blockade for postoperative pain, surgical plication of a nerve, implantation of nerve stimulator).
- Work with client *to prevent rather than "chase" pain.* Use flow sheet to document pain, therapeutic interventions, response, and length of time before pain recurs. Instruct client to report pain as soon as it begins, *because timely intervention is more likely to be successful in alleviating pain.*[2,11]
- Encourage verbalization of feelings about the pain *to evaluate coping abilities and to identify areas of additional concern.*[1,11]
- Review procedures/expectations and tell client when treatments will hurt. Discuss pain management methods that will be used *to reduce concerns of the unknown and muscle tension associated with anxiety/fear.*
- Use puppets/dolls for explanations/teaching when indicated, *to demonstrate procedures for child and enhance understanding to reduce level of anxiety/fear.*
- Provide/promote nonpharmacological pain management:
  Quiet environment, calm activities
  Comfort measures (e.g., back rub, change of position, use of heat/cold compresses)
  Use of relaxation exercises (e.g., focused breathing, visualization, guided imagery)
  Diversional/distraction activities, such as television/radio, socialization with others, commercial or individualized tapes (e.g., "white" noise, music, instructional)
  Presence of parent during painful procedures *to comfort child*
  Identification of ways to avoid/minimize pain; *splinting incision during cough, keeping body in good alignment and using proper body mechanics, and resting between activities can reduce occurrence of muscle tension/spasms or undue stress on incision*
- Establish collaborative approach for pain management based on client's understanding about, and acceptance of, available treatment options. *Pharmacological management is based on client's symptomatology and mechanism of pain, as well as tolerance for pain and for the various analgesics. Pain medications may include pills, injections, intravenous dosing/patient-controlled analgesia (PCA), or regional analgesia (e.g., epidural and spinal blocking).*[2–5,11,14,16]
- Administer analgesics to maximal dosage as needed *to maintain "acceptable" level of pain. The type of medication(s) ordered depends on the type and severity of pain (e.g., acetaminophen and nonsteroidal anti-inflammatory medications [NSAIDs] are commonly used to treat*

mild-to-moderate pain, while opiates [e.g., morphine, oxycodone and fentanyl] are used to treat moderate to severe pain). Note: Combinations of medications may be used on prescribed intervals.[5,12]

- Notify physician/healthcare provider if regimen is inadequate to meet pain control goal. Assist client to prevent (rather than treat pain) and alter drug regimen based on individual needs. *Once established, pain is more difficult to suppress. Increasing dosage, changing medication, or using a stepped program (e.g., switching from injection to oral route, or lengthening time interval between doses) helps in self-management of pain.*[4,7]
- Evaluate/document client's response to analgesics and assist in transitioning/altering drug regimen based on individual needs and planned interventions *to limit adverse effects and barriers to adequate use of analgesics.*[2]
- Evaluate for adverse medication effects (e.g., decrease in mental acuity, change in thought processes, confusion/delirium, urinary retention, severe nausea, vomiting, pruritus). *Intolerable symptoms that usually require change of medication(s).*[2,3,5,11,12]
- Demonstrate/monitor use of self-administration/patient-controlled analgesia (PCA) that involves client in plan *to administer own IV pain medication, or bolus additional dose when on continual basis drip.*[2–5,11,12]
- Provide information/monitor use of site-specific medications (e.g., spinal/epidural/regional anesthesia) *that might be used for certain procedures such as back surgery or amputation, labor/delivery).*[3,4,11,12]
- Instruct client in use of transcutaneous electrical stimulation (TENS) unit when ordered.

NURSING PRIORITY NO. 4 To promote wellness (Teaching/Discharge Considerations):

- Acknowledge the pain experience and convey acceptance of client's response to pain. *Reduces defensive responses, promotes trust, and enhances cooperation with regimen.*
- Involve client and SO/family in pain management program. *Provides additional support for the client and increases the likelihood of attaining goals when involved parties understand the process and feel a part of the solution.*
- Encourage adequate rest periods *to prevent fatigue that can impair ability to manage/cope with pain.*
- Review nonpharmacological measures for lessening pain. *Relaxation skills and techniques such as self-hypnosis, biofeedback, and Therapeutic Touch (TT) have no detrimental side effects.*
- Provide information/discuss pain management before planned procedures. *The primary concern of most clients/families is pain and discomfort following surgery/invasive procedure.*
- Address impact of pain on lifestyle/independence. *Understanding that pain can be manageable and that there are ways to maximize level of functioning promotes hope and cooperation with regimen.*
- Encourage performance of individualized physical therapy/exercise program. *Promotes active role in preventing muscle spasms/contractures, enhances sense of control.*
- Discuss ways SO(s) can assist client with pain management. *Helping to reduce precipitating factors that may cause or exacerbate pain (e.g., need to walk distances or climb stairs; strenuous activity, including household chores/yard work; noisy environment), supporting timely pain control, encouraging eating nutritious meals to enhance wellness, and providing gentle massage to reduce muscle tension facilitate recovery/pain control.*
- Identify specific signs/symptoms and changes in pain requiring evaluation by healthcare provider. *Provides opportunity to modify pain management regimen/allows for timely intervention for developing complications.*

⊕ Cultural   Collaborative   🏠 Community/Home Care   Diagnostic Studies   ∞ Pediatric/Geriatric/Lifespan   Medications

DOCUMENTATION FOCUS

Assessment/Reassessment

- Individual assessment findings, including client's description of response to pain, specifics of pain inventory, expectations of pain management, and acceptable level of pain.
- Locus of control and cultural beliefs affecting response to pain.
- Prior medication use; substance abuse.

Planning

- Plan of care and who is involved in planning.
- Teaching plan.

Implementation/Evaluation

- Response to interventions/teaching and actions performed.
- Attainment/progress toward desired outcome(s).
- Modifications to plan of care.

Discharge Planning

- Long-term needs, noting who is responsible for actions to be taken.
- Specific referrals made.

References

1. Engel, J. (2002). *Pocket Guide to Pediatric Assessment*. 4th ed. St. Louis, MO: Mosby, pp. 249, 259.
2. Young, D. (1999). Acute pain management. Iowa City, IA: University of Iowa Gerontological Nursing Interventions Research Center. Research Dissemination Core.
3. Information about Pain Management Options. Accessed July 2007 at www.seanesthesiology.com/handler.cfm?categoryID=35&ParentID=23.
4. Clinical practice guideline for the management of postoperative pain. Version 1.2. (2002). Washington, DC: Department of Defense, Veterans Health Administration. Accessed July 2007 at www.guidelines.gov.
5. Ameres, M. J., Yeh, B. (2001, update 2005). Pain after surgery. Accessed July 2007 at www.emedicine.com.
6. Smith, R., Curci, M., Silverman, A. (2002). Pain management: The global connection. *Nursing Management*, 33(6), 26–29.
7. Acute pain management: Operative or medical procedures and trauma. (Clinical Practice Guideline). (1992). Pub No. AHCPR 92-0019. Rockville, MD: Agency for Health Care Policy and Research, Public Health Service, U.S. Dept of Health and Human Services.
8. Porter, S. (2001). Pain, pain go away. (excerpt JCAHO 2001 Pain Standards.) American Academy of Family Physicans: FP Report, 7(3). Acessed July 2007 at www.aafp.org/fpr/20010300/.
9. Purnell, L. D., Paulanka, B. J. (1998). *Transcultural Health Care: A Culturally Competent Approach*. Philadelphia: F. A. Davis.
10. ND Pain, acute. In Doenges, M. E., Moorhouse, M. F., Geissler-Murr, A. C. (2002). *Nurse's Pocket Guide: Diagnoses, Interventions and Rationales*. 8th ed. Philadelphia: F. A. Davis.
11. Assessment and management of acute pain. (2002, update 2006). Bloomington, MN: Institute for Clinical Systems Improvement (ICSI). Available at www.guideline.gov.
12. Michael, J. A. (2002). Pain Medicine, Types. Accessed December 2003. Content available July 2007 in Managing Cancer Related Pain. Eastern Idaho Medical Center Web site. www.eirmc.org/.
13. Pasero, C., McCaffrey, M. (2005). No self-report means no pain-intensity rating. *AJN*, 105(10), 50–53.
14. Mann, A. R. (2006). Manage the power of pain. *Men in Nursing*, 1(4), 20–28.
15. D'Arcy, Y. (2007). Managing pain in a patient who's drug-dependent. *Nursing2007*, 37(3), 36–40.
16. Wheeler, M. S. (2006). Pain assessment and management in the patient with mild to moderate cogntive impairment. *Home Healthcare Nurse*, 24(6), 354–359.
17. Zwakhalen, S., Hamers, J., Abu-Saad, H., Berger, M. (2006). Pain in elderly people with severe dementia: A systematic review of behavioural pain assessment tools. *Geriatrics*, 6(3). Retrieved August 2007 at www.biomedcentral.com/1471-2318/6/3.

chronic Pain

Definition: Unpleasant sensory and emotional experience arising from actual or potential tissue damage or described in terms of such damage (International Association for the Study of Pain); sudden or slow onset of any intensity from mild to severe, constant or recurring without an anticipated or predictable end and a duration of greater than 6 months [Pain is a signal that something is wrong. Chronic pain may be recurrent and periodically disabling (e.g., migraine headaches) or may be unremitting. While chronic pain syndrome includes various learned behaviors, psychological factors become the primary contribution to impairment. It is a complex entity, combining elements from other NDs, such as risk for Disuse Syndrome; deficient Diversional Activity; interrupted Family Processes; Powerlessness; Self-Care Deficit.]

RELATED FACTORS
Chronic physical/psychosocial disability

DEFINING CHARACTERISTICS

Subjective
Verbal report of pain; coded report
Fear of reinjury
Altered ability to continue previous activities
Changes in sleep patterns; fatigue; anorexia
[Preoccupation with pain]
[Desperately seeks alternative solutions/therapies for relief/control of pain]

Objective
Observed protective/guarding behavior; irritability; restlessness
Facial mask; self-focusing
Reduced interaction with people; depression
Atrophy of involved muscle group
Sympathetic mediated responses (temperature, cold, changes of body position, hypersensitivity)

Sample Clinical Applications: Traumatic injuries, migraines, repetitive motion injury (carpal/cubital tunnel syndrome), rheumatoid arthritis, peripheral neuropathies in diabetes or AIDS, cancer, burns, endometriosis, neuralgia, gangrene

DESIRED OUTCOMES/EVALUATION CRITERIA
Sample NOC linkages:
Pain Control: Personal actions to control pain
Pain: Disruptive Effects: Severity of observed or reported disruptive effects of chronic pain on daily functioning
Pain: Adverse Psychological Response: Severity of observed or reported adverse cognitive and emotional responses to physical pain

Client Will (Include Specific Time Frame)

- Verbalize and demonstrate (nonverbal cues) relief or control of pain/discomfort.
- Verbalize recognition of interpersonal/family dynamics and reactions that affect the pain problem.

Cultural   Collaborative   Community/Home Care   Diagnostic Studies   Pediatric/Geriatric/Lifespan   Medications

- Demonstrate/initiate behavioral modifications of lifestyle and appropriate use of therapeutic interventions.

Sample NOC linkage:
Family Coping: Family actions to manage stressors that tax family resources

Family/SO(s) Will (Include Specific Time Frame)

- Cooperate in pain management program. (Refer to ND readiness for enhanced family Coping.)

ACTIONS/INTERVENTIONS

Sample NIC linkages:
Pain Management: Alleviation of pain or a reduction in pain to a level of comfort that is acceptable to the patient
Medication Management: Facilitation of safe and effective use of prescription and over-the-counter drugs
Simple Relaxation Therapy: Use of techniques to encourage and elicit relaxation for the purpose of decreasing undesirable signs and symptoms such as pain, muscle tension, or anxiety

NURSING PRIORITY NO. 1 To assess etiology/precipitating factors:

- Identify contributing factors (e.g., musculoskeletal trauma with lasting effects, chronic pancreatitis, cancers, osteoporosis, peripheral neuropathies from conditions such as diabetes or AIDS, fibromyalgia, overuse syndromes such as tendonitis, mechanical low back pain, spinal stenosis, amputation, urological disorders, ulcer disease, endometriosis, cardiovascular disease, poor circulation, arthritis, recurrent migraines, bipolar disorders, depression, personality disorders, etc.). *These conditions can cause/exacerbate pain that persists for longer than 6 months.*[2,13]
- Assist in diagnostic testing, including physical, neurological, psychological evaluation (e.g., Minnesota Multiphasic Personality Inventory [MMPI], pain inventory, psychological interview). *Chronic pain syndrome (CPS) is a common problem that presents a major challenge to healthcare providers because of its complex history, often unclear etiology, and poor response to therapy. The pathophysiology is multifactorial, and some believe that CPS is a learned behavioral syndrome that begins with a noxious stimulus causing pain that is then somehow reinforced internally or externally.*[2]
- Evaluate emotional/physical components of individual situation. *Individuals with certain psychological syndromes (e.g., major depression, somatization disorder, hypochondriasis) are prone to develop CPS. Many painful conditions cause or exacerbate emotional responses (e.g., depression, withdrawal, agitation, anger) that worsen over time. Persistent long-term pain (and/or pain medications) can unconsciously be used to avoid unpleasant situations or to obtain relief from emotions or responsibilities (e.g., guilt, anger; fear of work, sex, or relationships).*[2]
- Note client's locus of control (internal/external). *Individuals with external locus of control may take little or no responsibility for pain management.*
- Determine relevant cultural factors affecting pain response. *Pain is accepted and expressed in different ways (e.g., moaning aloud or enduring in stoic silence); some may magnify symptoms to convince others of reality of pain, or believe that suffering in silence helps atone for past wrongdoing.*[3]
- Note gender and age of client. *There may be differences between women and men as to how they perceive and/or respond to pain. Pain in children, ethnic minorities, or cognitively*

impaired persons is often underestimated and undertreated.[4] *While the prevalence of chronically painful conditions (e.g., arthritis) and illnesses (e.g., cancers) is common in the elderly, they may be reluctant to report pain.*[5,6]

• Evaluate current and past analgesic/narcotic drug use and nonprescription drug use (including alcohol). *Provides clues to options to try or avoid, identifies need for changes in medication regimen, as well as possible need for detoxification program.*

NURSING PRIORITY NO. 2 To determine client response to chronic pain situation:

• Evaluate pain behavior, noting past and current pain experience, using pain rating scale or pain diary. *Pain behaviors can include the same ones present in acute pain (e.g., crying, grimacing, withdrawal, narrowed focus), but may also include other behaviors (e.g., dramatization of complaints, depression, drug misuse). Pain complaints may be exaggerated, because of client's perception that pain is not believed, or because client believes caregivers are discounting reports of pain.*[12]

• Provide comprehensive assessment of pain problem, noting its duration, who has been consulted, and what therapies (including alternative/complementary) have been used. *The pathophysiology of chronic pain is multifactorial. If the condition causing the persistent pain is physiological and noncurable (e.g., terminal cancer), all diagnostics and treatments may have been exhausted, and pain management becomes the primary goal. If medical treatments are ongoing for painful conditions (e.g., spinal stenosis, pancreatitis, endometriosis, arthritis), consultations with specialists may be helpful in finding curative or palliative treatments. If pain is present without a clear etiology or continues unabated, complex rehabilitation techniques may be required, incorporating physical, occupational, psychological, and recreational therapies.*[1,2]

• Note lifestyle effects of pain. *Major effects of chronic pain on the client's life can include depressed mood, fatigue, weight loss or gain, sleep disturbances, reduced activity and libido, excessive use of drugs and alcohol, dependent behavior, and disability seemingly out of proportion to impairment.*[2,6]

• Assess degree of personal maladjustment of the client such as isolationism, anger, irritability, loss of work time/employment/school. *Chronic pain reduces client's coping abilities and psychological well-being, often resulting in problems with relationships and life functioning.*[12]

• Determine issues of secondary gain for the client/SO(s) (e.g., financial/insurance compensation pending, marital/family concern, school or work issues), *which may be present if there is marked discrepancy between claimed distress and objective findings, or there is a lack of cooperation during evaluation and in complying with prescribed treatment.*[7]

• Note codependent components, enabling behaviors of caregivers/family members *that support continuation of the status quo and may interfere with progress in pain management/resolution of situation.*

• Note availability/use of personal and community resources. *Client/SO may need many things (e.g., equipment, financial resources, vocational training, respite services, or placement in rehabilitation facility) in order to manage painful conditions and/or concerns or difficulties associated with condition.*[12]

• Make home visit when indicated, observing such factors as client's safety, equipment, adequate lighting, or family interactions *to note impact of home environment on the client and to determine changes that might be useful in improving client's life (e.g., grab bars in bathrooms and hallways, wider doors, ramps, assistance with activities of daily living, housekeeping, yard work).*

• Acknowledge and assess pain matter-of-factly, avoiding undue expressions of concern, as well as expressions of disbelief about client's suffering. *Conveying an attitude of empathic understanding of client's disabling distress can have a beneficial impact on client's perception of health.*[8]

Cultural Collaborative Community/Home Care Diagnostic Studies Pediatric/Geriatric/Lifespan Medications

NURSING PRIORITY NO. 3 To assist client to deal with pain:

- Encourage participation in multidisciplinary pain management plan. *Comprehensive team may include physical medicine specialist; physical, occupational, recreational, and vocational therapists; and emotional/behavioral therapists to address complex issues of unresolved pain issues, to set goals for pain relief, and to develop an individualized treatment and evaluation plan. Treatments could involve extended-relief oral pain medications or dermal patches; nerve blocking injections, implanted pump; massage and other hands-on therapies, as well as counseling and home exercise programs.*[12,13]

- Discuss pain management goals/review client expectations versus reality, *because it may be that while pain cannot be completely resolved, it can be significantly lessened or managed, to the degree that client can participate in desired/needed life activities, improving quality of life.*[12,13]

- Discuss the physiological dynamics of tension/anxiety and how this affects pain.

- Administer/encourage client use of analgesics, as indicated. *Different medications or combinations of drugs may be used such as opioids/narcotics, nonopioids (e.g., acetaminophen, Cox-2 inhibitors, and NSAIDs) and adjuvant medications (e.g., muscle relaxants, anticonvulsants, antidepressants) to manage persistent pain so that client may find relief and increase level of function.*[1,2,13]

- Provide consistent and sufficient medication for pain relief, especially in individuals who tend to be undermedicated (e.g., elderly, cognitively impaired, person with lifelong pain, those with terminal cancer). *Medications may need to be administered regularly (not just as needed), doses titrated either up or down, and dose maximized to optimize pain relief while managing side effects.*

- Recommend/employ nonpharmacological interventions, methods of pain control (e.g., heat/cold applications, progressive muscle relaxation, biofeedback, deep breathing, meditation, visualization/guided imagery, posture correction and muscle strengthening exercises, water therapy, electrical stimulation, massage/Therapeutic Touch [TT]) *to obtain comfort, improve healing, and decrease dependency on analgesics.*[12,14]

- Address medication misuse with client/SO and refer for appropriate counseling/interventions *when addiction is known or suspected to be interfering with client's well-being. Most people (if they don't already have a substance [drug or alcohol] abuse problem), don't become addicted to pain medications, even when used on a long-term basis. These individuals will take the pain medications in order to go about the business of their lives. Addicts may lie about their pain levels and about their activities in order to obtain pain medications or progressively higher doses of medications; and require specialized evaluation and interventions.*[1,2]

- Assist family in developing a program of coping strategies (e.g., staying active even when modified activities are required, living a healthy lifestyle. *Positive reinforcement, encouraging client to use own control can aid in focusing energies on more productive activities.*[15]

- Encourage limiting attention to pain behaviors, when appropriate (e.g., discussing pain for only a specified time; or acknowledging "I'm sorry your pain returned today, but you need to go to school"; or actively practicing relaxation or coping skills). *Reduces focus on pain, especially if client is highly dependent on pain for secondary gain issues or is addicted to medications.*[9]

- Encourage client to use positive affirmations: "I am healing." "I am relaxed." "I love this life." Have client be aware of internal-external dialogue. Say "cancel" when negative thoughts develop. *Negative thinking can exacerbate feelings of hopelessness, and replacing those thoughts with positive ones can be helpful to pain management.*[12]

- Encourage right-brain stimulation with activities such as love, laughter, and music. *These actions can release endorphins, enhancing sense of well-being.*[12]

chronic PAIN

- 🏠 • Encourage use of subliminal tapes *to bypass logical part of the brain by reinforcing: "I am becoming a more relaxed person." "It is all right for me to relax."*
- 💊 • Use tranquilizers, narcotics, and analgesics sparingly. *These drugs are physically and psychologically addicting and promote sleep disturbances, especially interference with deep REM—rapid eye movement—sleep. Client may need to be detoxified if many medications are currently used.*
- 🏠 • Be alert to changes in pain *that may indicate a new physical problem/developing complication.*

NURSING PRIORITY NO. 4 To promote wellness (Teaching/Discharge Considerations):

- • Provide anticipatory guidance to client with condition in which pain is common and educate about when, where, and how to seek intervention/treatments.
- ∞ • Discuss potential for developmental delays in child with chronic pain. Identify current level of function and review appropriate expectations for individual child.
- 💊 • Instruct client/SO in medication administration, including use of PCA pumps, as indicated. Review safe use of analgesics, including side effects requiring home management (e.g., constipation) or adverse effects requiring medical intervention (e.g., possible drug reactions). *Appropriate instruction in home management increases the accuracy and safety of medication administration.*[12]
- 🏠 • Encourage and assist family member/SO(s) to learn home-care interventions. *Massage and other nonpharmacological pain management techniques benefit the client through reduction of pain level and sense that client is not alone/has support of SO.*
- 🌐 • Incorporate desired folk healthcare practices and beliefs into regimen whenever possible. *Has been shown to increase compliance with pain management treatment plan.*[11]
- 💊 • Identify and discuss potential hazards of unproved or nonmedical therapies/remedies.
- 🏠 • Assist client and SO(s) to learn how to heal *by developing sense of internal control, by being responsible for own treatment, and by obtaining the information and tools to accomplish this.*
- 🏠 • Recommend that client and SO(s) take time for themselves. *Provides opportunity to reenergize and refocus on living/tasks at hand.*
- 🏠 • Address client's preferences and wishes for incurable pain or end-of-life pain management via advance directives *in order to assist family/SO in attending to client's needs.*[10]
- 🏠 • Identify community support groups/resources to meet individual needs (e.g., yard care, home maintenance, transportation). *Proper use of resources may reduce negative pattern of "overdoing" heavy activities, then spending several days in bed recuperating.*
- ⊗ • Refer for counseling (e.g., individual/family, marital therapy, Parent Effectiveness classes, etc.) as needed. *Presence of chronic pain affects all relationship/family dynamics.*[12]
- • Refer to NDs, compromised family Coping, ineffective Coping.

DOCUMENTATION FOCUS

Assessment/Reassessment

- • Individual findings, including duration of problem/specific contributing factors, previously/currently used interventions.
- • Perception of pain, effects on lifestyle, and expectations of therapeutic regimen.
- • Locus of control and cultural beliefs affecting response to pain.
- • Family's/SO's response to client, and support for change.
- • Availability/use of resources.

Planning

- • Plan of care and who is involved in planning.
- • Teaching plan.

Implementation/Evaluation

- Responses to interventions/teaching and actions performed.
- Attainment/progress toward desired outcome(s).
- Modifications to plan of care.

Discharge Planning

- Long-term needs and who is responsible for actions to be taken.
- Specific referrals made.

References

1. Farkas, H. (2002). Chronic pain. Accessed December 2003 at www.emedicine.com.
2. Singh, M. K., Patel, J., Gallagher, R. M. (2002, update 2005). Chronic pain syndrome. Accessed July 2007 at www.emedicine.com/pmr/topic32.htm.
3. Purnell, L. D., Paulanka, B. J. (1998). *Transcultural Health Care: A Culturally Competent Approach.* Philadelphia: F. A. Davis, p. 44.
4. Young, D. (1999). Acute pain management. Iowa City, IA: University of Iowa Gerontological Nursing Interventions Research Center. Research Dissemination Core.
5. McGuire, L. (1999). Pain management in older adults. In Stanley, M., Beare, P. G. *Gerontological Nursing: A Health Promotion/Prevention Approach.* 2d ed. Philadelphia: F. A. Davis.
6. The management of persistent pain in older persons. (2002). *J Am Geriatr Soc*, 50(6 Suppl), S205–S224. Accessed July 2007 at www.guideline.gov.
7. Bienenfeld, D. (2003, update 2005). Malingering. Accessed July 2007 at www.emedicine.com.
8. Smith, G. R., Rost, K., Kashner, T. M. (1995). A trial of the effect of a standardized psychiatric consultation on health outcomes and costs in somatizing patients. *Arch Gen Psychiatry*, 52(3), 238–243.
9. Spratt, E. G., DeMaso, D. (2002). Somatoform disorder: Somatization. Available at www. emedicine.com. Accessed January 2004.
10. American Medical Directors Association (AMDA). (1999, update 2003). Chronic pain management in the long-term care setting. Accessed July 2007. at www.guideline.gov.
11. Juarez, G., Ferrell, B., Borneman, T. (1998). Influence of culture on cancer pain management in Hispanic clients. *Cancer Practice*, 6(5), 262–269.
12. McCaffrey, M., Pasero, C. (1999). *Pain: Clinical Manual.* St. Louis, MO: Mosby.
13. D'Arcy, Y. (2005). Conquering PAIN: Have you tried these new techniques? *Nursing2005*, 35(3), 36–41.
14. Lark, S. (2005). The 21-day arthritis and pain miracle. Article for the Lark Letter: A Woman's Guide to Optimal Health and Balance, Special Report.
15. Warms, C. A., Marshal, J. M., Hoffman, A. J., et al. (2006). There are a few things you did not ask about my pain: Writing in the margins of a survey questionaire. *Rehabilitation Nursing*, 30(6), 248–256.

readiness for enhanced Parenting

Definition: A pattern of providing an environment for children or other dependent person(s) that is sufficient to nurture growth and development and can be strengthened

RELATED FACTORS
To be developed by nurse researchers and submitted to NANDA

DEFINING CHARACTERISTICS

Subjective
Expresses willingness to enhance parenting
Children or other dependent person(s) express(es) satisfaction with home environment

> **Objective**
> Emotional support of children[/dependent person(s)]; evidence of attachment
> Needs of children[/dependent person(s)] are met (e.g., physical and emotional)
> Exhibits realistic expectations of children [/dependent person(s)]

Sample Clinical Applications: As a health-seeking behavior, the client/family may be healthy or this diagnosis can be associated with any clinical condition

DESIRED OUTCOMES/EVALUATION CRITERIA
Sample NOC linkages:
Parenting Performance: Parental actions to provide a child with a nurturing and constructive physical, emotional, and social environment
Knowledge: Parenting: Extent of understanding conveyed about provision of a nurturing and constructive environment for a child from 1 year through 17 years of age
Parenting: Psychosocial Safety: Parental actions to protect a child from social contacts that might cause harm or injury

Client Will (Include Specific Time Frame)

- Verbalize realistic information and expectations of parenting role.
- Identify own strengths, individual needs, and methods/resources to meet them.
- Participate in activities to enhance parenting skills.
- Demonstrate improved parenting behaviors.

ACTIONS/INTERVENTIONS

Sample NIC linkages:
Parent Education: Childrearing Family: Assisting parents to understand and promote the physical, psychological, and social growth and development of their toddler, preschool, or school-age child/children
Parent Education: Infant: Instruction on nurturing and physical care needed during the first year of life
Parenting Promotion: Providing parenting information, support, and coordination of comprehensive services to high-risk families

NURSING PRIORITY NO. 1 To determine need/motivation for improvement:

- Ascertain motivation/expectations for change. *Motivation to improve and high expectations can encourage client to make changes that will improve skills. However, unrealistic expectations may hamper efforts.*
- Note family constellation: two-parent, single, extended family, or child living with other relative, such as grandparent/sibling; or relationship of dependent person (e.g., foster family). *Understanding makeup of the family provides information about needs to assist them in improving their family connections.*[1]
- Determine developmental stage of the family (e.g., new child, adolescent, child leaving/returning home, retirement). *These maturational crises bring changes in the family that can provide opportunity for enhancing parenting skills and improving family interactions.*[1]
- Assess family relationships and identify needs of individual members, noting any special concerns that exist, such as birth defects, illness, hyperactivity. *The family is a system, and*

Cultural   Collaborative   Community/Home Care   Diagnostic Studies   Pediatric/Geriatric/Lifespan   Medications

when members make decisions to improve parenting skills, the changes affect all parts of the system. Identifying needs, special situations, and relationships can help to develop plans to bring about effective change.[1]

 • Assess parenting skill level, taking into account the individual's intellectual, emotional, and physical strengths and weaknesses. *Identifies areas of need for education, skill training, and information on which to base plan for enhancing parenting skills.*[2,4]

• Observe attachment behaviors between parent(s) and child(ren), recognizing cultural background, which may influence expected behaviors. *Behaviors such as eye-to-eye contact, use of enface position, talking to infant in high-pitched voice are indicative of attachment behaviors in American culture but may not be appropriate in another culture. Failure to bond is thought to affect subsequent parent-child interactions.*[3,4]

• Determine presence/effectiveness of support systems, role models, extended family, and community resources available to the parent(s). *Parents desiring to enhance abilities and improve family life can benefit by role models that help them strengthen own style of parenting.*[2,3]

• Note cultural/religious influences on parenting, expectations of self/child, sense of success or failure. *Expectations may vary with different cultures, such as Arab Americans hold children to be sacred but childrearing is based on negative rather than positive reinforcements and parents are stricter with girls than boys. These beliefs may interfere with ability to improve parenting skills when there is conflict between the two.*[3,4]

NURSING PRIORITY NO. 2 To foster development of parenting skills:

• Create an environment in which relationships can be strengthened and needs of each individual family member can be met. *A safe environment in which individuals can freely express their thoughts and feelings optimizes learning and positive interactions among family members enhancing relationships.*[2,5]

• Make time for listening to concerns of the parent(s). *Promotes sense of importance and of being heard and identifies accurate information regarding needs of the family for enhancing relationships.*[2]

• Encourage expression of feelings, such as frustration, anger while setting limits on unacceptable behaviors. *Identification of feelings promotes understanding of self and enhances connections with others in the family. Unacceptable behaviors result in feelings of anger and diminished self-esteem and can lead to problems in the family relationships.*[3]

• Emphasize parenting functions rather than mothering/fathering skills. *By virtue of gender, each person brings something to the parenting role; however, nurturing tasks can be done by both parents, enhancing family relationships.*[5]

• Encourage attendance at skill classes, such as Parent Effectiveness Training. *Assists in developing communication skills of Active-listening, I-messages, and problem-solving techniques to improve family relationships and promote a win-win environment.*[2]

NURSING PRIORITY NO. 3 To promote optimum parenting skills/wellness:

• Involve all members of the family in learning. *The family system benefits from all members participating in learning new skills to enhance family relationships.*[1]

• Encourage parents to identify positive outlets for meeting their own needs. *Activities such as going out for dinner/dating, making time for their own interests and each other promotes general well-being, enhances family relationships, and improves family functioning.*[2]

• Provide information as indicated, including time management, stress-reduction techniques. *Learning about positive parenting skills, understanding growth and developmental expectations, and ways to reduce stress and anxiety promotes individual's ability to deal with problems that may arise in the course of family relationships.*[1,6]

- Discuss current "family rules," identifying areas of needed change. *Rules may be imposed by adults, rather than through a democratic process, involving all family members, leading to conflict and angry confrontations. Setting positive family rules with all family members participating can promote an effective, functional family.*[2,6]
- Discuss need for long-term planning and ways in which family can maintain desired positive relationships. *Each stage of life brings its own challenges, and understanding and preparing for each stage enables family members to move through them in positive ways, promoting family unity and resolving inevitable conflicts with win-win solutions.*[6]

DOCUMENTATION FOCUS

Assessment/Reassessment

- Individual findings, including parenting skill level, parenting expectations, family makeup, and developmental stages.
- Availability/use of support systems and community resources.
- Motivation and expectations for change.

Planning

- Plan for enhancement, who is involved in planning.

Implementation/Evaluation

- Family members' responses to interventions/teaching and actions performed.
- Attainment/progress toward desired outcome(s).
- Modifications to plan.

Discharge Planning

- Long-range needs and who is responsible for actions to be taken.
- Modification to plan.

References

1. Townsend, M. C. (2006). *Psychiatric Mental Health Nursing Concepts of Care*. 5th ed. Philadelphia: F. A. Davis.
2. Gordon, T. (2000). *Parent Effectiveness Training* (updated). New York: Three Rivers Press.
3. Doenges, M. E., Townsend, M. C., Moorhouse, M. F. (1998). *Psychiatric Care Plans Guidelines for Individualizing Care*. 3d ed. Philadelphia: F. A. Davis.
4. Lipson, J. G., Dibble, S. L., Minarik, P. A. (1999). *Culture & Nursing Care: A Pocket Guide*. San Francisco: UCSF Nursing Press.
5. Doenges, M. E., Moorhouse, M. F., Geissler-Murr, A. C. (2007). *Nurses' Pocket Guide, Diagnoses, Interventions, and Rationales*. 11th ed. Philadelphia: F. A. Davis.
6. Gordon, T. (1989). *Teaching Children Self-Discipline, At Home and At School*. New York: Random House.

risk for Poisoning

Definition: Accentuated risk of accidental exposure to, or ingestion of, drugs or dangerous products in doses sufficient to cause poisoning [or the adverse effects of prescribed medication/drug use]

Cultural   Collaborative   Community/Home Care   Diagnostic Studies   Pediatric/Geriatric/Lifespan   Medications

RISK FACTORS

Internal
Reduced vision
Lack of safety/drug education
Lack of proper precaution; [unsafe habits, disregard for safety measures, lack of
    supervision]
Verbalization that occupational setting is without adequate safeguards
Cognitive/emotional difficulties
[Age (e.g., young child, elderly person)]
[Chronic disease state, disability]
[Cultural or religious beliefs/practices]

External
Large supplies of drugs in house
Medicines stored in unlocked cabinets accessible to children/confused individuals
Availability of illicit drugs potentially contaminated by poisonous additives
Dangerous products placed within reach of children/confused individuals
[Therapeutic margin of safety of specific drugs (e.g., therapeutic versus toxic level, half-
    life, method of uptake and degradation in body, adequacy of organ function)]
[Use of multiple herbal supplements or megadosing]
NOTE: A risk diagnosis is not evidenced by signs and symptoms, as the problem has not
    occurred; rather, nursing interventions are directed at prevention.

Sample Clinical Applications: Substance abuse, dementia, cataracts/glaucoma, hepatitis,
    cirrhosis, renal failure, depression, suicidal ideation, developmental delay

DESIRED OUTCOMES/EVALUATION CRITERIA
Sample NOC linkages:
Risk Control: Drug Use: Personal actions to prevent, eliminate, or reduce drug use that
    poses a threat to health
Knowledge: Medication: Extent of understanding conveyed about the safe use of medication
Safe Home Environment: Physical arrangements to minimize environmental factors that
    might cause physical harm or injury in the home

Client/SO Will (Include Specific Time Frame)
- Verbalize understanding of dangers of poisoning.
- Identify hazards that could lead to accidental poisoning.
- Correct external hazards as identified.
- Demonstrate necessary actions/lifestyle changes to promote safe environment.

Refer to NDs Contamination and risk for Contamination for additional interventions related
    to poisoning associated with environmental contaminants.

ACTIONS/INTERVENTIONS

Sample NIC linkages:
Medication Management: Facilitation of safe and effective use of prescription and
    over-the-counter drugs

Environmental Management: Safety: Manipulation of the patient's surroundings for therapeutic benefit

Surveillance: Safety: Purposeful and ongoing collection and analysis of information about the patient and the environment for use in promoting and maintaining patient safety

NURSING PRIORITY NO. 1   To assess causative/contributing factors:

- Identify internal/external risk factors in client's environment (e.g., including infants/ young or frail elderly; confused or chronically ill person on multiple medications; person with suidical ideation; illicit drug use/dealing [e.g., marijuana, cocaine, heroin]; drug manufacture in home [e.g., methamphetamines]; access/exposure to dangerous chemicals).

∞ • Note age and cognitive status of client and care providers *to identify individuals who could be at higher risk for accidental poisoning. Babies, toddlers, and preschoolers are at risk because they are curious, like to put things into their mouths, and aren't aware of what's safe to eat. While school-age child can recognize danger and is at lower risk of unintentional poisoning, child is at risk for inadvertent overdose when taking medications without adequate supervision. The adolescent is at higher risk for experimentation due to natural inclination to take risks, peer pressure, and easy access to drugs and suicide attempts (with overdose of medications, and/or from illicit drug overdose/adverse reactions or alcohol toxicity).*[2,3,12,13] *Elderly persons are at risk because of the higher number of prescription and OTC medications they consume (polypharmacy) and because of visual and cognitive impairments, which can cause them to forget what medications have been consumed and in what amounts they were taken. Elderly persons are also likely to share medications. In addition, the presence of nutritional deficits and renal or hepatic degeneration can reduce ability to detoxify drugs.*[4,5]

- Assess mood, coping abilities, personality styles (e.g., temperament, impulsive behavior, level of self-esteem) *that may result in carelessness/increased risk-taking without consideration of consequences, or suicidal actions.* (Refer to ND risk for Suicide.)

- Determine client's allergies to medications/foods *in order to avoid exposure to substances causing potentially lethal reaction.*

- Ascertain client's knowledge and use of medications. *Some individuals (especially elderly) believe that medication offers the solution to every health problem, a belief bolstered by frequent television, radio, and written advertising promising relief from a multitude of conditions from colds to sexual vitality. This often leads to multiple drug use (polypharmacy) and contributes to potential for overdose, adverse reactions (e.g., digoxin toxicity), and drug interactions.*[6,12]

- Determine specific drug hazards:

  Use of prescription, OTC medications, and culturally based home remedies. *These have potential for intentional and accidental overdose, as well as dangerous interactions. Drugs that are therapeutic in small doses may be deadly when taken in excess (e.g., beta-blockers, warfarin, digoxin). One of the most common problems is inadvertent overdosage of acetaminophen (Tylenol), either by increased dosing or by taking it with a combination product also containing acetaminophen. In children, the most serious accidental poisonings occur with iron, methadone, and tricyclic antidepressants.*[1,5,7,14]

  Availability/regular use of vitamins and mineral and herbal supplements. *Vitamins (especially A and D) are toxic in large doses, and iron is especially harmful to children.*[8,14] *Herbal drugs can be a source of poisoning (usually when taken chronically), due to toxicity of individual ingredients or from contaminants (e.g., mercury, lead, and arsenic).*[1]

  Abuse of alcohol/other drugs (e.g., cocaine, methamphetamine, LSD, methadone). *These substances have potential for adverse reactions, cummulative affects with other substances, and risk for intentional and accidental overdose. Note: As little as 1 ounce of alcohol or a single dose of many drugs of abuse can cause serious injury/death in a small child.*[8,14]

- Identify environmental hazards:
  Storage of household chemicals (e.g., oven, toilet bowl, or drain cleaners; dishwasher products, bleach, hydrogen peroxide, flouride preparations, essential oils, furniture polish, lighter fluid, lamp oil, kerosene, paints, turpentine, rust remover, lubricant oils, bug sprays/powders, fertilizers) *are readily available toxins in various forms that are often improperly stored.*[1,7,8]
  Review employment/work site safety *for exposure to chemicals, including vapors/fumes.*
  Refer to ND risk for Contamination for environmental issues.
- Review results of laboratory tests/toxicology screening, as indicated. *Guides treatment when overdose or accidental poisoning is known or suspected.*

NURSING PRIORITY NO. 2 To assist in correcting factors that can lead to accidental poisoning:

- Discuss medication safety with client/SO according to individual needs:
  Prevent accidental ingestion: [4–10,14,18]
  Stress importance of supervising infant/child, frail elderly, or individuals with cognitive limitations.
  Keep medicines and vitamins out of sight/reach of children or cognitively impaired persons.
  Use child-resistant/tamper-resistant caps and locked medication cabinets.
  Recap medication containers immediately after obtaining current dosage. *Note: Many accidental poisonings occur when parent/caregiver steps away for a moment and child gets into product that was left out.*
  Code medicines for the visually impaired.
  Tell client to turn on light and put on glasses (if visually impaired) before taking or giving medications.
  Administer children's medications as drugs, not candy, *to prevent confusion.*
  Emphasize environmental safety regarding medications for all situations in which young child may be exposed (e.g., grandparents home, day care, preschool, etc.).[11]
  Discuss vitamin use (especially those containing iron) *that can be poisonous to children if taken in large doses.*[11–13]
  Prevent duplication/possible overdose:[4–10]
  Review analgesic safety (e.g., acetaminophen is an ingredient in many OTC medications, and unintentional overdose can occur).[15,17]
  Keep updated list of all medications (prescription, OTC, herbals, supplements) and review with healthcare providers when medications are changed, new ones added, or new healthcare providers are consulted.
  Keep prescription medication in original bottle with label. Do not mix with other medication/place in unmarked containers.
  Have responsible SO(s)/home health nurse supervise medication regimen/prepare medications for the cognitively or visually impaired, or obtain prefilled med boxes from pharmacy.
  Take prescription medications and OTC drugs as prescribed on label.
  Do not adjust medication dosage.
  Retain and read safety information that accompanies prescriptions about expected effects, nuisance side effects, reportable/adverse affects, and how to manage forgotten dose.
  Prevent taking medications that interact with one another or OTC/herbals/other supplements in an undesired or dangerous manner:[4–10]
  Keep list of/and reveal medication allergies, including type of reaction to healthcare providers/pharmacist.

Wear medical alert bracelet/necklace, as appropriate.

Do not take outdated/expired medications. Do not save partial prescriptions to use another time.

Encourage discarding outdated/unused drug safely (disposing in hazardous waste collection areas, not down drain/toilet).

Do not take medications prescribed for another person.

Avoid mixing alcohol with medications *(potentiates effects of many drugs)*.

Coordinate care when multiple healthcare providers are involved *to limit number of prescriptions/dosage levels*.

NURSING PRIORITY NO. 3 To promote wellness (Teaching/Discharge Considerations):

- Discuss general poison-prevention measures:[4–10]

Encourage parent/caregiver to place safety stickers on dangerous products (drugs/chemicals) *to warn children of harmful contents*.

Teach children about hazards of poisonous substances and to "ask first" before eating or drinking anything.

Review drug side effects/potential interactions and possibilities of misuse or overdosing (as with vitamin megadosing, etc.).[12]

Discuss issues regarding drug use in home (e.g., alcohol, marijuana, heroin) *to provide opportunity to address potential for client's/SO's accidental overdose or accidental ingestion by children when drugs/drug paraphernalia are in the home*.[13]

- Provide list of emergency numbers (i.e., local/national poison control numbers, physician office) to be placed by telephone *for use if poisoning occurs*.

- Instruct caregiver in event of poisoning, have product container on hand when contacting emergency provider.

- Discuss use of ipecac syrup in home. *The use of ipecac is controversial, as it may delay appropriate medical treatment (e.g., reduce the effectiveness of activated charcoal/oral antidotes) or be used inappropriately with adverse effects. Therefore, use in the home without direct advisement from poison control professionals is not recommended.*[16,17]

- Encourage client to obtain regular screening tests at prescribed intervals (e.g., prothrombin time/INR for Coumadin; drug levels for dilantin, digoxin; liver function studies when lipid-lowering agents [statins] are prescribed; or renal/thyroid function and serum glucose levels for antimanics [lithium] use) *to ascertain that circulating blood levels are within therapeutic range and absence of adverse effects*.

- Ask healthcare provider/pharmacist about any considered medications if pregnant, nursing, or planning to become pregnant, *as some drugs are dangerous to fetus or nursing infant*.

- Refer substance abuser to detoxification programs, inpatient/outpatient rehabilitation, counseling, support groups, and psychotherapy.

- Encourage participation in community awareness and education programs (e.g., CPR/first-aid class, home and workplace safety, hazardous materials disposal, access emergency medical personnel) *to assist individuals to identify and correct risk factors in environment, be prepared for emergency situation*.

DOCUMENTATION FOCUS

Assessment/Reassessment

- Identified risk factors noting internal/external concerns.

Planning

- Plan of care and who is involved in the planning.
- Teaching plan.

Implementation/Evaluation

- Response to interventions/teaching and actions performed.
- Attainment/progress toward desired outcome(s).
- Modification to plan of care.

Discharge Planning

- Long-term needs and who is responsible for actions to be taken.
- Specific referrals made.

References

1. Bates, N. (2000). What's your poison? Accessed July 2007 at www.dotpharmacy.com/uppoison.html.
2. Poisoning risk factors. (1997). Information sheet from Centers for Disease Control and Prevention. "What Affects a Child's Risk of Poisoning?" Adapted from recommendations in Injury Prevention and Injury Control for Children and Youth. Atlanta, GA: Committee on Injury and Poison Prevention of the American Academy of Pediatrics.
3. Barela, T. (2001). What affects a child's risk of poisoning? *TORCH* magazine. Accessed September 2003 at www.randolph.af.mil/se2/torch.
4. Stoehr, G. P. (1999). Pharmacology and older adults: The problem of polypharmacy. In Stanley, M., Beare, P. G. (eds). *Gerontological Nursing: A Health Promotion/Protection Approach.* 2d ed. Philadelphia: F. A. Davis, pp. 66–73.
5. Older adults are at risk for poisoning exposures. (2002). News release from Illinois Poison Control Center. Available at www.mchc.org. Accessed September 2003.
6. Nathan, M. S. (2001, update 2005). Poison proofing your home. Accessed July 2007 at www.emedicinehealth.com.
7. Cohen, J. S. (2001, update 2005). Poisoning. Accessed July 2007 at www.emedicinehealth.com.
8. Is my child at risk for poisoning during the holidays? (2003). Information sheet. Available at www.phoenixchildrens.com. Accessed September 2003.
9. Keep your children safe: Prevent accidental poisoning. Accessed July 2007 at www.cnn.com/HEALTH/library/HQ/01263.html.
10. American Society of Health-System Pharmacists Fact Sheet. (No date listed). Medicatons and you. Available at www.safemedication.com.
11. Children's Hospital Boston Fact sheet. (No date listed). Poisons. Available at www.childrenshospital.org/az/Site868.
12. Hingley, A. T. (2007). Preventing childhood poisoning. Retrieved April 2007 at www.kidsource.com/kidsource/content4/child.poison.fda.html.
13. Morris-Kukoski, C. L., Egland, A. G. (2006). Toxicity, deadly in a single dose. Article for Emedicine Web site. Accessed July 2007 at www.emedicine.com/ped/topic2726.htm.
14. National Women's Health Resource Center Fact Sheet. (2005). Medication safety. Available at www.healthywomen.org.
15. Smith, D. H. (2007). Managing acute acetaminophen toxicity. *Nursing2007,* 37(1), 58–63.
16. Manoguerra, A. S., Cobaugh, D. J. (2005). Guideline on the use of ipecac syrup in the out-of-hospital management of ingested poisons. *Clin Toxicol,* 43(1), 1–10.
17. American Academy of Clinical Toxicology: Position statement—Ipecac syrup. Retrieved April 2007 at www.clintox.org/Pos_Statements/Ipecac.html.
18. ND: Poisoning, risk for. In Doenges, M. E., Moorhouse, M. F., Geissler, Murr, A. C. (2004). *Nurse's Pocket Guide: Diagnoses, Interventions, and Rationales.* 9th ed. Philadelphia: F. A. Davis.

Post-Trauma Syndrome [specify stage]

Definition: Sustained maladaptive response to a traumatic, overwhelming event

POST-TRAUMA SYNDROME [specify stage]

Events outside the range of usual human experience
Serious threat to self/loved ones
Serious injury to self/loved ones; serious accidents (e.g., industrial, motor vehicle)
Abuse (physical and psychosocial); criminal victimization; rape
Witnessing mutilation/violent death; tragic occurrence involving multiple deaths
Disasters; sudden destruction of one's home/community; epidemics
Wars; being held prisoner of war; torture

DEFINING CHARACTERISTICS

Subjective
Intrusive thoughts/dreams; nightmares; flashbacks; [excessive verbalization of the
    traumatic event]
Palpitations; headaches [loss of interest in usual activities, loss of feeling of intimacy/
    sexuality]
Hopelessness; shame; guilt; [verbalization of survival guilt or guilt about behavior required
    for survival]
Anxiety; fear; grieving; depression
Reports of feeling numb
Gastric irritability; [change in appetite; sleep disturbance/insomnia; chronic fatigue/easy
    fatigability]
Difficulty in concentrating

Objective
Hypervigilance; exaggerated startle response; irritability; neurosensory irritability
Anger; rage; aggression
Avoidance; repression; alienation; denial; detachment; psychogenic amnesia
Altered mood states; [poor impulse control/explosiveness]; panic attacks; horror
Substance abuse; compulsive behavior
Enuresis (in children)
[Difficulty with interpersonal relationships; dependence on others; work/school failure]
[Stages:
Acute Subtype: Begins within 6 months and does not last longer than 6 months.
Chronic Subtype: Lasts more than 6 months.
Delayed Subtype: Period of latency of 6 months or more before onset of symptoms.]

Sample Clinical Applications: Traumatic injuries, physical/psychological abuse, dissociative disorder

DESIRED OUTCOMES/EVALUATION CRITERIA
Sample NOC linkages:
Fear Self-Control: Personal actions to eliminate or reduce disabling feelings of apprehension
    or uneasiness from an identifiable source
Abuse Protection: Protection of self or dependent others from abuse
Abuse Recovery: [specify Emotional or Physical]: Extent of healing of psychological/
    physical injuries due to abuse

Client Will (Include Specific Time Frame)

• Express own feelings/reactions, avoiding projection.

🌐 Cultural Collaborative 🏠 Community/Home Care Diagnostic Studies ∞ Pediatric/Geriatric/Lifespan Medications

- Verbalize a positive self-image.
- Report reduced anxiety/fear when memories occur.
- Demonstrate ability to deal with emotional reactions in an individually appropriate manner.
- Demonstrate appropriate changes in behavior/lifestyle (e.g., share experiences with others, seek/get support from SO[s] as needed, change in job/residence).
- Report absence of physical manifestations (such as pain, chronic fatigue).

Refer to ND Rape-Trauma Syndrome for additional outcomes when trauma is the result of rape.

ACTIONS/INTERVENTIONS

Sample NIC linkages:

Support System Enhancement: Facilitation of support to patient by family, friends, and community

Counseling: Use of an interactive helping process focusing on the needs, problems, or feelings of the patient and significant others to enhance or support coping, problem-solving, and interpersonal relationships

Anxiety Reduction: Minimizing apprehension, dread, foreboding, or uneasiness related to an unidentified source or anticipated danger

NURSING PRIORITY NO. 1 To assess causative factor(s) and individual reaction:

Acute
- Observe for/elicit information about physical or psychological injury and note associated stress-related symptoms (e.g., numbness, headache, tightness in chest, nausea, pounding heart). *Anxiety is viewed as a normal reaction to a realistic danger or threat, and noting these factors can identify the severity of the anxiety the client is experiencing in the circumstances.*[4]
- Identify such psychological responses as anger, shock, acute anxiety, confusion, denial. Note laughter, crying, calm or agitated, excited (hysterical) behavior; expressions of disbelief, guilt and/or self-blame, labile emotions. *Indicators of severe response to trauma that client has experienced and need for specific interventions.*[9]
- Assess client's knowledge of and anxiety related to the situation. Note ongoing threat to self (e.g., contact with perpetrator and/or associates) or perception of others as threatening. *Client may be aware but speak as though the incident is related to someone else. Flashbacks may occur with the individual reliving the incident/event.*[9]
- Note occupation (e.g., police, fire, rescue, emergency department staff, corrections officer, mental health worker, disaster responders, soldier or support personnel in combat zone, as well as family members). *These occupations carry a high risk for constantly being involved in traumatic events and the potential for exacerbation of stress response/block to recovery.*[1] *In addition, family members are also subjected to the same trauma, because they see the same events repeated on TV news channels/hear stories repeated by their loved one(s) who were directly involved.*
- Identify social aspects of trauma/incident (e.g., disfigurement, chronic conditions/permanent disabilities, loss of home or community) *that affect ability to return to normal involvement in activities/work.*[9]
- Ascertain ethnic background/cultural and religious perceptions and beliefs about the occurrence. *Client may believe occurrence is retribution from God or result of some indiscretion on his or her part; client may in some way also blame themselves for the incident/occurrence.*

Individual's view of how he or she is coping may be influenced by cultural background, religious beliefs, and family influence.[5,9]

🏠 • Determine degree of disorganization (e.g., task-oriented activity is not goal-directed, organized, or effective; individual is overwhelmed by emotion much of the time). *Presence of persistent frightening thoughts and memories, reliving the event, feeling emotionally numb and unable to be close to friends and family members, suffering from sleep and eating problems all interfere with ability to manage daily living, work, and relationships with others.*[9,14]

🏠 • Identify whether incident has reactivated preexisting or coexisting situations (physical/psychological). *Traumas or difficulties in client's life and how they were dealt with will affect how the client views the current trauma.*[7]

🏠 • Determine disruptions in relationships (e.g., family, friends, coworkers, SOs). *Support persons may not know how to deal with client/situation and may be oversolicitous or withdraw; either of these actions will be counterproductive to client's ability to cope with situation.*[9]

🏠 • Note withdrawn behavior, use of denial, and use of chemical substances or impulsive behaviors (e.g., chain-smoking, overeating). *Indicators of severity of anxiety and client's difficulty dealing with post-traumatic stress disorder (PTSD) and need for interventions to address these behaviors.*[9]

🏠 • Be aware of signs of increasing anxiety (e.g., silence, stuttering, inability to sit still). *Increasing anxiety may indicate risk for violence or need for medication or other measures to decrease anxiety and help client manage feelings.*[9]

🌐 • Note verbal/nonverbal expressions of guilt or self-blame when client has survived trauma in which others died. Validate congruency of observations with verbalizations. *Sense of own responsibility (blame) and guilt about not having done something to prevent incident or not having been "good enough" to deserve survival are strong beliefs, especially in individuals who are influenced by background, religious, and cultural factors.*[2]

🏠 • Assess signs/stage of grieving for self and others. *Identification and understanding of stages of grief assist with choice of interventions, planning of care, and movement toward resolution.*[2]

🏠 • Identify development of phobic reactions to ordinary articles (e.g., knives) and situations (e.g., walking in groups of people, strangers ringing doorbell). *These may trigger feelings from original trauma and need to be dealt with sensitively, accepting reality of feelings and stressing ability of client to deal with them.*[2]

Chronic (in addition to previous assessment)

🏠 • Evaluate continued somatic complaints. Investigate reports of new/changes in symptoms. *Reports of physical symptoms, such as gastric irritation, anorexia, insomnia, muscle tension, headache may accompany disorganization and need further evaluation and interventions.*[2]

🏠 • Note manifestations of chronic pain or pain symptoms in excess of degree of physical injury. *Psychological responses may magnify/exacerbate physical symptoms, indicating need for interventions to help client deal with pain.*[7]

🏠 • Be aware of signs of severe/prolonged depression; note presence of flashbacks, intrusive memories, nightmares, panic attacks, poor impulse control; and problems with memory/concentration, thoughts/perceptions, and conflict/agression/rage. *Symptoms are not uncommon following a trauma of such magnitude, although client may feel that he or she is "going crazy."*[4,13]

🏠 • Assess degree of dysfunctional coping (including substance use/abuse, suicidal ideation) and consequences. *Identifies needs/depth of interventions required. Individuals display different levels of dysfunctional behavior in response to stress, and often the choice of chemical substances/substance abuse is a way of deadening the psychic pain.*[2]

NURSING PRIORITY NO. 2 To assist client to deal with situation that exists:

Immediate post-incident

- Provide a calm, safe environment. *Promotes sense of trust and safety and can help client maintain control when anxiety is at a panic level.*[12]
- Assist with documentation for police report, as indicated, and stay with the client. *Developing accurate chain of evidence (maintaining sequencing and collection of evidence) and labeling each specimen and storing/packaging it properly provides important evidence for possibility of future prosecution.*[2]
- Listen to/investigate physical complaints. *Physical injuries may have occurred during incident, which may be masked by emotional reactions and limit client's ability to recognize them. These need to be identified and differentiated from anxiety symptoms so appropriate treatment may be instituted.*[2]
- Identify supportive persons (e.g., loved ones, spiritual advisor/pastor). *Having unconditional support from loving/caring others can help the client cope with the situation and move on to live more fully.*[2]
- Remain with client, listen as client recounts incident/concerns—possibly repeatedly. If client does not want to talk, accept silence. *Establishes trust, thus providing psychological support and allowing client opportunity to vent emotions.*[4]
- Provide nonthreatening, consistent environment in which client can talk freely about feelings, fear (including concerns about relationship with/response of SO), and experiences/sensations (e.g., loss of control, "near-death experience"). *Minimize stimuli, thereby reducing anxiety and calming individual, helping to break the cycle of anxiety/fear and encouraging them to express feelings and relive event.*[2]
- Help child to express feelings about event using techniques appropriate to developmental level (e.g., play for young child, stories/puppets for preschooler, peer group for adolescent). *Children are more likely to express in play what they may not be able to verbalize directly. Adolescents may benefit from such groups that help them gain knowledge, support, and a decreased sense of isolation and improved coping skills.*[3]
- Assist with practical realities (e.g., temporary housing, money, notifications of family members, or other needs). *Dealing with these issues is necessary and helps client remain connected to reality and maintain sense of control over daily living concerns.*[2]

Acute

- Allow the client to work through own kind of adjustment. If the client is withdrawn or unwilling to talk, do not force the issue. *Each person is an individual and has own ways of coping. Being there and allowing client to choose own path conveys sense of confidence in ability to deal with situation.*[10]
- Listen for expressions of fear of crowds or people. *May indicate continuing anxiety and difficulty reentering normal activities.*[9]
- Ascertain/monitor sleep pattern of children as well as adults. *Sleep disturbances/nightmares may develop, delaying resolution, impairing coping abilities, and interferring with return to desired lifstyle.*[7]
- Be aware of and assist client to use ego strengths in a positive way by acknowledging ability to handle what is happening. *Enhances self-concept and reduces sense of helplessness and powerlessness, thus enabling client to move on with life.*[3]
- Encourage client to learn stress-management techniques, such as deep breathing, meditation, relaxation, and exercise. *Reduces stress, enhancing coping skills and helping to resolve situation.*[11]
- Assist in dealing with practical concerns and effects of the incident, such as court appearances, altered relationships with SO(s), employment problems. *In the period immediately*

following the traumatic incident, individual is in a state of numbness and shock. Thinking becomes difficult, and assistance with practical matters will help manage necessary activities for the person to move through this time.[10]

- Identify employment, community resource groups. *Provides opportunity for ongoing support to deal with recurrent stressors as individual regroups/moves forward.*[12]
- Administer anti-anxiety or sedative/hypnotic medications with caution.

Chronic

- Continue listening to expressions of concern. *May have recurring symptoms, thus necessitating the need to continue talking about the incident.*[9]
- Permit free expression of feelings (may continue from the crisis phase). Do not rush client through expressions of feelings too quickly, and refrain from providing false reassurances. *Client may believe pain or anguish is misunderstood and may be depressed. Statements such as "You don't understand" or "You weren't there" are a defense—a way of pushing others away—and need to be responded to with empathy and concern.*[10]
- Encourage client to talk out experience when ready, expressing feelings of fear, anger, loss/grief. (Refer to NDs Grieving, complicated Grieving). *Client may need to repeat story over and over and needs to be accepted and assured that feelings are normal for the unusual event that has been experienced.*[9]
- Note whether feelings expressed appear congruent with events the client experienced. *Expressing feelings helps client recognize and identify them to enhance coping. Incongruency may indicate deeper conflict that can impede resolution.*[11]
- Encourage client to become aware and accepting of own feelings and reactions as being normal reactions in an abnormal situation. *There are no "bad" feelings, and awareness and acceptance enables client to deal with feelings once identified and move forward in recovery from traumatic event.*[6,14]
- Acknowledge reality of loss of self that existed before the incident. Assist client to move toward an acceptance of the potential for growth that exists within client. *Recognition that individual can never go back to being the person he or she was before the incident allows progress toward life as a different person.*[11]
- Continue to allow client to progress at own pace. *Taking own time to talk about what has happened, allowing feelings to be fully expressed, aids in the healing process. If rushed, client may believe he or she is not accepted or understood.*[2]
- Give "permission" to express/deal with anger at the assailant/situation in acceptable ways. *Being free to express anger appropriately allows it to be dissipated so underlying feelings can be identified and dealt with, thus strengthening coping skills.*[2]
- Avoid prompting discussion of issues that cannot be resolved. Keep discussion on practical and emotional level rather than intellectualizing the experience. *When feelings (the experience) are intellectualized, uncomfortable insights and/or awareness are avoided by the use of rationalization, blocking resolution of feelings and impairing coping abilities.*[2]
- Provide for sensitive, trained counselors/therapists and engage in therapies, such as psychotherapy in conjunction with medications, Implosive Therapy (flooding), hypnosis, relaxation, Rolfing, memory work, cognitive restructuring, Eye Movement Desensitization and Reprocessing (EMDR), physical and occupational therapies. *Although it is not necessary for the helping person to have experienced the same kind of trauma as the client, sensitivity and listening skills are important to helping the client confront fears and learn new ways to cope with what has happened. Therapeutic use of desensitization techniques (flooding, implosive therapy) provides for extinction through exposure to the fear. Body work can alleviate muscle tension. Some techniques (Rolfing) help to bring blocked emotions to awareness as sensations of the traumatic event are reexperienced.*[9]

- Discuss use of psychotropic medication. *May be used to decrease anxiety, lift mood, aid in management of behavior, and ensure rest until client regains control of own self. Lithium may be used to reduce explosiveness; low-dose psychotropics may be used when loss of contact with reality is a problem.*[8]

NURSING PRIORITY NO. 3 To promote wellness (Teaching/Discharge Considerations):

- Assist client to identify and monitor feelings while therapy is occurring. *Promotes awareness and helps client know that control of feelings as they arise will help move beyond traumatic episode.*[9]
- Provide information about what reactions client may expect during each phase. Let client know these are common reactions and phrase in neutral terms of "You may or you may not . . ." *Knowledge of what may be experienced helps reduce fear of the unknown, thereby enabling client to manage reactions if they occur. Use of neutral terms lets client understand that not all reactions may occur in own situation.*[3]
- Assist client to identify factors that may have created a vulnerable situation and that he or she may have power to change to protect self in the future. *While client is not responsible for event, may have unknowingly contributed to occurrence by their actions. Identifying those actions that are within their power to change provides sense of control over seemingly uncontrollable situations.*[9]
- Avoid making value judgments. *Client may be judging self and caregiver needs to convey non-judgmental stance to allow individual to deal with feelings of guilt and recrimination, accepting fact that he or she did the best they were capable of in the circumstances.*[3]
- Discuss lifestyle changes client is contemplating and how they may contribute to recovery. *Client needs to evaluate appropriateness of plans and look at long-range consequences (e.g., moving away from effective support group) to make the best choice for the future.*[4]
- Assist with learning stress-management techniques. *Deep breathing, counting to 10, reviewing the situation, reframing skills assist client in developing constructive ways to cope with feelings of powerlessness and to regain control of self. Reframing stressors/situation in other words or positive ideas can help client recognize and consider alternatives.*[4]
- Discuss drug regimen, potential side effects of prescribed medications and necessity of prompt reporting of untoward effects.
- Discuss recognition of and ways to manage "anniversary reactions," reinforcing normalcy of recurrence of thoughts and feelings at this time. *Understanding that these feelings are to be expected and planning for them helps client get through the anniversary of the event with the least difficulty.*[10]
- Suggest support group for SO(s). *Family members may not understand client's reactions and need help with understanding them and learning how to deal with client in the most helpful manner.*[2]
- Encourage psychiatric consultation. *May need additional therapy if client is unable to maintain control, is violent or inconsolable, or does not seem to be making an adjustment. Participation in a group may be helpful.*[2]
- Refer for long-term family/marital counseling, if indicated. *Additional/ongoing support or therapy may be needed to help family resolve crisis and look at potential for growth. Client problems affect others in family/relationships, and further counseling may help resolve issues of enabling behavior/communication problems.*[12]
- Refer to NDs ineffective Coping, Grieving; complicated Grieving; Powerlessness.

DOCUMENTATION FOCUS

Assessment/Reassessment

- Individual findings, noting current dysfunction and behavioral/emotional responses to the incident.

- Specifics of traumatic event.
- Reactions of family/SO(s).
- Cultural/religious beliefs and expectations.
- Availability/use of resources.

Planning

- Plan of care and who is involved in the planning.
- Teaching plan.

Implementation/Evaluation

- Responses to interventions/teaching and actions performed.
- Emotional changes.
- Attainment/progress toward desired outcome(s).
- Modifications to plan of care.

Discharge Planning

- Long-term needs and who is responsible for actions to be taken.
- Specific referrals made.

References

1. Doenges, M., Moorhouse, M., Geissler-Murr, A. (2002). *Nursing Care Plans, Guidelines for Individualizing Patient Care.* 6th ed. Philadelphia: F. A. Davis.
2. Doenges, M., Townsend, M., Moorhouse, M. (1998). *Psychiatric Care Plans: Guidelines for Individualizing Care.* 3d ed. Philadelphia: F. A. Davis.
3. Cox, H., et al. (2002). *Clinical Applications of Nursing Diagnoses.* 4th ed. Philadelphia: F. A. Davis.
4. Townsend, M. (2003). *Psychiatric Mental Health Nursing: Concepts of Care.* 4th ed. Philadelphia: F. A. Davis.
5. Lipson, J. G., Dibble, S. L., Minarik, P. A. (1996). *Culture & Nursing Care: A Pocket Guide.* San Francisco: School of Nursing, UCSF Nursing Press.
6. Stuart, G. W. (2001). Anxiety responses and anxiety disorders. In Stuart, G. W., Laraia, M. T. (eds). *Principles and Practice of Psychiatric Nursing.* 7th ed. St. Louis, MO: Mosby.
7. Kunert, P. K. (2002). Stress and adaptation. In Porth, C. M. (ed). *Pathophysiology: Concepts of Altered Health States.* Philadelphia: J.B. Lippincott.
8. Townsend, M. (2001). *Nursing Diagnoses in Psychiatric Nursing: Care Plans and Psychotropic Medications.* 5th ed. Philadelphia: F. A. Davis.
9. National Institute of Mental Health. (2000). Anxiety Disorders, NIH Publication No. 00-3879. Rockville, MD: author. Available at www.nimh.nih.gov.anxiety/anxiety.cfm. Accessed December 2003.
10. Harper, N. E. (1997). *Seven Choices.* Austin, TX: Centerpoint Press.
11. Harvard Mental Health Letter. (June 1996). Posttraumatic stress disorder—Part I. Boston, MA: Harvard Medical School Health Publications Group.
12. Harvard Mental Health Letter. (July 1996). Posttraumatic stress disorder—Part II. Boston, MA: Harvard Medical School Health Publications Group.
13. Gore, T. A., Richards-Reid, G. M. (2006). Posttraumatic stress disorder. Article for Emedicine Web site. Retrieved April 2007 at www.emedicine.com/med/topic1900.htm.
14. Lubit, R. (2005). Acute treatment of disaster survivors. Article for Emedicine Web site. Retrieved April 2007 at www.emedicine.com/med/topic3540.htm.

risk for Post-Trauma Syndrome

Definition: At risk for sustained maladaptive response to a traumatic, overwhelming event

🌐 Cultural   Ⓐ Collaborative   🏠 Community/Home Care   Diagnostic Studies   ∞ Pediatric/Geriatric/Lifespan   Medications

RISK FACTORS

Occupation (e.g., police, fire, rescue, corrections, emergency room staff, mental health worker, [and their family members])

Perception of event; exaggerated sense of responsibility; diminished ego strength

Survivor's role in the event

Inadequate social support; nonsupportive environment; displacement from home

Duration of the event

NOTE: A risk diagnosis is not evidenced by signs and symptoms, as the problem has not occurred; rather, nursing interventions are directed at prevention.

Sample Clinical Applications: Traumatic injuries, physical/psychological abuse, disssociative disorder

DESIRED OUTCOMES/EVALUATION CRITERIA

Sample NOC linkages:

Fear Level: Severity of manifested apprehension, tension, or uneasiness arising from an identifiable source

Fear Self-Control: Personal actions to eliminate or reduce disabling feelings of apprehension and tension from an identifiable source

Grief Resolution: Adjustment to actual or impending loss

Client Will (Include Specific Time Frame)

- Verbalizes absence of disabling apprehension.
- Demonstrate ability to deal with emotional reactions in an individually appropriate manner.
- Deal with practical aspects of situation (e.g., court appearances, temporary housing, funeral services, rebuilding life).
- Report relief/absence of physical manifestations (pain, nightmares/flashbacks, fatigue) associated with event.

ACTIONS/INTERVENTIONS

Sample NIC linkages:

Crisis Intervention: Use of short-term counseling to help the patient cope with a crisis and resume a state of functioning comparable to or better than the pre-crisis state

Coping Enhancement: Assisting a patient to adapt to perceived stressors, changes, or threats that interfere with meeting life demands and roles

Support System Enhancement: Facilitation of support to patient by family, friends, and community

NURSING PRIORITY NO. 1 To assess contributing factors and individual reaction:

- Identify client who survived or witnessed traumatic event (e.g., airplane/motor vehicle crash, mass shooting, fire destroying home and lands, robbery at gunpoint/other violent act) *to recognize individual at high risk for post-trauma syndrome.*
- Note occupation (e.g., police, fire, emergency services personnel/rescue workers, disaster responders, soldiers and support personnel in combat areas, and family members). *Studies reveal a moderate to high percentage of post-traumatic stress disorders develop in these populations when they have been exposed to one or more traumatic incidents.*[1,12] *In addition, family*

members are also at risk because they are subjected to the same trauma, as they see the events repeated on TV news channels/hear stories repeated by their loved one(s) who were directly involved.

- Assess client's knowledge of and anxiety related to potential for work-related trauma incident (e.g., shooting in line of duty or viewing body of murdered child); and number, duration, and intensity of recurring situations (e.g., EMT exposed to numerous on-the-job traumatic incidents; rescuers searching for victims of natural or man-made disasters). *Having information about these situations enables individuals to think about and plan for eventualities so anxiety can be dealt with in a positive manner.*[7]

- Ascertain ethnic background and cultural/religious perceptions and beliefs about the occurrence. *Client may believe occurrence is retribution from God, or result of some indiscretion on his or her part, or in some way blame themselves for the incident/occurrence. Individual's view of how he or she is coping may be influenced by cultural background, religious beliefs, and family influence.*[7]

- Identify how client's experiences may affect current situation. *Individual who has had previous experiences with traumatic events (i.e., fireman who deals with trauma on a regular basis or person who has been involved in a trauma herself or himself) may be more susceptible to PTSD and ineffective coping abilities.*[2]

- Listen for comments of guilt, humiliation, shame, or taking on responsibility (e.g., "I should have been more careful/gone back to get her"; "Don't call me a hero; I couldn't save my partner"; "My kids are the same age as the ones who died," etc.). *Expressing guilt for actions that individual might have taken can lead to ruminations about lack of responsible behavior, leading to anxiety and PTSD.*[9,12,13]

- Note verbal/nonverbal expressions of guilt or self-blame when client has survived trauma in which others died. *Sense of own responsibility (blame) and guilt about not having done something to prevent incident or not having been "good enough" to deserve surviving are strong beliefs, especially in individuals who are influenced by background, religious, and cultural factors.*[2]

- Evaluate for life factors/stressors currently or recently occurring, such as displacement from home due to catastrophic event (e.g., illness/injury, fire/flood/violent storm/earthquake) happening to individual whose child is dying of cancer or who suffered abuse as a child. *Cumulative effects of multiple events can put the individual at higher risk for developing PTSD (acute added to delayed onset reactions) and indicates need for preventive measures to be taken.*[4,12]

- Identify client's coping mechanisms. *Resolution of the posttrauma response is largely dependent on the coping skills the client has developed throughout own life and is able to bring to bear on current situation.*[4]

- Determine availability/usefulness of client's support systems, family, social, community, and so forth, being aware that family members themselves/community in general may also be at risk. *Having an effective available support system and talking with them about what is happening can help client and family members resolve feelings and move on with life in a positive manner.*[10]

NURSING PRIORITY NO. 2 To assist client to deal with situation that exists:

- Provide a calm, safe environment. *Client can deal with disruption of life more effectively when surrounded by quiet and by knowing he or she is safe.*[11]

- Encourage expression of feelings and reinforce that feelings/reactions to trauma are common and not indicators of weakness or failure. Note whether feelings expressed appear congruent with events the client experienced. *Expressing feelings helps client recognize and identify them to enhance coping. Incongruency may indicate deeper conflict that can impede resolution.*[7]

Cultural   Collaborative   Community/Home Care   Diagnostic Studies   Pediatric/Geriatric/Lifespan   Medications

- Help child to express feelings about event using techniques appropriate to developmental level (e.g., play for young child, stories/puppets for preschooler, peer group for adolescent). *Children are more likely to express in play what they may not be able to verbalize directly. Adolescents may benefit from groups, gaining knowledge, support, decreased sense of isolation and improved coping skills.*[3]

- Identify and discuss client's strengths (e.g., very supportive family, usually copes well with stress, etc.) as well as vulnerabilities (e.g., client tends toward alcohol/other drugs for coping, client has witnessed a murder, etc.). *Knowing one's strengths and weaknesses helps client know what actions to take to cope with and prevent anxiety from becoming overwhelming.*[9]

- Discuss how individual coping mechanisms have worked in past traumatic events. *Awareness of previous successful experiences can help client remember coping skills that can be used to deal with current situation in a positive manner.*[4]

- Evaluate client's perceptions of events and personal significance (e.g., policeman/parent investigating death of a child). *Individuals perceive events depending on their previous experiences, cultural and religious background and family of origin and will respond to any given trauma based on these factors. Incidents that touch a person's own life will be more difficult to deal with and may have a deeper effect.*[3]

- Provide emotional and physical presence *to strengthen client's coping abilities. Spending time with the client promotes trust and provides an opportunity for client to think about what will help in the current situation.*[4]

- Observe for signs and symptoms of stress responses, such as nightmares, reliving an incident, poor appetite, irritability, numbness and crying, family/relationship disruption. *These responses are normal in the early postincident time frame. If prolonged and persistent, the client may be experiencing post-traumatic stress disorder.*[9]

NURSING PRIORITY NO. 3 To promote wellness (Teaching/Discharge Considerations):

- Educate high-risk persons/families about signs/symptoms of posttrauma response, especially if it is likely to occur in their occupation/life. *Awareness allows individual to be proactive and seek support/timely intervention as needed.*

- Encourage client to identify and monitor feelings on an ongoing basis. *Promotes awareness of changes in ability to deal with stressors, allowing prompt intervention when necessary.*[5]

- Encourage learning stress-management techniques, such as deep breathing, meditation, relaxation, exercise. *Reduces stress, enhancing coping skills and helping to resolve situation.*[6]

- Recommend participation in debriefing sessions that may be provided following major events. *Dealing with the stressor promptly may facilitate recovery from event/prevent exacerbation. Debriefing is being used by many organizations who regularly deal with traumatic events to prevent the development of PTSD, although issues about best timing of debriefing continue to be debated.*[4]

- Explain that posttraumatic symptoms can emerge months or sometimes years after a traumatic experience and that help/support can be obtained when needed/desired if client begins to experience intrusive memories/other symptoms.

- Encourage individual to develop a survivor mentality. *People often have it within their means to head off life-threatening situations and even survive the worst when they plan for emergencies and think ahead about ways to survive, such as taking food, water, and protective gear on a day hike in case you get lost, fall and break a bone, or in other ways have to spend more time than anticipated.*[11]

⊛ • Identify employment, community resource groups (e.g., Assistance Support and Self Help in Surviving Trauma [ASSIST], employee peer assistance programs; Red Cross/other victim support services, Compasionate Friends, etc.). *Provides opportunity for ongoing support to deal with recurrent stressors as individual moves on with life.*[8,13]

⊛ • Refer for individual/family counseling, as indicated. *May need additional assistance to prevent continuation of anxiety and the onset of PTSD.*[7]

DOCUMENTATION FOCUS

Assessment/Reassessment

- Identified risk factors noting internal/external concerns.
- Client's perception of event and personal significance.
- Cultural/religious beliefs and expectations.

Planning

- Plan of care and who is involved in the planning.
- Teaching plan.

Implementation/Evaluation

- Response to interventions/teaching and actions performed.
- Attainment/progress toward desired outcome(s).

Discharge Planning

- Long-term needs and who is responsible for actions to be taken.
- Specific referrals made.

References

1. Doenges, M. E., Moorhouse, M .F., Geissler-Murr, A. C. (2002). *Nursing Care Plans, Guidelines for Individualizing Patient Care.* 6th ed. Philadelphia: F. A. Davis.
2. Doenges, M., Townsend, M., Moorhouse, M. (1998). *Psychiatric Care Plans: Guidelines for Individualizing Care.* 3d ed. Philadelphia: F. A. Davis.
3. Cox, H., et al. (2002). *Clinical Applications of Nursing Diagnoses.* 4th ed. Philadelphia: F. A. Davis.
4. Townsend, M. (2003). *Psychiatric Mental Health Nursing: Concepts of Care.* 4th ed. Philadelphia: F. A. Davis.
5. Stuart, G. W. (2001). Anxiety responses and anxiety disorders. In Stuart, G. W., Laraia, M. T. *Principles and Practice of Psychiatric Nursing.* 7th ed. St. Louis, MO: Mosby.
6. Kunert P. K. (2002). Stress and adaptation. In Porth, C. M. (ed). *Pathophysiology: Concepts of Altered Health States.* Philadelphia: J. B. Lippincott.
7. National Institute of Mental Health. (2000). Anxiety Disorders. NIH Publication No. 02-3879. Rockville, MD. Accessed July 2007 at www.nimh.nih.gov.anxiety/anxiety.cfm.
8. Harper, N. E. (1997). *Seven Choices.* 5th ed. Austin, TX: Centerpoint Press.
9. Harvard Mental Health Letter. (June 1996). Posttraumatic stress disorder—Part I. Boston, MA: Harvard Medical School Health Publications Group.
10. Harvard Mental Health Letter. (July 1996). Posttraumatic stress disorder—Part II. Boston, MA: Harvard Medical School Health Publications Group.
11. Kamier, K. (2004). *Surviving the Extremes: A Doctor's Journey to the Limits of Human Endurance.* Boston: St. Martin's.
12. Davis, N. (2003). (Short online summaries from) Multi-Sensory Trauma Processing, A Manual for Understanding and Treating PTSD and Job-Related Trauma. Retrieved April 2007 at www.rescue-workers.com/1.htm.
13. Galea, S., Nandi, A., Vlahov, D. (2005). The epidemiology of post-traumatic stress disorders after disasters. *Epidemiologic Reviews,* 27(1), 78–91.

⊕ Cultural   ⊛ Collaborative   🏠 Community/Home Care   ⚗ Diagnostic Studies   ∞ Pediatric/Geriatric/Lifespan   💊 Medications

readiness for enhanced Power

Definition: A pattern of participating knowingly in change that is sufficient for well-being and can be strengthened

RELATED FACTORS
To be developed by nurse researchers and submitted to NANDA

DEFINING CHARACTERISTICS

Subjective
Expresses readiness to enhance power; knowledge for participation in change; awareness of possible changes to be made; identification of choices that can be made for change
Expresses readiness to enhance freedom to perform actions for change; involvement in creating change; participation in choices for daily living and health
Note: Even though power (a response) and empowerment (an intervention approach) are different concepts, the literature related to both concepts supports the defining characteristics of this diagnosis.

Sample Clinical Applications: Any acute or chronic condition, or healthy individual looking to change life/improve well-being

DESIRED OUTCOMES/EVALUATION CRITERIA
Sample NOC linkages:
Personal Autonomy: Personal actions of a competent individual to exercise governance in life decisions
Decision-Making: Ability to make judgments and choose between two or more alternatives
Health Beliefs: Perceived Control: Personal conviction that one can influence a health outcome

Client Will (Include Specific Time Frame)

• Verbalize knowledge of what changes he or she want to make.
• Express awareness of own ability to be in charge of changes to be made.
• Participate in classes/group activities to learn new skills.
• State readiness to take power over own life.

ACTIONS/INTERVENTIONS

Sample NIC linkages:
Self-Responsibility Facilitation: Encouraging a patient to assume more responsibility for own behavior
Decision-Making Support: Providing information and support for a person who is making a decision regarding healthcare
Health System Guidance: Facilitating a patient's location and use of appropriate health services

NURSING PRIORITY NO. 1 To determine need/motivation for improvement:

• Determine current situation and circumstances that client is experiencing leading to desire to improve life. *Provides information to help client with planning for enhancing life.*[8]

- Ascertain motivation/expectations for change. *Motivation to improve and high expectations can encourage client to make changes that will improve his or her life. However, unrealistic expectations or motivation to please someone else may hamper efforts.*
- Identify emotional climate in which client and relationships live and work. *The emotional climate has a great impact between people. When a power differential exists in relationships, the atmosphere is largely determined by the person or people who have the power.*[4]
- Identify client locus of control: internal (expressions of responsibility for self and ability to control outcomes) or external (expressions of lack of control over self and environment). *Understanding locus of control can help client to work toward positive, internal control as he or she develops sense of ability to freely choose own actions.*[9]
- Determine cultural factors/religious beliefs influencing client's self-view. *These factors can be strong determinants in individual's ability to change/view self as powerful and may complicate growth process.*[9]
- Assess degree of mastery client has exhibited in his or her life. *Helps client to understand how he or she has functioned in the past and what is needed to improve.*
- Note presence of family/SOs that can or do act as support systems for client. *When family understands and supports client's desires and efforts, he or she is more likely to be successful.*[6]
- Determine whether client knows or uses assertiveness skills. *Learning and enhancing these skills will help client to improve ability to take personal responsibility for own self and relationships with others.*[1,3,5,7]

NURSING PRIORITY NO. 2 To assist client to clarify needs relative to ability to improve feelings of power:

- Discuss how client is currently involved in creating change in life. *Provides a baseline to measure growth and suggests possibilities for change.*[8]
- Listen to/Active-listen to client's perceptions and beliefs about the concept of power. *Enables client to identify underlying feelings and thoughts about this issue and how power can be gained in his or her life.*[8]
- Identify strengths/assets and past coping strategies that were successful. *These strategies can be built on to enhance feelings of control.*[6]
- Discuss the importance of assuming personal responsibility for life and relationships. *This requires one to be open to new ideas and experiences, different values, and beliefs and to be inquisitive.*
- Identify things client can and or cannot control. *Avoids wasting time on things that are not in the control of the client.*
- Treat expressed desires and decisions with respect. Avoid critical parenting expressions. *Individual may express thoughts and opinions that are creative and out of the ordinary, and critical parenting responses such as "That's a dumb idea," can crush person's brainstorming.*[9]

NURSING PRIORITY NO. 3 To promote optimum wellness, enhancing power (Teaching/Discharge Considerations):

- Assist client to set realistic goals for the future. *Even though client is thinking creatively and brainstorming ideas, goals need to be planned step by step to reach the desired outcome.*[6]
- Provide accurate verbal and written information about client's concerns/life situation. *Reinforces learning and promotes self-paced review.*[8]
- Assist client to learn/use assertive communication skills. *These techniques require practice, but as the client becomes more proficient, they will help to develop relationships that are more effective.*[2,3]

Cultural   Collaborative   Community/Home Care   Diagnostic Studies   Pediatric/Geriatric/Lifespan   Medications

- Use I-messages instead of You-messages. *I-messages acknowledge ownership of what is said, whereas You-messages suggest the other person is wrong or bad, fostering resentment and resistance instead of understanding and cooperation.*[8]
- Discuss importance of client paying attention to nonverbal communication. *Messages are often confusing/misinterpreted when verbal and nonverbal communications are not congruent.*[9]
- Help client learn to problem-solve differences. *Problem-solving process allows for each person involved to have input and promotes win-win solutions.*[8]
- Instruct and encourage use of stress-reduction techniques. *Relaxation helps individual to function more effectively, thus enhancing feelings of power.*[9]
- Refer to support groups/classes, as indicated, assertiveness training, effectiveness for women to "be your best." *Provides role models and allows individuals to learn from one another, thereby promoting problem-solving/enhancing learning.*[7]

DOCUMENTATION FOCUS

Assessment/Reassessment

- Individual findings, noting determination to improve sense of power, locus of control
- Motivation and expectations for change.
- Cultural/religious beliefs affecting self-view.
- Locus of control.

Planning

- Plan of care/interventions and who is involved in planning.
- Teaching plan.

Implementation/Evaluation

- Client's responses to interventions/teaching and actions performed.
- Attainment/progress toward desired outcome(s).
- Modifications to plan of care.

Discharge Planning

- Long-term needs and who is responsible for actions to be taken.
- Specific referrals made.

References

1. Self-help Brochures, Assertiveness, UIUC. Retrieved April 2007 at www.couns.uiuc.edu/Brochures/assertiv.htm.
2. Organizational Development & Training Tip Sheet (2002). Tufts University. Retrieved March 2007 at www.tufts.edu/hr/tips/assert.html.
3. Assertiveness Training Retrieved April 2007 at www.csusm.edu/caps/Assertiveness.html.
4. Adams, L. (December 2006). Working Together: Climate—the Emotional One That Is. Retrieved March 2007 at www.gordontraining.com/pdf/wt-200612-climate-the-emotional-one-that-is.pdf.
5. Adams, L. (April 2007). Taking Personal Responsibility. Available at www.gordontraining.com/work-free-resources.html.
6. Adams, L. (1989). Be Your Best (rev. ed.). Perigee Trade.
7. Alberte, R., Emmons, M. (1970). *Your Perfect Right.* San Luis Obispo, CA: Impact.
8. Family Effectiveness Training Program. (1997). Solana Beach, CA, Gordon Training International.
9. Townsend, M. (2006). *Psychiatric Mental Health Nursing Concepts of Care.* 5th ed. Philadelphia, F. A. Davis.

Powerlessness [specify level]

Definition: Perception that one's own action will not significantly affect an outcome; a perceived lack of control over a current situation or immediate happening

RELATED FACTORS

Healthcare environment [e.g., loss of privacy, personal possessions, control over therapies]
Interpersonal interaction [e.g., misuse of power, force; abusive relationships]
Illness-related regimen [e.g., chronic/debilitating conditions]
Lifestyle of helplessness [e.g., repeated failures, dependency]

DEFINING CHARACTERISTICS

Subjective

Low
Expressions of uncertainty about fluctuating energy levels
Moderate
Expressions of dissatisfaction/frustration over inability to perform previous tasks/activities
Expressions of doubt regarding role performance
Fear of alienation from caregivers
Reluctance to express true feelings; resentment; anger; guilt
Severe
Verbal expressions of having no control (e.g., over self-care, situation, outcome)
Depression over physical deterioration

Objective

Low
Passivity
Moderate
Dependence on others that may result in irritability
Inability to seek information regarding care
Passivity
Nonparticipation in care/decision making when opportunities are provided; does not monitor progress
Does not defend self-care practices when challenged
Severe
Apathy [withdrawal, resignation, crying]

Sample Clinical Applications: Chronic/debilitating conditions (e.g., COPD, MS), cancer, spinal cord injury, major depressive disorder, somatization disorders

DESIRED OUTCOMES/EVALUATION CRITERIA

Sample NOC linkages:
Personal Autonomy: Personal actions of a competent individual to exercise governance in life decisions
Health Beliefs: Perceived Control: Personal conviction that one can influence a health outcome
Participation in Healthcare Decisions: Personal involvement in selecting and evaluating healthcare options to achieve desired outcomes

Cultural   Collaborative   Community/Home Care   Diagnostic Studies   Pediatric/Geriatric/Lifespan   Medications

Client Will (Include Specific Time Frame)

- Express sense of control over the present situation and future outcome.
- Make choices related to and be involved in care.
- Identify areas over which individual has control.
- Acknowledge reality that some areas are beyond individual's control.

ACTIONS/INTERVENTIONS

Sample NIC linkages:

Self-Responsibility Facilitation: Encouraging a patient to assume more responsibility for own behavior

Health System Guidance: Facilitating a patient's location and use of appropriate health services

Decision-Making Support: Providing information and support for a person who is making a decision regarding healthcare

NURSING PRIORITY NO. I To assess causative/contributing factors:

- Identify situational circumstances (e.g., strange environment, immobility, diagnosis of terminal/chronic illness, lack of support system(s), lack of knowledge about situation) affecting the client at this time. *Knowing the specific situation of the client is essential to planning care and empowering the individual.*[4]

- Determine client's perception/knowledge of condition and treatment plan. *Identifying how client views and understands what is happening and what the plan of care entails is essential to begin to help client feel empowered.*[2]

- Ascertain client response to treatment regimen. Does client see reason(s) for and understand it is in the client's interest or is client compliant and helpless? *The manner in which the individual responds to the treatment indicates the depth of feelings of powerlessness and may interfere with progress.*[4]

- Identify client locus of control—internal (expressions of responsibility for self and ability to control outcomes—"I didn't quit smoking") or external (expressions of lack of control over self and environment—"Nothing ever works out"; "What bad luck to get lung cancer"). *Locus of control is a term used in reference to an individual's sense of mastery or control over events. Individuals view life change and stressful events differently. Those with internal locus of control tend to be more optimistic about their ability to deal with adversity even in the face of current difficulties. Individuals with external locus of control may attribute feelings of powerlessness to an external source perceiving it as beyond his or her control and will look to others to solve problems and take care of them.*[4,9]

- Note cultural/religious factors that may contribute to how client views self and is handling current situation. *One's values and beliefs may dictate gender roles and the individual's expectations of control, influencing the client's belief in ability to manage situation, participate in decision making, and direct own life.*[9,11]

- Assess degree of mastery client has exhibited in life. *How this individual has dealt with problems throughout life will help to understand feelings of powerlessness client is feeling during this crisis.*[4,5]

- Determine if there has been a change in relationships with SO(s). *Conflict in relationships may be contributing to sense of powerlessness. Domestic violence situations often leave the individuals involved feeling powerless to change what is happening.*[4]

• Note availability/use of resources. *Client who has few options for assistance or who is not knowledgeable about how to use resources needs to be given information and assistance to know how and where to seek help.*[3]

• Investigate healthcare providers and personal caregiver practices to determine if they support client control/responsibility. *Caregivers who do for the client what he or she is able to do for own self diminish client's sense of control. When client is given as much control as possible over self, sense of power is regained.*[3]

NURSING PRIORITY NO. 2 To assess degree of powerlessness experienced by the client:

• Listen to statements client makes: "They don't care"; "It won't make any difference"; "Are you kidding?" *Indicators of sense of powerlessness and hopelessness and need for specific interventions to provide sense of control over what is happening.*[2]

• Note expressions that indicate "giving up," such as "It won't do any good." *May indicate suicidal intent, indicating need for immediate evaluation and intervention.*[6]

• Note behavioral responses (verbal and nonverbal), including expressions of fear, interest or apathy, agitation, withdrawal. *These responses can show depth of anxiety, feelings of powerlessness over what is happening and indicate need for intervention to help client begin to look at situation with some sense of hope.*[6]

• Note lack of communication, flat affect, and lack of eye contact. *May indicate more severe state of mind, such as psychotic episode and need for immediate evaluation and treatment.*[4]

• Identify the use of manipulative behavior and reactions of client and caregivers. *Manipulation is used for management of powerlessness because of distrust of others, fear of intimacy, search for approval, and validation of sexuality.*[1,9]

NURSING PRIORITY NO. 3 To assist client to clarify needs relative to ability to meet them:

• Show concern for client as a person. *Communicates value of the individual, enhancing self-esteem.*[8]

• Make time to listen to/Active-listen to client's perceptions and concerns and encourage questions. *Provides time for client to explore views and understand what is happening in order to come to some decisions about situation, enhancing sense of control.*[8,10]

• Accept expressions of feelings, including anger and hopelessness. *Communicates empathy and understanding of reality of those feelings and provides a point of discussion to move toward sense of control.*[4]

• Avoid arguing or using logic with hopeless client. *Client will not accept that anything can make a difference. Arguing denies client's reality and may impede client-nurse relationship.*[2]

• Deal with manipulative behavior by being straightforward and honest with your communication and letting client know that this is a better way to get needs met. *When client makes a commitment to stop using manipulation in life, steps can be taken to recognize the behaviors and feelings and begin to change them. Keeping a journal can help to identify these issue.*[9]

• Express hope for the client. *Although client may not accept expressions of hope, there is always hope of something, and when options are explored, client may begin to see there is hope.*[8]

• Identify strengths/assets and past coping strategies that were successful. *Helps client to recognize own ability to deal with difficult situation, providing sense of power.*[5]

• Assist client to identify what he or she can do for self. Identify things the client can/cannot control. *Accomplishing something can provide a sense of control and helps client understand that there are things he or she can manage. Accepting that some things cannot be controlled helps client to stop wasting efforts and refocus energy.*[1]

🏠 • Encourage client to maintain a sense of perspective about the situation. *Discussing ways client can look at options and make decisions based on which ones will be best leads to the most effective solutions for situation.*[6]

NURSING PRIORITY NO. 4 To promote independence:

🏠 • Use client's locus of control to develop individual plan of care. *Tailoring care to the individual's ability will maximize effectiveness. For instance, client with internal control can take control of own care, and those with external control may need to begin with small tasks and add as tolerated, moving toward learning to take more control of care.*[6]

🏠 • Develop contract with client specifying goals agreed on. *When client is involved in planning, commitment to plan is enhanced, optimizing outcomes.*[2]

🏠 • Treat expressed decisions and desires with respect. Avoid critical parenting behaviors. *Listening to client and accepting what is said, no matter what the content, helps client hear own words and begin to process information and feelings. Comments that are heard as critical or condescending will block communication and growth.*[1,10]

🏠 • Provide client opportunities to control as many events as energy and restrictions of care permit. *Promotes sense of control over situation and helps client begin to feel more confident about own ability to manage what is happening.*[6,7]

🏠 • Discuss needs openly with client and set up agreed-on routines for meeting identified needs. *Minimizes use of manipulation. Manipulative behavior is often used to influence others to do what the person thinks he or she should do. Usually this results in defensiveness or outright rebellion against what is suggested, resulting in lack of trust and withdrawal on the part of the person being manipulated.*[9]

• Minimize rules and limit continuous observation to the degree that safety permits. *Provides sense of control for the client while maintaining a safe environment for the client.*[6]

🏠 • Support client efforts to develop realistic steps to put plan into action, reach goals, and maintain expectations. *Noting progress that is being made can provide a sense of control and diminish sense of powerlessness.*[6]

🏠 • Provide positive reinforcement for desired behaviors. *In Behavioral Therapy, the belief that when a behavior reinforces another behavior, the second behavior will recur is called a "positive reinforcer" and the function is called "positive reinforcement." By providing this reinforcement, the desired behaviors are more likely to continue.*[4]

🏠 • Direct client's thoughts beyond present state to future when appropriate. *Focusing on possibilities in small steps can help the client see that there can be hope in small things each day.*[1,8]

• Schedule frequent/regular contacts to check on client, deal with client needs, and let client know someone is available. *Communicates caring and concern for client and needs, reinforcing sense of worthiness.*[1]

🏠 • Involve SO(s) in client care as desired/appropriate. *Personal involvement by supportive family members can help client see the possibilities for resolving problems related to feelings of powerlessness.*[6]

NURSING PRIORITY NO. 5 To promote wellness (Teaching/Discharge Considerations):

🏠 • Instruct in/encourage use of anxiety and stress-reduction techniques. *Most individuals react to stress in predictable physiological and psychological ways. Feelings of powerlessness related to client's situation can be relieved by use of these techniques.*[5]

🏠 • Provide accurate verbal and written information about what is happening and discuss with client/SO(s). Repeat as often as necessary. *Providing information in different modalities allows better access and opportunity for increased understanding. People do not always hear every piece of information the first time it is presented because of anxiety and inattention, so repetition helps to fill in the missed information.*[6]

🏠 • Assist client to set realistic goals for the future. *Provides opportunity for client to decide what direction is desired and to gain confidence from completion of each goal.*[10]

🏠 • Assist client to learn/use assertive communication skills. *Practicing a new way of expressing thoughts and requests provides the client with a skill to achieve desires and improve relationships.*[10]

⊕ • Facilitate return to a productive role in whatever capacity possible for the individual. Refer to occupational therapist/vocational counselor as indicated. *Feelings of powerlessness may result from inability to engage in or resume previous activities, and learning new ways to be productive enhances self-esteem and reduces feelings of powerlessness.*[6]

🏠 • Encourage client to think productively and positively and take responsibility for choosing own thoughts. *Negative thinking can result in feelings of powerlessness, and learning to use positive thinking can reverse this pattern, promoting feelings of control and self-worth.*[6]

🏠 • Model problem-solving process with client/SO(s). *Learning a problem-solving method that results in a win-win solution improves family relationships and promotes feelings of self-worth in those involved.*[10]

🏠 • Suggest client periodically review own needs/goals. *It is easy to become discouraged as time goes on, and reviewing, thinking about needs, and how previously set goals are relevant in the present helps to either renew those goals or develop new goals to meet current situation.*[6,8]

⊕ • Refer to support groups, counseling/therapy, and so forth, as indicated. *May need additional assistance to resolve current problems/long-standing issues, troubled relationships.*[4]

DOCUMENTATION FOCUS

Assessment/Reassessment

• Individual findings, noting degree of powerlessness, locus of control, individual's perception of the situation.
• Specific cultural/religious factors.
• Availability/use of support system and resources.

Planning

• Plan of care and who is involved in the planning.
• Teaching plan.

Implementation/Evaluation

• Responses to interventions/teaching and actions performed.
• Specific goals/expectations.
• Attainment/progress toward desired outcome(s).
• Modifications to plan of care.

Discharge Planning

• Long-term needs and who is responsible for actions to be taken.
• Specific referrals made.

References

1. Doenges, M., Moorhouse, M., Geissler-Murr, A. (2002). *Nursing Care Plans, Guidelines for Individualizing Patient Care.* 6th ed. Philadelphia: F. A. Davis.

🌐 Cultural   ⊕ Collaborative   🏠 Community/Home Care   ⟋ Diagnostic Studies   ∞ Pediatric/Geriatric/Lifespan   Medications

2. Doenges, M., Townsend, M., Moorhouse, M. (1998). *Psychiatric Care Plans: Guidelines for Individualizing Care.* 3d ed. Philadelphia: F. A. Davis.
3. Cox, H., et al. (2002). *Clinical Applications of Nursing Diagnoses.* 4th ed. Philadelphia: F. A. Davis.
4. Townsend, M. (2006). *Psychiatric Mental Health Nursing: Concepts of Care.* 5th ed. Philadelphia: F. A. Davis.
5. Stuart, G. W. (2001). Anxiety responses and anxiety disorders. In Stuart, G. W., Laraia, M. T. *Principles and Practice of Psychiatric Nursing.* 7th ed. St. Louis, MO: Mosby.
6. Kunert, P. K. (2002). Stress and adaptation. In Porth, C. M. (ed) *Pathophysiology: Concepts of Altered Health States.* Philadelphia: J. B. Lippincott.
7. National Institute of Mental Health. (2000). Anxiety Disorders, NIH Publication No. 00–3879. Rockville, MD: author. Available at www.nimh.nih.gov.anxiety/anxiety.cfm. Accessed December 2003.
8. Neeld, E. H. (1997). *Seven Choices.* Austin, TX: Centerpoint Press.
9. Messina, J., Messina, C. Tools for Handling Control Issues Eliminating Manipulation. Retrieved April 2007 at www.coping.org/control/manipul.htm.
10. Gordon, T. (2000). *Parent Effectiveness Training* (updated ed). New York: Three Rivers Press.
11. Lipson, J. G., Dibble, S. L., Minarik, P. A. (1999). *Culture & Nursing Care: A Pocket Guide.* San Francisco: UCSF Nursing Press.

risk for Powerlessness

Definition: At risk for perceived lack of control over a situation and/or one's ability to significantly affect an outcome

RISK FACTORS

Physiological

Illness [hospitalization, intubation, ventilator, suctioning]; dying

Acute injury; progressive debilitating disease process (e.g., spinal cord injury, multiple sclerosis)

Aging [e.g., decreased physical strength, decreased mobility]

Psychosocial

Deficient knowledge (e.g., of illness or healthcare system)

Lifestyle of dependency

Inadequate coping patterns

Absence of integrality (e.g., essence of power)

Situational/chronic low self-esteem; disturbed body image

NOTE: A risk diagnosis is not evidenced by signs and symptoms, as the problem has not occurred; rather, nursing interventions are directed at prevention.

Sample Clinical Applications: New/unexpected diagnoses, chronic/debilitating conditions (e.g., COPD, MS), cancer, spinal cord injury, major depressive disorder, somatization disorders

DESIRED OUTCOMES/EVALUATION CRITERIA

Sample NOC linkages:

Personal Autonomy: Personal actions of a competent individual to exercise governance in life decisions

Health Beliefs: Perceived Control: Personal conviction that one can influence a health outcome

Participation in Healthcare Decisions: Personal involvement in selecting and evaluating healthcare options to achieve desired outcomes

Client Will (Include Specific Time Frame)

- Express sense of control over the present situation and hopefulness about future outcomes.
- Verbalize positive self-apprasial in current situation.
- Make choices related to and be involved in care.
- Identify areas over which individual has control.
- Acknowledge reality that some areas are beyond individual's control.

ACTIONS/INTERVENTIONS

Sample NIC linkages:

Self-Responsibility Facilitation: Encouraging a patient to assume more responsibility for own behavior

Health System Guidance: Facilitating a patient's location and use of appropriate health services

Decision-Making Support: Providing information and support for a person who is making a decision regarding healthcare

NURSING PRIORITY NO. I To assess causative/contributing factors:

- Identify situational circumstances (e.g., acute illness, sudden hospitalization, diagnosis of terminal or debilitating/chronic illness, very young or aging with decreased physical strength and mobility, lack of knowledge about illness, healthcare system). *Necessary information to develop individualized plan of care for this client.*[1]
- Determine client's perception/knowledge of condition and proposed treatment plan. *Identifying how client views and understands what is happening and what the plan of care entails is essential to help client feel empowered.*[7]
- Identify client locus of control—internal (expressions of responsibility for self and ability to control outcomes—"I didn't quit smoking") or external (expressions of lack of control over self and environment—"Nothing ever works out"; "What bad luck to get lung cancer"). *Locus of control is a term used in reference to an individual's sense of mastery or control over events. Individuals view life change and stressful events differently. Those with internal locus of control tend to be more optimistic about their ability to deal with adversity even in the face of current difficulties. Individuals with external locus of control may attribute feelings of powerlessness to an external source, perceiving it as beyond his or her control and will look to others to solve problems and take care of them.*[4,10]
- Note cultural/religious factors that may contribute to how client views self and is handling current situation. *One's values and beliefs may dictate gender roles and the individual's expectations of control, influencing the client's belief in ability to manage situation, participate in decision making, and direct own life.*[9,10]
- Assess client's self-esteem and degree of mastery client has exhibited in life situations. *Provides clues to client's ability to see self as in control and deal with current situation.*[7]
- Note availability and use of resources, relationship with SO/family and degree of support provided to client. *Presence of support system and ability to use resources appropriately facilitates problem-solving, enhancing sense of control. Client who has few options for assistance or who is not knowledgeable about how to use resources needs to be given information and assistance to know how and where to seek help.*[3]
- Listen to statements client makes that might indicate feelings of possiblility of loss of control (e.g., "They don't care"; "It won't make a difference"; "It won't do any good").

Cultural   Collaborative   Community/Home Care   Diagnostic Studies   Pediatric/Geriatric/Lifespan   Medications

Indicators of sense of powerlessness and hopelessness and need for specific interventions to provide sense of control over what is happening.[4]

- Determine congruency of responses (verbal and nonverbal) and note expressions of fear, disinterest or apathy, or withdrawal. *These responses can show depth of anxiety over what is happening and indicate need for intervention to help client begin to look at situation with sense of hope.*[5]
- Be alert for signs of manipulative behavior and note reactions of client and caregivers. *Manipulation may be used for management of powerlessness because of fear and distrust.*[4,10]

NURSING PRIORITY NO. 2 To assist client to clarify needs and ability to meet them:

- Show concern for client as a person. Encourage questions. *Communicates value of the individual, enhancing self-esteem. Questions may reveal lack of information or concerns client may have.*[8]
- Make time to listen to client's perceptions of the situation as well as concerns. *Provides time for client to explore views and understand what is happening to come to some decisions about situation, enhancing sense of control.*[5]
- Accept expressions of feelings, including anger and reluctance to try to work things out. *Communicates unconditional regard for the client and encourages individual to think about options even though situation may be difficult.*[5]
- Express hope for client and encourage review of past experiences with successful strategies. *Provides an opportunity for person to remember and accept that he or she has managed difficult situations before and can apply these strategies in current situation.*[4]
- Assist client to identify what he or she can do to help self and what situations cannot be controlled. *Accomplishing something can provide a sense of control and helps client understand that there are things he or she can manage. Accepting that some things cannot be controlled helps client to stop wasting efforts and refocus energy.*[1,2]

NURSING PRIORITY NO. 3 To promote wellness (Teaching/Discharge Considerations):

- Encourage client to be active in own healthcare management and to take responsibility for choosing own actions and reactions. *Discussing ways client can look at options and make decisions based on which ones will be best leads to the most effective solutions for situation.*[6,7]
- Involve client/SO(s) in planning process, using client's locus of control. *Tailoring care to the individual's ability will maximize effectiveness. For instance, client with internal control can take control of own care, and those with external control may need to begin with small tasks and add as tolerated, moving toward learning to take more control of care.*[6]
- Model problem-solving process with client and SOs. *Learning a problem-solving method that results in a win-win solution improves family relationships and promotes feelings of self-worth in those involved.*[8]
- Support client efforts to develop realistic steps to put plan into action, reach goals, and maintain expectations. *Noting progress that is being made can enhance sense of control.*[6]
- Provide accurate verbal and written instructions about what is happening and what realistically might happen. Providing information in different modalities allows better access and opportunity for increased understanding to support decision-making process.[6]
- Identify resource books/classes for assertiveness training and stress-reduction, as appropriate. *Reinforces learning and promotes self-paced review.*[8]
- Suggest client periodically review own needs/goals. *Reviewing needs and how previously set goals are relevant in the present helps to either renew those goals or develop new goals to meet current situation.*[5]

- Refer to support groups for chronic conditions/disability (e.g., MS Society, Easter Seals, Alzheimer's, Al-Anon) or counseling/therapy, as appropriate. *May need additional assistance to manage difficulties of current situation.*[4]

DOCUMENTATION FOCUS

Assessment/Reassessment

- Individual findings, noting potential for powerlessness, locus of control, individual's perception of the situation.
- Cultural values/religious beliefs.
- Locus of control.
- SO/family involvement and support.
- Availability/use of resources.

Planning

- Plan of care and who is involved in the planning.
- Teaching plan.

Implementation/Evaluation

- Responses to interventions/teaching and actions performed.
- Specific goals/expectations.
- Modifications to plan of care.

Discharge Planning

- Long-term needs and who is responsible for actions to be taken.
- Specific referrals made.

References

1. Doenges, M. E., Moorhouse, M. F., Geissler-Murr, A. C. (2002). *Nursing Care Plans, Guidelines for Individualizing Patient Care.* 6th ed. Philadelphia: F. A. Davis.
2. Doenges, M., Townsend, M., Moorhouse, M. (1998). *Psychiatric Care Plans: Guidelines for Individualizing Care.* 3d ed. Philadelphia: F. A. Davis.
3. Cox, H., et al. (2002). *Clinical Applications of Nursing Diagnoses.* 4th ed. Philadelphia: F. A. Davis.
4. Townsend, M. (2006). *Psychiatric Mental Health Nursing: Concepts of Care.* 5th ed. Philadelphia: F. A. Davis.
5. Stuart, G. W. (2001). Anxiety responses and anxiety disorders. In Stuart, G. W., Laraia, M. T. *Principles and Practice of Psychiatric Nursing.* 7th ed. St. Louis, MO: Mosby.
6. Kunert, P. K. (2002). Stress and adaptation. In Porth, C. M. (ed). *Pathophysiology: Concepts of Altered Health States.* Philadelphia: J. B. Lippincott.
7. National Institute of Mental Health. (2000). Anxiety Disorders. NIH Publication No. 00-3879. Rockville, MD: author. Available at www.nimh.nih.gov.anxiety/anxiety.cfm. Accessed January 2004.
8. Gordon, T. (2000). *Parent Effectiveness Training* (updated ed). New York: Three Rivers Press.
9. Lipson, J. G., Dibble, S. L., Minarik, P. A. (1996). *Culture & Nursing Care: A Pocket Guide.* San Francisco: School of Nursing, UCSF Nursing Press.
10. Messina, J., Messina, C. Tools for Handling Control Issues Eliminating Manipulation. Retrieved April 2007 at www.coping.org/control/manipul.htm.

ineffective Protection

Definition: Decrease in the ability to guard self from internal or external threats such as illness or injury

Cultural Collaborative Community/Home Care Diagnostic Studies Pediatric/Geriatric/Lifespan Medications

RELATED FACTORS

Extremes of age

Inadequate nutrition

Alcohol abuse

Abnormal blood profiles (e.g., leukopenia, thrombocytopenia, anemia, coagulation)

Drug therapies (e.g., antineoplastic, corticosteroid, immune, anticoagulant, thrombolytic)

Treatments (e.g., surgery, radiation)

Cancer; immune disorders

DEFINING CHARACTERISTICS

Subjective

Neurosensory alterations

Chilling

Itching

Insomnia; fatigue; weakness

Anorexia

Objective

Deficient immunity

Impaired healing; altered clotting

Maladaptive stress response

Perspiring [inappropriately]

Dyspnea; cough

Restlessness; immobility

Disorientation

Pressure sores

Sample Clinical Applications: Cancer, AIDS, systemic lupus, substance abuse, tuberculosis, dementia/Alzheimer's disease, anorexia/bulimia nervosa, diabetes mellitus, thrombophlebitis, conditions requiring long-term steroid use (e g., COPD, asthma, renal failure), major surgery

Authors' note: The purpose of this diagnosis seems to combine multiple NDs under a single heading for ease of planning care when a number of variables may be present. Outcomes/evaluation criteria and interventions are specifically tied to individual related factors that are present, such as:

Extremes of age: Includes concerns regarding body temperature/thermoregulation; memory or thought process/sensory-perceptual alterations; impaired mobility, risk for falls, sedentary lifestyle, self-care deficits; risk for trauma, suffocation, or poisoning; risk for skin/tissue integrity and fluid volume imbalances.

Inadequate nutrition: Brings up issues of nutrition (less or more than body requirements), risk for unstable blood glucose; risk for infection, delayed surgical recovery; impaired swallowing; disturbed thought processes, impaired skin/tissue integrity; trauma, ineffective coping, and interrupted family processes.

Alcohol [other drug] abuse: May be situational or chronic with problems ranging from ineffective breathing patterns, decreased cardiac output, impaired liver function, and fluid volume deficit to nutritional problems, infection, trauma, disturbed thought processes, and coping/family process difficulties.

Abnormal blood profile: Suggests possibility of fluid volume deficit, decreased tissue perfusion, impaired gas exchange, activity intolerance, or risk for infection or injury.

Drug therapies, treatments, and disease concerns: Includes ineffective tissue perfusion, activity intolerance; cardiovascular, respiratory, and elimination concerns; risk for infection, fluid volume imbalances, impaired skin/tissue integrity, impaired liver function; pain, nutritional problems, fatigue/sleep deprivation, ineffective therapeutic regimen management; and emotional responses (e.g., anxiety, sorrow/grief, coping, etc.).

- It is suggested that the user refer to specific NDs based on identified related factors and individual concerns for this client to find appropriate outcomes and interventions.

Sample NOC linkages:
Cognition: Ability to execute complex mental processes
Blood coagulation: Extent to which blood clots within normal period of time
Immune Status: Natural and acquired appropriately targeted resistance to internal and external antigens

Sample NIC linkages:
Postanesthesia Care: Monitoring and management of the patient who has recently undergone general or regional anesthesia
Infection Protection: Minimizing the acquisition and transmission of infectious agents
Surveillance: Safety: Purposeful and ongoing collection and analysis of information about the patient and the environment for use in promoting and maintaining patient safety

Rape-Trauma Syndrome [specify]

Definition: Sustained maladaptive response to a forced, violent sexual penetration against the victim's will and consent [Rape is not a sexual crime, but a crime of violence and identified as sexual assault. Although attacks are most often directed toward women, men also may be victims.]
NOTE: This syndrome includes the following three subcomponents: [A] Rape-Trauma; [B] Compound Reaction; and [C] Silent Reaction. [All three are presented here.]

RELATED FACTORS
Rape [actual/attempted forced sexual penetration]

DEFINING CHARACTERISTICS

[a] Rape-Trauma
Acute phase

Subjective
Embarrassment; humiliation; shame; guilt; self-blame
Loss of self-esteem; helplessness; powerlessness
Shock; fear; anxiety; anger; revenge
Nightmare and sleep disturbances
Change in relationships; sexual dysfunction

Objective
Physical trauma [e.g., bruising, tissue irritation]; muscle tension/spasms
Confusion; disorganization; impaired ability to make decisions
Agitation; hyperalertness; aggression
Mood swings; vulnerability; dependence; depression

Cultural   Collaborative   Community/Home Care   Diagnostic Studies   Pediatric/Geriatric/Lifespan   Medications

Substance abuse; suicide attempts

Denial; phobias; paranoia; dissociative disorders

[b] Compound Reaction

Definition: Forced violent sexual penetration against the victim's will and consent; trauma syndrome that develops from this attack or attempted attack includes an acute phase of disorganization of the victim's lifestyle and a long-term process of reorganization of lifestyle

RELATED FACTORS

To be developed by nurse researchers and submitted to NANDA

DEFINING CHARACTERISTICS

Subjective

Acute Phase

Emotional reactions (e.g., anger, embarrassment, fear of physical violence and death, humiliation, self-blame, revenge)

Multiple physical symptoms (e.g., gastrointestinal irritability, genitourinary discomfort, muscle tension, sleep pattern disturbance)

Reactivated symptoms of previous conditions (e.g., physical/psychiatric illness); substance abuse

Long-Term Phase

Changes in lifestyle (e.g., changes in residence, dealing with repetitive nightmares and phobias, seeking family/social network support)

[c] Silent Reaction

Definition: Forced violent sexual penetration against the victim's will and consent; trauma syndrome that develops from this attack or attempted attack includes an acute phase of disorganization of the victim's lifestyle and a long-term process of reorganization of lifestyle

RELATED FACTORS

To be developed by nurse researchers and submitted to NANDA

DEFINING CHARACTERISTICS

Subjective

Increase in nightmares

Abrupt changes in relationships with men

Pronounced changes in sexual behavior

Objective

Increasing anxiety during interview (e.g., blocking of associations, long periods of silence; minor stuttering, physical distress)

No verbalization of the occurrence of rape

Sudden onset of phobic reactions

Sample Clinical Applications: Sexual assault, abuse

RAPE-TRAUMA SYNDROME [specify]

DESIRED OUTCOMES/EVALUATION CRITERIA
Sample NOC linkages:
Abuse Recovery: Physical: Extent of healing of physical injuries due to sexual abuse
Abuse Recovery: Emotional: Extent of healing of psychological injuries due to abuse
Coping: Personal actions to manage stressors that tax an individual's resources

Client Will (Include Specific Time Frame)

- Report absence of physical complications, pain, and discomfort.
- Deal appropriately with emotional reactions as evidenced by behavior and expression of feelings.
- Verbalize a positive self-image.
- Verbalize recognition that incident was not of own doing.
- Identify behaviors/situations within own control that may reduce risk of recurrence.
- Deal with practical aspects (e.g., court appearances).
- Demonstrate appropriate changes in lifestyle (e.g., change in job/residence) that contribute to recovery and seek/obtain support from SO(s), as needed.
- Interact with individuals/groups in desired and acceptable manner.

ACTIONS/INTERVENTIONS

Sample NIC linkages:
Rape-Trauma Treatment: Provision of emotional and physical support immediately following a reported rape
Crisis Intervention: Use of short-term counseling to help the patient cope with a crisis and resume a state of functioning comparable to or better than the precrisis state
Counseling: Use of an interactive helping process focusing on the needs, problems, or feelings of the patient and significant others to enhance or support coping, problem-solving, and interpersonal relationships

NURSING PRIORITY NO. I To assess trauma and individual reaction, noting length of time since occurrence of event:

- Observe for and elicit information about physical injury and assess stress-related symptoms such as numbness, headache, tightness in chest, nausea, pounding heart, and so forth. *Indicators of degree of/reaction to trauma experienced by the client, which may occur immediately and in the days or weeks following the attack.*[3,4]
- Identify psychological responses: anger, shock, acute anxiety, confusion, denial. Note laughter, crying, calm or agitated, excited (hysterical) behavior, expressions of disbelief or self-blame. *Victim may exhibit expressed response pattern (Compound reaction), displaying these feelings openly and freely as manifestations of experiencing the trauma of rape/sexual assault, and the accompanying feelings of fear of death, violation, powerlessness and helplessness. On the other hand, may exhibit controlled (Silent) response pattern with little or no emotion expressed. Any emotion is appropriate, as each person responds in own individual way; however, inappropriate behaviors/acting out may require intervention.*[1,4] (Refer to NDs risk for self/other-directed Violence.)
- Note silence, stuttering, inability to sit still. *May be signs of increasing anxiety, thus indicating need for further evaluation and intervention. Anxiety is suppressed and client does not talk about the trauma, resulting in an overwhelming emotional burden.*[1]

Cultural Collaborative Community/Home Care Diagnostic Studies Pediatric/Geriatric/Lifespan Medications

- Determine degree of disorganization. *Initially, the individual may be in shock and disbelief, which is a normal response to the incident. The person may respond by withdrawing and be unable to manage activities of daily living, especially when the incident was particularly brutal, requiring assistance and treatment to enable her or him to recover and move on.*[4]
- Identify whether incident has reactivated preexisting or coexisting situations (physical/psychological). *The presence of these factors can affect how the client views the current trauma. Previous traumatic incidents that have not been effectively resolved may compound the current incident.*[1]
- Ascertain cultural values/religious beliefs that may affect how client views incident, self, and expectations of SO/family reaction. *Client may believe incident will bring shame on the family, blame self, or that family will blame client, thus affecting client's ability to reach out to others for support.*[6]
- Determine disruptions in relationships with men and with others (e.g., family, friends, coworkers, SO[s]). *Many women find that they react to men in general in a different way, seeing them as reminders of the assault.*[1]
- Identify development of phobic reactions to ordinary articles (e.g., knives) and situations (e.g., walking in groups of people, strangers ringing doorbell). *These are manifestations of extreme anxiety, and client will need to continue treatment to learn how to manage feelings.*[4]
- Note degree of intrusive repetitive thoughts, sleep disturbances. *Survivor may notice disruptions in activities of daily living, reliving the attack, thoughts of recrimination, self-blame ("Why didn't I . . .?"), nightmares. Although these factors are distressing and upsetting, they are part of the normal healing process.*[4]
- Assess degree of dysfunctional coping. *Client may turn to use of alcohol, other drugs, suicidal/homicidal ideation, marked change in sexual behavior in an attempt to cope with traumatic event.*[4]

NURSING PRIORITY NO. 2   To assist client to deal with situation that exists:

- Explore own feelings (nurse/caregiver) regarding rape/incest issue prior to interacting with the client. *Since the feelings related to these incidents are so pervasive, the individual involved in caregiving needs to recognize own biases to prevent imposing them on the client.*[1]

Acute phase/immediate care
- Stay with the client/do not leave child unattended. Listen but do not probe. Tell client you are sorry this has happened and that she or he is safe now. *During this phase, the client experiences a complete disruption of life as she or he has known it, and presence of caregiver provides reassurance/sense of safety.*[2,4]
- Involve rape or sexual assault response team (SART), or sexual assault nurse examiner (SANE) when available. Provide same-sex examiner when appropriate. *Presence of the response team who has been trained to collect evidence appropriately and sensitively provides assurance to the survivor that she or he is being taken care of. Client may react to someone who is the sex of the attacker and use of a same-sex examiner communicates sensitivity to her or his feelings at this difficult time.*[4,7]
- Be sensitive to cultural factors that may affect specifics of examination process. *For example, some cultures do not allow women to be examined without a male family member being present. These issues need to be considered when treating the survivor.*[6]
- Evaluate infant/child/adolescent as dictated by age, gender, and developmental level. *Age of the survivor is an important consideration in deciding plan of care and appropriate interventions.*[4,8]
- Assist with documentation of incident for police/child-protective services reports, explaining each step of the procedure. Maintain sequencing and collection of evidence (chain of

evidence), label each specimen, and store/package properly. Be careful to use nonjudgmental language. *It is crucial to maintain chain of evidence to provide accurate information to law enforcement for potential legal proceedings when perpetrator is charged. Words can carry legal implications that may affect subsequent proceedings.*[1]

- Provide environment in which client can talk freely about feelings and fears. *Client needs to talk about the incident and concerns such as issues of relationship with/response of SO(s), pregnancy, sexually transmitted diseases so they may be dealt with in a positive manner.*[4]
- Provide information about emergency birth control and prophylactic treatment for STDs and assist with finding resources for follow-through. *Promotes client's peace of mind and opportunity to prevent these conditions.*[4,8]
- Provide psychological support by listening and remaining with client. If client does not want to talk, accept silence. *May indicate Silent Reaction to the occurrence in which the individual contains their emotions, using all their energy to maintain composure.*[4]
- Listen to/investigate physical complaints. Assist with medical treatments, as indicated. *Emotional reactions may limit client's ability to recognize physical injury.*[4]
- Assist with practical realities. *Client may be so emotionally distraught that she or he may not be able to attend to needs for such things as safe temporary housing, money, or other issues that may need to be addressed. Assistance helps individual maintain contact with reality.*[4,5]
- Determine client's ego strengths and help him or her use them in a positive way by acknowledging client's ability to handle what is happening. *Validation of belief that person can deal with what has happened and move forward with life promotes self-acceptance and helps client begin this process.*[4,9]
- Identify supportive persons for this individual. *Client needs to know she or he can go to a strong system of friends, family, or advocate who will respond with empathy.*[4]

Postacute phase

- Allow the client to work through own kind of adjustment. If client is withdrawn or unwilling to talk (Silent reaction), do not force the issue. *Individuals react in many ways to the traumatic event of rape, and no response is abnormal. Factors that influence how the survivor deals with the situation are personality, support system, existing life problems and prior sexual victimization, relationship with the offender, degree of violence used, social and cultural influences, and ability to cope with stress.*[2,4]
- Listen for expressions of fear of crowds, men, and so forth. *May reveal developing phobias needing evaluation and appropriate interventions, ongoing therapy.*[2,4]
- Discuss specific concerns/fears. Identify appropriate actions and provide information as indicated. *May need diagnostic testing for pregnancy, sexually transmitted diseases, or other resources. Meeting these needs and providing information will help client begin the process of recovery.*[4]
- Include written instructions that are concise and clear regarding medical treatments, crisis support services, and so on. Encourage return for follow-up. *Reinforces teaching, provides opportunity to deal with information at own pace. Follow-up appointment provides opportunity for determining how client is managing feelings and what needs may not have been met.*[4]

Long-term phase

- Continue listening to expressions of concern. Note persistence of somatic complaints, (e.g., nausea, anorexia, insomnia, muscle tension, headache). *May need to continue to talk about the assault. Repeating the story helps client to move on, but continued somatic concerns may indicate developing PTSD.*[4,8]
- Permit free expression of feelings (may continue from the crisis phase). Refrain from rushing client through expressions of feelings too quickly and avoid reassuring inappropriately. *Client may believe pain and/or anguish is misunderstood and depression may limit responses.*[1]

- Acknowledge reality of loss of self that existed before the incident. Assist client to move toward an acceptance of the potential for growth that exists within individual. *Following this traumatic event, the individual will not be able to go back to the person they were before. Life will always have the memory of what happened, and client needs to accept that reality and move on in the best way possible.*[2]

- Continue to allow client to progress at own pace. *The process of grieving is a very individual one, and each person needs to know that she or he can take whatever time needed to resolve her or his feelings and move on with life.*[4] (Refer to ND Grieving for additional interventions.)

- Give "permission" to express/deal with anger at the perpetrator/situation in acceptable ways. Set limits on destructive behaviors. *Facilitates resolution of feelings without diminishing self-concept.*[5]

- Keep discussion on practical and emotional level rather than intellectualizing the experience. *When the person talks about the incident intellectually, instead of identifying and talking about feelings, client avoids dealing with the feelings, thus inhibiting recovery.*[1]

- Assist in dealing with ongoing concerns about and effects of the incident, such as court appearance, sexually transmitted disease, relationship with SO(s), and so forth. *Depending on degree of disorganization, client will need help to deal with these practical and emotional issues.*[4]

- Provide for sensitive, trained counselors, considering individual needs. *Male/female counselors may be best determined on an individual basis, as counselor's gender may be an issue for some clients, affecting ability to disclose and deal with feelings.*[1]

NURSING PRIORITY NO. 3 To promote wellness (Teaching/Discharge Considerations):

- Provide information about what reactions client may expect during each phase. Let client know these are common reactions and phrase in neutral terms of "You may or may not . . ." *Be aware that, although male rape perpetrators are usually heterosexual, the male victim may be concerned about his own sexuality and may exhibit a homophobic response. Such information helps client anticipate and deal with reactions if they are experienced.*[1]

- Assist client to identify factors that may have created a vulnerable situation and that she or he may have power to change to protect self in the future. *While client needs to be assured that she or he is not to blame for incident, the circumstances of the incident need to be assessed to identify factors that are within the individual's control to avoid a similar incident occurring.*[4]

- Avoid making value judgments. *The survivor is usually blaming self about the incident and agonizing over the circumstances; therefore, nonjudgmental language is very important to help the person accept that the fault is not hers or his.*[1]

- Discuss lifestyle changes client is contemplating and how they will contribute to recovery. *Helps client evaluate appropriateness of plans. In the anxiety of the moment, the individual may believe that changing residence, job, or other aspects of her or his environment will be healing. In reality, these changes may not help and may make matters worse.*[4]

- Encourage psychiatric consultation if client is violent, inconsolable, or does not seem to be making an adjustment. Participation in a group may be helpful. *May need intensive professional help to come to terms with the assault.*[1]

- Refer to family/marital counseling, as indicated. *When relationships with family members are affected by the incident, counseling may be needed to resolve the issues.*[1,9]

- Refer to NDs Anxiety, ineffective Coping, Fear, complicated Grieving, and Powerlessness, as appropriate.

DOCUMENTATION FOCUS

Assessment/Reassessment

- Individual findings, including nature of incident, individual reactions/fears, degree of trauma (physical/emotional), effects on lifestyle.
- Cultural/religious factors.
- Reactions of family/SO(s).
- Samples gathered for evidence and disposition/storage (chain of evidence).

Planning

- Plan of action and who is involved in planning.
- Teaching plan.

Implementation/Evaluation

- Responses to interventions/teaching and actions performed.
- Attainment/progress toward desired outcome(s).
- Modifications to plan of care.

Discharge Planning

- Long-term needs and who is responsible for actions to be taken.
- Specific referrals made.

References

1. Townsend, M. C. (2003). *Psychiatric Mental Health Nursing Concepts of Care.* 4th ed. Philadelphia: F. A. Davis.
2. Dealing with Rape—Rape Trauma Syndrome. Available at www.rapecrisis.org.za/dealing/trauma.htm. Accessed January 2004.
3. Cox, H. C., et al. (2002). *Clinical Applications of Nursing Diagnosis: Adult, Child, Women's, Psychiatric, Gerontic, and Home Health Considerations.* 4th ed. Philadelphia: F. A. Davis.
4. Rape Trauma Syndrome. Accessed August 2007 at www.rapevictimadvocates.org/trauma.html.
5. Doenges, M. E., Moorhouse, M. F., Geissler-Murr, A. C. (2004). *Nurses' Pocket Guide, Diagnoses, Interventions, and Rationales.* 9th ed. Philadelphia: F. A. Davis.
6. Lipson, J., Dibble, S., Minarik, P. (1996). *Culture & Nursing Care: A Pocket Guide.* San Francisco: UCSF Nursing Press.
7. Menna, A. Rape Trauma Syndrome; The Journey to Healing Belongs to Everyone. Retrieved August 2007 at www.giftfromwithin.org/html/journey.html.
8. The Rape, Abuse, & Incest National Network (RAINN). Prevention section. Retrieved August 2007 at www.rainn.org/get-information/index.html.
9. Lauer, T. Rape Trauma. American Association for Marriage and Family Therapy. Retrieved August 2007 at www.aamft.org/families/Consumer_Updates/RapeTrauma.asp.

impaired Religiosity

Definition: Impaired ability to exercise reliance on beliefs or participate in rituals of a particular faith tradition

[NANDA] recognizes that the term "religiosity" may be culture-specific; however, the term is useful in the United States and is well supported in the U.S. literature.

RELATED FACTORS

Developmental and Situational

Life transitons; aging; end-stage life crises

Cultural   Collaborative   Community/Home Care   Diagnostic Studies   Pediatric/Geriatric/Lifespan   Medications

Physical
Illness; pain

Psychological Factors
Ineffective support/coping
Anxiety; fear of death
Personal crisis [/disaster]; lack of security
Use of religion to manipulate

Sociocultural
Cultural/environmental barriers to practicing religion
Lack of social integration/sociocultural interaction

Spiritual
Spiritual crises; suffering

DEFINING CHARACTERISTICS

Subjective
Expresses emotional distress because of separation from faith community
Expresses a need to reconnect with previous belief patterns/customs
Questions religious belief patterns/customs
Has difficulty adhering to prescribed religious beliefs and rituals (e.g., religious cere-
monies, dietary regulations, clothing, prayer, worship/religious services, private reli-
gious behaviors/reading religious materials/media, holiday observances, meetings with
religious leaders)

Sample Clinical Applications: Any acute or chronic condition, palliative care, end-of-life

DESIRED OUTCOMES/EVALUATION CRITERIA
Sample NOC linkages:
Spiritual Health: Connectedness with self, others, higher power, all life, nature, and the uni-
verse that transcends and empowers the self

Client Will (Include Specific Time Frame)

- Express ability to once again participate in beliefs and rituals of desired religion.
- Discuss beliefs/values about spiritual/religious issues.
- Attend religious/worship services of choice, as desired.
- Verbalize concerns about end-of-life issues and fear of death.

ACTIONS/INTERVENTIONS

Sample NIC linkages:
Spiritual Growth Facilitation: Facilitation of growth in patient's capacity to identify,
connect with, and call upon the source of meaning, purpose, comfort, and hope in his or
her life
Spiritual Support: Assisting the patient feel balance and connection with a greater power

NURSING PRIORITY NO. 1 To assess causative/contributing factors:

- Determine client's usual religious/spiritual beliefs, values, past spiritual commitment. *Provides a baseline for understanding current problem.* [5]
- Note client's/SO's reports and expressions of anger/concern, alienation from God, sense of guilt or retribution. *Perception of guilt may cause spiritual crisis/suffering resulting in rejection of religious symbols, anger toward God.* [6]
- Determine sense of futility, feelings of hopelessness, lack of motivation to help self. *Indicators that client may see no, or only limited, options/alternatives or personal choices, and treatment needs to be directed at finding what has happened in client's life to bring about these feelings.* [5]
- Assess extent of depression client may be experiencing. *Some studies suggest that a focus on religion may protect against depression.* [7]
- Note recent changes in behavior (e.g., withdrawal from others/religious activities, dependence on alcohol or medications). *Lack of connectedness with self/others impairs ability to trust others or feel worthy of trust from others/God.* [6,7]
- Identify cultural values/expectations regarding religious beliefs or practices. *Individuals grow up in a family that instills a value system within them. As the person grows up, ideas/values/expectations may change or be strengthened by new information, different questioning, and alternative viewpoints, which may affect current situation.* [3]
- Note socioeconomic status of individual/family. *Women who are poor may have high levels of personal religiosity, yet participate less in organized religion because they may feel stigmatized by their situation (e.g., single mothers, those receiving public assistance, or those engaging in a lifestyle that conflicts with church norms).* [2]

NURSING PRIORITY NO. 2 To assist client/SOs to deal with feelings/situation:

- Use therapeutic communication skills of reflection and Active-listening. *Communicates acceptance and enables client to find own solutions to concerns as situation is discussed and deeper meanings are discovered.* [4]
- Encourage expression of feelings about illness/condition, death. *As people age, they become more concerned about their own mortality, and others often see them as in poor health and as spiritual and religious. If they have been diagnosed with a terminal illness, they may be feeling more angry and rejecting of God than seeking his help.* [5,8]
- Discuss personal beliefs that may hinder participation in religious activities. *Provides opportunity for self-reflection, such as own worthiness and ability to forgive self for past decisions/life choices.*
- Discuss differences between grief and guilt and help client to identify and deal with each. Point out consequences of actions based on guilt. *Individuals often feel guilty about the "what if's" of life. "If only I had done this!" "If only I had paid more attention!" "If only I had made him go to the doctor!" Most of these guilty feelings are not based on reality and, when they are acted on, the individual does not get the release he or she seeks.* [5]
- Suggest use of journaling/reminiscence. *Promotes life review and can assist in clarifying values/ideas, recognizing and resolving feelings/situation.* [4]
- Encourage client to identify individuals who can provide needed support (e.g., spiritual advisor, parish nurse). *When client is seeking to restore reliance on religious beliefs, these providers can often be helpful.* [6]
- Review client's religious affiliation, associated rituals, and beliefs. *Helps client examine what has been important in the past and may trigger some desire to reconnect with these previous beliefs.* [6]

- Provide opportunity for nonjudgmental discussion of philosophical issues related to religious belief patterns and customs. *Open communication can assist client to check reality of perceptions and identify personal options and willingness to resume desired activities.*[1]
- Discuss desire to continue/reconnect with previous belief patterns and customs and perceived barriers. *As client begins to think about current feelings of alienation from previous religious connections, these discussions can help to clarify and allow client to think about how these beliefs can be regained.*[5]
- Identify ways to strengthen spiritual/religious expression. *There are multiple options for enhancing participation in faith community (e.g., joining womens/mens group or prayer/study group, volunteering time to community projects, singing in the choir, reading spiritual writings).*
- Involve client in refining heathcare goals and therapeutic regimen, as appropriate. *Identifies role illness/condition is playing in current concerns about ability to/appropriateness of participating in desired religious activities.*[7]

NURSING PRIORITY NO. 3 To promote wellness (Teaching/Discharge Considerations):

- Help client identify spiritual counselor who could be helpful (e.g., minister, priest, spiritual advisor who has qualifications/experience) in dealing with specific concerns of client. *Provides answers to spiritual questions, assists in the journey of self-discovery, and can help client learn to accept/forgive self.*[6]
- Provide privacy for meditation/prayer, performance of rituals, as appropriate. *Many individuals prefer to pray/meditate in private so they can concentrate without interruption or questions from others.*
- Explore alternatives/modifications of ritual based on setting and individual needs/limitations. *Individual may not be able to go to a church or temple, so providing another setting—chapel in the hospital or quiet room with appropriate religious artifacts/material—can provide the setting desired.*[6]
- Provide bibliotherapy, list of relevant resources/Web sites *for later reference/self-paced learning and ongoing support.*[4]

DOCUMENTATION FOCUS

Assessment/Reassessment

- Individual findings, including nature of spiritual conflict, effects of participation in treatment regimen.
- Physical/emotional responses to conflict.

Planning

- Plan of care and who is involved in planning.
- Teaching plan.

Implementation/Evaluation

- Responses to interventions/teaching and actions performed.
- Attainment/progress toward desired outcomes(s).
- Modifications to plan of care.

Discharge Planning

- Long-term needs and who is responsible for actions to be taken.
- Available resources, specific referrals made.

References

1. Burkhardt, L. (2005). A click away: Documenting spiritual care. *JCN*, 22(1), 6–12. Retrieved August 2007 at http://ncf.intervarsity.org/jcn/archive/05wi/lb612.pdf.
2. Sullivan, S. (2006). Faith and Poverty: Personal Religiosity and Organized Religion in the Lives of Low-Income Urban Mothers. Retrieved August 2007 at www.bc.edu/bc_org/research/rapl/events/abstract_sullivan.html.
3. Lipson, J. G., Dibble, S. L., Minarik, P. A. (1999) *Culture & Nursing Care: A Pocket Guide.* San Francisco: School of Nursing, UCSF Nursing Press.
4. Townsend, M. (2006). Psychiatric Mental Health Nursing Concepts of Care. 5th ed. Philadelphia: F. A. Davis.
5. Doenges, M., Moorhouse, M., Murr, A. (2006). *Nursing Care Plans, Guidelines for Individualizing Patient Care.* 7th ed. Philadelphia: F. A. Davis.
6. Doenges, M., Moorhouse, M., Murr, A. (2008). *Nurse's Pocket Guide: Diagnoses, Prioritized Interventions, and Rationales.* 11th ed. Philadelphia: F. A. Davis.
7. Murray-Swank, A., et al. (2006). Religiosity, Psychosocial Adjustment, and Subjective Burden of Persons Who Care for Those with Mental Illness. Psychiatric Services, American Psychiatric Association: Arlington, VA.
8. Mills, J. (2006). The Ontology of Religiosity: The Oceanic Feeling and the Value of the Lived Experience. Huumanists. Retrieved April 2007 at www.huumanists.org/rh/mills.html.

readiness for enhanced Religiosity

Definition: Ability to increase reliance on religious beliefs or participate in rituals of a particular faith tradition

[NANDA] recognizes that the term "religiosity" may be culture-specific; however, the term is useful in the United States and is well supported in the U.S. literature.

RELATED FACTORS
To be developed by nurse researchers and submitted to NANDA

DEFINING CHARACTERISTICS

Subjective
Expresses desire to strengthen religious belief patterns/customs that had provided comfort/religion in the past

Requests assistance to increase participation in prescribed religious beliefs (e.g., religious ceremonies, dietary regulations/rituals, clothing, prayer, worship/religious services, private religious behaviors, reading religious materials/media, holiday observances)

Requests assistance to expand religious options/religious materials/experiences

Requests meeting with religious leaders/facilitators

Requests forgiveness/reconciliation

Questions/rejects belief patterns/customs that are harmful

Sample Clinical Applications: As a health-seeking behavior, the client/family may be healthy or this diagnosis can be associated with any clinical condition

DESIRED OUTCOMES/EVALUATION CRITERIA
Sample NOC linkages:

Spiritual Health: Connectedness with self, others, higher power, all life, nature, and the universe that transcends and empowers the self

Client Will (Include Specific Time Frame)

- Acknowledge need to strengthen religious affiliations and continue/resume previously comforting rituals.

Cultural Collaborative Community/Home Care Diagnostic Studies Pediatric/Geriatric/Lifespan Medications

- Verbalize willingness to seek help to enhance desired religious beliefs.
- Become involved in spiritually based programs of own choice.
- Recognize the difference between belief patterns and customs that are helpful and those that may be harmful.

ACTIONS/INTERVENTIONS

Sample NIC linkages:

Spiritual Growth Facilitation: Facilitation of growth in patient's capacity to identify, connect with, and call upon the source of meaning, purpose, comfort, and hope in his or her life

Spiritual Support: Assisting the patient to feel balance and connection with a greater power

NURSING PRIORITY NO. 1 To determine spiritual state/motivation for growth:

- Determine client's current thinking about desire to learn more about religious beliefs and actions.
- Ascertain religious beliefs/cultural values of family of origin and climate in which client grew up. *Early religious training deeply affects children and is carried on into adulthood. Conflict between family's beliefs and client's current learning may need to be addressed.*[7]
- Identify cultural values/expectations regarding religious beliefs and/or practices. *Individuals grow up in a family that instills a value system within them. As the person grows up, ideas/values/expectations may change or be strengthened by new information, different questioning, and alternative viewpoints.*[3]
- Note socioeconomic status of individual/family. *Women who are poor may have high levels of personal religiosity, yet participate less in organized religion because they may feel stigmatized by their situation (e.g., single mothers, those receiving public assistance, or those engaging in a lifestyle that conflicts with church norms).*[2]
- Discuss client's spiritual commitment, beliefs, and values. *Enables examination of these issues and helps client learn more about self and what he or she desires/believes.*[7]
- Explore how spirituality/religious practices have affected client's life. *Some philosophers believe that the value of religiosity is the deepened sense of quality of life associated with practicing one's beliefs/tenets.*[8]
- Ascertain motivation and expectations for change. *The client's motivation needs to be for self and not for others, and client needs to understand own expectations to move forward with desire to improve status.*[4]

NURSING PRIORITY NO. 2 To assist client to integrate values and beliefs to strengthen sense of wholeness and achieve optimum balance in daily living:

- Establish nurse-client relationship in which dialogue can occur. *Client can feel safe in this relationship to say anything and know it will be accepted.*[5]
- Identify barriers and beliefs that may hinder growth or self-discovery. *Provides opportunity for self-reflection such as own worthiness and ability to forgive self for past decisions/life choices. Previous practices and beliefs may need to be considered and accepted or discarded in new search for religious beliefs.*[8]
- Discuss cultural beliefs of family of origin and how they have influenced client's religious practices. *As client expands options for learning new/other religious beliefs and practices, these influences will provide information for comparing/contrasting new information.*[7]

🏠 • Explore connection of desire to strengthen belief patterns and customs to daily life. *Becoming aware of how these issues affect the individual's daily life can enhance ability to incorporate them into everything he or she does.*[1]

🏠 • Identify ways in which individual can develop a sense of harmony with self and others. *Client may have some new beliefs that may or may not be shared with others, and discussing these can clarify understanding by each individual.*[1]

NURSING PRIORITY NO. 3 To enhance optimum wellness:

🏠 • Encourage client to seek out and experience different religious beliefs, services, and ceremonies, as desired. *Trying out different religions will give client more information to contrast and compare what will fit his or her belief system.*[6]

🏠 • Provide bibliotherapy/reading materials pertaining to spiritual issues. *Client may be interested in learning about new spiritual ideas and finding resources that clarify thinking will help to develop own beliefs.*[4]

🏠 • Encourage client to engage in stress-reducing activities, such as meditation, relaxation exercises, or Mindfulness (method of being in the moment). *Promotes general well-being and sense of control over self and ability to choose desired religious activities.*[5]

🏠 • Encourage participation in religious activities, worship/religious services, reading religious materials/media, prayer/study groups, volunteering in church choir, or other needed duties. *Enhances client's knowledge and promotes connectedness with self/others/higher power.*[4]

⊛ • Refer to community resources (e.g., parish nurse, religion classes, other support groups).

DOCUMENTATION FOCUS

Assessment/Reassessment

• Assessment findings, including client perception of needs and desire/expectations for growth/enhancement.
• Motivation/expectations for change.

Planning

• Plan for growth and who is involved in planning.

Implementation/Evaluation

• Response to activities/learning and actions performed.
• Attainment/progress toward desired outcome(s).
• Modifications to plan.

Discharge Planning

• Long-range needs/expectations and plan of action.
• Specific referrals made.

References

1. Burkhardt, L. (2005). A click away: Documenting spiritual care. *JCN*, 22(1), 6–12. Retrieved August 2007 at http://ncf.intervarsity.org/jcn/archive/05wi/lb612.pdf.
2. Sullivan, S. (2006). Faith and Poverty: Personal Religiosity and Organized Religion in the Lives of Low-Income Urban Mothers. Retrieved August 2007 www.bc.edu/bc_org/research/rapl/events/abstract_sullivan.html.

3. Lipson, J. G., Dibble, S. L., Minarik, P. A. (1999). *Culture & Nursing Care: A Pocket Guide*. San Francisco: School of Nursing, UCSF Nursing Press.
4. Townsend, M. (2006). *Psychiatric Mental Health Nursing Concepts of Care*. 5th ed. Philadelphia: F. A. Davis.
5. Doenges, M., Moorhouse, M., Murr, A. (2006). *Nursing Care Plans, Guidelines for Individualizing Patient Care*. 7th ed. Philadelphia: F. A. Davis.
6. Doenges, M., Moorhouse, M., Murr, A. (2008). *Nurse's Pocket Guide Diagnoses, Prioritized Interventions, and Rationales*. 11th ed. Philadelphia: F. A. Davis.
7. Murray-Swank, A., et al. (2006). Religiosity, Psychosocial Adjustment, and Subjective Burden of Persons Who Care for Those with Mental Illness. Psychiatric Services, American Psychiatric Association: Arlington, VA.
8. Mills, J. (2006). The Ontology of Religiosity: The Oceanic Feeling and the Value of the Lived Experience. Huumanists. Retrieved April 2007 at www.huumanists.org/rh/mills.html.

risk for impaired Religiosity

Definition: At risk for an impaired ability to exercise reliance on religious beliefs and/or participate in rituals of a particular faith tradition

[NANDA] recognizes that the term "religiosity" may be culture-specific; however, the term is useful in the United States and is well-supported in the U.S. literature.

RISK FACTORS

Developmental
Life transitions

Environmental
Lack of transportation
Barriers to practicing religion

Physical
Illness; hospitalization; pain

Psychological
Ineffective support/coping/caregiving
Depression
Lack of security

Sociocultural
Lack of social interaction; social isolation
Cultural barrier to practicing religion

Spiritual
Suffering

NOTE: A risk diagnosis is not evidenced by signs and symptoms, as the problem has not occurred; rather, nursing interventions are directed at prevention.

Sample Clinical Applications: Any acute or chronic condition, palliative care, end-of-life

DESIRED OUTCOMES/EVALUATION CRITERIA
Sample NOC linkages:
Spiritual Health: Connectedness with self, others, higher power, all life, nature, and the universe that transcends and empowers the self

Client Will (Include Specific Time Frame)

- Express understanding of relation of situation/health status to thoughts and feelings of concern about ability to participate in desired religious activities.
- Seek solutions to individual factors that may interfere with reliance on religious beliefs/ participation in religious rituals.
- Identify and use resources appropriately.

ACTIONS/INTERVENTIONS

Sample NIC linkages:

Spiritual Growth Facilitation: Facilitation of growth in patient's capacity to identify, connect with, and call upon the source of meaning, purpose, comfort, and hope in his or her life

Spiritual Support: Assisting the patient to feel balance and connection with a greater power

NURSING PRIORITY NO. 1 To assess causative/contributing factor:

- Ascertain current situation (e.g., illness, hospitalization, prognosis of death, depression, lack of support systems, financial concerns). *Identifies problems client is dealing with in the moment that may be affecting desire to be involved with religious activities.*[1]
- Note client's concerns/expressions of anger, belief that illness/condition is result of lack of faith. *Individual may blame own self for what has happened and could reject religious beliefs and/or God.*[6]
- Determine client's usual religious/spiritual beliefs, past or current involvement in specific church activities. *Provides an understanding of how client saw religion in own life before current disruption.*[1]
- Identify cultural values/expectations regarding religious beliefs and/or practices. *Individuals grow up in a family that instills a value system within them. As the person grows up, ideas/values/expectations may change or be strengthened by new information, different questioning, and alternative viewpoints, which may affect current situation.*[3]
- Note quality of relationships with significant others and friends. *Individual may withdraw from others in relation to the stress of illness, pain, and suffering. Others may be encouraging client to rely on religious beliefs at a time when individual is questioning own beliefs in the current situaion.*[1]
- Note socioeconomic status of individual/family. *Women who are poor may have high levels of personal religiosity, yet participate less in organized religion because they may feel stigmatized by their situation (e.g., single mothers, those receiving public assistance, or those engaging in a lifestyle that conflicts with church norms).*[2]
- Assess lack of transportation/environmental barriers to participation in desired religious activities. *These barriers can be realistic in the face of such issues as poor bus systems, inability of individual to get to bus stop (physical problems of walking or distance to the bus stop), or inablility to drive a car.*[2]
- Ascertain substance use/abuse. *Individuals often turn to use of various substances in distress, and this can affect the ability to deal with problems in a positive manner.*[7]

NURSING PRIORITY NO. 2 To assist client to deal with feelings/situation:

- Develop nurse-client relationship. *Individual can express feelings and concerns freely when he or she feels safe to do so.*[5]

- Discuss personal beliefs that may hinder participation in religious activities. *Provides opportunity for self-reflection such as own worthiness and ability to forgive self for past decisions/life choices.*
- Use therapeutic communication skills of Active-listening, reflection, and I-messages. *Helps client to find own solutions to problems/concerns and promotes sense of control.*[4]
- Have client identify and prioritize current/immediate needs. *Dealing with current needs is easier than trying to predict the future. Also, it is important to take care of basic needs before moving on to higher needs.*[4]
- Provide time for nonjudgmental discussion of individual's spiritual beliefs and fears about impact of current illness and/or treatment regimen. *Helps to clarify thoughts and promote ability to deal with stresses of what is happening.*[6]
- Review with client past difficulties in life and coping skills that were used at that time. *Recalling problems with family/bosses can help client to remember how those were handled and how those skills could be used in current situation.*
- Encourage client to discuss feelings about death and end-of-life issues when illness/prognosis is grave. *People are often afraid to talk about the possibility of their own death for fear it will bring reality to self and upset family.*[1]

NURSING PRIORITY NO. 3 To promote wellness (Teaching/Discharge Considerations):

- Have client identify support systems available. *Individual will usually know who can provide the best support for him or her in present situation. Family may not be the most supportive if they don't want to accept the reality of client's illness/situation.*[5]
- Help client learn relaxation techniques, meditation, guided imagery, and Mindfulness (living in the moment and enjoying it). *Learning to relax can help client to process information and make decisions in a more positive manner.*[4]
- Take the lead from the client in initiating participation in religious activities, prayer, other activities. *Client may be vulnerable in current situation and needs to be allowed to decide own participation in these actions. Living and participating in desired religious activities will help client to understand the tenets of his or her choice.*[8]
- Refer to appropriate resources such as crisis counselor, governmental agencies, spiritual advisor (who has qualifications/experience dealing with specific problems such as death/dying, relationship problems, substance abuse, suicide), hospice, psychotherapy, Alcoholics/Narcotics Anonymous. *May need additional help to deal with current situation.*[4,6,7]

DOCUMENTATION FOCUS

Assessment/Reassessment

- Individual findings, including risk factors, nature of current distress.
- Physical/emotional response to distress.
- Access to/use of resources.

Planning

- Plan of care and who is involved in planning.
- Teaching plan.

Implementation/Evaluation

- Responses to interventions/teaching and actions performed.
- Attainment/progress toward desired outcome(s).
- Modifications to plan of care.

Discharge Planning

- Long-term needs and who is responsible for actions to be taken.
- Available resources, specific referrals made.

References

1. Burkhardt, L. A Click Away: Documenting Spiritual Care. Available at http://ncf.intervarsity.org/jcn/archive/05wi/lb612.pdf.
2. Sullivan, S. Faith and Poverty: Personal Religiosity and Organized Religion in the Lives of Low-Income Urban Mothers. Available at www.bc.edu/bc_org/research/rapl/events/abstract_sullivan.html.
3. Lipson, J. G., Dibble, S. L., Minarik, P. A. (1999). *Culture & Nursing Care: A Pocket Guide.* San Francisco: School of Nursing, UCSF Nursing Press.
4. Townsend, M. (2006). *Psychiatric Mental Health Nursing Concepts of Care.* 5th ed. Philadelphia: F. A. Davis.
5. Doenges, M., Moorhouse, M., Murr, A. (2006). *Nursing Care Plans, Guidelines for Individualizing Patient Care.* 7th ed. Philadelphia: F. A. Davis.
6. Doenges, M., Moorhouse, M., Murr, A. (2008). *Nurse's Pocket Guide Diagnoses, Prioritized Interventions, and Rationales.* 11th ed. Philadelphia: F. A. Davis.
7. Murray-Swank, A., et al. (2006). Religiosity, Psychosocial Adjustment, and Subjective Burden of Persons Who Care for Those with Mental Illness. Psychiatric Services, American Psychiatric Association: Arlington, VA.
8. Mills, J. (2006). The Ontology of Religiosity: The Oceanic Feeling and the Value of the Lived Experience. Huumanists. Retrieved April 2007 at www.huumanists.org/rh/mills.html.

Relocation Stress Syndrome

Definition: Physiological and/or psychosocial disturbance following transfer from one environment to another

RELATED FACTORS

Losses; feeling of powerlessness

Lack of adequate support system; lack of predeparture counseling; unpredictability of experience

Isolation; language barrier

Impaired psychosocial health; passive coping

Decreased health status

DEFINING CHARACTERISTICS

Subjective

Anxiety (e.g., separation); anger

Insecurity; worry; fear

Loneliness; depression

Unwillingness to move; concern over relocation

Sleep disturbance

Objective

Move from one environment to another

Increased [frequency of] verbalization of needs

Pessimism; frustration

Increased physical symptoms/illness

Withdrawal; aloneness; alienation; [hostile behavior/outbursts]

Loss of identity/self-worth/self-esteem; dependency

[Increased confusion/cognitive impairment]

Cultural   Collaborative   Community/Home Care   Diagnostic Studies   Pediatric/Geriatric/Lifespan   Medications

Sample Clinical Applications: Chronic conditions (e.g., MS, asthma, cystic fibrosis), brain injury/stroke, dementia, schizophrenia, developmental delay, end-of-life/hospice care

DESIRED OUTCOMES/EVALUATION CRITERIA

Sample NOC linkages:

Psychosocial Adjustment: Life Change: Adaptation psychosocial response of an individual to a significant life change

Quality of Life: Extent of positive perception of current life circumstances

Coping: Personal actions to manage stressors that tax an individual's resources

Client Will (Include Specific Time Frame)

- Verbalize understanding of reason(s) for change.
- Demonstrate appropriate range of feelings and lessened fear.
- Participate in routine and special/social events, as able.
- Verbalize acceptance of situation.
- Experience no catastrophic event.

ACTIONS/INTERVENTIONS

Sample NIC linkages:

Coping Enhancement: Assisting a patient to adapt to perceived stressors, changes, or threats that interfere with meeting life demands and roles

Hope Instillation: Facilitation of the development of a positive outlook in a given situation

Family Involvement Promotion: Facilitating family participation in the emotional and physical care of the patient

NURSING PRIORITY NO. 1 To assess degree of stress as perceived/experienced by client and determine issues of safety:

- Determine situation/cause for relocation (e.g., planned move for new job; change in marital status; loss of home/community due to natural or manmade disaster; deterioration in health status/ability to care for self; caregiver burnout; elderly parent being requested to move closer to adult child). *Although nursing research has not currently validated the defining characteristics of relocation stress syndrome as a nursing diagnosis,[1,11] the belief that stress associated with relocation can be extreme is widely accepted in society. The effects of relocation can be minimal and transient, or very troubling and persistent.[2]*
- Note client's age, developmental level, role in family. *Age and position in life cycle makes a difference in the impact of issues involved in relocating. For example, children can be traumatized by transfer to new school, loss of friends and familiar surroundings[3] elderly persons may be affected by loss of their long-term home with its memories, neighborhood setting, and support persons.[12,13]*
- Identify cultural or religious concerns that may affect client's coping or impact social interactions, expectations. *Cultural norm may be that elders are cared for by family—not placed in a facility—causing client to feel abandoned; or individual may be required to defer to family decision maker and feel powerless in determining own destiny.[2,12,13]*
- Note ethnic ties/primary language spoken and read. *During times of stress, individuals may lapse into language of childhood. This affects healthcare providers who must try to reduce the client's feelings of alienation/confusion while communicating with client of another primary language, or client who is displaced from cultural attachments.[6]*

- Ascertain if client participated in the decision to relocate and perceptions about change(s), expectations for the future. *A forced relocation is much more stressful than one that is desired.*[4] *Client may be concerned that temporary placement will deplete savings or be fearful of being a burden on family members.*

- Determine involvement of family/SO(s). Note availability/use of support systems and resources. Ascertain presence/absence of comprehensive information and planning (e.g., when/how move took place, if the environment for the client is similar or greatly changed, etc.). *These factors can greatly affect client's ability to adjust to change.*[4]

- Note signs of increased stress in client recently relocated: *Client may report/demonstrate irritability, withdrawal, crying, moodiness, problems sleeping, or fatigue; "new" physical discomfort/pain (e.g., stomaches, headaches, back pain); change in appetite, increased use of alcohol/other drugs, or greater susceptablilty to colds.*[2,5,12,13]

- Observe behavior, noting presence of increasing anxiety, suspiciousness/paranoia, defensiveness. Compare with SO's/staff's description of customary responses. *Relocation may temporarily exacerbate mental deterioration (cognitive inaccessibility) and impair communication (social inaccessibility).*

- Identify issues of safety that may be involved, such as difficulty adjusting to new environment (e.g., navigating streets/choosing correct bus; locating dining hall/bathroom in facility), concerns of elopement/running away.

NURSING PRIORITY NO. 2 To assist client to deal with situation/changes:

- Collaborate in treatment of underlying conditions (e.g., chronic confusional states, brain injury, posttrauma rehabilitation, etc.) and physical stress symptoms *that are potentially exacerbating relocation stress or that may affect the length of time that relocation is required.*

- Encourage free expression of feelings about reason for relocation, including venting of anger, grief, loss of personal space/belongings/friends, financial strains, powerlessness, and so forth. Acknowledge reality of situation and maintain hopeful attitude regarding move/change. *Bringing feelings out into the open helps clarify emotion and make feelings easier to deal with.*[10,14] Refer to NDs relating to client's particular situation (e.g., impaired Adjustment, ineffective Coping, Grieving, etc.) for additional interventions

- Anticipate variety of emotions and reactions. *May vary from insomnia and loss of appetite to becoming involved with alcohol/other drugs, or exacerbation of health problems/onset of serious illness or behavioral problems.*[8]

- Identify strengths/successful coping behaviors the individual has used previously. *Incorporating these into problem-solving builds on past successes.*

- Encourage client to maintain contact with friends (e.g., telephone, letters, e-mail, video/audio tapes, arranged visits) *to reduce sense of isolation.*[9]

- Provide client with information/list of organizations/community services (Welcome Wagon, senior citizens or teen clubs, churches, singles' groups, sports leagues, etc.) *to provide contacts for client to develop new relationships and learn more about the new setting.*[10]

- Obtain interpreter (where language differences exist) *to exchange information with the client/SO regarding residence/relocation wishes and to make helpful referrals.*[6]

- Suggest/refer to professionals (e.g., social worker, financial resources, mental healthcare provider, minister/spiritual advisor) if serious difficulties develop (e.g., depression, alcohol/drug abuse, deteriorating behavior of children) *if client has special needs and/or persistent problems with adaptation.*[5,15]

- Take practical steps to alleviate stress for child. Encourage parents to walk with child to school/rehearse boarding the school bus, visit new classroom, contact friends child left behind, drive past places of interest to child, find a safe play place, unpack child's favorite toys, invite neighborhood children to a get-acquainted party, etc. *Helps child to maintain ties and develop new ones, thus reducing sense of loss and shifting focus to the future.*[3]

- Facilitate client's adjustment to new environment/facility:[4,7,9,13,16]

Determine client's usual schedule of activities and incorporate into facility routine, as possible. *Reinforces sense of importance of individual.*

Orient to surroundings/schedules and repeat directions, as needed.

Introduce to new staff members, roommate/residents.

Provide clear, honest information about actions/events.

Provide consistency in daily routine; maintain same staff with client in new facility, as possible, during adjustment phase.

Address ways to preserve lifestyle (e.g., usual bath/bedtimes in new facility, involvement in church activities). *Helps reduce the sense of loss associated with move.*

Encourage individual/family to personalize area with pictures, own belongings, and the like as soon as possible. *Enhances sense of belonging, self-expression, and creation of personal space.*

Introduce socialization and diversional activities, such as meals with new acquantainces, art therapy, music, movies, etc. *Involvement increases opportunity to interact with others/form new friendships, thus decreasing isolation and stress reactions.*

Encourage hugging and use of touch unless client is paranoid or agitated at the moment. *Human connection reaffirms acceptance of individual.*

Place in private room, if appropriate, and include SO(s)/family in care activities, mealtime, etc. *Keeping client secluded may be needed under some circumstances (e.g., advanced Alzheimer's disease with fear or aggressive reactions) to decrease the client's stress reactions to new environment.*

Deal with aggressive behavior by imposing calm, firm limits. Control environment and protect others from client's disruptive behavior. *Promotes safety for client/others.*

Remain calm, place in a quiet environment, provide time-out, *to prevent escalation of disruptive behaviors (e.g., panic state, violence).*

- Anticipate and address feelings of distress in family/caregivers when placing loved one in a different environment (e.g., nursing home, foster care). *Support and referrals may be needed to help SOs in practical issues and adjustment.*

NURSING PRIORITY NO. 3 To promote wellness (Teaching/Discharge Considerations):

- Involve client in formulating goals and plan of care when possible. *Supports independence and commitment to achieving outcomes.*
- Encourage communication between client/family/SO *to provide mutual support and problem-solving opportunities.*[5]
- Discuss benefits of adequate nutrition, rest, and exercise *to maintain physical well-being and reduce adverse effects of stressful situation.*
- Instruct in anxiety- and stress-reduction activities (e.g., meditation/other relaxation techniques, exercise, group socialization), as able, *to enhance psychological well-being and coping abilities.*
- Encourage participation in activities/hobbies/personal interactions, as appropriate. *Promotes creative endeavors, stimulating the mind.*
- Identify community support/cultural or ethnic groups client can access.
- Support self-responsibility and coping strategies *to foster sense of control and self-worth.*

DOCUMENTATION FOCUS

Assessment/Reassessment

- Assessment findings, individual's perception of the situation/changes, specific behaviors.

- Cultural/religious concerns.
- Safety issues.

Planning

- Note plan of care, who is involved in planning, and who is responsible for proposed actions.
- Teaching plan.

Implementation/Evaluation

- Response to interventions (especially time-out/seclusion)/teaching and actions performed.
- Sentinel events.
- Attainment/progress toward desired outcome(s).
- Modifications to plan of care.

Discharge Planning

- Long-term needs and who is responsible for actions to be taken.
- Specific referrals made.

References

1. Mallick, M. J., Whipple, T. W. (2000). Validity of the nursing diagnosis of relocation stress syndrome. *Nurs Res,* 49(2), 97–100.
2. Conquering relocation stress. (2001). Public information article by the U.S. Army for military families. Available at www.usarec.army. Accessed September 2003.
3. Chiaro, C. (2003). Preventing relocation stress, easing children's transition. Special report for the *Colorado Springs Business Journal.*
4. Health impacts of relocation. (2002). Summary Evidence Review Series: No. 11. Health Impact Assessment. Accessed September 2003 at http://online.northumbria.ac.uk/faculties/hswe/hia/evidence/eleven.htm.
5. Solomon, A. (2000). Relocation stress: The warning signs. Article for Psych Bytes. Accessed July 2007 at www.therapyinla.com/psych/psych0100.html.
6. Purnell's Model for Cultural Competence. In Purnell, L. D., Paulanka, B. J. (1998). *Transcultural Health Care: A Culturally Competent Approach.* Philadelphia: F. A. Davis, pp. 11, 14.
7. Nypaver, J. M., Titus, M., Brugler, C. J. (1996). Patient transfer to rehabilitation: Just another move? Relocation stress syndrome. *Rehabil Nurs,* 21(2), 94–97.
8. Stress. Article for Youth Center, Army Community Services. Accessed January 2004 at www.armycommunity-services.org. [supported with 12 or 14]
9. ND. (2002). Relocation Stress Syndrome, risk for. In Cox, H. C., et al. *Clinical Applications of Nursing Diagnosis: Adult, Child, Women's, Psychiatric, Gerontic, and Home Health Considerations.* 4th ed. Philadelphia: F. A. Davis.
10. Puskar, K. R., Dvorsak, K. G. (1991). Relocation stress in adolescents: Helping teenagers cope with a moving dilemma. *Pediatr Nurs,* 17(3), 298–297.
11. Walker, C. A., Curry, L. C., Hogstel, M.O. (2007). Relocation stress syndrome in older adults transitioning from home to long term care facility: Myth or reality? *J Psychosoc Nurs Ment Health Serv,* 45(1), 38–45.
12. Helpful moving tips: Family relocation checklist. (2004). Retrieved July 2007 from MyArmyLifeToo Web site. Available at www.myarmylifetoo.com/.
13. Mintz, T. G. (2005). Relocation stress syndrome in older adults. *Social Work Today,* 5(6), 38.
14. Dion, R. (2005). Overcoming relocation stress. Article provided by Military OneSource., PTSD Support Services. Available at www.ptsdsupport.net/relocation_stress.html.
15. Murphy, K. (2005). Anxiety: When is it too much? *Nursing Made Incredibly Easy!* 3(5), 22–31.
16. Munche, J. A., McCarty. (2006). Geriatric rehabilitation. Article for Emedicine. Retrieved April 2007 at www.emedicine.com/pmr/topic164.htm.

risk for Relocation Stress Syndrome

Definition: At risk for physiological and/or psychosocial disturbance following transfer from one environment to another

Cultural   Collaborative   Community/Home Care   Diagnostic Studies   Pediatric/Geriatric/Lifespan   Medications

RISK FACTORS

Move from one environment to another

Moderate to high degree of environmental change [e.g., physical, ethnic, cultural]

Lack of adequate support system/group; lack of predeparture counseling

Passive coping; feelings of powerlessness; losses

Moderate mental competence

Unpredictability of experiences

NOTE: A risk diagnosis is not evidenced by signs and symptoms, as the problem has not occurred; rather, nursing interventions are directed at prevention.

Sample Clinical Applications: Chronic conditions (e.g., MS, asthma, cystic fibrosis), brain injury/stroke, dementia, schizophrenia, developmental delay

DESIRED OUTCOMES/EVALUATION CRITERIA

Sample NOC linkages:

Psychosocial Adjustment: Life Change: Psychosocial adaptation of an individual to a life change

Quality of Life: An individual's expressed satisfaction with current life circumstances

Grief Resolution: Adjustment to actual or impending loss

Client Will (Include Specific Time Frame)

- Verbalize understanding of reason(s) for change.
- Express feelings and concerns openly and appropriately.
- Experience no catastrophic event.

ACTIONS/INTERVENTIONS

Sample NIC linkages:

Discharge Planning: Preparation for moving a patient from one level of care to another within or outside the current healthcare agency

Emotional Support: Provision of reassurance, acceptance, and encouragement during times of stress

Socialization Enhancement: Facilitation of another persons's ability to interact with others

NURSING PRIORITY NO. 1   To identify risk/contributing factors:

- Determine situation/cause for relocation (e.g., planned move for new job, change in marital status, loss of home/community due to natural or man-made disaster; deterioration in health status/ability to care for self, caregiver burnout; elderly parent being requested to move closer to adult child). *Although nursing research has not currently validated the defining characteristics of relocation stress syndrome as a nursing diagnosis,[1,5] the belief that stress associated with relocation can be extreme is widely accepted in society. The effects of relocation can be minimal and transient, or very troubling and persistent.[2]*
- Note client's age, developmental level, role in family. *Age and position in life cycle makes a difference in the impact of issues involved in relocating. For example, children can be traumatized by transfer to new school, loss of friends and familiar surroundings;[3] elderly persons may be affected by loss of their long-term home with its memories, neighborhood setting, and support persons.[4,6,7]*

- Identify cultural and/or religious concerns that may affect client's coping or impact social interactions, expectations. *Cultural norm may be that elders are cared for by family—not placed in a facility—causing client to feel abandoned; or individual may be required to defer to family decision maker and feel powerless in determining own destiny.*[2,6,7]

- Note ethnic ties/primary language spoken and read. *During times of stress, individuals may lapse into language of childhood. This affects healthcare providers who must try to reduce client's feelings of alienation while communicating, with client of another primary language, or client who is displaced from cultural, familial attachments.*[2,8]

- Ascertain if client has participated in the decision to relocate, perceptions about change(s), and expectations for the future. *Decision may have been made with/without client's input or understanding of event or consequences, which can impact adjustment. A forced relocation is much more stressful than one that is desired.*[4,7] *Client may be concerned that temporary placement will deplete savings or fearful of being a burden on family members and felt pressured to move.*

- Note whether relocation will be temporary (e.g., extended care for rehabilitation therapies, moving in with family while house being repaired after fire, etc.) or long-term/permanent (e.g., move from home of many years, placement in nursing home). *To some degree, a temporary relocation is usually easier to cope with than a permanent relocation. However, any anticipated disruption of the client's usual way of living is upsetting, and emotional responses aren't always congruent with the magnitude of the event.*

- Determine involvement of family/SO(s). Note availability/use of support systems and resources. Ascertain presence/absence of comprehensive information and planning (e.g., when/how move will take place, if the environment for the client will be similar or greatly changed, etc.). *These factors can greatly affect client's ability to cope with change.*[4]

NURSING PRIORITY NO. 2 To prevent/minimize adverse response to change:

- Collaborate in treatment of underlying conditions (e.g., chronic confusional states, brain injury, posttrauma rehabilitation, etc.) and physical stress symptoms *that could exacerbate relocation stress or that affects length of time that relocation may be needed.*

- Provide information to client/SO as early in process as possible *to eliminate misconceptions and facilitate decision-making process. This can include obtaining audiovisual materials/Web sites about the new home/city/region/country.*[8,9]

- Discuss relocation/move with child. *Information for child must be aimed at level of understanding and interest.*[3] *Child lacks ability to put problem into perspective, so minor mishap may seem catastrophic. Also, child is more vulnerable to stress because he or she has less control over environment than most adults.*[2,9]

- Avoid moving adolescent in middle of school year, when possible. *Adolescent is vulnerable to emotional, social, and cognitive dysfunction because of the great importance of peer group and loss of friends and social standing caused by relocation.*[9]

- Involve client in placement choices when possible (e.g., move to nursing home or adult foster care) *to provide client with some control over the situation.*

- Encourage visit to new community/surroundings/school before transfer when possible. *Provides opportunity to "get acquainted" with new situation, reducing fear of unknown.*

- Suggest contact with someone (friend, family, business associate) who has been to/lived in new area where move is being planned *to absorb some of their experience and knowledge.*[8,9]

- Take practical steps to alleviate stress for child. Encourge parents to walk with child to school/rehearse boarding the school bus, visit new classroom, contact friends child left behind, drive past places of interest to child, find a safe play place, unpack child's favorite toys, invite neighborhood children to a get-acquainted party, etc.; *helps child to maintain ties and develop new ones, reducing sense of loss and shifting focus to the future.*[3]

Cultural Collaborative Community/Home Care Diagnostic Studies Pediatric/Geriatric/Lifespan Medications

🏠 • Encourage free expression of feelings about reason for relocation. Acknowledge reality of situation and maintain hopeful attitude regarding move/change. *Bringing feelings out into the open helps clarify emotion and make feelings easier to deal with.*[9,10]

NURSING PRIORITY NO. 3 To promote wellness (Teaching/Discharge Considerations):

🏠 • Involve client in formulating goals and plan of care when possible. *Fosters sense of control and self-worth, supports independence and commitment to achieving outcomes.*

🏠 • Encourage client/SO to accept that relocation is an adjustment and that it takes time to adapt to new circumstances/environment.

🏠 • Instruct in anxiety- and stress-reduction activities (e.g., meditation/other relaxation techniques, exercise, group socialization) as able *to enhance psychological well-being and coping abilities.*

🏠 • Provide client with information/list of organizations/community services (e.g., Welcome Wagon, senior citizens or teen clubs, churches, singles' groups, sports leagues, etc.) *to provide contacts for client to develop new relationships and learn more about the new setting.*[10]

🏠 • Discuss safety issues regarding new environment *(e.g., how to navigate streets/choose correct bus; locate dining hall/bathroom in facility),* concerns of elopement/running away.

🏠 • Anticipate variety of emotions and reactions. *May vary from insomnia and loss of appetite to becoming involved with alcohol/other drugs, or exacerbation of health problems/onset of serious illness or behavioral problems. Awareness provides opportunity for timely intervention.*[6,9]

• Refer to ND Relocation Stress Syndrome for additional interventions.

DOCUMENTATION FOCUS

Assessment/Reassessment

• Assessment findings, individual's perception of the situation/changes, specific behaviors.
• Cultural/religious concerns.
• Safety issues.

Planning

• Note plan of care, who is involved in planning, and who is responsible for proposed actions.
• Teaching plan.

Implementation/Evaluation

• Response to interventions (especially time-out/seclusion)/teaching and actions performed.
• Sentinel events.
• Attainment/progress toward desired outcome(s).
• Modifications to plan of care.

Discharge Planning

• Long-term needs and who is responsible for actions to be taken.
• Specific referrals made.

References

1. Mallick, M. J., Whipple, T. W. (2000). Validity of the nursing diagnosis of relocation stress syndrome. *Nurs Res,* 49(2), 97–100.

2. Conquering relocation stress. (2001). Public information article by the U.S. Army for military families. Accessed September 2003 at www.usarec.army.
3. Chiaro, C. (2003). Preventing relocation stress, easing children's transition. Special report for the *Colorado Springs Business Journal.*
4. Health impacts of relocation. (2002). Summary Evidence Review Series: No. 11. Health Impact Assessment. Accessed September 2003 at http://online.northumbria.ac.uk/faculties/hswe/hia/evidence/eleven.htm.
5. Walker, C. A., Curry, L. C., Hogstel, M. O. (2007). Relocation stress syndrome in older adults transitioning from home to long term care facility: Myth or reality? *J Psychosoc Nurs Ment Health Serv,* 45(1), 38–45.
6. Helpful moving tips: Family relocation checklist. (2004). Retrieved July 2007 from MyArmyLifeToo Web site. Available at www.myarmylifetoo.com/.
7. Mintz, T. G. (2005). Relocation stress syndrome in older adults. *Social Work Today,* 5(6), 38.
8. Solomon, A. (2000). Relocation stress: The warning signs. Article for Psych Bytes. Accessed July 2007 at www.therapyinla.com/psych/psych0100.html.
9. Dion, R. (2005). Overcoming relocation stress. Article provided by Military OneSource, PTSD Support Services. Accessed July 2007 at www.ptsdsupport.net/relocation_stress.html.
10. ND. (2002). Relocation Stress Syndrome, risk for. In Cox, H. C., et al. *Clinical Applications of Nursing Diagnosis: Adult, Child, Women's, Psychiatric, Gerontic, and Home Health Considerations.* 4th ed. Philadelphia: F. A. Davis.

ineffective Role Performance

Definition: Patterns of behavior and self-expression that do not match the environmental context, norms, and expectations

[Note: There is a typology of roles: sociopersonal (friendship, family, marital, parenting, community), home management, intimacy (sexuality, relationship building), leisure/exercise/recreation, self-management, socialization (developmental transitions), community contributor, and religious.]

RELATED FACTORS

Knowledge
Inadequate/lack of role model
Inadequate role preparation (e.g., role transition, skill rehearsal, validation)
Lack of education
[Developmental transitions]
Unrealistic role expectations

Physiological
Body image alteration; cognitive deficits; neurological deficits; physical illness; mental illness, depression; low self-esteem
Fatigue; pain; substance abuse

Social
Inadequate role socialization [e.g., role model, expectations, responsibilities]
Young age, developmental level
Lack of resources; low socioeconomic status
Stress; conflict; job schedule demands
[Family conflict]; domestic violence
Inadequate support system; lack of rewards
Inappropriate linkage with the healthcare system

DEFINING CHARACTERISTICS

Subjective
Altered role perceptions; change in self-/other's perception of role
Change in usual patterns of responsibility/capacity to resume role
Inadequate opportunities for role enactment
Role dissatisfaction/overload/denial
Discrimination [by others]; powerlessness

Objective
Deficient knowledge; inadequate role competency/skills
Inadequate adaptation to change; inappropriate developmental expectations
Inadequate confidence/motivation/self-management/coping
Inadequate external support for role enactment
Role strain/conflict/confusion/ambivalence; [failure to assume role]
Uncertainty; anxiety; depression; pessimism
Domestic violence; harassment; system conflict

Sample Clinical Applications: Chronic conditions (e.g., MS, pain, fatigue syndrome), cancer, substance abuse, brain/spinal cord injury, major surgery, major depression, bipolar disorder, borderline personality disorder, schizophrenia

DESIRED OUTCOMES/EVALUATION CRITERIA
Sample NOC linkages:
Role Performance: Congruence of an individual's role behavior with role expectations
Coping: Personal actions to manage stressors that tax an individual's resources
Psychosocial Adjustment: Life Change: Adaptive psychosocial response of an individual to a significant life change

Client Will (Include Specific Time Frame)
- Verbalize realistic perception and acceptance of self in changed role.
- Verbalize understanding of role expectations/obligations.
- Talk with family/SO(s) about situation and changes that have occurred and limitations imposed.
- Develop realistic plans for adapting to new role/role changes.

ACTIONS/INTERVENTIONS

Sample NIC linkages:
Role Enhancement: Assisting a patient, significant other, or family to improve relationships by clarifying and supplementing specific role behaviors
Normalization Promotion: Assisting parents and other family members of children with chronic diseases or disabilities in providing normal life experiences for their children and families
Values Clarification: Assisting another to clarify her or his own values in order to facilitate effective decision making

NURSING PRIORITY NO. 1 To assess causative/contributing factors:

- Identify type of role dysfunction. *Life changes such as developmental (adolescent to adult); situational (husband to father, change in employment status, gender identity); health-illness transitions can affect how client functions in usual role. This information is important to developing a plan of care and appropriate interventions and goals.*[1,3]

🏠 • Determine client role in family constellation. *How client has functioned in the past (i.e., husband/father, wife/mother), provides a beginning point of reference for understanding changes that have occurred due to health alterations (mental or physical), lack of knowledge about role/role skills, lack of role model, or what other situation has occurred to bring about a role change.*[1]

🏠 • Identify how client sees self as a man/woman in usual lifestyle/role functioning. *Each person has a perception of self that is important to know to understand changes that may be occurring.*[1]

🏠 • Ascertain client's view of sexual functioning. *Changes such as the loss of childbearing ability following hysterectomy, erectile dysfunction following prostate surgery can affect how client views self in role as male or female and may need specific interventions to resolve feelings of loss.*[1]

🌐 • Identify cultural factors relating to individual's gender roles. *Varies with the culture; for instance, for American Indians who are in matrilineal clans or band, women may make important decisions, male roles include ritual to protect family and community well-being. In Arab American families, men are expected to be responsible for financial affairs, and women typically assume subservient and caregiving roles.*[4]

🏠 • Determine client's perceptions/concerns about current situation. *May believe current role is more appropriate for the opposite sex (e.g., passive role of the "client" may be somewhat less threatening for women).*[2]

🏠 • Interview SO(s) regarding their perceptions and expectations. *The beliefs of the individuals who will be directly involved with the client and the situation (such as parent's bringing a new baby home from the hospital, adult child assuming responsibility for elder parent) are important to understanding the new roles the individuals are undertaking. Conflicts can arise when expectations vary from individual to individual.*[5]

🏠 • Determine client's socioeconomic status, linkage to the healthcare system. *People who are poor may not have healthcare insurance or access to care and perceive themselves as unworthy.*[1]

🏠 • Identify availability/use of resources. *Individual may be unaware or have difficulty accessing community support/assistance programs.*

🏠 • Investigate history of incidents of domestic violence in the family. *Neither individual in this situation sees self as worthy and both have poor self-esteem. The perpetrator does not get what he or she wants through the use of violence, and the survivor (the battered person) often believes she or he deserves this treatment. The roles of perpetrator and survivor are difficult to alter without intensive therapy as well as support for other family members/children.*[1,7]

NURSING PRIORITY NO. 2 To assist client to deal with existing situation:

🏠 • Discuss perceptions and significance of the situation as seen by client. *Provides opportunity to clarify any misperceptions and discuss changes client may have to make in regard to what has happened (e.g., loss of a limb, disfiguring surgery).*[3]

🏠 • Maintain positive attitude toward the client. *Promotes safe relationship in which client can discuss changes that are occurring and plan for a positive future.*[1]

🏠 • Provide opportunities for client to exercise control over as much of situation as possible. *Enhances self-concept and promotes commitment to goals.*[1]

🏠 • Offer realistic assessment of situation and communicate hope. *Client may or may not accept reality, but opportunity to discuss issues and have a sense of hope can help client begin to accept reality.*[6]

🌐 • Discuss and assist the client/SO(s) to develop strategies for dealing with changes in role related to past transitions, cultural expectations, and value/belief challenges. *Helps those involved deal with differences between individuals (e.g., adolescent task of separation in which parents clash with child's choices).*[2,4,8]

- Acknowledge reality of situation related to role change and help client to express feelings of anger, sadness, grief, and depression. Encourage celebration of positive aspects of change and expressions of feelings. *Changes in role necessitated by illness/accident, changes in family structure (new baby, child leaving home for college, elderly parent needing care), or any other circumstance, results in a sense of loss and need to deal with the feelings that accompany the change.*[1,5]
- Provide open environment for client to discuss concerns about sexuality. *Embarrassment can block discussion of sensitive subject and potentially impede progress.* (Refer to NDs Sexual Dysfunction; ineffective Sexuality Pattern.)[7]
- Educate about role expectations using written and audiovisual materials. *Using different modalities enables client to review material at leisure and begin to incorporate information into own thinking.*[2]
- Identify role model for the client. *Promotes opportunity for client to observe how someone else functions in a role that is new to him or her.*[2]
- Use techniques of role rehearsal to practice new role. *Provides opportunity for the client to try on and develop new skills to cope with anticipated changes.*[7]

NURSING PRIORITY NO. 3 To promote wellness (Teaching/Discharge Considerations):

- Make information available (including bibliotherapy, appropriate Web sites) for client to learn about role expectations/demands that may occur. *Provides opportunity to be proactive in dealing with changes, such as classes to help new parents learn about new roles, credible Web sites for additional information regarding individuals' specific concerns.*[5]
- Discuss use of medication, as appropriate. *Client may benefit from antidepressants to combat depression, or psychotropic medications may be required to address other mental health issues.*[1,7]
- Accept client in changed role. Encourage and give positive feedback for changes and goals achieved. *Provides reinforcement and facilitates continuation of efforts.*[7]
- Refer to support groups, employment counselors, Parent Effectiveness classes, counseling/psychotherapy, as indicated by individual need(s). *Provides ongoing support to sustain progress.*[6]
- Refer to NDs impaired Parenting; Self-Esteem [specify], as appropriate.

DOCUMENTATION FOCUS

Assessment/Reassessment

- Individual findings, including specifics of predisposing crises/situation, perception of role change.
- Cultural/religious factors.
- Expectations of SO(s).
- Availability/use of resources.

Planning

- Plan of care and who is involved in planning.
- Teaching plan.

Implementation/Evaluation

- Responses to interventions/teaching and actions performed.
- Attainment/progress toward desired outcome(s).
- Modifications of plan of care.

Discharge Planning

• Long-term needs and who is responsible for actions to be taken.
• Specific referrals made.

References

1. Townsend, M. C. (2003). *Psychiatric Mental Health Nursing Concepts of Care.* 4th ed. Philadelphia: F. A. Davis.
2. Cox, H. C., et al. (2002). *Clinical Applications of Nursing Diagnosis: Adult, Child, Women's, Psychiatric, Gerontic, and Home Health Considerations.* 4th ed. Philadelphia: F. A. Davis.
3. Doenges, M. E., Moorhouse, M. F., Geissler-Murr, A. C. (2002). *Nurses' Pocket Guide, Diagnoses, Interventions, and Rationales.* 8th ed. Philadelphia: F. A. Davis.
4. Lipson, J. G., Dibble, S. L., Minarik, P. A. (1996). *Culture & Nursing Care: A Pocket Guide.* San Francisco: UCSF Nursing Press.
5. Gjerdingen, D. (2000). Expectant parents' anticipated changes in workload after the birth of their first child. *J Fam Pract*, 49(11), 993–997.
6. Rice, J., Hicks, P. B., Wiche, V. (2000). Life care planning: A role for social workers. *Soc Work Health Care*, 31(1), 85–94.
7. Doenges, M. E., Townsend, M. C., Moorhouse, M. F. (1998). *Psychiatric Care Plans Guidelines for Individualizing Care.* 3d ed. Philadelphia: F. A. Davis.
8. Cultural Awareness Self Concept. Retrieved April 2007 at http://academic.cuesta.edu/atorrey/culture.pdf.

readiness for enhanced Self-Care

Definition: A pattern of performing activities for oneself that helps to meet health-related goals and can be strengthened

RELATED FACTORS
To be developed by nurse researchers and submitted to NANDA

DEFINING CHARACTERISTICS

Subjective
Expresses desire to enhance independence in maintaining life/health/personal development/well-being
Expresses desire to enhance knowledge for strategies for self-care/responsibility for self-care/self-care
[Note: Based on the definition and defining characteristics of this ND, the focus appears to be broader than simply meeting routine basic ADLs and addresses independence in maintaining overall health, personal development, and general well-being.]

Sample Clinical Applications: Presence of chronic physical or psychological conditions, or any individual seeking improved well-being/independence in meeting own needs

DESIRED OUTCOMES/EVALUATION CRITERIA
Sample NOC linkages:
Self-Care Status: Ability to perform basic personal care activities and household tasks
Self-Care: Instrumental Activities of Daily Living (IADL): Ability to perform activities to function in the home or community independently with or without assistive device
Self-Direction of Care: Care recipient actions taken to direct others who assist with or perform physical tasks and personal care

Cultural   Collaborative   Community/Home Care   Diagnostic Studies   Pediatric/Geriatric/Lifespan   Medications

Client Will (Include Specific Time Frame)

- Maintain responsibility for planning and achieving self-care goals/general well-being.
- Demonstrate proactive management of chronic conditions/potential complications or changes in capabilities.
- Identify/use resources appropriately.
- Remain free of preventable complications.

ACTIONS/INTERVENTIONS

Sample NIC linkages:

Self-Care Assistance: IADL: Assisting and instructing a person to perform instrumental activites of daily living (IADL) needed to function in the home or community

Self-Modification Assistance: Reinforcement of self-directed change initiated by the patient to achieve personally important goals

NURSING PRIORITY NO. 1 To determine current self-care status and motivation for growth:

- Determine individual strengths and skills of the client *to incorporate into plan of care, enhacing likelihood of achieving outcomes.*[1]
- Ascertain motivation and expectations for change. *Motivation to improve and high expectations can encourage client to make changes that will improve his or her life. However, unrealistic expectations may hamper efforts.*
- Note availability/use of resources, supportive person(s) *to ascertain that client has means for sharing common concerns, needs, and wishes as well as has access to social support and approval (e.g., support group participants, family members, professionals).*[2]
- Determine age/developmental issues and presence of medical conditions resulting in very specific deficits (e.g., loss of visual/spatial orientation affecting driving, muscular weakness affecting fine motor coordination, peripheral neuropathy impairing sensory interpretation, etc.) *that could impact potential for growth/interrupt client's ability to meet own needs.*[1,3]
- Assess for potential challenges to enhanced participation in self-care (e.g., language barrier with healthcare providers, lack of information, insufficient time for discussion; sudden/progressive change in health status, catastrophic events, etc.).

NURSING PRIORITY NO. 2 To assist client/SO plan to meet individual needs:

- Discuss client's understanding of situation *to determine areas that can be clarified or strengthened.*
- Provide accurate/relevant information regarding current/future needs *so that client can incorporate into self-care plans while minimizing problems (e.g., stress, resistance) often associated with change.*[2]
- Promote client/SO participation in problem identification and decision making. *Optimizes outcomes and supports health promotion.*[4]
- Review coping skills (e.g., assertiveness, interpersonal relations, decision making, problem-solving, stigma management, and time management) *that are useful in managing a wide range of stressful conditions. Encourage client to ask for assistance, as needed/desired.*[2]
- Active-listen to client's/SO('s) concerns. *Exhibits regard for client's values and beliefs and provides opportunity to support positive responses and address questions/concerns.*[3]

• Encourage communication among those who are involved in the client's health promotion. *Periodic review provides clarification of issues, reinforcement of successful interventions, and possiblity for early intervention, where needed, to manage chronic conditions.*

NURSING PRIORITY NO. 3 To promote optimum wellness (Teaching/Discharge considerations):

• Assist client to set realistic goals for the future. *Enhances likelihood of success and commitment to behavioral changes.*

• Support client in making health-related decisions and pursuit of self-care practices that promote health *to foster self-esteem and support positive self-concept.*

• Identify reliable reference sources (including Web sites) regarding individual needs/strategies for self-care. *Reinforces learning and promotes self-paced review.*

• Provide for ongoing evaluation of self-care program *to identify progress and needed changes for continuation of health, adaptation in management of limiting conditions.*

• Review safety concerns and modification of medical therapies or activities/environment, as needed, *to prevent injury and enhance successful functioning.*

• Refer to home-care provider, social services, physical/occupational therapy, rehabilitation, and counseling resources, as indicated/requested, *for education, assistance, and adaptive devices and modifications that may be desired.*[1]

• Identify additional community resources (e.g., senior services, handicap transportation van for appointments, accessible/safe locations for social/sports activities, Meals on Wheels, etc.) *to obtain additional forms of assistance that may improve client's independence and self-care.*[1]

DOCUMENTATION FOCUS

Assessment/Reassessment

• Individual findings, including strengths, health status, and any limitation(s).
• Availability/use of resources/support person(s), assistive devices.
• Motivation and expectations for change.

Planning

• Plan of care/interventions and who is involved in planning.
• Teaching plan.

Implementation/Evaluation

• Client's responses to interventions/teaching and actions performed.
• Attainment/progress toward desired outcome(s).
• Modifications to plan.

Discharge Planning

• Long-term needs and who is responsible for actions to be taken.
• Type of and source for assistive devices.
• Specific referrals made.

References:

1. ND: Self-Care Deficit: Bathing/hygeine, dressing/grooming, feeding, toileting. In Doenges, M. E., Moorhouse, M. F., Geissler-Murr, A. C. (2005). *Nursing Diagnosis Manual: Planning, Individualizing, and Documenting Client Care.* Philadelphia. F. A. Davis.

Cultural   Collaborative   Community/Home Care   Diagnostic Studies   Pediatric/Geriatric/Lifespan   Medications

2. Livneh, H., Antonak, R. F. (2005). Psychosocial adaptation to chronic illness and disability: A primer for counselors (practice & theory). *Journal of Counseling and Development.* Excerpt accessed July 2007 at www.accessmylibrary.com/coms2/summary_0286-19174530_ITM.
3. Baldwin, K. M. (2006). Stroke: It's a knock-out punch. *Nursing Made Incredibly Easy!*, 4(2), 10–23.
4. Singleton, J. K. (No date listed). Nurses' perspectives of encouraging client's care-of-self in a short-term rehabilitation unit within a long-term care facility. CE offering for ARN Web site. Accessed August 2007 at www.rehabnurse.org/ce/010200/010200_a.htm.

Self-Care Deficit: bathing/hygiene, dressing/grooming, feeding, toileting

Definition: Impaired ability to perform or complete feeding, bathing/hygiene, dressing and grooming, or toileting activities for oneself [on a temporary, permanent, or progressing basis] (Specify level of independence using a standardized functional scale.)

[**Note:** Self-Care also may be expanded to include the practices used by the client to promote health, the individual responsibility for self, a way of thinking. Refer to NDs ineffective Health Maintenance; impaired Home Maintenance.]

RELATED FACTORS
Weakness; fatigue; decreased motivation
Neuromuscular/musculoskeletal impairment
Environmental barriers
Severe anxiety
Pain, discomfort
Perceptual/cognitive impairment
Inability to perceive body part/spatial relationship [bathing/hygiene]
Impaired transfer ability [self-toileting]
Impaired mobility status [self-toileting]
[Mechanical restrictions such as cast, splint, traction, ventilator]

DEFINING CHARACTERISTICS

Self-Feeding Deficit
Inability to:
Prepare food for ingestion; open containers
Handle utensils; get food onto utensil; bring food from a receptacle to the mouth
Ingest food safely; manipulate food in mouth; chew/swallow food
Pick up cup or glass
Use assistive device
Ingest sufficient food; complete a meal
Ingest food in a socially acceptable manner

Self-Bathing/Hygiene Deficit
Inability to:
Get bath supplies
Wash body
Obtain water source; regulate bath water
Access bathroom [tub]
Dry body

Self-Dressing/Grooming Deficit

Impaired ability to obtain clothing, put on/take off necessary items of clothing, fasten
  clothing

Inability to:

Choose clothing, pick up clothing

Put clothing on upper/lower body, put on socks/shoes, remove clothes

Use zippers/assistive devices

Maintain appearance at a satisfactory level

Self-Toileting Deficit

Inability to:

Get to toilet or commode

Manipulate clothing for toileting

Sit on/rise from toilet or commode

Carry out proper toilet hygiene

Flush toilet or [empty] commode

Sample Clinical Applications: Arthritis, neuromuscular impairment (e.g., MS, brain
  injury/stroke, Parkinson's disease, spinal cord injury), chronic pain, chronic fatigue
  syndrome, depression, dementia, autism, developmental delay, end-of-life/hospice care

DESIRED OUTCOMES/EVALUATION CRITERIA

Sample NOC linkages:

Self-Care Status: Ability to perform basic personal care activities and household tasks

Self-Care: Bathing: Ability to cleanse own body independently with or without assistive device

Self-Care: Dressing: Ability to dress self independently with or without assistive device

Self-Care: Eating: Ability to prepare and ingest food and fluid independently with or
  without assistive device

Self-Care: Toileting: Ability to toilet self independently with or without assistive device

Client Will (Include Specific Time Frame)

- Identify individual areas of weakness/needs.
- Verbalize knowledge of healthcare practices.
- Demonstrate techniques/lifestyle changes to meet self-care needs.
- Perform self-care activities within level of own ability.
- Identify personal/community resources that can provide assistance.

ACTIONS/INTERVENTIONS

Sample NIC linkages:

Self-Care Assistance: [specify]: Assisting another to perform activities of daily living

Bathing: Cleaning of the body for the purpose of relaxation, cleanliness, and healing

Dressing: Choosing, putting on, and removing clothes for a person who cannot do this for self

Hair Care [or] Nail Care: Promotion of neat, clean, attractive hair/nails and prevention of
  skin lesions related to improper care of nails

Feeding: Providing nutritional intake for patient who is unable to feed self

Bowel/Urinary Elimination Management: Establishment and maintenance of a regular
  pattern of bowel elimination/maintenance of an optimum urinary elimination pattern

Cultural Collaborative Community/Home Care Diagnostic Studies Pediatric/Geriatric/Lifespan Medications

NURSING PRIORITY NO. 1 To identify causative/contributing factors:

- Determine age/developmental issues and existing conditons (e.g., heart/renal failure, spinal cord injury, malnutrition, pain, trauma, surgery) and cognitive/psychological factors (e.g., mental illness, brain injury, CVA, MS, Alzheimer's disease, etc.) *affecting ability of individual to care for own needs. Assists in setting realistic goals and creates baseline for evaluating effectiveness of interventions.*[3,10]
- Identify other etiological factors present, including language barriers, speech impairment, visual acuity, loss of visual/spatial orientation, hearing problem, emotional instability/lability *that can both affect and be affected by self-care needs and deficits.* Refer to NDs impaired verbal Communication; impaired Environmental Interpretation; risk for unilateral Neglect, disturbed Sensory Perception (specify) for related interventions.
- Review medication regimen *for possible effects on alertness/mentation, energy level, balance, perception. Note: All prescribed and OTC medications have the potential for side effects, adverse effects, and interactions that may be harmful to the client or affect client's ability to provide self-care.*
- Assess barriers to participation in regimen *that can limit use of resources/choice of options (e.g., lack of information, insufficient time for discussion; psychological or intimate family problems that may be difficult to share, fear of appearing stupid or ignorant, social/economic limitations, work/home environment problems).*[1]

NURSING PRIORITY NO. 2 To assess degree of disability:

- Identify degree of individual impairment/functional level according to a functional scale as below:[1]

0—Completely independent
1—Requires use of equipment or device
2—Requires help from another person for assistance, supervision, or teaching
3—Requires help from another person and equipment device
4—Dependent, does not participate in activity

- Note anticipated duration of disruption/intensity of care required. *A wide variety of factors can impact self-care, some of which may be (1) invariable or permanent (e.g., quadriplegia or advanced dementia), (2) temporary (e.g., fractures requiring immobilization, or mild stroke with potential for good recovery), and (3) variable (e.g., person having episode of severe depression or episodes of remitting/exacerbating type MS).*[1]
- Assess cognitive functioning (memory, intelligence, concentration, ability to attend to task, etc.) *to determine client's ability to participate in care, potential to return to normal functioning, or to learn/relearn tasks.*[1]
- Determine individual strengths and skills of the client *to incorporate into plan of care enhancing likelihood of achieving outcomes.*

NURSING PRIORITY NO. 3 To assist in correcting/dealing with deficit(s) in general:

- Collaborate in treatment of underlying conditions *to enhance client's capabilities, maximize rehabilitation potential.*[1]
- Promote communication among all those involved in caring for/assisting the client. *Enhances coordination and continuity of care.*
- Active-listen to client's/SO('s) concerns. *Exhibits regard for client's values and beliefs, clarifies barriers to participation in self-care, provides opportunity to work on problem-solving solutions, and to provide encouragement/support.*[1,10,12]

- Provide accurate/relevant information regarding current/future needs *so that client can incorporate into self-care plans while minimizing problems (e.g., heightened anxiety, depression, resistance) often associated with change.*[2,11]
- Promote client/SO participation in problem identification and desired outcomes. *Can ease frustration of current loss of independence, enhancing recovery, optimizing outcomes, and supporting health promotion.*[2,12]
- Establish "contractual" partnership with client/SO(s) if appropriate/indicated for motivation/behavioral modification.
- Practice and promote short-term goal-setting and achievment *to recognize that today's success is as important as any long-term goal, accepting ability to do one thing at a time, and conceputalization of self-care in a broader sense.*
- Instruct in/review appropriate skills necessary for self-care, using terms understandable to client (e.g., child, adult, cognitively impaired person) and with sensitivity to developmental needs for practice, repetition, or reluctance. *Individualized teaching best affords reinforcement of learning. Sensitivity to special needs attaches value to the client's needs.*[3]
- Encourage client to use eye glasses/contacts and hearing aides as appropriate. *Improves reception and interpretation of sensory input to facilitate self-care.*
- Perform/assist with meeting client's needs when he or she is unable to meet own needs (*e.g., personal care assistance is part of nursing care and should not be neglected while promoting and integrating self-care independence*).
- Anticipate needs and begin with familiar, easily accomplished tasks *to encourage client and build on successes.*
- Cue client, as indicated. *Cognitively impaired or forgetful client can often successfully participate in many activities with cueing, which can enhance self-esteem and potentiate learning/relearning of self-care tasks.*[1,3]
- Maintain a supportive attitude and allow sufficient time for client *to accomplish tasks to fullest extent of ability.*
- Refrain from unnecessary conversation/interruptions *that divert focus from the task at hand and can contribute to client's level of frustration.*
- Avoid doing things for client that client can do for self, but provide assistance as needed. *Client may be fearful or dependent, and although assistance is helpful in preventing frustration (and sometimes easier for the caregivers in terms of their time), it is important for client to do as much as possible for self to regain/maintain self-esteem, reduce helplessness, and promote optimal recovery.*[2]
- Review coping skills (e.g., assertiveness, interpersonal relations, decision making, problem-solving, stigma management, and time management) *that are useful in managing a wide range of stressful conditions. Encourage client to ask for assistance as needed/desired.*[2,11]
- Schedule activities *to conform to client's normal schedule as much as possible (e.g., bathing at a relaxing time for client, rather than on a set routine).*[1]
- Plan activities to prevent/accommodate fatigue and/or exacerbation of pain *to conserve energy and promote maximum participation in self-care.*[2]
- Identify energy-saving behaviors (*e.g., sitting instead of standing when possible, organizing needs before beginning tasks*). (Refer to NDs Activity Intolerance; Fatigue for additional interventions.)
- Review medication needs (e.g., vitamins, nutritional supplements, pain reliever, antidepressants, etc.) *that may improve general well-being/ability to participate in self-care.*[1]
- Refer/arrange for home visit, as indicated, *to assess environmental concerns that can impact client's abilities to care for self in home. If necessary modifications are not feasible/cannot be made, client may require temporary/long-term relocation or regular home-care assistance.*[2]

⊕ Cultural ⊗ Collaborative 🏠 Community/Home Care ⬳ Diagnostic Studies ∞ Pediatric/Geriatric/Lifespan 💊 Medications

• Consult with/refer to rehabilitation professionals to identify/obtain assistive devices (e.g., modified eating utensils, modified clothing), mobility aids (e.g., rolling commode/shower chair), and home modification as necessary (e.g., adequate lighting; cutout under kitchen/bathroom sink; lowering cabinets/closet rods; handheld shower, raised toilet seat/grab bars for bathroom) *to optimize self-care efforts.*[1,3,10,12]

• Note availability/use of resources, supportive person(s) *to ascertain that client has means for sharing common concerns, needs, and wishes, as well as access to social support and approval (e.g., support group participants, family members, professionals).*[11]

NURSING PRIORITY NO. 4 To meet specific self-care needs:

🏠 Self-feeding deficit:

• Assess client's need/ability to prepare food as indicated (including shopping, cooking, cutting food, opening containers, etc.). *Identifies specific assistance required.*

• Encourage food/fluid choices reflecting individual likes and abilities and that meet nutritional needs *to maximize food intake.*[4]

• Ascertain that client can swallow safely, checking gag and swallow reflexes, as indicated. (Refer to ND impaired Swallowing for related interventions.)

• Provide food/fluid of appropriate consistency *to facilitate swallowing.* Cut food into bite-size pieces *to prevent overfilling mouth/reduce risk of choking.*

• Assist client to handle utensils or in guiding utensils to mouth. *May require specialized equipment (e.g., rocker knife, plate guard, built-up handles) to increase independence, or assistance with movement of arms/hands.*[3]

• Assist client with cup/glass/bottle for liquids, using straw or adaptive lids as indicated *to enhance fluid intake while reducing spills.*

• Allow client time for intake of sufficient food *for feeling satisfied or completing a meal.*[1]

• Assist client with social graces when eating with others; provide privacy *when manners might be offensive to others or client could be embarrassed.*

• Collaborate with nutritionist/physician *for special diets or feeding methods necessary to provide adequate nutrition.*[2]

• Feed client allowing adequate time for chewing and swallowing, *when client is not able to obtain nutrition by self-feeding.* Avoid providing fluids until client has swallowed food/mouth is clear. *Prevents "washing down" foods, reducing risk of choking.*[1]

🏠 Self-bathing/hygiene deficit:

• Ask client/SO for input on bathing habits/cultural bathing preferences. *Creates opportunities for client to (1) keep long-standing routines (e.g., bathing at bedtime to improve sleep), and (2) exercise control over situation. This enhances self-esteem, while respecting personal and cultural preferences.*[5]

• Bathe or assist client in bathing, providing for any/all hygiene needs, as indicated. *Type (e.g., bed bath, towel bath, tub bath, shower) and purpose (e.g., cleansing, removing odor, or simply soothing agitation) of bath is determined by individual need.*[1]

• Obtain hygiene supplies (soap, toothpaste, toothbrush, mouthwash, lotion, shampoo, razor, towels, etc.) for specific activity to be performed and place in client's easy reach *to provide visual cues and facilitate completion of activity.*

• Ascertain that all safety equipment is in place/properly installed (e.g., grab bars, anti-slip strips, shower chair, hydraulic lift) and that client/caregiver(s) can safely operate equipment *to prevent injury to client and caregivers.*[6]

• Instruct client to request assistance when needed/place call device within easy reach, *so client can summon help if bathing alone;* or stay with client *as dictated by safety needs.*

∞ • Provide for adequate warmth (e.g., covering client during bed bath or warming bathroom). *Certain individuals (especially infants, the elderly, and very thin or debilitated persons) are prone to hypothermia and can experience evaporative cooling during and after bathing.*[7]

• Determine that client can perceive water temperature, adjust water temperature safely, or that water is correct temperature for client's bath or shower *to prevent chilling or burns. This step requires that client is cognitively and physically able to perceive hot and cold and to adjust faucets safely; otherwise, adequate supervision must be provided at all times.*[7]

• Assist client in/out of shower/tub as indicated. *Needs are variable (e.g., client may need to get into tub before running water; may require a shower chair, may be independent with one fixture and not another), requiring assessment of individual situations.*[1]

• Assist with/encourage client to complete hygiene steps (oral care, lotion application, applying deodorant, washing/styling hair, etc.). *These steps may be completed at same or different time as bathing but are usually part of a daily routine that is necessary for client's physical well-being and emotional/social comfort.*[1]

🏠 Self-dressing/grooming deficit:

• Ascertain that appropriate clothing is available. *Client may not have sufficient clothing, clothing may be inadequate for situation or weather conditions, or clothing may need to be modified for client's particular medical condition or physical limitations.*[2]

• Assist client in choosing clothing, or lay out clothing as indicated. *May be needed when client has cognitive, physical, or psychiatric conditions affecting ability to choose appropriate pieces of clothing or to maintain a satisfactory appearance.*[3]

• Dress client/assist with dressing, as indicated. *Client may need assistance in putting on or taking off items of clothing (e.g., shoes and socks, or over-the-head shirt), or may require partial or complete assistance with fasteners (e.g., buttons, snaps, zippers, shoelaces).*[1,2]

• Allow sufficient time for dressing/undressing *because tasks may be tiring, painful, and difficult to complete.*

• Use adaptive clothing as indicated (e.g., clothing with front closure, wide sleeves and pant legs, Velcro or zipper closures).

• Teach client to dress affected side first, then unaffected side (when client has paralysis or injury to one side of body) *to allow for easier manipulation of clothing.*[2]

• Provide for/assist with grooming activities (e.g., shaving, hair care, cleaning and clipping nails, makeup) on a routine, consistent basis. Encourage participation, guiding client's hand through tasks, as indicated. *Experiencing the normal process of a task through established routine and guided practice facilitates optimal relearning.*[8]

🏠 Self-toileting deficit:

• Provide mobility assistance to bathroom or commode; or place on bedpan or offer urinal, as indicated. *Client might be impaired because of age, cognitive problems, weakness, acute injury or illness, requiring a range of interventions from complete care to help with walking.*[1,2]

• Direct cognitively impaired client to bathroom, if needed. *May need directions to the facilities, or reminders to use the bathroom, etc.*[8]

• Observe for behaviors such as pacing, fidgeting, holding crotch *that may be indicative of need for prompt toileting.*[8]

• Provide privacy *to enhance self-esteem and improve ability to urinate/defecate.*[3]

• Assist with manipulation of clothing if needed, *to decrease incidence of functional incontinence caused by difficulty removing clothing/underwear.*[9]

• Observe need for/assist in obtaining modified clothing or fasteners *to assist client in manipulation of clothing, fostering independence in self-toileting.*

🌐 Cultural Ⓐ Collaborative 🏠 Community/Home Care Diagnostic Studies ∞ Pediatric/Geriatric/Lifespan Medications

- Provide/assist with use of assistive equipment (e.g., raised toilet seat, support rails, spill-proof urinals, fracture pans, bedside commode) *to promote independence and safety in sitting down or arising from toilet, or for aiding elimination when client unable to go to bathroom.*[1,2]
- Keep toilet paper/wipes and hand-washing items within client's easy reach *to enhance self-cleansing efforts.*
- Implement bowel or bladder training/retraining programs as indicated. *This may include developing a schedule for toileting and other interventions as seen in NDs Bowel Incontinence, Constipation, impaired Urinary Elimination, Urinary Incontinence, [specify].*[1,2]

NURSING PRIORITY NO. 5 To promote wellness (Teaching/Discharge Considerations):

- Assist the client to become aware of rights and responsibilities in health/healthcare and to assess own health strengths—physical, emotional, and intellectual.
- Support client *in making health-related decisions and assist in developing self-care practices and goals that promote health.*
- Instruct in relaxation techniques (e.g., deep breathing, meditation, music, yoga) *to reduce frustration/enhance coping.*
- Provide for ongoing evaluation of self-care program *to note progress, identify changes in needs.*
- Modify program periodically *to accommodate changes in client's abilities. Assists client to adhere to plan of care to fullest extent.*
- Encourage keeping a journal *to note progress/identify factors affecting ability to perform self-care activities and to foster self-care and self-determination.*[1,3,11]
- Review safety concerns. Modify activities/environment *to reduce risk of injury and promote successful community functioning.*
- Refer to home-care provider, social services, physical/occupational therapy, rehabilitation and counseling resources as indicated.
- Identify/arrange consult with community resources (e.g., Meals on Wheels, home care/visiting nurse service, senior services, nutritionist) *to provide long-term support/additional forms of assistance that may improve client's independence and self-care.*[2,3]
- Review instructions from other members of the healthcare team and provide written copy. *Provides clarification, reinforcement, and for periodic review by client/caregivers.*[1]
- Discuss respite/other care options with family. *Allows them free time away from the care situation to renew themselves, enhances coping abilities.* (Refer to ND Caregiver Role Strain for related interventions.)
- Assist/support family with alternative placements as necessary. *Enhances likelihood of finding individually appropriate situation to meet client's needs.*
- Be available for discussion of feelings (e.g., grieving, anger, frustration). *Provides opportunity for client/family to get feelings out in the open, realize the feelings are normal, and begin to problem-solve solutions as indicated.*
- Refer to NDs ineffective Coping; compromised family Coping; risk for Disuse Syndrome; risk for Falls/Injury/Trauma; impaired physical Mobility; Powerlessness; situational low Self-Esteem, as appropriate.

DOCUMENTATION FOCUS

Assessment/Reassessment

- Individual findings, functional level, and specifics of limitation(s).
- Needed resources/adaptive devices.
- Availability/use of community resources.
- Who is involved in care/provides assistance.

Planning

- Plan of care and who is involved in planning.
- Teaching plan.

Implementation/Evaluation

- Response to interventions/teaching and actions performed.
- Attainment/progress toward desired outcome(s).
- Modifications of plan of care.

Discharge Planning

- Long-term needs and who is responsible for actions to be taken.
- Type of and source for assistive devices.
- Specific referrals made.

References

1. ND: Self-Care Deficit: Bathing/hygiene, dressing/grooming, feeding, toileting. In Doenges, M. E., Moorhouse, M. F., Geissler-Murr, A. C. (2004). *Nurse's Pocket Guide: Diagnoses, Interventions, and Rationales.* 9th ed. Philadelphia: F. A. Davis.
2. ND: Self-Care Deficit (specify). In Doenges, M. E., Moorhouse, M. F., Geissler, Murr, A. C. (2002). *Nursing Care Plans: Guidelines for Individualizing Patient Care.* 6th ed. Philadelphia: F. A. Davis, pp. 238, 291, 545, 729.
3. ND: Self Care Deficit (Feeding, Bathing-Hygiene, Dressing-Grooming, Toileting). In Cox, H. C., et al. (2002). *Clinical Applications of Nursing Diagnosis: Adult, Child, Women's Psychiatric, Gerontic, and Home Health Considerations.* 4th ed. Philadelphia: F. A. Davis, pp. 331–335.
4. Kayser-Jones, J., Schell, E. (1997). The mealtime experience of a cognitively impaired elder: Ineffective and effective strategies. *J Gerontol Nurs, 23*(7), 33.
5. Freeman, E. (1997). International perspectives on bathing. *J Gerontol Nurs, 22*(1), 40–44.
6. Schemm, R. L., Gitlin, L. N. (1998). How occupational therapists teach older patients to use bathing and dressing devices in rehabilitation. *Am J Occup Ther, 52*(4), 276–282.
7. Miller, M. (1997). Physically aggressive resident behavior during hygienic care. *J Gerontol Nurs, 23*(5), 24–39.
8. Sloane, P., et al. (1995). Bathing the Alzheimer's patient in long term care: Results and recommendation from three studies. *Am J Alzheimer's Dis, 10*(4), 3–11.
9. Penn, C., et al. (1996). Assessment of urinary incontinence. *J Gerontol Nurs, 22*, 8.
10. Baldwin, K. M. (2006). Stroke: It's a knock-out punch. *Nursing Made Incredibly Easy!, 4*(2), 10–23.
11. Livneh, H., Antonak, R. F. (2005). Psychosocial adaptation to chronic illness and disability: A primer for counselors (practice & theory). *Journal of Counseling and Development.* Excerpt accessed July 2007 at www.accessmylibrary.com/coms2/summary_0286-19174530_ITM.
12. Singleton, J. K. (No date listed). Nurses' perspectives of encouraging client's care-of-self in a short-term rehabiltiation unit within a long-term care facility. CE offering for ARN Web site. Accessed July 2007 at www.rehabnurse.org/ce/010200/010200_a.htm.

readiness for enhanced Self-Concept

Definition: A pattern of perceptions or ideas about the self that is sufficient for well-being and can be strengthened

RELATED FACTORS
To be developed by nurse researchers and submitted to NANDA

DEFINING CHARACTERISTICS

Subjective
Expresses willingness to enhance self-concept

Cultural   Collaborative   Community/Home Care   Diagnostic Studies   Pediatric/Geriatric/Lifespan   Medications

Accepts strengths/limitations
Expresses confidence in abilities
Expresses satisfaction with thoughts about self/sense of worthiness
Expresses satisfaction with body image/personal identity/role performance

Objective
Actions are congruent with expressed feelings and thoughts

Sample Clinical Applications: As a health-seeking behavior, the client may be healthy or this diagnosis can occur in any clinical condition

DESIRED OUTCOMES/EVALUATION CRITERIA
Sample NOC Linkages:
Self-Esteem: Personal judgment of self-worth
Hope: Optimism that is personally satisfying and life-supporting
Personal Autonomy: Personal actions of a competent individual to exercise governance in life decisions

Client Will (Include Specific Time Frame)

- Verbalize understanding of own sense of self-worth.
- Participate in programs and activities to enhance self-esteem.
- Demonstrate behaviors/lifestyle changes to promote positive self-esteem.
- Participate in family/group/community activities to enhance self-concept.

ACTIONS/INTERVENTIONS

Sample NIC Linkages:
Self-Modification Assistance: Reinforcement of self-directed change initiated by the patient to achieve personally important goals
Self-Esteem Enhancement: Assisting a patient to increase his or her personal judgment of self-worth
Hope Instillation: Facilitation of the development of a positive outlook in a given situation

NURSING PRIORITY NO. 1 To assess current situation and desire to enhance self-concept:

- Determine current status of individual's belief about self. *Self-concept consists of the physical self (body image), personal self (identity) and self-esteem and information about client's current thinking about self provides a beginning for making changes to improve self.*[1,2]
- Determine availability/quality of family/SO(s) support. *Presence of supportive people who reflect positive attitudes regarding the individual promotes a positive sense of self.*[1]
- Identify family dynamics, present and past. *Self-esteem begins in early childhood and is influenced by the perceptions of how the individual is viewed by significant others. Provides information about family functioning that will help to develop plan of care for enhancing client's self-concept.*[1,2]
- Note willingness to seek assistance, motivation for change. *Individuals who have a sense of their own self-image and are willing to look at themselves realistically will be better able to achieve desired growth.*[1]
- Determine client's concept of self in relation to cultural/religious ideals/beliefs. *Culture and religion play a major role in view individual has of self in relation to self-worth.*[3]

- Observe nonverbal behaviors and note congruence with verbal expressions. Discuss cultural meanings of nonverbal communication. *Incongruence between verbal and nonverbal communication requires clarification. Interpretation of nonverbal expressions is culturally determined and needs to be identified to avoid misinterpretation.*[1,3]

NURSING PRIORITY NO. 2 To promote client sense of self-esteem:

- Develop therapeutic relationship. Be attentive, validate client's communication, maintain open communication, use skills of Active-listening and I-messages. *Promotes trusting situation in which client is free to be open and honest with self and others.*[2–4]
- Accept client's perceptions/view of current status. *Avoids threatening existing self-esteem and provides opportunity for client to develop realistic plan for improving self-concept.*[3]
- Be aware that people are not programmed to be rational. *Individuals must seek information, choosing to learn, to think rather than merely accepting/reacting in order to have respect for self, facts, honesty, and to develop positive self-regard.*[3,7]
- Discuss client perception of self, confronting misconceptions and identifying negative self-talk. Address distortions in thinking, such as self-referencing (beliefs that others are focusing on individuals' weaknesses/limitations); filtering (focusing on negative and ignoring positive); catastrophizing (expecting the worst outcomes). *Addressing these issues openly allows client to identify things that may negatively affect self-concept and provides an opportunity for change.*[3,7,8]
- Have client list current/past successes and strengths. *Emphasizes fact that client is and has been successful in many actions taken.*[1,8]
- Use positive I-messages rather than praise. *Praise is a form of external control, coming from outside sources, whereas I-messages allow the client to develop internal sense of self-worth.*[4,5]
- Discuss what behavior does for client (positive intention). Ask what options are available to the client/SO(s). *Encourages thinking about what inner motivations are and what actions can be taken to enhance self-esteem.*[3]
- Provide reinforcement for progress noted. *Positive words of encouragement support development of effective coping behaviors, promotes continuation of efforts and personal growth.*[3,6]
- Allow client to progress at own rate. *Adaptation to a change in self-concept depends on its significance to the individual and disruption to lifestyle.*[3]
- Involve in activities/exercise program of choice, promote socialization. *Enhances sense of well-being/can help to energize client.*[3,6,8]

NURSING PRIORITY NO. 3 To promote enhanced sense of personal worth and happiness:

- Assist client to identify personally achievable goals. Provide positive feedback for verbal and behavioral indications of improved self-view. *Increases likelihood of success and commitment to change.*[3,6]
- Refer to vocational/employment counselor, educational resources, as appropriate. *Assists with improving development of social/vocational skills.*[3]
- Encourage participation in classes/activities/hobbies that client enjoys or would like to experience. *Provides opportunity for learning new information/skills that can enhance feelings of success, improving self-concept.*[3,5]
- Reinforce that current decision to improve self-concept is ongoing. *Continued work and support are necessary to sustain behavior changes/personal growth.*[3,5]
- Discuss ways to develop optimism. *Optimism is a key ingredient in happiness and can be learned.*[7]

• Suggest enrolling in assertiveness training classes. *Promotes learning to assist with developing new skills of voice control, posture, eye contact, or expression of feelings in an assertive, rather than aggressive or passive manner to promote self-esteem.*[3]

• Emphasize importance of grooming and personal hygiene and assist in developing skills to improve appearance and dress for success. *Looking your best improves sense of self-worth, and presenting a positive appearance enhances how others see you. While these things are important, having an adequate foundation for the experience of competence and worth is essential to maintaining one's self-concept.*[1,6]

DOCUMENTATION FOCUS

Assessment/Reassessment

• Individual findings, including evaluations of self and others, current and past successes.
• Interactions with others/lifestyle.
• Cultural/religious influences.
• Motivation for/willingness to change.

Planning

• Plan of care and who is involved in planning.
• Educational plan.

Implementation/Evaluation

• Responses to interventions/teaching and actions performed.
• Attainment/progress toward desired outcome(s).
• Modifications to plan of care.

Discharge Planning

• Long-term needs and who is responsible for actions to be taken.
• Specific referrals made.

References

1. Townsend, M. C. (2003). *Psychiatric Mental Health Nursing Concepts of Care.* 4th ed. Philadelphia: F. A. Davis.
2. Doenges, M. E., Townsend, M. C., Moorhouse, M. F. (1998). *Psychiatric Care Plans Guidelines for Individualizing Patient Care.* 3d ed. Philadelphia: F. A. Davis.
3. Doenges, M. E., Moorhouse, M. F., Geissler-Murr, A. C. (2004). *Nurse's Pocket Guide Diagnoses, Interventions, and Rationales.* 9th ed. Philadelphia: F. A. Davis.
4. Gordon, T. Family Effectiveness Training, Video Home Program
5. Gordon, T. (2000). *Parent Effectiveness Training* (updated ed). New York: Three River Press.
6. FAQ's about Self Esteem. National Association of Self-Esteem. Available at www.self-esteem-nase.org.
7. Schuman, W. Keeping your sunny side up. Retrieved April 2007 at www.beliefnet.com/story/147/story_14745_1.html.
8. Beland, N. (April–May 2005). Special report: The pursuit of happiness. Women's Health. Retrieved April 2007 at http://womenshealthmag.com/article/0,6176,s1-3-72-111-2,00.html.

chronic low Self-Esteem

Definition: Long-standing negative self-evaluation/feelings about self or self-capabilities

RELATED FACTORS

To be developed by nurse researchers and submitted to NANDA

[Fixation in earlier level of development]

[Continual negative evaluation of self/capabilities from childhood]

[Personal vulnerability]

[Life choices perpetuating failure; ineffective social/occupational functioning]

[Feelings of abandonment by SO; willingness to tolerate possibly life-threatening domestic violence]

[Chronic physical/psychiatric conditions; antisocial behaviors]

DEFINING CHARACTERISTICS

Subjective

Self-negating verbalization

Expressions of shame/guilt

Evaluates self as unable to deal with events

Rejects positive/exaggerates negative feedback about self

Objective

Hesitant to try new things/situations

Frequent lack of success in work/life events

Overly conforming; dependent on others' opinions

Lack of eye contact

Nonassertive; passive; indecisive

Excessively seeks reassurance

Sample Clinical Applications: Chronic health conditions, degenerative diseases, eating disorders, substance abuse, depressive disorders, personality disorders, pervasive developmental disorders

DESIRED OUTCOMES/EVALUATION CRITERIA

Sample NOC linkages:

Self-Esteem: Personal judgment of self-worth

Personal Autonomy: Personal actions of a competent individual to exercise governance in life decisions

Hope: Optimism that is personally satisfying and life-supporting

Client Will (Include Specific Time Frame)

• Verbalize understanding of negative evaluation of self and reasons for this problem.
• Participate in treatment program to promote change in self-evaluation.
• Demonstrate behaviors/lifestyle changes to promote positive self-image.
• Verbalize increased sense of self-worth in relation to current situation.
• Participate in family/group/community activities to enhance change.

ACTIONS/INTERVENTIONS

Sample NIC linkages:

Self-Esteem Enhancement: Assisting a patient to increase his or her personal judgment of self-worth

Cultural   Collaborative   Community/Home Care   Diagnostic Studies   Pediatric/Geriatric/Lifespan   Medications

Emotional Support: Provision of reassurance, acceptance, and encouragement during times of stress

Body Image Enhancement: Improving a patient's conscious and unconscious perceptions and attitudes toward his or her body

NURSING PRIORITY NO. 1 To assess causative/contributing factors:

- Determine factors of low self-esteem that may have been exacerbated by current situation, noting age and developmental level of individual. *Occurrences such as family crises, physical disfigurement from an accident or illness, feelings of abandonment by SO resulting in social isolation are important to identify to develop plan of care and choose appropriate interventions to help client develop a sense of self-worth.*[1]

- Assess content of negative self-talk. Note client's perceptions of how others view him or her. *Constant repetition of negative words and thoughts reinforce idea that individual is worthless and belief that others view him or her in a negative manner. Identifying these negative ruminations and bringing them to the client's awareness enables person to begin to replace them with positive thoughts.*[1]

- Note nonverbal behavior (e.g., nervous movements, lack of eye contact). *Incongruencies between verbal/nonverbal communication require clarification to ensure accuracy of interpretation.*[1,6]

- Determine availability/quality of family/SO(s) support. *Family is an important component of how an individual views self. The development of a positive sense of self depends on how the person relates to members of the family, as they are growing up and in the current situation.*[1,3]

- Identify family dynamics, present and past. *How family members interact affects an individual's development and sense of self-esteem. If family members are negative and nonsupportive, or positive and supportive, affects the needs of the client at this time.*[4,5]

- Be alert to client's concept of self in relation to cultural/religious ideal(s). *Composition and structure of nuclear family influences individual's sense of who they are in relation to others in the family and in society. Mexican American culture dictates that family comes first, the father is the authority in the family, and the behavior of the individual reflects on the entire family.*[10]

- Determine degree of participation and cooperation with therapeutic regimen. *Maintaining scheduled medications, such as antidepressants/antipsychotics, and other aspects of the plan of care indicates need for additional evaluation and possibility of change in regimen.*[1,2]

- Note willingness to seek assistance, motivation for change. *Determines client's degree of participation in adhering to therapeutic regimen.*[1,11]

NURSING PRIORITY NO. 2 To promote client's sense of self-esteem in dealing with situation:

- Develop therapeutic relationship. Be attentive, validate client's communication, provide encouragement for efforts, maintain open communication, use skills of Active-listening and I-messages. *Promotes trusting situation in which client is free to be open and honest with self and therapist so current situation can be dealt with most effectively.*[1,4,5]

- Collaborate in addressing presenting medical/safety concerns. *Client's self-esteem may be affected by physical changes of current medical situation. Changes in body, such as weight loss/gain, chronic illness, amputation will affect how client sees self as a person. Attitude may contribute to feelings of depression and lack of attention to personal safety requiring evaluation and assistance.*[1,3,8]

- Accept client's perceptions/view of situation. Avoid threatening existing self-esteem. *Promotes trust and allows client to begin to look at options for improving self-esteem.*[2,9]

- Be aware that people are not programmed to be rational. *They must seek information—choosing to learn, to think rather than merely accepting/reacting—in order to have respect for self, facts, honesty, and to develop positive self-esteem.*[1,3]
- Discuss client perceptions of self related to what is happening; confront misconceptions and negative self-talk. Address distortions in thinking, such as self-referencing (belief that others are focusing on individual's weaknesses/limitations), filtering (focusing on negative and ignoring positive), catastrophizing (expecting the worst outcomes). *Addressing these issues openly provides opportunity for change.*[1,3,11]
- Emphasize need to avoid comparing self with others. Encourage client to focus on aspects of self that can be valued. *Changing negative thinking can be effective in developing positive self-talk to enhance self-esteem.*[2,6]
- Have client list current/past successes and strengths. *Often in the depths of despair and sense of failure in current situation, individual forgets these positive aspects of his or her life, and bringing them to mind can remind client of these successes, enhancing sense of self-esteem.*[3–5]
- Use positive I-messages rather than praise. *Praise may be heard as manipulative and insincere and be rejected. Use of positive I-messages communicates a feeling that is genuine and real and allows client to feel good about himself or herself, developing internal sense of self-esteem.*[4–6]
- Discuss what behavior does for client (positive intention) and what options are available to the client/SO(s). *Helping client begin to look at what rewards are gained from current actions and what actions might be taken to achieve the same rewards in a more positive way can provide a realistic and accurate self-appraisal, enhancing sense of competence and self-worth.*[1,3,11]
- Assist client to deal with sense of powerlessness. (Refer to ND Powerlessness.)
- Set limits on aggressive or problem behaviors such as acting out, suicide preoccupation, or rumination. Put self in client's place using empathy not sympathy. *Preventing undesirable behavior prevents feelings of worthlessness. Suicidal thoughts need further evaluation and intervention. Use of empathy helps caregiver to understand client's feelings better.*[1,2]
- Give reinforcement for progress noted. *Positive words of encouragement promote continuation of efforts, supporting development of coping behaviors.*[2,4,5,12]
- Encourage client to progress at own rate. *Adaptation to a change in self-concept depends on its significance to individual, disruption to lifestyle, and length of crisis/condition.*[1,2,6]
- Assist client to recognize and cope with events, alterations, and sense of loss of control. *Incorporating changes accurately into self-concept enhances sense of self-worth.*[1,2,8]
- Involve in activities/exercise program, promote socialization. *Enhances sense of well-being/can help energize client.*[1,6]

NURSING PRIORITY NO. 3 To promote wellness (Teaching/Discharge Considerations):

- Discuss inaccuracies in self-perception with client/SO(s). *Enables client and significant others to begin to look at misperceptions and accept reality and look at options for change to improve sense of self-worth.*[1,7,9]
- Model behaviors being taught, involving client in goal-setting and decision making. *Facilitates client's developing trust in their own unique strengths.*
- Prepare client for events/changes that are expected, when possible. *Providing time to adapt to changes allows client to prepare self and feel more confident in ability to manage the changes, enhancing sense of self-worth.*[1,2,8]
- Provide structure in daily routine/care activities. *Knowing what to expect promotes a sense of control and ability to deal with activities as they occur.*[1,2,]
- Emphasize importance of grooming and personal hygiene. Assist in developing skills as indicated (e.g., makeup classes, dressing for success). *People feel better about themselves when they present a positive outer appearance.*[1,3,6]

Cultural   Collaborative   Community/Home Care   Diagnostic Studies   Pediatric/Geriatric/Lifespan   Medications

• Assist client to identify goals that are personally achievable. Provide positive feedback for verbal and behavioral indications of improved self-view. *Increases likelihood of success and commitment to change.*[6,12]

• Refer to vocational/employment counselor, educational resources as appropriate. *Assists with development of social/vocational skills, promoting sense of competence and self-responsibility.*[1,2,4,6]

• Encourage participation in classes/activities/hobbies that client enjoys or would like to experience. *Meaningful accomplishment, assuming self-responsibility, and participating in new activities engenders one's sense of competence and self-worth.*[9,13]

• Reinforce that this therapy is a brief encounter in overall life of the client/SO(s), with continued work and ongoing support being necessary to sustain behavior changes/personal growth. *Provides individual with information and encouragement to build on for the future.*[1,7,8]

• Refer to classes to assist with learning new skills (e.g., assertiveness training, positive self-image, communication skills). *These skills can help client develop a sense of competence through realistic and accurate self-appraisal promoting self-esteem.*[11]

• Refer to counseling/therapy, mental health or other special needs support groups as indicated. *May need additional intervention to develop needed changes.*[1,11,12]

DOCUMENTATION FOCUS

Assessment/Reassessment

• Individual findings, including early memories of negative evaluations (self and others), subsequent/precipitating failure events.
• Effects on interactions with others/lifestyle.
• Specific medical/safety issues.
• Cultural/religious factors.
• Motivation for/willingness to change.

Planning

• Plan of care and who is involved in planning.
• Teaching plan.

Implementation/Evaluation

• Responses to interventions/teaching and actions performed.
• Attainment/progress toward desired outcome(s).
• Modifications to plan of care.

Discharge Planning

• Long-term needs and who is responsible for actions to be taken.
• Specific referrals made.

References

1. Townsend, M. C. (2006). *Psychiatric Mental Health Nursing Concepts of Care.* 5th ed. Philadelphia: F. A. Davis.
2. Doenges, M. E., Townsend, M. C., Moorhouse, M. F. (1998). *Psychiatric Care Plans Guidelines for Individualizing Patient Care.* 3d ed. Philadelphia: F. A. Davis.
3. Doenges, M. E., Moorhouse, M. F., Geissler-Murr, A. C. (2004). *Nurse's Pocket Guide Diagnoses, Interventions, and Rationales.* 9th ed. Philadelphia: F. A. Davis.

4. Gordon, T. Family Effectiveness Training, Video Home Program
5. Gordon, T. (2000). *Parent Effectiveness Training* (updated ed). New York: Three River Press.
6. FAQ's about Self Esteem. National Association of Self-Esteem. Available at www.self-esteem-nase.org.
7. Vasconcellos, J., Reasoner, R., Borba, M., Duhl, L., Canfield, J. In Defense of Self-Esteem. National Association for Self-Esteem. Accessed January 2004 at www.self-esteem-nase.org.
8. Battle, J. (1990). *Self-Esteem: The New Revolution.* Edmonton, Alberta, Canada: James Battle & Associates.
9. Reasoner, R. (2000). *The True Meaning of Self-Esteem.* Palo Alto, CA: Consulting Psychologists Press.
10. Lipson, J. G., Dibble, S. L, Minarik, P. A. (1996). *Culture & Nursing Care: A Pocket Guide.* San Francisco: UCSF Nursing Press.
11. Peden, A. R., Hall, L. A., Rayens, M. K., et al. (2000). Reducing negative thinking and depressive symptoms in college women. *J Nurs Scholar, 32,* 145–151. Accessed August 2007 at [Medline]
12. Seligman, M., Reivich, K., Jaycox, L. H., Gillham, J. (2005). *The Optimistic Child.* Houghton, Mifflin: New York.
13. Branden, N. (1995). *The Six Pillars of Self-Esteem.* Bantam Book: New York.

situational low Self-Esteem

Definition: Development of a negative perception of self-worth in response to a current situation (specify)

RELATED FACTORS

Developmental changes [e.g., maturational transitions, adolescence, aging]

Functional impairment; disturbed body image

Loss [e.g., loss of health status, body part, independent functioning; memory deficit/cognitive impairment]

Social role changes

Failures/rejections; lack of recognition[/rewards; feelings of abandonment by SO]

Behavior inconsistent with values

DEFINING CHARACTERISTICS

Subjective
Verbally reports current situational challenge to self-worth
Expressions of helplessness/uselessness
Evaluation of self as unable to deal with situations or events

Objective
Self-negating verbalizations
Indecisive/nonassertive behavior

Sample Clinical Applications: Traumatic injuries, surgery, pregnancy, newly diagnosed conditions (e.g., diabetes mellitus), adjustment disorders, substance use, stroke, dementia

DESIRED OUTCOMES/EVALUATION CRITERIA

Sample NOC linkages:

Self-Esteem: Personal judgment of self-worth

Psychosocial Adjustment: Life Change: Adaptive psychosocial response of an individual to a significant life change

Abuse Recovery: Emotional: Extent of healing of psychological injuries due to abuse

Client Will (Include Specific Time Frame)

• Verbalize understanding of individual factors that precipitated current situation.

Cultural Collaborative Community/Home Care Diagnostic Studies Pediatric/Geriatric/Lifespan Medications

- Identify feelings and underlying dynamics for negative perception of self.
- Express positive self-appraisal.
- Demonstrate behaviors to restore positive self-image.
- Participate in treatment regimen/activities to correct factors that precipitated crisis.

ACTIONS/INTERVENTIONS

Sample NIC linkages:

Self-Esteem Enhancement: Assisting a patient to increase his or her personal judgment of self-worth

Coping Enhancement: Assisting a patient to adapt to perceived stressors, changes, or threats that interfere with meeting life demands and roles

Support System Enhancement: Facilitation of support to patient by family, friends, and community

NURSING PRIORITY NO. 1 To assess causative/contributing factors:

- Determine individual situation (e.g., family crisis, termination of a relationship, loss of employment, physical disfigurement) related to low self-esteem in the present circumstances. *Many factors are involved in a person's self-esteem, and this information is essential for planning accurate care.*[1]
- Identify basic sense of self-esteem of client; image client has of self—existential, physical, and psychological. *The components of self-concept consist of the physical self or body image, the personal self or personal identity, and the self-esteem. Each aspect plays a role in the client's ability to deal with current situation/crisis.*[1]
- Assess degree of threat/perception of client concerning crisis. *How individuals perceive themselves is based on the self-judgments they make. How the client sees the current situation in relation to ability to cope will affect his or her sense of self-worth and needs to be acknowledged and planned for to help client deal with feelings of low self-esteem.*[1,2]
- Ascertain sense of control client has (or perceives to have) over self and situation. *Client's locus of control/degree of control client believes or perceives he or she has may be a critical factor in ability to deal with current situation/crisis. Individuals with internal locus of control tend to be more optimistic about their ability to deal with adversity even in the face of current difficulties. Individuals with external locus of control will look to others to solve problems and take care of them.*[1–3]
- Determine client's awareness of own responsibility for dealing with situation, personal growth, and so forth. *These factors enhance the ability of the client to effectively manage situation in a positive manner.*[4]
- Assess family/SO(s) dynamics and support of client. *How family members interact affects an individual's development and sense of self-esteem. Effective interactions among family members usually lead to positive support for the client in current situation. Dysfunctional interactions may be detrimental to client's ability to deal with what is happening.*[2,3]
- Verify client's concept of self in relation to cultural/religious ideals. *Self-esteem is developed by many factors, including genetics and environment. Cultural and religious influences during the individual's life affect beliefs about self, measure of worth, and ability to deal with current situation/crisis.*[1,5]
- Determine past coping skills in relation to current episode. *Trust is built over time, and past experiences with failure or success will affect client's expectations regarding the eventual outcome of dealing with current illness/crisis.*[8,9]

- Assess negative attitudes or self-talk. *An individual who is feeling unimportant, incompetent, and not in control often is unconsciously saying negative things to himself or herself that contribute to a loss of self-esteem and an attitude of despair, affecting current situation.*[1,7]
- Note nonverbal body language. *Incongruencies between verbal/nonverbal communication require clarification to assure accuracy of interpretation.*[1,2]
- Assess for self-destructive/suicidal thoughts or behavior. *Client who believes situation is hopeless often begins to consider suicide as an option.* (Refer to ND risk for Suicide as appropriate.)[1]
- Identify previous adaptations to illness/disruptive events in life. *May be predictive of current ability to deal with situation and suggest eventual outcome.*[1]
- Note availability/use of resources to address specific need (e.g., rehabilitation services, home-care support, job placement). *Individual may be unaware or have difficulty accessing community supports/assistance programs.*

NURSING PRIORITY NO. 2 To assist client to deal with loss/change and recapture sense of positive self-esteem:

- Assist with treatment of underlying condition when possible. *For example, cognitive restructuring and improved concentration in mild brain injury often result in restoration of positive self-esteem.*[1]
- Encourage expression of feelings, anxieties. Facilitate grieving the loss. *As client expresses feelings and anxieties, he or she begins to deal with the realities of the current situation and the loss that occurs with the changes of illness.*[1] (Refer to ND Grieving as appropriate.)
- Active-listen to client's concerns/negative verbalizations without comment or judgment. *Conveys a message of acceptance and confidence in client's ability to deal with whatever occurs.*[6]
- Identify individual strengths/assets and aspects of self that remain intact, can be valued. Reinforce positive traits, abilities, self-view. *Client may not see these in the anxiety and hopelessness of the immediate situation, and reminding client of own positive attributes can help him or her recover hope and develop a positive attitude about situation.*[1,7]
- Help client identify own responsibility and control or lack of control in situation. *Accepting responsibility enables client to look realistically at what is under own control and what is not. When client stops expending energy on issues that cannot be controlled, energy is freed up to concentrate on more productive avenues.*[1,8]
- Assist client to problem-solve situation, developing plan of action and setting goals to achieve desired outcome. *Personal involvement enhances commitment to plan, optimizing outcomes.*[6]
- Convey confidence in client's ability to cope with current situation. *Validation helps client accept own ability to deal with what is happening.*[1]
- Mobilize support systems; identify individuals in similar circumstances. *Feeling hopeless and alone lowers client's ability to manage care and concentrate on healing. Support systems can provide role modeling and the help needed to engender hope and enhance self-esteem.*[1,3]
- Provide opportunity for client to practice alternative coping strategies, including progressive socialization opportunities. *Involvement with others provides client with situation in which new actions can be tried out and validated or discarded to enhance feelings of self-worth.*[1,3]
- Encourage use of visualization, guided imagery, and relaxation. *These strategies promote a positive sense of self and general well-being, enhancing client's coping ability.*[1]
- Provide feedback about client's self-negating remarks/behavior, using I-messages. *Allows client to experience a different view. I-messages are a nonjudgmental way to let individual understand how behavior is perceived/affecting others and self.*[6]

Cultural   Collaborative   Community/Home Care   Diagnostic Studies   Pediatric/Geriatric/Lifespan   Medications

- Encourage involvement in decisions about care when possible. *Promotes sense of control over what is happening, enhancing feelings of self-worth.*[1,8]
- Give reinforcement for progress noted. *Positive words of encouragement promote continuation of efforts, supporting development of coping behaviors.*[6,10]

NURSING PRIORITY NO. 3 To promote wellness (Teaching/Discharge Considerations):

- Assist client to identify personally achievable goals. *Increases likelihood of client's success and commitment to change.*[2,10]
- Encourage client to look to the future and set long-range goals for achieving necessary lifestyle changes. *Supports view that this is an ongoing process, providing client with hope for the future.*[1,3]
- Support independence in ADLs/mastery of therapeutic regimen. *Individuals who are confident are more secure and positive in self-appraisal.*[1,2]
- Promote attendance in therapy/support group as indicated. *Provides opportunity to discuss own situation and hear how others are dealing with similar problems, promoting new ideas about own ability to deal with issues.*[1,9,10]
- Involve extended family/SO(s) in treatment plan as appropriate. *Enhances their understanding of what client wishes to accomplish, increasing likelihood they will provide appropriate support to client.*[1]
- Provide information/bibliotherapy/reliable Web sites. *Reinforces learning, allowing client to progress at own pace. Promotes opportunity for making informed decisions and improving ability to deal with situation.*[1,7]
- Refer to vocational/employment counselor, educational resources, as appropriate. *Assists with development of social/vocational skills, promoting sense of competence and self-responsibility.*[1,2]
- Suggest participation in group/community activities (e.g., assertiveness classes, volunteer work, support groups). *Provides opportunities for learning new information and being appreciated for contributions, enhancing sense of self-worth.*[1,2]
- Refer to counseling/therapy, mental health, or other special-needs support groups, as indicated. *May need additional support to deal with crisis.*[1,10]

DOCUMENTATION FOCUS

Assessment/Reassessment

- Individual findings, noting precipitating crisis, client's perceptions, effects on desired lifestyle/interaction with others.
- Cultural values/religious beliefs, locus of control.
- Family support, availability/use of resources.

Planning

- Plan of care and who is involved in planning.
- Teaching plan.

Implementation/Evaluation

- Responses to interventions/teaching, actions performed, and changes that may be indicated.
- Attainment/progress toward desired outcome(s).
- Modifications to plan of care.

Discharge Planning

- Long-term needs/goals and who is responsible for actions to be taken.
- Specific referrals made.

References

1. Townsend, M. C. (2003). *Psychiatric Mental Health Nursing Concepts of Care.* 4th ed. Philadelphia: F. A. Davis.
2. FAQs, National Association for Self-Esteem. Available at www.self-esteem-nase.org.
3. Battle, J. (1990). *Self-Esteem: The New Revolution.* Edmonton, Alberta, Canada: James Battle & Associates.
4. Reasoner, R. (2000). *The True Meaning of Self Esteem.* Palo Alto, CA: Consulting Psychologists Press.
5. Lipson, J. G., Dibble S. L., Minarik, P. A. (1996). *Culture & Nursing Care: A Pocket Guide.* San Francisco: UCSF Nursing Press.
6. Gordon, T. (2000). *Parent Effectiveness Training.* New York: Three Rivers Press.
7. Peden, A., et al. (2000). Reducing negative thinking and depressive symptoms in college women. *J Nurs Scholarsh, 32,* 2.
8. Munson, P. J. (1991). Life's Decisions—by Chance or by Choice? Adapted from Winning Teachers, Teaching Winners. Santa Cruz, CA: ETR Associates.
9. Vasconcellos, J., Reasoner, R., Borba, M., Duhl, L., Canfield, J. In Defense of Self-Esteem. National Association for Self-Esteem. Accessed January 2004 at www.self-esteem-nase.org.
10. Seligman, M., Reivich, K., Jaycox, L. H., Gillham, J. (1995). *The Optimistic Child.* Houghton, Mifflin: New York.

risk for situational low Self-Esteem

Definition: At risk for developing negative perception of self-worth in response to a current situation (specify)

RISK FACTORS

Developmental changes

Disturbed body image; functional impairment

Loss [e.g., loss of health status, body part, independent functioning; memory deficit/cognitive impairment]

Social role changes

Unrealistic self-expectations; history of learned helplessness

History of neglect/abuse/abandonment

Behavior inconsistent with values

Lack of recognition; failures; rejections

Decreased control over environment

Physical illness

NOTE: A risk diagnosis is not evidenced by signs and symptoms, as the problem has not occurred; rather, nursing interventions are directed at prevention.

Sample Clinical Applications: Traumatic injuries, surgery, pregnancy, newly diagnosed conditions (e.g., diabetes mellitus, hypertension), adjustment disorders, substance use, stroke, dementia

DESIRED OUTCOMES/EVALUATION CRITERIA

Sample NOC linkages:

Self-Esteem: Personal judgment of self-worth

Psychosocial Adjustment: Life Change: Adaptive psychosocial response of an individual to a significant life change

Abuse Recovery: Emotional: Extent of healing of psychological injuries due to abuse

Cultural   Collaborative   Community/Home Care   Diagnostic Studies   Pediatric/Geriatric/Lifespan   Medications

Client Will (Include Specific Time Frame)

- Acknowledge factors that lead to possibility of feelings of low self-esteem.
- Verbalize view of self as a worthwhile, important person who functions well both interpersonally and occupationally.
- Demonstrate self-confidence by setting realistic goals and actively participating in life situation.

ACTIONS/INTERVENTIONS

Sample NIC linkages:

Self-Esteem Enhancement: Assisting a patient to increase his or her personal judgment of self-worth

Coping Enhancement: Assisting a patient to adapt to perceived stressors, changes, or threats that interfere with meeting life demands and roles

Support System Enhancement: Facilitation of support to patient by family, friends, and community

NURSING PRIORITY NO. 1 To assess causative/contributing factors:

- Determine individual factors that may contribute to diminished self-esteem. *Proactive information allows identification of appropriate interventions to deal with current situation.*[1,2]
- Identify basic sense of self-worth of client, image client has of self—existential, physical, psychological. *The components of self-concept consist of the physical self or body image, the personal self or personal identity, and the self-esteem with each aspect playing a role in the client's ability to deal with anticipated changes.*[1]
- Note client's perception of threat to self in current situation. *Perception is more important than reality of what is happening. Some individuals view a potentially severe situation as something easily handled while another may view a minor problem with anxiety and catastrophizing.*[2,3]
- Ascertain sense of control client has (or perceives to have) over self and situation. *Individual with internal locus of control tends to perceive self in control of what is happening and will participate more actively in care and feel more sense of self-worth.*[7,8]
- Determine client awareness of own responsibility for dealing with situation, personal growth and so forth. *Acceptance of responsibility for self enables client to feel more comfortable with treatment regime and participate more fully, promoting self-esteem.*[1,9]
- Assess family/SO(s) dynamics and support of client. *How family interacts with one another affects not only the development of self-esteem but also the maintenance of a sense of self-worth when client is facing an illness or crisis. Dysfunctional interactions may be detrimental to client's ability to deal with what is happening.*[1,5]
- Verify client's concept of self in relation to cultural/religious ideals. *Culture and religion play a major role in view individual has of self in relation to self-worth. Illness may interfere with this view; for instance, males in Mexican American culture are seen as the head of the household, and giving up this role because of illness can diminish self-esteem.*[4]
- Assess negative attitudes and/or self-talk. *Contributes to view of situation as hopeless, difficult.*[3,6]
- Listen for self-destructive/suicidal thoughts or behaviors. *Indicates high level of stress, need for further evaluation and referral for mental health services.*[1,6] (Refer to ND risk for Suicide as appropriate.)

- Note nonverbal body language. *Incongruencies between verbal/nonverbal communications require clarification to assure accuracy of interpretation.*[1]
- Identify previous adaptations to illness/disruptive events in life. *Provides information about how client handled those situations and may be predictive of current outcome.*[1]
- Determine availability/use of support systems. *Feeling hopeless and alone lowers client ability to manage care and concentrate on healing. Support systems can provide role modeling and the help needed to engender hope and enhance self-esteem.*[1]
- Note availability/use of resources to address specific need (e.g., rehabilitation services, home-care support, job placement). *Individual may be unaware or have difficulty accessing community supports/ assistance programs.*
- Refer to NDs situational low Self-Esteem, and chronic low Self-Esteem as appropriate for additional nursing priorities/interventions.

DOCUMENTATION FOCUS

Assessment/Reassessment

- Individual findings, including individual expressions of lack of self-esteem, effects on interactions with others/lifestyle.
- Underlying dynamics and duration (situational or situational exacerbating chronic).
- Cultural values/religious beliefs, locus of control.
- Family support, availability/use of resources.

Planning

- Plan of care and who is involved in planning.
- Teaching plan.

Implementation/Evaluation

- Responses to interventions/teaching, actions performed, and changes that may be indicated.
- Attainment/progress toward desired outcome(s).
- Modifications to plan of care.

Discharge Planning

- Long-term needs/goals and who is responsible for actions to be taken.
- Specific referrals made.

References

1. Townsend, M. C. (2003). *Psychiatric Mental Health Nursing Concepts of Care.* 4th ed. Philadelphia: F. A. Davis.
2. Battle, J. (1990). *Self-Esteem: The New Revolution.* Edmonton, Alberta, Canada: James Battle & Associates.
3. Reasoner, R. (2000). *The True Meaning of Self Esteem.* Palo Alto, CA: Consulting Psychologists Press.
4. Lipson, J. G., Dibble, S. L., Minarik, P. A. (1996). *Culture & Nursing Care: A Pocket Guide.* San Francisco: UCSF Nursing Press.
5. Gordon, T. (2000). *Parent Effectiveness Training.* New York: Three Rivers Press.
6. Peden, A., et al. (2000). Reducing negative thinking and depressive symptoms in college women. *J Nurs Scholarsh, 32,* 2.
7. Munson, P. J. (1991). Life's Decisions—by Chance or by Choice? Adapted from Winning Teachers, Teaching Winners. Santa Cruz, CA: ETR Associates.
8. Vasconcellos, J., Reasoner, R., Borba, M., Duhl, L., Canfield, J. In Defense of Self-Esteem. National Association for Self-Esteem. Accessed January 2004 at www.self-esteem-nase.org.
9. FAQs, National Association for Self-Esteem. Available at www.self- esteem-nase.org.

Cultural   Collaborative   Community/Home Care   Diagnostic Studies   Pediatric/Geriatric/Lifespan   Medications

Self-Mutilation

Definition: Deliberate self-injurious behavior causing tissue damage with the intent of causing nonfatal injury to attain relief of tension

RELATED FACTORS

Adolescence; peers who self-mutilate; isolation from peers

Dissociation; depersonalization; psychotic state (e.g., command hallucinations); character disorder; borderline personality disorders; emotionally disturbed; developmentally delayed/autistic individual

History of self-injurious behavior, inability to plan solutions, inability to see long-term consequences

Childhood illness/surgery/sexual abuse; battered child

Disturbed body image; eating disorders

Ineffective coping; perfectionism

Negative feelings (e.g., depression, rejection, self-hatred, separation anxiety, guilt, depersonalization); low self-esteem; unstable self-esteem/body image

Poor communication between parent and adolescent; lack of family confidant

Feels threated with loss of significant relationship [loss of parent/parental relationship]

Disturbed interpersonal relationships; use of manipulation to obtain nurturing relationship with others

Family alcoholism/divorce; violence between parental figures; family history of self-destructive behaviors

Living in nontraditional settings (e.g., foster, group, or institutional care); incarceration

Inability to express tension verbally; mounting tension that is intolerable; needs quick reduction of stress

Irresistible urge to cut/damage self; impulsivity; labile behavior

Sexual identity crisis

Substance abuse

DEFINING CHARACTERISTICS

Subjective
Self-inflicted burns (e.g., eraser, cigarette)
Ingestion/inhalation of harmful substances/objects

Objective
Cuts/scratches on body
Picking at wounds
Biting; abrading; severing
Insertion of object(s) into body orifice(s)
Hitting
Constricting a body part

Sample Clinical Applications: Borderline personality, dissociative disorders, bipolar disorder, developmental delay, autism, eating disorders, substance abuse, physical/psychological abuse, gender identity crisis

DESIRED OUTCOMES/EVALUATION CRITERIA

Sample NOC linkages:

Self-Mutilation Restraint: Personal actions to refrain from intentional self-inflected injury (nonlethal)

Impulse Self-Control: Self-restraint of compulsive or impulsive behaviors

Distorted Thought Self-Control: Self-restraint of disruption in perception, thought processes, and thought content

Client Will (Include Specific Time Frame)

- Verbalize understanding of reasons for occurrence of behavior.
- Identify precipitating factors/awareness of arousal state that occurs prior to incident.
- Express increased self-concept/self-esteem.
- Seeks help when feeling anxious and having thoughts of harming self.

ACTIONS/INTERVENTIONS

Sample NIC linkages:

Behavior Management: Self-Harm: Assisting the patient to decrease or eliminate self-mutilating or self-abusive behavior

Environmental Management: Safety: Manipulation of the patient's surroundings for therapeutic benefit

Limit Setting: Establishing the parameters of desirable and acceptable patient behavior

NURSING PRIORITY NO. 1   To assess causative/contributing factors:

- Determine underlying dynamics of individual situation as listed in Related Factors. Note previous episodes of self-mutilation behavior. *Although some body piercing (e.g., ears) is generally accepted as decorative, piercing of multiple sites often is an attempt to establish individuality, addressing issues of separation and belonging, but it is not considered as self-injury behaviors.*[1,7]

- Identify previous history of self-mutilative behavior and relationship to stressful events. *Self-injury is considered an attempt to alter a mood state, an outlet for negative emotions such as anger, shame. Information about previous behavior and precipitating factors is important to understanding and planning care in current situation.*[1,7,9]

- Determine presence of inflexible, maladaptive personality traits that reflect personality/character disorder. *Identification of impulsive, unpredictable, or inappropriate behaviors, intense anger, or lack of control of anger is important for planning appropriate interventions and plan of care. Clients who have been diagnosed as borderline personality disorder are often unstable and prone to self-injury and need a specific treatment plan to diminish these behaviors.*[1,9]

- Evaluate history of mental illness (e.g., borderline personality, identity disorder, bipolar disorder). *These illnesses may be the underlying cause of the self-injurious behavior.*[1,2]

- Note beliefs, cultural/religious practices that may be involved in choice of behavior. *Growing up in a family that did not allow feelings to be expressed, individual may believe that feelings are wrong or bad. Family dynamics may come out of religious or cultural expectations that support strict punishment for transgressions. Individuals may believe mental illness is the result of unacceptable actions, and feelings of guilt may lead to anxiety and subsequent self-injurious behaviors.*[4]

- Note use/abuse of addicting substances. *May be indicative of attempt to treat self and needs further evaluation and additional intervention.*[2,6]

- Review laboratory findings (e.g., blood alcohol, polydrug screen, glucose, and electrolyte levels). *Helpful for identifying drug use or medical problems that may be affecting behavior negatively.*[1]

🌐 Cultural   Ⓐ Collaborative   🏠 Community/Home Care   ✏️ Diagnostic Studies   ∞ Pediatric/Geriatric/Lifespan   💊 Medications

NURSING PRIORITY NO. 2 To structure environment to maintain client safety:

- Assist client to identify feelings leading up to desire for self-mutilation. *Early recognition of recurring feelings provides opportunity to seek other ways of coping.*[5]
- Provide external controls/limit setting. *Decreasing the opportunity to self-mutilate helps the client learn to stop the behavior.*[4,8]
- Encourage appropriate expression of feelings. *Helps client to identify feelings and promote understanding of what leads to development of tension and subsequent injurious behavior.*[2]
- Keep client in continuous staff view and do special observation checks during inpatient stay. *Promotes safety by recognizing escalating behaviors and providing timely intervention.*[2,5]
- Structure inpatient milieu to maintain positive, clear, open communication among staff and clients, with an understanding that "secrets are not tolerated" and will be confronted. *Prevents manipulative behavior, so client does not pit one staff member against another to fulfill own desires.*[1,4,5]
- Note feelings of healthcare providers/family, such as frustration, anger, defensiveness, need to rescue. *Client may be manipulative, evoking defensiveness and conflict. These feelings need to be identified, recognized, and dealt with openly with staff/family and client.*[4]
- Provide care for client's wounds, when self-mutilation occurs, in a matter-of-fact manner. Refrain from offering sympathy or additional attention. *A matter-of-fact approach can convey empathy/concern but not undue concern that could provide reinforcement for maladaptive behavior and encourage its repetition.*[2]
- Discuss use of medication, such as clozapine. *This medication has been shown to reduce acts of self-injurious behavior and help client maintain a more stable mood.*[3]
- Develop schedule of/refer to alternative healthy, success-oriented activities. *Groups such as Overeaters Anonymous (OA) or similar 12-step program based on individual needs, self-esteem activities, including positive affirmations, visiting with friends, and exercise helps client to practice new behaviors in a supportive environment.*[7]

NURSING PRIORITY NO. 3 To promote movement toward positive changes:

- Encourage client involvement in formulating plan of care and developing goals for preventing undesired behavior. *Being involved in own decisions can help to reestablish ego boundaries, enhances commitment to goals, optimizing outcomes and enhancing self-esteem.*[2,5]
- Develop a contract between client and counselor to enable the client to stay physically safe, such as "I will not cut or harm myself for the next 24 hours." Renew contract on a regular basis and have both parties sign and date each contract. *Making a commitment in writing helps client to think before acting and can prevent new incidents of self-injury.*[4]
- Provide avenues of communication for times when client needs to talk. *Having an opportunity to discuss anxieties helps client to avoid cutting or damaging self.*[4,6]
- Assist client to learn assertive behavior. Include the use of effective communication skills, focusing on developing self-esteem by replacing negative self-talk with positive comments. *Low self-esteem is a factor in this behavior, and by learning new ways of expressing self, client can begin to feel better and deal with anxieties in a more positive manner.*[2]
- Choose interventions that help the client to reclaim power in own life (e.g., experiential and cognitive). *Beginning to think in a positive manner and then translating that into action provides reinforcement for using power to stop injurious behaviors and develop a more productive lifestyle.*[2]

NURSING PRIORITY NO. 4 To promote wellness (Teaching/Discharge Considerations):

* Discuss commitment to safety and ways in which client will deal with precursors to undesired behavior. *Identifies specific precursors for individual and provides a plan for client to follow when anxiety becomes overwhelming.*[2,8]

* Promote the use of healthy behaviors, identifying the consequences and outcomes of current actions. *As client develops a more positive attitude and accepts the idea that current actions are being destructive to desired lifestyle, new behaviors can help make needed changes.*[2]

* Identify support systems. *Knowing who client can turn to when anxiety becomes a problem helps to avoid injurious behavior.*[1]

* Discuss living arrangements when client discharged from inpatient program. *May need assistance with transition to changes required to avoid recurrence of self-mutilating behaviors.*[2]

* Involve family/SO(s) in planning for discharge and involve in group therapies as appropriate. *Promotes coordination and continuation of plan, commitment to goals.*[2,6]

* Discuss the role neurotransmitters play in predisposing individual to beginning this behavior. *It is believed that problems in the serotonin system may make the person more aggressive and impulsive, combined with a home where they learned that feelings are bad or wrong leads to turning aggression on self.*[8]

* Provide information and discuss the use of medication as appropriate. *Antidepressant medications may be useful, but they need to be weighed against the potential for overdosing.*[1,3]

* Refer to NDs Anxiety; Self-Esteem (specify); impaired Social Interaction.

DOCUMENTATION FOCUS

Assessment/Reassessment

* Individual findings, including risk factors present, underlying dynamics, prior episodes.
* Cultural/religious practices.
* Laboratory test results.
* Substance use/abuse.

Planning

* Plan of care and who is involved in planning.
* Teaching plan.

Implementation/Evaluation

* Response to interventions/teaching and actions performed.
* Attainment/progress toward desired outcome(s).
* Modifications to plan of care.

Discharge Planning

* Long-range needs and who is responsible for actions to be taken.
* Community resources, referrals made.

References

1. Townsend, M. C. (2006). *Psychiatric Mental Health Nursing Concepts of Care.* 5th ed. Philadelphia: F. A. Davis.
2. Doenges, M. E., Townsend, M. C., Moorhouse, M. F. (1998). *Psychiatric Care Plans Guidelines for Individualizing Care.* 3d ed. Philadelphia: F. A. Davis.
3. Chengappa, K. N., et al. (1999). Clozapine reduces severe self-mutilation and aggression in psychotic patients with borderline personality disorder. *J Clin Psychiatry,* 60(7), 477–484.

🌐 Cultural   Ⓐ Collaborative   🏠 Community/Home Care   Diagnostic Studies   ∞ Pediatric/Geriatric/Lifespan   Medications

4. Clarke, L., Whittaker, M. (1998). Self-mutilation: Culture, contexts, and nursing responses. *J Clin Nurs*, 7(2), 129–137.
5. Dallam, S. J. (1997). The identification and management of self-mutilating patients in primary care. *Nurs Pract*, 22(5), 151–153, 159–165.
6. Selekman, M. D. (2004). Adolescent self-harm: A growing epidemic. *Family Therapy Magazine*, 1(2), 34–40.
7. Cox, et al. (2002). *Clincal Applications of Nursing Diagnosis: Adult, Child, Women's Psychiatric, Gerontic and Home Health Considerations*. 4th ed. Philadelphia: F. A. Davis.
8. Focus Adolescent Services: Self-Injury. (2001). Retrieved August 2007 at www.focusas.com/SelfInjury.html.
9. Frey, R. (2002, updated 2006). Self-mutilation. Gale Encyclopedia of Medicine. Retrieved August 2007 at www.healthatoz.com/healthatoz/Atoz/common/standard/transform.jsp?requestURI=/healthatoz/Atoz/ency/self-mutilation.jsp.

risk for Self-Mutilation

Definition: At risk for deliberate self-injurious behavior causing tissue damage with the intent of causing nonfatal injury to attain relief of tension

RISK FACTORS

Adolescence; peers who self-mutilate; isolation from peers

Dissociation; depersonalization; psychotic state (e.g., command hallucinations); character disorders; borderline personality disorders; emotionally disturbed child; developmentally delayed/autistic individuals

History of self-injurious behavior, inability to plan solutions, inability to see long-term consequences

Childhood illness/surgery/sexual abuse; battered child

Disturbed body image; eating disorders

Ineffective coping; loss of control over problem-solving situations; perfectionism

Negative feelings (e.g., depression, rejection, self-hatred, separation anxiety, guilt); low/unstable self-esteem

Feels threatened with loss of significant relationship; loss of significant relationship; lack of family confidant

Disturbed interpersonal relationships; use of manipulation to obtain nurturing relationship with others

Family alcoholism/divorce; violence between parental figures; family history of self-destructive behaviors

Living in nontraditional settings (e.g., foster, group, or institutional care); incarceration

Inability to express tension verbally; mounting tension that is intolerable; needs quick reduction of stress; irresistible urge to damage self; impulsivity

Sexual identity crisis

Substance abuse

NOTE: A risk diagnosis is not evidenced by signs and symptoms, as the problem has not occurred; rather, nursing interventions are directed at prevention.

Sample Clinical Applications: Borderline personality, dissociative disorders, bipolar disorder, developmental delay, autism, eating disorders, substance abuse, physical/psychological abuse, gender identity crisis

DESIRED OUTCOMES/EVALUATION CRITERIA

Sample NOC linkages:

Self-Mutilation Restraint: Personal actions to refrain from intentional self-inflicted injury (nonlethal)

Impulse Self-Control: Self-restraint of compulsive or impulsive behaviors
Distorted Thought Self-Control: Self-restraint of disruption in perception, thought
processes, and thought content

Client Will (Include Specific Time Frame)

- Verbalize understanding of reasons for occurrence of behavior.
- Identify precipitating factors/awareness of arousal state that occurs prior to incident.
- Express increased self-concept/self-esteem.
- Demonstrate self-control as evidenced by lessened (or absence of) episodes of self-mutilation.
- Engage in use of alternative methods for managing feelings/individuality.

ACTIONS/INTERVENTIONS

Sample NIC linkages:
Behavior Modification: Promotion of a behavior change
Calming Technique: Reducing anxiety in patient experiencing acute distress
Behavior Management: Self-Harm: Assisting the patient to decrease or eliminate self-mutilating or self-abusive behavior

NURSING PRIORITY NO. I To assess causative/contributing factors:

- Determine underlying dynamics of individual situation as listed in Risk Factors. Note the presence of conditions that may interfere with ability to control own behavior (e.g., psychotic state, mental retardation, autism) *that may lead to incidents of self-injury.*[1]
- Asses for inflexible, maladaptive personality traits. *May reflect personality/character disorder (e.g., impulsive, unpredictable, inappropriate behaviors, intense anger or lack of control of anger) that may lead to self-mutilative behaviors.*[1]
- Evaluate history of mental illness (e.g., borderline personality, identity disorder, bipolar disorder). *These illnesses may be the underlying cause of the self-injurious behavior.*[1,2]
- Identify previous episodes of self-mutilating behavior (e.g., cutting, scratching, bruising). *Self-injury is considered an attempt to alter a mood state, an outlet for negative emotions such as anger, shame. Information about previous behavior and precipitating factors is important to understanding and planning care in current situation.*[1,7,9] *Note: Although some body piercing (e.g., ears) is generally accepted as decorative, and while piercing of multiple sites often is an attempt to establish individuality, addressing issues of separation and belonging, it is not considered self-injury behaviors.*[2]
- Note beliefs, cultural/religious practices that may be involved in choice of behavior. *Growing up in a family that did not allow feelings to be expressed, individual may believe that feelings are wrong or bad. Family dynamics may come out of religious or cultural expectations that support strict punishment for transgressions. Individuals may believe mental illness is the result of unacceptable actions, and feelings of guilt may lead to anxiety and subsequent self-injurious behaviors.*[4]
- Determine use/abuse of addictive substances, including alcohol. *Individuals often use these substances to self-medicate feelings of anxiety and may increase the risk of suicide by sixfold.*[2,8]
- Note degree of impairment in social and occupational functioning. *May dictate treatment setting (e.g., specific outpatient program, or short-stay inpatient when client is experiencing extreme anxiety).*[1,5]

Cultural Collaborative Community/Home Care Diagnostic Studies Pediatric/Geriatric/Lifespan Medications

- Review laboratory findings (e.g., blood alcohol, polydrug screen, glucose, electrolyte levels). *Helpful for identifying drug use or medical problems that may be affecting behavior negatively.*[1]

NURSING PRIORITY NO. 2 To structure environment to maintain client safety:

- Assist client to identify feelings and behaviors that precede desire for self-mutilation. *Early recognition of recurring feelings provides client opportunity to seek other ways of coping, including asking for help.*[2,6]
- Provide external controls/limit setting as indicated. *Decreases the opportunity to injure self and helps client think about reasons for actions and learn different ways to deal with them.*[1]
- Encourage client to recognize and appropriately express feelings verbally. *Learning to express feelings enables client not only to recognize them, but also to begin to find acceptable/appropriate ways to deal with them.*[6,7]
- Note feelings of healthcare providers/family, such as frustration, anger, defensiveness, distraction, despair and powerlessness, need to rescue. *Client may be manipulating/splitting providers/family members, which evokes defensiveness and resultant conflict. These feelings need to be identified, recognized, and dealt with openly with staff/family and client.*[1]
- Refer to alternative healthy, success-oriented activities. *Groups such as Overeaters Anonymous (OA) or similar 12-step program based on individual needs, self-esteem activities including positive affirmations, visiting with friends, and exercise helps client to practice new behaviors in a supportive environment.*[6]

NURSING PRIORITY NO. 3 To promote movement toward positive actions:

- Encourage client involvement in formulating plan of care and developing goals for preventing undesired behavior. *Being involved in own decisions can help to reestablish ego boundaries, enhances commitment to goals, optimizing outcomes and enhancing self-esteem.*[2,5]
- Develop a contract between client and counselor to enable the client to stay physically safe, such as "I will not cut or harm myself for the next 24 hours." Renew contract on a regular basis, signed and dated by both parties. *Discussing the contract gets issues out in the open and conveys a sense of acceptance of the client, while placing some of the responsibility for safety on the client.*[1,2]
- Provide avenues of communication for times when client needs to talk. *Having an opportunity to discuss anxieties helps client to avoid cutting or damaging self.*[4,6]
- Choose interventions that help the client to reclaim power in own life (e.g., experiential and cognitive). *As client experiences new ways of interacting with others, he or she can begin to think more positively about self-worth and changing behaviors.*[2]
- Identify the consequences and outcomes of current actions: "Does this get you what you want?" "How does this behavior help you achieve your goals?" *Provides client with opportunity to look at own behaviors in a different way and begin to understand how they are harmful rather than helpful. Contrasting healthy behaviors versus current actions can help client decide to change them. Dialectic Behavior therapy is effective in reducing injurious behavior along with the use of medication.*[1,3,6]
- Assist client to learn assertive behavior rather than nonassertive/aggressive behavior. Include use of effective communication skills, focusing on developing self-esteem by replacing negative self-talk with positive comments. *By learning these new skills, client interacts with others and gets needs met in positive, acceptable ways, promoting self-worth and lessening anxiety and risk of injurious actions.*[1,9]

🏠 • Discuss with client/family normalcy of adolescent task of separation and ways of achieving. *Helps individual members understand these actions and begin to recognize the normal from the ones that are of concern and need intervention.*[1,6]

⊕ • Involve client/family in group therapies as appropriate. *Group setting aids in promoting diffusion of anger; provides insight as to how negative, aggressive behavior affects others, making feedback easier to digest and understand.*[2]

NURSING PRIORITY NO. 4 To promote wellness (Teaching/Discharge Considerations):

🏠 • Discuss commitment to safety and ways in which client will deal with precursors to undesired behavior. *Helps client verbalize anger and anxiety and understand how these feelings lead to desire to injure self and actions that can be taken to prevent this behavior.*[4,6]

🏠 • Mobilize support systems. *These individuals often come from abusive families, and unresolved feelings of abandonment remain into adulthood. Positive support by many people in their lives can help them begin to overcome these feelings.*[1,8]

🏠 • Arrange for continued involvement in group therapy after discharge from program. *Remaining in this supportive environment can help client maintain new behaviors as he or she begins to increase responsibility for self/own action.*[2]

💊 • Discuss and provide information about the use of medication as appropriate. *Antidepressant medications may be useful, but use needs to be weighed against potential for overdosing. (Note: The antidepressant Effexor can cause hostility, suicidal ideas, and self-harm in adolescent/young adults.) Medications that stabilize moods, ease depression, and calm anxiety may be tried to reduce the urge to self-harm.*[1,3]

• Refer to NDs Anxiety; Self-Esteem (specify), impaired Social Interaction.

DOCUMENTATION FOCUS

Assessment/Reassessment

• Individual findings, including risk factors present, underlying dynamics, prior episodes.
• Cultural/religious practices.
• Laboratory test results.
• Substance use/abuse.

Planning

• Plan of care and who is involved in planning.
• Teaching plan.

Implementation/Evaluation

• Response to interventions/teaching and actions performed.
• Attainment/progress toward desired outcome(s).
• Modifications to plan of care.

Discharge Planning

• Long-range needs and who is responsible for actions to be taken.
• Community resources, referrals made.

References

1. Townsend, M. C. (2006). *Psychiatric Mental Health Nursing Concepts of Care.* 4th ed. Philadelphia: F. A. Davis.

⊕ Cultural   ⊕ Collaborative   🏠 Community/Home Care   ✎ Diagnostic Studies   ∞ Pediatric/Geriatric/Lifespan   💊 Medications

2. Doenges, M. E., Townsend, M. C., Moorhouse, M. F. (1998). *Psychiatric Care Plans Guidelines for Individualizing Care*. 3d ed. Philadelphia: F. A. Davis.
3. Chengappa, K. N., et al. (1999). Clozapine reduces severe self-mutilation and aggression in psychotic patients with borderline personality disorder. *J Clin Psychiatry*, 60(7), 477–484.
4. Clarke, L., Whittaker, M. (1998). Self-mutilation: Culture, contexts, and nursing responses. *J Clin Nurs*, 7(2), 129–137.
5. Dallam, S. J. (1997). The identification and management of self-mutilating patients in primary care. *Nurs Pract*, 22(5), 151–153, 159–165.
6. Cox, et al. (2002). *Clinical Applications of Nursing Diagnosis: Adult, Child, Women's Psychiatric, Gerontic and Home Health Considerations*. 4th ed. Philadelphia: F. A. Davis.
7. Selekman, M. D. (2004). Adolescent self-harm: A growing epidemic. *Family Therapy Magazine*, 1(2), 34–40.
8. Focus Adolescent Services: Self-Injury. (2001). Retrieved August 2007 at www.focusas.com/SelfInjury.html.
9. Frey, R. (2002, updated 2006). Self-mutilation. Gale Encyclopedia of Medicine. Retrieved August 2007 at www.healthatoz.com/healthatoz/Atoz/common/standard/transform.jsp?requestURI=/healthatoz/Atoz/ency/self-mutilation.jsp.

disturbed Sensory Perception (specify: visual, auditory, kinesthetic, gustatory, tactile, olfactory)

Definition: Change in the amount or patterning of incoming stimuli accompanied by a diminished, exaggerated, distorted, or impaired response to such stimuli

RELATED FACTORS

Insufficient environmental stimuli: [therapeutically restricted environments (e.g., isolation, intensive care, bedrest, traction, confining illnesses, incubator); socially restricted environment (e.g., institutionalization, homebound, aging, chronic/terminal illness, infant deprivation), stigmatized (e.g., mentally ill/developmentally delayed/handicapped)]

Excessive environmental stimuli: [excessive noise level, such as work environment, client's immediate environment (ICU with support machinery)]

Altered sensory reception/transmission/integration: [neurological disease, trauma, or deficit; altered status of sense organs]

Biochemical imbalances [e.g., elevated BUN, elevated ammonia, hypoxia]; electrolyte imbalance; [drugs, e.g., stimulants or depressants, mind-altering drugs]

Psychological stress; [sleep deprivation]

DEFINING CHARACTERISTICS

Subjective

[Reported] change in sensory acuity [e.g., photosensitivity, hypoesthesias/hyperesthesias, diminished/altered sense of taste, inability to tell position of body parts (proprioception)]

Sensory distortions

Objective

[Measured] change in sensory acuity

Change in usual response to stimuli [e.g., rapid mood swings, exaggerated emotional responses, anxiety/panic state]

Change in behavior pattern; restlessness; irritability

Change in problem-solving abilities; poor concentration

Disorientation; hallucinations; [illusions]; [bizarre thinking]

Impaired communication

[Motor incoordination, altered sense of balance/falls (e.g., Ménière's syndrome)]

disturbed SENSORY PERCEPTION (specify: visual, auditory, kinesthetic, gustatory, tactile, olfactory)

Sample Clinical Applications: Glaucoma, cataract, brain tumor/stroke, traumatic injury, amputation, surgery, immobility, peripheral neuropathy (e.g., diabetes), substance abuse, schizophrenia, developmental delay

DESIRED OUTCOMES/EVALUATION CRITERIA

Sample NOC linkages:

Sensory Function Status: Extent to which an individual correctly perceives skin stimulation, sounds, proprioception, taste and smell, and visual images

Distorted Thought Self-Control: Self-restraint of disruptions in perception, thought processes, and thought content

Risk Control: Personal actions to prevent, eliminate, or reduce modifiable health threats

---

Client Will (Include Specific Time Frame)

- Regain/maintain usual level of cognition.
- Recognize and correct/compensate for sensory impairments.
- Verbalize awareness of sensory needs and presence of overload and/or deprivation.
- Identify/modify external factors that contribute to alterations in sensory/perceptual abilities.
- Use resources effectively and appropriately.
- Be free of injury.

ACTIONS/INTERVENTIONS

Sample NIC linkages:

Communication Enhancement: Hearing [or] Vision Deficit: Assistance in accepting and learning alternative methods for living with diminished hearing [or] vision

Peripheral Sensation Management: Prevention or minimization of injury or discomfort in the patient with altered sensation

Hallucination [or] Delusion Management: Promoting the comfort, safety, and reality orientation of a patient experiencing hallucinations [or] false, fixed beliefs that have little or no basis in reality

Environmental Management: Manipulation of the patient's surroundings for therapeutic benefit, sensory appeal, and psychological well-being

NURSING PRIORITY NO. 1 To assess causative/contributing factors:

- Identify client with condition that can affect sensing, interpreting, and communicating stimuli, as noted in Related Factors. *Specific clinical concerns (e.g., neurological disease or trauma, intensive care unit confinement, surgery, pain, biochemical imbalances, psychosis, substance abuse, toxemia) have the potential for altering one or more of the senses, with resultant change in the reception, sensitivity, or interpretation of sensory input.*[1]
- Be aware of current diagnosis or treatments *(e.g., glaucoma, surgery, immobility, recent stroke, diabetes, mental illness; drug toxicity or side effects [e.g., halos around lights, ringing in ears]; middle-ear disturbances [altered sense of balance]) that can cause/exacerbate sensory problems.*
- ∞ • Note age and developmental stage. *Problems with sensory perception may be known to client/caregiver (e.g., child wearing hearing aid, elderly adult with known macular degeneration), where compensatory interventions are in place. Screening/evaluation may be required if*

⊕ Cultural   ⊛ Collaborative   🏠 Community/Home Care   ⟋ Diagnostic Studies   ∞ Pediatric/Geriatric/Lifespan   💊 Medications *sensory impairments are suspected, but not obvious, as might occur when an infant is not progressing developmentally or an older individual has a gradual loss of sensory discrimination associated with aging; or sensory changes associated with a sudden neurological event.*[2,3,9]

- Evaluate medication regimen and determine possible use/misuse of drugs (prescription, OTC, illicit) *to identify effects, side effects, adverse effects or drug interactions that may be causing/exacerbating sensory/perceptual problems.*
- Review results of sensory/motor neurological testing and laboratory studies (e.g., cognitive testing or laboratory values, such as electrolytes, chemical profile, ABGs, serum drug levels) *to note presence/possible cause of changes in response to sensory stimuli.*

NURSING PRIORITY NO. 2 To determine degree of impairment:

- Assess ability to speak, hear, interpret, and respond to simple commands *to obtain an overview of client's mental/cognitive status and ability to interpret stimuli.*
- Evaluate sensory awareness (e.g., hot/cold, dull/sharp, smell, taste, visual acuity and hearing, gait/mobility, and location/function of body parts). *Screening can be done in clinic or facility may identify problems requiring more extensive evaluation.*
- Determine response to touch and painful stimuli *to note whether response is appropriate to stimulus and whether it is immediate or delayed. The sense of touch is usually maintained throughout life and may become more important if other senses are diminished. Different types of touch/contact are associated with different meanings (including communication of ideas, information, and emotion).*[3]
- Observe for behavioral responses (e.g., illusions/hallucinations, delusions, withdrawal, hostility, crying, inappropriate affect, confusion/disorientation) *that may indicate mental/emotional problems or chemical toxicity (as might occur with digoxin or other drug overdose/reaction) or be associated with brain/neurological trauma or infection.*
- Note inattention to body parts, segments of environment; lack of recognition of familiar objects/persons. *Loss of comprehension of auditory, visual, or other sensations may be indicative of unilateral neglect/inability to recognize and respond to environmental cues.*[10]
- Ascertain client's perception of problem/changes. Note SO(s) observations of changes that have occurred and client's responses to changes. *Client may or may not be aware of changes (e.g., diabetic with neuropathy may not realize he or she has lost discrimination for pain in feet; or parents may notice child's problem with coordination or difficulty with words).*
- Refer to additional NDs Anxiety; acute/chronic Confusion; disturbed Thought Processes; unilateral Neglect, as appropriate and based on findings.

NURSING PRIORITY NO. 3 To promote normalization of response to stimuli:

General interventions:
- Note degree of alteration/involvement (single/multiple senses) *to determine scope/complexity of condition and needed interventions.*
- Ascertain/validate client's perceptions. Listen to and respect client's expressions of deprivation *to assist in planning of appropriate care, to identify inconsistencies in reception and integration of stimuli, and to provide compassionate regard for client's feelings.*[4]
- Provide means of communication as indicated by client's current situation.
- Document perceptual deficit in chart and code on wall in client's room, if needed, *so caregivers are aware of specific needs/limitations.*
- Avoid isolating client, physically or emotionally, *to prevent sensory deprivation/limit confusion.*
- Address client by name and have personnel wear name tags/reintroduce self, as needed, *to preserve client's sense of identity and orientation.*

- Reorient to time, place, and situation/events, as necessary, *to reduce confusion and provide sense of normalcy to client's daily life.*
- Explain procedures/activities, expected sensations, and outcomes. *Helpful in reducing anxiety associated with altered interpretation of environment.*
- Promote a stable environment with assignment of same personnel as much as possible *to promote continuity of care/limit confusion.*
- Provide appropriate sensory stimulation, including familiar smells/sounds, tactile stimulation with a variety of objects, changing of light intensity and other cues (e.g., clocks, calendars).
- Eliminate extraneous noise/stimuli, including nonessential equipment, alarms/audible monitor signals when possible. *Reduces anxiety and exaggerated emotional responses/ confusion associated with sensory overload.*[4]
- Provide feedback *to assist client to separate reality from fantasy/altered perception.*
- Protect from bodily harm (e.g., falls, burns, positioning problems), *as client may not perceive pain/have impaired sense of position, thereby increasing the risk for falls.*
- Provide undisturbed rest/sleep periods *to reduce anxiety, agitation, or psychosis that can accompany sleep deprivation, particularly when client is confined to bed (e.g., intensive care unit).*
- Plan care with client/SO(s), as appropriate. *Enhances commitment to and continuation of plan, thus optimizing outcomes.*
- Encourage SO(s) to bring in familiar objects and to talk with and touch the client. *Client often can experience positive response to loved ones, thus enhancing recovery.*
- Collaborate with/involve other health-team members in providing rehabilitative therapies and stimulating modalities (e.g., music therapy, sensory training, remotivation therapy) *to achieve maximal gains in function and psychosocial well-being.*[11]
- Limit/carefully monitor use of sedation, especially in older population *who are more sensitive to side effects.*
- Identify and encourage use of resources/prosthetic devices (e.g., hearing aids, computerized visual aid/glasses with a level plumb line for balance). *Useful for augmenting senses.*

Visual deficits:
- Note particular vision problem (e.g., loss of visual field, change in depth perception, double vision, blindness) *that affects client's ability to perceive environment and learn/relearn motor skills.*[3]
- Speak to visually impaired or unresponsive client frequently, especially when entering room/client's presence *to provide auditory stimulation and prevent startle reflex.*
- Approach from visually intact side, position objects to take advantage of intact visual field, and use eye patch, when needed, *to decrease sensory confusion when client has loss of vision or field of vision in one eye.*[3]
- Provide/encourage listening to music, radio, TV, talking books, and use of talking timepieces and computers, as appropriate.
- Supply adequate lighting for reading and activities.
- Place glasses/contacts where they can be easily found and encourage client to wear corrective lenses during waking hours.
- Arrange bed, personal articles, and food trays to take advantage of functional vision. *Enhances independence and safety.*
- Describe food and placement, feeding or assisting client as necessary (e.g., cooking, cutting food, offering finger food, placing food in clock-position on plate, etc.), *when vision impairments could hinder nutritional intake or cause social discomfort.*
- Assist client with picking out clothing *if problems with color discrimination causes mismatching.*[3]
- Color-code doors and drawers to assist client with low vision *in locating belongings, or a particular site (e.g., bathroom).*

Auditory deficits:

- Determine if client reads lips and turn toward/face client, enunciating words clearly.
- Encourage client's use of hearing aid when one is available.
- Refer for periodic evaluation by audiologist *to note changes in acuity, determine if client might benefit from a hearing aid.*[3]
- Lower the pitch of the voice and speak in tone that does not include shouting *(which increases the pitch of the voice).*[3]
- Speak slowly and distinctly; use simple sentences. Avoid asking multiple questions at one time *to enhance client's comprehension and ability to respond.*
- Use touch to get the client's attention, if needed.
- Be aware/careful of facial expressions.
- Pay attention to background noise and reduce it to a minimum when attempting conversation. *Background noise is often amplified, causing misinterpretation of conversation/inability to hear words, and often results in overstimulation of senses.*[3]

Kinesthetic and tactile deficits:

- Encourage proper body positioning/alignment *to prevent muscle strain or injury.*
- Provide firm mattress/chair *to maintain positioning and good posture.*
- Assist with/recommend period weight shifts *to enhance circulation and relieve tissue pressure, reducing risk of tissue damage.*
- Provide tactile stimulation as care is given, and when communicating with client (respecting cultural and personal preferences). *Communicates presence/connection with other human being, because touching is an important part of caring, and the need for touch is a deep psychological need.*
- Be aware that older clients may be more interested in touching *because they have lost loved ones, their appearance may not be as attractive as it once was, and the attitude of the public toward older adults does not encourage physical contact with them.*[3]
- Stimulate sense of touch (e.g., give client objects to touch, grasp; have client practice touching walls/other boundaries). *Aids in retraining sensory pathways to integrate reception and interpretation of stimuli.*[4]
- Provide touch, using level of appropriate intensity (e.g., light, moderate, deep, strong), *depending on the need (e.g., light touch to get client's attention, stroking to convey love to infant).*[3,5]
- Teach client/SO to frequently inspect skin and extremities for pressure points/skin trauma *when client is unable to sense pain and prone to tissue injury.*[4,6]

Taste and smell:

- Note taste and smell dysfunction (loss or distortion of function) that may be associated with chronic conditions (e.g., cystic fibrosis, chronic sinusitis, hypothyroidism, MS, Alzheimer's disease, head trauma) or may suggest a new/developing problem (e.g., zinc deficiency, dental conditions, allergies).[7]
- Evaluate client's medications *if reporting changes in tastes of foods (foods taste or smell odd), ability to salivate, or loss of appetite.*[3,8]
- Encourage variety of food colors and textures, flavor enhancers (in addition to good chewing) *to maximize taste sensation.*[3,8]
- Assist client in observing for offensive or dangerous odors (e.g., body odor, spoiled foods, or propane gas or smoke) *if sense of smell is diminished.*[3]
- Remove offensive odors from client's presence, especially *when client is immobile, debilitated, and/or suffering from oversensitivity to odors, nausea, or vomiting.*[4]

NURSING PRIORITY NO. 4 To prevent injury/complications:

- Place call bell/other communication device within reach and be sure client knows where it is/how to use it.

---

disturbed SENSORY PERCEPTION (specify: visual, auditory, kinesthetic, gustatory, tactile, olfactory)

- Provide safety measures (e.g., side rails/grab poles, bed in low position, adequate lighting, use of vision/hearing devices; clearing of obstacles; assistance with walking, providing basic and specific information [e.g., I am on your right side; this water is hot; swallow now; stand up, etc.]) *to protect client from injury or enhance client's ability to interpret stimuli.*[11]
- Monitor use of heating pads/lights, ice packs; temperature of bath water, etc. *Reduces risk of thermal injury.*
- Position doors, rugs, and furniture so they are out of travel path, ambulate with assistance or strategically place grab bars *to aid in maintaining balance, reduce risk for falls.*
- Refer for evaluation of vocational abilities/driving skills. *Changes in sensory reception/integration may impair ability to perform complicated tasks, putting client and others at risk for injury.*
- Refer to NDs risk for Falls; risk for Injury; risk for Trauma.

NURSING PRIORITY NO. 5 To promote wellness (Teaching/Discharge Considerations):

- Provide explanations of and plan care with client, involving SO(s) as much as possible. *Enhances commitment to and continuation of plan, optimizing outcomes.*
- Review ways to prevent/limit exposure to conditions affecting sensory functions (e.g., how exposure to loud noise and toxins can impair hearing; early childhood screening for speech and language disorders; vaccines to prevent measles, mumps, menengitis, once known to be major causes of hearing loss).[12]
- Assist client/SO(s) *to learn effective ways of coping with and managing sensory disturbances, anticipating safety needs according to client's sensory deficits and developmental level.*
- Demonstrate use/care of sensory prosthetic devices (e.g., assistive vision or listening devices, etc.).
- Review home safety measures pertinent to deficits.
- Identify resources/community programs for acquiring and maintaining assistive devices.
- Discuss need for regular evaluation of drug regimen, noting possible toxic side effects/interactions of both prescription and OTC drugs. *Prompt recognition of side effects allows for timely intervention/change in drug regimen.*
- Promote meaningful socialization and diversional activities as able (e.g., TV/radio, conversation, large print or talking books). Refer to NDs deficient Diversional Activity; Social Isolation for related interventions.
- Refer to helping resources such as Society for the Blind, Self-Help for the Hard of Hearing (SHHH), or local support groups, screening programs, etc., as indicated.
- Refer to additional NDs Anxiety; acute/chronic Confusion; disturbed Thought Processes; unilateral Neglect, as appropriate.

DOCUMENTATION FOCUS

Assessment/Reassessment

- Individual findings, noting specific deficit/associated symptoms, perceptions of client/SO(s).
- Safety issues.
- Assistive device needs.
- Availability/use of resources.

Planning

- Plan of care, including who is involved in planning.
- Teaching plan.

Cultural   Collaborative   Community/Home Care   Diagnostic Studies   Pediatric/Geriatric/Lifespan   Medications

Implementation/Evaluation

- Responses to interventions/teaching and actions performed.
- Attainment/progress toward desired outcome(s).
- Modifications to plan of care.

Discharge Planning

- Long-term needs and who is responsible for actions to be taken.
- Available resources; specific referrals made.

References

1. ND: Sensory Perception, disturbed. In Cox, H.C. et al. (2002). *Clinical Applications of Nursing Diagnosis: Adult, Child, Women's, Psychiatric, Gerontic, and Home Health Considerations*. 4th ed. Philadelphia: F. A. Davis, pp. 431–438.
2. Engel, J. (2002). *Pocket Guide to Pediatric Assessment*. 4th ed. St. Louis, MO: Mosby.
3. Gallman, L., Elfervig, L. S. (1995). The aging sensory system. In Stanley, M., Beare, P. G. *Gerontological Nursing: A Health Promotion/Protection Approach*. 2d ed. Philadelphia: F. A. Davis, pp. 93–101.
4. NDs: Sensory Perception, disturbed (specify). In Doenges, M. E., Moorhouse, M. F., Geissler-Murr, A. C. (2002). *Nursing Care Plans: Guidelines for Individualizing Patient Care*. 6th ed. Philadelphia: F. A. Davis, pp. 236, 272, 395, 773, 789.
5. D'Apolito, K., McGrath, J., O'Brien, A. (2000). *Infant and family centered developmental care guidelines. In National Association of Neonatal Nurses Clinical Practice Guidelines*. 3d ed. Des Plaines, IL: National Association of Neonatal Nurses.
6. Mayfield, J. A., et al. (1998). Preventative foot care in people with diabetes (Technical Review). *Diabetes Care*, 21, 2161–2177.
7. Henkin, R. I. (2000–2007). Taste and Smell Clinic Research and Clinical Overview. Accessed July 2007 at www.tasteandsmell.com/clinical.htm.
8. Glezos, S. P. Taste and smell loss: Risk for disease? Seminar presentation for the NIH Office of Behavioral and Social Sciences Research (OBSSR). Accessed July 2007 at http://obssr.od.nih.gov.
9. Whiteside, M. M., Wallhagen, M. I., Pettengill, E. (2006). Sensory impairment in older adults: Part 2: Vision loss. *AJN*, 106(11), 52–61.
10. Baldwin, K. M. (2006). Stroke: It's a knock-out punch. *Nursing Made Incredibly Easy!*, 4(2), 10–23.
11. Muche, J. A., McCarty, S. (2006). Geriatric rehabilitation. Article for Emedicine Web site. Retrieved April 2007 at www.emedicine.com/neuro/topic164.htm.
12. National Institute on Deafness and Other Communication Disorders (NIDCD). (2006). Strategic plan: Plain language version FY 2003–2005. Retrieved August 2007 at www.nidcd.nih/.

Sexual Dysfunction

Definition: The state in which an individual experiences a change in sexual function during the sexual response phases of desire, excitation, and/or orgasm, which is viewed as unsatisfying, unrewarding, or inadequate.

RELATED FACTORS

Ineffectual/absent role models; lack of SO

Lack of privacy

Misinformation or lack of knowledge

Vulnerability

Physical abuse; psychosocial abuse (e.g., harmful relationships)

Altered body function/structure (e.g., pregnancy, recent childbirth, drugs, surgery, anomalies, disease process, trauma, radiation, [effects of aging])

Biopsychosocial alteration of sexuality

Values conflict

DEFINING CHARACTERISTICS

Subjective

Verbalization of problem [e.g., loss of sexual desire, disruption of sexual response patterns such as premature ejaculation, dyspareunia, vaginismus]; alterations in achieving percieved sex role

Actual/perceived limitation imposed by disease/therapy

Alterations in achieving sexual satisfaction; inability to achieve desired satisfaction

Perceived deficiency of sexual desire/alteration in sexual excitation

Seeking confirmation of desirability [concern about body image]

Change of interest in self/others; [alteration in relationship with SO]

Sample Clinical Applications: Arthritis, cancer, major surgery, heart disease, hypertension, diabetes mellitus, spinal cord injury, traumatic injury, pregnancy/childbirth, abuse, depression

DESIRED OUTCOMES/EVALUATION CRITERIA

Sample NOC linkages:

Sexual Functioning: Integration of physical, socioemotional, and intellectual aspects of sexual expression and performance

Physical Aging: Normal physical changes that occur with the natural aging process

Abuse Recovery: Sexual: Extent of healing of physical and psychological injuries due to sexual abuse or exploitation

Client Will (Include Specific Time Frame)

- Verbalize understanding of sexual anatomy/function and alterations that may affect function.
- Verbalize understanding of individual reasons for sexual problems.
- Identify stressors in lifestyle that may contribute to the dysfunction.
- Identify satisfying/acceptable sexual practices and some alternative ways of dealing with sexual expression.
- Discuss concerns about body image, sex role, desirability as a sexual partner with partner/SO.

ACTIONS/INTERVENTIONS

Sample NIC linkages:

Sexual Counseling: Use of an interactive helping process focusing on the need to make adjustments to sexual practice or to coping with a sexual event/disorder

Teaching: Sexuality: Assisting individuals to understand physical and psychosocial dimensions of sexual growth and development

Values Clarification: Assisting another to clarify her or his own values in order to facilitate effective decision making

NURSING PRIORITY NO. 1 To assess causative/contributing factors:

- Perform a complete history and physical, including a sexual history, noting usual pattern of functioning and level of desire, issues of rape/abuse. *Establishes a database from which an individualized plan of care can be formulated.*[15]

Cultural   Collaborative   Community/Home Care   Diagnostic Studies   Pediatric/Geriatric/Lifespan   Medications

- Note vocabulary and style of communication used by the individual/SO. *Maximizes communication/understanding of words and meaning in an area that individual may find difficult to discuss. Knowing that male and female brains are organized differently may help with recognizing different styles of communication.*[4]

- Have client describe problem in own words. *Sexual dysfunction is divided into four categories—sexual desire (decreased libido), arousal (erectile dysfunction or aversion/avoidance of sex), orgasm (delay/absence), or sexual pain disorders (dyspareunia/vaginismus).*[13,15] *Client's perception of the problem may differ from the care provider's, and plan of care needs to be based on client's perceptions for maximum effectiveness.*[1,9]

- Be alert to comments of client. *Sexual concerns are often disguised as humor, sarcasm, or off-hand remarks. Many people are uncomfortable talking about sexual issues but want to discuss them with care provider, so they use this method to bring up the subject. It is important for the caregiver to recognize and acknowledge client's concern.*[2,5]

- Determine importance of sex to individual/partner and client's motivation for change. *Both individuals may have differing levels of desire and expectations that may create conflict in relationship.*[3,15]

- Assess client's/SO's knowledge of sexual anatomy/function and effects of current situation/condition (e.g., client's concern about penis size, failure with performance). *Basic knowledge is essential for understanding the problem and how it is affecting the individual. Lack of knowledge may impact client's understanding of situation and expectation for return to previous norm or change for the future.*[3,7]

- Determine preexisting problems/conditions (e.g., illness/surgery/trauma) that may affect current situation/perception of individual/SO. *Physical conditions (e.g., arthritis, MS, hypertension, diabetes mellitus, fatigue, presence of a colostomy, urinary incontinence) can directly affect sexual functioning, or individual can believe that condition precludes sexual activity, such as recent myocardial infarction or heart surgery.*[3,6,7,13,16]

- Identify stress factors in individual situation (e.g., *marital/job stress, role conflicts). Interpersonal problems (marital and relationship), lack of trust and open communication between partners can contribute to difficulties. These factors may be producing enough anxiety to cause depression or other psychological reaction(s) that would cause physiological symptoms.*[5,11]

- Observe behavior/stage of grieving when related to body changes, loss of a body part, or change in function (e.g., pregnancy, obesity, amputation, mastectomy, hysterectomy/menopause). *A change in body image can affect how individual views body in many aspects, but particularly in the sensitive area of sexual functioning and indicates need for information and additional support.*[7]

- Discuss cultural values/religious beliefs or conflicts present. *Client may feel guilt or shame about sexual desires/difficulties because of family beliefs about sex and genital area of the body, and how sexuality was communicated to the client as he or she was growing up, or through religious teachings.*[1,2]

- Explore with client the meaning of client's behavior. *Masturbation, for instance, may have many meanings/purposes, such as for relief of anxiety, sexual deprivation, pleasure, a nonverbal expression of need to talk, a way of alienating.*[3] *Or, client's inhibitions may be decreased by changes in cognition.*[12]

- Review medication regimen/drug use (prescription, OTC, illegal, alcohol) and cigarette use. *Antihypertensives may cause erectile dysfunction; MAO inhibitors and tricyclics can cause erection/ejaculation problems and anorgasmia in women; SSRI antidepressants can cause decreased libido or orgasm disorders; antihistamines may cause temporary vaginal dryness (dyspareunia); narcotics/alcohol produce erectile dysfunction and inhibit orgasm; smoking creates vasoconstriction and may be a factor in erectile dysfunction. Evaluation of drug and individual response is important to determine accurate intervention.*[1,10,13,15]

- Review lab results (e.g., hormone levels, serum glucose, red blood cell count, drug levels). *Testing may reveal undiagnosed conditions such as diabetes resulting in erectile dysfunction in men; anemia affecting arousal. Inappropriate drug levels or hormone deficiencies—decreased estrogen in women and decreased testosterone in men and women may result in decreased libido; hypothyroidism may impair sexual arousal.*[15]

- Assist with/review diagnostic studies to determine cause of erectile dysfunction. *More than half of the cases have a physical cause such as diabetes, vascular problems, and so on. Monitor penile tumescence during REM sleep to determine physical ability. Men are embarrassed to bring up the subject with their healthcare provider even when they are seeing him or her for other conditions; unless the provider specifically asks, the subject is not addressed.*[6,8,9,13]

- Assist with/review diagnostic studies for female sexual disorders (e.g., vaginal photo-plethysmography *to assess vaginal blood flow/engorgement*, vaginal pH *to identify infection or diminished secretions*, biothesiometer *to test sensitivity of clitoris and labia*).[16]

NURSING PRIORITY NO. 2 To assist client/SO(s) to deal with individual situation:

- Establish therapeutic nurse-client relationship. *Promotes treatment and facilitates sharing of sensitive information/feelings in a safe environment.*[1]

- Avoid making value judgments. *They do not help the client to cope with the situation. Nurse needs to be aware of and be in control of own feelings and response to client expressions and/or concerns. Client needs to be free to express concerns in whatever way is comfortable to individual.*[3] *And even clients with limited cognition have a right to engage in intimate behaviors.*[12]

- Assist with treatment of underlying medical conditions, including changes in medication regimen, weight management, cessation of smoking, and so forth. *Many conditions (e.g., cardiovascular, diabetes, arthritis) can affect sexual functioning, as well as medication side effects that may affect sexual ability.*[7,13–15]

- Collaborate with physical therapist to identify mechanical aides that may be useful for clients with physical conditions/disabilities.[15]

- Provide factual information about individual condition (e.g., premature ejaculation, female problems of dysparunia; low sexual desire). *Accurate information helps client make informed decisions about own situation.*[2,8,10,15]

- Determine what client wants to know to tailor information to client needs. *Providing too much information may be overwhelming and result in client not remembering something that is essential. Information affecting client safety/consequences of actions may need to be reviewed/reinforced.*[1,7,9]

- Encourage and accept expressions of concern, anger, grief, fear. *Individuals need to be free to express these feelings and be accepted so they can begin to deal with situation and move on in a positive way.*[6,10,13]

- Assist client to be aware/deal with stages of grieving for loss/change. *Sexual dysfunction is often a result of losses such as breast cancer treatment, prostate surgery, and need to be addressed in the context of the whole. Healthcare providers need to be willing to help client understand grieving issues.*[2,7,11]

- Encourage client to share thoughts/concerns with partner and to clarify values/impact of condition on relationship. *Helps to identify issues in the relationship that may be related to the sexual dysfunction.*[3,11,15]

- Provide for/identify ways to obtain privacy to allow for sexual expression for individual or between partners without embarrassment or objections of others. *Often caregivers do not think about the importance of providing this basic need for couples, but in any setting, privacy may be difficult to provide unless it is thought about and planned for.*[6,12]

⊕ Cultural   Collaborative   🏠 Community/Home Care   Diagnostic Studies   ∞ Pediatric/Geriatric/Lifespan   Medications

- Discuss client's rights regarding intimacy in residential/extended care settings with SO/family. Review appropriateness of home visits or provision for privacy for intimate contact. *Family members may not realize that the need for sexual expression is not limited by advancing age, declining cognition, or marital status. And they may be unaware that client has a right to engage in appropriate intimate behaviors.*[12]
- Assist client/SO(s) to problem-solve alternative ways of sexual expression. *When illness/condition, such as arthritis, paraplegia interfere with a couple's usual sexual activities, couple needs to learn new ways to achieve satisfaction.*[3]
- Discuss use of medications such as papaverine, sildenafil (Viagra), or vardenafil (Levitra) *for erectile dysfunction*, or lubricating gels/hormone creams or possibly hormonal replacement therapy *for vaginal dryness/dyspareunia* as appropriate.[15,16]
- Provide information about availability of corrective measures such as reconstructive surgery (e.g., penile/breast implants), Eros Therapy (handheld device used to improve blood flow to clitoris and external labia to increase sensitivity of tissues), or behavioral therapies (e.g., self-stimulation, sensate focus exercises, Masters & Johnson treatment strategies), when indicated. *Sexual problems, such as erectile dysfunction, female orgasmic disorders, female sexual arousal disorders may respond to these interventions, providing more satisfactory sexual life.*[8,10,14–16]
- Refer to appropriate resources as need indicates (e.g., healthcare coworker with greater comfort level and/or knowledgeable clinical nurse specialist or professional sex therapist, family counseling). *Not all professionals are knowledgeable or comfortable dealing with sexual issues, and referrals to more appropriate resources can provide client/couple with accurate assistance.*[2,6,12]

NURSING PRIORITY NO. 3 To promote wellness (Teaching/Discharge Considerations):

- Provide sex education, explanation of normal sexual functioning when necessary. *Many individuals are not knowledgeable about these areas, and often providing accurate information can help assuage anxiety about unknowns, such as normal changes of aging, or provide an accurate basis for understanding problems being experienced.*[6,15,16]
- Provide written material appropriate to individual needs. Include bibliotherapy and reliable Internet resources related to client's concerns. *Provides reinforcement for client to read/access at his or her leisure, when ready to deal with sensitive materials.*[3,6,7]
- Encourage ongoing dialogue and take advantage of teachable moments that occur. *Within a therapeutic relationship, comfort is achieved and individual is encouraged to ask questions and be receptive to continuing conversation about sexual issues.*[1,2]
- Demonstrate and assist client to learn relaxation or visualization techniques. *Stress is often a component of sexual dysfunction, and using these skills can help with resolution of problems.*[2,5]
- Identify resources for assistive devices/sexual "aids." *These aids can enhance sex life of couple and prevent/help with problems of dysfunction.*[3,6]
- Stress importance of engaging in regular self-examination as indicated (e.g., breast/testicular examinations). *Encourages client to participate in own health prevention activities, become more aware of potential problems, and become more comfortable with sexual self.*[3,5]
- Identify community resources for further assistance, such as Reach for Recovery, CanSurmount, Ostomy Association.[11]
- Refer for further professional assistance concerning relationship difficulties, low sexual desire/other sexual concerns such as premature ejaculation, vaginismus, painful intercourse. *May need additional/continuing help to deal with individual situation/associated depression.*[3,15] Note: *Referral to counselor expert in trauma may be preferred to assist sexual abuse survivors overcome sexual difficulties.*[15]

DOCUMENTATION FOCUS

Assessment/Reassessment

- Individual findings, including nature of dysfunction, predisposing factors, perceived effect on sexuality/relationships.
- Cultural/religious factors, conflicts.
- Response of SO(s).
- Motivation for change.

Planning

- Plan of care and who is involved in planning.
- Teaching plan.

Implementation/Evaluation

- Response to interventions/teaching and actions performed.
- Attainment/progress toward desired outcome(s).
- Modifications to plan of care.

Discharge Planning

- Long-term needs/referrals and who is responsible for actions to be taken.
- Community resources, specific referrals made.

References

1. Townsend, M. C. (2003). *Psychiatric Mental Health Nursing Concepts of Care*. 4th ed. Philadelphia: F. A. Davis.
2. Doenges, M. E., Townsend, M. C., Moorhouse, M. F. (1998). *Psychiatric Care Plans Guidelines for Individualizing Care*. 3rd ed. Philadelphia: F. A. Davis.
3. Hyde, J., DeLamater, J. (2002). *Understanding Human Sexuality*. 7th ed. New York: McGraw-Hill.
4. Moir, A., Jessel, D. (1991). *Brain Sex, the Real Difference Between Men & Women*. New York: Dell.
5. New Our Bodies, Ourselves: Boston Women's Health Staff. (1998). Boston: Smith, Peta.
6. Sexuality in Midlife and Beyond: A Special Health Report. (2003). Harvard Medical School.
7. Stanley, M., Beare, P. G. (1999). *Gerontological Nursing*. 2d ed. Philadelphia: F. A. Davis.
8. Carver, C. (1998). Premature ejaculation: A common and treatable concern. *J Am Psy Nurs Assoc*, 4(6), 199–204.
9. McEnany, G. (1998). Sexual dysfunction in the pharmacologic treatment of depression: When "don't ask, don't tell" is an unsuitable approach to care. *J Am Psy Nurs Assoc*, 4(1), 24–29.
10. Phillips, N. A. (2000). Female sexual dysfunction: Evaluation and treatment. *Am Family Phys*, 62(1), 127–136, 141–142.
11. Cox, H. C., et al. (2002). *Clinical Applications of Nursing Diagnosis: Adult, Child, Women's, Psychiatric, Gerontic and Home Health Considerations*. 4th ed. Philadelphia: F. A. Davis.
12. Sexuality in the nursing home. (1997). The Legal Center for People with Disabilities and Older People.
13. McDaniel, N.D. (2007). Beyond Viagra: The Hidden Roots and Risks of Eretile Dysfunction. Retrieved August 2007 at www.lifescript.com/channels/healthy_living/Mens_Health/beyond_viagra_the_hidden_roots_and_risks_of_erectile_dysfunction.asp.
14. Male Sexual Health (2005). Retrieved August 2007 at www.moderntherapy.com/male/sexual-health.html.
15. Ballas, P. (2006). Sexual problems overview. Retrieved August 2007 at MedlinePlus: www.nlm.nih.gov/medlineplus/ency/article/001951.htm.
16. Female sexual dysfunction. (2003). Retrieved August 2007 at www.womenshealthchannel.com/fsd/index.shtml.

ineffective Sexuality Pattern

Definition: Expressions of concern regarding own sexuality

Cultural   Collaborative   Community/Home Care   Diagnostic Studies   Pediatric/Geriatric/Lifespan   Medications

RELATED FACTORS

Knowledge/skill deficit about alternative responses to health-related transitions, altered body function or structure, illness or medical treatment

Lack of privacy

Impaired relationship with an SO; lack of SO

Ineffective/absent role models

Conflicts with sexual orientation or variant preferences

Fear of pregnancy/acquiring a sexually transmitted disease

DEFINING CHARACTERISTICS

Subjective

Reported difficulties/limitations/changes in sexual behaviors/activities

Alteration in relationship with SO

Alterations in achieving perceived sex role

Conflicts involving values

[Expressions of feeling alienated, lonely, loss, powerless, angry]

Sample Clinical Applications: Spinal cord injury, brain injury/stroke, sexually transmitted disease, cancer, mastectomy, hysterectomy, menopause, prostatectomy, gender reassignment

DESIRED OUTCOMES/EVALUATION CRITERIA

Sample NOC linkages:

Sexual Identity: Acknowledgment and acceptance of own sexual identity

Child Development: Adolescence: Milestones of physical, cognitive, and psychosocial progression from 12 years through 17 years of age

Role Performance: Congruence of an individual's role behavior with role expectations

Client Will (Include Specific Time Frame)

• Verbalize understanding of sexual anatomy and function.
• Verbalize knowledge and understanding of sexual limitations, difficulties, or changes that have occurred.
• Verbalize acceptance of self in current (altered) condition.
• Demonstrate improved communication and relationship skills.
• Identify individually appropriate method of contraception.

ACTIONS/INTERVENTIONS

Sample NIC linkages:

Sexual Counseling: Use of an interactive helping process focusing on the need to make adjustments to sexual practice or to coping with a sexual event/disorder

Teaching: Sexuality: Assisting individuals to understand physical and psychosocial dimensions of sexual growth and development

Teaching: Safe Sex: Providing instruction concerning sexual protection during sexual activity

Support System Enhancement: Facilitation of support to patient by family, friends, and community ineffective SEXUALITY PATTERN

NURSING PRIORITY NO. 1 To assess causative/contributing factors:

- Obtain complete physical and sexual history, as indicated, including perception of normal function. *Sexuality is multifaceted beginning with one's body, biological sex, and gender (biological, social, and legal status as girls/boys, women/men).*
- Note use of vocabulary (assessing basic knowledge) and comments/concerns about sexual identity. *Components of sexual identity include one's gender identity (how one feels about his or her gender) as well as one's sexual orientation (straight, lesbian, gay, bisexual, transgendered).*[12]
- Determine importance of sex and a description of the problem in the client's own words. Be alert to comments of client/SO (e.g., discount of overt or covert sexual expressions such as "He's just a dirty old man"). *Sexual concerns are often disguised as sarcasm, humor, or in offhand remarks.*[1,2] *Information about client's perception of the problem is essential to planning appropriate care to meet client's needs.*
- Note cultural values/religious beliefs and conflicts that may exist. Elicit impact of perceived problem on SO/family. *Individuals are encultured as they grow up and, depending on particular family views and taboos, these factors may create conflicts regarding variant sexual practices with resultant feelings of shame and guilt.*[3,8]
- Assess stress factors in client's environment that might cause anxiety or psychological reactions. *Sexual variant behaviors, power issues involving SO, adult children, aging, employment, loss of prowess related to illness/condition are often associated with stress in the client's life.*[1,11]
- Explore knowledge of effects of altered body function/limitations precipitated by illness or medical treatment of alternative sexual responses and expressions (e.g., reassignment procedure). *Client needs to understand when conditions, such as undescended testicle in young male, gender change, mutilating cancer surgery have an effect on sexuality.*[10]
- Review substance use history (prescription medication, OTC drugs, alcohol, and illicit drugs). *Substance/prescription drug use may affect sexual functioning or be used to relieve anxiety of sexually deviant behavior.*[2]
- Explore issues and fears associated with sex. *Possibility of pregnancy, acquiring sexually transmitted diseases, trust/control issues, inflexible beliefs, preference confusion, altered performance need to be addressed so they may be understood and resolved.*[3,13]
- Determine client's interpretation of the altered sexual activity or behavior. *May be a way of controlling, provide relief of anxiety, pleasure, lack of partner. These behaviors, when related to body changes, including pregnancy or weight loss/gain, or loss of body part, may reflect a stage of grieving.*[3]
- Assess life-cycle issues, such as adolescence, young adulthood, menopause, aging. *All people are sexual beings from birth to death. Stage of maturation/transition bring changes that affect sexual self, and understanding of the normalcy can help individual grow with them.*[3,7]

NURSING PRIORITY NO. 2 To assist client/SO to deal with individual situation:

- Provide atmosphere in which discussion of sexual problems is encouraged/permitted. *Sense of trust/comfort enhances ability to discuss sensitive matters and begin to resolve issues.*[5]
- Avoid value judgments. *They do not help the client to cope with the situation. Nurse needs to be aware of and in control of own feelings and responses to the client's expressions and/or concerns.*[9]
- Provide information about individual situation, determining client needs and desires. *Lack of knowledge may contribute to current situation, and providing desired information conveys message of importance and self-responsibility.*[3]
- Encourage discussion of individual situation and open expression of feelings without judgment. *Sexuality includes feelings, attitudes, relationships, self-image, ideals, and behaviors,*

Cultural   Collaborative   Community/Home Care   Diagnostic Studies   Pediatric/Geriatric/Lifespan   Medications

and influences how one experiences the world.[12] *Talking about sexual practices, concerns about sexual identity, or sexual issues related to illness/condition provides opportunity for resolution.*[1,2]

- Provide specific suggestions about interventions directed toward the identified problems. *Being specific about actions client can take, such as alternate sexual positions when arthritis prevents movement, masturbation when no partner is available, use of condoms when infection is a concern, positive discussion of normalcy of sexual behavior when identity is being questioned, can lead discussion in appropriate direction to begin to look for options/solutions.*[3,5]

- Identify alternative forms of sexual expression that might be acceptable to both partners. *Being able to communicate satisfactorily with partner and identifying ways to achieve sexual satisfaction for both is important to the relationship.*[1,2]

- Discuss ways to manage individual devices/appliances. *Change in body image/medical condition may require the use of devices such as an ostomy bag, breast prostheses, a urinary collection device that may affect how client views sexual activity. Providing information about ways to deal with these issues helps client to refocus attention on achieving satisfactory sexual experience.*[6,7]

- Discuss use of performance-enhancing medications, such as sildenafil (Viagra), vardenafil (Levitra), tadalafil (Cialis). *Erectile dysfunction is a common occurrence as men age, and while frequently caused by an underlying physical condition/prescribed medication, psychological issues often accompany this problem. While an accurate diagnosis is necessary, there are many treatments available.*[2,3] *Prescription drugs are popular, but the individual needs to feel desire and be sexually stimulated for them to work.*[6]

- Determine concerns of older client regarding sexuality. *Myths abound regarding sexual activity as people grow older, and individual may believe he or she is no longer attractive or a satisfying sex life is no longer possible; accurate information can correct misperceptions.*[6,7]

- Provide anticipatory guidance about losses that are to be expected. *Surgical procedures resulting in a major change in body image, whether planned as in transsexual surgery, or unplanned as in emergency bowel resection with resultant colostomy, or traumatic amputation, result in a loss of known self, which needs specific intervention to integrate change.*[3,9]

- Introduce client to individuals who have successfully managed a similar problem, when possible. *Provides a positive role model and support for problem-solving.*[9]

NURSING PRIORITY NO. 3 To promote wellness (Teaching/Discharge Considerations):

- Provide factual information about problem(s) as identified by the client. *Specific facts about individual situation will provide client with knowledge needed to deal with what is happening, such as conflict with sexual orientation or variant preferences or impaired relationship with SO.*[9]

- Engage in ongoing dialogue with the client and SO(s) as situation permits. *As communication continues, new insights arise and understanding is enhanced.*[2,4]

- Discuss methods/effectiveness/side effects of contraceptives if indicated. *Assists individual/couple to make an informed decision on a method that meets own values/religious beliefs and allows client to meet needs and desires to plan for and/or prevent pregnancy.*[1,5]

- Refer to community resources as indicated. *May need additional information and support that can be obtained at resources such as planned parenthood, gender identity clinic, social services, others.*[8,9]

- Refer for intensive individual/group psychotherapy, which may be combined with couple/family and/or sex therapy, as appropriate.

- Refer to NDs disturbed Body Image; Self-Esteem (specify); Sexual Dysfunction.

DOCUMENTATION FOCUS

Assessment/Reassessment

- Individual findings, including nature of concern, perceived difficulties/limitations or changes, specific needs/desires.
- Cultural/religious beliefs, conflicts.
- Response of SO(s).

Planning

- Plan of care and who is involved in the planning.
- Teaching plan.

Implementation/Evaluation

- Response to interventions/teaching and actions performed.
- Attainment/progress toward desired outcome(s).
- Modifications to plan of care.

Discharge Planning

- Long-term needs/teaching and referrals and who is responsible for actions to be taken.
- Community resources, specific referrals made.

References

1. Townsend, M. C. (2003). *Psychiatric Mental Health Nursing Concepts of Care.* 4th ed. Philadelphia: F. A. Davis.
2. Doenges, M. E., Townsend, M. C., Moorhouse, M. F. (1998). *Psychiatric Care Plans Guidelines for Individualizing Care.* 3rd ed. Philadelphia: F. A. Davis.
3. Hyde, J., DeLamater, J. (2002). *Understanding Human Sexuality.* 7th ed. New York: McGraw-Hill.
4. Moir, A., Jessel, D. (1991). *Brain Sex: the Real Difference Between Men & Women.* New York: Dell.
5. New Our Bodies, Ourselves: Boston Women's Health Staff. (1998). Boston: Smith, Peta.
6. Sexuality in Midlife and Beyond: A Special Health Report. (2003). Harvard Medical School.
7. Stanley, M., Beare, P. G. (1999). *Gerontological Nursing* 2d ed. Philadelphia: F. A. Davis.
8. Saunders, P., Pickering, R. (1997). The causes of homosexuality. Available at www.cmf.org.uk/index.htm?pubs/pubs.htm. Accessed March 2002.
9. Becker, J. V., Johnson, B. R., Kavoussi, R. J. (1999). Sexual and gender identity disorders. In Hales, R. E., Yudofsky, S. C. (eds). (1999). *Essentials of Clinical Psychiatry.* Washington, DC: American Psychiatric Press.
10. Bell, R. (1998). *Changing Bodies, Changing Lives.* 3rd ed. New York: Random House.
11. Issues and Answers: Fact Sheet on Sexuality Education. (2001). *Siecus Report,* 29(6). Retrieved August 2007 at www.siecus.org/pubs/fact/fact0007.html.
12. Planned Parenthood. (2006). Sexual Health, Sexuality. Retrieved August 2007 at http://plannedparenthood.org/sexual-health/sexual-health-relationship/sexuality.htm.
13. Kaplan, H. S. (1995). *Sexual Desire Disorders: Dysfunctional Regulation of Sexual Motivation.* Levittown, PA: Brunner/Mazel.

impaired Skin Integrity

Definition: Altered epidermis and/or dermis

RELATED FACTORS

External
Hyperthermia; hypothermia
Chemical substance; radiation; medications
Physical immobilization

Cultural Collaborative Community/Home Care Diagnostic Studies Pediatric/Geriatric/Lifespan Medications

Humidity; moisture; [excretions/secretions]

Mechanical factors (e.g., shearing forces, pressure, restraint), [trauma: injury/surgery]

Extremes in age

Internal

Imbalanced nutritional state (e.g., obesity, emaciation); impaired metabolic state; changes in fluid status

Skeletal prominence; changes in turgor; [presence of edema]

Impaired circulation/sensation; changes in pigmentation

Developmental factors

Immunological deficit

[Psychogenic factors (e.g., obsessive compulsive behaviors)]

DEFINING CHARACTERISTICS

Subjective

[Reports of itching, pain, numbness of affected/surrounding area]

Objective

Disruption of skin surface [epidermis]

Destruction of skin layers [dermis]

Invasion of body structures

Sample Clinical Applications: Arteriosclerosis, venous insufficiency, hypertension, obesity, diabetes mellitus, malignant neoplasms, traumatic injury, surgery, chronic steroid use (e.g., COPD, asthma), renal failure, burns, radiation therapy, malnutrition

DESIRED OUTCOMES/EVALUATION CRITERIA

Sample NOC linkages:

Tissue Integrity: Skin & Mucous Membranes: Structural intactness and normal physiological function of skin and mucous membranes

Wound Healing: Primary Intention: Extent of regeneration of cells and tissues following intentional closure

Wound Healing: Secondary Intention: Extent of regeneration of cells and tissues in an open wound

Client Will (Include Specific Time Frame)

• Display timely healing of skin lesions/wounds/pressure sores without complication.

• Maintain optimal nutrition/physical well-being.

• Participate in prevention measures and treatment program.

• Verbalize feelings of increased self-esteem and ability to manage situation.

ACTIONS/INTERVENTIONS

Sample NIC linkages:

Wound Care: Prevention of wound complications and promotion of wound healing

Incision Site Care: Cleansing, monitoring, and promotion of healing in a wound that is closed with sutures, clips, or staples

Pressure Ulcer Care: Facilitation of healing in pressure ulcers

NURSING PRIORITY NO. 1   To assess causative/contributing factors:

🏠 • Identify underlying condition/pathology involved. *Skin integrity problems can be the result of (1) disease processes that affect circulation and perfusion of tissues (e.g., arteriosclerosis, venous insufficiency, hypertension, obesity, diabetes, malignant neoplasms); (2) medications (e.g., anticoagulants, corticosteroids, immunosuppressives, antineoplastics) that adversely affect/impair healing;(3) burns/radiation (can break down internal tissues as well as skin); and (4) nutrition and hydration (e.g., malnutrition deprives the body of protein and calories required for cell growth and repair, and dehydration impairs transport of oxygen and nutrients). Disruption in skin integrity can be intentional (e.g., surgical incision) or unintentional (accidental trauma; drug effect/alleric reaction, etc.), and closed (e.g., contusion, abrasion, rash) or open (e.g., laceration, penetrating wound, ulcerations).*[1,2,13]

🏠 • Note general health. *Many factors (e.g., debilitation; immobility; use of restraints; extremes of age; mental status; dehydration or malnutrition; presence of chronic disease; occupational, treatment, and environmental hazards) can all affect the ability of the skin to perform its functions (e.g., protection, sensation, movement and growth, chemical synthesis, immunity, thermoregulation and excretion).*[3,4]

∞ • Determine client's age and developmental factors/ability to care for self. *Newborn/infant's skin is thin, provides ineffective thermal regulation and nails are thin.*[5] *Babies and children are prone to skin rashes associated with viral, bacterial, and fungal infections and allergic reactions. In adolescence, hormones stimulate hair growth and sebaceous gland activity. In adults, it takes longer to replenish epidermis cells, resulting in increased risk of skin cancers and infection. In older adults, there is decreased epidermal regeneration, fewer sweat glands, less subcutaneous fat, elastin, and collagen, causing skin to become thinner, drier, and less responsive to pain sensations.*[1,3,4,6,7]

🏠 • Evaluate client's skin care practices and hygiene issues. *Individual's skin may be oily, dry, or sensitive and is affected by bathing frequency (or lack of bathing), temperature of water, types of soap and other cleansing agents. Incontinence (urinary or bowel) and ineffective hygiene can result in serious skin impairment and discomfort.*

🏠 • Note presence of compromised vision, hearing, or speech *that may impact client's self-care as relates to skin care (e.g., diabetic with impaired vision probably cannot satisfactorily examine own feet).*[11]

🏠 • Ascertain allergy history. *Individual may be sensitive or allergic to substances (e.g., insects, grasses, medications, lotions, soaps, foods) that can adversely affect the skin.*

🏠 • Note distribution and scarcity of hair *(e.g., loss of hair on lower legs may indicate peripheral vascular disease). (Refer to ND risk for Peripheral Vascular Dysfunction for additional interventions.)*[5,14]

🏠 • Assess blood supply (e.g., capillary return time, color, and warmth) and sensation of skin surfaces/affected area on a regular basis *to provide comparative baseline and opportunity for timely intervention when problems are noted.*[3,9]

✏️ • Calculate ankle-brachial index *to evaluate actual/potential for impairment of circulation to lower extremities. Result less than 0.9 indicates need for close monitoring/more aggressive intervention (e.g., tighter blood glucose and weight control in diabetic client).*[15]

• Determime treatment-related skin/tissue conditions (e.g., surgical incision, IV/invasive line insertion site, use of restraints). Assess surgical sites *for signs of infection (e.g., swelling, redness, pain);* assess IV site *for infiltration (e.g., swelling, erythema, coolness, and pain, failure of infusion) or evidence of extravasation (e.g., blistering, blanching, skin sloughing).*[4] Evaluate skin surrounding restraints for abrasions, contusions, skin breaks, or skin color/temperature changes distal to restraints *suggesting impaired circulation.*

✏️ • Review laboratory results (e.g., Hb/Hct, blood glucose, blood and/or wound culture/sensitivities for infectious agents [viral/bacterial/fungal], albumin/protein) *to evaluate causative* *factors or ability to heal. Note: Albumin <3.5 correlates to decreased wound healing/increased pressure ulcers.*[1,15,16]

NURSING PRIORITY NO. 2 To assess extent of involvement/injury:

∞ • Obtain a complete history of current skin condition(s) (especially in children where recurrent rash/lesions are common), including age at onset, date of first episode, duration, original site, characteristics of lesions, and any changes that have occurred. *Common skin manifestations of sensitivity/allergies are hives, eczema, and contact dermatitis. Contagious rashes include measles, rubella, roseola, chickenpox, and scarlet fever. Bacterial, viral, and fungal infections can also cause skin problems (e.g., impetigo, cellulitis, cold sores, shingles, athlete's foot, and candidiasis diaper rashes).*[6]

🏠 • Perform routine skin inspections describing observed changes. Note color, temperature, surface changes, texture, and contours. Evaluate color changes in areas of least pigmentation (e.g., sclera, conjunctiva, nail beds, buccal mucosa, tongue, palms, and soles of feet). *Systematic inspection can identify improvement/changes for timely intervention.*[8]

🏠 **General wounds/lesions:**

• Describe rash/lesion, noting color, location, significant characteristics (e.g., flat or raised rash, weeping or painful blisters, itching wheal, etc.) and surrounding information (e.g., exposure to contagious disease, reaction to medication, recent insect bite, ingrown toenail, sexually transmitted disease, etc.) *to assist in diagnosing problem and needed interventions.*

• Determine anatomic location and depth of skin/tissue injury/damage (e.g., epidermis, dermis, and/or underlying issues) and describe (e.g., partial or full-thickness burn) *to provide baseline/document changes.*[3,10]

• Photograph lesion(s) as appropriate *to document status/provide visual baseline for future comparisons.*

• Note character and color of drainage, when present (e.g., blood, bile, pus, stoma effluent), *which can cause skin irritation/excoriation.*

Pressure ulcers/decubitus:

• Determine/document (1) dimensions and depth in centimeters; (2) exudates—color, odor, and amount; (3) margins—fixed or unfixed; (4) tunneling/tracts; (5) evidence of necrosis (e.g., color gray to black) or healing (e.g., pink/red granulation tissue) *to establish comparative baseline/evaluate effectiveness of interventions.*[8,16,17]

• Classify pressure ulcer(s) using tool such as Waterlow, Braden, Norton (or similar) Ulcer Classification System. *Provides consistent terminology for assessment and documentation of pressure sores.*[8,16,17]

• Remeasure wound(s) regularly and periodically photograph, and observe incisions/wounds for complications *to monitor progress/failure of healing.*

NURSING PRIORITY NO. 3 To determine impact of condition:

🏠 • Determine if wound is acute (e.g., injury from surgery or trauma) or chronic (e.g., venous/arterial insufficiency), *which affects healing time and the client's emotional and physical responses. For example, an acute and noninfected wound can heal in about 4 weeks, while a chronic wound often does not progress through phases of healing in an orderly or timely fashion.*[10]

🏠 • Determine client's level of discomfort (e.g., can vary widely from minor itching or aching, to deep pain with burns, or excoriation associated with drainage) *to clarify intervention needs and priorities.*

- Ascertain attitudes of individual/SO(s) about condition (e.g., cultural values, stigma). Obtain/review psychological assessment of client's emotional status, noting potential or sexual problems arising from presence of condition. *The healthy wholeness and beauty of skin impacts the client's body image and self-esteem. Lesions or wounds that disfigure can be especially devastating.*

NURSING PRIORITY NO. 4 To assist client with correcting/minimizing condition and achieving optimal healing:

- Practice and instruct client/caregiver(s) in scrupulous hand washing and clean or sterile technique *to reduce incidence of contamination or infection.*
- Provide optimum nutrition (including adequate protein, lipids, calories, trace minerals and multivitamins [e.g., A, C, D, E]) *to promote skin health/healing and to maintain general good health.*
- Provide adequate hydration (oral, tube feeding, IV, ambient room humidity, etc.) *to reduce/replenish transepidermal water loss.*
- Encourage client to verbalize feelings and discuss how/if condition affects self-concept. (Refer to NDs disturbed Body Image, situational low Self-Esteem.)
- Assist client to work through stages of grief and feelings associated with individual condition.
- Use touch, facial expressions, and tone of voice *to lend psychological support and acceptance of client.*

Promote wound healing:[1,5,9,12,14,17]
- Keep surgical area(s) clean/dry; carefully dress wounds; support incision (e.g., use of Steri-Strips, splinting when coughing) and stimulate circulation to surrounding areas *to assist body's natural process of repair.*
- Consult with physician/wound specialist as indicated *to assist with developing plan of care for problematic or potentially serious wounds.*
- Assist with debridement/enzymatic therapy as indicated (e.g., burns, severe pressure sores) to remove nonviable, contaminated or infected tissue.[18]
- Use body-temperature physiological solutions (e.g., isotonic saline) *to clean or irrigate wounds and prevent washout of electrolytes.*
- Cleanse wound with irrigation syringe or gauze squares, avoiding cotton balls or other products *that shed fibers.*
- Maintain appropriate moisture environment for particular wound (e.g., expose lesions/ulcer to air and light if excess moisture is impeding healing, or use occlusive dressings to maintain a moist environment for autolytic debridement of wound) as indicated.[18]
- Use appropriate barrier dressings or wound coverings (e.g., semipermeable, occlusive, wet-to-damp, DuoDerm, Tegaderm, hydrocolloid, hydrofiber or gel; hydropolymers, etc.), drainage appliances, and skin-protective agents for open/draining wounds and stomas *to protect wound and surrounding tissues from excoriating secretions/drainage, and to promote wound healing.*[18]
- Apply/administer topical/systemic drugs as indicated *for* individual situation.

Prevent skin impairment:[3–5,7,9,12,14,17]
- Maintain/instruct in overall skin hygiene (e.g., wash thoroughly, pat dry, gently massage with lotion or appropriate cream) *to provide barrier to infection, reduce risk of dermal trauma, improve circulation, and enhance comfort.*
- Cleanse skin after incontinent or diaphoretic episodes *to restore normal skin pH and flora and limit potential for infection.*

Cultural   Collaborative   Community/Home Care   Diagnostic Studies   Pediatric/Geriatric/Lifespan   Medications

- Use proper turning/transfer techniques. Avoid movements *that cause friction/shearing (e.g., pulling client with parallel force, dragging movements, etc.).*
- Encourage early ambulation/mobilization. *Reduces risks associated with immobility.*
- Develop regularly timed repositioning schedule for client with mobility and sensation impairments, using turn sheet as needed; encourage/assist with periodic weight shifts for client in chair *to reduce stress on pressure points and encourage circulation to tissues.*
- Use appropriate padding devices (e.g., air/water mattress, egg crate/gel pads, heel rolls, foam boots) when indicated *to reduce pressure on/enhance circulation to compromised tissues.*
- Limit/avoid use of plastic material (e.g., rubber sheet, plastic-backed linen savers), and remove wet/wrinkled linens promptly. *Moisture potentiates skin breakdown and increases risk for infection.*
- Remove adhesive products with care, removing on horizontal plane, and using mineral oil or Vaseline for softening, if needed, *to prevent abrasions or tearing of skin.*
- Secure dressings with tape (e.g., elastic, paper tape, nonadherent dressings), or Montgomery straps when frequent dressing changes are required. Use stockinette, tubular/gauze wrap, or similar product instead of tape to secure dressings and drains *to limit dermal injury.*[13]
- Apply hot and cold applications judiciously *to reduce risk of dermal injury in persons with circulatory and neurosensory impairments.*
- Avoid use of latex products *when client has known or suspected sensitivity.* (Refer to ND latex Allergy Response.)

NURSING PRIORITY NO. 5 To promote wellness (Teaching/Discharge Considerations):

- Discuss importance of skin and measures to maintain proper skin functioning. *The integumentary system is the largest multifunctional organ of the body and thus merits special care.*
- Review/stress benefits of following medical regimen. *Enhances commitment to plan, optimizing outcomes.*
- Encourage regular inspection/monitoring of skin for changes or failure to heal. *Early detection and reporting to healthcare providers promotes timely evaluation and intervention.*
- Identify safety measures for client with persistent sensation impairments. *Proper care of skin/extremities during cold or hot weather (e.g., wearing gloves, boots, clean/dry socks, properly fitting shoes/boots, face protection, etc.) reduces risk of injury.*[11,15]
- Encourage/maintain mobility, activity, and range of motion *to enhance circulation and promote health of skin and other organs.*
- Discuss avoidance of products containing perfumes, dyes, preservatives *(may cause dermatitis reactions)* or alcohol, povidone-iodine, hydrogen peroxide *(may hinder wound healing).*
- Encourage restriction/abstinence from tobacco, *which can cause vasoconstriction.*
- Review measures *to avoid spread/reinfection of communicable conditions.*
- Discuss proper/safe use of equipment/appliances (e.g., heating pad, ostomy appliances, padding straps of braces).
- Emphasize wisdom of limiting lengthy/unnecessary sun exposure, using high SPF sun block, and avoiding tanning beds.
- Assist client to learn stress reduction and alternate therapy techniques *to control feelings of helplessness and enhance coping ability.*
- Refer to dietitian or certified diabetes educator as appropriate *to manage general well-being, enhance healing, reduce risk of recurrence of diabetic ulcers*

DOCUMENTATION FOCUS

Assessment/Reassessment

- Characteristics of lesion(s)/condition, ulcer classification.

- Causative/contributing factors.
- Impact of condition.

Planning

- Plan of care and who is involved in planning.
- Teaching plan.

Implementation/Evaluation

- Responses to interventions/teaching and actions performed.
- Attainment/progress toward desired outcome(s).
- Modifications to plan of care.

Discharge Planning

- Long-term needs/referrals and who is responsible for actions to be taken.
- Specific referrals made.

References

1. Llewellyn, S. (2002). Skin integrity and wound care (lecture materials). Chapel Hills, NC: Cape Fear Community College Nursing Program.
2. Colburn, L. (2001). Prevention for chronic wounds. In Krasner, D., Rodeheaver, G., Sibbald, R. G. *Chronic Wound Care: A Clinical Source Book for Healthcare Professionals*. 2d ed. Wayne, PA: HMP Communications.
3. Calianno, C. (2002). Patient hygiene, part 2—Skin care: Keeping the outside healthy. *Nursing2002*, 32(6), June Clinical Supp.
4. Lund, C. H., Osborne, J. W., Culler, J., et al. (2001). Neonatal skin care: Clinical Outcomes of the AWHONN/NANN evidence-based clinical practice guideline. *JONN*, 30(1), 30–40.
5. McGovern, C. (2003). Skin, hair and nail assessment. Unit 2 (lecture materials). Villanova, PA: Villanova University College of Nursing. Accessed July 2007 at www.homepage.villanova.edu/.
6. Engel, J. (2002). *Pocket Guide to Pediatric Assessment*. 4th ed. St. Louis, MO: Mosby, pp. 99–112.
7. Wiersema, L. A., Stanley, M. (1999). The aging integumentary system. In Stanley, M., Beare, P. G. *Gerontological Nursing: A Health Promotion/Protection Approach*. 2d ed. Philadelphia: F. A. Davis, pp. 102–111.
8. Krasner, D., Rodeheaver, G., Sibbald, R. G. (2001). Advanced wound caring for a new millennium. In Krasner, D., Rodeheaver, G., Sibbald, R. G. *Chronic Wound Care: A Clinical Source Book for Healthcare Professionals*. 2d ed. Wayne, PA: HMP Communications.
9. ND: Skin Integrity, impaired. In Doenges, M. E., Moorhouse, M. F., Geissler-Murr, A. C. (2002). *Nursing Care Plans: Guidelines for Individualizing Patient Care*. 6th ed. Philadelphia: F. A. Davis.
10. Hahn, J. F., et al. Wounds: Nursing care and product selection—Part 1 (CE offering). Nursing Spectrum. Available at http://nsweb.nursingspectrum.com/ce/ce80.htm. Accessed September 2003.
11. Lawrance, D. P. DIABETES FYI-Foot Care (Monograph 5 in series). Champaign, IL: University of Illinois, McKinley Diabetes Team.
12. No author listed. Risk factors and prevention. Geriatric Syndromes: Pressure Ulcers. Novartis Foundation for gerontology. Available at http://geriatricsyllabus.com. Accessed February 2004.
13. Baranoski, S. (2003). Skin tears: Staying on guard against the enemy of frail skin. *Nursing2003*, 33(10), Suppl-Travel Nursing, pp. 14–20.
14. Hess, C. (2002). *Clinical Guide to Wound Care*. 4th ed. Philadelphia. Lippincott Williams & Wilkins.
15. Carrington, A. L., et al. (2001). Peripheral vascular and nerve function associated with lower limb amputation in people with and without diabetes. *Clin Sci*, 101, 261–266.
16. Catania, K., Huang, C., James, P., Ohr, M. (2007). PUPPI: The pressure ulcer prevention protocol interventions. *AJN*, 107(4), 44–51.
17. Reddy, M., Gill, S. S., Rochon, P. A. (2006). Preventing pressure ulcers: A systematic review. *JAMA*, 296, 974–984.
18. Okan, K., Woo, K., Ayello, E. A., et al. (2007). The role of moisture balance in wound healing. *Advances for Skin & Wound Care: The Journal for Prevention and Healing*, 20(1), 39–53.

risk for impaired Skin Integrity

Definition: At risk for skin being adversely altered
Note: Risk should be determined by the use of a standardized risk assessment tool [e.g., Braden, Norton (or similar) Scale]

RISK FACTORS

External
Chemical substance; radiation
Hypothermia; hyperthermia
Physical immobilization
Excretions; secretions; humidity; moisture
Mechanical factors (e.g., shearing forces, pressure, restraint)
Extremes of age

Internal
Medications
Imbalanced nutritional state (e.g., obesity, emaciation), impaired metabolic state, [changes in fluid status]
Skeletal prominence; changes in skin turgor; [presence of edema]
Impaired circulation/sensation; change in pigmentation
Developmental factors
Psychogenic factors [e.g., obsessive compulsive behaviors]
Immunological factors

NOTE: A risk diagnosis is not evidenced by signs and symptoms, as the problem has not occurred; rather, nursing interventions are directed at prevention.

Sample Clinical Applications: Arteriosclerosis, venous insufficiency, hypertension, obesity, diabetes mellitus, systemic lupus, malignant neoplasms, chronic steroid use (e.g., COPD, asthma), renal failure, malnutrition

DESIRED OUTCOMES/EVALUATION CRITERIA
Sample NOC linkages:
Risk Control: Personal actions to prevent, eliminate, or reduce modifiable health threats
Immobility Consequences: Physiological: Severity of compromise in physiological functioning due to impaired physical mobility
Tissue Integrity: Skin & Mucous Membranes: Structural intactness and normal physiological function of skin and mucous membranes

Client Will (Include Specific Time Frame)

• Identify individual risk factors.
• Verbalize understanding of treatment/therapy regimen.
• Demonstrate behaviors/techniques to prevent skin breakdown.

ACTIONS/INTERVENTIONS

Sample NIC linkages:

Skin Surveillance: Collection and analysis of patient data to maintain skin and mucous membrane integrity

Pressure Management: Minimizing pressure to body parts

Pressure Ulcer Prevention: Prevention of pressure ulcers for a patient at high risk for developing them

NURSING PRIORITY NO. 1 To assess causative/contributing factors:

- Identify client with underlying conditions/problems that have potential for *skin integrity problems such as (1) disease processes that affect circulation and perfusion of tissues (e.g., arteriosclerosis, venous insufficiency, hypertension, obesity, diabetes, malignant neoplasms); (2) medications (e.g., anticoagulants, corticosteroids, immunosuppressives, antineoplastics) that adversely affect/impair healing; (3) radiation (can break down internal tissues as well as skin); and (4) nutrition and hydration (e.g., malnutrition deprives the body of protein and calories required for cell growth and repair, and dehydration impairs transport of oxygen and nutrients).*[1–5]

- Note general health. *Many factors (e.g., debilitation, immobility, use of restraints, extremes of age, mental status, dehydration or malnutrition, presence of chronic disease; occupational, treatment, and environmental hazards) can all affect the ability of the skin to perform its functions (e.g., protection, sensation, movement and growth, chemical synthesis, immunity, thermoregulation and excretion).*[1,6]

- Determine client's age and developmental factors/ability to care for self. *Newborn/infant's skin is thin. Babies and children are prone to skin rashes associated with viral, bacterial, and fungal infections and allergic reactions. In adolescence, hormones stimulate hair growth and sebaceous gland activity. In adults, it takes longer to replenish epidermis cells, resulting in increased risk of skin cancers and infection. In older adults there is decreased epidermal regeneration, fewer sweat glands, and less subcutaneous fat and elastin and collagen, causing skin to become thinner, drier, and less responsive to pain sensations.*[1,3,4,7–9]

- Perform risk assessment using a standardized tool (e.g., Braden Scale) *to determine pressure sore risk and appropriate interventions. Provides baseline for periodic comparison to note changes in risk status and need for alterations in the plan of care.*

- Evaluate client's skin care practices and hygiene issues. *Individual's skin may be oily, dry, or sensitive and is affected by bathing frequency (or lack of bathing), temperature of water, and types of soap and other cleansing agents. Incontinence (urinary or bowel) and ineffective hygiene can result in serious skin impairment and discomfort.*

- Note presence of compromised vision, hearing, or speech *that may impact client's self-care as relates to skin care (e.g., diabetic with impaired vision probably cannot satisfactorily examine own feet).*[10]

- Ascertain allergy history. *Individual may be sensitive or allergic to substances (e.g., insects, grasses, medications, lotions, soaps, foods) that can adversely affect the skin.*

- Assess blood supply (e.g., capillary return time, color, and warmth) and sensation of skin surfaces/affected area on a regular basis *to provide comparative baseline and opportunity for timely intervention when problems are noted.*[11]

- Calculate ankle-brachial index *to evaluate actual/potential for impairment of circulation to lower extremities. Result less than 0.9 indicates need for close monitoring/more aggressive intervention (e.g., tighter blood glucose and weight control in diabetic client).*[12,13]

- Review laboratory results (e.g., Hb/Hct, blood glucose, albumin/protein) *to evaluate causative factors or ability to heal. Note: Albumin <3.5 correlates to decreased wound healing/increased incidence of pressure ulcers.*[14]

🌐 Cultural   Collaborative   🏠 Community/Home Care   ✎ Diagnostic Studies   ∞ Pediatric/Geriatric/Lifespan   💊 Medications

NURSING PRIORITY NO. 2 To maintain optimal skin integrity:[1,2,9,11]

- Perform routine skin inspections, assessing color, temperature, surface changes, texture, and contours. Evaluate color changes in areas of least pigmentation (e.g., sclera, conjunctiva, nail beds, buccal mucosa, tongue, palms, and soles of feet). Report potential problem areas (e.g., reddened/blanched areas or rashes) promptly. *Systematic inspection can identify developing problems; also promotes early intervention, thus reducing likelihood of progression to skin breakdown.*[15]

- Handle client gently (particularly infant, young child, elderly frail). *Epidermis of infants and very young children is thin and lacks subcutaneous depth that will develop with age. Skin of the older client is also thin, less elastic, and prone to injury, such as bruising and skin tears.*[5]

- Practice and instruct client/caregiver(s) in scrupulous hand washing and clean or sterile technique, as appropriate, *to reduce incidence of contamination or infection.*

- Maintain/instruct in good skin hygiene (e.g., wash thoroughly, pat dry, gently massage with lotion or appropriate cream) *to reduce risk of dermal trauma, improve circulation, and promote comfort.*

- Provide preventative skin care to incontinent client: change continence pads/diapers frequently; cleanse perineal skin daily and after each incontinence episode; apply skin protectant ointment *to minimize contact with irritants (urine, stool, excessive moisture).*[16]

- Cleanse skin after diaphoretic episodes *to maintain normal skin pH and flora and limit potential for infection.*

- Develop regularly timed repositioning schedule for client with mobility and sensation impairments, using turn sheet, as needed; encourage/assist with periodic weight shifts for client in chair *to reduce stress on pressure points and encourage circulation to tissues.*

- Use proper turning/transfer techniques. *Avoids movements that cause friction/shearing (e.g., pulling client with parallel force, dragging movements, etc.).*

- Pay special attention to bony prominences and other pressure points (e.g., heels, toes, elbows) when positioning client *to prevent pressure trauma and impaired circulation.*

- Provide foam/flotation/alternating pressure/air mattress *to reduce pressure on skin/tissues and lesions, decreasing tissue ischemia.*

- Use appropriate padding devices (e.g., air/water mattress, egg crate/gel pads, heel rolls/foam boots) when indicated *to reduce pressure on/enhance circulation to compromised tissues.*

- Encourage early ambulation. *Promotes circulation and reduces risks associated with immobility.*

- Provide for safety measures during ambulation and other therapies *to reduce risk of dermal injury (e.g., assistive devices or sufficient personnel, grab bars, clear pathways, safe chairs, properly fitting hose/footwear, use of heating pads/lamps, restraints).*

- Limit/avoid use of plastic material (e.g., rubber sheet, plastic-backed linen savers), and remove wet/wrinkled linens promptly. *Moisture potentiates skin breakdown and increases risk for infection.*

- Use paper tape or a nonadherent dressing on frail skin and remove it gently, or use stockinette, tubular/gauze wrap, or other similar product instead of tape to secure dressings and drains *to limit dermal injury.*[5]

- Avoid use of latex products *when client has known or suspected sensitivity.* (Refer to ND latex Allergy Response.)

- Apply hot and cold applications judiciously *to reduce risk of dermal injury in persons with circulatory and neurosensory impairments.*

- Provide adequate clothing/covers; protect from drafts *to prevent vasoconstriction and reduction of circulation to skin.*

- Keep bedclothes dry, use nonirritating materials, and keep bed free of wrinkles, crumbs, and so forth *to prevent skin irritation.*

- 🏠 Try colloidal bath, application of lotions, or careful use of ice pack *to decrease irritable itching.*
- 🏠 Keep nails cut short, encouraging client *to refrain from scratching* or suggest use of/obtain order for mittens (considered a restraint), if necessary, *to prevent dermal injury from scratching.*
- Refer to ND impaired Skin Integrity for additional interventions, as indicated.

NURSING PRIORITY NO. 3 To promote wellness (Teaching/Discharge Considerations):

- 🏠 Discuss importance of skin and measures to maintain proper skin functioning. *The integumentary system is the largest multifunctional organ of the body and thus merits special care.*
- 🔬 Stress importance of regular inspection/monitoring of skin for changes and effective skin care in preventing skin problems. *Early detection and reporting to healthcare providers promotes timely evaluation and intervention.*
- 🏠 Counsel diabetic and neurologically impaired client regarding the necessity of meticulous skin care, especially of lower extremities. *Healing of lower-extremity injuries tends to be more problematic in this population, resulting in increased incidence of amputation.*
- 🏠 Avoid products containing perfumes, dyes, preservatives *(may cause dermatitis reactions)* or alcohol, povidone-iodine, hydrogen peroxide *(may hinder healing).*
- 🏠 Instruct in care of skin/extremities during cold or hot weather (e.g., wearing gloves, boots, clean/dry socks, properly fitting shoes/boots, face protection) *to reduce risk of tissue damage, especially in clients with impaired sensation.*
- 🏠 Recommend elevation of lower extremities when sitting *to enhance venous return and reduce edema formation.*
- 🏠 Encourage continuation of regular exercise program (active/assistive) *to enhance circulation.*
- 🏠 Discuss need for adequate nutritional intake (including adequate protein, lipids, calories, trace minerals, and multivitamins) *to promote skin health/healing and to maintain general good health.*
- 🏠 Determine fluid needs/sources for hydration (e.g., oral, tube feeding, ambient room humidity, etc.) *to reduce/replenish transepidermal water loss.*
- 🏠 Encourage restriction/abstinence from tobacco, *which can cause vasoconstriction.*
- 🏠 Discuss importance of limiting lengthy/unnecessary sun exposure and avoiding use of tanning beds. Stress necessity of avoiding exposure to sunlight in specific conditions (e.g., systemic lupus, tetracycline/psychotropic drug use, radiation therapy) as well as potential for development of skin cancer.
- Advise use of high SPF sunblock/sunscreen, particularly on young child, client with fair skin [prone to burn], and client using multiple medications, etc., *to limit skin damage (immediate and over time) associated with sun exposure.*

DOCUMENTATION FOCUS

Assessment/Reassessment

- Individual findings, including individual risk factors.

Planning

- Plan of care and who is involved in planning.
- Teaching plan.

Implementation/Evaluation

- Responses to interventions/teaching and actions performed.

🌐 Cultural 🔬 Collaborative 🏠 Community/Home Care Diagnostic Studies ∞ Pediatric/Geriatric/Lifespan Medications

- Attainment/progress toward desired outcome(s).
- Modifications to plan of care.

Discharge Planning

- Long-term needs and who is responsible for actions to be taken.

References

1. Calianno, C. (2002). Patient hygiene, part 2—Skin care: Keeping the outside healthy. *Nursing2002*, 32(6), June Clinical Supp.
2. Neonatal skin care. Evidence-based clinical practice guideline. (2001). Washington DC: Association of Women's Health, Obstetric and Neonatal Nurses (AWHONN). Available at www.guideline.gov. Accessed September 2003.
3. Llewellyn, S. (2002). Skin integrity and wound care (lecture materials). Chapel Hills, NC: Cape Fear Community College Nursing Program.
4. Colburn, L. (2001). Prevention for chronic wounds. In Krasner, D., Rodeheaver, G., Sibbald, R. G. *Chronic Wound Care: A Clinical Source Book for Healthcare Professionals.* 2d ed. Wayne, PA: HMP Communications.
5. Baranoski, S. (2003). Skin tears: Staying on guard against the enemy of frail skin. *Nursing2003*, 33(10), Suppl-Travel Nursing, pp. 14–20.
6. Lund, C. H., Osborne, J. W., Culler, J., et al. (2001). Neonatal skin care: Clinical Outcomes of the AWHONN/NANN. Evidence-based clinical practice guideline. *JONN*, 30(1), 30–40.
7. McGovern, C. (2003). Skin, hair and nail assessment. Unit 2 (lecture materials). Villanova, PA: Villanova University College of Nursing. Accessed July 2007 at www.homepage.villanova.edu/.
8. Engel, J. (2002). *Pocket Guide to Pediatric Assessment.* 4th ed. St. Louis, MO: Mosby, pp. 99–112.
9. Wiersema, L. A., Stanley, M. (1999). The aging integumentary system. In Stanley, M., Beare, P. G. *Gerontological Nursing: A Health Promotion/Protection Approach.* 2d ed. Philadelphia: F. A. Davis, pp. 102–111.
10. Lawrance, D. P. DIABETES FYI-Foot Care (Monograph 5 in series). Champaign, IL: University of Illinois, McKinley Diabetes Team.
11. ND: Skin Integrity, impaired. In Doenges, M. E., Moorhouse, M. F., Geissler-Murr, A. C. (2002). *Nursing Care Plans: Guidelines for Individualizing Patient Care.* 6th ed. Philadelphia: F. A. Davis
12. Murabito, J. M., Evans, J. C., Larson, M. G., et al. (2003). The ankle-brachial index in the elderly and risk of stroke, coronary disease and death. *Arch Intern Med*, 163, 1939–1942.
13. Carrington, A. L., et al. (2001). Peripheral vascular and nerve function associated with lower limb amputation in people with and without diabetes. *Clin Sci*, 101, 261–266.
14. Catania, K., Huang, C., James, P., Ohr, M. (2007). PUPPI: The pressure ulcer prevention protocol interventions. *AJN*, 107(4), 44–51.
15. Krasner, D., Rodeheaver, G., Sibbald, R. G. (2001). Advanced wound caring for a new millennium. In Krasner, D., Rodeheaver, G., Sibbald, R. G. *Chronic Wound Care: A Clinical Source Book for Healthcare Professionals.* 2d ed. Wayne, PA: HMP Communications.
16. Gray, M., Bliss, D. Z., Doughty, D. B., et al. (2007). Incontinence-associated dermatitis: A consensus. *Journal of Wound, Ostomy and Continence Nursing*, 34(1), 45–54.

readiness for enhanced Sleep

Definition: A pattern of natural, periodic suspension of consciousness that provides adequate rest, sustains a desired lifestyle, and can be strengthened

RELATED FACTORS
To be developed by nurse researchers and submitted to NANDA

DEFINING CHARACTERISTICS

Subjective
Expresses willingness to enhance sleep
Expresses a feeling of being rested after sleep
Follows sleep routines that promote sleep habits

Objective
Amount of sleep and REM sleep is congruent with developmental needs
Occasional or infrequent use of medications to induce sleep

Sample Clinical Applications: Postoperative recovery, chronic pain, pregnancy—prenatal/postpartal period, sleep apnea

DESIRED OUTCOMES/EVALUATION CRITERIA
Sample NOC Linkages:
Sleep: Natural periodic suspension of consciousness during which the body is restored
Rest: Quantity and pattern of diminished activity for mental and physical rejuvenation
Comfort Level: Extent of positive perception of physical and psychological ease

Client Will (Include Specific Time Frame)

- Identify individually appropriate interventions to promote sleep.
- Verbalize feeling rested after sleep.
- Adjust lifestyle to accommodate routines that promote sleep.

ACTIONS/INTERVENTIONS

Sample NIC Linkages:
Sleep Enhancement: Facilitation of regular sleep/wake cycles
Simple Relaxation Therapy: Use of techniques to encourage and elicit relaxation for the purpose of decreasing undesirable signs and symptoms such as pain, muscle tension, or anxiety
Environmental Management: Manipulation of the patient's surroundings for therapeutic benefit

NURSING PRIORITY NO. 1   To determine motivation for continued growth:

- Listen to client's reports of sleep quantity and quality. Determine client's perception of adequate sleep. *Reveals client's experience and expectations regarding sleep. Provides opportunity to address misconceptions/unrealistic expectations and plan for interventions.*
- Observe or obtain feedback from client/SO(s) regarding usual bedtime, number of hours of sleep, time of arising *to determine usual sleep pattern and provide comparative baseline for improvements.*
- Ascertain movitation and expectation for change. *Motivation to improve and high expectations can encourage client to make changes that will improve his or her life. However, unrealistic expectations may hamper efforts.*
- Note client report of potential for alteration of habitual sleep time (e.g., change of work pattern/rotating shifts) or change in normal bedtime (e.g., hospitalization). *Helps identify circumstances that are known to interrupt sleep patterns and that could disrupt the person's biological rhythms.*[1,2,8]

NURSING PRIORITY NO. 2   To assist client to enhance sleep/rest:

- Review client's usual bedtime rituals and routines and environmental needs. *Provides information on client's management of the situation and identifies areas that might be modified when the need arises.*

- Discuss/implement effective age-appropriate bedtime rituals for infant/child (e.g., rocking, story reading, cuddling, favorite blanket/toy). *Rituals can enhance ability to fall asleep, reinforce that bed is a place to sleep, and promote sense of security for child.*[3]
- Provide quiet environment and comfort measures (e.g., back rub, washing hands/face, cleaning and straightening sheets) for client in facility. *Promotes relaxation and readiness for sleep.*
- Arrange care *to provide for uninterrupted periods for rest.* Explain necessity of disturbances for monitoring vital signs or other care when client is hospitalized. Do as much care as possible during night without waking client. *Allows for longer periods of uninterrupted sleep, especially during night.*
- Suggest limiting fluid intake in evening if nocturia or bed-wetting is a problem *to reduce need for nighttime elimination.*
- Assist client/provide instruction in use of necessary equipment. *Client may use oxygen or CPAP system to improve sleep/rest in presence of hypoxia or sleep apnea.*
- Discuss dietary matters, such as limiting chocolate, heavy meals, caffeine/alcoholic beverages prior to bedtime, *which are substances known to impair falling or staying asleep. Use of alcohol at bedtime may help individual fall asleep, but ensuing sleep is then fragmented.*[4]
- Explore/implement use of warm bath, intake of light protein snack before bedtime, comfortable room temperature, soothing music, favorite calming television show. *Nonpharmaceutical aids may enhance falling asleep without the undesired side effects associated with medications.*
- Investigate use of sleep mask, darkening shades/curtains, earplugs, low-level background (white) noise in situations where sleep might not come easily/be disturbed by environmental factors.
- Recommend continuing same schedule for sleep throughout week—including days off. *Maintaining sleep pattern helps sustain biological rhythms.*

NURSING PRIORITY NO. 3 To promote optimum wellness:

- Assure client that occasional sleeplessness should not threaten health. *Knowledge that occasional insomnia is universal and usually not harmful may promote relaxation and relief from worry.*[5]
- Encourage regular exercise during day *to aid in stress control/release of energy. Note: Exercise at bedtime may stimulate rather than relax client and may actually interfere with sleep.*[7]
- Assist to develop individual program of relaxation (e.g., biofeedback, self-hypnosis, visualization, progressive muscle relaxation). *Reduces sympathetic response and stress to aid in inducing sleep.*[6]
- Address sleep management techniques that may be useful during stressful conditions/lifestyle changes (e.g., pregnancy, new baby, menopause, medical procedures, new job, moving, change in relationship, grief, etc.).
- Recommend periodic review of medications. *Many prescription and OTC drugs can disrupt sleep.*
- Advise using prescription or OTC sleep medications sparingly. These medications, while useful for promoting sleep in the short-term, can interfere with REM sleep.

DOCUMENTATION FOCUS

Assessment/Reassessment

- Assessment findings, including specifics of sleep pattern and effects on lifestyle/level of functioning.
- Any medications/interventions, previous therapies.
- Motivation and expectations for change

Planning

- Plan of care and who is involved in planning.
- Teaching plan.

Implementation/Evaluation

- Client's response to interventions/teaching and actions performed.
- Attainment/progress toward desired outcome(s).
- Modifications to plan of care.

Discharge Planning

- Long-term needs and who is responsible for actions to be taken.
- Specific referrals made.

References

1. Cochran, H. (2003). Diagnose and treat primary insomnia. *Nurse Practitioner, 28*(9), 13–27.
2. Spenceley, S. M. (1993). Sleep inquiry: A look with fresh eyes. *Image, 25*(3), 249–255.
3. Mindell, J. (1997). *Sleeping Through the Night: How Infants, Toddlers, and Their Parents Can Get a Good Night's Sleep.* HarperCollins.
4. Bahr, Sr. R. T. (1999). Sleep Disturbances. In Stanley, M., Beare, P. G. *Gerontological Nursing: A Health Promotion/Protection Approach.* 2d ed. Philadelphia: F. A. Davis, pp. 335–341.
5. Brain basics: Understanding sleep. National Institute of Neurological Disorders and Stroke (NINDS). Accessed July 2007 at www.ninds.nih.gov.
6. ND: Sleep Pattern, disturbed. In Cox, H. C., et al. (2002). *Clinical Applications of Nursing Diagnosis: Adult, Child, Women's, Psychiatric, Gerontic, and Home Health Considerations.* 4th ed. Philadelphia: F. A. Davis, pp. 375–380.
7. Grandjean, C. K., Gibbons, S. W. (2000). Assessing ambulatory geriatic sleep complaints. *Nurse Practitioner: Am J Prim Health Care, 25*(9), 25.
8. Pronitis-Ruotolo, D. (2001). Surviving the night shift: Making Zeitgeber work for you. *AJN, 101*(7), 63.

Sleep Deprivation

Definition: Prolonged periods of time without sleep (sustained natural, periodic suspension of relative consciousness)

RELATED FACTORS

Sustained environmental stimulation/uncomfortable sleep environment

Inadequate daytime activity; sustained circadian asynchrony; aging-related sleep stage shifts; non–sleep-inducing parenting practices

Sustained inadequate sleep hygiene; prolonged use of pharmacological or dietary antisoporifics

Prolonged discomfort (e.g., physical, psychological); periodic limb movement (e.g., restless leg syndrome, nocturnal myoclonus); sleep-related enuresis/painful erections

Nightmares; sleepwalking; sleep terror

Sleep apnea

Sundowner's syndrome; dementia

Idiopathic CNS hypersomnolence; narcolepsy; familial sleep paralysis

DEFINING CHARACTERISTICS

Subjective

Daytime drowsiness; decreased ability to function

Malaise; lethargy; fatigue

Anxiety

Perceptual disorders (e.g., disturbed body sensation, delusions, feeling afloat); heightened sensitivity to pain

Cultural   Collaborative   Community/Home Care   Diagnostic Studies   Pediatric/Geriatric/Lifespan   Medications

Objective

Restlessness; irritability
Inability to concentrate; slowed reaction
Listlessness; apathy
Fleeting nystagmus; hand tremors
Acute confusion; transient paranoia; agitation; combativeness; hallucinations

Sample Clinical Applications: COPD, heart failure (nocturia), chronic pain, sleep apnea, pregnancy/postpartum, colic, dementia/Alzheimer's disease, anxiety disorders, post-traumatic stress disorder

DESIRED OUTCOMES/EVALUATION CRITERIA
Sample NOC linkages:
Sleep: Natural periodic suspension of consciousness during which the body is restored
Rest: Quantity and pattern of diminished activity for mental and physical rejuvenation
Pain Control: Personal actions to control pain

Client Will (Include Specific Time Frame)

• Identify individually appropriate interventions to promote sleep.
• Verbalize understanding of sleep disorder.
• Adjust lifestyle to accommodate chronobiological rhythms.
• Report improvement in sleep/rest pattern.

Sample NOC linkages:
Family Coping: Family actions to manage stressors that tax an individual's resources

Family Will (Include Specific Time Frame)

• Deal appropriately with parasomnias.

ACTIONS/INTERVENTIONS

Sample NIC linkages:
Sleep Enhancement: Facilitation of regular sleep/wake cycles
Anxiety Reduction: Minimizing apprehension, dread, foreboding, or uneasiness related to an unidentified source or anticipated danger
Environmental Management: Comfort: Manipulation of the patient's surroundings for promotion of optimal comfort

NURSING PRIORITY NO. 1   To assess causative/contributing factors:

∞ • Note client's age and developmental stage. *The average adult requires 7 to 8 hours sleep; pregnant women and new mothers, while needing more sleep, usually are sleep-deprived; studies show that sleep disorders occur in 35% to 45% of children age 2 to 18 years;[16] adolescents and young adults don't get enough sleep, have irregular sleep patterns, and are at risk for problem sleepiness;[18] menopausal women often report interrupted sleep because of hot flashes/hormonal influences; elderly persons sleep fewer hours, report less restful sleep and need for more sleep.[1–5,15,16]*
• Determine presence of physical or psychological stressors: *These include multiple, varying factors, such as night-shift work hours/rotating shfits; pain (acute and chronic), current/recent*

illness, hospitalization, especially in intensive care unit; death of a spouse, loss of a job; new baby in the home, inadequate sleep-promoting behaviors; etc.

- Note presence of diagnoses *that are known to affect sleep (e.g., mental confusion/dementias, certain brain infections [e.g., encephalitis], brain injury, narcolepsy, obsessive/compulsive disorder, anxiety, depression, and other major psychological disorders; drug or alcohol abuse; restless leg syndrome; sleep-induced respiratory disorders/obstructive sleep apnea, childhood snoring with sleep apnea).*[6,7]

- Evaluate medication regimen for products affecting sleep. *Diet pills/other stimulants, sedatives, antidepressants, antihypertensives, diuretics, narcotics, agents with anticholinergic effects, and need for medications requiring nighttime dosing can inhibit getting to sleep or remaining asleep.*[8,9,20]

- Note environmental factors affecting sleep *(e.g., unfamiliar or uncomfortable sleep environment, excessive noise and light, frequent checking of vital signs, uncomfortable temperature, roommate irritations/actions—snoring, watching television late at night, etc.). Note: Clients in critical care units are known to experience lack of sleep or frequent disruptions, often compounding their illness.*[9]

- Determine presence of parasomnias: nightmares/terrors, sleepwalking/talking, or other complex behaviors during sleep. *May occur at any age, with as many as 30% of children (peak age 4 to 8 years) having a sleep disorder at some time.*[20] Note reports of terror, brief periods of paralysis, sense of body being disconnected from the brain. *Occurrence of sleep paralysis, though not widely recognized in the United States, has been well documented elsewhere and may result in feelings of fear/reluctance to go to sleep. May require more extensive evaluation for serious sleep disorders.*[10,17]

NURSING PRIORITY NO. 2 To assess degree of impairment:

- Assess client's usual sleep patterns and current sleep disturbance, relying upon client/SO report of problem. Incorporate screening information into in-depth sleep diary or testing if needed. *Usual sleep patterns are individual, but sleep loss has been shown to be the most common complaint reported in primary care settings;*[4,11] *therefore, screening for the problem should be routine. Data collected from a comprehensive assessment is needed to determine etiology of challenging sleep disturbances, including the stage of sleep that is impaired.*[9,12]

- Ascertain quality of sleep for bed partner/family members. *Loud irregular snoring (sleep apnea), periodic nightmares/sleep terrors or sleep talking, sleepwalking, or involuntary muscle activity can interfere with sleep of bed partner/entire family.*[20]

- Determine client's sleep expectations. *Individual may have faulty beliefs/attitudes about sleep and unrealistic sleep expectations (e.g., "I must get 8 hours of sleep every night, or I can't accomplish anything").*[11]

- Ascertain duration of current problem and effect on life/functional ability. *Client may not get enough sleep and not realize that life functioning is being impaired (e.g., can't concentrate in school, falls asleep when stopped at a light while driving).*[11]

- Listen to subjective reports of sleep quality (e.g., "short, interrupted") and response from lack of good sleep (feeling foggy, sleepy, and woozy, fighting sleep, fatigue, etc.). *Helps clarify client's perception of sleep quantity/quality and response to inadequate sleep.*[11]

- Observe for physical signs of fatigue. *Client may display restlessness, irritability, disorientation, frequent yawning, and/or other changes in mood/behavior or performance (e.g., inability to tolerate stress, problems with concentration or learning). Fatigue, daytime sleepiness, and functional impairment have been reported as significant problem in teens.*[3,4,11,15,20]

- Determine interventions client has tried to date. *Helps identify appropriate options and may reveal additional interventions that can be attempted.*

- Distinguish client's beneficial bedtime habits from detrimental ones (*e.g., drinking late-evening milk versus late-evening coffee*).
- Instruct client and/or bed partner to keep a sleep-wake log *to document symptoms and identify factors that are interfering with sleep.*
- Obtain a chronological chart *to determine client's peak performance rhythms.*
- Investigate anxious feelings *to help determine basis and appropriate anxiety-reduction techniques/behavioral therapy needs.*[20]

NURSING PRIORITY NO. 3 To assist client to establish optimal sleep pattern:[2,4,5,8,9,11,13,14]

- Review medications being taken and their effect on sleep, suggesting modifications in regimen, *if medications are found to be interfering.*
- Encourage client to restrict caffeine and other stimulating substances from late-afternoon/evening intake. Recommend avoidance of bedtime alcohol. *Both alcohol and some medications can produce immediate sleep followed by early awakening/difficulty remaining asleep.*
- Avoid eating large evening/late-night meals.
- Recommend light bedtime snack (protein, simple carbohydrate, and low fat) and/or glass of warm milk for individuals who feel hungry, ingested 15 to 30 minutes before retiring. *Sense of fullness and satiety can encourage sleep.*
- Limit evening fluid intake if nocturia is present *to reduce need for nighttime elimination.*
- Promote adequate physical exercise activity during day, finishing workout at least 3 hours before bedtime. *Enhances expenditure of energy/release of tension so that client feels ready for sleep/rest. Note: Rigorous exercise close to bedtime can delay onset of sleep.*
- Suggest abstaining from daytime naps, or napping in the morning *to improve ability to fall asleep at night.*
- Recommend quiet relaxing activities prior to bedtime such as reading, listening to soothing music, meditation *to reduce stimulation and promote relaxation.*
- Discuss/implement effective age-appropriate bedtime rituals (*e.g., going to bed at same time each night, brushing teeth, reading, drinking warm milk, rocking, story reading, cuddling, favorite blanket/toy*) *to enhance client's ability to fall asleep, reinforce that bed is a place to sleep, and promote sense of security for child.*
- Provide back massage/other therapeutic touch, as appropriate. *Touch can be relaxing and emotionally pleasing, given that the client has SO's undivided attention for a few moments.*
- Provide calm, quiet environment for hospitalized client, *to manage controllable sleep-disrupting factors (e.g., reduce noise and talking, dim lights, shut room door, adjust room temperature as needed, silence/reduce volume on phones, beepers, alarms, television, radios).*
- Administer pain medication first *to make sure client is pain-free*, and then sedatives/other sleep medications (*so that hypnotic will be more effective*) when indicated, noting client's response. Time pain medications for peak effect/duration *to reduce need for redosing during prime sleep hours.*
- Discuss appropriate use of benzodiazepines when indicated. *May be useful in some clients for reducing risk of injury associated with sleepwalking or for management of severe sleep terrors.*[20]
- Instruct client to get out of bed, leave bedroom, engage in relaxing activities *if unable to fall asleep,* and not return to bed until feeling sleepy.
- Recommend/instruct client in relaxation techniques (*e.g., visualization, breathing, yoga*).
- Refer for biofeedback, cognitive therapy, etc., *when measures that are more intensive are needed/desired to cope with stressors and promote relaxation.*
- Refer client/collaborate with healthcare team for evaluation/treatment of more serious sleep problems (*e.g., obstructive sleep apnea, narcolepsy, sleep paralysis, bed-wetting, nocturnal leg cramps, restless leg syndrome, etc.*).[16,17,19,20]

- Review with the client the physician's recommendations for managing obstructive sleep apnea such as medical or surgical treatment of obesity; medications, structural surgery (e.g., alteration of facial structures; removal of tonsils and adnoids in children),[19] or apnea/oxygenation therapy—continuous positive airway pressure (CPAP) such as Respironics—*when sleep apnea is severe as documented by sleep-disorder studies.*

NURSING PRIORITY NO. 4 To promote wellness (Teaching/Discharge Considerations):

- Review possibility of next-day drowsiness/"rebound" insomnia and temporary memory loss *that may be associated with sleep disorders and/or prescription sleep medications.*
- Discuss short-term use/appropriateness of OTC sleep medications/herbal supplements. Note possible side effects and drug interactions.
- Identify appropriate safety precautions (e.g., securing doors/windows and stairways, placing client bedroom on first floor), and attaching audible alarm to bedroom door *to alert parents when child is sleepwalking.*[19]
- Refer to support group/counselor *to help deal with psychological stressors (e.g., grief, sorrow).* (Refer to NDs Grieving, chronic Sorrow.)
- Encourage family counseling as indicated *to help deal with concerns arising from parasomnias (e.g., sleep talking, sleepwalking, night terrors, etc.).*
- Refer to sleep specialist/laboratory for sleep studies *when problem is unresponsive to customary interventions.*

DOCUMENTATION FOCUS

Assessment/Reassessment

- Assessment findings, including specifics of sleep pattern (current and past) and effects on lifestyle/level of functioning.
- Medications/interventions, previous therapies.
- Family history of similar problem.
- Effects of sleep disturbance on SO/family.

Planning

- Plan of care and who is involved in planning.
- Teaching plan.

Implementation/Evaluation

- Client's response to interventions/teaching and actions performed.
- Attainment/progress toward desired outcome(s).
- Modifications to plan of care.

Discharge Planning

- Long-term needs and who is responsible for actions to be taken.
- Specific referrals made.

References

1. ND: Sleep Deprivation (developmental considerations). In Cox, H. C., et al. (2002). *Clinical Applications of Nursing Diagnosis: Adult, Child, Women's, Psychiatric, Gerontic, and Home Health Considerations.* 4th ed. Philadelphia: F. A. Davis, pp. 368–369.
2. Mindell, J. (1997). *Sleeping Through the Night: How Infants, Toddlers, and Their Parents Can Get a Good Night's Sleep.* New York: HarperCollins.

Cultural   Collaborative   Community/Home Care   Diagnostic Studies   Pediatric/Geriatric/Lifespan   Medications

3. No author listed. Adolescent sleep needs and patterns: Research report and resource guide. National Sleep Foundation. Accessed July 2007 at www.sleepfoundation.org.
4. No author listed. Women and sleep. National Sleep Foundation. Accessed July 2007 at www.sleepfoundation.org.
5. Bahr, Sr. R. T. (1999). Sleep disturbances. In Stanley, M., Beare, P. G. *Gerontological Nursing: A Health Promotion/Protection Approach.* 2d ed. Philadelphia: F. A. Davis, pp. 337–341.
6. Sateia, M. J., et al. (2000). Evaluation of chronic insomnia: An American Academy of Sleep Medicine review. *Sleep,* 23(2), 243–308.
7. Clinical practice guideline: Diagnosis and management of childhood obstructive sleep apnea syndrome. (2002). *Pediatrics,* 109(4), 704–712. Accessed July 2007 at http://aappolicy.aappublications.org/cgi/content/full/pediatrics;109/4/704.
8. Barroso, J. (2003). Living with illness: HIV-related fatigue. *AJN,* 102(5), 83.
9. Honkus, V. L. (2003). Sleep deprivation in critical care units. *Crit Care Nurs Quart,* 26(3), 179–191.
10. Cardinal, F. (2004). Sleep disorders—the basics. (Monographs). Accessed July 2007 at http://sleepdisorders.about.com.
11. Cochran, H. (2003). Diagnose and treat primary insomnia. *Nurse Practitioner,* 28(9), 13–27.
12. Spenceley, S. M. (1993). Sleep inquiry: A look with fresh eyes. *Image,* 25(3), 249–255.
13. Pronitis-Ruotolo, D. (2001). Surviving the night shift: Making Zeitgeber work for you. *AJN,* 101(7), 63.
14. Cmiel, C. A., et al. (2004). Noise control: A nursing team's approach to sleep promotion. *AJN,* 104(2), 40–48.
15. National Ag Safety Database (NASD). (2002). Sleep deprivation: Cause and consequences. Fact sheet for Nebraska Rural Health and Safety Coalition. Retrieved August 2007 at www.cdc.gov/nasd/docs/d000701-d000800/d000705/d000705.html.
16. Connelly, K. P. (2006). Sleep disorders: Nightmares. Article (excerpt) for Emedicine Web site. Retrieved July 2007 at www.emedicine.com/ped/topic1609.htm.
17. Bruis, M. J. (2004, editorial review 2005). Sleep Disorders: Parsomnias. Article for MedicineNet.com Web site. Accessed July 2007 at www.medicinenet.com/script/main/art.asp?articlekey=47489.
18. National Sleep Foundation Sleep and Teens Task Force. (2000). Adolescent Sleep Needs and Patterns: Research Report and Resource Guide, pp. 2–4.
19. Garcia, J., Wills, L. (2002). Sleep disorders in children and teens: Helping patients and their families get some sleep. *Postgraduate Medicine,* 107(3). Retrieved August 2007 at www.postgradmed.com/issues/2000/03_00/garcia.htm.
20. Schenck, C. H., Mahowald, M. W.(2002). Parasomnias: Managing bizarre sleep-related behavior disorders. *Postgrauate Medicine,* 107(3). Retrieved August 2007 at www.postgradmed.com/issues/2000/03_00/schenck.htm.

impaired Social Interaction

Definition: Insufficient or excessive quantity or ineffective quality of social exchange

RELATED FACTORS

Deficit about ways to enhance mutuality (e.g., knowledge, skills)

Communication barriers [including head injury, stroke, other neurological conditions affecting ability to communicate]

Self-concept disturbance

Absence of significant others

Limited physical mobility [e.g., neuromuscular disease]

Therapeutic isolation

Sociocultural dissonance

Environmental barriers

Disturbed thought processes

DEFINING CHARACTERISTICS

Subjective

Discomfort in social situations

Inability to communicate/receive a satisfying sense of social engagement (e.g., belonging, caring, interest, or shared history)

Family report of changes in interaction (e.g., style, pattern)

Objective
Use of unsuccessful social interaction behaviors
Dysfunctional interaction with others

Sample Clinical Applications: Brain injury/stroke, cancer, neuromuscular disease (e.g., MS), cerebral palsy, substance abuse, Alzheimer's disease, schizophrenia, autism

DESIRED OUTCOMES/EVALUATION CRITERIA
Sample NOC linkages:
Social Interaction Skills: Personal behaviors that promote effective relationships
Child Development: (specify age): Milestones of physical, cognitive, and psychosocial progression by [specify] months/years of age
Role Performance: Congruence of an individual's role behavior with role expectations

Client Will (Include Specific Time Frame)

- Verbalize awareness of factors causing or promoting impaired social interactions.
- Identify feelings that lead to poor social interactions.
- Express desire/be involved in achieving positive changes in social behaviors and interpersonal relationships.
- Give self positive reinforcement for changes that are achieved.
- Develop effective social support system; use available resources appropriately.

ACTIONS/INTERVENTIONS

Sample NIC linkages:
Socialization Enhancement: Facilitation of another person's ability to interact with others
Behavior Modification: Social Skills: Assisting the patient to develop or improve interpersonal social skills
Complex Relationship Building: Establishing a therapeutic relationship with a patient who has difficulty interacting with others

NURSING PRIORITY NO. 1 To assess causative/contributing factors:

- Review social history with client/SO(s) and go back far enough in time to note when changes in social behavior or patterns of relating occurred/began. *For example, loss or long-term illness of loved one; failed relationships; loss of occupation, financial, or political (power) position; change in status in family hierarchy (job loss, aging, illness); poor coping/adjustment to developmental stage of life, as with marriage, birth/adoption of child, or children leaving home are situations that may affect quality of social exchange.[1]*
- Ascertain ethnic/cultural or religious implications for the client. *These factors can dictate choice of behaviors, may even script interactions with others. Client may perceive behaviors as normal because of belief system or may have conflict regarding behaviors that are not accepted by larger society, such as homosexuality or gender identity disorder.[1,5,6]*
- Review medical history, noting stressors of physical/long-term illness (e.g., stroke, cancer, MS, head injury, Alzheimer's disease), mental illness (e.g., schizophrenia), medications/substance use, debilitating accidents, learning disabilities (e.g., sensory integration difficulties, Asperger's disorder, autism spectrum disorder), and emotional disabilities. *Conditions such as these can isolate individual who feels disconnected from others, resulting in difficulty relating in social situations.[3,4]*

- Note presence of visual or hearing impairments. *Individuals with these conditions may find communication barriers are increased, social interaction is affected, and interventions need to be designed to promote involvement with others in positive ways.*[1,3]
- Determine family patterns of relating and social behaviors. Explore possible family scripting of behavioral expectations in the children and how the client was affected. *Parents are important in teaching their children social skills (e.g., sharing, taking turns, and allowing others to talk without interrupting). Family may not have effective patterns of relating to others, and the child learns these skills in this setting. Often child reflects family expectations rather than own desires and may result in conforming or rebellious behaviors.*[2,6,9]
- Observe client while relating to family/SO(s) and note observations of prevalent patterns. *Identification of patterns will help with plan for change.*[2]
- Encourage client to verbalize feeling of discomfort about social situations. Note any causative factors, recurring precipitating patterns, and barriers to using support systems. *Identifies areas of concern and suggests possible ways to learn new skills.*[2]

NURSING PRIORITY NO. 2 To assess degree of impairment:

- Encourage client to verbalize perceptions of reasons for problems. Active-listen noting indications of hopelessness, powerlessness, fear, anxiety, grief, anger, feeling unloved/unlovable; problems with sexual identity; hate (directed or not). *These feelings arise from the anxiety that comes with the need to participate with others in social situations and begin to interfere with work, friendships, and life in general.*[5,7]
- Observe and describe social/interpersonal behaviors in objective terms, noting speech patterns, body language (1) in the therapeutic setting and (2) in normal areas of daily functioning (if possible): family, job, social/entertainment settings. *Provides information about extent of anxiety client experiences in different settings and suggests possible interventions.*[5,7]
- Determine client's use of coping skills and defense mechanisms. *Symptoms associated with social anxiety affect ability to be involved in social situations, making client's life miserable and seriously interfering with work, friendships, and family life.*[5,7]
- Evaluate possibility of client being the victim of or using destructive behaviors against self or others. (Refer to ND [actual/]risk for other-directed/self-directed Violence.) *Problems of poor communication lead to frustration and anger, leaving the individual with few coping skills and may result in destructive behaviors.*[1,2]
- Interview family, SO(s), friends, spiritual leaders, coworkers, as appropriate. *Obtaining observations of client's behavioral changes from others associated with the individual provides a broader view of actual problems and how behavior affects client's life/others.*[5]

NURSING PRIORITY NO. 3 To assist client/SO(s) to recognize/make positive changes in impaired social and interpersonal interactions:

- Establish therapeutic relationship using positive regard for the person, Active-listening and providing safe environment for self-disclosure. *Client who is having difficulty interacting in social situations needs to feel comfortable and accepted before he or she is willing to talk about self and concerns.*[1,2]
- Have client list behaviors that cause discomfort. *Anxiety usually has physical symptoms such as a racing heart, dry mouth, shaky voice, blushing, sweating, and nausea, and once recognized, client can choose to begin treatment to change.*[5,7]
- Have family/SO(s) list client's behaviors that are causing discomfort for them. *Anxiety is contagious, and by identifying specific behaviors, all members of the family can begin to deal appropriately with them so they are diminished.*[5,7]

- 🏠 • Review/list negative behaviors observed previously by caregivers, coworkers, and so forth. *Others may see behaviors and the problems associated with them, such as unwillingness to participate in necessary activities (eating in a public place, interviewing for a job) and may provide additional information needed to develop an appropriate plan of care.*[1]
- 🏠 • Compare lists and validate reality of perceptions. Help client prioritize those behaviors needing change. *Each individual may have a different view of what constitutes a problem, and by comparing lists, each person hears how others view the problems, enabling the client/family to identify behaviors/concerns to be dealt with.*[1,7]
- 🏠 • Explore with client and role-play means of making agreed upon changes in social interactions/behaviors (as determined earlier). *Client needs to learn social skills, because they have never learned the elements of interacting with others in social settings. Role-playing one-on-one is less threatening and can help individual identify with another and practice new social skills.*[5]
- ⊕ • Role-play random social situations in therapeutically controlled environment with "safe" therapy group. Have group note behaviors, both positive and negative, and discuss these and any changes needed. *Having client participate in a controlled group environment provides opportunities to try out different behaviors in a built-in social setting where members can make friends and provide mutual advice and comfort.*[1,5]
- 🏠 • Role-play changes and discuss impact. Include family/SO(s) as indicated. *Provides opportunity for person to recognize changes in feelings and behavior and enhances comfort with new behaviors.*[4]
- 🏠 • Provide positive reinforcement for improvement in social behaviors and interactions. *Encourages continuation of desired behaviors/efforts for change.*[5]
- ⊕ • Participate in multidisciplinary client-centered conferences *to evaluate progress.* Involve everyone associated with client's care, family members, SO(s), and therapy group. *These conferences have the advantage of providing information from and to each participant in an atmosphere of trust where questions can be asked, decisions can be made, and goals for the future can be agreed on.*[1]
- 🏠 • Work with the client to alleviate underlying negative self-concepts *because they often impede positive social interactions. By replacing negative thoughts with positive messages, client can reduce anxiety and develop a positive sense of self-esteem. While this is not an easy process, the rewards are great when client is willing to practice consistently.*[2]
- ⊕ • Involve neurologically impaired client in individual or group interactions as situation allows. *Individual may not be able to interact appropriately because of disabilities, but involvement in the group provides an opportunity to practice and relearn skills to enable reintegration into social situations.*[1,8]
- ⊕ • Refer for family therapy as indicated. *Social behaviors and interpersonal relationships involve more than the individual, and family may need additional help to resolve ongoing family problems.*[1,2]

NURSING PRIORITY NO. 4 To promote wellness (Teaching/Discharge Considerations):

- 🏠 • Encourage client to keep a daily journal in which social interactions of each day can be reviewed and the comfort/discomfort experienced noted with possible causes/precipitating factors. *Helps client to identify specific problem areas and begin to choose to take responsibility for own behavior(s).*[5,7]
- 🏠 • Assist the client to develop positive social skills through practice of skills in real social situations accompanied by a support person. Provide positive feedback with the use of I-messages during interactions with client. *Cognitive and behavioral methods can help individuals overcome fears with the help of a trusted person. I-messages convey a positive message, individual does not feel criticized, and is encouraged to continue new thinking and behaviors.*[1,5]

- Discuss the use of medications when indicated and monitor for effectiveness and side effects. *Several kinds of drugs have been found to be effective in the treatment of social anxiety problems, selective serotonin reuptake inhibitors (SSRIs), such as paroxetine (Paxil) and sertraline (Zoloft), are usually the first choice. Anti-anxiety drugs, such as clonazepam (Klonopin) and alprazolam (Xanax), can reduce anxiety and may be used alone or in conjunction with SSRIs. Propranolol (Inderal) has been found to be useful for performance anxiety, and when taken an hour before the scheduled event, may suppress the physical symptoms of anxiety.*[5,7]
- Seek community programs for client involvement that promote positive behaviors the client is striving to achieve. *Encouraging reading materials, attending classes, community support groups, and lectures for self-help can help to alleviate negative self-concepts that lead to impaired social interactions.*[2,5]
- Involvement in a music-based program, if available (e.g., the Listening Program). *There is a direct correlation between the musical portion of the brain and the language area, and the use of these programs may result in better communication skills.*[10]
- Encourage ongoing family or individual therapy as long as it is promoting growth and positive change. *Be alert to possibility of therapy being used as a crutch. While therapy groups can be useful, individuals can become dependent on the process and not move on to managing on their own.*[1]
- Provide for occasional follow-up for reinforcement of positive behaviors after professional relationship has ended. *Change is difficult and identifying problems that may arise during these contacts can enhance maintenance and enable client/family to continue to progress.*[2]
- Refer to/involve psychiatric clinical nurse specialist when indicated. *May need additional assistance to promote long-term change.*[1]

DOCUMENTATION FOCUS

Assessment/Reassessment

- Individual findings, including factors affecting interactions, nature of social exchanges, specifics of individual behaviors, type of learning disability present.
- Cultural/religious beliefs and expectations.
- Perceptions/response of others.

Planning

- Plan of care and who is involved in the planning.
- Teaching plan.

Implementation/Evaluation

- Responses to interventions/teaching and actions performed.
- Attainment/progress toward desired outcome(s).
- Modifications to plan of care.

Discharge Planning

- Long-term needs and who is responsible for actions to be taken.
- Community resources, specific referrals made.

References

1. Townsend, M. C. (2003). *Psychiatric Mental Health Nursing Concepts of Care*. 4th ed. Philadelphia: F. A. Davis.
2. Doenges, M. E., Townsend, M. C., Moorhouse, M. F. (1998). *Psychiatric Care Plans Guidelines for Individualizing Care*. 3rd ed. Philadelphia: F. A. Davis.

3. Cox, H., Hinz, M., Lubno, M. A., Newfield, S., Scott-Tilley, D., Slater, M., Sridaromont, K. (2002). *Clinical Applications of Nursing Diagnosis Adult, Child, Women's Psychiatric, Gerontic and Home Health Considerations.* 4th ed. Philadelphia: F. A. Davis.
4. Drew, N. (1991). Combating the social isolation of chronic mental illness. *J Psychosocial Nurs*, 29(6), 14–17.
5. Beyond shyness and stage fright: Social anxiety disorder. (October 2003). Harvard Mental Health Letter.
6. Lipson, J. G., Dibble, S. L, Minarik, P, A. (1996). *Culture & Nursing Care: A Pocket Guide.* San Francisco: School of Nursing, UCSF Nursing Press.
7. National Institute of Mental Health. (2000). Anxiety Disorders. NIH Publication No. 00–3879. Retrieved August 2007 at www.medhelp.org/NIHlib/GF-222.html.
8. Bellis, T. J. (2002). *When the Brain Can't Hear: Unraveling the Mystery of Auditory Processing Disorder.* New York: Atria Books.
9. No author or pub date listed. The Development of Social Skills. Retrieved August 2007 at www.incrediblehorizons.com/social-skills.htm.
10. The Listening Program. Retrieved August 2007 at www.thelisteningprogram.com/How_TLP_Works.asp.

Social Isolation

Definition: Aloneness experienced by the individual and perceived as imposed by others and as a negative or threatened state

RELATED FACTORS

Factors contributing to the absence of satisfying personal relationships (e.g., delay in accomplishing developmental tasks); immature interests
Alterations in physical appearance/mental status
Altered state of wellness
Unaccepted social behavior/values
Inadequate personal resources
Inability to engage in satisfying personal relationships
[Traumatic incidents or events causing physical or emotional pain]

DEFINING CHARACTERISTICS

Subjective
Expresses feelings of aloneness imposed by others/rejection
Insecurity in public
Inability to meet expectations of others; inadequate purpose in life
Developmentally inappropriate interests
Experiences feelings of differences from others; expresses values unacceptable to the dominant cultural group

Objective
Absence of supportive significant other(s)—[family, friends, group]
Sad/dull affect; uncommunicative; withdrawn; no eye contact
Evidence of handicap (e.g., physical/mental); illness
Developmentally inappropriate behaviors; repetitive/meaningless actions
Seeks to be alone; preoccupation with own thoughts
Shows behavior unaccepted by dominant cultural group; exists in a subculture; projects hostility

Sample Clinical Applications: Traumatic injuries, facial scarring/acne, chemotherapy, AIDS, dementia, major depression, conduct disorder, developmental delay, paranoid disorders, schizophrenia

DESIRED OUTCOMES/EVALUATION CRITERIA
Sample NOC linkages:
Social Involvement: Social interactions with persons, groups, or organizations
Loneliness Severity: Severity of emotional, social, or existential isolation response
Social Support: Perceived availability and actual provision of reliable assistance from others

Client Will (Include Specific Time Frame)

- Identify causes and actions to correct isolation.
- Verbalize willingness to be involved with others.
- Participate in activities/programs at level of ability/desire.
- Express increased sense of self-worth.

ACTIONS/INTERVENTIONS

Sample NIC linkages:
Socialization Enhancement: Facilitation of another person's ability to interact with others
Visitation Facilitation: Promoting beneficial visits by family and friends
Normalization Promotion: Assisting parents and other family members of children with chronic diseases or disabilities in providing normal life experiences for their children and families

NURSING PRIORITY NO. 1 To assess causative/contributing factors:

- Determine presence of factors as listed in Related Factors and other concerns (e.g., elderly, female, adolescent, ethnic/racial minority, economically/educationally disadvantaged, hearing or visually impaired). *Identifying individual factors allows for developing an accurate plan of care for the client.*[5]
- Perform physical exam, paying particular attention to any illnesses identified. *Individuals who are isolated appear to be susceptible to health problems, especially coronary heart disease, although little is understood about why that is.*[10]
- Note onset of physical/mental illness and whether recovery is anticipated or condition is chronic/progressive. *Individual may withdraw from activities because of concern about how others view changes that occur due to illness, concern with own thoughts, alterations in physical appearance/mental status. Anticipated length of illness may dictate choice of interventions.*[1,4]
- Identify blocks to social contacts. *Reluctance to engage in social activities may be the result of problems such as physical immobility, sensory deficits, housebound for any reason, incontinence, financial constraints, transportation difficulties. Individual may be afraid of what others might think of her or him, be concerned of embarrassing self, or of not having money or means of transportation for desired activities.*[1]
- Ascertain implications of cultural values/religious beliefs for the client *that may dictate choice of behaviors, may even script interactions with others. Client may perceive behaviors as normal because of belief system, or may have conflict regarding behaviors that may be unacceptable to the larger society, such as homosexuality or gender identity disorder.*[1,5,6]
- Assess factors in client's life that may contribute to sense of helplessness. *Losses, such as a spouse, parent, or other, or presence of chronic pain/other disabling conditions may cause individual to withdraw, desire to be alone, and refuse to participate in therapeutic activities.*[1,3]
- Listen to comments of client regarding sense of isolation. Differentiate isolation from solitude and loneliness *that may be acceptable or by choice. Provides clues to what client is*

thinking and feeling about current situation. Client who chooses to be alone and is satisfied may not need further intervention.[2,5]

- Assess client's feelings about self, sense of ability to control situation, sense of hope, and coping skills. *If client is isolating self because of negative feelings, lack of hope, etc., measures to promote self-esteem will need to be taken.*[5]

- Identify support systems available to the client, including presence of/relationship with extended family. *People with social anxiety often do not have support systems because of their withdrawal from contact with others. Often the family of origin may be anxious and does not provide the encouragement and support needed by a temperamentally inhibited child or may be too helpful, enabling client to withdraw further. It is difficult for these individuals to ask for help, because they are afraid to meet new people and often find support only when they seek help for other conditions, such as depression.*[4,9]

- Identify behavior response of isolation. *Individual may display behaviors such as excessive sleeping/daydreaming, which also may potentiate isolation.*[7,10]

- Note drug use (legal/illicit). *Individual may begin to use drugs such as alcohol or cocaine to control anxiety in social situations.*[7]

- Review history and elicit information about traumatic events that may have occurred. (Refer to ND Post-Trauma Syndrome.) *While little is known about the origins of social anxiety disorders, clients who have experienced a traumatic event may withdraw from contact and suffer from anxiety when faced with having to deal with social situations.*[1,5]

NURSING PRIORITY NO. 2 To alleviate conditions that contribute to client's sense of isolation:

- Establish therapeutic nurse-client relationship. *Promotes trust and acceptance, allowing client to feel safe and free to discuss sensitive matters without being judged.*[2]

- Spend time interacting with client and identify other resources available. *Getting to know client and identifying concerns about being involved in activities with others can lead to appropriate interventions. Other people such as a volunteer, social worker, chaplain may be able to spend time with client, enhancing circle of trusted people.*[4]

- Develop plan of action with client: Look at available resources; support risk-taking behaviors, financial planning, appropriate medical care/self-care, and so forth. *Helping client to learn how to manage these issues of daily living can increase self-confidence and help individual to feel more comfortable in social settings.*[5]

- Introduce client to those with similar/shared interests and other supportive people. *Provides role models and encourages getting to know others who share feelings of anxiety, providing an opportunity to develop social skills and learn some ways of problem-solving to deal with anxiety.*[2,5]

- Promote participation in recreational/special-interest activities in setting that client views as safe. *These activities have the advantage of providing physical and mental stimulation for client who feels isolated and anxious in social settings.*[2,9]

- Provide positive reinforcement when client makes move(s) toward other(s). *Acknowledges and encourages continuation of efforts, helping client toward independence.*[1,7]

- Identify foreign language resources for client who speaks another language. *A professional interpreter is important to ensure accuracy of interpretation; newspaper, radio programming in appropriate foreign language helps client feel connected with own community.*[6,8]

- Assist client to problem-solve solutions to short-term/imposed isolation. *Conditions such as communicable disease measures, including compromised host, may require individual to be isolated from others for his or her protection as well as others', and working together to decide how to manage loneliness can promote successful outcome.*[1,3]

- Encourage open visitation when possible and/or telephone contacts. *Maintains involvement with others, promoting social involvement, especially when client is unable to go out to activities.*[3]

🌐 Cultural Collaborative 🏠 Community/Home Care Diagnostic Studies ∞ Pediatric/Geriatric/Lifespan Medications

• Provide environmental stimuli when client is confined. *Open curtains in room, display pictures of family or views of nature, promote television and radio listening, Internet access to help client feel less isolated.*[3]

 • Provide for placement in sheltered community when necessary. *The individual who is mentally impaired may be unable to learn to participate in society and display socially acceptable behaviors, and will benefit from an environment that offers structure and assistance.*[3]

NURSING PRIORITY NO. 3 To promote wellness (Teaching/Discharge Considerations):

• Assist client to learn social skills as needed. *Enhancing problem-solving, communication, social skills, and learning skills to manage ADLs will improve sense of self-esteem.*[4]

• Encourage and assist client to enroll in classes as appropriate. *Assertiveness, vocational, sex education classes may provide skills to improve ability to engage more effectively in social situations.*[5]

• Involve children and adolescents in age-appropriate programs/activities, as indicated. *Promotes socialization skills and peer contact to enable young person to learn by interacting with others.*[5]

• Help client differentiate between isolation and loneliness or aloneness and discuss how to avoid slipping into an undesired state. *Time for the individual to be alone is important to the maintenance of mental health, but the sadness created by isolation and loneliness needs different interventions.*[2]

• Involve client in programs directed to correction and prevention of identified causes of problem. *Activities such as senior citizen services, daily telephone contact, house sharing, pets, day-care centers, church resources can help individual move out of isolation and become involved in life.*[5,10]

• Discuss use of medications, as indicated. *Prescribed medications, such as SSRIs, can be very effective in treating social disorders.*[3,7]

• Refer to counselor/therapist, as appropriate. *Facilitates grief work, promotes relationship building, and provides opportunity to work toward improvement of individual issues affecting social interactions.*[1]

DOCUMENTATION FOCUS

Assessment/Reassessment

• Individual findings, including precipitating factors, effect on lifestyle/relationships, and functioning.
• Client's perception of situation.
• Cultural/religious factors.
• Availability/use of resources and support systems.

Planning

• Plan of care and who is involved in planning.
• Teaching plan.

Implementation/Evaluation

• Responses to interventions/teaching and actions performed.
• Attainment/progress toward desired outcome(s).
• Modifications to plan of care.

Discharge Planning

• Long-term needs/referrals and who is responsible for actions to be taken.
• Available resources, specific referrals made.

References

1. Townsend, M. C. (2003). *Psychiatric Mental Health Nursing Concepts of Care.* 4th ed. Philadelphia: F. A. Davis.
2. Doenges, M. E., Townsend, M. C., Moorhouse, M. F. (1998). *Psychiatric Care Plans Guidelines for Individualizing Care.* 3d ed. Philadelphia: F. A. Davis.
3. Cox, H., Hinz, M., Lubno, M. A., Newfield, S., Scott-Tilley, D., Slater, M., Sridaromont, K. (2002). *Clinical Applications of Nursing Diagnosis: Adult, Child, Women's Psychiatric, Gerontic and Home Health Considerations.* 4th ed. Philadelphia: F. A. Davis.
4. Drew, N. (1991). Combating the social isolation of chronic mental illness. *J Psychosoc Nurs,* 29(6), 14–17.
5. Harvard Mental Health Letter. Beyond shyness and stage fright: Social anxiety disorder. October 2003.
6. Lipson, J. G., Dibble, S. L., Minarik, P. A. (1996). *Culture & Nursing Care: A Pocket Guide.* San Francisco: School of Nursing, UCSF Nursing Press.
7. National Institute of Mental Health. (2000). Anxiety Disorders. NIH Publication No. 00-3879. Retrieved August 2007 at www.medhelp.org/NIHlib/GF-222.html.
8. Andrulis, D. P. (2002). What a Difference an Interpreter Can Make, Health Care Experiences of Uninsured with Limited English Proficiency. The Access Project. Boston, MA: Brandeis University.
9. McPherson, M., Smith-Lovin, L., Brashears, M. (June 2006). Social isolation in U.S.: Changes in core discussion networks over two decades. *American Sociological Review,* 71, 353–375. Retrieved May 2007 at www.asanet.org/galleries/default-file/June06ASRFeature.pdf.
10. House, J. (2001). Social isolation kills, but how and why? *Psychosomatic Medicine,* 63, 273–274. Retrieved May 2007 at www.psychosomaticmedicine.org/cgi/content/full/63/2/273.

chronic Sorrow

Definition: Cyclical, recurring, and potentially progressive pattern of pervasive sadness experienced (by a parent or caregiver, individual with chronic illness or disability) in response to continual loss, throughout the trajectory of an illness or disability

RELATED FACTORS
Death of a loved one
Experiences chronic illness/disability (e.g., physical or mental); crises in management of the illness
Crises related to developmental stages; missed opportunities/milestones
Unending caregiving

DEFINING CHARACTERISTICS

Subjective
Expresses negative feelings (e.g., anger, being misunderstood, confusion, depression, disappointment, emptiness, fear, frustration, guilt, self-blame, helplessness, hopelessness, loneliness, low self-esteem, recurring loss, overwhelmed)
Expresses feelings of sadness (e.g., periodic, recurrent)

Objective
Expresses feelings that interfere with ability to reach highest level of personal/social well-being

Sample Clinical Applications: Cancer, MS, Parkinson's disease, AIDS, ALS, prematurity, genetic/congenital defects, infertility, dementia/Alzheimer's disease, bipolar disorder, schizophrenia, developmental delay

DESIRED OUTCOMES/EVALUATION CRITERIA
Sample NOC linkages:

Cultural Collaborative Community/Home Care Diagnostic Studies Pediatric/Geriatric/Lifespan Medications

Depression Level: Severity of level of melancholic mood and loss of interest in life events
Depression Self-Control: Personal actions to minimize melancholy and maintain interest in life events
Hope: Optimism that is personally satisfying and life-supporting

Client Will (Include Specific Time Frame)

- Acknowledge presence/impact of sorrow.
- Demonstrate progress in dealing with loss(es) as evidenced by recognizing positive aspects of situation.
- Participate in work and/or self-care ADLs as able.
- Verbalize a sense of progress toward resolution of sorrow and hope for the future.

ACTIONS/INTERVENTIONS

Sample NIC linkages:
Mood Management: Providing for safety, stabilization, recovery, and maintenance of a patient who is experiencing dysfunctionally depressed or elevated mood
Grief Work Facilitation: Assistance with the resolution of a significant loss
Hope Instillation: Facilitation of the development of a positive outlook in a given situation

NURSING PRIORITY NO. 1 To assess causative/contributing factors and effect on life:

- Determine current/recent events or conditions contributing to client's state of mind, as listed in Related Factors (e.g., death of loved one, chronic physical or mental illness or disability, etc.). *Individual information is necessary when formulating a plan of care to address appropriate issues.*[1]
- Note cues of sadness. *Expressions of feelings of loss, such as sighing, faraway looks, unkempt appearance, inattention to conversation, and refusing food can be indicators of sorrow that is not being dealt with. Note: Chronic sorrow may be cyclical—at times deepening versus times of feeling somewhat better.*[4,5]
- Be aware of use of avoidance behaviors. *Anger, withdrawal, denial are part of the grieving process and may be used to avoid dealing with the reality of what has happened. However, in a situation that is unchangeable, such as developmentally disabled child or a child with diabetes, sorrow is seen as a normal response and will continue to be a factor even as the family copes with the condition.*[5,7]
- Identify cultural values/religious beliefs and possible conflicts. *Expressions of sorrow are influenced by these beliefs and may result in conflicts. For instance, the Mexican American culture believes genetic defects are the will of God, but individual may be angry at God because of occurrence. Or, individual/family may have difficulty living up to the expectations of others (e.g., "God does not give us more than we can handle.")*[6]
- Ascertain response of family/SOs to client's situation and support provided. *Parents who have chronically ill children or premature babies, adults who have multiple sclerosis, elderly caregivers of spouses with dementia may continue to have feelings of sorrow even though they seem to be managing fairly well but due to cyclic nature of sorrow will require ongoing support/assistance from others to cope.*[4,7]
- Determine level of functioning, ability to care for self/others. Assess needs of family/SO. *Individual who is coping with chronic illnesses such as Parkinson's, MS, HIV/AIDS may exhibit chronic sorrow related to the illness, fear of death, poverty, and isolation associated with these conditions, which may lead to difficulty managing ADLs for self or meeting needs of family.*[2,3]
- Refer to NDs Caregiver Role Strain, ineffective Coping, complicated Grieving, as appropriate.

NURSING PRIORITY NO. 2 To assist client to move through sorrow:

- Encourage verbalization about situation. Active-listen feelings and be available for support/assistance. *Helpful in beginning resolution and acceptance. Individuals involved, client, and caregivers benefit from being able to talk freely about the situation. Active-listening conveys a message of acceptance and helps individual come to own resolution.*[1,5]

- Encourage expression of anger/fear/anxiety. (Refer to appropriate NDs.) *Individual needs to deal with these feeling before she or he can move forward.*[1]

- Acknowledge reality of feelings of guilt/blame, including hostility toward spiritual power. (Refer to ND Spiritual Distress.) *It was believed that grief had an end stage, but research has shown that individuals in chronic conditions, such as diabetes mellitus, multiple sclerosis, disabling conditions, continue to experience chronic sorrow and lifelong recurring sadness. Understanding this can help individual accept that these feelings are real, and when they are validated, they can be dealt with.*[5,11,12]

- Provide comfort and availability as well as caring for physical needs. *The way healthcare professionals respond to families is important to helping them cope with the situation as physical care is given.*[5,9]

- Discuss ways individual has dealt with past losses and reinforce use of previously effective coping skills. *As client begins to look at how they have handled previous situations, effective coping skills can be recalled and applied to current situation.*[2,9,10]

- Instruct/encourage use of visualization and relaxation skills. *Learning these stress-management skills can help the individual relax, enhancing ability to deal with feelings of sorrow regarding the long-term situation.*[5,8]

- Discuss use of medication when depression is interfering with ability to manage life. *Client may benefit from the short-term use of an antidepressant medication to help with dealing with situation.*[1]

- Assist SOs to cope with client response. *Family/SO may not be dysfunctional but may be intolerant and lack understanding of individual responses to long-term illness. Grief is unique to each individual and may not always follow a particular course to resolution that may not be understood by all.*[4,5,12]

- Include family/SO in setting realistic goals for meeting individual needs. *Inclusion of all family members ensures they all have the same information and are all working toward effective coping strategies.*[4,5]

NURSING PRIORITY NO. 3 To promote wellness (Teaching/Discharge Considerations):

- Discuss healthy ways of dealing with difficult situations. *Providing information about effective communication skills, understanding condition they are dealing with, and expectations of the course of the illness/condition can promote personal growth and lead to a positive outcome for the family.*[7,8]

- Have client identify familial, religious, and cultural factors that have meaning for him or her. *May help bring loss or distressing situation into perspective and promote grief/sorrow understanding.*[6]

- Encourage involvement in usual activities, exercise, and socialization within limits of physical and psychological state. *Energy is restored and individuals can go on with their lives when they are willing and able to continue activities.*[5,7]

- Introduce concept of mindfulness (living in the moment), and encourage client to recognize and embrace moments of joy in own life. *Promotes feelings of capability and belief that this moment can be dealt with/enjoyed.*[8,12]

- Refer to other resources (e.g., pastoral care, counseling, psychotherapy, respite care providers, support groups). *Provides additional help when needed to resolve situation, continue grief work, and move on with life.*[3]

⊕ Cultural ⊛ Collaborative 🏠 Community/Home Care ⟋ Diagnostic Studies ∞ Pediatric/Geriatric/Lifespan ⬗ Medications

Assessment/Reassessment

- Individual findings, including nature of sorrow, effects on participation in treatment regimen.
- Physical/emotional response to conflict, expressions of sadness.
- Cultural issues/religious conflicts.
- Reactions of family/SO.

Planning

- Plan of care and who is involved in planning.
- Teaching plan.

Implementation/Evaluation

- Response to interventions/teaching, and actions performed.
- Attainment/progress toward desired outcome(s).
- Modifications to plan of care.

Discharge Planning

- Long-term needs and who is responsible for actions to be taken.
- Available resources, specific referrals made.

References

1. Doenges, M. E., Moorhouse, M. F., Geissler-Murr, A. C. (2004). *Nurse's Pocket Guide Diagnoses, Interventions and Rationales.* 9th ed. Philadelphia: F. A. Davis.
2. Lindgren, C. L. (1996). Chronic sorrow in persons with Parkinson's and their spouse caregivers. *Scholarly Inquiry for Nursing Practice: An International Journal,* 10(4), 351–366.
3. Lichtensten, B., Laska, M. K., Clair, J. M. (2002). Chronic sorrow in the HIV-positive patient: Issues of race, gender, and social support. Birmingham, AL Department of Sociology, University of Alabama at Birmingham.
4. Kearney, P. (2003). Chronic Grief (or Is It Periodic Grief?). Available at www.indiana.edu/~famlygrf/units/chronic.html. Accessed February 2004.
5. Lowes, L., Lyne, P. (2000). Chronic sorrow in parents of children with newly diagnosed diabetes: A review of the literature and discussion of the implications for nursing practice. *J Advanced Nurs,* 32(1), 41–48.
6. Lipson, J. G., Dibble, S. L., Minarik, P. A. (1996). *Culture & Nursing Care: A Pocket Guide.* San Francisco: School of Nursing, UCSF Nursing Press.
7. Mallow, G. E., Bechtel, G. A. (1999). Chronic sorrow: The experience of parents with children who are developmentally disabled. *J Psychosoc Nurs,* 17(7), 31–43.
8. Kabat-Zinn, J. (1994). *Wherever You Go There You Are.* New York: Hyperion.
9. Kearney, P. M., Griffin, T. (2001). Between joy and sorrow: Being a parent of a child with a developmental disability. *Journal of Advanced Nursing,* 34, 582–592.
10. Olansky, S. (1962). Chronic sorrow: A response to having a mentally defective child. *Social Casework,* 43, 190–193.
11. Hobdell, E. (2004). Chronic sorrow and depression in parents of children with neural tube defects. *J Neurosci Nurs,* 36(2), 82–88, 94. Retrieved May 2007 at www.medscape.com/viewarticle/474596_1.
12. Kearney, P. (Updated 2006). Chronic Grief (or Is It Periodic Grief?). Grief in a Family Context. Retrieved May 2007 at www.indiana.edu/~famlygrf/units/chronic.html

Spiritual Distress

Definition: Impaired ability to experience and integrate meaning and purpose in life through a person's connectedness with self, others, art, music, literature, nature, and/or a power greater than oneself

RELATED FACTORS

Active dying

Loneliness; social alienation; self-alienation; sociocultural deprivation

Anxiety; pain

Life change

Chronic illness [of self or others]; death

[Challenged belief/value system (e.g., moral/ethical implications of therapy)]

DEFINING CHARACTERISTICS

Subjective

Connections to Self

Expresses lack of hope, meaning/purpose in life, serenity (e.g., peace), love, acceptance, forgiveness of self, courage

[Expresses] anger; guilt

Connections with Others

Refuses interactions with significant other(s)/spiritual leaders

Verbalizes being separated from support system

Expresses alienation

Connections with Art, Music, Literature, Nature

Inability to express previous state of creativity (e.g., singing/listening to music/writing)

Disinterested in nature/reading spiritual literature

Connections with Power Greater Than Self

Sudden changes in spiritual practices

Inability to pray/participate in religious activities/to experience the transcendent

Expresses hopelessness/suffering/having anger toward God

Expresses being abandoned

Request to see a religious leader

Objective

Connections to Self

Poor coping

Connections with Power Greater Than Self

Inability to be introspective

Sample Clinical Applications: Chronic conditions (e.g., rheumatoid arthritis, MS, systemic lupus erythematosus, ALS), cancer, traumatic brain injury/vegetative state, fetal demise, infertility, SIDS

DESIRED OUTCOMES/EVALUATION CRITERIA

Sample NOC Linkages:

Spiritual Health: Connectedness with self, others, higher power, all life, nature, and the universe that transcends and empowers the self

Hope: Optimism that is personally satisfying and life-supporting

Psychosocial Adjustment: Life Change: Adaptive psychosocial response of an individual to a significant life change

Client Will (Include Specific Time Frame)

• Verbalize increased sense of connectedness and hope for future.

• Demonstrate ability to help self/participate in care.

Cultural   Collaborative   Community/Home Care   Diagnostic Studies   Pediatric/Geriatric/Lifespan   Medications

- Participate in activities with others, actively seek relationships.
- Discuss beliefs/values about spiritual issues.
- Verbalize acceptance of self as not deserving illness/situation: "No one is to blame."

ACTIONS/INTERVENTIONS

Sample NIC Linkages:
Spiritual Support: Assisting the patient to feel balance and connection with a greater power
Hope Instillation: Facilitation of the development of a positive outlook in a given situation
Grief Work Facilitation: Assistance with the resolution of a significant loss

NURSING PRIORITY NO. 1 To assess causative/contributing factors:

- Determine client's religious/spiritual orientation, current involvement, presence of conflicts. *Identification of individual spiritual practices/restrictions that may affect client care or create conflict between spiritual beliefs and treatment provide for more accurate interventions.*[1]
- Listen to client's/SO(s') reports/expressions of concern, anger, alienation from God, belief that illness/situation is a punishment for wrongdoing, and so forth. *Indicates depth of grieving process and possible need for spiritual advisor or other resource to address client's belief system if desired.*[2]
- Assess for influence of cultural beliefs and spiritual values that affect individual in this situation. *Circumstances of illness/situation may conflict with client's view of self, cultural background, and distress over values. For instance, many Mexican Americans are Catholic with strong beliefs in the relationship of illness and religious practices.*[5]
- Note recent changes in behavior (e.g., withdrawal from others/creative or religious activities, dependence on alcohol/medications). *Helpful in determining severity/duration of situation and possible need for additional referrals such as substance withdrawal.*[1,7]
- Assess sense of self-concept, worth, ability to enter into loving relationships. *Lack of connectedness with self/others impairs client's ability to trust others or feel worthy of trust from others, leading to difficulties in relationships with others.*[1,7]
- Observe behavior indicative of poor relationships with others (e.g., manipulative, nontrusting, demanding). *Manipulation is used for management of client's sense of powerlessness because of distrust of others, interfering with relationships with others.*[3,6]
- Determine support systems available to client/SO(s) and how they are used. *Provides insight to client's willingness to pursue outside resources.*[1,4]
- Determine sense of futility, feelings of hopelessness and helplessness, lack of motivation to help self. *Indicators that client may see no, or only limited, options/alternatives or personal choices available, lacks energy to deal with situation and need for further evaluation.*[1]
- Note expressions of inability to find meaning in life, reason for living. Evaluate suicidal ideation. *Crisis of the spirit/loss of will to live places client at increased risk for inattention to personal well-being/harm to self. Indicates need for referral to mental health professional for evaluation/intervention.*[1,7]

NURSING PRIORITY NO. 2 To assist client/SO(s) to deal with feelings/situation:

- Develop therapeutic nurse-client relationship. Ascertain client's views as to how care provider(s) can be most helpful. Convey acceptance of client's spiritual beliefs/concerns. *Promotes trust and comfort, encouraging client to be open about sensitive matters.*[6]

- Establish environment that promotes free expression of feelings and concerns. *Provides opportunity for client to explore own thoughts and make appropriate decisions regarding spiritual issues.*[4]
- Provide calm, peaceful setting when possible. *Promotes relaxation and enhances opportunity for reflection on situation/discussions with others, meditation.*[3]
- Encourage life-review by client. Support client in finding a reason for living. *Promotes sense of hope and willingness to continue efforts to improve situation.*[3]
- Be aware of influence of care provider's own belief system. *It is still possible to be helpful to client while remaining neutral/not espousing own beliefs, because client's beliefs and needs are what is important.*[6]
- Identify inappropriate coping behaviors currently being used and associated consequences and discuss with client. *Recognizing negative consequences of actions may enhance desire to change.*[2]
- Set limits on acting-out behavior that is inappropriate/destructive. *Promotes safety for client/others and helps prevent loss of self-esteem.*[2,7]
- Ascertain past successes and coping behaviors. *Helps to determine approaches used previously that may be effective in dealing with current situation, providing encouragement.*[6]
- Problem-solve solutions/identify areas for compromise. *May be useful in resolving conflicts that arise from feelings of anxiety regarding questioning of beliefs and current illness/situation.*[3]
- Assist in developing coping skills *to deal with stressors of illness/necessary changes in lifestyle.*[7,9]

NURSING PRIORITY NO. 3 To facilitate setting goals and moving forward:

- Use therapeutic communication skills of reflection and Active-listening. *Conveys message of competence and helps client find own solutions to concerns.*[7]
- Involve client in refining healthcare goals and therapeutic regimen as appropriate. *Promotes feelings of control over what is happening, enhancing commitment to plan and optimizing outcomes.*[3]
- Encourage client/family to ask questions. *Demonstrates support for individual's willingness to learn.*
- Discuss difference between grief and guilt and help client to identify and deal with each. Point out consequences of actions based on guilt. *Aids client in assuming responsibility for own actions and avoids acting out of false guilt.*[6]
- Identify role models (e.g., individual experiencing similar situation). *Provides opportunities for sharing of experiences/hope and identifying new options to deal with situation.*[7]
- Assist client to learn use of meditation, mindfulness, and prayer, if desired. *Provides avenue for learning forgiveness to heal past hurts and developing a sense of peace.*[3,8]
- Provide information that anger with God is a normal part of the grieving process. *Realizing these feelings are not unusual can reduce sense of guilt, encourage open expression, and facilitate resolution of grief.*[3,7]
- Provide time and privacy to engage in spiritual growth/religious activities as desired (e.g., prayer, meditation, scripture reading, listening to music). *Allows client to focus on self and seek connectedness with spiritual beliefs and values.*[6]
- Encourage/facilitate outings to neighborhood park/nature walks. *Sunshine, fresh air, and activity can stimulate release of endorphins, promoting sense of well-being and encouraging connection with nature.*[6]
- Provide play therapy for child that encompasses spiritual data. *Interactive pleasurable activity promotes open discussion and enhances retention of information. Child will act out feelings in play therapy easier than talking. Provides opportunity for child to practice what has been learned and for therapist to evaluate child's progress.*[3]

🌐 Cultural Ⓐ Collaborative 🏠 Community/Home Care ⚗ Diagnostic Studies ∞ Pediatric/Geriatric/Lifespan 💊 Medications

- Abide by parents' wishes in discussing and implementing child's spiritual support. *Limits confusion for child and prevents conflict of values/beliefs.*[3]
- Refer to appropriate resources (e.g., pastoral/parish nurse or religious counselor, crisis counselor, hospice; psychotherapy; Alcoholics/Narcotics Anonymous). *Useful in dealing with immediate situation and identifying long-term resources for support to help foster sense of connectedness.*[7,8]
- Refer to NDs ineffective Coping, Powerlessness, Self-Esteem (specify), Social Isolation, risk for Suicide for additional interventions as indicated.

NURSING PRIORITY NO. 4 To promote wellness (Teaching/Discharge Considerations):

- Make time for nonjudgmental discussion of philosophical issues/questions about spiritual impact of illness/situation and/or treatment regimen. *Open communication can assist client in reality checks of perceptions and help to identify personal options.*[6]
- Assist client to develop long-term goals for dealing with future/illness situation. *Involvement in planning for desired outcomes enhances commitment to goal, optimizing outcomes.*[7]
- Suggest use of journaling. *Provides opportunity to write feelings and happenings; reviewing them over time can assist in clarifying values/ideas, recognizing and resolving feelings/situation.*[6,10]
- Assist client to identify SO(s)/others who could provide support as needed. *Ongoing support is important to enhance sense of connectedness and continue progress toward goals.*[6]
- Identify spiritual resources that could be helpful (e.g., contact spiritual advisor who has qualifications/experience in dealing with specific problems such as death/dying, relationship problems, substance abuse, suicide). *Provides answers to spiritual questions, assists in the journey of self-discovery, and can help client learn to accept and forgive self.*[6]

DOCUMENTATION FOCUS

Assessment/Reassessment

- Individual findings, including nature of spiritual conflict, effects of participation in treatment regimen.
- Physical/emotional responses to conflict.

Planning

- Plan of care and who is involved in planning.
- Teaching plan.

Implementation/Evaluation

- Responses to interventions/teaching and actions performed.
- Attainment/progress toward desired outcome(s).
- Modifications to plan of care.

Discharge Planning

- Long-term needs and who is responsible for actions to be taken.
- Available resources, specific referrals made.

References

1. Fallot, R. D. (1998). Assessment of spirituality and implications for service planning. *New Directions in Mental Health Services, 80,* 13–23.

2. Moller, M. D. (1999). Meeting spiritual needs on an inpatient unit. *J Psychosoc Nurs,* 37(11), 5–10.
3. Baldacchino, D., Draper, P. (2001). Spiritual coping strategies: A review of the nursing research literature. *J Adv Nurs,* 34(6), 833–841.
4. Cox, H. C., et al. (2002). *Clinical Applications of Nursing Diagnosis.* 4th ed. Philadelphia: F. A. Davis.
5. Lipson, J. G., Dibble, S. L., Minarik, P. A. (1996). *Culture & Nursing Care: A Pocket Guide.* San Francisco: UCSF Nursing Press.
6. Ross, L. A. (1994). Spiritual aspects of nursing. *J Adv Nurs,* 19, 439–447.
7. Townsend, M. C. (2003). *Psychiatric Mental Health Nursing Concepts of Care.* 4th ed. Philadelphia: F. A. Davis.
8. Hospital and Palliative Nurses Association: Spiritual Distress-Patient/Family Teaching Sheets, 2005. Retrieved May 2007 at www.hpna.org/pdf/PatientSheet_SpiritualDistress.pdf.
9. Savrock, J. (2006). Counseling Distressed Students May Be Improved by Religious Discussion. Retrieved May 2007 at www.ed.psu.edu/news/spiritual.asp.
10. Johnson, C. V., Hayes, J. A. (2003). Troubled spirits: Prevalence and predictors of religious and spiritual concerns among university students and counseling center clients. *J of Counseling Psychology,* 50, 409–419.

risk for Spiritual Distress

Definition: At risk for an impaired ability to experience and integrate meaning and purpose in life through connectedness with self, others, art, music, literature, nature, and/or a power greater than oneself

RISK FACTORS

Physical
Physical/chronic illness, substance abuse

Psychosocial
Stress; anxiety; depression
Low self-esteem; poor relationships; blocks to experiencing love; inability to forgive; loss; separated support systems; racial/cultural conflict
Change in religious rituals/spiritual practices

Developmental
Life changes

Environmental
Environmental changes; natural disasters
NOTE: A risk diagnosis is not evidenced by signs and symptoms, as the problem has not occurred; rather, nursing interventions are directed at prevention.

Sample Clinical Applications: Chronic conditions (e.g., rheumatoid arthritis, MS, systemic lupus erythematosus, ALS), cancer, traumatic brain injury/vegetative state, fetal demise, infertility, SIDS

DESIRED OUTCOMES/EVALUATION CRITERIA
Sample NOC linkages:
Spiritual Health: Connectedness with self, others, higher power, all life, nature, and the universe that transcends and empowers the self
Hope: Optimism that is personally satisfying and life-supporting
Psychosocial Adjustment: Life Change: Adaptive psychosocial response of an individual to a significant life change

Cultural Collaborative Community/Home Care Diagnostic Studies Pediatric/Geriatric/Lifespan Medications

Client Will (Include Specific Time Frame)

- Identify meaning and purpose in own life that reinforces hope, peace, and contentment.
- Verbalize acceptance of self as being worthy, not deserving of illness/situation, and so forth.
- Identify and use resources appropriately.

ACTIONS/INTERVENTIONS

Sample NIC linkages:

Spiritual Support: Assisting the patient to feel balance and connection with a greater power

Coping Enhancement: Promotion of deep inhalation by the patient with subsequent generation of high intrathoracic pressures and compression of underlying lung parenchyma for the forceful expulsion of air

Forgiveness Facilitation: Assisting an individual to forgive and/or experience forgiveness in relationship with self, others, and higher power

NURSING PRIORITY NO. I To assess causative/contributing factors:

- Ascertain current situation (e.g., natural disaster, death of a spouse, personal injustice). *Identification of circumstances that put the individual at risk for loss of connectedness with spiritual beliefs is essential to plan for appropriate interventions.*[8]
- Listen to client's/SO('s) reports/expressions of anger/concern, belief that illness/situation is a punishment for wrongdoing, and so forth. *Identifies need for client to talk about and be listened to in regard to concerns about potential loss of control over his or her life.*[3]
- Note reason for living and whether it is directly related to situation. *Tragic occurrences such as home and business washed away in a flood/lost in a fire, parent whose only child is terminally ill, loss of a spouse can cause individual to question previous beliefs, and how he or she has coped in the past/will cope in future.*[1,3]
- Determine client's religious/spiritual orientation, current involvement, presence of conflicts, especially in current circumstances. *Client may be a member of a religious organization, and whether he or she is active or whether conflicts have risen in relation to current illness/situation will indicate need for assistance from spiritual advisor, pastor, or other resource client would accept.*[1,9]
- Assess sense of self-concept, worth, ability to enter into loving relationships. *Lack of connectedness with self and others impairs client's ability to trust others or feel worthy of trust from others.*[1,7]
- Observe behavior indicative of poor relationships with others. *Client may be manipulative, nontrusting, and demanding because of distrust of self and others, interfering with relationships with others, indicating need for learning positive ways to interact with others.*[2,4]
- Determine support systems available to, and used by, client/SO(s). *Provides insight into individual's willingness to pursue outside resources.*[6,11]
- Ascertain substance use/abuse. *Complicates situation, affects ability to deal with problems in a positive manner, and identifies need for referral to appropriate treatment programs.*[4,10]
- Assess for influence of cultural beliefs and spiritual values that affect individual in this situation. *Circumstances of illness/situation may conflict with client's view of self, cultural background, and distress over values. For instance, many Mexican Americans are Catholic with strong beliefs in the relationship of illness and religious practices.*[5]

NURSING PRIORITY NO. 2 To assist client/SO(s) to deal with feelings/situation:

🏠 • Establish environment that promotes free expression of feelings and concerns. *Provides opportunity for client to explore own thoughts and make appropriate decisions regarding spiritual issues and conflicts.*[7,11]

🏠 • Use therapeutic communication skills of reflection and Active-listening. *Communicates confidence in client's ability to find own solutions to concerns.*[7]

🏠 • Have client identify and prioritize current/immediate needs. *Helps client focus on what needs to be done and identifies manageable steps to take to achieve goals.*[6]

🏠 • Discuss client's interest in the arts, music, and literature. *Provides insight into meaning of these issues and how they are integrated into individual's life.*

🏠 • Make time for nonjudgmental discussion of philosophical issues/questions about spiritual impact of illness/situation and/or treatment regimen. *Open communication can assist client to make reality checks of perceptions and begin to identify personal options.*[6]

🏠 • Discuss difference between grief and guilt and help client to identify and deal with each. *Helps client to assume responsibility for own actions, become aware of the consequences of acting out of false guilt.*[6]

🏠 • Review coping skills used and their effectiveness in current situation. *Identifies strengths to incorporate into plan and techniques needing revision.*[6]

🏠 • Identify role model (e.g., individual experiencing similar situation/disease). *Sharing of experiences/hope provides opportunity for client to look at options as modeled by others and to begin to deal with reality.*[7]

∞ • Provide play therapy for child that encompasses spiritual data. *Interactive pleasurable activity promotes open discussion and enhances retention of information. Child will act out feelings in play therapy easier than talking. Provides opportunity for child to practice what has been learned and for therapist to evaluate child's progress.*[3]

∞ • Abide by parents' wishes in discussing and implementing child's spiritual support. *Limits confusion for child and prevents conflict of values/beliefs.*[3]

🔗 • Refer to appropriate resources (e.g., crisis counselor, governmental agencies; pastoral/parish nurse or spiritual advisor who has qualifications/experience dealing with specific problems such as death/dying, relationship problems, substance abuse, suicide; hospice, psychotherapy, Alcoholics/Narcotics Anonymous). *Useful in dealing with immediate situation and identifying long-term resources for support to help foster sense of connectedness.*[7,9]

NURSING PRIORITY NO. 3 To promote wellness (Teaching/Discharge Considerations):

🏠 • Role-play new coping techniques. *Provides opportunity to practice and enhances integration of new skills/necessary lifestyle changes.*[4]

🏠 • Assist client to learn use of meditation, mindfulness, and prayer, if desired. *Provides avenue for learning forgiveness to heal past hurts and developing a sense of peace.*[3,9]

🏠 • Suggest use of journaling. *Provides opportunity to write feelings and happenings; reviewing them over time can assist in clarifying values/ideas, recognizing and resolving feelings/situation.*[6,10]

🏠 • Encourage individual to become involved in cultural activities of their choosing. *Art, music, plays, and other cultural activities provide a means of connecting with self and others.*

🔗 • Discuss possibilities of taking classes and becoming involved in discussion groups or community programs.

🔗 • Assist client to identify SO(s) and individuals/support groups who could provide ongoing support. *This is a daily need requiring lifelong commitment, and having sufficient support can help client maintain spiritual resolve.*[6]

🌐 Cultural 🔗 Collaborative 🏠 Community/Home Care ✏ Diagnostic Studies ∞ Pediatric/Geriatric/Lifespan 💊 Medications

- Discuss benefit of family counseling as appropriate. *Issues of this nature (e.g., situational losses, natural disasters, difficult relationships) affect family dynamics, and family may find it useful to discuss and resolve problems they are experiencing.*[7]

DOCUMENTATION FOCUS

Assessment/Reassessment

- Individual findings, including risk factors, nature of current distress.
- Physical/emotional responses to distress.
- Access to/use of resources.

Planning

- Plan of care and who is involved in planning.
- Teaching plan.

Implementation/Evaluation

- Responses to interventions/teaching and actions performed.
- Attainment/progress toward desired outcome(s).
- Modifications to plan of care.

Discharge Planning

- Long-term needs and who is responsible for actions to be taken.
- Available resources, specific referrals made.

References

1. Fallot, R. D. (1998). Assessment of spirituality and implications for service planning. *New Directions in Mental Health Services, 80*, 13–23.
2. Moller, M. D. (1999). Meeting spiritual needs on an inpatient unit. *J Psychosoc Nurs, 37*(11), 5–10.
3. Baldacchino, D., Draper, P. (2001). Spiritual coping strategies: A review of the nursing research literature. *J Adv Nurs, 34*(6), 833–841.
4. Cox, H. C., et al. (2002). *Clinical Applications of Nursing Diagnosis: Adult, Child, Women's, Psychiatric, Gerontic, and Home Health Considerations.* 4th ed. Philadelphia: F. A. Davis.
5. Lipson, J. G., Dibble, S. L., Minarik, P. A. (1999). *Culture & Nursing Care: A Pocket Guide.* San Francisco: UCSF Nursing Press.
6. Ross, L. A. (1994). Spiritual aspects of nursing. *J Adv Nurs, 19*, 439–447.
7. Townsend, M. C. (2003). *Psychiatric Mental Health Nursing Concepts of Care.* 4th ed. Philadelphia: F. A. Davis.
8. Doenges, M. E., Moorhouse, M. F., Murr, A. C. (2008). *Nurse's Pocket Guide Diagnoses, Interventions, and Rationales.* 11th ed. Philadelphia: F. A. Davis.
9. Hospital and Palliative Nurses Association. (2005). Spiritual Distress-Patient/Family Teaching Sheets. Retrieved May 2007 at www.hpna.org/pdf/PatientSheet_SpiritualDistress.pdf.
10. Savrock, J. (2006). Counseling Distressed Students May Be Improved by Religious Discussion. Retrieved May 2007 at www.ed.psu.edu/news/spiritual.asp.
11. Johnson, C. V., Hayes, J. A. (2003). Troubled spirits: Prevalence and predictors of religious and spiritual concerns among university students and counseling center clients. *J of Counseling Psychology, 50*, 409–419.

readiness for enhanced Spiritual Well-Being

Definition: Ability to experience and integrate meaning and purpose in life through connectedness with self, others, art, music, literature, nature, and/or a power greater than oneself that can be strengthened

RELATED FACTORS
To be developed by nurse researchers and submitted to NANDA

DEFINING CHARACTERISTICS

Subjective

Connections to Self
Expresses desire for enhanced: acceptance, coping, courage, forgiveness of self, hope, joy, love, meaning/purpose in life, satisfying philosophy of life, surrender
Expresses lack of serenity (e.g., peace)
Meditation
Connections with Others
Requests interactions with significant others/spiritual leaders
Requests forgiveness of others
Connections with Powers Greater Than Self
Participates in religious activities; prays
Expresses reverence/awe; reports mystical experiences

Objective

Connections with Others
Provides service to others
Connections with Art, Music, Literature, Nature
Displays creative energy (e.g., writing, poetry, singing); listens to music; reads spiritual literature; spends time outdoors

Sample Clinical Applications: As a health-seeking behavior, the client may be healthy or this diagnosis can occur in any clinical condition

DESIRED OUTCOMES/EVALUATION CRITERIA
Sample NOC linkages:
Spiritual Health: Connectedness with self, others, higher power, all life, nature, and the universe that transcends and empowers the self
Hope: Optimism that is personally satisfying and life-supporting
Quality of Life: Extent of positive perception of current life circumstances

Client Will (Include Specific Time Frame)

* Acknowledge the stabilizing and strengthening forces in own life needed for balance and well-being of the whole person.
* Identify meaning and purpose in own life that reinforces hope, peace, and contentment.
* Verbalize a sense of peace/contentment and comfort of spirit.
* Demonstrate behavior congruent with verbalizations that lend support and strength for daily living.

ACTIONS/INTERVENTIONS

Sample NIC linkages:
Spiritual Growth Facilitation: Facilitation of growth in patient's capacity to identify, connect with, and call upon the source of meaning, purpose, comfort, strength, and hope in his or her life

Religious Ritual Enhancement: Facilitating participation in religious practices

Meditation Facilitation: Facilitating a person to alter his or her level of awareness by focusing specifically on an image or thought

NURSING PRIORITY NO. 1   To determine spiritual state/motivation for growth:

- Ascertain client's perception of current state/degree of connectedness and expectations. *Provides insight as to where client is currently and specific hopes for the future.*[1]
- Ascertain motivation/expectations for change. *Motivation to improve and high expectations can encourage client to make changes that will improve his or her life. However, unrealistic expectations may hamper efforts.*
- Review spiritual/religious history, activities/rituals, and frequency of participation. *Determines basis to build on for growth/change.*[1]
- Determine relational values of support systems to client's spiritual centeredness. *The client's family of origin may have differing beliefs from those espoused by the individual that may be a source of conflict for the client. Comfort can be gained when family and friends share client's beliefs and support the search for spiritual knowledge.*[2]
- Explore meaning/interpretation and relationship of spirituality, life/death, and illness to life's journey. *This information helps client strengthen personal belief system, enabling him or her to move forward and live life to the fullest.*[2,3]
- Clarify the meaning of client's spiritual beliefs/religious practice and rituals to daily living. *Discussing these issues allows client to explore spiritual needs and decide what fits own view of the world to enhance life.*[6]
- Explore ways that spirituality/religious practices have affected client's life and given meaning and value to daily living. Note consequences as well as benefits. *Promotes understanding and appreciation of the difference between spirituality and religion and how each can be used to enhance client's journey of self-discovery.*[3]
- Discuss life's/God's plan (when this is the person's belief) for the individual. *Helpful in determining individual goals/choosing specific options.*[2]

NURSING PRIORITY NO. 2   To assist client to integrate values and beliefs to achieve a sense of wholeness and optimum balance in daily living:

- Explore ways beliefs give meaning and value to daily living. *As client develops understanding of these issues, they will provide support for dealing with current/future concerns.*[4]
- Clarify reality/appropriateness of client's self-perceptions and expectations. *Necessary to provide firm foundation for growth. Unrealistic ideas can impede desired improvement.*[2]
- Determine influence of cultural beliefs/values. *Most individuals are strongly influenced by the spiritual/religious orientation of their family of origin, which can be a very major determinate for client's choice of activities/receptiveness to various options.*[5]
- Discuss the importance and value of connections to client's daily life. *The contacts that one has with others maintains a feeling of belonging and connection and promotes feelings of wholeness and well-being.*[4,6]
- Identify ways to achieve connectedness or harmony with self, others, nature, higher power (e.g., meditation, prayer, talking/sharing self with others; being out in nature/gardening/walking; attending religious activities). *This is a highly individual and personal decision, and no action is too trivial to be considered.*[4]

NURSING PRIORITY NO. 3   To enhance optimum wellness:

- Encourage client to take time to be introspective in the search for peace and harmony. *Finding peace within oneself will carry over to relationships with others and own outlook on life.*[1]

Nursing Diagnoses in Alphabetical Order

- Discuss use of relaxation/meditative activities (e.g., yoga, tai chi, prayer). *Helpful in promoting general well-being and sense of connectedness with self/nature/spiritual power.*[4,6]
- Suggest attendance/involvement in dream-sharing group *to develop/enhance learning of the characteristics of spiritual awareness and facilitate the individual's growth.*[1]
- Identify ways for spiritual/religious expression. *There are multiple options for enhancing spirituality through connectedness with self/others (e.g., volunteering time to community projects, mentoring, singing in the choir, painting, or spiritual writings).*[3,4]
- Encourage participation in desired religious activities, contact with minister/spiritual advisor. *Validating one's beliefs in an external way can provide support and strengthen the inner self.*[1,3]
- Discuss and role-play, as necessary, ways to deal with alternative view/conflict that may occur with family/SO(s)/society or cultural group. *Provides opportunity to try out different behaviors in a safe environment and be prepared for potentialities.*[3]
- Provide bibliotherapy, list of relevant resources (e.g., study groups, parish nurse, poetry society), and reliable Web sites *for later reference/self-paced learning and ongoing support.*[3]

DOCUMENTATION FOCUS

Assessment/Reassessment

- Assessment findings, including client perception of needs and desire/expectations for growth/enhancement.
- Cultural values/religious beliefs.
- Motivation/expectations for change.

Planning

- Plan for growth and who is involved in planning.

Implementation/Evaluation

- Response to activities/learning and actions performed.
- Attainment/progress toward desired outcome(s).
- Modifications to plan.

Discharge Planning

- Long-range needs/expectations and plan of action.
- Specific referrals made.

References

1. Fallot, R. D. (1998). Assessment of spirituality and implications for service planning. *New Directions in Mental Health Services*, 80, 13–23.
2. Moller, M. D. (1999). Meeting spiritual needs on an inpatient unit. *J of Psychosoc Nurs*, 37(11), 5–10.
3. Baldacchino, D., Draper, P. (2001). Spiritual coping strategies: A review of the nursing research literature. *J Adv Nurs*, 34(6), 833–841.
4. Cox, H. C., et al. (2002). *Clinical Applications of Nursing Diagnosis.* 4th ed. Philadelphia: F. A. Davis.
5. Lipson, J. G., Dibble, S. L., Minarik, P. A. (1996). *Culture & Nursing Care: A Pocket Guide.* San Francisco: UCSF Nursing Press.
6. Ross, L. A. (1994). Spiritual aspects of nursing. *J Adv Nurs*, 19, 439–447.

Stress Overload

Definition: Excessive amounts and types of demands that require action

RELATED FACTORS

Inadequate resources (e.g., financial, social, education/knowledge level)
Intense, repeated stressors (e.g., family violence, chronic illness, terminal illness)
Multiple coexisting stressors (e.g., environmental threats/demands; physical threats/demands; social threats/demands)

DEFINING CHARACTERISTICS

Subjective
Expresses difficulty in functioning/problems with decision making
Expresses a feeling of pressure/tension
Expresses increased feelings of impatience/anger
Reports negative impact from stress (e.g., physical symptoms, psychological distress, feeling of "being sick" or of "going to get sick")
Reports situational stress as excessive (e.g., rates stress level as a 7 or above on a 10-point scale)

Objective
Demonstrates increased feelings of impatience/anger

Sample Clinical Applications: Chronic illness (e.g., MS, diabetes, Parkinson's), terminal illness (e.g., ovarian cancer, ALS), abusive situations, bipolar disorder, depression, social phobia

DESIRED OUTCOMES/EVALUATION CRITERIA
Sample NOC linkages:
Stress Level: Severity of manifested physical or mental tension resulting from factors that alter an existing equilibrium
Anxiety Self-Control: Personal actions to eliminate or reduce feelings of apprehension, tension, or uneasiness from an unidentifiable source
Leisure Participation: Use of relaxing, interesting, and enjoyable activities to promote well-being

Client Will (Include Specific Time Frame)

- Assess current situation accurately.
- Identify ineffective stress-mangagment behaviors and consequences.
- Meet psychological needs as evidenced by appropriate expression of feelings, identification of options, and use of resources.
- Verbalize or demonstrate reduced stress reaction.

ACTIONS/INTERVENTIONS

Sample NIC linkages:
Emotional Support: Provision of reassurance, acceptance, and encouragement during times of stress

Coping Enhancement: Assisting a patient to adapt to perceived stressors, changes, or threats that interfere with meeting life demands and roles

Resiliency Promotion: Assisting individuals, families, and communities in development, use, and strengthening of protective factors to be used in coping with environmental and societal stressors

NURSING PRIORITY NO. 1   To identify causative/precipitating factors and degree of impairment:

- Ascertain what events have occurred (e.g., family violence, death of loved one; separation from living partner/parent; change in financial status or living conditions; chronic/terminal illness, work place stress, loss of job/retirement; major trauma; catastrophic natural or man-made event) over remote and recent past *to assist in determining number, duration, and intensity of events causing perception of overwhelming stress.*
- Evaluate client's report of physical/emotional problems (e.g., fatigue, aches and pains, irritable bowel, skin rashes, frequent colds, sleeplessnes, crying spells, anger, feeling overwhelmed or numb, compulsive behaviors, etc.) *that can be representing body's response to stress.*[1]
- Determine client's/SO's understanding of events, noting differences in viewpoints.
- Note client's gender, age, and developmental level of functioning. *Women, children, young adults, divorced and separated persons tend to have higher stress levels. Multiple stressors can weaken immune system and tax physical and emotional coping mechanisms of persons of any age, but particulary the elderly.*[1–3]
- Note cultural values/religious beliefs *that may affect client's expectation for self in dealing with situation, ability to ask for help from others, and expectations placed on client by SO/ family.*[7]
- Identify client locus of control: internal (expressions of responsibility for self and ability to control outcomes—"I didn't quit smoking") or external (expressions of lack of control over self and environment—"Nothing ever works out"). *Knowing client's locus of control will help in developing a plan of care reflecting client's ability to realistically make changes that will help to manage stress better.*[7]
- Assess emotional responses and coping mechanisms being used.
- Determine stress feelings and self-talk client is engaging in. *Negative self-talk, all or nothing/pessimistic thinking, exaggeration, unrealistic expectations will contribute to stress overload.*[2]
- Assess degree of mastery client has exhibited in life. *Passive individual may have more difficulty being assertive and standing up for rights.*
- Determine presence/absence/nature of resources (e.g., whether family/SO are supportive, lack money, problems with relationship/social functioning).
- Note change in relationships with SO(s). *Conflict in the family, loss of a family member, divorce can result in a change in support client is accustomed to and impair ability to manage situation.*
- Evaluate stress level using appropriate tool (e.g., Stress & Depression, Self-Assessment Tool) to help identify areas of most distress. *While most stress seems to come from disasterous events in individual's life, positive events can also be stressful.*
- Review lab results to identify physiological conditions (e.g., thryoid/other hormone imbalance, anemia, unstable glucose levels, kidney/liver disease) *that may be causing/exacerbating stress.*[1]

NURSING PRIORITY NO. 2 To assist client to deal with current situation:

- Discuss situation/condition in simple, concise manner. *May help client to express emotions, grasp situation, and feel more in control.*
- Active-listen to concerns and provide empathetic presence, using talk and silence as needed.
- Deal with the immediate issues first (e.g., treatment of physical injury, meet safety needs, removal from traumatic/violent environment).
- Collaborate in treatment of underlying conditions (e.g., diabetes, hormone imbalance, depression).[1]
- Provide/encourage restful environment where possible.
- Assist client in determining whether or not he or she can change stressor or response. *May help client to sort out things over which he or she has control and determine responses that can be modified.*
- Allow client to react in own way without judgment. Provide support and diversion as indicated.
- Help client to set limits on acting-out behaviors and learn ways to express emotions in an acceptable manner. *Promotes internal locus of control, enabling client to maintain self-concept and feel more positive about self.*
- Address use of ineffective/dangerous coping mechanisms (e.g., substance use/abuse, self/other-directed violence) and refer for counseling as indicated.

NURSING PRIORITY NO. 3 To promote wellness (Teaching/Discharge Considerations):

- Use client's locus of control to develop individual plan of care *(e.g., for client with internal control, encourage client to take control of own care; for those with external control, begin with small tasks and add as tolerated).*[4]
- Incorporate strengths/assets and past coping strategies that were successful for client. *Reinforces that client is able to deal with difficult situations.*
- Encourage strengthening of positive SO/family routines and interactions *that support and provide assistance in managing stress.*[5]
- Provide information about stress and exhaustion phase, which occurs when person is experiencing chronic/unresolved stress. *Release of cortisol can contribute to reduction in immune function, resulting in physical illness, mental disability, and life dysfunction.*
- Review stress management/coping skills that client can use:[1,2,4-6]
  Practice behaviors that may help *reduce negative consequences*—change thinking by focusing on positives, reframing thoughts, changing lifestyle.
  Learn to read own body signs (e.g., shakiness, irritability, sleep disturbances, fatigue, etc.).
  Take a step back, reduce obligations; simplify life; learn to say no *to reduce sense of being overwhelmed.*
  Practice exchanging stresses (i.e., when a new stress comes into play, eliminate or postpone another stress) *to keep total stress level below overstress level.*
  Seek help/assistance in meeting obligations, delegate tasks as appropriate.
  Learn to control and redirect anger.
  Develop and practice positive self-esteem skills.
  Rest, sleep, and exercise on regular/set times *to recuperate and rejuvenate self.*
  Postpone changes in living situation (e.g., moving, remodeling) if possible.
  Particpate in self-help actions (e.g., deep breathing, find time to be alone, get involved in recreation or desired activity; plan something fun/develop humor) *to actively relax.*
  Eliminate possible food or environmental allergens and toxins.

Eat nutritious meals; avoid junk food/excessive sugars.

Avoid excessive caffeine, alcohol/other drugs, and nicotine *to balance body chemicals and support general health.*

Take a multivitamin, mineral, trace element preparation.

Develop spiritual self (e.g., meditate/pray; block negative thoughts, learn to give and take, speak and listen, forgive and move on).

Interact socially, reach out, nurture self and others *to reduce loneliness/sense of isolation.*

- Review proper medication use *to manage exacerbating conditions (e.g., depression, mood disorders).*

- Identify community resources (e.g., vocational counseling, educational programs, child/elder care, WIC/food stamps, home/respite care) *that can help client manage lifestyle/environmental stress.*

- Refer for therapy, as indicated (e.g., medical treatment, psychological counseling; hypnosis, massage, biofeedback).

DOCUMENTATION FOCUS

Assessment/Reassessment

- Individual findings, noting specific stressors, individual's perception of the situation, locus of control.
- Specific cultural/religious factors.
- Availability/use of support systems and resources.

Planning

- Plan of care and who is involved in planning.
- Teaching plan.

Implementation/Evaluation

- Responses to interventions/teaching and actions performed.
- Attainment/progress toward desired outcome(s).
- Modifications to plan of care.

Discharge Planning

- Long-term needs/referrals and who is responsible for actions to be taken.
- Specific referrals made.

References

1. Burns, S. L. (1997). The medical basis of stress, depression, anxiety, sleep problems and drug use. Retrieved August 2007 at www.teachhealth.com/.
2. Klimes, R. (2007). Managing stress: Living without stress overload. CE offering for Learn.Well.org Web site. Retrieved April 2007 at www.learnwell.org/stress.htm.
3. Woolston, C. (2006). Stress and aging. Retrieved July 2007 at www.yourhealthconnection.com/topic/stressaging.
4. Cummings, B. (2003). Managing stress: Coping with life's challenges. In *Health: The Basics.* 5th ed. Pearson Education, Inc.
5. Beckett, C. (2000). Family Theory as a Framework for Assessment. Retrieved August 2007 at http://jan.ucc.nau.edu/~nur350-c/class/2_family/theory/lesson2-1-3.html.
6. No author listed. (2007). Taking Control of Stress. Harvard Health Publications: Big Sandy, TX, 1, Special Supplement.
7. Lipson, J. G., Dibble. S. L., Minarik, P. A. (1996). *Culture & Nursing Care: A Pocket Guide.* San Francisco: School of Nursing, UCSF Nursing Press.

risk for Suffocation

Definition: Accentuated risk of accidental suffocation (inadequate air available for inhalation)

RISK FACTORS

Internal
Reduced olfactory sensation
Reduced motor abilities
Lack of safety education/precautions
Cognitive/emotional difficulties [e.g., altered consciousness/mentation]
Disease/injury process

External
Pillow/propped bottle placed in an infant's crib
Hanging a pacifier around infant's neck
Playing with plastic bags; inserting small objects into airway
Leaving children unattended in water
Discarded refrigerators without removed doors
Vehicle warming in closed garage [faulty exhaust system]; use of fuel-burning heaters not
    vented to outside
Household gas leaks; smoking in bed
Low-strung clothesline
Eating large mouthfuls [or pieces] of food
NOTE: A risk diagnosis is not evidenced by signs and symptoms, as the problem has not
    occurred; rather, nursing interventions are directed at prevention.

Sample Clinical Applications: Substance use/abuse, spinal cord injury, crushing chest
    injury, obesity, near-drowning, burn/inhalation injury, sleep apnea, seizure disorder

DESIRED OUTCOMES/EVALUATION CRITERIA
Sample NOC linkages:
Risk Control: Personal actions to prevent, eliminate, or reduce modifiable health threats
Aspiration Prevention: Personal actions to prevent the passage of fluid and solid particles
    into the lung
Personal Safety Behavior: Personal actions of an adult to control behaviors that can cause
    physical injury

Client/Caregiver Will (Include Specific Time Frame)

- Verbalize knowledge of hazards in the environment.
- Identify interventions appropriate to situation.
- Correct hazardous situations to prevent/reduce risk of suffocation.
- Demonstrate CPR skills and how to access emergency assistance.

ACTIONS/INTERVENTIONS

Sample NIC linkages:
Airway Management: Facilitation of patency of air passages

Aspiration Precautions: Prevention or minimization of risk factors in the patient at risk for aspiration

Teaching Infant Safety: Instruction on safety during first year of life

NURSING PRIORITY NO. 1   To assess causative/contributing factors:

- Determine client's/SO's knowledge of individual safety concerns/environmental hazards present *to identify misconceptions and educational needs. Suffocation can be caused by (1) spasm of airway (e.g., food or water going down wrong way, irritant gases, asthma; (2) airway obstruction (e.g., foreign body, tongue falling back in unconscious person, or swelling of tissues from burn injury/allergic reaction); (3) airway compression (e.g., tying rope/band tightly around neck, hanging, throttling, or smothering); (4) conditions affecting the respiratory mechanism (e.g., epilepsy, tetanus, rabies, nerve diseases causing paralysis of chest wall or diaphragm); (5) conditions affecting respiratory center in brain (e.g., electric shock, stroke/other brain trauma; medications such as morphine, barbiturates); and (6) compression of the chest (e.g., crushing as might occur with cave-in, auto crash, pressure in a massive crowd).*[1,7,8]
- Identify level of concern/awareness and motivation of client/SO(s) to correct safety hazards and improve individual situation. *Lack of commitment may limit growth/willingness to make changes, placing dependent individuals at risk.*
- Determine age, developmental level, and mentation (e.g., infant/young child, frail elder, person with developmental delay, altered level of consciousness, or cognitive impairments/dementia) *to identify individuals unable to be responsible for/protect self.*
- Assess neurological status/note history of conditions such as stroke, cerebral palsy, MS, ALS, *that have potential to compromise airway or affect ability to swallow.*[4]
- Determine presence of seizure disorder, noting use of antiepileptics and how well condition is controlled. *Seizure activity (and especially status epilepticus) is a major risk factor for respiratory inhibition/arrest.*[4]
- Note reports of sleep disturbance and daytime fatigue. *May be indicative of sleep apnea (airway obstruction) requiring referral for evaluation.* (Refer to NDs Insomnia, Sleep Deprivation.)
- Review medication regimen *to note potential for oversedation and respiratory failure (e.g., central nervous system depressants, analgesics, sedatives, antidepressants).*[10]
- Assess for allergies to medications, foods, environmental factors *that could result in severe/anaphylactic reaction resulting in respiratory arrest.*
- Be alert to/carefully monitor those individuals who are severely depressed, mentally ill, or aggressive and in restraints. *These individuals could be at risk for suicide by suffocation (e.g., inhaled carbon monoxide or death by strangling or hanging).*[2] (Refer to ND risk for Suicide.)
- Note signs of respiratory distress (e.g., cough, stridor, wheezing, increased work of breathing) *that could indicate swelling/obstruction of airways.*[3] (Refer to NDs ineffective Airway Clearance, risk for Aspiration, ineffective Breathing Pattern, impaired spontaneous Ventilation, as appropriate, for additional interventions.)

NURSING PRIORITY NO. 2   To reverse/correct contributing factors:

- Discuss with client/SO(s) identified environmental/work-related safety hazards and problem-solve methods for resolution (e.g., need for smoke/carbon monoxide alarms, vents for household heater, clean chimney, properly strung clothesline, proper venting of machinery exhaust, monitoring of stored chemicals, bracing trench walls when digging).
- Protect airway at all times, especially if client unable to protect self:[2,4,7,11]
  Use proper positioning, suctioning, use of airway adjuncts, as indicated, *for comatose/cognitively impaired individual or client with swallowing impairment or obstructive sleep apnea.*

Cultural   Collaborative   Community/Home Care   Diagnostic Studies   Pediatric/Geriatric/Lifespan   Medications

Provide seizure precautions and antiseizure medication, as indicated.

Administer medications when client is sitting or standing upright and can swallow without difficulty.

Stress importance of chewing carefully, taking small amounts of food, and using caution *to prevent aspiration when talking or drinking while eating.*

Provide diet modifications as indicated by specific needs (e.g., developmental level; presence/degree of swallowing disability, impaired cognition) *to reduce risk of aspiration.*

Avoid physical and mechanical restraints, including vest/waist restraint, side rails, choke hold. *Increases agitation and risk of partial escape, resulting in entrapment of head/hanging.*

- Emphasize with client/SO the importance of getting help when beginning to choke or feel respiratory distress (e.g., staying with people instead of leaving table, make gestures across throat; making sure someone recognizes the emergency) *in order to provide timely intervention such as abdominal thrusts and calling 911*

- Refrain from smoking in bed; supervise smoking materials (use, disposal, and storage) for impaired individuals. Keep smoking materials out of reach of children.

- Avoid idling automobile (or using fuel-burning heaters) in closed or unvented spaces.

- Emphasize importance of periodic evaluation and repair of gas appliances/furnace, automobile exhaust system *to prevent exposure to carbon monoxide.*

- Review child protective measures:[2,5,6,9,11]

Place infant in supine position for sleep. (Refer to ND sudden infant Death Syndrome.)

Do not prop baby bottles in infant crib.

Attach pacifier to clothing—not around neck; remove bib before putting baby in bed.

Store/dispose of plastic bags (e.g., shopping, garbage, dry cleaning, and shipping) out of reach of infants/young children.

Avoid use of plastic mattress or crib covers.

Avoid placing infant to sleep on soft surfaces (e.g., beanbag chair, basket with soft sides, soft pillow/comforter, water bed) *that baby can sink into or be unable to free face.*

Use a crib with slats that are no more than 2 3/8 inches apart *so that baby cannot get head trapped or slip body through slats.*

Refrain from bedsharing with infant/young child *to prevent accidental smothering.*

Provide constant supervision of young children in bathtub or swimming pool.

Make certain that blind and curtain cords, drawstrings on clothing, etc., are out of reach of small children *to prevent accidental hanging.*

Observe young child/impaired individual for objects put in mouth (e.g., food such as raw carrots, nuts, seeds, popcorn, hot dogs; toy parts, buttons, balloons, batteries, coins, etc.) *that can get lodged in airway/cause choking.*

Lock/remove lid or door of chests, trunks, old refrigerators/freezers *to prevent child from being trapped in airless environment.*

NURSING PRIORITY NO. 3 To promote wellness (Teaching/Discharge Considerations):

- Review safety factors identified in individual situation and methods for remediation.
- Develop plan with client/caregiver for long-range management of situation to avoid risks. *Enhances commitment to plan, optimizing outcomes.*
- Discuss possibility of choking resulting from relaxation of throat muscle and impaired judgment *when combining drinking alcohol with eating.*
- Involve family members in learning and practicing rescue techniques (e.g., treating of choking or breathing problems, and CPR) *to deal with emergency situations (especially when at-home client is at risk on a regular basis).*

🏠 • Encourage individuals to read package labels and identify and remove safety hazards such as toys with small parts, and monitor Web sites for product recalls.

🏠 • Promote water/swimming pool safety, vigilance, and use of approved flotation equipment, fencing/locked gates, alarm system, etc.

🏠 • Discuss fire safety and concerns regarding use of heaters, household gas appliances, old/discarded appliances. Encourage home fire safety drills yearly.

🏠 • Promote public education in techniques for clearing blocked airways (e.g., Heimlich maneuver, CPR).

🏠 ∞ • Collaborate in community public health education regarding hazards for children (e.g., appropriate toy size for young child; discussing dangers of "huffing" [inhalants] and playing choking/hanging games with pre-teens; how to spot potential for depression/risk of suicidal gestures in adolescent) *to reduce potential for accidental/intentional suffocation.*[12]

DOCUMENTATION FOCUS

Assessment/Reassessment

• Individual risk factors, including individual's cognitive status and level of knowledge.
• Level of concern/motivation for change.
• Equipment/airway adjunct needs.

Planning

• Plan of care and who is involved in planning.
• Teaching plan.

Implementation/Evaluation

• Responses to interventions/teaching and actions performed.
• Attainment/progress toward desired outcome(s).
• Modifications to plan of care.

Discharge Planning

• Long-term needs/referrals, appropriate preventive measures, and who is responsible for actions to be taken.
• Specific referrals made.

References

1. No author listed. Suffocation and artificial respiration. (2000). Fact sheet for WebHealthCentre. Retrieved July 2007 at http://webhealthcentre.com.
2. Summary of the practice parameter for the prevention and management of aggressive behavior in child and adolescent psychiatric institutions with special reference to seclusion and restraint. (February 2002). *J Am Acad Child Adoles Psychiatry,* 41(2Suppl), 4S–25S. Retrieved July 2007 at www.guideline.gov.
3. Kline, A. (2003). Pinpointing the cause of pediatric respiratory distress. *Nursing,* 33(9), 58–63.
4. ND: Suffocation, risk for in Seizure Disorders. In Doenges, M. E., Moorhouse, M. F., Geissler-Murr, A. C. (2002). *Nursing Care Plans: Guidelines for Individualizing Patient Care.* 6th ed. Philadelphia: F. A. Davis, pp. 201–203.

🌐 Cultural   Ⓐ Collaborative   🏠 Community/Home Care   Diagnostic Studies   ∞ Pediatric/Geriatric/Lifespan   💊 Medications

5. Task Force on Infant Sleep Position and Sudden Infant Death Syndrome. Changing concepts of sudden infant death syndrome: Implications for infant sleeping environment and sleep position. (2000). *Pediatr*, 105(3), 650–656.

6. No author listed. Suffocation. Doctors Book of Home Remedies for Children. Retrieved July 2007 at www.mothernature.com.

7. Green, P. M. (1993). High risk for suffocation. In McFarland, G. K., McFarlane, E. A. (eds). *Nursing Diagnosis and Interventions.* St. Louis, MO: Mosby.

8. No author listed. Suffocation. Health Sciences Centre, Winnipeg, Manitoba. Retrieved July 2007 at www.hsc.mb.ca/impact/suffocation.htm.

9. No author listed. Preventing strangulation and suffocation among infants and children. SAFEUSA. Retrieved July 2007 at http://safeusa.org.

10. *Apnea: Handbook of Signs and Symptoms,* 3rd ed. Retrieved July 2007 at www.wrongdiagnosis.com/s/suffocation/book-diseases-5a.htm.

11. Homeir, B. P. (2004). Household safety: Preventing suffocation. Article for KidsHealth Web site. Retrieved April 2007 at www.kidshealth.org/parent/positive/family/safety_suffocation.html.

12. Dowshen, S. (2005). Kids and dangerous "suffocation games." Article for KidsHealth Web site. Retrieved April 2007 at www.kidshealth.org/research/suffocation.html.

risk for Suicide

Definition: At risk for self-inflicted, life-threatening injury

RISK FACTORS

Behavioral
History of prior suicide attempt
Buying a gun; stockpiling medicines
Making/changing a will; giving away possessions
Sudden euphoric recovery from major depression
Impulsiveness; marked changes in behavior/attitude/school performance

Demographic
Age (e.g., elderly, young adult males, adolescents)
Race (e.g., Caucasian, Native American)
Male gender
Divorced; widowed

Physical
Physical/terminal illness; chronic pain

Psychological
Family history of suicide; abuse in childhood
Substance use/abuse
Psychiatric illness/disorder (e.g., depression, schizophrenia, bipolar disorder)
Guilt
Gay or lesbian youth

Situational
Living alone; retired; economic instability; relocation; institutionalization
Loss of autonomy/independence

Presence of gun in home

Adolescents living in nontraditional settings (e.g., juvenile detention center, prison, half-way house, group home)

Social

Loss of important relationship; disrupted family life; poor support systems; social isolation

Grief, loneliness

Hopelessness; helplessness

Legal/disciplinary problems

Cluster suicides

Verbal

Threats of killing oneself; states desire to die/[end it all]

NOTE: A risk diagnosis is not evidenced by signs and symptoms, as the problem has not occurred; rather, nursing interventions are directed at prevention.

Sample Clinical Applications: Acute/chronic brain syndrome, hormonal imbalances (e.g., PMS, postpartum psychosis), substance use/abuse, chronic/terminal illness (e.g., ALS, cancer), major depression, schizophrenia, bipolar disorder, panic state

DESIRED OUTCOMES/EVALUATION CRITERIA

Sample NOC linkages:

Suicide Self-Restraint: Personal actions to refrain from gestures and attempts at killing self

Coping: Personal actions to manage stressors that tax an individual's resources

Hope: Optimism that is personally satisfying and life-supporting

Client Will (Include Specific Time Frame)

- Acknowledge difficulties perceived in current situation.
- Identify current factors that can be dealt with.
- Be involved in planning course of action to correct existing problems.
- Make decision that suicide is not the answer to perceived/real problems.

ACTIONS/INTERVENTIONS

Sample NIC linkages:

Suicide Prevention: Reducing the risk for self-inflicted harm with intent to end life

Behavior Management: Self-Harm: Assisting the patient to decrease or eliminate self-mutilating or self-abusive behavior

Client Contracting: Negotiating an agreement with a patient that reinforces a specific behavior change

NURSING PRIORITY NO. 1   To assess causative/contributing factors and degree of risk:

- Identify degree of risk/potential for suicide and seriousness of threat. Use a scale of 1 to 10 and prioritize according to severity of threat, availability of means. *Most people who are contemplating suicide send a variety of signals indicating their intent, and recognizing these warning signs allows for immediate intervention.*[4]

🌐 Cultural   Ⓐ Collaborative   🏠 Community/Home Care   Diagnostic Studies   ∞ Pediatric/Geriatric/Lifespan   Medications

- Note behaviors indicative of intent. *Individual may not make statements of intent, but gestures, presence of means such as guns, threats, giving away possessions, previous attempts, and presence of hallucinations or delusions may provide clues to intent.*[3,6]

- Ask directly if person is thinking of acting on thoughts/feelings to determine intent. *Most individuals want someone to see what desperate straits they are in, and by bringing the issue into the open, discussion can begin and plans made to keep the person safe.*[3,7]

- Note withdrawal from usual activities, lack of social interactions. *These are classic behaviors of the individual who is feeling depressed and sad and may be having negative thoughts of worthlessness.*[6]

- Identify losses client has experienced and meaning of those losses. *Unresolved issues may be contributing to thoughts of hopelessness, feelings of despair, and suicidal ideation.*[3,6]

- Note age and gender. While women talk about suicide more frequently, men usually succeed more often. Risk of suicide is greater in teens and the elderly, but there is a rising awareness of risk in early childhood.[4,8,10]

- Determine cultural/religious beliefs that may be affecting client's thinking about life and death. *Family of origin and culture in which individual grew up influence attitudes toward taking one's own life; for instance Protestants commit suicide more frequently than Catholics or Jews, and whites are at highest risk, followed by Native Americans, African Americans, Hispanic Americans, and Asian Americans.*[2,3,10]

- Identify conditions such as acute/chronic brain syndrome, panic state, hormonal imbalance (e.g., PMS, postpartum psychosis, drug-induced). *These conditions may interfere with ability to control own behavior leading to impulsive actions that may put client at risk.*[1,10]

- Review laboratory results (e.g., blood alcohol, serum glucose, ABGs, electrolytes, renal function tests). *Identifies factors that may affect reasoning ability interfering with ability to think clearly about issues that are leading to thoughts of suicide.*[1,3,5]

- Assess physical complaints. *Sleeping difficulties, lack of appetite can be indicators of depression and suicidal ideation requiring further evaluation.*[3,4]

- Review family history for suicidal behavior. *Individual risk is increased when other family members have committed suicide or exhibited symptoms of depression. Studies have shown a possible genetic link toward suicidal behavior.*[3]

- Assess coping behaviors presently used. *Client's current negative thinking may preclude looking at positive behaviors that have been used in the past that would help in the current situation. Client may believe there is no alternative except suicide.*[6,7]

- Ascertain presence of SO(s)/friends available for support. *Individuals who have positive support systems whom they can rely on during a crisis situation are less likely to commit suicide and are more apt to return to a successful life.*[3]

- Determine drug use/"self" medication. *The use of alcohol, especially the combination of alcohol and barbiturates, increases the risk of suicide.*

- Note history of disciplinary problems/involvement with judicial system. *Feelings of despair over problems with the legal system and lack of hope about outcome can lead to belief that the only solution is suicide.*[3,10]

NURSING PRIORITY NO. 2 To assist clients to accept responsibility for own behavior and prevent suicide:

- Develop therapeutic nurse-client relationship, providing consistent care provider. *Promotes sense of trust, allowing individual to discuss feelings openly. Collaborating with the client to better understand the problem affirms the client's ability to solve the current situation.*[3,6]

- Maintain straightforward communication. *By being direct and honest and acknowledging need for attention, care provider can avoid reinforcing manipulative behavior.*[6]

- Explain concern for safety and willingness to help client stay safe. *Clients often believe their concerns will not be taken seriously, and stating clearly that they will be listened to sends a clear message of support and caring.*[6]
- Encourage expression of feelings and make time to listen to concerns. *Acknowledges reality of feelings and that they are okay. Helps individual sort out thinking and begin to develop understanding of situation.*[3,6]
- Give permission to express angry feelings in acceptable ways and let client know someone will be available to assist in maintaining control. *Promotes acceptance and sense of safety while client is regaining own control.*[3,4]
- Acknowledge reality of suicide as an option. Discuss consequences of actions if they follow through on intent. Ask how it will help individual to resolve problems. *Can help client to focus on consequences of actions and begin to discuss the possibility of other options.*[5,7]
- Help client identify more appropriate solutions/behaviors. *Alternative activities, such as exercise, can lessen sense of anxiety and associated physical manifestations.*[3]
- Maintain observation of client and check environment for hazards that could be used to commit suicide. *Increases client safety/reduces risk of impulsive behavior when client is hospitalized.*[3]
- Discuss use of antidepressant medications, especially when there may be a significant organic component to the suicidal ideation. *While the use of medications may be helpful in the short term, there are some drawbacks, namely, the length of time it takes for most medications to take effect, and the potential for giving a client a means of suicide because of the possibility of a lethal overdose.*[6,9,10]
- Reevaluate potential for suicide periodically at key times (e.g., mood changes, increasing withdrawal), as well as when client is feeling better and planning for discharge becomes active. *The highest risk is when the client has both suicidal ideation and sufficient energy with which to act.*[5,6]

NURSING PRIORITY NO. 3 To assist client to plan course of action to correct/deal with existing situation:

- Gear interventions to individual involved. *Age, relationships, and current situation determine what is needed to help client deal with feelings of despair and hopelessness.*[6,10]
- Negotiate contract with client regarding willingness not to do anything lethal for a stated period of time. Specify what care provider will be responsible for and what client responsibilities are. *Making a contract in which the individual agrees to stay alive for a specified period of time, from day one through the entire course of treatment and written and signed by each party, may help the client to follow through with therapy to find reason for living. Although there is little research on the effectiveness of these contracts, they are frequently used.*[6]
- Specify alternative actions necessary if client is unwilling to negotiate contract. *Client may be willing to agree to other actions (i.e., calling therapist if feelings are overwhelming), even though he or she is not willing to commit to a contract.*[6]
- Provide directions for actions client can take, avoiding negative statements such as "do nots." *Providing opportunity for client to have control over circumstances can promote a positive attitude and give client some hope for the future.*[3,5]

NURSING PRIORITY NO. 4 To promote wellness (Teaching/Discharge Considerations):

- Promote development of internal control. *Helping the client look at new ways to deal with problems can provide a sense of own ability to solve problems, improve situation, and hope for the future.*[3]

🌐 Cultural 🅐 Collaborative 🏠 Community/Home Care ⟋ Diagnostic Studies ∞ Pediatric/Geriatric/Lifespan 💊 Medications

- Assist with learning problem-solving, assertiveness training, and social skills. *By learning these new skills, client can begin to feel more confidence in own ability to handle problems that arise and deal with the current situation.*[3,5]
- Engage in physical activity programs. *Promotes release of endorphins and feelings of self-worth, improving sense of well-being and giving client hope.*[3]
- Determine nutritional needs and help client to plan for meeting them. *Enhances general well-being and energy level.*[1,10]
- Review use of antidepressants noting that it takes 4 to 8 weeks for effects of medication to be observed, and different medications may need to be tried to obtain maximum benefit. Stress importance of continuing medication after symptoms of depression resolve. *Studies of older adults age 70 and over reveal significant decrease in relapse when antidepressant continued for 2 years beyond becoming symptom-free.*[10]
- Involve family/SO in planning. *Improves understanding and support when family knows the facts and has a part in planning for rehabilitation efforts for the client.*[1,5]
- Refer to formal resources as indicated. *May need assistance with referrals to individual/group/marital psychotherapy, substance abuse treatment program, or social services when situation involves mental illness, family disorganization.*[3,5,10]

DOCUMENTATION FOCUS

Assessment/Reassessment

- Individual findings, including nature of concern (e.g., suicidal/behavioral risk factors and level of impulse control, plan of action/means to carry out plan).
- Client's perception of situation, motivation for change.
- Cutural/religious beliefs influencing attitudes about life/suicide.
- Availability of family/support system.

Planning

- Plan of care and who is involved in the planning.
- Details of contract regarding suicidal ideation/plans.
- Teaching plan.

Implementation/Evaluation

- Actions taken to promote safety.
- Response to interventions/teaching and actions performed.
- Attainment/progress toward desired outcome(s).
- Modifications to plan of care.

Discharge Planning

- Long-range needs and who is responsible for actions to be taken.
- Available resources, specific referrals made.

References

1. Cox, H. C., et al. (2002). *Clinical Applications of Nursing Diagnosis: Adult, Child, Women's, Psychiatric, Gerontic, and Home Health Considerations.* 4th ed. Philadelphia: F. A. Davis.
2. Lipson, J. G., Dibble, S. L., Minarik, P. A. (1996). *Culture & Nursing Care: A Pocket Guide.* San Francisco: UCSF Nursing Press.
3. Townsend, M. C. (2003). *Psychiatric Mental Health Nursing Concepts of Care.* 4th ed. Philadelphia: F. A. Davis.

4. Doenges, M. E., Moorhouse, M. F., Murr, A. G. (2004). *Nurse's Pocket Guide Diagnoses, Interventions, and Rationales.* 9th ed. Philadelphia: F. A. Davis.
5. Doenges, M., Townsend, M., Moorhouse, M. (1998). *Psychiatric Care Plans: Guidelines for Individualizing Care.* 3d ed. Philadelphia: F. A. Davis.
6. Jurich, A. P. (2003). The Nature of Suicide. Clinical Update (insert in *Family Therapy Magazine*), 3(6), 1–8.
7. Gettinger-Dinner, L. (April 30, 2007). Suicide Risk Assessment: What Providers Need to Know. Retrieved May 2007 at http://news.nurse.com/apps/pbcs.dll/article?AID=/20070430/CA09/304300012&SearchID=73281745058190.
8. Whetstone, L., Morrissey, S. (2007). Children at risk: The association between perceived weight status and suicidal thoughts and attempts in middle school youth. *J School Health,* 77(2), 59–66.
9. Sherman, C. (2002). Antisuicidal Effect of Psychotropics Remains Uncertain. *Clin Psychiatry News,* 30(8). Retrieved May 2007 at www.namiscc.org/Research/2002/AntipsychoticSuicideRisk.htm.
10. National Institute of Mental Health. (April 2007). Older adults: Depression & suicide facts. NIH pub no. 4593. Retrieved May 2007 at www.nimh.nih.gov/publicat/elderlydepsuicide.cfm.

delayed Surgical Recovery

Definition: Extension of the number of postoperative days required to initiate and perform activities that maintain life, health, and well-being

RELATED FACTORS
Extensive/prolonged surgical procedure
Pain
Obesity
Preoperative expectations
Postoperative surgical site infection

DEFINING CHARACTERISTICS

Subjective
Perception that more time is needed to recover
Report of pain/discomfort; fatigue
Loss of appetite with or without nausea
Postpones resumption of work/employment activities

Objective
Evidence of interrupted healing of surgical area (e.g., red, indurated, draining, immobilized)
Difficulty in moving about; requires help to complete self-care

Sample Clinical Applications: Major surgical procedures, traumatic injuries with surgical intervention, chronic conditions (e.g., diabetes mellitus, cancer, HIV/AIDS, COPD)

DESIRED OUTCOMES/EVALUATION CRITERIA
Sample NOC linkages:
Wound Healing: Primary: Extent of regeneration of cells and tissues following intentional closure
Self-Care: Activities of Daily Living (ADL): Ability to perform the most basic physical tasks and personal care activities independently with or without assistive device
Endurance: Capacity to sustain activity

Client Will (Include Specific Time Frame)

- Display complete healing of surgical area.
- Perform desired self-care activities.
- Report increased energy, able to participate in usual (work/employment) activities.

Cultural · Collaborative · Community/Home Care · Diagnostic Studies · Pediatric/Geriatric/Lifespan · Medications

ACTIONS/INTERVENTIONS

Sample NIC linkages:

Self-Care Assistance: Assisting another to perform activities of daily living

Energy Management: Regulating energy use to treat or prevent fatigue and optimize function

Wound Care: Prevention of wound complications and promotion of wound healing

NURSING PRIORITY NO. 1   To assess causative/contributing factors:

- Identify factors affecting ability to care for self/meet own needs (e.g., low socioeconomic status/poverty; lack of insurance, inadequate transportation, family/support system; severe trauma/prolonged hospitalization with multiple complicating factors; client with severe anxiety about diagnosis/outcome, etc.) *that increase risk for adverse outcomes.*[7]

- Determine age/developmental level and general state of health *to help determine time that may be required for client to resume ADLs and other activities, or expectation of time needed for healing. Note: The older adult undergoing surgical treatment is at greater risk for delayed recovery because of age-related changes in numerous systems and protective mechanisms that increase the potential for complications.*[1,8]

- Note underlying condition/pathology (e.g., cancer, burns, diabetes, hypothyroidism, obesity, steroid therapy, major trauma, infections, radiation therapy, cardiopulmonary disorders, debilitating illness) *that can adversely affect healing and prolong recuperation time.*[4,9]

- Determine the length of operative procedure/time under anesthesia (e.g., typical or lengthy); type/severity of perioperative complications (e.g., trauma/other conditions requiring multiple surgeries; heavy bleeding during procedure); type of surgical wound (e.g., clean, clean-contaminated, or grossly contaminated/acutely infected); and development of postoperative complications (e.g., surgical site infection, suture reactions, dehiscence, ventilator-associated pneumonia, deep vein thrombosis) *that can affect the pace of healing or prolong recovery.*[3,4]

- Assess circulation and sensation in surgical area *to evaluate for (1) internal bleeding that compromises wound integrity; or (2) loss of blood flow to area, resulting in decreased oxygen supply to tissues, or nerve damage delaying healing.*[2,3]

- Note use of plastics (e.g., incontinence pads/moisture barriers) or latex materials. *Plastics retain heat and enhance growth of pathogens in wound. Client sensitivity to latex can cause skin/tissue reactions that delay healing.* (Refer to ND latex Allergy Response.)

- Review client's preoperative medication regimen *to ascertain that none could impede healing processes (e.g., aspirin and NSAIDs increase bleeding time, alcohol—a potent vasodilator—and some herbals such as garlic and ginkgo biloba can also be associated with bleeding complications)*[3]

- Determine nutritional status and current intake *to ascertain if nutrition is adequate to support healing. Client may have preexisting nutritional concerns (e.g., elderly person with anorexia, person with morbid obesity) or may have been fasting for several days perioperatively or experienced nausea, vomiting, and loss of appetite postoperatively, depending on the surgical procedure performed and client's reactions to medications (e.g., pain medications, antibiotics).*[2,3,8]

- Note lifestyle factors (e.g., obesity, cigarette smoking, sedentary lifestyle) *that may impede recovery.*

- Perform pain assessment *to ascertain whether pain management is adequate to meet client's needs during recovery.*

- Review results of laboratory tests (e.g., CBC, blood/wound cultures, serum glucose, etc.) *to assess for presence/type of infections, metabolic/endocrine dysfunction/other conditions affecting body's ability to heal.*

- Evaluate client's cognitive and emotional state, noting presence of postoperative changes, including confusion, depression, apathy, expressions of helplessness *to determine need for further assessment of possible physical or psychological interferences.*
 • Ascertain attitudes/cultural values of individual about condition. *Family beliefs and cultural values, stress and fear related to surgery (and the reason for it), possible stigma about relative condition/disease or change in body image, or motivation to return to usual role/activities all impact rate and expectations for sick role and recovery.*[6]

NURSING PRIORITY NO. 2 To determine impact of delayed recovery:

- Note length of illness/hospitalization, time of discharge, and progress to date *to compare with general expectations for procedure and situation.*
- Determine client's/SO's expectations for recovery and specific stressors related to delay (e.g., return to work/school, home responsibilities/child care, financial difficulties, limited support system).
- Determine energy level and current participation in ADLs *to compare with usual level of function.*
- Ascertain whether client usually requires assistance in home setting and who provides it/current availability and capability.
- Note client/SO reports of helplessness/inability to cope with situation.
- Obtain psychological assessment of client's emotional status, noting potential problems arising from current situation.

NURSING PRIORITY NO. 3 To promote optimal recovery:

- Practice and instruct client/caregiver(s) in proper handwashing and aseptic technique for incisional care *to reduce incidence of contamination and infection.*[5]
- Administer/discuss use of medications to manage postoperative discomforts (e.g., pain, nausea/vomiting) and other concurrent or underlying conditions, such as diabetes, osteoporosis, heart failure, COPD. *Client may require antibiotics, insulin to support tissue repair, or management of chronic pain to improve mobility and tissue recovery.*[2]
- Instruct client/SO in necessary self-care of incisions and specific symptom managment. *With short hospital stays, client/SO are usually expected to provide a great deal of postoperative care and monitoring at home.*[7]
- Provide wound care expectations and instructions in verbal and written forms *to facilitate self-care and reduce likelihood of misinterpretation of information when client/SO is providing care at home.*[3]
- Instruct client/SO in routine inspection of incision/wound and to report changes in wound indicative of failure to heal (e.g., deepening wound, local or systemic fever, exudates [noting color, amount, and odor], loss of approximation of wound edges) *to establish comparative baseline and allow for early intervention (e.g., antimicrobial therapy, wound irrigation/packing, and so forth).*
- Limit/avoid use of plastics or latex materials in wound care, as appropriate. *Can delay healing/cause skin breakdown.*
- Collaborate in treatment/assist with wound care, as indicated. *May require surgical debridement, barrier dressings, skin-protective agents for open/draining wounds. Include wound care specialist/stomal therapist, as appropriate, to troubleshoot healing difficulties.*
- Provide optimal nutrition with adequate protein *to provide a positive nitrogen balance, which aids in healing and contributes to general good health.*

Cultural Collaborative Community/Home Care Diagnostic Studies Pediatric/Geriatric/Lifespan Medications

- Encourage adequate fluid and electrolyte intake *to avoid dehydration of tissues and to promote optimal cellular/organ function.*[2]
- Encourage early ambulation/regular exercise *to promote circulation, improve muscle strength and overall endurance, and reduce risks associated with immobility.*[2]
- Recommend pacing (alternating activity with adequate rest periods) *to reduce fatigue and allow weakened muscles/tissues to recuperate.*[2]
- Employ nonpharmacological healing measures, as indicated (e.g., breathing exercises, listening to music, relaxation tapes, biofeedback, hot or cold applications) *to promote relaxation of muscles and tissue healing as well as improve coping and outlook for positive healing experience.*[2]
- Refer for outpatient/follow-up care, as indicated (e.g., telephone monitoring, home visit, wound care clinic, pain management program, and so forth).

NURSING PRIORITY NO. 4   To promote wellness (Teaching/Discharge Considerations):

- Discuss reality of recovery process and client's/SO's expectations. *Individuals are often unrealistic regarding energy and time required for healing and own abilities/responsibilities to facilitate process.*
- Involve client/SO(s) in setting incremental goals. *Enhances commitment to plan and reduces likelihood of frustration, thus blocking progress.*
- Demonstrate self-care skills, provide client/SO with health-related information and psychosocial support *to manage symptoms and pain, thus enhancing well-being.*
- Refer to physical/occupational therapist, as indicated *to address exercise program and home-care needs and identify assistive devices to facilitate independence in ADLs.*
- Identify suppliers for dressings/wound care items and assistive devices, as needed.
- Consult nutritionist for individual dietary plan *to meet increased nutritional needs that reflect personal situation/resources.*
- Evaluate home situation (e.g., lives alone, bedroom/bathroom on second floor, availability of assistance). *Identifies necessary adjustments, such as moving bedroom to first floor, arranging for commode during recovery, and obtaining an in-home emergency call system.*
- Discuss alternative placement (e.g., convalescent/rehabilitation center, as appropriate). *Brief stay with concentrated support/therapy may speed recovery/return to home.*
- Identify community resources (e.g., visiting nurse, home healthcare agency, Meals on Wheels, respite care). *Facilitates adjustment to home setting.*
- Refer for counseling/support. *May need additional help to overcome feelings of discouragement, deal with changes in life.*

DOCUMENTATION FOCUS

Assessment/Reassessment

- Assessment findings, including individual concerns, family involvement, and support factors/availability of resources.
- Cultural expectations.
- Assistive device use/need.

Planning

- Plan of care and who is involved in planning.
- Teaching plan.

Implementation/Evaluation

- Responses of client/SO(s) to plan/interventions/teaching and actions performed.
- Attainment/progress toward desired outcome(s).
- Modifications to plan of care.

Discharge Planning

- Long-range needs and who is responsible for actions to be taken.
- Specific referrals made.

References

1. ND: Surgical Recovery, delayed. In Cox, H. C., et al. (2002). *Clinical Applications of Nursing Diagnosis: Adult, Child, Women's, Psychiatric, Gerontic, and Home Health Considerations.* 4th ed. Philadelphia: F. A. Davis.
2. No author listed. Post-surgical rehabilitation and healing: benefits of RECOVERY. (Monograph). Surgery, Treatments and Wound Healing with Biostructural Medicine. Accessed July 2007 at www.recoverymedicine.com/post_surgical_healing.htm.
3. Semchyshyn, N., Sengelmann, R. D. (2002, update 2006). Surgical complications. Accessed July 2007 at www.emedicine.com/derm/topic829.htm.
4. Odom-Forren, J. (2006). Preventing surgical site infections. *Nursing2006,* 36(6), 59–63.
5. Stadelmann, W. K., Degenis, A. G., Tobin, G. R. (1998). Impediments to wound healing. *Am J Surg,* 176 (2A suppl), 39S.
6. Purnell, L., Paulanka, B. (1998). *Transcultural Health Care: A Culturally Diverse Approach.* 2d ed. Philadelphia: F. A. Davis.
7. Pieper, B., Sieggreen, M., Freeland, B., et al. (2006). Discharge information needs of patients after surgery. *J Wound, Ostomy and Continence Nursing,* 33(3), 281–290.
8. Dunn, D. (2006). Age-smart care: Preventing perioperative complications in older adults. *Nursing Made Incredibly Easy!,* 4(3), 30–39.
9. Dunn, D. (2005). Preventing preoperative complications in special populations. *Nursing2005,* 35(1), 36–43.

impaired Swallowing

Definition: Abnormal functioning of the swallowing mechanism associated with deficits in oral, pharyngeal, or esophageal structure or function

RELATED FACTORS

Congenital Deficits
Upper airway anomalies; mechanical obstruction (e.g., edema, tracheostomy tube, tumor); history of tube feeding
Neuromuscular impairment (e.g., decreased or absent gag reflex, decreased strength or excursion of muscles involved in mastication, perceptual impairment, facial paralysis); conditions with significant hypotonia
Respiratory disorders; congenital heart disease
Behavioral feeding problems; self-injurious behavior
Failure to thrive; protein energy malnutrition

Neurological Problems
Nasal/nasopharyngeal cavity defects; oropharynx/laryngeal anomalies; tracheal/laryngeal/esophageal defects

Gastroesophageal reflux disease; achalasia
Traumas; acquired anatomic defects; cranial nerve involvement; traumatic head injury
Prematurity; developmental delay; cerebral palsy

DEFINING CHARACTERISTICS

Subjective
Esophageal Phase Impairment
Complaints [reports] of "something stuck"; odynophagia
Food refusal; volume limiting
Heartburn; epigastric pain
Nighttime coughing/awakening

Objective
Oral Phase Impairment
Weak suck resulting in inefficient nippling
Slow bolus formation; lack of tongue action to form bolus; premature entry of bolus
Incomplete lip closure; food pushed out of/falls from mouth
Lack of chewing
Coughing/choking/gagging before a swallow
Piecemeal deglutition; abnormality in oral phase of swallow study
Inability to clear oral cavity; pooling in lateral sulci; nasal reflux; sialorrhea or drooling
Long meals with little consumption
Pharyngeal Phase Impairment
Food refusal
Altered head positions; delayed/multiple swallows
Inadequate laryngeal elevation; abnormality in pharyngeal phase by swallow study
Choking; coughing; gagging; nasal reflux; gurgly voice quality
Unexplained fevers; recurrent pulmonary infections
Esophageal Phase Impairment
Observed evidence of difficulty in swallowing (e.g., stasis of food in oral cavity, coughing/choking); abnormality in esophageal phase by swallow study
Hyperextension of head (e.g., arching during or after meals)
Repetitive swallowing; bruxism
Unexplained irritability surrounding mealtime
Acidic-smelling breath; regurgitation of gastric contents (wet burps); vomitus on pillow; vomiting; hematemesis

Sample Clinical Applications: Brain injury/stroke, neuromuscular conditions (e.g., muscular dystrophy, cerebral palsy, Parkinson's disease, ALS, Guillain-Barré syndrome), facial trauma, head/neck cancer, radical neck surgery/laryngectomy, cleft lip/palate, tracheoesophageal fistula, gastroesophageal reflux disease, dementia

DESIRED OUTCOMES/EVALUATION CRITERIA
Sample NOC linkages:
Swallowing Status: Safe passage of fluids and solids from the mouth to the stomach
Self-Care: Eating: Ability to prepare and ingest food and fluid independently with or without assistive device

---

Client Will (Include Specific Time Frame)

- Pass food and fluid from mouth to stomach safely.
- Maintain adequate hydration as evidenced by good skin turgor, moist mucous membranes, and individually appropriate urine output.
- Achieve or maintain desired body weight.

Sample NOC linkage:
Risk Control: Personal actions to prevent, eliminate, or reduce modifiable health threats

Client/Caregiver Will (Include Specific Time Frame)

- Verbalize understanding of causative/contributing factors.
- Identify individually appropriate interventions/actions to promote intake and prevent aspiration.
- Demonstrate feeding methods appropriate to the individual situation.
- Demonstrate emergency measures in the event of choking.

ACTIONS/INTERVENTIONS

Sample NIC linkages:
Swallowing Therapy: Facilitating swallowing and preventing complications of impaired swallowing
Aspiration Precautions: Prevention or minimization of risk factors in the patient at risk for aspiration
Airway Suctioning: Removal of airway secretions by inserting a suction catheter into the patient's oral airway or trachea

NURSING PRIORITY NO. 1 To assess causative/contributing factors and degree of impairment:

- ∞ Evaluate client's potential for swallowing problems, noting age and medical conditions (e.g., Parkinson's, multiple sclerosis, myasthenia gravis/other neuromuscular conditions). *Swallowing disorders are especially common in elderly, possibly due to coexistence of variety of neurological, neuromuscular, or other conditions. Infants at risk include those born prematurely, or with tracheoesophageal fistula, or lip and palate malformation. Persons with traumatic brain injuries often exhibit swallowing impairments, regardless of gender or age.*[1-4]
- Determine current situation (e.g., intubation, surgery of head/neck/jaw; cervical spine injury, vocal cord paralysis, problems with saliva production or management; pain with swallowing; mental or anxiety disorder).[12]
- Assess client's cognitive and sensory-motor functional status. *Sensory awareness, orientation, concentration, and motor coordination affect desire and ability to swallow safely and effectively.*[7]
- Note voice quality and speech. *Abnormal voice (dysphonia) and abnormal speech patterns (dysarthria) are signs of motor dysfunction of structures involved in oral and pharyngeal swallowing.*[1]
- Note symmetry of facial structures/muscle tone. Assess strength and excursion of muscles involved in chewing and swallowing. Evaluate ability to swallow using small sips of water.
- Note hyperextension of head/arching of neck during/after meals, or repetitive swallowing, *which suggests inability to complete swallowing process.*

- Determine infant's ability to initiate/sustain effective suck. *Weak suck results in inefficient nippling, suggesting ineffective movement of tongue and mouth muscles, impairing ability to swallow.*
- Ascertain presence and strength of cough and gag reflex. *Although absence of gag reflex is not necessarily predictive of client's eventual ability to swallow safely, it does increase client's potential for aspiration (overt or silent).*[1,4] *Coughing, drooling, double swallowing, decreased ability to move food in mouth, and throat clearing with/after swallowing is indicative of swallowing dysfunction and increases risk for aspiration.*[1,8,9]
- Auscultate breath sounds *to evaluate the presence of aspiration, especially if client is coughing with intake or has a "gurgly or gargly" voice.*[8]
- Inspect oropharyngeal cavity for edema, inflammation, altered integrity of oral mucosa/structures (e.g., lesions or tumors of the mouth/oral cavity and throat).[1,6]
- Evaluate state of detention (e.g., poor/missing teeth, ill-fitting dentures) and adequacy of oral hygiene.
- Review medications *that may affect oropharyngeal function (e.g., benzodiazapines, neuroleptics, anticonvulsants, anticholinergics, opioids, antidepessants, antineoplastics, diuretics), thus impairing swallowing by means of sedation, pharyngeal weakness, dry mouth, etc.*[1,5]
- Review laboratory test results for underlying problems (e.g., *candida*/other infections; Cushing's disease/other metabolic conditions) *that can affect swallowing.*[5]
- Prepare for/assist with diagnostic testing of swallowing activity (e.g., transnasal or esophageal endoscopy, videofluorographic swallow studies [VFSS]; fiber-optic endoscopic examination of swallowing techniques [FEEST]) *to identify the pathophysiology of swallowing disorder.*[1,6,13]

NURSING PRIORITY NO. 2 To prevent aspiration and maintain airway patency:

- Withhold oral feedings until appropriate diagnostic workup is completed *to determine client's individual factors causing impaired swallowing and identify specific needs.*
- Consult with physician/dietitian regarding meeting current nutritional needs. *May need enteral (preferably by gastrostomy [PEG] tube) or parenteral feedings in order to obtain nutrition, while reducing risk of aspiration that could accompany nasogastric feedings.*[10]
- Move client to chair for meals, snacks, and drinks when possible; if client must be in bed, raise head of bed as upright as possible with head in anatomic alignment and slightly flexed forward during feeding. Keep HOB elevated for 30 to 45 minutes after feeding, if possible, *to reduce risk of regurgitation/aspiration.*[12,14]
- Instruct client to cough and expectorate *when secretion management is of concern.*
- Have suction equipment available during initial feeding attempts and as indicated. Suction oral cavity if client cannot clear secretions *to prevent aspiration.*
- Instruct client in self-suctioning techniques, when appropriate (e.g., for drooling, frequent choking, structural changes in mouth/throat). *Promotes independence/sense of control.*

NURSING PRIORITY NO. 3 To enhance swallowing ability to meet fluid and caloric body requirements:

- Consult with physician/speech pathologist/dysphagia specialist/gastroenterologist/rehabilitation team, as indicated. *Therapies may consist of dietary modification, compensatory movements, medical or surgical procedures, etc. For example, medications may help with underlying condition (e.g., swallowing problem associated with Parkinson's disease), surgery (e.g., reconstructive facial surgery following trauma or to correct structural defect in infant), or esophageal dilatation when impaired sphincter function or esophageal strictures impede swallowing. Client/SO may learn specific retraining or compensatory techniques (e.g., modifying head and neck posture, strengthening of swallowing muscles, or techniques of food placement in mouth).*[1,6,13–15]

🏠 • Encourage a rest period before meals *if fatigue is interfering with efforts.*

🏠 • Provide analgesics (with caution) before feeding, as indicated, *to enhance comfort, but avoiding decreasing awareness/sensory perception.*

🏠 • Implement dietary modifications as indicated:[1,6,13–15]

Provide proper consistency of food/fluid. *Foods that can be formed into a bolus before swallowing such as gelatin desserts prepared with less water than usual, pudding, and custard; thickened liquids (addition of thickening agent, or yogurt, cream soups prepared with less water), thinned purees (hot cereal with water added) or thick drinks such as nectars or fruit juices that have been frozen into "slush" consistency, medium-soft boiled or scrambled eggs, canned fruit, soft-cooked vegetables are most easily swallowed.*

Feed one consistency or texture of food at a time. *Single textured foods (e.g., pudding, hot cereal, pureed food) should be tolerated well before advancing to soft table foods.*[10]

Avoid milk products and chocolate, *which may thicken oral secretions and impair swallowing,* and sticky foods (e.g., peanut butter, white bread) *that are difficult to swallow or need fluids to completely swallow.*[10]

Ensure temperature (hot or cold versus tepid) of foods/fluid, *which will stimulate sensory receptors.*

Avoid pouring liquid into the mouth or "washing food down" with liquid. *May cause client to lose control of food bolus, increasing risk of aspiration. Note: To avoid posterior head tilting while drinking, some people find drinking from a straw easier than sipping from a cup (if a straw is easier, consider using a flexible one-way straw); if a cup is easier, consider using a "nosey" cup that is double handled and made of durable plastic.*

Feed smaller, more frequent meals *to limit fatigue associated with eating efforts and to promote adequate nutritional intake.*

Determine food preferences of client and present foods in an appealing, attractive manner. *Client may make effort to overcome swallowing problems when food is appealing and desired.*

🏠 • Provide/encourage proper food placement, chewing, and swallowing techniques:[1,6,13–15]

Provide cognitive cues and specific directions (e.g., remind client to "open mouth, chew, or swallow now"), as indicated, *to enhance concentration and performance of swallowing sequence.*

Focus attention on feeding/swallowing activity by decreasing environmental stimuli, *which may be distracting during feeding. Also, if client is talking or laughing while eating, risk of aspiration is increased.*[11]

Position client on the unaffected side when appropriate, placing food in this side of mouth and having client use the tongue *to assist with managing the food when one side of the mouth is affected (e.g., hemiplegia).*

Manage size of bites—use a small spoon/cut all solid foods into small pieces (e.g., *small bites 1/2 tsp. or less are usually easier to swallow).*

Place food midway in oral cavity *to adequately trigger the swallowing reflex.*

Massage the laryngopharyngeal musculature (sides of trachea and neck) gently *to stimulate swallowing.*

Observe oral cavity after each bite and have client check around cheeks with tongue for remaining/unswallowed food *to prevent overloading mouth with food/reduce risk of aspiration.*

Allow ample time for eating (feeding). Incorporate client's eating style and pace when feeding *to avoid fatigue and frustration with process.*

Remain with client during meal *to reduce anxiety and provide assistance if needed.*

Provide positive feedback for client's efforts. *Encourages continuation of efforts/attainment of goals.*

Discontinue feeding and remove any food from mouth if client choking/unable to swallow *to reduce potential for aspiration.*

- Provide oral hygiene following each feeding. *To clear mouth of retained food particles, reduce risk of infection/dental carries.*
- Monitor intake, output, and body weight *to evaluate adequacy of fluid and caloric intake and need for changes to therapeutic regimen.*
- Discuss use of tube feedings/parenteral solutions as indicated *for the client unable to achieve adequate nutritional intake.*
- Refer to lactation counselor/support group (e.g., La Leche League) *for breastfeeding guidance/problem-solving.* (Refer to NDs ineffective Breastfeeding; ineffective Infant Feeding Pattern for additional interventions for infants.)

NURSING PRIORITY NO. 4 To promote wellness (Teaching/Discharge Considerations):

- Consult with nutritionist *to establish optimum dietary plan considering specific pathology, nutritional needs, available resources.* (Refer to ND risk for imbalanced Nutrition: less than body requirements.)
- Establish routine schedule for obtaining weight (same time of day/clothes) and specific weight loss/gain to be reported to primary care provider. *Facilitates timely intervention to change regimen as needed.*
- Consult with pharmacist *to determine if pills may be crushed or if liquids/capsules are available.* Administer medication in gelatin, jelly, or puddings as appropriate.
- Instruct client and/or SO in specific feeding/swallowing techniques. *Enhances client safety and independence.*
- Demonstrate/instruct client/SO in emergency measures in event of choking *to prevent aspiration/more serious complications.*
- Encourage continuation of facial exercise program *to maintain/improve muscle strength.*
- Recommend avoiding food intake within 3 hours of bedtime, eliminating alcohol and caffeine intake, reducing weight if needed, using stress-reduction techniques, and elevating head of bed during sleep *to limit potential for gastric reflux and aspiration.*

DOCUMENTATION FOCUS

Assessment/Reassessment

- Individual findings, including degree/characteristics of impairment, current weight/recent changes.
- Effects on lifestyle/socialization and nutritional status.

Planning

- Plan of care and who is involved in planning.
- Teaching plan.

Implementation/Evaluation

- Response to interventions/teaching and actions performed.
- Attainment/progress toward desired outcome(s).
- Modifications to plan of care.

Discharge Planning

- Long-term needs and who is responsible for actions to be taken.
- Available resources and specific referrals made.

References

1. Palmer, J. B., Drennan, J. C., Baba, M. (2000). Evaluation and treatment of swallowing impairments. Accessed July 2007 at www.aafp.org/afp/20000415/2453.html.
2. Engel, J. (2002). *Pocket Guide to Pediatric Assessment*. 4th ed. St. Louis, MO: Mosby, p. 158.
3. Kosta, J. C., Mitchell, C. A. (1998). Current procedures for diagnosing dysphagia in elderly clients. *Geriatr Nurs*, 19(4), 195.
4. Leder, S. B. (1999). Fiberoptic endoscopic evaluation of swallowing in patients with acute traumatic brain injury. *J Head Trauma Rehabil*, 14(5), 448–453.
5. American Gastroenterological Association. (1999). Medical position statement on management of oropharyngeal dysphagia.. *Gastroenterology*, 116(2), 452–454.
6. No author listed. Swallowing problems (dysphagia). College of Physicians and Surgeons, Department of Otolaryngology/Head and Neck Surgery. Accessed July 2007 at www.entcolumbia.org/dysphag.htm.
7. Poertner, L. C., Coleman, R. F. (1998). Swallowing therapy in adults. *Otolaryngol Clin North Am*, 31(3), 56.
8. Lugger, K. E. (1994). Dysphagia in the elderly stroke patient. *J Neurosci Nurs*, 26, 78.
9. Baker, D. M. (1993). Assessment and management of impairments in swallowing. *Nurs Clin North Am*, 28, 793.
10. Fine, R., Ackley, B. J. (2002). ND: Impaired Swallowing. In Ackley, B. J., Ladwig, G. B. *Nursing Diagnosis Handbook: A Guide to Planning Care*. 5th ed. St. Louis, MO: Mosby, pp. 735, 736.
11. Galvan, T. J. (2001). Dysphagia: Going down and staying down. *Am J Nurs*, 101(1), 37–42.
12. Haines, C. (2006). Digestive diseases: Swallowing problems. Article for Medicinenet. Retrieved April 2007 at www.medicinetnet.com/swallowing/.
13. National Institute for Neurological Disorders and Stroke (NINDS). (2007). Swallowing disorders information page. Retrieved April 2007 at www.ninds.nih.gov/.
14. Searle, J. (No date listed). Eating and swallowing: Fact sheet regarding Huntington's disease. Retrieved April 2007 at http://huntingtondisease.tripod.com/swallowing/id22.html.
15. McCarron, K. (2006). The shakedown on Parkinson's disease. *Nursing Made Incredibly Easy!*, 4(6), 40–49.

effective Therapeutic Regimen Management

Definition: Pattern of regulating and integrating into daily living a program for treatment of illness and its sequelae that is satisfactory for meeting specific health goals

RELATED FACTORS

To be developed by nurse researchers and submitted to NANDA

[Complexity of healthcare management; therapeutic regimen]

[Added demands made on individual or family]

[Adequate social supports]

DEFINING CHARACTERISTICS

Subjective

Verbalizes desire to manage the treatment of illness/prevention of sequelae

Verbalizes intent to reduce risk factors for progression of illness and sequelae

Objective

Appropriate choices of daily activities for meeting the goals of a treatment or prevention program

Illness symptoms that are within a normal range of expectation

Cultural   Collaborative   Community/Home Care   Diagnostic Studies   Pediatric/Geriatric/Lifespan   Medications

Sample Clinical Applications: Chronic conditions (e.g., asthma, arthritis, systemic lupus), genetic/congenital conditions (e.g., sickle cell anemia, spina bifida)

DESIRED OUTCOMES/EVALUATION CRITERIA

Sample NOC linkages:

Symptom Control: Personal actions to minimize perceived adverse changes in physical and emotional functioning

Knowledge: Treatment Regimen: Extent of understanding conveyed about a specific treatment regimen

Participation in Healthcare Decisions: Personal involvement in selecting and evaluating healthcare options to achieve desired outcome

Client Will (Include Specific Time Frame)

- Develop plan to address individual risk factors for progression of illness/sequelae.
- Demonstrate effective problem-solving in integrating changes of therapeutic regimen into lifestyle.
- Identify/use available resources.
- Remain free of preventable complications/progression of illness and sequelae.

ACTIONS/INTERVENTIONS

Sample NIC linkages:

Health System Guidance: Facilitating a patient's location and use of appropriate health services

Health Education: Developing and providing instruction and learning experiences to facilitate voluntary adaptation of behavior conducive to health in individuals, families, groups, or communities

Anticipatory Guidance: Preparation of patient for an anticipated developmental or situational crisis

NURSING PRIORITY NO. 1 To assess situation and individual needs:

- Ascertain client's knowledge/understanding of condition and treatment needs. Note specific health goals. *Provides a basis for determining direction client wants to go and planning individualized care.*[1]
- Identify individual's perceptions of adaptation to treatment/anticipated changes. *How client sees the situation is important to discussing what is happening in regard to the treatment regimen and planning for the future.*[1]
- Note treatments added to present regimen and client's/SO's associated learning needs. *As changes are made, client needs to understand what the new medication/treatment is for and what to expect, as well as how it fits into the current regimen. Understanding these issues helps client feel confident in incorporating new treatments.*[3]
- Determine client's/family's health goals, patterns of healthcare, and associated cultural/religious beliefs. *Provides information about current behaviors, possible misperceptions, and areas of potential conflict such as values, cultural mores, religious beliefs, or financial concerns.*[1]
- Discuss present resources used by client, and possible need for change. *Continuing to monitor needs, such as hours of home-care assistance, access to case manager, and making changes as indicated, supports complex/long-term program.*[3]

NURSING PRIORITY NO. 2 To assist client/SO(s) in developing strategies to meet increased demands of therapeutic regimen:

- Identify steps necessary to reach desired health goal(s). *Promotes understanding that goal(s) can only be reached by knowing what needs to be done as treatment regimen progresses.*[5]
- Accept client's evaluation of own strengths/limitations while working together to improve abilities. *Promotes sense of self-esteem and confidence to continue efforts.*[3]
- Provide information about individual healthcare needs, using client's/SO's perferred learning style and tools (e.g., books, articles, television reports, pictures, audiovideo, computer databases). *Promotes sense of control and confidence in own ability to be able to learn about illness/condition and be in charge of own treatment regimen.*[5]
- Encourage client/SO to ask questions, check information with their own healthcare provider, who can recommend articles/books or reliable Internet sites. *Remind client that not all information is written by qualified medical experts.*[6]
- Acknowledge individual's efforts, capabilities, and skills to acquire/maintain interpersonal, self-care, and coping skills. *Reinforces client's movement toward attainment of desired outcomes.*[5,7]

NURSING PRIORITY NO. 3 To promote wellness (Teaching/Discharge Considerations):

- Promote client/caregiver choices and involvement in planning and implementing added tasks/responsibilities. *Individuals gain self-esteem by being involved in the daily planning of care when they have sufficient support and are given options about what they can do.*[3]
- Provide for follow-up contact (e.g., clinic/home visit; telephone/e-mail) as appropriate. *Encourages continuation of therapeutic regimen and opportunity to help client/family identify needs and solutions as they arise, preventing untoward complications.*[3,7]
- Assist in implementing strategies for monitoring progress/responses to therapeutic regimen. *Promotes proactive problem-solving to maintain effectiveness of regimen.*[5]
- Mobilize support systems, including peers, family/SO(s), social, financial, etc. *When client gets the support needed to master and sustain self-management, there are potential benefits for individual health and the overall healthcare system. When these issues are managed well, client/family can attend to the process of recovery or (in the case of chronic illness) learn to live well with situation.*[1,4,8]
- Refer to community support systems, as indicated, *for assistance with lifestyle/relationship issues, finances, housing, or legal concerns (e.g., advance directives, healthcare choices).*[2]

DOCUMENTATION FOCUS

Assessment/Reassessment

- Findings, including dynamics of individual situation.
- Individual strengths/additional needs.
- Cultural/religious beliefs and expectations.

Planning

- Plan of care and who is involved in planning.
- Teaching plan.

Cultural   Collaborative   Community/Home Care   Diagnostic Studies   Pediatric/Geriatric/Lifespan   Medications

Implementation/Evaluation

- Response to interventions/teaching and actions performed.
- Attainment/progress toward desired outcome(s).
- Modifications to plan of care.

Discharge Planning

- Short-range and long-range needs and who is responsible for actions.
- Available resources, specific referrals made

References

1. Cox, H. C., et al. (2002). *Clinical Applications of Nursing Diagnosis: Adult, Child, Women's, Psychiatric, Gerontic, and Home Health Considerations.* 4th ed. Philadelphia: F A. Davis.
2. Healthy People 2010 Toolkit, A Field Guide to Health Planning. (2002). Washington, DC: Public Health Foundation.
3. Stuifbergen, A. (1997). Health promotion: An essential component of rehabilitation for persons with chronic disabling conditions. *ADV Nurs Sci*, 19(4), 147–148.
4. Larsen, L. S. (1998). Effectiveness of counseling intervention to assist family caregivers of chronically ill relatives. *J Psychosoc Nurs*, 36(8), 26.
5. Lai, S. C., Cohen, M. N. (1999). Promoting lifestyle changes. *AJN*, 99(4), 63.
6. NIAMS. How to Find Medical Information. National Instiute of Arthritis and Musculoskelatal and Skin Diseases. Accessed July 2007 at www.niams.nih.gov/hi/topics/howto/howto.htm.
7. New York State Office of Mental Health Wellness. Self-management: Evidenced based practices: Accessed July 2007 at www.omh.state.ny.us/omhweb/ebp/adult_wellness.htm.
8. Heisler, M. (2006). Building peer support programs to manage chronic disease: Seven models for success. Article for Chronic Disease Care Web site. Accessed July 2007 at www.chcf.org/topics/chronicdisease/index.cfm?itemID=127997.

ineffective Therapeutic Regimen Management

Definition: Pattern of regulating and integrating into daily living a program for treatment of illness and the sequelae of illness that is unsatisfactory for meeting specific health goals

RELATED FACTORS
Complexity of healthcare system/therapeutic regimen
Decisional conflicts
Economic difficulties
Excessive demands made (e.g., individual or family); family conflict
Family patterns of healthcare
Inadequate number and types of cues to action
Knowledge deficits
Mistrust of regimen/healthcare personnel
Perceived seriousness/susceptibility/barriers/benefits
Powerlessness
Social support deficits

DEFINING CHARACTERISTICS

Subjective
Verbalizes desire to manage the illness
Verbalizes difficulty with prescribed regimen

Objective
Failure to include treatment regimens in daily routines/take action to reduce risk factors
Makes choices in daily living ineffective for meeting the health goals
[Unexpected acceleration of illness symptoms]

Sample Clinical Applications: Chronic conditions (e.g., COPD, MS, arthritis, chronic pain, end-stage liver/renal failure) or new diagnoses necessitating lifestyle changes

DESIRED OUTCOMES/EVALUATION CRITERIA
Sample NOC linkages:
Treatment Behavior: Illness or Injury: Personal actions to palliate or eliminate pathology
Health Beliefs: Personal convictions that influence health behaviors
Adherence Behavior: Self-initiated actions to promote wellness, recovery, and rehabilitation

Client Will (Include Specific Time Frame)

- Verbalize acceptance of need/desire to change actions to achieve agreed-on health goals.
- Verbalize understanding of factors/blocks involved in individual situation.
- Participate in problem-solving of factors interfering with integration of therapeutic regimen.
- Demonstrate behaviors/changes in lifestyle necessary to maintain therapeutic regimen.
- Identify/use available resources.

ACTIONS/INTERVENTIONS

Sample NIC linkages:
Self-Modification Assistance: Reinforcement of self-directed change initiated by the patient to achieve personally important goals
Health System Guidance: Facilitating a patient's location and use of appropriate health services
Client Contracting: Negotiating an agreement with a patient that reinforces a specific behavior change

NURSING PRIORITY NO. 1 To identify causative/contributing factors:

- Ascertain client's knowledge/understanding of condition and treatment needs. *Provides a baseline so planning care can begin where the client is in relation to condition/illness and current regimen.*[1]
- Determine client's/family's health goals and patterns of healthcare. *Provides information about current behaviors/misperceptions that may be potential areas of conflict, values, or financial considerations.*[1]
- Identify cultural values/religious beliefs affecting client's view of situation and willingness to make necessary changes. *Expectations of others may dictate client's adaptation to situation and willingness to modify life.*[8]
- Identify client locus of control. *Those with an internal locus of control (e.g., expressions of responsibility for self and ability to control outcomes, such as "I didn't quit smoking") are more likely to take charge of situation, whereas individuals with an external locus of control (e.g., expressions of lack of control over self and environment, such as "Nothing ever works out" or "What bad luck to get lung cancer") may perceive difficulties as beyond his or her control and will look to others/external source to solve his or her problems and take care of them.*[7,8]

- Identify individual perceptions and expectations of treatment regimen. *May reveal misinformation, unrealistic expectations, or other factors that may be interfering with client's willingness to follow therapeutic regimen.*[1]
- Determine issues of secondary gain for the client/SO(s). *Marital/family concern or attention, school/work issues, or financial considerations may subconsciously prolong recovery and interfere with complying with prescribed treatment.*
- Review complexity of treatment regimen (e.g., number of expected tasks, such as taking medication four times/day or once/day), and evaluate how difficult tasks might be for client (e.g., must stop smoking or must follow strict dialysis diet even when feeling well, etc.). *These factors are often involved in lack of participation in treatment plan.*
- Note availability/use of resources for assistance, caregiving/respite care. *Client may not have, be aware of, or know how to access resources that may be available.*[6]

NURSING PRIORITY NO. 2 To assist client/SO(s) to develop strategies to improve management of therapeutic regimen:

- Use therapeutic communication skills to assist client to problem-solve solution(s). *Active-listening promotes accurate identification of the problem, ensuring that problem-solving is directed to the correct solution.*[7]
- Explore client involvement in or lack of mutual goal-setting. *Understanding client's willingness to be involved or not provides insight into the reasons for these actions and appropriate interventions.*[7]
- Have client identify consequences of current behaviors/ineffective management of condition. *May help client visualize the "cost" of lack of commitment to therapeutic regimen.*
- Use client's locus of control to develop individual plan to adapt regimen (*e.g., for client with internal control, encourage client to take control of own care and for those with external control, begin with small tasks and add as tolerated*).[7]
- Identify steps necessary to reach desired goal(s). *Specifying steps to take requires discussion and the use of critical thinking skills to determine how to best reach the agreed-on goals.*[4]
- Contract with the client for participation in care. *By making a contract, client commits self to therapeutic regimen and is more likely to follow through because of commitment.*[6]
- Accept client's evaluation of own strengths/limitations while working together to improve abilities. State belief in client's ability to cope and/or adapt to situation. *Individuals often minimize own strengths and exaggerate limitations when faced with the difficulties of a chronic illness. By helping in concrete ways, client can begin to accept reality of strengths. Stating your belief in positive terms lets client hear someone else's evaluation and begin to accept that he or she can manage the situation.*[3]
- Acknowledge individual efforts/capabilities. Positive reinforcement *encourages continuation of desired behaviors and facilitates movement toward attainment of desired outcomes.*[5,7]
- Provide information as well as help client to know where and how to find it on own. Reinforce previous instructions and rationale, using a variety of learning modalities, including role-playing, demonstration, written materials, and so forth. *Incorporating multiple modalities promotes retention of information. Developing client's skill at finding own information encourages self-sufficiency and sense of self-worth.*[2]

NURSING PRIORITY NO. 3 To promote wellness (Teaching/Discharge Considerations):

- Emphasize importance of client knowledge and understanding of the need for treatment/medication as well as consequences of actions/choices. *Reinforces client's role in success of therapeutic regimen, encouraging continuation of competent behaviors.*[1]

Nursing Diagnoses in Alphabetical Order

• Promote client/caregiver/SO(s) participation in planning and evaluating process. *Enhances commitment to plan, optimizing outcomes.*[1]

• Assist client to develop strategies for monitoring therapeutic regimen. *Promotes early recognition of changes, allowing proactive response.*[5]

• Mobilize support systems, including family/SO(s), social, financial, and so on. *Success of therapeutic regimen is enhanced by using support systems effectively, avoiding stress and worry of dealing with unresolved problems.*[2]

• Refer to counseling/therapy (group and individual) as indicated. *May need additional help to deal with stress and anxiety of chronic condition/illness.*[1]

• Identify home- and community-based nursing services. *Provides services for assessment, follow-up care, and education in client's home to promote continuation of effective management of therapeutic regimen.*[1]

DOCUMENTATION FOCUS

Assessment/Reassessment

• Findings, including underlying dynamics of individual situation, client's perception of problem/needs, locus of control.
• Cultural values, religious beliefs.
• Family involvement/needs.
• Individual strengths/limitations.
• Availability/use of resources.

Planning

• Plan of care and who is involved in planning.
• Teaching plan.

Implementation/Evaluation

• Response to interventions/teaching and actions performed.
• Attainment/progress toward desired outcome(s).
• Modifications to plan of care.

Discharge Planning

• Long-range needs and who is responsible for actions to be taken.
• Available resources, specific referrals made.

References

1. Cox, H. C., et al. (2002). *Clinical Applications of Nursing Diagnosis: Adult, Child, Women's, Psychiatric, Gerontic, and Home Health Considerations.* 4th ed. Philadelphia: F. A. Davis.
2. Healthy People 2010 Toolkit: A Field Guide to Health Planning. (2002). Washington, DC: Public Health Foundation.
3. Stuifbergen, A. (1997). Health promotion: An essential component of rehabilitation for persons with chronic disabling conditions. *ADV Nurs Sci,* 19(4), 147–148.
4. Larsen L. S. (1998). Effectiveness of counseling intervention to assist family caregivers of chronically ill relatives. *J Psychosoc Nurs,* 36(8), 26.
5. Lai, S. C., Cohen, M. N. (1999). Promoting lifestyle changes. *AJN,* 99(4), 63.
6. Miller, J. F. (1999). *Coping with Chronic Illness: Overcoming Powerlessness.* 3d ed. Philadelphia: F. A. Davis.
7. Townsend, M. C. (2003). *Psychiatric Mental Health Nursing Concepts of Care.* 4th ed. Philadelphia: F. A. Davis.
8. Lipson, J. G., Dibble, S. L., Minarik, P. A. (1996). *Culture & Nursing Care: A Pocket Guide.* San Francisco: UCSF Nursing Press.

⊕ Cultural   Ⓐ Collaborative   🏠 Community/Home Care   ✎ Diagnostic Studies   ∞ Pediatric/Geriatric/Lifespan   💊 Medications

ineffective community Therapeutic Regimen Management

Definition: Pattern of regulating and integrating into community processes programs for treatment of illness and the sequelae of illness that are unsatisfactory for meeting health-related goals

RELATED FACTORS

To be developed by nurse researchers and submitted to NANDA
[Lack of safety for community members]
[Economic insecurity]
[Healthcare not available]
[Unhealthy environment]
[Education not available for all community members]
[Lack of means to meet human needs for recognition, fellowship, security, and membership]

DEFINING CHARACTERISTICS

Subjective
[Community members/agencies verbalize overburdening of resources/inability to meet therapeutic needs of all members]

Objective
Deficits in advocates for aggregates
Deficit in community activities for prevention
Illness symptoms above the norm expected for the population; unexpected acceleration of illness
Insufficient healthcare resources (e.g., people, programs); unavailable healthcare resources for illness care
[Deficits in community for collaboration and development of coalitions to address needs]

Sample Clinical Applications: HIV/AIDS, substance abuse, sexually transmitted diseases, teen pregnancy, prematurity, acute lead poisoning, influenza, SARS

DESIRED OUTCOMES/EVALUATION CRITERIA

Sample NOC linkages:

Community Competence: Capacity of a community to collectively problem-solve to achieve community goals

Community Health Status: General state of well-being of a community or population

Community Risk Control: Communicable Disease: Community actions to eliminate or reduce the spread of infectious agents that threaten public health

Community Will (Include Specific Time Frame)

• Identify both strengths and limitations affecting community treatment programs for meeting health-related goals.
• Participate in problem-solving of factors interfering with regulating and integrating community programs.
• Report unexpected acceleration/illness symptoms near norm expected for the incidence or prevalence of disease(s).

ACTIONS/INTERVENTIONS

Sample NIC linkages:

Community Health Development: Facilitating members of a community to identify a community's health concerns, mobilize resources, and implement solutions

Program Development: Planning, implementing, and evaluating a coordinated set of activities designed to enhance wellness, or to prevent, reduce, or eliminate one or more health problems of a group or community

Health Policy Monitoring: Surveillance and influence of government and organization regulations, rules, and standards that affect nursing systems and practices to ensure quality care of patients

NURSING PRIORITY NO. 1   To identify causative/precipitating factors:

- Evaluate community healthcare resources for illness/sequelae of illness. *Identifying current available resources provides a starting point to determine needs of the community and plan for future needs.*[1]
- Note reports from members of the community regarding ineffective/inadequate community functioning. *Provides feedback from people who live in the community and avail themselves of resources, thus presenting a realistic picture of problem areas.*[2]
- Determine areas of conflict among members of community. *Cultural/religious beliefs, values, social mores, and lack of a shared vision may limit dialogue or creative problem-solving if not addressed.*[4]
- Investigate unexpected acceleration of illness in the community. *Prompt identification of illness, such as West Nile virus, or HIV allows community to develop plan of care and intervene to prevent further spread with possibility of becoming epidemic.*[2]
- Identify strengths/limitations of community resources and community commitment to change. *Knowledge of these factors is important for developing a plan for community improvement. Without this information, any plan will have difficulty succeeding.*[2]
- Ascertain effect of related factors on community activities. *Issues of safety, poor air quality, lack of education/information, lack of sufficient healthcare facilities affect citizens and how they view their community—whether it is a healthy, positive environment in which to live or lacks adequate healthcare/safety resources.*[1]
- Determine knowledge/understanding of treatment regimen. *Citizens need to know and understand what is being proposed to correct the identified deficiencies, before they are willing to be involved and actively support goals of the treatmemt regimen.*[1]
- Note use of resources available to community for developing/funding programs. *May require creative program planning to utilize resources to meet multiple needs.*

NURSING PRIORITY NO. 2   To assist community to develop strategies to improve community functioning/management:

- Foster cooperative spirit of community without negating individuality of members/groups. *As individuals feel valued and respected, they are more willing to work together with others to develop plan for identifying and improving healthcare for the community.*[2]
- Involve community in determining healthcare goals and prioritizing them to facilitate planning process. *The goal is healthy people in a healthy community, and as community members*

become involved and see that by prioritizing the identified goals, progress can be seen as individuals become healthier and needed services become readily available.[2]

 • Plan together with community health and social agencies to problem-solve solutions identified and anticipated problems/needs. *Working together promotes a sense of involvement and control, helping people implement more effective problem-solving.*[3]

• Identify specific populations at risk or underserved to actively involve them in process. *Populations, such as low-income/poor families, migrant, immigrant, and homeless as well as racial and ethnic minorities need to be involved in problem identification and solutions, because they are closely involved in the issues they face on a daily basis and can provide important facts to be considered. Being part of the solution empowers these groups and promotes continued participation in the process.*[3,5]

• Create teaching plan/form speakers' bureau. *Disseminating information to community members regarding value of treatment/preventive programs helps people know and understand the importance of these actions and be willing to support the programs.*[3]

NURSING PRIORITY NO. 3 To promote wellness (Teaching/Discharge Considerations):

• Assist community to develop a plan for continued assessment of community needs and functioning (e.g., access to adequate healthcare; education regarding disease prevention, public health threats, and immunization; local warning system and evacuation plan in event of disaster; emergency contact numbers; planning for community members with special needs [including elderly, handicapped, low-income]; violence prevention, personal/property protection; water/sanitation/toxic substance management, mobilization of local/state/national resources, etc.). *Promotes proactive approach in planning for the future and continuation of efforts to improve healthy behaviors and necessary services.*[1,5]

• Encourage community to form partnerships within the community and between the community and the larger society. *Aids in long-term planning for anticipated/projected needs/concerns to assure the quality and accessibility of health services.*[1]

DOCUMENTATION FOCUS

Assessment/Reassessment

• Assessment findings, including members' perceptions of community problems, healthcare resources
• Community use of available resources.

Planning

• Plan and who is involved in planning process.
• Teaching plan.

Implementation/Evaluation

• Community's response to plan/interventions and actions performed.
• Attainment/progress toward desired outcome(s).
• Modifications to plan.

Discharge Planning

• Long-range goals and who is responsible for actions to be taken.
• Specific referrals made.

Nursing Diagnoses in Alphabetical Order

References

1. Environmental Health Competency Project: Draft Recommendations for Non-Technical Competencies at the Local Level. Washington, DC: American Public Health Association. Accessed July 2007 at www.apha.org/programs/standards/healthcompproject/.
2. Public Health in America. (September 1994). Washington, DC: American Public Health Association. July 2007. Available at www.health.gov/phfunctions/public.
3. Healthy People 2010 Toolkit: A Field Guide to Health Planning. (2002). Washington, DC: Public Health Foundation.
4. Cox, H. C., et al. (2002). *Clinical Applications of Nursing Diagnosis: Adult, Child, Women's, Psychiatric, Gerontic, and Home Health Considerations.* 4th ed. Philadelphia: F. A. Davis.
5. U.S. Department of Human Services. Centers for Disease Control and Prevention. CDC Health Protection Goals Accessed July 2007 at www.cdc.gov/index.htm.

ineffective family Therapeutic Regimen Management

Definition: Pattern of regulating and integrating into family processes a program for treatment of illness and the sequelae of illness that is unsatisfactory for meeting specific health goals

RELATED FACTORS
Complexity of therapeutic/healthcare system
Decisional conflicts
Economic difficulties
Excessive demands; family conflicts

DEFINING CHARACTERISTICS

Subjective
Verbalizes difficulty with therapeutic regimen
Verbalizes desire to manage the illness

Objective
Inappropriate family activities for meeting health goals
Acceleration of illness symptoms of a family member
Failure to take action to reduce risk factors; lack of attention to illness

Sample Clinical Applications: Chronic conditions (e.g., COPD, MS, arthritis, chronic pain, substance abuse, end-stage liver/renal failure) or new diagnoses necessitating lifestyle changes

DESIRED OUTCOMES/EVALUATION CRITERIA
Sample NOC linkages:
Family Health Status: Overall health and social competence of family unit
Family Participation in Professional Care: Family involvement in decision making, delivery, and evaluation of care provided by healthcare personnel
Family Functioning: Capacity of the family to meet the needs of its members during developmental transitions

Family Will (Include Specific Time Frame)

• Identify individual factors affecting regulation/integration of treatment program.
• Participate in problem-solving of identified factors.

Cultural   Collaborative   Community/Home Care   Diagnostic Studies   Pediatric/Geriatric/Lifespan   Medications

- Verbalize acceptance of need/desire to change actions to achieve agreed-on outcomes or health goals.
- Demonstrate behaviors/changes in lifestyle necessary to maintain therapeutic regimen.

ACTIONS/INTERVENTIONS

Sample NIC linkages:

Family Involvement Promotion: Facilitating family participation in the emotional and physical care of the patient

Family Mobilization: Utilizing family strengths to influence patient's health in a positive direction

Health System Guidance: Facilitating a patient's location and use of appropriate health services

NURSING PRIORITY NO. 1 To identify causative/precipitating factors:

- Ascertain family's perception of efforts to date. *Perceptions are more important than facts, and by getting family's point of view, realistic goals can be set and family can look to the future.*[2]
- Evaluate family functioning/activities as related to appropriateness. *Looking at frequency/effectiveness of family communication, promotion of autonomy, adaptation to meet changing needs, health of home environment/lifestyle, problem-solving abilities, ties to community provides information about current problem areas and need for specific interventions.*[1]
- Note family health goals and agreement of individual members. *Presence of conflict interferes with problem-solving and needs to be addressed before family can move forward to meet goals.*[2]
- Determine understanding and value of the treatment regimen to the family. *Individual members may misunderstand either the cause of the illness or the prescribed regimen and may disagree with what is happening, thereby promoting dissension within the family group and causing distress for the identified client.*[1]
- Identify cultural values/religious beliefs affecting view of situation and willingness to make necessary changes. *May affect choice of interventions.*
- Identify availability and use of resources. *Knowing who is available to help and support the family will help in planning care to maximize positive outcomes.*[2]

NURSING PRIORITY NO. 2 To assist family to develop strategies to improve management of therapeutic regimen:

- Provide information to aid family in understanding the value of the treatment program. *Accurate information helps individuals make decisions based on that knowledge, see the connection between illness and treatment, and may improve adherence to therapeutic regimen.*[3]
- Assist family members to recognize inappropriate family activities. Help the members identify both togetherness and individual needs and behavior. *Effective interactions can be enhanced and perpetuated when these factors are identified and used to improve family behaviors.*[2]
- Make a plan jointly with family members to deal with complexity of healthcare regimen/system and other related factors. *Enhances commitment to plan, optimizing outcomes when family and caregivers work together to plan therapeutic regimen.*[2,5]
- Identify community resources as needed using the three strategies of education, problem-solving, and resource-linking to address specific deficits. *Providing information, helping family members learn effective problem-solving techniques, and how to access needed resources can help them deal successfully with the chronically ill family member.*[4]

NURSING PRIORITY NO. 3 To promote wellness as related to future health and well-being of family members:

 • Help family identify criteria to promote ongoing self-evaluation of situation/effectiveness and family progress. *Involvement promotes sense of control and provides the opportunity to be proactive in meeting needs.*[2]

• Make referrals to and/or jointly plan with other health/social and community resources. *Problems often are multifaceted, requiring involvement of numerous providers/agencies to plan appropriate regimen to meet family/individual needs.*[3]

• Provide contact person/case manager for one-on-one assistance, as needed. *Having a single contact to coordinate care, provide support, and assist with problem-solving maintains continuity and prevents misunderstandings and errors in managing the family's regimen.*[1]

• Refer to NDs Caregiver Role Strain, ineffective Therapeutic Regimen Management, as indicated.

DOCUMENTATION FOCUS

Assessment/Reassessment

• Individual findings, including nature of problem/degree of impairment, family values/health goals, and level of participation and commitment of family members.
• Cultural values, religious beliefs.
• Availability and use of resources.

Planning

• Plan of care and who is involved in planning.
• Teaching plan.

Implementation/Evaluation

• Response to interventions/teaching and actions performed.
• Attainment/progress toward desired outcome(s).
• Modifications of plan of care.

Discharge Planning

• Long-term needs, plan for meeting and who is responsible for actions.
• Specific referrals made.

References

1. Cox, H. C., et al. (2002). *Clinical Applications of Nursing Diagnosis: Adult, Child, Women's, Psychiatric, Gerontic, and Home Health Considerations.* 4th ed. Philadelphia: F.A. Davis.
2. Healthy People 2010 Toolkit: A Field Guide to Health Planning. (2002). Washington, DC: Public Health Foundation.
3. Stuifbergen, A. (1997). Health promotion: An essential component of rehabilitation for persons with chronic disabling conditions. *ADV Nurs Sci,* 19(4), 147–148.
4. Larsen. L. S. (1998). Effectiveness of counseling intervention to assist family caregivers of chronically ill relatives. *J Psychosoc Nurs,* 36(8), 26.
5. Gance-Cleveland, B. (2005). Motivational interviewing as a strategy to increase families' adherence to treatment regimens. *Journal for Specialists in Pediatric Nursing,* 10(3), 151–155.

🌐 Cultural ⊛ Collaborative 🏠 Community/Home Care ✎ Diagnostic Studies ∞ Pediatric/Geriatric/Lifespan 💊 Medications

readiness for enhanced Therapeutic Regimen Management

Definition: A pattern of regulating and integrating into daily living a program for treatment of illness and its sequelae that is sufficient for meeting health-related goals and can be strengthened

RELATED FACTORS
To be developed by nurse researchers and submitted to NANDA

DEFINING CHARACTERISTICS

Subjective
Expresses desire to manage the illness (e.g., treatment, prevention)
Expresses little difficulty with prescribed regimens
Describes reduction of risk factors

Objective
Choices of daily living are appropriate for meeting goals (e.g., treatment, prevention)
No unexpected acceleration of illness symptoms

Sample Clinical Applications: Diabetes mellitus, CHF, COPD/asthma, MS, systemic lupus, HIV positive/AIDS, prematurity

DESIRED OUTCOMES/EVALUATION CRITERIA
Sample NOC linkages:
Symptom Control: Personal actions to minimize perceived adverse changes in physical and emotional functioning
Knowledge: Treatment Regimen: Extent of understanding conveyed about a specific treatment regimen
Participation in Healthcare Decisions: Personal involvement in selecting and evaluating healthcare options to achieve desired outcomes

Client Will (Include Specific Time Frame)

- Assume responsibility for managing treatment regimen.
- Demonstrate proactive management by anticipating and planning for eventualities of condition/potential complications.
- Identify/use additional resources, as appropriate.
- Remain free of preventable complications/progression of illness and sequelae.

ACTIONS/INTERVENTIONS

Sample NIC linkages:
Health System Guidance: Facilitating a patient's location and use of appropriate health services
Health Education: Developing and providing instruction and learning experiences to facilitate voluntary adaptation of behavior conducive to health in individuals, families, groups, or communities
Anticipatory Guidance: Preparation of patient for an anticipated developmental or situational crisis

NURSING PRIORITY NO. 1 To determine motivation for continued growth:

🏠 • Verify client's level of knowledge/understanding of therapeutic regimen. Note specific health goals. *Provides opportunity to assure accuracy and completeness of knowledge base for future learning.*[1]

🏠 • Determine individual's perceptions of adaptation to treatment/anticipated changes. *How client sees the situation is important to discussing what is happening in regard to the treatment regimen and planning for the future.*[1]

🏠 • Identify individual's expectations of long-term treatment needs/anticipated changes. *Knowing expectations identifies understanding and acceptance of what is realistic for own situation.*[3]

🏠 • Discuss resources presently used by client. *Noting whether changes can be arranged (e.g., increased hours of home-care assistance; access to case manager to support complex/long-term program) helps with planning for improved therapeutic regimen.*[3]

🌐 • Determine influence of cultural beliefs on client/caregiver(s) participation in regimen. *For instance, some Mexican Americans may not believe in usual health maintenance and prevention because of their traditional present-time orientation and belief that the future is in God's hands and so may have difficulty adhering to a long-term healthcare regimen.*[7]

NURSING PRIORITY NO. 2 To assist client/SO(s) to develop plan to meet individual needs:

🏠 • Identify steps necessary to reach desired health goal(s). *Understanding the process enhances commitment and the likelihood of achieving the goals.*[4]

🏠 • Accept client's evaluation of own strengths/limitations while working together to improve abilities. *Promotes sense of self-esteem and confidence to continue efforts to manage therapeutic regimen, such as diabetes, multiple sclerosis, more effectively.*[6]

🌐 • Incorporate client's cultural values/religious beliefs that support attainment of health goals. Problem-solve conflicts *to facilitate growth.*

🏠 • Provide information/bibliotherapy. Help client/SO(s) identify and evaluate resources they can access on their own. *Promotes sense of confidence in own ability to learn about illness/ condition. When referencing the Internet or nontraditional/unproven resources, the individual must exercise some restraint and determine the reliability of the source/information provided before acting on it.*[5]

🏠 • Acknowledge individual's efforts, capabilities, and skills to acquire/maintain interpersonal, self-care, and coping skills. *Provides positive reinforcement, encouraging continued progress toward desired goals to enhance therapeutic regimen.*[3,5,8]

🏠 • Acknowledge individual efforts/capabilities *to reinforce movement toward attainment of desired outcomes.*[3]

NURSING PRIORITY NO. 3 To promote optimum well-being:

🏠 • Promote client/caregiver choices and involvement in planning for and implementing added tasks/responsibilities. *Being involved in planning and knowing that he or she can make own choices promotes commitment to program and enhances probability that client will follow through with change.*[1,8]

🏠 • Assist in implementing strategies for monitoring progress/responses to therapeutic regimen. *Promotes proactive problem-solving, enabling client/caregiver to identify problems as they arise and deal appropriately with them so regimen is maintained.*[1,8]

🏠 • Identify additional community resources/support groups. *Provides additional opportunities for role-modeling, skill training, anticipatory problem-solving, etc.*[2,6]

🌐 Cultural   🅐 Collaborative   🏠 Community/Home Care   🧪 Diagnostic Studies   ∞ Pediatric/Geriatric/Lifespan   💊 Medications

DOCUMENTATION FOCUS

Assessment/Reassessment

- Findings, including dynamics of individual situation.
- Individual strengths/additional needs.
- Cultural values, religious beliefs.

Planning

- Plan of care and who is involved in planning.
- Teaching plan.

Implementation/Evaluation

- Response to interventions/teaching and actions performed.
- Attainment/progress toward desired outcome(s).
- Modifications to plan of care.

Discharge Planning

- Short-range and long-range needs and who is responsible for actions.
- Available resources, specific referrals made.

References

1. Cox, H. C., et al. (2002). *Clinical Applications of Nursing Diagnosis: Adult, Child, Women's, Psychiatric, Gerontic, and Home Health Considerations.* 4th ed. Philadelphia: F. A. Davis.
2. Healthy People 2010 Toolkit: A Field Guide to Health Planning. (2002). Washington, DC: Public Health Foundation.
3. Stuifbergen, A. (1997). Health promotion: An essential component of rehabilitation for persons with chronic disabling conditions. *ADV Nurs Sci,* 19(4), 147–148.
4. Larsen L. S. (1998). Effectiveness of counseling intervention to assist family caregivers of chronically ill relatives. *J Psychosoc Nurs,* 36(3), 26.
5. Lai, S. C., Cohen, M. N. (1999). Promoting lifestyle changes. *AJN,* 99(4), 63.
6. Miller, J. F. (1999). *Coping with Chronic Illness: Overcoming Powerlessness.* 3rd ed. Philadelphia: F. A. Davis.
7. Lipson, J. G., Dibble, S. L., Minarik, P. A. (1996). *Culture & Nursing Care: A Pocket Guide.* San Francisco: UCSF Nursing Press.
8. New York State Office of Mental Health Wellness. Self-management: Evidenced based practices: Accessed July 2007 at www.omh.state.ny.us/omhweb/ebp/adult_wellness.htm.

ineffective Thermoregulation

Definition: Temperature fluctuation between hypothermia and hyperthermia

RELATED FACTORS

Trauma; illness [e.g., cerebral edema, CVA, intracranial surgery, or head injury]
Immaturity; aging [e.g., loss/absence of brown adipose tissue]
Fluctuating environmental temperature
[Changes in hypothalamic tissue causing alterations in emission of thermosensitive cells and regulation of heat loss/production]
[Changes in metabolic rate/activity; changes in level/action of thyroxine and catecholamines]
[Chemical reactions in contracting muscles]

DEFINING CHARACTERISTICS

Objective
Fluctuations in body temperature above and below the normal range
Tachycardia
Reduction in body temperature below normal range; cool skin; moderate pallor; mild shivering; piloerection; cyanotic nail beds; slow capillary refill; hypertension
Warm to touch; flushed skin; increased respiratory rate; seizures

Sample Clinical Applications: Prematurity, brain injury/CVA/intracranial surgery (cerebral edema), infections/sepsis, major surgical procedures

DESIRED OUTCOMES/EVALUATION CRITERIA
Sample NOC linkages:
Thermoregulation: Balance among heat production, heat gain, and heat loss
Thermoregulation: Newborn: Balance among heat production, heat gain, and heat loss during the first 28 days of life

Client/Caregiver Will (Include Specific Time Frame)

- Verbalize understanding of individual factors and appropriate interventions.
- Demonstrate techniques/behaviors to correct underlying condition/situation.
- Maintain body temperature within normal limits.

ACTIONS/INTERVENTIONS

Sample NIC linkages:
Temperature Regulation: Attaining or maintaining body temperature within a normal range
Temperature Regulation: Intraoperative: Attaining or maintaining body temperature within a normal range
Fever Treatment: Management of a patient with hyperpyrexia caused by nonenvironmental factors

NURSING PRIORITY NO. 1 To identify causative/contributing factors:

- Obtain history concerning present symptoms, correlate with previous episodes/family history, and diagnostic studies. *Thermoregulation is a controlled process that maintains the body's core temperature in the range at which most biochemical processes work best (99°F to 99.6°F).*[1,2] *Exercise, behavioral impulses, metabolic and hormonal changes influence changes in body temperature, leading to loss or gain of heat.*
- Determine specific factors involved in current temperature fluctuation (e.g., environmental factors, surgery, infectious process, effects of drugs/toxins, brain/spinal cord injury). *Thermoregulation is affected in two ways: (1) endogenous factors (via diseases or conditions of body/organ systems) and (2) exogenous factors (via enviromental exposures, medications, and nutrition).*[2] *Helps to determine the scope of interventions that may be needed (e.g., simple addition of warm blankets after surgery, or hypothermia therapy following brain trauma).*[4,6]
- ∞ Note client's age (e.g., premature neonate, young child, or aging individual), *as it can directly impact ability to maintain/regulate body temperature and respond to changes in environment.*[3,5]

⊕ Cultural   Ⓐ Collaborative   🏠 Community/Home Care   ✎ Diagnostic Studies   ∞ Pediatric/Geriatric/Lifespan   💊 Medications

- Review laboratory results (e.g., tests indicative of infection, thyroid/other endocrine tests, drug screens) *to identify potential internal causes of temperature imbalances.*

NURSING PRIORITY NO. 2 To assist with measures to correct/treat underlying cause:

- Monitor temperature by appropriate route (e.g., tympanic, rectal, oral), noting variation from client's usual/normal temperature. *Rectal and tympanic temperatures most closely approximate core temperature; however, shell temperatures (oral, axillary, touch) are often measured at home and are predictive of fever or subnormal temperatures. Rectal temperature measurement may be the most accurate but is not always expedient (e.g., client declines, is agitated, has rectal lesions or surgery, etc.). Abdominal temperature monitoring may be done in the premature neonate.*
- Have cooling and warming equipment/supplies readily available during and following procedures/surgery.
- Initiate emergent or immediate interventions, such as cooling or warming measures, fluids, electrolytes, nutrients, and medications (e.g., antipyretics, antibiotics, neoplastics), as indicated, *to restore or maintain body temperature within normal range and optimize organ function.*[1-8]
- Maintain ambient temperature in comfortable range *to prevent/compensate for client's heat production or heat loss (e.g., may need to add or remove clothing or blankets, avoid drafts, reduce or increase room temperature/humidity).*
- Place newborn infant under radiant warmer, cover infant's head with cap, use layers of lightweight blankets. *Newborns/infants can have temperature instability. Heat loss is greatest through the head and by evaporation and convection.*[5]
- Refer to NDs risk for imbalanced Body Temperature, Hypothermia, or Hyperthermia for additional interventions.

NURSING PRIORITY NO. 3 To promote wellness (Teaching/Discharge Considerations):

- Review causative/related factors with client/SO(s). *Provides information about what, if any, measures can be implemented to protect client from harm or limit potential for problems associated with ineffective thermoregulation.*
- Discuss with client/caregivers dressing appropriately, such as:[1]
  Wearing layers of clothing that can be removed or added as needed
  Donning hat and gloves in cold weather
  Using water-resistant outer gear to protect from wet weather chill
  Dressing in light, loose protective clothing in hot weather
- Review home management of temperature fluctuations in special population (e.g., newborn infant, person with spinal cord injury, frail elder). *Measures could include use of heating pads, ice bag; heaters or fans; adding/removing clothing or blankets, cool or warm liquids and bathwater; skin-to-skin contact in newborn, etc.).*[5-8]
- Provide oral and written information concerning client's disease processes, current therapies, and postdischarge precautions, as appropriate to situation. *Allows for early intervention and implementation of preventive or corrective measures.*
- Refer to teaching section in NDs risk for imbalanced Body Temperature, Hypothermia, or Hyperthermia, as appropriate.

DOCUMENTATION FOCUS

Assessment/Reassessment

- Individual findings, including nature of problem, degree of impairment/fluctuations in temperature.

Planning

- Plan of care and who is involved in planning.
- Teaching plan.

Implementation/Evaluation

- Responses to interventions/teaching actions performed.
- Attainment/progress toward desired outcome(s).
- Modifications to plan of care.

Discharge Planning

- Long-term needs and who is responsible for actions to be taken.
- Specific referrals made.

References

1. Worfolk, J. (1997). Keep frail elders warm! *Geriatr Nurs*, 18(1), 7–11.
2. Kneis, R. C. (1996). Geriatric trauma: What you need to know. *Int J Traum Nurs*, 2(3), 85–91.
3. Cox, H. C., et al. (2002). *Clinical Applications of Nursing Diagnosis: Adult, Child, Women's, Psychiatric, Gerontic, and Home Health Considerations*. 4th ed. Philadelphia: F. A. Davis.
4. ND: Surgical Intervention. In Doenges, M. E., Moorhouse, M. F., Geissler-Murr, A. C. (2002). *Nursing Care Plans: Guidelines for Individualizing Patient Care*. 6th ed. Philadelphia: F. A. Davis.
5. Suggested guidelines for early discharge of term, healthy newborns. (Revised 1998). Accessed July 2007 at http://depts.washington.edu/nicuweb/NICU-WEB/earlydis.stm.
6. Hoppe, J., Sinert, R. (2006). Heat exhaustion and heatstroke. Article for Emedicine Web site. Retrieved March 2007 at www.emedicine.com/emerg/topic236.htm.
7. Galligan, M. (2006). Proposed guidelines for skin-to-skin treatment of neonatal hypothermia. *MCN, the Amer J Maternal/Child Nurs*, 31(5), 298–304.
8. Jones, T. S. (2005). A bolt out of the blue: Dealing with the aftermath of spinal cord injury. *Nursing Made Incredibly Easy!*, 3(6), 14–15, 17–28.

disturbed Thought Processes

Definition: Disruption in cognitive operations and activities

RELATED FACTORS
To be developed by nurse researchers and submitted to NANDA
[Physiological changes, aging, hypoxia, head injury, malnutrition, infections]
[Biochemical changes, medications, substance abuse]
[Sleep deprivation]
[Psychological conflicts, emotional changes, mental disorders]

DEFINING CHARACTERISTICS

Subjective
[Ideas of reference, hallucinations, delusions]

Objective
Inaccurate interpretation of environment
Inappropriate thinking; egocentricity

Cultural Collaborative Community/Home Care Diagnostic Studies Pediatric/Geriatric/Lifespan Medications

Memory deficit; [confabulation]

Hypervigilance; hypovigilance

Cognitive dissonance [decreased ability to grasp ideas, make decisions, problem-solve, use abstract reasoning or conceptualize, calculate; disordered thought sequencing]

Distractibility; [altered attention span]

[Inappropriate social behavior]

Sample Clinical Applications: Brain injury/CVA, CNS infections, anorexia nervosa, substance abuse, septicemia, cirrhosis of liver, delirium, dementia, schizophrenia, dissociative disorders, paranoid disorder, obsessive-compulsive disorder

DESIRED OUTCOMES/EVALUATION CRITERIA

Sample NOC linkages:

Distorted Thought Self-Control: Self-restraint of disruptions in perception, thought processes, and thought content

Cognition: Ability to execute complex mental processes

Memory: Ability to cognitively retrieve and report previously stored information

---

Client Will (Include Specific Time Frame)

- Recognize changes in thinking/behavior.
- Verbalize understanding of causative factors when known/able.
- Identify interventions to deal effectively with situation.
- Demonstrate behaviors/lifestyle changes to prevent/minimize changes in mentation.
- Maintain usual reality orientation.

ACTIONS/INTERVENTIONS

Sample NIC linkages:

Dementia Management: Provision of a modified environment for the patient who is experiencing a chronic confusional state

Delusion Management: Promoting the comfort, safety, and reality orientation of a patient experiencing false, fixed beliefs that have little or no basis in reality

Environmental Management: Safety: Manipulation of the patient's surroundings for therapeutic benefit

NURSING PRIORITY NO. 1 To assess causative/contributing factors:

- Identify underlying condition. *Disturbances in thinking can be the result of a wide variety of conditions (e.g., recent stroke, CNS infections; dementias, retardation; traumatic brain injury with increased intracranial pressure, anoxic event; acute urinary infections [especially in elderly]; malnutrition, metabolic problems [e.g., acid-base imbalances, diabetes, renal/hepatic failure]; sensory deprivation or overstimulation; toxins, including drug interactions/reactions, drug overdose, accidental exposures; emotional/psychiatric illness [e.g., schizophrenia]).*[2,8–10]
- Interview SO(s)/caregiver(s) to determine client's usual cognitive ability, changes in behavior, length of time problem has existed, and other pertinent information *to provide baseline for comparison.*[6,10]
- Determine alcohol/other drug use (prescription/OTC/illicit/herbal). *Drugs can have direct effects on the brain or have dose-related effects that alter thought processes and sensory perception.*[2,8,9]

• Note schedule of medication administration. *May be significant when evaluating cumulative effects/interactions.*

 • Assess for presence/severity of pain, as well as use of or need for analgesics. *Both pain and the treatments for pain can diminish the acuity of client's thinking processes. Untreated pain can increase confusion and agitation.*[1,7]

• Assess dietary intake/nutritional status. *Good nutrition is essential for optimal brain functioning. Persons with anorexia, major depression, substance use, and chronic debilitating conditions may have problems with thinking related to deficits in nutrients, vitamins, electrolytes, and minerals.*[2,8–10]

• Evaluate impact of environment. *Excessive noise, multiple people in client's surroundings, chaotic lifestyle, rapid changes in routines, etc., can result in overstimulation/confusion, clouding client's thinking and impairing coping abilities.*

• Monitor laboratory values. *Abnormalities such as metabolic alkalosis, hypokalemia, anemia, elevated ammonia levels, infections, drug toxicity, etc., may be affecting thought processes.*

• Assist with/review results of diagnostic testing (e.g., MRI, CT scan, spinal tap) *to help identify etiology of thinking impairment.*

NURSING PRIORITY NO. 2 To assess degree of impairment:

• Evaluate mental status using appropriate tools *(establishes baseline and comparative functional level according to age, developmental stage, and neurological status)*, noting:[5,11]

extent of impairment in thinking ability. *Varies widely, with impairments being overt or difficult to identify. Long time periods and sophisticated neuropsychiatric testing may be required to more fully identify nature of this impairment.*

remote/recent memory. *Remote memory is often intact, while recent/short-term memory may be lost or impaired.*

orientation to person/place/time. *Confusion may be short-term, long-term, or permanent and can be stable or progressive.* (Refer to NDs acute/chronic Confusion.)

insight and judgment. *Client may/may not be aware of changes in these areas, but family, friends or colleagues may report concerns.*[8,11]

changes in personality or response to stimuli. *Can range from lethargy and withdrawal to anger, agitation, and violent responses.*[9,10]

attention span/distractibility and ability to make decisions or problem-solve. *Determines ability to participate in planning/executing care.*

ability to receive, send, and appropriately interpret communications. Note absence of speech or changes in speech patterns (e.g., slowing and/or slurring of speech, problems with word finding, presence of aphasia, etc.). *Speech and communication difficulties are both indicators and consequences of impaired thought processes.*[9]

client's anxiety level (from mild to panic level) *that both causes and potentiates alterations in thought processes.*[2,9,10] (Refer to ND Anxiety.)

occurrence of paranoia and delusions, hallucinations. *Can occur with brain injury, mental illness, metabolic and electrolyte disturbances, alcohol/other drug use/overdose, dementias, etc., reflecting escalation of thought disturbances.*[2]

• Assist with in-depth testing of specific cognitive abilities/executive brain functions, as appropriate.

NURSING PRIORITY NO. 3 To prevent further deterioration, maximize level of function:

• Perform periodic neurological/behavioral assessments as indicated and compare with baseline. Note changes in level of consciousness and cognition (e.g., increased lethargy, confusion, drowsiness, irritability; changes in ability to communicate or appropriateness of thinking and behavior). Have client write name periodically; keep this record for comparison and report differences. *Early recognition of changes promotes proactive modifications to plan of care.*[2]

- Assist with treatment for underlying problems such as anorexia, brain injury/increased intracranial pressure, sleep disorders, biochemical imbalances. *Cognition/thinking often improves with treatment/correction of medical/psychiatric problems.*[6]
- Establish alternate means for self-expression if unable to communicate verbally. *Provides way of determining thinking ability if unable to communicate verbally.* (Refer to ND impaired verbal Communication.)
- Reorient to person/place/time as needed *to reinforce/maintain reality of the moment. Note: Inability to maintain orientation is a sign of deterioration.*
- Encourage family/SO(s) to participate in reorientation and provide ongoing input (e.g., current news and family happenings). *Promotes sense of normalcy, maintains contact with family.*
- Stay with client when agitated, frightened. *Support may provide calming effect, reducing anxiety and risk of injury.*[2]
- Note behavior indicative of potential for violence and take appropriate actions *to prevent harm to client/others. Clients with brain injuries often have lowered impulse control, problems with anger management, and the potential for violent outbursts, requiring specific interventions designed to help the client learn to control these behaviors.*[7] (Refer to ND risk for other-directed Violence.)
- Provide safety measures (e.g., side rails, padding as necessary; bed in low position/on floor, close supervision, seizure precautions) as indicated. *May help to prevent accidents/injury to client.*[2]
- Schedule structured activity and rest periods. *Provides stimulation without undue fatigue, helping to maintain orientation and sense of reality.*[3]
- Encourage/provide opportunities for adequate sleep. *Sleep deprivation can increase confusion. Regular sleep routine reinforces the idea of bedtime, and adequate rest can enhance clarity of thinking.*[6] (Refer to ND Sleep Deprivation.)
- Monitor medication regimen, limit use of sedatives and drugs affecting the nervous system *that have shown correlation with episodes of confusion.*[1–3,8]
- Refer to appropriate rehabilitation providers. *Cognitive retraining program, speech therapist, psychosocial resources, biofeedback, counselor may help client to enhance degree of functioning.*[6]

NURSING PRIORITY NO. 4 To create therapeutic milieu and assist client/SO(s) to develop coping strategies (especially when condition is irreversible):

- Provide opportunities for SO(s)/caregiver(s) to ask questions and obtain information. *SOs frequently have difficulty accepting and dealing with client's aberrant behavior and may require assistance in understanding and coping with the situation.*[2]
- Listen with regard to client's verbalizations in spite of speech pattern/content *to convey interest and worth to individual, enhancing self-esteem and encouraging continued efforts.*[3]
- Maintain a pleasant, quiet environment and approach client in a slow, calm manner. *Client may respond with anxious or aggressive behaviors if startled or overstimulated.*
- Maintain reality-oriented relationship and environment. *Using aids such as clocks, calendars, personal items, and seasonal decorations helps individual maintain current reality.*[6]
- Present reality concisely and briefly and do not challenge illogical thinking. *Helps client stay focused on the present. Client may react defensively if thinking is challenged.*[6]
- Give simple directions, using short words and simple sentences. *Provides for processing of basic communication when thinking is impaired.*[3]

- Reduce provocative stimuli, negative criticism, arguments, and confrontations *to avoid triggering fight/flight responses.*
- Refrain from forcing activities and communications. *Client may feel threatened and may withdraw or rebel.*
- Respect individuality and personal space. *Conveys concern for the person regardless of the circumstances.*[3]
- Use touch judiciously, respecting personal needs/cultural beliefs, but keeping in mind physical and psychological importance of touch. *Touch is a powerful communication tool and can have positive and negative reactions, and the appropriateness of its use is culturally determined.*[5]
- Provide nutritionally well-balanced diet incorporating client's preferences as able. Encourage client to eat, provide pleasant environment, and allow sufficient time to eat. *Enhances intake, improving nutritional status and general well-being.*[6]
- Provide ample time for client to respond to questions/comments and make simple decisions. *Processing information takes more time when thinking is impaired, and allowing more time promotes communication and client's sense of self-esteem.*[6]
- Inform family/caregiver of the meaning of/reasons for common behaviors observed in client with disturbed thought processes, as well as the probable course of disease process and plan of care. *Helps them to understand and cope with situation and assists them in providing a safe environment for the client.*[4]
- Support client/SO(s) with grieving for loss of self/abilities, as in Alzheimer's disease. *Progressive loss of mental abilities is difficult for family members to deal with as they grieve the loss of the person they knew. Providing opportunity for individuals to talk about feelings of grief will promote coping abilities.*[4] (Refer to ND Grieving.)
- Encourage participation in resocialization activities/groups as appropriate. *Can help the individual maintain/regain some degree of social skills. Even in conditions of dementia, client can benefit from these activities.*[6]

NURSING PRIORITY NO. 5 To promote wellness (Teaching/Discharge Considerations):

- Assist in identifying ongoing treatment needs/rehabilitation program for the individual *to maintain gains and continue progress if able.*[6]
- Emphasize importance of cooperation with therapeutic regimen. *Client and SOs benefit from maintaining regimen as agreed on, and working together benefits everyone.*[6]
- Promote socialization within individual limitations. *Client may have difficulty tolerating large or even small groups of people, unfamiliar or noisy surroundings.* (Refer to ND disturbed Sensory Perception.)
- Identify problems related to aging that are remediable and assist client/SO(s) to seek appropriate assistance/access resources. *Encourages problem-solving to improve condition when possible rather than accept the status quo.*
- Help client/SO(s) develop plan of care when problem is progressive/long-term. *Advance planning addressing home care, transportation, assistance with care activities, support and respite for caregivers enhances management of client in home setting.* (Refer to NDs risk for Caregiver Role Strain; Self-Care Deficit (specify) for related interventions.)
- Refer to community resources (e.g., social services, day-care programs, support groups, drug/alcohol rehabilitation; mental health treatment program) *to provide assistance and support for client/caregivers.*
- Refer to NDs acute Confusion, chronic Confusion; impaired Environmental Interpretation Syndrome; Grieving; impaired Memory; Self-Care Deficit; disturbed Sensory Perception as appropriate for additional interventions.

⊕ Cultural Ⓐ Collaborative 🏠 Community/Home Care Diagnostic Studies ∞ Pediatric/Geriatric/Lifespan Medications

DOCUMENTATION FOCUS

Assessment/Reassessment

- Individual findings, including nature of problem, current and previous level of function, effect on independence and lifestyle.
- Results of tests/diagnostic studies, and mental status/cognitive evaluations.
- SO/family support and participation.
- Availability/use of resources.

Planning

- Plan of care and who is involved in planning.
- Teaching plan.

Implementation/Evaluation

- Response to interventions/teaching and actions performed.
- Attainment/progress toward desired outcome(s).
- Modifications to plan of care.

Discharge Planning

- Long-term needs/referrals and who is responsible for actions to be taken.
- Available resources, specific referrals made.

References

1. Foreman, M. (1989). Complexities of acute confusion. *Geriatr Nurs, 3*, 136.
2. ND: Thought Processes, disturbed. In Doenges, M. E., Moorhouse, M. F., Geissler-Murr. (2002). *Nursing Care Plans: Guidelines for Individualizing Patient Care.* 6th ed. Philadelphia: F. A. Davis, pp. 217, 369, 410, 535, 715, 773.
3. Dellasaga, C., Strickllin, M. L. (1993). Cognitive impairment in the elderly home health clients. *Home Health Care Serve Q*, 14, 81
4. Smart, G., Sundeen, S. (1991). *Pocket Guide to Psychiatric Assessment.* St. Louis, MO: Mosby.
5. Doenges, M. E., Townsend, M. C., Moorhouse, M. F. (1998). *Psychiatric Care Plans Guidelines for Individualizing Care.* 3d ed. Philadelphia: F. A. Davis.
6. Cox, H. C., et al. (2002). *Clinical Applications of Nursing Diagnosis: Adult, Child, Women's, Psychiatric, Gerontic, and Home Health Considerations.* 4th ed. Philadelphia: F. A. Davis.
7. Johnson, G. (1998). Traumatic brain injury survival guide. Retrieved July 2007 at www.tbiguide.com.
8. Naylor, M. D., Stephens, C. Bowles, K. H., et al. (2005). Cognitively impaired older adults. *AJN*, 105(2), 52–61.
9. Palmer, R. M. (2006). Management of common clinical disorders in geriatric patients: Delerium. Article for Medscape Web site. Retrieved May 2007 at www.medscape.com/viewarticle/53466.
10. Simon, J. H. (2004). Schizophrenia. CME article for Hardin Memorial Hospital Web site. Retrieved May 2007 at www.hmh.net/adam/patientreports/000047.htm.
11. Holm, K., Foreman, M. (2006). Analysis of measures of functional and cognitive ability for aging adults with cardiac and vascular disease. *J of Cardiovascular Nursing*, 21(5-Suppl), 40–45.

impaired Tissue Integrity

Definition: Damage to mucous membrane, corneal, integumentary, or subcutaneous tissues

RELATED FACTORS
Altered circulation
Nutritional factors (e.g., deficit or excess); [metabolic/endocrine dysfunction]
Fluid deficit/excess

Knowledge deficit
Impaired physical mobility
Chemical irritants (including body excretions, secretions, medications); radiation (including therapeutic radiation)
Temperature extremes
Mechanical (e.g., pressure, shear, friction), [surgery]
Knowledge deficit
[Infection]

DEFINING CHARACTERISTICS

Objective
Damaged tissue (e.g., cornea, mucous membrane, integumentary, subcutaneous)
Destroyed tissue

Sample Clinical Applications: Trauma, burns, diabetes mellitus, peripheral vascular disease, venous insufficiency, AIDS, cancer, radiation therapy, sickle cell crisis, cocaine use, scleroderma, infections, borderline personality or obsessive-compulsive disorders

DESIRED OUTCOMES/EVALUATION CRITERIA
Sample NOC linkages:
Tissue Integrity: Skin & Mucous Membranes: Structural intactness and normal physiological function of skin and mucous membranes
Tissue Perfusion: Peripheral: Adequacy of blood flow through the small vessels of the extremities to maintain tissue function

Client/Caregiver Will (Include Specific Time Frame)

- Verbalize understanding of condition and causative factors.
- Identify interventions appropriate for specific condition.
- Demonstrate behaviors/lifestyle changes to promote healing and prevent complications/recurrence.

Sample NOC linkage:
Wound Healing: Secondary Intention: Extent of regeneration of cells and tissues in an open wound

Client Will (Include Specific Time Frame)

- Display progressive improvement in wound/lesion healing.

ACTIONS/INTERVENTIONS

Sample NIC linkages:
Wound Care: Prevention of wound complications and promotion of wound healing
Incision Site Care: Cleansing, monitoring, and promotion of healing in a wound that is closed with sutures, clips, or staples
Pressure Ulcer Care: Facilitation of healing in pressure ulcers

Cultural   Collaborative   Community/Home Care   Diagnostic Studies   Pediatric/Geriatric/Lifespan   Medications

NURSING PRIORITY NO. 1   To identify causative/contributing factors:

- Identify underlying condition/pathology involved in tissue injury (e.g., diabetic neuropathies, peripheral arterial disorders; sensory/perceptual deficits; cognitive impairments/developmental delay; frail elder; emotional/psychological problems; surgery/traumatic injuries; debilitating illness/long-term immobility). *Suggests treatment options, desire/ability to protect self, and potential for recurrence of tissue damage.*
- Assess skin/tissue color, temperature, and sensation *for adequacy of blood supply and nerve innervation.*
- Observe trauma/surgical client for tissue bleeding or spread of hematoma formation in injured areas, *which can result in compressed blood vessels and impaired circulation, aggravating injury to tissues.*[1,2]
- Assess for individual factors *that increase risk of circulatory insufficiency/occlusion and can impede healing; for example: (1) trauma to extremity that causes internal tissue damage (e.g., burns, high-velocity and penetrating trauma); fractures (especially long-bone fractures) with hemorrhage;(2) external pressures (e.g., from tight dressings, splints or casting, burn eschar); (3) immobility (e.g., long-term bedrest, traction/cast); (4) presence of conditions affecting peripheral circulation and sensation (e.g., atherosclerosis, diabetes, venous insufficiency); (5) lifestyle factors (e.g., smoking, obesity, and sedentary lifestyle); (6) use of medications (e.g., anticoagulants, corticosteroids, immunosuppressives, antineoplastics) that adversely affect healing; (7) vigorous sports/exercise;(8) malnutrition (deprives the body of protein and calories required for cell growth and repair); and (9) dehydration (impairs transport of oxygen and nutrients).*[1-5,11,14,17]
- Evaluate skin/mucous membranes for hydration status; note presence/degree of edema (1+ to 4+), urine characteristics and output. *Determines presence of fluid deficit or overload that can adversely affect cell/tissue strength and organ function. Note: Edematous tissues are prone to breakdown.* (Refer to ND risk for imbalanced Fluid Volume.)
- Evaluate pulses/calculate ankle-brachial index *to evaluate actual/potential for impairment of circulation to lower extremities. Result less than 0.9 indicates need for close monitoring/more aggressive intervention (e.g., tighter blood glucose and weight control in diabetic client).*[7]
- Determine race/ethnic background, family history for genetic factors *that may make individual vulnerable to particular conditions (e.g., sickle cell anemia impairs circulation),* and cultural/religious beliefs and practices regarding use of folk remedies/practices *that may damage tissues or impact choice of treatment options.*
- Determine nutritional status/impact of malnutrition on situation (e.g., pressure points on emaciated or elderly client, obesity, lack of activity, slow healing/failure to heal).
- Evaluate client's health/safety practices noting lack of cleanliness, poor oral care, lack of foot/toenail care, unsafe sexual practices, failure to use safety equipment for occupational or sports-related activities, and unprotected exposure to sun or toxic substances *that can place client at risk for injury to tissues or impaired function.*
- Note use of prosthetic, diagnostic, or external devices (e.g., artificial limbs, contacts, dentures, endotracheal airways, indwelling catheters, esophageal dilators, etc.), *which can cause pressure on/injure delicate tissues or provide entry point for infectious agents.*

NURSING PRIORITY NO. 2   To assess degree of impairment:

- Obtain a history of condition (e.g., pressure, venous, or diabetic wound; eye or oral lesions, etc.), including whether condition is acute or recurrent; original site/characteristics of wound; and duration of problem and changes that have occurred over time.

Nursing Diagnoses in Alphabetical Order

- Assess skin/tissues, bony prominences, and pressure areas, noting color, texture, and turgor. Note: Assess areas of least pigmentation for color changes (e.g., sclera, conjunctiva, nailbeds, buccal mucosa, tongue, palms, and soles of feet).
- Assess wound/lesion, documenting (1) location; (2) dimensions and depth in cm; (3) exudates—color, odor, and amount; (4) margins-fixed or unfixed; (5) tunneling/tracts—*(full extent of lesions of mucous membranes or subcutaneous tissue may not be visually discernible)*; (6) evidence of necrosis (e.g., color gray to black) or healing (e.g., pink/red granulation tissue) *in order to clarify treatment needs and establish a comparative baseline.*[4,5]
- Classify pressure ulcer(s) using such tools as Waterlow, Braden, Norton (or similar) Ulcer Classification System. *Provides consistent terminology for assessment and documentation of pressure ulcers.*[6]
- Remeasure/photograph wound(s) periodically *to evaluate progress, development of complications/delayed healing.*
- Review diagnostic studies (e.g., x-rays, imaging scans, biopsies). *May be necessary to determine cause for/extent of impairment.*
- Obtain specimens of wound exudate/lesions for culture/sensitivity, when appropriate, *to identify effective antimicrobial therapies.*
- Monitor laboratory studies (e.g., CBC, electrolytes, glucose, cultures) *for systemic changes indicative of infection/other sytemic complications.*
- Determine psychological effects of condition on the client and family. *Can be devastating for client's body/self-image and esteem—especially if condition is severe/disfiguring/chronic—as well as costly and burdensome for SO/caregiver.*

NURSING PRIORITY NO. 3   To facilitate healing:

General:[10,11,13,14]

- Modify/eliminate factors contributing to condition, if possible. Assist with treatment of underlying condition(s), as appropriate.
- Provide/encourage optimum nutrition (including adequate protein, lipids, calories, trace minerals, and multivitamins) *to promote tissue health/healing* and adequate hydration *to reduce/replenish cellular water loss and enhance circulation.*
- Encourage adequate periods of rest and sleep *to promote healing and meet comfort needs.*
- Promote early mobility. Assist with/encourage position changes, active/passive and assistive exercises *to promote circulation and prevent excessive tissue pressure.*

Incisions/wounds:[10,11,13–15]

- Inspect lesions/wounds daily for changes (e.g., signs of infection/complications or healing). *Promotes timely intervention/revision of plan of care.*
- Keep surgical area(s) clean/dry, change dressings/drainage appliances frequently, as indicated, *to prevent accumulation of secretions/excretions that can cause skin/tissue excoriation.*
- Practice aseptic technique for cleansing/dressing/medicating wounds or lesions. *Reduces risk of cross-contamination.*
- Protect incision/wound approximation (e.g., use of Steri-Strips, splinting when coughing) and stimulate circulation to surrounding areas *to assist body's natural process of repair.*
- Collaborate with other healthcare providers (e.g., physician, wound specialist, or ostomy nurse), as indicated, *to assist with developing plan of care for problematic or potentially serious wounds.*
- Apply appropriate barrier dressings or wound coverings (e.g., semipermeable, occlusive, wet-to-damp, hydrocolloid, hydrogel), drainage appliances, and skin-protective agents for

open/draining wounds and stomas *to protect the wound and surrounding tissues from excoriating secretions/drainage and to enhance healing.*[14,16]

- Assist with debridement/enzymatic therapy, as indicated (e.g., burns, severe pressure ulcer).
- Provide appropriate protective and healing devices (e.g., eye pads/goggles; heel protectors, padding/cushions/gel pads; therapeutic beds and mattresses; splints, chronic ulcer dressings, compression wrap, etc.).
- Refer to NDs dependent on individual situation (e.g., risk for perioperative positioning Injury, impaired physical/bed Mobility, impaired Skin Integrity, disturbed visual Sensory Perception, ineffective Tissue Perfusion, risk for Trauma, risk for Infection) *for related interventions.*

NURSING PRIORITY NO. 4 To correct hazards/minimize impairment:[4–6, 8–12]

- Assess IV sites on regular basis for erythema, edema, tenderness, burning, etc., *which indicate infiltration or phlebitis, requiring immediate discontinuation of site use or interventions to heal the area.*
- Use appropriate catheter (e.g., peripheral or central venous) when infusing anticancer or other toxic drugs, and ascertain that IV is patent and infusing well *to prevent infiltration and extravasation with resulting tissue damage.*
- Inspect skin/tissues routinely around incisions and cast edges and traction devices *to ensure proper application/function; note possible development of pressure points.*
- Remove adhesive products with care, removing on horizontal plane and using mineral oil or Vaseline for softening, if needed, *to prevent abrasions or tearing of skin/damage to underlying tissues.*
- Monitor for correct placement of tubes, catheters, and other devices, and assess skin tissues around these devices for effects of tape/fasteners or pressure from the devices *to prevent damage to skin and tissues as a result of pressure, friction, or shear forces.*
- Develop regularly timed repositioning schedule for client with mobility and sensation impairments, using turn sheet as needed; encourage/assist with periodic weight shifts for client in chair *to reduce stress on pressure points and encourage circulation to tissues.*
- Use/demonstrate proper turning and transfer techniques *to avoid movements that cause friction/shearing (e.g., pulling client with parallel force, dragging movements).*
- Provide foam/flotation/alternating pressure/air mattress and appropriate padding devices (e.g., foam boots, heel protectors, ankle rolls), when indicated, *to reduce tissue pressure and enhance circulation to compromised tissues.*[16]
- Limit use of plastic material (e.g., rubber sheet, plastic-backed linen savers), and remove wet/wrinkled linens promptly. *Moisture potentiates skin/underlying tissues, increasing risk of breakdown/infection.*
- Restrict/avoid use of restraints; use adequate padding and evaluate circulation, movement, and sensation of extremity frequently, when restraints are required. *Reduces risk of impaired circulation/tissue ischemia.*
- Elevate linens over affected extremity with bed cradle *to reduce pressure on/irritation of compromised tissues.*
- Encourage physical activity/exercise *to stimulate circulation, enhance organ function, and prevent/limit potential complications of immobility.*
- Provide/assist with oral care (e.g., oral/dental hygiene, avoiding extremes of hot or cold, change position of ET/NG tubes, lubricate lips, etc.) *to prevent damage to oral mucous membranes.* (Refer to ND impaired Oral Mucous Membrane for additional interventions.)
- Encourage use of adequate clothing/covers; protect from drafts *to prevent vasoconstriction that can compromise circulation.*

∞ 🏠 • Provide/instruct in proper care of extremities during cold or hot weather. *Individuals with impaired sensation or young children/individuals unable to verbalize discomfort require special attention to deal with extremes in weather (e.g., dressing in layers, wearing gloves, boots, clean/dry socks, properly fitting shoes/boots, face mask in winter; or use of sunscreen and light clothing to protect from dermal injury in summer).*

🏠 • Advise smoking cessation/refer for resources, if indicated. *Smoking causes vasoconstriction/interferes with healing.*

NURSING PRIORITY NO. 5 To promote wellness (Teaching/Discharge Considerations):

🏠 • Encourage verbalizations of feelings and expectations regarding condition and potential for recovery of structure and function.

🏠 • Help client and family to identify/implement successful coping skills *to reduce pain/discomforts and to improve quality of life.*

🏠 • Discuss importance of follow-up care (e.g., diabetic foot care clinic, wound care specialist, enterostomal therapist) as appropriate, self-monitoring and reporting of changes in condition/pain characteristics. *Promotes early intervention/reduces potential for complications.*

⊕ • Review medical regimen (e.g., proper use of topical sprays, creams, ointments, soaks, or irrigations).

🏠 • Instruct in dressing changes (technique and frequency) and proper disposal of soiled dressings *to prevent spread of infectious agent.*

🏠 • Identify required changes in lifestyle, occupation, or environment *necessitated by limitations imposed by condition or to avoid causative factors.*

⊕ • Refer to community/governmental resources as indicated (e.g., Public Health Department, OSHA, National Association for the Prevention of Blindness) *for information regarding specific conditions/to report hazards.*

DOCUMENTATION FOCUS

Assessment/Reassessment

- Individual findings, including history of condition, characteristics of wound/lesion, evidence of other organ/tissue involvement.
- Impact on functioning/lifestyle.
- Availability/use of resources.

Planning

- Plan of care and who is involved in planning.
- Teaching plan.

Implementation/Evaluation

- Responses to interventions/teaching, actions performed.
- Attainment/progress toward desired outcome(s).
- Modifications to plan of care.

Discharge Planning

- Long-term needs/referrals and who is responsible for actions to be taken.
- Specific referrals made.

References

1. Fort, C. W. (2003). How to combat 3 deadly trauma complications. *Nursing*, 33(5), 58–63.
2. Paula, R. (2002, update 2006). Compartment syndrome, extremity. Accessed July 2007 at www.emedicine.com/emerg/topic739.htm.
3. Peripheral vascular disease. (Public information sheet). Available at http://ivillagehealth.com. Accessed January 2004.
4. Llewellyn, S. (2002). Skin integrity and wound care. (Lecture materials). Chapel Hills, NC: Cape Fear Community College Nursing Program.
5. Colburn, L. (2001). Prevention for chronic wounds. In Krasner, D., Rodeheaver, G., Sibbald, R. G. *Chronic Wound Care: A Clinical Source Book for Healthcare Professionals*. 2d ed. Wayne, PA: HMP Communications.
6. No author listed. Risk factors and prevention. Geriatric Syndromes: Pressure Ulcers. Accessed February 2004 at http://geriatricsyllabus.com.
7. Murabito, J. M., Evans, J. C., Larson, M. G., et al. (2003). The ankle-brachial index in the elderly and risk of stroke, coronary disease and death. *Arch Intern Med*,163, 1939–1942.
8. Calianno, C. (2002). Patient hygiene, part 2—Skin care: Keeping the outside healthy. *Nursing*, 32(6), June Clinical Supp.
9. Wiersema, L. A., Stanley, M. (1999). The aging integumentary system. In Stanley, M., and Beare, P. G. *Gerontological Nursing: A Health Promotion/Protection Approach*. 2d ed. Philadelphia: F. A. Davis, pp. 102–111.
10. NDs: Skin Integrity, impaired and Tissue Integrity, impaired. In Doenges, M. E., Moorhouse, M. F., Geissler-Murr, A. C. (2002). *Nursing Care Plans: Guidelines for Individualizing Patient Care*. 6th ed. Philadelphia: F. A. Davis.
11. McGovern, C. (2003). Skin, hair and nail assessment. Unit 2. (Lecture materials). Villanova, PA: Villanova University College of Nursing. Accessed July 2007 at www.homepage.villanova.edu/.
12. Faller, N., Beitz, J. (2001). When a wound isn't a wound: Tubes, drains, fistulas and draining wounds. In Krasner, D., Rodeheaver, G., Sibbald, R. G. *Chronic Wound Care: a Clinical Source Book for Healthcare Professionals*. 2d ed. Wayne, PA: HMP Communications.
13. Peripheral Arterial Occlusive Disease. (Fact sheet). Available at www.fpnotebook.com. Accessed January 2004.
14. Guideline for management of wounds in patients with lower-extremity arterial disease. (2002). Wound Ostomy and Continence Nurses Society (WOCN), Clinical practice guideline series; No 1. Accessed July 2007 at www.guideline.gov/summary/summary.aspx?doc_id=3290.
15. Okan, K., Woo, K., Ayello, E. A., et al. (2007). The role of moisture balance in wound healing. *Advances for Skin & Wound Care: J for Prevention and Healing*, 20(1), 39–53.
16. Sieggreen, N. Y. (2006). Getting a leg up on managing venous ulcers. *Nursing Made Incredibly Easy!*, 4(6), 52–60.
17. Stotts, N. A., Wipke-Tevis, D. D., Hopf, H. W. (2007). Cofactors in impaired wound healing (excerpts). In *Chronic Wound Care*. 4th edition excerpts. Retrieved August 2007 at www.chronicwoundcarebook.com/

ineffective Tissue Perfusion (specify type: renal, cerebral, cardiopulmonary, gastrointestinal, peripheral)

Definition: Decrease in oxygen resulting in the failure to nourish the tissues at the capillary level. [Tissue perfusion problems can exist without decreased cardiac output; however, there may be a relationship between cardiac output and tissue perfusion.]

RELATED FACTORS
Hypervolemia; hypovolemia
Interruption of blood flow
Decreased hemoglobin concentration in blood; enzyme poisoning
Altered affinity of hemoglobin for oxygen; impaired transport of oxygen
Mismatch of ventilation with blood flow; exchange problems
Hypoventilation

DEFINING CHARACTERISTICS

Subjective
Cardiopulmonary
Chest pain

Dyspnea

Sense of "impending doom"

Gastrointestinal

Nausea

Abdominal pain or tenderness

Peripheral

Claudication

Objective

Renal

Altered blood pressure outside of acceptable parameters

Oliguria; anuria; hematuria

Elevation in BUN/creatine ratio

Cerebral

Altered mental status; speech abnormalities

Behavioral changes; [restlessness]

Changes in motor response; extremity weakness; paralysis

Changes in pupillary reactions

Difficulty in swallowing

Cardiopulmonary

Arrhythmias

Capillary refill >3 sec

Altered respiratory rate outside of acceptable parameters

Use of accessory muscles; chest retraction; nasal flaring

Bronchospasms

Abnormal arterial blood gases

[Hemoptysis]

Gastrointestinal

Hypoactive/absent bowel sounds

Abdominal distention

[Vomiting]

Peripheral

Altered skin characteristics (e.g., hair, nails, moisture)

Skin temperature changes

Skin discolorations; skin color pales on elevation, color does not return on lowering the leg

Altered sensations

Blood pressure changes in extremities; weak/absent pulses; diminished arterial pulsations; bruits

Edema

Delayed healing

Positive Homans' sign

Sample Clinical Applications: Atherosclerosis, coronary artery disease, CHF, myocardial infarction, pulmonary embolus, anemia, Raynaud's disease, peripheral vascular disease, brain injury/CVA, trauma/compartment syndrome, thrombophlebitis, diabetes mellitus, necrotizing enterocolitis

DESIRED OUTCOMES/EVALUATION CRITERIA

Sample NOC linkages:

Urinary Elimination: Collection and discharge of urine

Cultural   Collaborative   Community/Home Care   Diagnostic Studies   Pediatric/Geriatric/Lifespan   Medications

Tissue Perfusion: Cerebral: Adequacy of blood flow through the cerebral vasculature to maintain brain function

Tissue Perfusion: Cardiac: Adequacy of blood flow through the coronary vasculature to maintain heart function

Tissue Perfusion: Pulmonary: Adequacy of blood flow through pulmonary vasculature to perfuse alveoli/capillary unit

Tissue Perfusion: Abdominal Organs: Adequacy of blood flow through the small vessels of the abdominal viscera to maintain organ function

Tissue Perfusion: Peripheral: Adequacy of blood flow through the small vessels of the extremities to maintain tissue function

Client Will (Include Specific Time Frame)

- Verbalize understanding of condition, therapy regimen, side effects of medications, and when to contact healthcare provider.
- Demonstrate behaviors/lifestyle changes to improve circulation (e.g., cessation of smoking; use of relaxation techniques, exercise/dietary program).
- Demonstrate increased perfusion as individually appropriate (e.g., skin warm/dry, peripheral pulses present/strong, vital signs within client's normal range, alert/oriented, balanced intake/output, absence of edema, free of pain/discomfort).

ACTIONS/INTERVENTIONS

Sample NIC linkages:

Fluid/Electrolyte Management: Promotion of fluid/electrolyte balance and prevention of complications resulting from abnormal or undesired fluid/serum electrolyte levels

Cerebral Perfusion Promotion: Promotion of adequate perfusion and limitation of complications for a patient experiencing or at risk for inadequate cerebral perfusion

Cardiac Care: Limitation of complications resulting from an imbalance between myocardial oxygen supply and demand for a patient with symptoms of impaired cardiac function

Gastrointestinal Intubation: Insertion of a tube into the gastrointestinal tract

Circulatory Care: Arterial/Venous Insufficiency: Promotion of arterial/venous circulation

NURSING PRIORITY NO. 1 To assess causative/contributing factors:

- Determine history of conditions associated with thrombus or emboli (e.g., stroke, DVT, fractures [especially long bones/pelvis]; Raynaud's or Buerger's disease); or conditions that can affect multiple body systems (e.g., congestive heart failure, major trauma, sickle cell anemia; pheochromocytoma/Addison's disease/other endocrine imbalances; pancreatitis; intraperitoneal hemorrhage) *to identify client at higher risk for vascular occlusion or decreased systemic circulation resulting in ineffective tissue perfusion.*
- Note high-risk behaviors (e.g., smoking, prolonged periods of immobility). *Places client at greater risk for developing peripheral vascular disease (PVD) or complications of PVD.*[4,10]
- Evaluate for signs of infection especially when immune system is compromised, *as sepsis/septic shock can occur, resulting in decreased cardiac output/systemic perfusion with multiple organ involvement and critical consequences.*
- Review laboratory results *for conditions (e.g., hyperlipidemia, hypercholesterolemia, hypercoagulation) that can impair/occlude circulation.*

NURSING PRIORITY NO. 2 To note degree of impairment/organ involvement:

General assessments:

- Note customary baseline data (e.g., usual BP, weight, mentation, cardiac and respiratory status; oxygen saturation/ABGs, and other appropriate laboratory studies). *Provides comparison with usual findings.*
- Note presence, location, intensity, duration of pain, *which is typically associated with tissue ischemia anywhere in the body.*
- Review results of diagnostic studies (e.g., x-rays, ultrsound/CT/angiography/other imaging scans, organ pressure measurements, endoscopy, etc.) *to determine location/severity of condition.*
- Ascertain impact on functioning/lifestyle. *For example, leg pain may prevent client from shopping for groceries; impaired sensation or decreased mentation may place client at risk for falls; or reduced cardiac circulation may lead to angina with exertion.*

Body systems assessments:

Renal[1]

- Determine usual voiding pattern *to note changes (e.g., low output such as may occur with hypovolemia or disease/injury to kidneys; or need for diuretics, etc.).*
- Note characteristics of urine (e.g., concentrated, dilute) and measure specific gravity *to evaluate kidney's ability to concentrate the urine.*
- Measure urine output on a regular schedule. *Intake may be calculated against output to monitor renal function and to determine replacement needs.*
- Weigh daily or on regular basis *to ascertain if fluid is being retained.*
- Observe for dependent/generalized edema. *Edema (on scale of +1 to +4) occurs primarily in dependent tissues (hands, feet, lumbosacral area) and becomes generalized over body as kidneys fail.*
- Note mentation and behavior. *Adverse changes may be the consequence of fluid shifts, accumulation of toxins, acidosis, electrolyte imbalances, or increased BUN/Cr.*
- Auscultate BP, ascertain client's usual range. *Hypotension (and hypovolemia) can result in decreased glomerular filtration rate (GFR) that initially may increase rennin and raise BP, before shock state causes BP to fall.*
- Review laboratory studies (e.g., BUN/Cr levels, protein, specific gravity, electrolytes) *to assess status of renal function; evaluate progression of renal dysfunction/failure and effects on body/organ function.*

Cerebral[1]

- Determine presence of changes in cognition, vision, or sensory/motor responses, hemiparesis, headache, problems with speech and swallowing; behavioral changes *indicative of ineffective cerebral perfusion (e.g., brain trauma, TIA, or CVA from hemorrhage or clot).*
- Interview SO(s) regarding their perception of situation/changes in behavior.
- Note history of syncope, brief/intermittent periods of confusion/blackout. *Suggests conditions such as orthostatic hypotension, syncope, TIA.*
- Evaluate blood pressure. *Blood pressure can be indicative of certain perfusion impairments. For example, chronic or severe acute hypertension can precipitate cerebrovascular spasm and stroke. Low blood pressure/severe hypotension causes inadequate perfusion of brain, with adverse changes in consciousness/mentation.[2]*

Cultural Collaborative Community/Home Care Diagnostic Studies Pediatric/Geriatric/Lifespan Medications

- Monitor fluid and electrolyte status. *Imbalances have a direct bearing on brain perfusion and function.*
- Review medication, noting use of anticoagulants/antiplatelet agents/other drugs *that could cause intracranial bleeding.*

Cardiopulmonary[1]

- Investigate reports of chest pain/angina; note changes in vital signs and characteristics of pain *to evaluate for potential myocardial ischemia or inadequate systemic oxygenation/perfusion of organs.*
- Determine cardiac rhythm, presence of dysrhythmias. *Can be caused by inadequate myocardial perfusion, electrolyte imbalances, or be associated with brain injury (e.g., bradycardia can accompany traumatic injury, or stroke can be precipitated by dysrhythmias).*
- Investigate reports of difficulty breathing; note respiratory rate outside of acceptable parameters, use of accessory muscles to breath. *Indicative of oxygen exchange problems or ventilation/perfusion mismatch.*[3]
- Inspect for pallor, mottling, cool/clammy skin, and diminished pulses. *Systemic vasoconstriction resulting from reduced cardiac output may be evidenced by poor skin/tissue perfusion and diminished pulses.*
- Observe for sudden onset of chest pain, cyanosis, respiratory distress, hemoptysis, diaphoresis, hypoxia, anxiety, restlessness. *Signs of pulmonary emboli requiring prompt evaluation/intervention.*
- Review diagnostic studies (e.g., ECG, echocardiogram, angiography, Doppler ultrasound, chest radiography; pulse oximetry/oxygen saturation/capnometry/ABGs, electrolytes, BUN/Cr, cardiac enzymes) *to identify conditions requiring treatment, or to evaluate response to therapies.*[1-3,6]

Gastrointestinal[1]

- Note reports of nausea/vomiting along with problems with elimination. *May reflect hypoperfusion of the gastrointestinal tract, which is particularly vulnerable to even small decreases in circulating volume.*[2]
- Ascertain location/type/intensity/timing of abdominal pain (e.g., midepigastric pain following meals and lasting several hours suggests abdominal angina reflecting atherosclerotic occlusive disease).[7]
- Investigate reports of pain out of proportion to degree of injury after trauma. *May reflect developing abdominal compartment syndrome.*[8]
- Auscultate bowel sounds. *May be hypoactive or absent as result of surgery, or ileus/other obstruction, or hyperactive as might occur with GI bleeding.*
- Measure abdominal girth and compare with client's customary waist size/belt length *to monitor development/progression of distention, possibly reflecting intra-abdominal bleeding, infection, or edema associated with toxins.*
- Note changes in stool characteristics/presence of blood. *May indicate breakdown of mucosa due to ischemia/necrotizing enterocolitis.*
- Review laboratory tests/diagnostic studies (e.g., metabolic panel, complete blood count, amylase and lipase; clotting studies; x-rays, CT/other abdominal scans, endoscopy, etc.).[9]

Peripheral

- Ascertain characteristics of extremity pain (e.g., with/without activity, temperature/color changes, paresthesia; timing [day/night] that symptoms are worse; precipitating/aggravating events [e.g., walking] and relieving factors [e.g., rest, sitting down]) *to help isolate and differentiate problems (e.g., intermittent claudication versus loss of function and pain due to ischemia related to loss of perfusion).*[4]

- Palpate for presence and quality of pulses. Note pulselessness, paralysis, paresthesia, pain, and pallor *suggestive of peripheral vascular disease.*[4]

- Measure capillary refill *to determine adequacy of systemic circulation.* Calculate ankle-brachial index (ABI) as appropriate (diabetic clients or others with impaired circulation to lower extremities). *Result less than 0.9 indicates need for more aggressive preventive interventions to manage peripeheral vascular disease.*[11]

- Inspect lower extremities for skin texture (e.g., atrophic, shiny appearance), lack of hair, dry/scaly, reddened skin, and skin breaks/ulcerations *that often accompany diminished peripheral circulation.*[4]

- Auscultate for systolic/continuous bruits below obstruction in extremity.

- Check for calf tenderness or pain on dorsiflexion of foot (Homans' sign), swelling, and redness. *Indicators of deep vein thrombosis (DVT), although DVT can be present without a positive Homans' sign.*[1]

- Measure circumference of extremities as indicated. *Useful in identifying edema in involved extremity.*[1]

- Investigate reports of pain out of proportion to degree of injury, especially when combined with pallor, parasthesia, paralysis, and pulselessness. *May reflect developing compartment syndrome.*

- Review laboratory studies (e.g., clotting times, Hb/Hct, renal/cardiac function tests) and diagnostic studies (e.g., Doppler ultrasound, MRI/other scan, venogram, angiography) *to evaluate effectiveness of perfusion and determine degree of impairment.*[4,5]

NURSING PRIORITY NO. 3 To maximize tissue perfusion:

General:

- Collaborate in treatment of underlying conditions (e.g., stent placement, surgical reperfusion procedures, medications, fluids, nutrients, treatment of sepsis, etc.) as indicated *to improve tissue perfusion/organ function.*

Renal[1]

- Administer medication (e.g., antihypertensive agents, diuretics, anticoagulants in presence of thrombosis, steroids in membranous nephropathy) as indicated *to treat underlying condition.*

- Provide for fluid and diet restrictions, as indicated, while providing adequate calories and hydration *to meet the body's needs without overtaxing kidney function.*

- Provide psychological support for client/SO(s), especially when progression of disease and resultant treatment (dialysis) may be long-term. *Enhances coping skills and promotes adjustment to changes in lifestyle.*

- Refer to NDs deficient/excess Fluid Volume, impaired Urinary Elimination for additional interventions.

Cerebral[1]

- Elevate HOB (e.g., 10 degrees) and maintain head/neck in midline or neutral position *to promote circulation/venous drainage.*

- Administer medications as indicated to treat underlying condition. *For example, steroids/diuretics may be used to decrease edema, anticoagulants may be required for cerebral embolus.*

Cultural   Collaborative   Community/Home Care   Diagnostic Studies   Pediatric/Geriatric/Lifespan   Medications

- Assist with/monitor hypothermia therapy *that may be used to decrease metabolic and oxygen needs associated with hypermetabolic state/hyperthermia.*
- Prepare client for surgery as indicated (e.g., carotid endarterectomy, evacuation of hematoma/space-occupying lesion).
- Refer to NDs decreased Cardiac Output, decreased Intracranial Adaptive Capacity for additional interventions.

Cardiopulmonary[1,6]

- Administer medications (e.g., antihypertensive agents, antidysrhythmics, fibrinolytic agents) *to treat underlying condition.*
- Monitor vital signs, hemodynamic pressures, heart sounds, and cardiac rhythm *to monitor response to therapies.*
- Encourage quiet, restful atmosphere. *Conserves energy/lowers tissue O_2 demands.*
- Caution client to avoid strenuous activities *that increase cardiopulmonary workload (e.g., straining at stool, heavy lifting).*
- Provide perfusion support as indicated (e.g., oxygen by appropriate delivery method; IV fluids, blood) *to increase circulating volume and oxygenation.*
- Prepare for/assist with emergency procedures (e.g., arteriography, placement of cardiac stents, CABG surgery, thrombectomy, placement of vena cava filter) as indicated *to treat underlying/life-threatening conditions.*[3]
- Refer to NDs ineffective Breathing Pattern, decreased Cardiac Output, impaired Gas Exchange for additional interventions.

Gastrointestinal[1]

- Maintain gastric/intestinal decompression; when indicated, measure output periodically and note characteristics of drainage.
- Provide small/easily digested food and fluids when oral intake tolerated.
- Encourage rest after meals *to maximize blood flow to digestive system.*
- Prepare client for surgery as indicated. *May be a surgical emergency; for example, gastric resection, bypass graft, mesenteric endarterectomy.*
- Refer to NDs Nausea, imbalanced Nutrition: Less than body requirements for additional interventions.

Peripheral[1,16]

- Encourage early ambulation when possible. *Enhances venous return.*
- Discourage sitting/standing for long periods, wearing constrictive clothing, crossing legs *that can restrict circulation and lead to edema.*
- Elevate the legs when sitting, avoiding sharp angulation of the hips or knees or use of knee gatch on bed; elevate entire foot as indicated *to enhance venous return/minimize edema formation.*
- Provide air mattress, foam/gel padding, bed/foot cradle *to reduce excessive tissue pressure that could lead to skin breakdown.*
- Apply/instruct client/SO in application/periodic removal of antithromboembolic devices/hose to lower extremities *to limit venous stasis, improve venous return, and reduce risk of DVT in client who is limited in activity.*
- Avoid massaging the leg *in presence of thrombosis to reduce risk for embolus.*
- Exercise caution in use of hot water bottles or heating pads. *Tissues may have decreased sensitivity due to ischemia, increasing risk of dermal injury. Heat also increases the metabolic demands of already compromised tissues.*

---

ineffective TISSUE PERFUSION (specify type: renal, cerebral, cardiopulmonary, gastrointestinal, peripheral)

- Monitor circulation/movement/sensation above and below casts/traction device. Apply ice cautiously and elevate injured limb as appropriate *to reduce edema.*
- Perform assistive/active range-of-motion exercises (Buerger and Buerger-Allen).
- Emphasize necessity for smoking cessation *to reduce vasoconstrictive effects.*
- Assist with/prepare for medical procedures (e.g., sympathectomy, vein graft) *to improve peripheral circulation.*
- Discuss care of dependent limbs, body hygiene, foot care as appropriate. *When circulation is impaired, changes in sensation place client at risk for development of lesions/ulcerations that are often slow to heal.*
- Assist with/prepare for surgical procedures (e.g., sympathectomy, vein graft, fasciotomy) *to improve peripheral circulation, relieve excessive tissue pressure.*
- Monitor closely for signs of shock when sympathectomy is done *(result of unmediated vasodilation).*
- Administer medications with caution (e.g., vasodilators, papaverine, antilipemics, anticoagulants). *Drugs used to improve tissue perfusion also carry risk of adverse responses (e.g., altered drug response, changes in half-life/drug clearance, problems with interactions).*
- Refer to ND risk for Peripheral Neurovascular Dysfunction for additional interventions.

NURSING PRIORITY NO. 4 To promote wellness (Teaching/Discharge Considerations):

- Discuss individual risk factors (e.g., family history, obesity, age, smoking, hypertension, diabetes, clotting disorders) and potential outcomes of atherosclerosis (e.g., systemic and peripheral vascular disease conditions). *Information necessary for client to make informed choices about remediating risk factors and committing to lifestyle changes as appropriate to prevent onset of complications/manage symptoms when condition present.)*[12,13]
- Encourage discussion of feelings regarding prognosis/long-term effects of condition. *Major/unplanned life changes can strain coping abilities, impairing functioning and jeopardizing relationships, and may even result in depression.*
- Identify necessary changes in lifestyle and assist client to incorporate disease management into ADLs. *Promotes independence, enhances self-concept regarding ability to deal with change and manage own needs.*
- Instruct in home blood pressure monitoring; advise purchase of home monitoring equipment, refer to community resources as indicated *Facilitates management of hypertension, which is a major risk factor for damage to blood vessels/organ function.*[14]
- Encourage smoking cessation, refer to Smoke-out, other stop-smoking programs. *Smoking causes vasoconstriction, compromising perfusion.*
- Demonstrate/encourage use of relaxation activities, exercises/techniques *to decrease tension level.*
- Establish regular exercise program *to enhance circulation, reduce/maintain weight, and promote general well-being.*[15]
- Review specific dietary changes/restrictions with client (e.g., reduction of cholesterol and triglycerides, high or low protein intake, avoidance of rye in Buerger's disease).
- Emphasize importance of avoiding use of aspirin, some OTC drugs, vitamins containing potassium, mineral oil, or alcohol *when taking anticoagulants.*
- Review appropriate safety measures. *For example, use of electric razor for shaving, wearing gloves for gardening, or avoiding forceful blowing of nose when taking anticoagulants to decrease risk of trauma resulting in prolonged bleeding.*
- Refer to specific support groups, counseling as appropriate *to assist with problem-solving, provide role model, enhance coping ability.*

🌐 Cultural Ⓐ Collaborative 🏠 Community/Home Care ⚗ Diagnostic Studies ∞ Pediatric/Geriatric/Lifespan 💊 Medications ineffective TISSUE PERFUSION (specify type: renal, cerebral, cardiopulmonary, gastrointestinal, peripheral)

DOCUMENTATION FOCUS

Assessment/Reassessment

- Individual findings, noting nature/extent and duration of problem, effect on independence/lifestyle.
- Characteristics of pain, precipitators, and what relieves pain.
- Vital signs, cardiac rhythm/dysrhythmias.
- Pulses/BP, including above/below suspected lesion as appropriate.
- I/O and weight as indicated.

Planning

- Plan of care and who is involved in planning.
- Teaching plan.

Implementation/Evaluation

- Response to interventions/teaching, actions performed.
- Attainment/progress toward desired outcome(s).
- Modifications to plan of care.

Discharge Planning

- Long-term needs and who is responsible for actions to be taken.
- Available resources, specific referrals made.

References

1. ND: Tissue Perfusion, ineffective (specify). In Doenges, M. E., Moorhouse, M. F., Geissler-Murr, A. C. (2002). *Nursing Care Plans: Guidelines for Individualizing Patient Care.* 6th ed. Philadelphia: F. A. Davis.
2. Schulman, C. (2002). End points of resuscitation: Choosing the right parameters to monitor. *Dimens Crit Care Nurs,* 21(1), 2–10.
3. Task Force on Pulmonary Embolism, European Society of Cardiology. (2000). Guidelines on diagnosis and management of acute pulmonary embolism. Accessed July 2007 at www.idealibrary.com.
4. Stephens, E. (2003, update 2007). Peripheral vascular disease. Accessed July 2007 at www.emedicine.com/emerg/topic862.htm.
5. No author listed. (1999). Antithrombotic therapy: A national clinical guideline. Scottish Intercollegiate Guidelines Network (SIGN). Accessed July 2007 at www.sign.ac.uk/guidelines/fulltext/36/index.html.
6. Goldrich, G. (2006). Understanding the 12-lead ECG, part I. *Nursing2006,* 36(11), 36–41.
7. Scott-Conner, C. E. H., Ballinger, B. (2005). Abdominal angina. Retrieved May 2007 at www.emedicine.com/med/topic2.htm.
8. Rasul, A. T. (2005). Compartment Syndrome. Retrieved May 2007 at www.emedicine.com/pmr/topic33.htm.
9. Paula, R. (2006). Compartment syndrome, abdominal. Article for Emedicine Web site. Retrieved April 2007 at www.emedicine.com/emerg/topic935.htm.
10. Nieves, J., Capone-Swearer, D. (2006). The clot that changes lives. *Nursing2006Critical Care,* 1(3), 18–28.
11. Sieggreen, M. (2006). A contemporary approach to peripheral arterial disease. *Health Practitioner: The American J of Primary Health Care,* 31(7), 14–25.
12. Sieggreen, M. Y. (2006). Getting a leg up on managing venous ulcers. *Nursing Made Incredibly Easy!,* 4(6), 52–60.
13. Baldwin, K. M. (2006). Stroke: It's a knock-out punch. *Nursing Made Incredibly Easy!* 4(2), 10–23.
14. Sauerbeck, L. R. (2006). Primary stroke prevention. *AJN,* 106,11, 40–49.
15. Frost, K. L., Topp, R. (2006). A physical activity RX for the hypertensive patient. *Nurse Practitioner: The American J of Primary Health Care,* 31(4), 29–37.
16. Bartley, M. K. (2006). Keep venous thromboembolism at bay. *Nursing2006,* 36(10), 36–41.

impaired Transfer Ability

Definition: Limitation of independent movement between two nearby surfaces

RELATED FACTORS

Insufficient muscle strength; deconditioning; neuromuscular impairment; musculoskeletal impairment (e.g., contractures)

Impaired balance

Pain

Obesity

Impaired vision

Lack of knowledge; cognitive impairment

Environment constraints (e.g., bed height, inadequate space, wheelchair type, treatment equipment, restraints)

DEFINING CHARACTERISTICS

Subjective or Objective

Inability to transfer from bed to chair/chair to bed; from chair to car/car to chair; from chair to floor/floor to chair; on or off a toilet/commode; in or out of tub/shower; from bed to standing/standing to bed; from chair to standing/standing to chair; from standing to floor/floor to standing; between uneven levels

Note: Specify level of independence using a standardized functional scale—[refer to ND impaired physical Mobility for suggested functional level classification]

Sample Clinical Applications: Arthritis, fractures, amputation, neuromuscular diseases (e.g., MS, ALS, Guillian-Barré syndrome), paralysis, glaucoma, macular degeneration, dementias

DESIRED OUTCOMES/EVALUATION CRITERIA

Sample NOC linkages:

Transfer Performance: Ability to change body location independently with or without assistive device

Balance: Ability to maintain body equilibrium

Body Positioning: Self-Initiated: Ability to change own body position independently with or without assistive device

Client/Caregiver Will (Include Specific Time Frame)

- Verbalize understanding of situation and appropriate safety measures.
- Master techniques of transfer successfully.
- Make desired transfer safely.

ACTIONS/INTERVENTIONS

Sample NIC linkages:

Transport: Moving a patient from one location to another

Body Mechanics Promotion: Facilitating the use of posture and movement in daily activities to prevent fatigue and musculoskeletal strain or injury

Cultural   Collaborative   Community/Home Care   Diagnostic Studies   Pediatric/Geriatric/Lifespan   Medications

Exercise Promotion: Strength Training: Facilitating regular physical exercise to maintain or advance to a higher level of fitness and health

NURSING PRIORITY NO. 1 To assess causative/contributing factors:

• Determine presence of conditions that contribute to transfer problems. *Neuromuscular and musculoskeletal problems, such as MS, fractures, back injuries, knee/hip replacement surgery, amputation, quadriplegia/paraplegia, contractures/spastic muscles, agedness (arthritis, decreased muscle mass/tone/strength), and effects of dementias, brain injury, etc., can seriously impact balance and physical and psychological well-being.*[1,5]

• Evaluate perceptual/cognitive impairments and ability to follow directions. *Plan of care/choice of interventions is dependent upon nature of condition—acute, chronic, progressive; for example, client with severe brain injury may have permanent limitations because of impaired cognition affecting memory, judgment, problem-solving, and motor coordination, requiring more intensive inpatient and long-term care.*

• Note factors complicating current situation. *Recent surgery, traction apparatus; debilitating illness, weakness; mechanical ventilation, multiple IV/indwelling tubings can restrict movement.*

• Review medication regimen/schedule *to determine possible side effects or drug interactions impairing balance and/or muscle tone.*

NURSING PRIORITY NO. 2 To assess functional ability:

• Perform "Get-up and Go" test, as indicated, *to assess client's basic ability to transfer and ambulate safely. In this test, the client is asked to get up from a seated position in a chair, stand still momentarily, walk forward 10 feet, turn around, walk back to the chair, turn, and sit down. Factors assessed include sitting balance, ability to transfer from sitting to standing and back to sitting, the pace and stability of ambulation, and the ability to turn without staggering. If the client is not safe with ambulation, assistance may also be required with transfers.*[2] *Note: Client may perform this test adequately and still have difficulty with some transfers such as in/out of a car or bathtub, or from floor to chair.*

• Determine degree of impairment in relation to 0 to 4 scale, noting muscle strength and tone, joint mobility, cardiovascular status, balance, and endurance. *Identifies strengths and deficits (e.g., ability to ambulate with assistive devices or problems with balance, failure to attend to one side, inability to bear weight [client is nonweight-bearing or partial weight-bearing]) and may provide information regarding potential for recovery.*[5]

• Observe movement when client is unaware of observations *to note any incongruence with reported abilities.*

• Note emotional/behavioral responses of client/SO to problems of immobility. *Restrictions or limitations imposed by immobility can cause physical, social, emotional, and financial difficulties for everyone.*

NURSING PRIORITY NO. 3 To promote optimal level of movement:

• Assist with treatment of underlying condition causing dysfunction. *Treatment of condition (e.g., surgery for hip replacement, therapy for unilateral neglect following stroke) can alleviate or improve difficulties with transfer activity.*

• Consult with PT/OT/rehabilitation team *to develop general and specific muscle strengthening and range-of-motion (ROM) exercises, transfer training and techniques, as well as recommendations/provision of balance, gait, and mobility aids/adjunctive devices.*[2]

- Position devices (e.g., call light, bed-positioning switch) in easy reach on the bed/chair. *Facilitates transer/allows client to obtain assistance for transfer as needed.*
- Use appropriate number of people to assist with transfers and correct equipment *to safely transfer the client in a particular situation (e.g., chair to bed, chair to car, in/out of shower/tub, etc.).*[6,7]
- Demonstrate/assist with use of siderails/stand pole, overhead trapeze, transfer/sit-to-stand hoist; specialty slings; cane, walker, wheelchair, crutches, as necessary, *to protect client or care providers from injury during transfers/movements.*[6,7]
- Provide instruction/reinforce information for client and caregivers regarding body and equipment positioning *to improve/maintain balance during transfers.*
- Monitor body alignment, posture, and balance and encourage wide base of support *when standing to transfer.*
- Use full-length mirror, as needed, *to facilitate client's view of own postural alignment.*

NURSING PRIORITY NO. 4 To promote wellness (Teaching/Discharge Considerations):

- Instruct client/caregiver in appropriate safety measures. *Proper use of transfer board, locking wheels on bed/chair; correct placement of equipment for optimal body mechanics of client and caregivers(s); use of gait belt, supportive/nonslip footwear, good lighting, clearing floor of clutter, and so forth is important to facilitating transfers and reducing the possibility of fall and subsequent injury to client and caregiver.*[3]
- Discuss need for and sources of care/supervision. *Home-care agency, before- and after-school programs, elderly day care, personal companions, etc., may be required to assist with/monitor activity.*[4]
- Refer to appropriate community resources *for evaluation and modification of environment (e.g., roll-in-shower/tub, correction of uneven floor surfaces/steps, installation of ramps, use of standing tables/lifts, etc.).*
- Refer also to NDs impaired bed/physical/wheelchair Mobility, unilateral Neglect, or impaired Walking for additional interventions.

DOCUMENTATION FOCUS

Assessment/Reassessment

- Individual findings, including level of function/ability to participate in desired transfers.
- Mobility aides/transfer devices used.

Planning

- Plan of care and who is involved in the planning.
- Teaching plan.

Implementation/Evaluation

- Responses to interventions/teaching and actions performed.
- Attainment/progress toward desired outcome(s).
- Modifications to plan of care.

Discharge Planning

- Discharge/long-range needs, noting who is responsible for each action to be taken.
- Specific referrals made.
- Sources of/maintenance for assistive devices.

Cultural   Collaborative   Community/Home Care   Diagnostic Studies   Pediatric/Geriatric/Lifespan   Medications

References

1. Mass, M. L. (1989). Impaired physical mobility. (Unpublished manuscript). Cited in research article for National Institutes for Health.
2. Cruise, C. M., Koval, K. J. (1998). Rehabilitation of the elderly. *Arch Am Acad Orthop Surg, 2*(1), 103–107.
3. No author listed. (2000). Patient safety during transfers. Policy/Operations Manual. UTMB Department of Rehabilitation Services.
4. Hogue, C. C. (1984). Falls and mobility late in life. An ecological model. *J Am Geriatr Soc, 32,* 858–861.
5. Tinetti, M. E. Williams, T. F., Mayewski, R. (1986). Fall risk index for elderly patients based on number of chronic disabilities. *Am J Med, 80,* 429–434.
6. Parsons, K. S., Galinsky, T. L., Waters, T. (2006). Suggestions for preventing musculoskeletal disorders in home healthcare workers, Part 1: Lift and transfer assistance for partially weight-bearing home care patients. *Home Healthcare Nurse,* 24(3), 158–164.
7. Parsons, K. S., Galinsky, T. L., Waters, T. (2006). Suggestions for preventing musculoskeletal disorders in home healthcare workers, Part 2: Lift and transfer assistance for non-weight-bearing home care patients. *Home Healthcare Nurse,* 24(4), 227–233.

risk for Trauma

Definition: Accentuated risk of accidental tissue injury (e.g., wound, burn, fracture)

RISK FACTORS

Internal
Weakness; balancing difficulties; reduced muscle/hand/eye coordination
Poor vision
Reduced sensation
Lack of safety education/precautions
Insufficient finances
Cognitive/emotional difficulties
History of previous trauma

External [includes but is not limited to]:
Slippery floors (e.g., wet or highly waxed); unanchored rugs/electric wires
Bathtub without antislip equipment
Use of unsteady ladder/chairs
Obstructed passageways; entering unlighted rooms
Inadequate stair rails; children playing without gates at top of stairs
High beds; inappropriate call-for-aid mechanisms for bedresting client
Unsafe window protection in homes with young children
Pot handles facing toward front of stove; bathing in very hot water (e.g., unsupervised bathing of young children)
Potential igniting gas leaks; delayed lighting of gas appliances
Wearing flowing clothes around open flames; flammable children's clothing/toys
Smoking in bed/near oxygen; grease waste collected on stoves
Children playing with dangerous objects; accessibility of guns
Playing with explosives; experimenting with chemicals; inadequately stored combustibles (e.g., matches, oily rags)/corrosives (e.g., lye); contact with corrosives
Overloaded fuse boxes; faulty electrical plugs; frayed wires; defective appliances; overloaded electrical outlets
Exposure to dangerous machinery; contact with rapidly moving machinery
Struggling with restraints

Contact with intense cold; lack of protection from heat source; overexposure to radiation

Large icicles hanging from the roof

Use of cracked dishware; knives stored uncovered

High-crime neighborhood

Driving a mechanically unsafe vehicle; driving at excessive speeds; driving without necessary visual aids; driving while intoxicated

Children riding in the front seat of car; nonuse/misuse of seat restraints

Unsafe road/walkways; physical proximity to vehicle pathways (e.g., driveways, lanes, railroad tracks)

Misuse[/nonuse] of necessary headgear [e.g., for bicycles, motorcycles, skateboarding, skiing]

NOTE: A risk diagnosis is not evidenced by signs and symptoms, as the problem has not occurred; rather, nursing interventions are directed at prevention.

Sample Clinical Applications: Substance intoxication/abuse, peripheral neuropathy, cataracts/glaucoma/macular degeneration, Parkinson's disease, seizure disorder, dementia, major depression, developmental delay

DESIRED OUTCOMES/EVALUATION CRITERIA

Sample NOC linkages:

Physical Injury Severity: Severity of injuries from accidents and trauma

Abuse Protection: Protection of self or dependent others from abuse

Knowledge: Personal Safety: Extent of understanding conveyed about prevention of unintentional injuries

Client/Caregiver Will (Include Specific Time Frame)

- Identify and correct potential risk factors in the environment.
- Demonstrate appropriate lifestyle changes to reduce risk of injury.
- Identify resources to assist in promoting a safe environment.
- Recognize need for/seek assistance to prevent accidents/injuries.

ACTIONS/INTERVENTIONS

This ND is a compilation of a number of situations that can result in injury. Refer to specific NDs, such as risk for imbalanced Body Temperature; risk for Contamination; impaired Environmental Interpretation Syndrome; risk for Falls; impaired Home Maintenance; Hyperthermia; Hypothermia; risk for Injury; impaired physical Mobility; risk for impaired Parenting; risk for Poisoning; disturbed Sensory Perception; impaired Skin Integrity; risk for Suffocation; disturbed Thought Processes; impaired Tissue Integrity; risk for self-/other-directed Violence; impaired Walking, as appropriate, for more specific interventions.

Sample NIC linkages:

Environmental Management: Safety: Manipulation of the patient's surroundings for therapeutic benefit

Environmental Management: Worker Safety: Monitoring and manipulation of the work-site environment to promote safety and health of workers

Teaching: Infant/Toddler Safety: Instruction on safety during first/second and third years of life

Surveillance: Safety: Purposeful and ongoing collection and analysis of information about the patient and the environment for use in promoting and maintaining patient safety

Cultural · Collaborative · Community/Home Care · Diagnostic Studies · Pediatric/Geriatric/Lifespan · Medications

NURSING PRIORITY NO. 1 To assess causative/contributing factors:

- Determine factors related to individual situation and extent of risk for trauma. *Influences scope and intensity of interventions to manage threats to safety, which are dynamic and constants in every life and situation. Clients interfacing with the healthcare system are at higher risk for trauma for any number of reasons (e.g., illness state, cognitive function, family structure, information and training, etc.), and require protection in numerous ways.*[1]
- Note client's age/gender/developmental stage, decision-making ability, level of cognition/competence *to determine client's ability to recognize danger and to protect self.*
- Ascertain client's/SO's knowledge of safety needs/injury prevention and ways of looking at and improving own environment. *Lack of appreciation of significance of individual hazards increases risk of traumatic injury.*[1]
- Assess influence of stressors (e.g., physical, mental, work-related, financial, etc.) *that can impair judgment/greatly increase client's potential for injury.*
- Assess mood, coping abilities, personality styles (i.e., temperament, aggression, impulsive behavior, level of self-esteem). *May result in careless/increased risk-taking without consideration of consequences.*[13,14]
- Evaluate individual's emotional and behavioral response to violence in surroundings (e.g., neighborhood, television, peer group). *May affect client's view of and regard for own/others' safety.*[13–15]
- Evaluate environment (home/work/transportation) *for obvious safety hazards, as well as situations that can exacerbate injury or adversely affect client's well-being. Unsafe factors include a vast array of possibilities (e.g., unsafe heating appliances, smoking materials, toxic substances and chemicals, open flames, knives, improperly stored guns, overloaded electrical outlets, dangerous neighborhoods, unsupervised children).*[1]
- Review potential occupational risk factors (e.g., works with dangerous tools and machinery, electricity, explosives, etc.; police/fire/EMS officers; working with hazardous chemicals/various inhalants/radiation, etc.).
- Note history of accidents during specific period of time, noting circumstances of the accident (e.g., time of day that falls occur, activities going on, who was present). *Investigation of such events can provide clues for client's risk for subsequent events and potential for enhanced safety by a change in the people or environment involved (e.g., client may need assistance when getting up at night, or increased playground supervision may be required).*
- Determine potential for abusive behavior by family members/SO(s)/peers. *Anyone, but especially child/frail elder, may require placement if incurring repeated injuries in family/community setting.*
- Note socioeconomic status/availability and use of resources. *Lack of resources, including financial, may limit ability to meet safety needs (e.g., proper child safety seat, appliance repairs, window grates, etc.).*
- Review diagnostic studies/laboratory results, noting impairments/imbalances *that may result in/exacerbate conditions, such as confusion, tetany, pathological fractures, etc.*

NURSING PRIORITY NO. 2 To enhance safety in healthcare environment:

- Perform thorough assessments regarding safety issues when planning for client care/discharge. *Failure to accurately assess and intervene or refer regarding these issues can place the client at needless risk and creates negligence issues for the healthcare practitioner.*[12]
- Monitor client's therapeutic regimen on a continual basis (e.g., client's vital signs, medications, treatment modalaties, infusions, nutrition, physical environment) *to prevent healthcare-related injuries.*[12]

• Collaborate in treatment of underlying medical/surgical/psychiatric conditions *to improve cognition/thinking processes, musculoskeletal function, awareness of own safety needs, and general well-being.*

 • Refer to physical or occupational therapist as appropriate *to identify high-risk tasks, conduct site visits, select/create/modify equipment, and provide education about body mechanics and musculoskeletal injuries, as well as provide needed therapies.*[3]

• Emphasize with client importance of obtaining assistance when weak/sedated and when problems of balance, coordination, or postural hypotension are present *to reduce risk of syncope/falls.*

• Provide quiet environment and reduced stimulation as indicated. *Helps limit confusion or over-stimulation for clients at risk for such conditions as seizures, tetany, autonomic hyperreflexia.*

• Demonstrate/encourage use of techniques to reduce/manage stress and vent emotions such as anger, hostility *to reduce risk of violence to self/others.*

• Provide for routine safety needs:[2–11]

Provide adequate supervision and frequent observation.

Place young children, confused client/person with dementia near nurses' station

Provide for appropriate communication tools (e.g., call light, writing implements and paper; alphabet picture board, etc.).

Demonstrate use and place call bell/light within client's reach.

Orient/reorient client to environment as needed.

Encourage client's use of corrective vision and hearing aids.

Keep bed in low position or place mattress on floor as appropriate.

Maintain correct body alignment and mechanics.

Provide positioning as required by situation (e.g., immobilization of fractures).

Implement appropriate measures to maintain skin and tissue health.

Protect client with sensory impairments from injury due to heat and cold.

Provide seizure precautions when indicated.

Lock wheels on bed/wheelchair/movable furniture.

Assist with activities and transfers as needed.

Provide well-fitting, nonskid footwear.

Demonstrate/monitor use of assistive devices, such as cane, walker, crutches, wheelchair, safety bars.

Clear travel paths, pick up small items from floor; keep furniture in one place and door in one position (completely open or closed).

Provide adequate area lighting.

Follow facility protocol/closely monitor use of restraints when required (e.g., vest, limb, belt, mitten).

 Administer treatments, medications and therapies in a therapeutic manner.

Dispose of sharp implements in appropriate container.

NURSING PRIORITY NO. 3 To enhance safety for client in community care setting:

• Provide information to caregivers regarding client's specific disease/condition(s) and associated risks. *For example, postural hypotension, muscle weakness (e.g., MS), dementia, osteoporosis, head injury can impair function or cognition, impacting client's ability to protect self.*

• Identify interventions/safety devices to promote safe physical environment and individual safety:[7,8,11–14]

Recommend wearing visual/hearing aids *to maximize sensory input.*

Ensure availability of communication devices (telephone, computer, alarm system/medical emergency alert device, etc.).

Install/maintain electrical and fire safety devices, extinguishers, and alarms.

Review oxygen safety rules.

Identify environmental needs (e.g., decals on glass doors *to show when they are closed*, adequate lighting of stairways, handrails, ramps, bathtub safety tapes *to reduce risk of falls*; lowering temperature on hot water heater *to prevent accidental burns*; creation of ergonomic workstation.

Obtain seat raisers for chairs; ergonomic beds/chairs.

Encourage participation in back-safety classes; injury-prevention exercises, mobility/transfer device training.

Install childproof cabinets for medications/toxic household substances, use tamper-proof medication containers.

Review proper storage/disposal of volatile liquids; installation of proper ventilation for use when mixing/using toxic substances; use of safety glasses/goggles.

Stress importance of appropriate use of car restraints, bicycle/skating/skiing helmets.

Discuss swimming pool fencing and supervision; attending first-aid/CPR classes.

Obtain trigger locks/gun safes for firearms.

- Initiate appropriate teaching *if reckless behavior is occurring/likely to occur* (e.g., *smoking in bed, driving without safety belts, working with chemicals without safety goggles, etc.*).
- Encourage participation in self-help programs *to address individual risks* (e.g., *assertiveness training, positive self-image to enhance self-esteem, smoking cessation, weight management*).
- Refer to counseling/psychotherapy, as need indicates, *especially when individual is "accident-prone" or self-destructive behavior is noted*. Refer to NDs [actual/]risk for self-directed Violence.

NURSING PRIORITY NO. 4 To promote wellness (Teaching/Discharge Considerations):

- Discuss importance of self-monitoring of conditions/emotions that can contribute to occurrence of injury to self/others (e.g., fatigue, anger, irritability). *Client/SO may be able to modify risk through monitoring of actions, or postponement of certain actions, especially during times when client is likely to be highly stressed.*
- Review expectations caregivers have of children, cognitively impaired, or elderly family members *to identify needed information, required assistance with care, follow-up that may be needed to provide safe environment for client.*
- Problem-solve with client/parent *to provide adequate child supervision after school, during working hours, and on school holidays.*
- Discuss need for/sources of adult supervision (e.g., elderly day care, home health aide or companion, etc.).
- Encourage client's family to identify neighbors or friends willing *to assist elderly/individuals with disabilities in providing such things as checking on client who lives alone, or snow and ice removal from walks and steps, assist with structural maintenance, etc.*
- Explore behaviors related to use of alcohol, tobacco, and recreational drugs and other substances. *Provides opportunity to review consequences of previously determined risk factors (e.g., increase in oral cancer among teenagers using smokeless tobacco, potential consequences of illegal activities, effects of smoking on health of family members as well as fire danger; occurrence of spontaneous abortion, fetal alcohol syndrome/neonatal addiction in prenatal women using tobacco, alcohol, and other drugs).*[13-15]
- Encourage development of fire safety program. *Participation in family fire drills, use of smoke detectors, yearly chimney cleaning, purchase of fire-retardant clothing (especially children's nightwear), fireworks safety, safe use of in-home oxygen/propane sources, etc., enhances home safety.*

- Recommend use of seat belts, approved infant seat, fitted helmets for cyclists, wearing necessary visual aids; driver training course for new and mature drivers; avoidance of hitchhiking; substance abuse program as indicated *to promote transportation safety.*
- Identify community resources (e.g., financial, volunteer) *to assist with necessary home improvements/equipment purchases.*
- Refer to other resources as indicated (e.g., counseling/psychotherapy, parenting classes, budget counseling).
- Provide client/caregiver with emergency contact numbers as individually indicated (e.g., doctor, 911, poison control, police).
- Provide client/caregiver with bibliotherapy/written resources *for later review and self-paced learning.*
- Encourage involvement in community awareness programs and problem-solving of identified community needs:

  Participate in self-help programs (e.g., Neighborhood Watch, Helping Hand, after-school activities). *Programs based on identified needs enhances support of community members and potential funding sources.*

  Promote educational opportunities *geared toward increasing awareness of safety measures (e.g., firearms safety) and resources available to the individual.*

  Seek out/involve businesses in volunteer outreach activities such as building safe playgrounds, community/street cleanup, home repair/improvement for frail elders, etc.

  Advocate for/promote solutions for problems of design of buildings, equipment, transportation, and workplace practices *that contribute to accidents.*

DOCUMENTATION FOCUS

Assessment/Reassessment

- Individual risk factors, past/recent history of injuries, awareness of safety needs.

Planning

- Plan of care and who is involved in the planning.
- Teaching plan.

Implementation/Evaluation

- Responses to interventions/teaching, actions performed.
- Attainment/progress toward desired outcome(s).
- Modifications to plan of care.

Discharge Planning

- Long-term needs and who is responsible for actions to be taken.
- Available resources, specific referrals made.

References

1. Ebright, P. R., Patterson, E. S., Render, M. L. (2002). The "New Look" approach to patient safety: A guide for clinical specialist leadership. *Clin Nurs Spec,* 16(5), 247–253.
2. ND: Trauma, risk for. In Doenges, M. E., Moorhouse, M. F., Geissler-Murr, A. C. (2002). *Nurse's Pocket Guide: Diagnoses, Interventions, and Rationales.* 8th ed. Philadelphia: F. A. Davis.
3. Nelson, A., et al. (2003). Safe patient handling & movement. *AJN,* 103(3), 32–43.
4. Walton, J. (2001). Helping high-risk surgical patients beat the odds. *Nursing,* 31(3), 54.

Cultural   Collaborative   Community/Home Care   Diagnostic Studies   Pediatric/Geriatric/Lifespan   Medications

5. Mion, L. C., Mercurio, A. T. (1992). Methods to reduce restraints: Process, outcomes and future directions. *J Gerontol Nurs*, 20(10), 5.

6. Wright, A. (1998). Nursing interventions with advanced osteoporosis. *Home Health Nurs*, 16(3), 145.

7. Kedlaya, D., Kuang, T. (2002, update 2007). Assistive devices to improve independence. Accessed July 2007 at www.emedicine.com/pmr/topic210.htm.

8. Safety for older consumers' home safety checklist. Available at Consumer Product Safety Commission (CPSC). Accessed July 2007 at www.cpsc.gov.

9. Nursing Care Plan: Extended Care, Falls, risk for. In Doenges, M. E., Moorhouse, M. F., Geissler-Murr, A. C. (2002). *Nursing Care Plans: Guidelines for Individualizing Patient Care.* 6th ed. (CD-ROM). Philadelphia: F. A. Davis.

10. Daus, C. (1999). Maintaining mobility: Assistive equipment helps the geriatric population stay active and independent. *Rehab Management*, 12(5), 58–61.

11. Horn, L. B. (2000). Reducing the risk of falls in the elderly. *Rehab Management*, 13(3), 36–38.

12. Keepnews, D., Mitchell, P. H. (2003). Health Systems' Accountability for patient safety. *Online J of Issues in Nursing*, 8(2). Manuscript 2. Retrieved March 2007 at http://nursingworld.org/ojin/topic22/tpc22_2.htm.

13. Gorman-Smith, D., Tolan, P. (1998). The role of exposure to community violence and developmental problems among inner city youth. *Dev Psychopathol*, 10(1), 101.

14. Youth Violence in the United States. National Center for Injury Prevention and Control. Accessed July 2007 at www.cdc.gov/ncipc/factsheets/yvfacts.htm.

15. Schwebel, D. C., Barton, B. K. (2005). Contributions of multiple risk factors to child injury. *J of Pediatr Psychol*, 30(7), 553–561.

impaired Urinary Elimination

Definition: Dysfunction in urine elimination

RELATED FACTORS

Multiple causality; sensory motor impairment; anatomical obstruction; UTI; [mechanical trauma; fluid/volume states; psychogenic factors; surgical diversion]

DEFINING CHARACTERISTICS

Subjective
Frequency; urgency
Hesitancy
Dysuria
Nocturia, [enuresis]

Objective
Incontinence
Retention

Sample Clinical Applications: Urinary tract infection, prostate disease (BPH), bladder cancer, spinal cord injury, MS, pregnancy/childbirth, pelvic trauma, abdominal surgery, dementia/Alzheimer's disease

DESIRED OUTCOMES/EVALUATION CRITERIA

Sample NOC linkages:

Urinary Elimination: Collection and drainage of urine
Urinary Continence: Control of the elimination of urine from the bladder
Self-Care: Toileting: Ability to toilet self independently with or without assistive device

Client Will (Include Specific Time Frame)

- Verbalize understanding of condition.
- Identify specific causative factors.
- Achieve normal elimination pattern or participate in measures to correct/compensate for defects.
- Demonstrate behaviors/techniques to prevent urinary infection.
- Manage care of urinary catheter, or stoma and appliance following urinary diversion.

ACTIONS/INTERVENTIONS

Sample NIC linkages:
Urinary Elimination Management: Maintenance of an optimum urinary elimination pattern
Urinary Catheterization: Insertion of a catheter into the bladder for temporary or permanent drainage of urine
Perineal Care: Maintenance of perineal skin integrity and relief of perineal discomfort

NURSING PRIORITY NO. 1 To assess causative/contributing factors:

- Note presence of physical diagnoses that may be involved, such as urinary tract infection, dehydration; surgery (including urinary diversion); neurological conditions (e.g., MS, stroke, Parkinson's disease; paraplegia/tetraplegia); mental/emotional dysfunction (e.g., impaired cognition, delirium/confusion, depression, Alzheimer's disease); prostate disorders; recent/multiple pregnancies; pelvic trauma.[1]
- Determine pathology of bladder dysfunction relative to identified medical diagnosis (e.g., in neurological/demyelinating diseases, such as MS, problem may be failure to store urine, empty bladder, or both). *Identifies direction for further evaluation/treatment options to discover specifics of individual situation.*[2,3,9]
- Note client's age and gender. Incontinence and urinary tract infections are more prevalent in women and older adults; painful bladder syndrome/interstitial cystitis (PBS/IC) is more common in women.[5,10]
- Assist with/perform physical examination (e.g., cough test *for incontinence*, palpation *for bladder retention/masses,* prostate size, observation for urethral stricture, etc.).[11]
- Investigate pain, noting location, duration, intensity; presence of bladder spasms, back or flank pain *to assist in differentiating between bladder and kidney cause of dysfunction. Note: Bladder pain located suprapubically, vaginally, in the perineum, low back, or in the medial aspects of the thighs that is relieved by voiding and often recurs with bladder filling suggests presence of PBS/IC.*[10]
- Have client complete standardized self-report tool, such as Pelvic Pain and Urgency/Frequency (PUF) client symptom survey, as indicated. *Helpful in evaluating the presence and severity of PBS/IC symptoms.*[10]
- Note reports of exacerbations (flare-ups) and spontaneous remissions of symptoms of urgency and frequency, which may/may not be accompanied by pain, pressure, or spasm. *Clients with PBS/IC void approximately 16 times per day with voided volumes usually less than normal.*[10]
- Determine client's usual daily fluid intake (both amount and beverage choices/use of caffeine). Note condition of skin and mucous membranes, color of urine *to determine level of hydration.*[5]

🌐 Cultural 🅐 Collaborative 🏠 Community/Home Care ⟋ Diagnostic Studies ∞ Pediatric/Geriatric/Lifespan 💊 Medications

• Review medication regimen to identify drugs that can alter bladder or kidney function (e.g., some antihypertensive agents [e.g. ACE inhibitors, beta-blockers]; anticholinergics [e.g. antihistamines, antiparkinsonian drugs]; antidepressants/antipsychotics, sedative/hypnotics/opioids; caffeine, and alcohol).[12]

• Send urine specimen (midstream clean-voided or catheterized) for culture and sensitivities in presence of signs of urinary tract infection—cloudy, foul odor; bloody urine.

• Obtain specimen for antibody-coated bacteria assay. *Diagnosis of bacterial infection of the kidney or prostate is important for immediate treatment to prevent damage to these organs.*[3]

• Strain all urine for calculi and describe stones expelled or send to laboratory for analysis. *Retrieval of calculi allows identification of type of stone and influences choice of therapy.*[3]

• Review laboratory tests *for hyperglycemia/hyperparathyroidism/other metabolic conditions; changes in renal function, presence of infection/sexually transmitted disease (STD), cytology revealing cancer.*

• Rule out gonorrhea in men. *This infection needs to be considered when urethritis with a penile discharge is present and there are no bacteria in the urine.*[3]

• Assist with/perform potassium sensitivity test (instillation of potassium solution into bladder). *Eighty percent of clients with PBS/IC will react positively.*[10]

• Review results of other diagnostic studies (e.g., uroflowmetry, cystometogram, postvoid residual, pressure flow and leak point pressure measurement, videourodynamics, electromyography, kidneys/ureters/bladder[KUB] imaging, etc.) *to identify presence/type of elimination problem.*[13]

NURSING PRIORITY NO. 2 To assess degree of interference/disability:

• Ascertain client's previous pattern of elimination and compare with current situation. Ask about/note reports of problems (e.g., frequency, urgency, painful urination; leaking/incontinence; changes in size/force of urinary stream; problems emptying bladder completely; nocturia/enuresis) *to assist identification/treatment of particular dysfunction.*

• Ascertain client's/SO's perception of problem/degree of disability and impact on self-image (e.g., client may be restricting social/employment/travel activities; having sexual/relationship difficulties; experiencing depression).

• Note influence of culture/ethnicity or gender on client's view of problems of incontinence. *Limited evidence exists to understand and help people cope with the physical and psychosocial consequences of this chronic, socially isolating, and potentially devastating disorder.*[6]

• Have client keep a voiding diary for 3 days to record fluid intake, voiding times, precise urine output, and dietary intake. *Helps determine baseline symptoms, the severity of frequency/urgency; and whether diet is a factor if symptoms worsen.*

NURSING PRIORITY NO. 3 To assist in treating/preventing urinary alteration:

• Encourage fluid intake up to 2000 to 3000 mL/day (within cardiac tolerance), including cranberry juice. *Maintains renal function, prevents infection and formation of urinary stones, avoids encrustation around indwelling catheter, or may be used to flush urinary diversion appliance.*[5]

• Discuss possible dietary restrictions (e.g., especially coffee, alcohol, carbonated drinks, citrus, tomatoes, and chocolate) based on individual symptoms.[10]

• Assist with developing toileting routines (e.g., timed voiding, bladder training, prompted voiding, habit retraining) as appropriate. *For adults who are cognitively intact and physically capable of self-toileting, bladder training, timed voiding, and habit retraining may be beneficial.*[5,14] *However, bladder retraining is not recommended for clients with PBS.*[10]

Nursing Diagnoses in Alphabetical Order

- Encourage client to verbalize fear/concerns (e.g., disruption in sexual activity, inability to work, concern about involvement in social activities). *Open expression allows client to talk about, deal with feelings, and begin to solve the identified problems.*[6]
- Implement/monitor interventions for specific elimination problem (e.g., pelvic floor exercises/other bladder retraining modalities; medication regimen, antimicrobials [single dose is frequently being used for UTI], sulfonamides, antispasmodics). Evaluate client's response *to modify treatment as needed.*[3]
- Discuss possible surgical procedures and medical regimen as indicated (e.g., client with benign prostatic hypertrophy, bladder/prostatic cancer, PBS/IC, etc.). *For example, cystoscopy with bladder hydrodistention for PBS/IC, or an electrical stimulator may be implanted to treat chronic urinary urge incontinence, nonobstructive urinary retention, and symptoms of urgency and frequency.*[6,10]
- Refer to specific NDs Urinary Incontinence (specify); [acute/chronic] Urinary Retention for additional interventions/treatment regimens.

NURSING PRIORITY NO. 4   To assist in management of long-term urinary alterations:

- Keep bladder deflated by use of an indwelling catheter connected to closed drainage. Investigate alternatives when possible. *Measures such as intermittent catheterization, surgical interventions, urinary drugs, voiding maneuvers, condom catheter may be preferable to the indwelling catheter to provide more effective control and prevent possibility of recurrent infections.*[3,7]
- Provide latex-free catheter and care supplies. *Reduces risk of developing sensitivity to latex, which can develop in individuals requiring frequent catheterization or who have long-term indwelling catheters.*[8]
- Check frequently for bladder distention and observe for overflow. *Requires immediate intervention to reduce risk of infection or autonomic hyperreflexia.*[3]
- Maintain acidic environment of the bladder by the use of agents such as vitamin C, Mandelamine when appropriate. *There is some evidence that the acidic environment discourages bacterial growth by preventing bacteria from adhering to the bladder wall.*[3]
- Adhere to a regular bladder/diversion appliance emptying schedule. *Avoids accidents and prevents embarrassment to the individual.*[4]
- Provide for routine diversion appliance care, and assist client to recognize and deal with problems such as alkaline salt encrustation, ill-fitting appliance, malodorous urine, infection, etc. *Provides information and promotes competence in care, increasing self-confidence in dealing with appliance on a regular basis.*[4]

NURSING PRIORITY NO. 5   To promote wellness (Teaching/Discharge Considerations):

- Emphasize importance of keeping perineal area clean and dry. *Reduces risk of infection or skin breakdown.*[3]
- Instruct female clients with urinary tract infection to drink large amounts of fluid, void immediately after intercourse, wipe from front to back, promptly treat vaginal infections, and take showers rather than tub baths as appropriate. *These measures can limit risk of/avoid reinfection.*[5]
- Recommend smoking cessation program as appropriate. *Cigarette smoking can also be a source of bladder irritation.*
- Encourage SO(s) who participate in routine care to recognize complications (including latex allergy) necessitating medical follow-up. *Client may be too embarrassed to discuss symptoms, and caregivers need to be alert to changes that necessitate evaluation and treatment.*[6]

- Instruct in proper application and care of appliance for urinary diversion. Encourage liberal fluid intake, avoidance of foods/medications that produce strong odor, use of white vinegar or deodorizer in pouch to promote odor control. *These measures help to ensure patency of device and prevent embarrassing situations for client.*[4]
- Identify sources for supplies, programs/agencies providing financial assistance. *Lack of access to necessities can be a barrier to management of incontinence and having help to obtain needed equipment can assist with daily care.*[6]
- Recommend avoidance of gas-forming foods in presence of ureterosigmoidostomy. *Flatus can cause urinary incontinence.*[2]
- Recommend use of silicone catheter. *These catheters are more comfortable and have fewer problems with infection when permanent/long-term catheterization is required.*[3]
- Demonstrate proper positioning of catheter drainage tubing and bag. *Facilitates drainage/prevents reflux and complications of infection.*[2]
- Refer client/SO(s) to appropriate community resources such as ostomy specialist, support group, sex therapist, psychiatric clinical nurse specialist, and so on. *May be necessary to deal with changes in body image/function.*[6]

DOCUMENTATION FOCUS

Assessment/Reassessment

- Individual findings, including previous and current pattern of voiding, nature of problem, effect on desired lifestyle.
- Cultural factors/concerns.

Planning

- Plan of care and who is involved in planning.
- Teaching plan.

Implementation/Evaluation

- Response to interventions/teaching, actions performed.
- Attainment/progress toward desired outcome(s).
- Modifications to plan of care.

Discharge Planning

- Long-term needs and who is responsible for actions to be taken.
- Available resources/specific referrals made.
- Individual equipment needs and sources.

References

1. ND: Urinary Elimination, impaired. In Doenges, M. E., Moorhouse, M. F., Murr, A. C. (2004). *Nurse's Pocket Guide: Diagnoses, Interventions, and Rationales.* 9th ed. Philadelphia: F. A. Davis.
2. Cox, H. C., et al. (2002). *Clinical Applications of Nursing Diagnosis: Adult, Child, Women's, Psychiatric, Gerontic, and Home Health Considerations.* 4th ed. Philadelphia: F. A. Davis.
3. ND: Urinary Elimination, impaired. In Doenges, M. E., Moorhouse, M. F., Geissler-Murr, A. C. (2002). *Nursing Care Plans, Guidelines for Individualizing Patient Care.* 6th ed. Philadelphia: F. A. Davis.
4. Colwell, J. C., et al. (2001). The state of the standard diversion. *J Wound Ostomy Continence Nurs*, 28(1), 6–17.
5. Wyman, J. F. (2003). Treatment of urinary incontinence in men and older women. In Newman, D. K., Palmer, M. H. (eds). The state of the science on urinary incontinence. *Am J Nurs*, 293, 3(suppl), 20.
6. Newman, D. K., Palmer, M. H. (eds). (2003). The state of the science on urinary incontinence. *Am J Nurs*, 293, 3(suppl), 20

7. Beers, M. H., Berkow, R. (eds). (1999). *The Merck Manual of Diagnosis and Therapy.* 17th ed. Whitehouse Station, NJ: Merck Research Laboratories.
8. Statement on natural latex allergies and SB latex. Accessed July 2007 at www.regnet.com/sblc/html/body_sbvsnat.html.
9. Gray, M. (2005). Overactive bladder: An overview. *Journal of Wound, Ostomy and Continence Nursing,* 32(3), Suppl, 1–5.
10. Panzera, A. K. (2007). Interstitial cystitis/painful bladder syndrome. *Urol Nurs,* 27(1), 13–19. Retrieved May 2007 at www.medscape.com/viewarticle/555699?src=mp.
11. Bates, B. (February 15, 2007). Simple questions can help uncover urinary incontinence. (Womens Health). *Family Practice News.* Retrieved May 2007 at www.highbeam.com/doc/1G1-160480576.html.
12. Newman, D. K. (2005). Assessment of the patient with an overactive bladder. *Journal of Wound, Ostomy and Continence Nursing,* 32(3), Suppl, 5–10.
13. Albo, M., Richter, H. E. (2006). Urodynamic testing. Fact sheet for National Kidney and Urologic Diseases Information Clearinghouse. Retrieved August 2007 at http://kidney.niddk.nih.gov/kudiseases/pubs/urodynamic/index.htm.
14. Milne, J. L., Krissovich, M. (2004). Behavioral therapies at the primary care level: The current state of knowledge. *Journal of Wound, Ostomy and Continence Nursing,* 31(6), 367–376.

readiness for enhanced Urinary Elimination

Definition: A pattern of urinary functions that is sufficient for meeting eliminatory needs and can be strengthened

RELATED FACTORS
To be developed by nurse researchers and submitted to NANDA

DEFINING CHARACTERISTICS

Subjective
Expresses willingness to enhance urinary elimination
Positions self for emptying of bladder

Objective
Urine is straw-colored/odorless
Amount of output/specific gravity is within normal limits
Fluid intake is adequate for daily needs

Sample Clinical Applications: Spinal cord injury, MS, pregnancy/childbirth, pelvic trauma, abdominal surgery, prostate disease

DESIRED OUTCOMES/EVALUATION CRITERIA
Sample NOC Linkages:
Urinary Continence: Control of the elimination of urine from the bladder
Knowledge: Disease Process: Extent of understanding conveyed about a specific disease process
Urinary Elimination: Collection and drainage of urine

Client Will (Include Specific Time Frame)

- Verbalize understanding of condition that has potential for altering elimination.
- Achieve normal/acceptable elimination pattern, emptying bladder/voiding in appropriate amounts.
- Alter lifestyle/environment to accommodate individual needs.

🌐 Cultural   Collaborative   🏠 Community/Home Care   Diagnostic Studies   ∞ Pediatric/Geriatric/Lifespan   Medications

ACTIONS/INTERVENTIONS

Sample NIC Linkages:

Urinary Elimination Management: Maintenance of an optimum urinary elimination pattern

Prompted Voiding: Promotion of urinary continence through the use of timed verbal toileting reminders and positive social feedback for successful toileting

Urinary Habit Training: Establishing a predictable pattern of bladder emptying to prevent incontinence for persons with limited cognitive ability who have urge, stress, or functional incontinence

NURSING PRIORITY NO. 1   To assess situation and adaptive skills being used by client:

- Note presence of physical diagnoses (e.g., surgery, childbirth, recent/multiple pregnancies, pelvic trauma, neurogenic bladder from central nervous disorders or neuropathies [stroke/spinal cord injury, diabetes], mental/emotional dysfunction, prostate disease/surgery) *that can impact client's elimination patterns.*[1]
- Determine client's usual/previous pattern of elimination and compare with current situation *to determine how pattern can be improved.*[1]
- Observe current voiding pattern and time, color and amount voided, as indicated (e.g., postsurgical client), *to document normalization of elimination.*[1]
- Ascertain methods of self-management (e.g., limiting or increasing liquid intake, acting on urge in timely manner, establishing voiding schedule, regularly spaced catheterization) *to identify strengths/areas of concern in elimination management.*[2]
- Determine client's usual daily fluid intake. *Both amount and beverage choices are important in managing elimination.*[2–4]
- Ascertain motivation/expectations for change. *Motivation to improve and high expectations can encourage client to make changes that will improve his or her life. However, unrealistic expectations may hamper efforts.*

NURSING PRIORITY NO. 2   To assist client to strengthen management of urinary elimination:

- Encourage fluid intake, including water and cranberry juice, *to help maintain renal function, prevent infection.*[1]
- Regulate liquid intake at prescheduled times *to promote predictable voiding pattern.*[2,3]
- Suggest restricting fluid intake 2 to 3 hours before bedtime *to reduce voiding during the night.*[2,4,5]
- Assist with modifying current routines, as appropriate. *Client may benefit from additional information, such as regarding cues/urge to void, adjusting schedule of voiding/catheterization (shorter or longer), relaxation or distraction techniques, standing or sitting upright during voiding, to ensure that bladder is completely empty, or practicing pelvic muscle strengthening exercises.*[2,4–6]
- Provide assistance/devices, as indicated. *Having means of summoning assistance; placement of bedside commode, urinal, or bedpan within client's reach; use of elevated toilet seats or mobility devices enhances client's ability to maintain urinary function.*[5]
- Modify/recommend dietary changes, if indicated. *Client may benefit from reduction of caffeine because of its bladder-irritant effect or weight loss may help reduce overactive bladder symptoms and incontinence by decreasing pressure on the bladder.*[2,4–6]
- Modify medication regimens, as appropriate. For example, administer prescribed diuretics in the morning *to lessen nighttime voiding;* reduce or eliminate use of hypnotics, if possible, *as client may be too sedated to recognize/respond to urge to void.*[5]

- Refer to appropriate resources (e.g., medical supply company, ostomy nurse, rehabilitation team) *for assistance, as desired/needed, to promote self-care.*

NURSING PRIORITY NO. 3 To promote optimum wellness:

- Encourage continuation of successful toileting program and identify possible alterations to meet individual needs (e.g., use of adult briefs for extended outing or travel with limited access to toilet). *Promotes proactive problem-solving and supports self-esteem and normalization of social interactions/desired lifestyle activities.*[7]
- Instruct client/SO/caregivers in cues that client needs (e.g., voiding on routine schedule; showing client location of the bathroom; providing adequate room lighting, signs, color coding of door) *to assist client in continued continence, especially when in unfamiliar surroundings.*[3–5]
- Review expectations/prognosis of underlying condition (e.g., MS, prostate disease). *Provides information to assist client/SO to make informed decisions and plan for possible changes.*
- Review with client/SO the signs/symptoms of urinary complications and need for medical follow-up. *Promotes timely intervention to limit or prevent adverse events.*

DOCUMENTATION FOCUS

Assessment/Reassessment

- Findings/adaptive skills being used.
- Motivation/expectation for change.

Planning

- Plan of care and who is involved in planning.
- Teaching plan.

Implementation/Evaluation

- Responses to treatment plan/interventions and actions performed.
- Attainment/progress toward desired outcome(s).
- Modifications to plan of care.

Discharge Planning

- Available resources, equipment needs/sources.

References

1. ND: Urinary Elimination, readiness for enhanced. In Doenges, M. E., Moorhouse, M. F., Murr, A. C. (2004). *Nurse's Pocket Guide: Diagnoses, Interventions and Rationales.* 9th ed. Philadelphia: F. A. Davis.
2. Sampselle, C. M. (2003). Behavioral interventions in young and middle-age women. In Newman, D. K., Palmer, M. H. (eds). The state of the science on urinary incontinence. *AJN,* 293(suppl), 9–19.
3. Lyons, S. S., Specht, J. K. P. (1999). Prompted voiding for persons with urinary incontinence. University of Iowa Gerontological Nursing Interventions Research Center. Available at www.guideline.gov. Accessed June 2003.
4. Wyman, J. F., et al. (1998). Comparative efficacy of behavioral interventions in the management of female urinary incontinence. *Am J Obstet Gynecol,* 179(4), 999–1007.
5. Wyman, J. F. (2003). Treatment of urinary incontinence in men and older women. In Newman, D. K., Palmer, M. H. (eds). The state of the science on urinary incontinence. *AJN,* 293(suppl), 26–35.
6. Burgio, K. L., et al. (1989). Behavioral training for post-prostatectomy urinary incontinence. *J Urol,* 141(2), 303–306.
7. Pringle-Specht, J. K. (2005). Nine myths of incontinence in older adults. *AJN,* 105(6), 58–68.

functional Urinary Incontinence

Definition: Inability of usually continent person to reach toilet in time to avoid unintentional loss of urine

RELATED FACTORS

Altered environmental factors [e.g., poor lighting or inability to locate bathroom]
Neuromuscular limitations
Weakened supporting pelvic structures
Impaired vision/cognition
Psychological factors; [impaired cognition/dementia; reluctance to request assistance/use bedpan]
[Increased urine production]

DEFINING CHARACTERISTICS

Subjective
Senses need to void
[Voiding in large amounts]

Objective
Loss of urine before reaching toilet; amount of time required to reach toilet exceeds length of time between sensing urge and uncontrolled voiding
Able to completely empty bladder
May only be incontinent in early morning

Sample Clinical Applications: Diabetes mellitus, congestive heart failure (diuretic use), arthritis, bladder prolapse/cystocele, stroke

DESIRED OUTCOMES/EVALUATION CRITERIA
Sample NOC linkages:
Urinary Elimination: Collection and drainage of urine
Urinary Continence: Control of the elimination of urine from the bladder
Self-Care: Toileting: Ability to toilet self independently with or without assistive device

Client/Caregiver Will (Include Specific Time Frame)

• Verbalize understanding of condition and identify interventions to prevent incontinence.
• Alter environment to accommodate individual needs.
• Report voiding in individually appropriate amounts.
• Void at acceptable times and places.

ACTIONS/INTERVENTIONS

Sample NIC linkages:
Prompted Voiding: Promotion of urinary continence through the use of timed verbal toileting reminders and positive social feedback for successful toileting
Urinary Habit Training: Establishing a predictable pattern of bladder emptying to prevent incontinence for persons with limited cognitive ability who have urge, stress, or functional incontinence
Self-Care Assistance: Toileting: Assisting another with elimination

NURSING PRIORITY NO. 1 To assess causative/contributing factors:

- Identify/differentiate client with functional incontinence (e.g., bladder and urethra are functioning normally, but client either cannot get to toilet or has impaired mental function that interferes with recognizing need to urinate and getting to toilet on time) from other types of incontinence.[5]
- Determine if client is voluntarily postponing urination. *Often the demands of the work setting, either because of restrictions on bathroom breaks, working alone (e.g., pharmacist, nurse, teacher), demands of the job (heavy workload and unable to find time for a bathroom break) make it difficult for individuals to go to the bathroom when the need arises, resulting in frequent urinary tract infections and incontinence.*[1]
- Evaluate cognition. *Disease process/medications can affect mental status/orientation to place, recognition of urge to void, or its significance.*[1]
- Note presence/type of functional impairments (e.g., poor eyesight, mobility problems, dexterity problems/self-care deficits) *that can hinder ability to get to bathroom.*[6]
- Identify environmental conditions that interfere with timely access to bathroom/successful toileting process. *Unfamiliar surroundings, poor lighting, improperly fitted chair walker, low toilet seat, absence of safety bars, and travel distance to toilet may affect self-care ability.*
- Review medical history for conditions known to increase urine output or alter bladder tone. *For example, diabetes mellitus, prolapsed bladder, MS can affect frequency of urination and ability to hold urine until individual can reach the bathroom.*[1]
- Note use of medications or agents that can increase urine formation. *Diuretics, alcohol, caffeine are several factors that can increase amount and frequency of voiding.*
- Test urine for presence of glucose. *Hyperglycemia can cause polyuria and overdistention of the bladder, resulting in problem with continence.*

NURSING PRIORITY NO. 2 To assess degree of interference/disability:

- Determine the frequency and timing of continent/incontinent voids. *Information will be used to plan program to manage incontinence.*[3]
- Initiate voiding diary. Note time of day/night when incontinence occurs as well as timing issues (e.g., difference between the time it takes to get to bathroom/remove clothing and involuntary loss of urine).
- Measure/estimate amount of urine voided or lost with incontinent episodes *to help determine options for managing problem.*
- Ascertain effect on lifestyle (including socialization and sexuality) and self-esteem. *There is a general belief that incontinence is an inevitable result of aging and that nothing can be done about it. However, those with incontinence problems are often embarrassed, withdraw from social activities and relationships, and hesitate to discuss the problem—even with their healthcare provider.*[1]

NURSING PRIORITY NO. 3 To assist in treating/preventing incontinence:

- Remind client to void when needed and schedule voiding times (e.g., cognitive decline, client who ambulates slowly because of physical limitations, etc.) *to reduce incontinence episodes/promote comfort.*[6]
- Administer prescribed diuretics in the morning. *The effect of these medications diminishes by bedtime, thus resulting in less nighttime voidings.*[2]
- Reduce or eliminate use of hypnotics, if possible. *Client may be too sedated to recognize/respond to urge to void.*[4]

⊕ Cultural   Ⓐ Collaborative   🏠 Community/Home Care   Diagnostic Studies   ∞ Pediatric/Geriatric/Lifespan   Medications

- Provide means of summoning assistance. *Ready placement of a call light when hospitalized or a bell in the home setting enables client to obtain toileting help, as needed.*[4]
- Use night-lights to mark bathroom location. *Elderly person may become confused upon arising and be unable to locate bathroom in the dark, and lighting will facilitate access, reducing the possibility of accidents.*[4]
- Provide cues such as adequate room lighting, signs, and color coding of door. *Assists disoriented client to find the bathroom.*[4]
- Remove throw rugs, excess furniture in travel path to bathroom. *Reduces risk of falls, facilitates access to bathroom, and avoids loss of urine.*[4]
- Adapt clothes for quick removal. *Velcro fasteners, full skirts, crotchless panties or no panties, suspenders or elastic waists instead of belts on pants facilitate toileting once urge to void is noted.*[4]
- Raise chair or toilet seat or provide bedside commode, urinal, or bedpan as indicated. *Facilitates toileting when individual has difficulty with movement.*[1]
- Schedule voiding on regular time schedule (e.g., every 3 hours). *Emptying bladder on a regular schedule minimizes pressure, reducing overflow voiding.*[1]
- Restrict fluid intake 2 to 3 hours before bedtime. *Reduces need to waken to void during the night.*[1]
- Include physical/occupational therapist in determining ways to alter environment, appropriate assistive devices. *Useful in meeting individual needs of client.*[1]

NURSING PRIORITY NO. 4 To promote wellness (Teaching/Discharge Considerations):

- Discuss with client/SO need for prompted and scheduled voidings *to manage continence when client is unable to respond immediately to urge to void.*[1]
- Suggest limiting intake of coffee, tea, and alcohol. *Diuretic effect of these substances impacts voiding pattern and can contribute to incontinence.*[1]
- Maintain positive regard when incontinence occurs. *Reduces embarrassment associated with incontinence, need for assistance, use of bedpan.*[1]
- Promote participation in developing long-term plan of care. *Encourages involvement in follow-through of plan, thus increasing possibility of success and confidence in own ability to manage program.*[1]
- Refer to NDs reflex/stress/total/or urge Urinary Incontinence for additional interventions, as appropriate.

DOCUMENTATION FOCUS

Assessment/Reassessment

- Current elimination pattern/assessment findings and effect on lifestyle and self-esteem.

Planning

- Plan of care and who is involved in planning.
- Teaching plan.

Implementation/Evaluation

- Response to interventions/teaching and actions performed.
- Attainment/progress toward desired outcome(s).
- Modifications to plan of care.

Discharge Planning

- Long-term needs and who is responsible for actions to be taken.
- Specific referrals made.

References

1. Newman, D. K., Palmer, M. H. (eds). (2003). The state of the science on urinary incontinence. *Am J Nurs*, 293, 3(suppl), 20
2. Doenges, M. E., Moorhouse, M. F., Geissler-Murr, A. C. (2002). *Nursing Care Plans: Guidelines for Individualizing Patient Care*. 6th ed. Philadelphia: F. A. Davis.
3. Wyman, J. F. (2003). Treatment of urinary incontinence in men and older women. In Newman, D. K., Palmer, M. H. (eds). The state of the science on urinary incontinence. *Am J Nurs*, 293, 3(suppl), 20.
4. Cox, H. C., et al. (2002). *Clinical Applications of Nursing Diagnosis: Adult, Child, Women's, Psychiatric, Gerontic, and Home Health Considerations*. 4th ed. Philadelphia: F. A. Davis.
5. American Geriatrics Society Foundation for Health in Aging. (2004): Incontinence. In Eldercare at Home, Chapter 10. Retrieved August 2007 at http://healthinaging.org/public_education/eldercare/10.xml.
6. Pringle-Specht, J. K. (2005). Nine myths of incontinence in older adults. *AJN*, 105(6), 58–68.

overflow Urinary Incontinence

Definition: Involuntary loss of urine associated with overdistention of the bladder

RELATED FACTORS

Bladder outlet obstruction; fecal impaction
Urethral obstruction; severe pelvic prolapse
Detrusor external sphincter dyssynergia; detrusor hypocontractility
Side effects of anticholinergic/decongestant medications; calcium channel blockers

DEFINING CHARACTERISTICS

Subjective
Reports involuntary leakage of small volumes of urine
Nocturia

Objective
Bladder distention
High postvoid residual volume
Observed involuntary leakage of small volumes of urine

Sample Clinical Applications: Uterine prolapse, benign prostatic hypertrophy, diabetes mellitus, MS, spinal cord injury, pelvic fractures, urinary stones

DESIRED OUTCOMES/EVALUATION CRITERIA

Sample NOC linkages:
Urinary Continence: Control of elimination of urine from the bladder
Urinary Elimination: Collection and drainage of urine
Knowledge: Disease Process: Extent of understanding conveyed about a specific disease process

Client Will (Include Specific Time Frame)

• Verbalize understanding of causative factors and appropriate interventions for individual situation.
• Demonstrate techniques/behaviors to alleviate/prevent overflow incontinence.
• Void in sufficient amounts with no palpable bladder distention; experience no postvoid residuals greater than 50 mL; have no dribbling/overflow.

Cultural   Collaborative   Community/Home Care   Diagnostic Studies   Pediatric/Geriatric/Lifespan   Medications

ACTIONS/INTERVENTIONS

Sample NIC linkages:

Urinary Incontinence Care: Assistance in promoting continence and maintaining perineal skin integrity

Urinary Catheterization: Intermittent: Regular periodic use of a catheter to empty the bladder

NURSING PRIORITY NO. 1 To assess causative/contributing factors:

- Review client's history for (1) bladder outlet obstruction (e.g., prostatic hypertrophy, urethral stricture, urinary stones or tumors); (2) nonfunctioning detrusor muscle (i.e., sensory or motor paralytic bladder due to underlying neurological disease); or (3) atonic bladder that has lost its muscular tone (i.e., chronic overdistention) *to identify potential for/presence of conditions associated with overflow incontinence.*[5]
- Note client's age and gender. *Urinary incontinence due to overflow bladder is more common in older men because of the prevalence of obstructive prostate gland enlargement.*[1,4,5]
- Review medication regimen *for drugs that can cause/exacerbate retention and overflow incontinence (e.g., anticholinergics, calcium channel blockers, psychotropics, anesthesia, opiates, sedatives, alpha- and beta-blockers, antihistamines, neuroleptics).*[2–4,6]

NURSING PRIORITY NO. 2 To determine degree of interference/disability:

- Note client reports of symptoms common to overflow incontinence:[3,4]
  Feeling no need to urinate, while simultaneously losing urine
  Feeling the urge to urinate but not being able to
  Feeling as though the bladder is never completely empty
  Passing a dribbling stream of urine, even after spending a long time at the toilet
  Frequently getting up at night to urinate
- Prepare for/assist with urodynamic testing (e.g., uroflowmetry *to assess urine speed and volume;* cystometrogram *to measure bladder pressure and volume;* bladder scan *to measure retention or postvoid residual, leak point pressure, etc.).*[1]

NURSING PRIORITY NO. 3 To assist in treating/preventing overflow incontinence:

- Collaborate in treatment of underlying conditions (e.g., medications or surgery for prostatic hypertrophy; use of medication, such as terazosin, to relax urinary sphincter; altering dose/discontinuing medications contributing to retention). *If the underlying cause of the overflow problem can be treated or eliminated, client may be able to return to normal voiding pattern.*
- Demonstrate/instruct client/SO(s) in use of gentle massage over bladder (Credé's maneuver). *May facilitate bladder emptying when cause is detrusor weakness.*
- Implement intermittent or continuous catheterization. *Short-term use may be required while acute conditions are treated (e.g., infection, surgery for enlarged prostate); long-term use is required for permanent conditions (e.g., spinal cord injury/other neuromuscular conditions resulting in permanent bladder dysfunction).*
- Refer to NDs urge Urinary Incontinence, stress Urinary Incontinence, [acute/chronic] Urinary Retention for additional interventions.

NURSING PRIORITY NO. 4 To promote wellness (Teaching/Discharge Considerations):

- Establish regular schedule for bladder emptying whether voiding or using catheter.

🏠 • Stress need for adequate fluid intake, including use of acidifying fruit juices or ingestion of vitamin C *to discourage bacterial growth and stone formation.*

🔗 • Instruct client/SO(s) in clean intermittent self-catheterization (CISC) techniques *to prevent reflux/increased renal pressures and enhance independence.*

🔗 • Review signs/symptoms of complications requiring prompt medical evaluation *to promote timely intervention/prevent complications.*

DOCUMENTATION FOCUS

Assessment/Reassessment

• Current elimination pattern/assessment findings and effect on lifestyle/sleep.

Planning

• Plan of care and who is involved in planning.
• Teaching plan.

Implementation/Evaluation

• Response to interventions/teaching and actions performed.
• Attainment/progress toward desired outcome(s).
• Modifications to plan of care.

Discharge Planning

• Long-term needs and who is responsible for actions to be taken.
• Specific referrals made.

References

1. Weiss, B. D. (1998). Diagnostic evaluation of urinary incontinence in geriatric patients. *American Family Physician, 57*(11). Retrieved May 2007 at www.aafp.org/afp/980600ap/weiss.html.
2. National Association for Continence (NAFC). (2005). Fact Sheet. The four basic types of urinary incontinence. Retrieved August 2007 at www.nafc.org/about_incontinence/types/htm.
3. Gray, M. (2005). Overactive bladder: An overview. *Journal of Wound, Ostomy and Continence Nursing, 32*(3), Suppl, 1–5.
4. American Geriatrics Society Foundation for Health in Aging. (2004). Incontinence. In Eldercare at Home, Chapter 10. Retrieved August 2007 at http://healthinaging.org/public_education/eldercare/10.xml.
5. No author listed. (1995–2007). Urinary incontinence. The Merck Manual of Health & Aging (online), Section 3, Chapter 57. Retrieved August 2007 at www.merck.com/pubs/mmanual_ha/sec3/ch57/ch57a.html.
6. Goode, P. S., Burgio, K. L. (2004). In Kursh, E. D., Ulchaker, J. C. (eds). *Office Urology: The Clinicians Guide.* Totawa, NJ: Humana Press.

reflex Urinary Incontinence

Definition: Involuntary loss of urine at somewhat predictable intervals when a specific bladder volume is reached

RELATED FACTORS

Tissue damage (e.g., due to radiation cystitis, inflammatory bladder conditions, radical pelvic surgery)

Neurological impairment above level of sacral or pontine micturition center

🌐 Cultural 🔗 Collaborative 🏠 Community/Home Care ✏️ Diagnostic Studies ∞ Pediatric/Geriatric/Lifespan 💊 Medications

DEFINING CHARACTERISTICS

Subjective
No sensation of bladder fullness/urge to void/voiding
Sensation of urgency without voluntary inhibition of bladder contraction
Sensations associated with full bladder (e.g., sweating, restlessness, abdominal discomfort)

Objective
Predictable pattern of voiding
Inability to voluntarily inhibit or initiate voiding
Complete emptying with [brain] lesion above pontine micturition center
Incomplete emptying with [spinal cord] lesion above sacral micturition center

Sample Clinical Applications: Spinal cord injury, MS, bladder/pelvic cancer, Parkinson's disease, dementia

DESIRED OUTCOMES/EVALUATION CRITERIA
Sample NOC linkages:
Urinary Continence: Control of the elimination of urine from the bladder
Neurological Status: Autonomic: Ability of the autonomic nervous system to coordinate visceral and hemostatic function
Urinary Elimination: Collection and discharge of urine

Client Will (Include Specific Time Frame)

- Verbalize understanding of condition/contributing factors.
- Establish bladder regimen appropriate for individual situation.
- Demonstrate behaviors/techniques to control condition and prevent complications.
- Void at acceptable times and places.

ACTIONS/INTERVENTIONS

Sample NIC linkages:
Urinary Bladder Training: Improving bladder function for those with urge incontinence by increasing the bladder's ability to hold urine and the patient's ability to suppress urination
Urinary Catheterization: Intermittent: Regular periodic use of a catheter to empty the bladder
Urinary Incontinence Care: Assistance in promoting continence and maintaining perineal skin integrity

NURSING PRIORITY NO. 1 To assess degree of interference/disability:

- Identify pathology of problem (e.g., pelvic cancer, central nervous system disorder/spinal cord injury, stroke, Parkinson's disease, brain tumor) *that results in either hypotonic or spastic neurogenic bladder, thereby affecting bladder storage, emptying, and control.*[1,7–9]
- Note whether client experiences any sense of bladder fullness or awareness of incontinence. *Individuals with reflex incontinence have little to no awareness of need to void. Loss of sensation of bladder filling can result in overfilling, inadequate emptying (retention), and/or constant dribbling.*[2,3,6 9] (Refer to NDs [acute/chronic] Urinary Retention and overflow Urinary Incontinence for additional interventions.)

- Review voiding diary, if available, or record frequency and time of urination. Compare timing of voidings, particularly in relation to liquid intake and medications. *Aids in targeting interventions to meet individual situation.*[4]
- Measure amount of each voiding. *Incontinence often occurs once a specific bladder volume is reached and may indicate need for insertion of a permanent/intermittent catheter.*[5]
- Evaluate for concomitant urinary retention; determine actual bladder volume (via bladder scan) in client with incomplete emptying/on scheduled catheterization *when attempting toilet training and to avoid unnecessary catheterizations.*[10] *Note: Often the bladder is not completely emptied, because there is no voluntary control of the bladder.*[2]
- Measure/scan postvoid residuals/catheterization volumes. *Determines frequency for emptying bladder and reduces incontinence episodes.*[10]
- Evaluate client's ability to manipulate/use urinary collection device or catheter. *Type and degree of neurological impairment (i.e., spinal cord injury, multiple sclerosis, dementia) may interfere with client's ability to be self-sufficient.*[3]
- Determine availability/use of resources or assistance.
- Refer to urologist/appropriate specialist *for testing. Urinalysis, ultrasound, radiographs, and urine flowmetry to measure urine flow is standard. A urodynamic evaluation measuring bladder capacity, pressure, and rate of urinary flow may also be indicated.*[6]

NURSING PRIORITY NO. 2 To assist in managing incontinence:

- Collaborate in treatment of underlying cause/management of incontinence. *Degree of impairment, potential for improvement, client's capabilities and availability of assistance, if needed, must be considered in order to develop a comprehensive plan.*
- Involve client/SO/caregiver in creating plan of care *to develop mutually agreed upon goals and ensure individual needs are met, enhancing commitment to plan.*
- Encourage minimum of 1500 to 2000 mL of fluid intake daily. Regulate liquid intake at prescheduled times (with and between meals). *Promotes a predictable voiding pattern to help with treatment regimen.*[6]
- Restrict fluids 2 to 3 hours before bedtime. *Can reduce need to void during the night, preventing incontinence/interruption of sleep.*[6]
- Instruct client to void/or take to toilet before the expected time of incontinence *in an attempt to stimulate the reflex for voiding.*[4]
- Instruct in measures such as pouring warm water over perineum, running water in sink, stimulating/massaging tissues over bladder, lower abdomen, thighs. *May stimulate voiding reflexes and voiding, preventing loss of urine at unpredictable times.*[7]
- Set alarm to awaken during night to maintain schedule, or use external catheter/collection device, as appropriate. *Developing a regular time for voiding will empty the bladder, preventing incontinence during the night.*[3,6]
- Implement continuous or intermittent catheterization schedule, if condition indicates, *to prevent overdistention and detrusor muscle damage.*[4,8]

NURSING PRIORITY NO. 3 To promote wellness (Teaching/Discharge Considerations):

- Encourage continuation of regular toileting or bladder program. *May be able to establish a schedule that takes advantage of whatever ability remains, even though the neurological impairment is affecting bladder sensation.*[6]
- Suggest use of incontinence pads/pants during day and with social contact, if appropriate. *Depending on client's activity level, amount of urine loss, manual dexterity, and cognitive ability, these devices provide security and comfort and protect the skin and clothing from urine leakage, reduce odor, and are generally unnoticeable under clothing.*[6]

Cultural · Collaborative · Community/Home Care · Diagnostic Studies · Pediatric/Geriatric/Lifespan · Medications

- Stress importance of perineal care following voiding and frequent changing of incontinence pads, if used. *Maintains cleanliness and prevents skin irritation/breakdown and odor.*[6]
- Encourage limited intake of coffee, tea, and alcohol. *Diuretic effect of these substances may affect predictability of voiding pattern.*[2]
- Instruct in proper care of catheter and cleaning techniques. *Reduces risk of infection.*[3]
- Review signs/symptoms of urinary complications and need for medical follow-up. *Provides immediate attention preventing exacerbation of problem or extension of infection into kidneys.*

DOCUMENTATION FOCUS

Assessment/Reassessment

- Findings/degree of disability and effect on lifestyle.
- Availability of resources/support person.

Planning

- Plan of care and who is involved in planning.
- Teaching plan.

Implementation/Evaluation

- Responses to treatment plan/interventions and actions performed.
- Attainment/progress toward desired outcome(s).
- Modifications to plan of care.

Discharge Planning

- Long-term needs and who is responsible for actions to be taken.
- Available resources, equipment needs/sources.

References

1. ND: Urinary Incontinence, reflex. In Doenges, M. E., Moorhouse, M. F., Murr, A. C. (2004). *Nurse's Pocket Guide: Diagnoses, Interventions, and Rationales.* 9th ed. Philadelphia: F. A. Davis.
2. WebMD. (Updated 2006). Incontinence/Overactive Bladder. Retrieved August 2007 at www.webmd.com/urinary-incontinence-oab/womens-guide/Urinary-Incontinence-in-Women-Topic-Overview.
3. Doenges, M. E., Moorhouse, M. F., Geissler-Murr, A. C. (2002). *Nursing Care Plans, Guidelines for Individualizing Patient Care.* 6th ed. Philadelphia: F. A. Davis.
4. Newman, D. K., Palmer, M. H. (eds). (2003). The state of the science on urinary incontinence. *Am J Nurs,* 293, 3(suppl), 20.
5. Cox, H. C., et al. (2002). *Clinical Applications of Nursing Diagnosis: Adult, Child, Women's, Psychiatric, Gerontic, and Home Health Considerations.* 4th ed. Philadelphia: F. A. Davis.
6. Urinary Incontinence. Penn State Health and Disease information: A–Z topics. Accessed August 2007 at www.hmc.psu.edu/healthinfo/uz/urinaryincontinence.htm.
7. Beers, M. H., Berkow, R. (eds). (1999). *The Merck Manual of Diagnosis and Therapy.* 17th ed. Whitehouse Station, NJ: Merck Research Laboratories.
8. Gray, M. (2005). Assessment and management of urinary incontinence. *Nurse Pract,* 30(7), 32–43.
9. Rackley, R., Vasavada, S. P. (2006). Incontinence, urinary: Nonsurgical therapies. Article for Emedicine Web site. Retrieved April 2007 at www.emedicine.com/med/topic3085.htm.
10. Newman, D. K. (2006). Using the BladderScan™ for bladder volume assessment. Retrieved May 2007 at www.seekwellness.com/incontinence/using_the_bladderscan.htm.

stress Urinary Incontinence

Definition: Sudden leakage of urine with activities that increase intra-abdominal pressure

RELATED FACTORS
Degenerative changes in pelvic muscles; weak pelvic muscles
High intra-abdominal pressure [e.g., obesity, gravid uterus]
Intrinsic urethral sphincter deficiency

DEFINING CHARACTERISTICS

Subjective
Reported involuntary leakage of small amounts of urine on exertion [e.g., lifting, impact aerobics]; with sneezing, laughing, or coughing; in the absence of detrusor contraction/an overdistended bladder

Objective
Observed involuntary leakage of small amounts of urine on exertion [e.g., lifting, impact aerobics]; with sneezing, laughing, or coughing; in the absence of detrusor contraction/an overdistended bladder

DESIRED OUTCOMES/EVALUATION CRITERIA
Sample NOC linkages:
Urinary Continence: Control of elimination of urine from the bladder
Symptom Control: Personal actions to minimize perceived adverse changes in physical and emotional functioning

Client Will (Include Specific Time Frame)

- Verbalize understanding of condition and interventions for bladder conditioning.
- Demonstrate behaviors/techniques to strengthen pelvic floor musculature.
- Remain continent even with increased intra-abdominal pressure.

ACTIONS/INTERVENTIONS

Sample NIC linkages:
Pelvic Muscle Exercise: Strengthening and training the levator ani and urogenital muscles through voluntary repetitive contraction to decrease stress, urge, or mixed types of urinary incontinence
Urinary Incontinence Care: Assistance in promoting continence and maintaining perineal skin integrity
Urinary Habit Training: Establishing a predictable pattern of bladder emptying to prevent incontinence for persons with limited cognitive ability who have urge, stress, or functional incontinence

NURSING PRIORITY NO. 1   To assess causative/contributing factors:

- Identify physiological causes of increased intra-abdominal pressure (e.g., obesity, gravid uterus; repeated heavy lifting [occupational risk]); contributing history, such as multiple births, bladder or pelvic trauma/fractures; surgery (e.g., radical prostatectomy, bladder/other pelvic surgeries that may damage sphincter muscles); and participation in high-impact athletic or military field activities (particularly women). *Identification of specifics of individual situation provides for developing an accurate plan of care.*[1,4,10,15]

- Assess for urine loss (usually in small amounts) with coughing, sneezing, or sports activities; relaxed pelvic musculature and support, noting inability to start/stop stream while voiding, bulging of perineum when bearing down. *Severity of symptoms may indicate need for more specialized evaluation.*
- Review client's medications for those that may cause/exacerbate stress incontinence (e.g., alpha-blockers, angiotension converting ezyme (ACE) inhibitors, loop diruectcs).[16]
- Assess for mixed incontinence (consisting of two or more kinds of incontinence), noting whether bladder irritability, reduced bladder capacity, or voluntary overdistention is present. *Concomitant urge or reflex incontinence often occurs with stress incontinence and impacts treatment choices.*[6] (Refer to NDs Urinary Incontinence [specify urge, reflex], [acute/chronic] Urinary Retention.)

NURSING PRIORITY NO. 2 To assess degree of interference/disability:

- Observe voiding patterns, time and amount voided, and note the stimulus provoking incontinence. Review voiding diary if available. *Provides information that can help determine type of incontinence and type of treatment indicated.*[6]
- Prepare for/assist with testing/refer to urology specialist as indicated. *Diagnosing urinary incontinence often requires comprehensive evaluation (e.g., measuring bladder filling and capacity, leak-point pressure, rate of urinary flow, pelvic ultrasound, cystogram/other scans) to differentiate stress incontinence from other types* [2–4,7,17]
- Determine effect on lifestyle (including daily activities, participation in sports/exercise and recreation, socialization, sexuality) and self-esteem. *Untreated incontinence can have emotional and physical consequences. Client may limit or abstain from sports/recreational activities. Urinary tract infections, skin rashes, and sores can occur. Self-esteem is affected and the client may suffer from depression and withdraw from social functions.*[6,15]
- Ascertain methods of self-management. *Client may already be limiting liquid intake, voiding before any activity, or using undergarment protection.*[6]
- Perform bladder scan to determine postvoid residuals as indicated. *Presence of volumes greater than 100 ml (or 150 ml in elder clients) suggests incomplete emptying of bladder, requiring further evaluation.*[17]

NURSING PRIORITY NO. 3 To assist in treating/preventing incontinence:

- Suggest/implement self-help techniques:
  Practice timed voidings (e.g., every 3 hours during the day) *to keep bladder relatively empty.*
  Delay voiding to 3- to 4-hour intervals between voids. *May improve bladder capacity/retention time and acceptable time between bathroom breaks.*[6]
  Restrict fluid intake 2 to 3 hours before bedtime. *Decreasing the amount of evening fluid intake reduces the need for awakening to void, resulting in more restful sleep.*[5]
  Limit use of coffee/tea and alcohol. *Diuretic effect of these substances may lead to bladder distention, increasing likelihood of incontinence.*[12]
  Encourage weight loss as indicated *to reduce pressure on intra-abdominal and pelvic organs.*[7]
  Void before physical exertion such as exercise/sports activites *to reduce potential for incontinence.*[18]
  Encourage regular pelvic floor strengthening exercises (Kegel exercises). *These exercises involve tightening the muscles of the pelvic floor and need to be done numerous times throughout the day.*[6,10]
  Avoid/limit heavy lifting, high-impact aerobics/sports *to decrease incontinence associated with elevated intra-abdominal pressures.*[12]

Incorporate "bent-knee sit-ups" into exercise program. *Increasing abdominal muscle tone can help relieve stress incontinence.*[11]

 • Assist with medical treatment of underlying urological condition, as indicated. *Stress incontinence may be treated with surgical intervention (e.g., bladder neck suspension, pubo-vaginal sling to reposition bladder/strengthen pelvic musculature; or prostate surgery) and nonsurgical therapies (e.g., use of pessary, vaginal cones; electrical stimulation; biofeedback, etc.).*[8,9,18–20]

• Administer medications, as indicted, such as sympathomimetics (propantheline or Pro-Banthine); antispasmodics (oxybutynin or Ditropan). *May improve bladder tone and increase effectiveness of bladder sphincter/proximal urethra contractions.*[6,9,14]

NURSING PRIORITY NO. 4 To promote wellness (Teaching/Discharge Considerations):

• Suggest use of incontinence pads/pants as needed. *Considering client's activity level, amount of urine loss, physical size, manual dexterity, and cognitive ability to determine specific product choices best suited to individual situation and needs may be necessary when leakage continues to occur in spite of other measures.*[9,13]

• Emphasize importance of perineal care following voiding and frequent changing of incontinence pads. Recommend application of oil-based emollient. *Prevents infection and protects skin from irritation.*[13]

• Discuss participation in/incontinence management for activities such as heavy lifting, strenuous sports activities that increase intra-abdominal pressure. *Substituting swimming, bicycling, or low-impact exercise if possible may help reduce frequency of incontinence/maintain active life.*

• Recommend/refer for behavioral training/support, as indicated. *Research indicates that combining pelvic floor muscle exercises with biofeedback is more effective than simple verbal/written instructions.*[21]

DOCUMENTATION FOCUS

Assessment/Reassessment

• Findings/pattern of incontinence and physical factors present.
• Effect on lifestyle and self-esteem.
• Client understanding of condition.

Planning

• Plan of care and who is involved in the planning.
• Teaching plan.

Implementation/Evaluation

• Responses to interventions/teaching, actions performed, and changes that are identified.
• Attainment/progress toward desired outcome(s).
• Modifications to plan of care.

Discharge Planning

• Long-term needs, referrals, and who is responsible for specific actions.
• Specific referrals made.

References

1. Doenges, M. E., Moorhouse, M. F., Geissler-Murr, A. C. (2004). *Nurse's Pocket Guide: Diagnoses, Interventions, and Rationales.* 9th ed. Philadelphia: F. A. Davis.
2. Urinary Incontinence. Penn State Health & Disease Information. Accessed July 2007 at www.hmc.psu.edu/healthinfo/uz/urinaryincontinence.htm.
3. No author listed. (1996). Urinary incontinence. American Medical Directors Association (AMDA). Available at www.guidleine.gov. Accessed September 2003.
4. Guerrero, P., Sinert, R. (2002, update 2006). Urinary incontinence. Accessed August 2007 at www.emedicine.com/emerg/topic791.htm.
5. Doenges, M. E., Moorhouse, M. F., Geissler-Murr, A. C. (2002). *Nursing Care Plans: Guidelines for Individualizing Patient Care.* 6th ed. Philadelphia: F. A. Davis.
6. Ford-Martin, P. A. (1999, update 2002). Urinary catheterization. Gale Encyclopedia of Medicine. Gale Research. Accessed August 2007 at www.lifesteps.com/gm/Atoz/ency/urinary_catheterization.jsp.
7. Beers, M. H., Berkow, R. (eds). (1999). *The Merck Manual of Diagnosis and Therapy.* 17th ed. Whitehouse Station, NJ: Merck Research Laboratories.
8. Choe, J. M. (2003). Incontinence, urinary: Surgical therapies. Accessed July 2007 at www.emedicine.com/emerg/topic3084.htm.
9. Choe, J. M. (2002). Incontinence, urinary: Nonsurgical therapies. Accessed July 2007 at www.emedicine.com/emerg/topic3085.htm.
10. Wyman, J. F. (2003). Treatment of urinary incontinence in men and older women. In Newman, D. K., Palmer, M. H. (eds). The state of the science on urinary incontinence. *Am J Nurs,* 293, 3(suppl), 20.
11. ND: Urinary Incontinence, stress. In Cox, H. C., et al. (2002). *Clinical Applications of Nursing Diagnosis: Adult, Child, Women's, Psychiatric, Gerontic, and Home Health Considerations.* 4th ed. Philadelphia: F. A. Davis.
12. Newman, D. K., Palmer, M. H. (eds). (2003). The state of the science on urinary incontinence. *Am J Nurs,* 293, 3(suppl), 20.
13. What is urinary incontinence? Accessed September 2003 at http://ourworld.compuserve.com/homepages/nacs/INCONT.HTM.
14. Booth, C. (2002). Introduction to Urinary Incontinence. *Hosp Pharmacist,* 9(3), 65–68.
15. Carls, C. (2007). The prevalence of stress urinary incontinence in high school and college-age female athletes in the Midwest: Implications for education and prevention. *Urol Nurs,* 27(1), 21–24, 39. Retrieved May 2007 at www.medscape.com/viewarticle/555700?src=mp.
16. Resnick, N. M. (2003). Urinary Incontinence. In Cassel, C. K., Leipzig, R. M., Cohen, H. J., et al. (eds). *Geriatric Medicine: An Evidence-Based Approach.* New York: Springer.
17. Newman, D. K. (2006). Using the BladderScan™ for bladder volume assessment. Retrieved May 2007 at www.seekwellness.com/incontinence/using_the_bladderscan.htm.
18. Bray, B., Van Sell, S. L., Miller-Anderson, M. (2007). Stress incontinence: It's no laughing matter. *RN,* 70(4), 25–29.
19. Rackley, R., Vasavada, S. P. (2006). Incontinence, urinary: Nonsurgical therapies. Article for Emedicine Web site. Retrieved May 2007 at www.emedicine.com/med/topic3085.htm.
20. National Kidney and Urologic Diseases Information Clearing House (NKUDIC). (2003). Treatments for urinary incontinence in women. Accessed August 2007 at http://kidney.niddk.nih.gov/kudiseases/pubs/treatmentsuiwomen/index.htm.
21. Bump, R. C., Hurt, W. G., Fantl, J. A. (1991). Assessment of Kegel pelvic muscle exercise performance after brief verbal instruction. *Am J Obstet Gynecol,* 165, 322–327.

total Urinary Incontinence

Definition: Continuous and unpredictable loss of urine

RELATED FACTORS

Neuropathy preventing transmission of reflex [signals to the reflex arc] indicating bladder fullness

Neurological dysfunction [e.g., cerebral lesions]

Independent contraction of detrusor reflex

Trauma/disease affecting spinal cord nerves [destruction of sensory or motor neurons below the injury level]

Anatomic (fistula)

DEFINING CHARACTERISTICS

Subjective
Constant flow of urine at unpredictable times without uninhibited bladder
   contractions/spasm or distention
Nocturia
Lack of bladder/perineal filling [awareness]
Unawareness of incontinence

Objective
Unsuccessful incontinence refractory treatments

Sample Clinical Applications: Spinal cord injury/nerve compression, spina bifida,
   myelomeningocele, Guillain-Barré syndrome, brain injury/stroke, hydrocephalus, MS,
   cerebral palsy, Parkinson's disease, diabetes mellitus, abdominal trauma, dementia

DESIRED OUTCOMES/EVALUATION CRITERIA
Sample NOC linkages:
Urinary Continence: Control of elimination of urine from the bladder
Self-Care: Toileting: Ability to toilet self independently with or without assistive device
Tissue Integrity: Skin & Mucous Membranes: Structural intactness and normal
   physiological function of skin and mucous membranes

Client/Caregiver Will (Include Specific Time Frame)

- Verbalize awareness of causative/contributing factors.
- Establish bladder regimen for individual situation.
- Demonstrate behaviors, techniques to manage condition and to prevent complications.
- Manage incontinence so that social functioning is regained/maintained.

ACTIONS/INTERVENTIONS

Sample NIC linkages:
Urinary Incontinence Care: Assistance in promoting continence and maintaining perineal
   skin integrity
Urinary Catheterization: Insertion of a catheter into the bladder for temporary or perma-
   nent drainage of urine
Perineal Care: Maintenance of perineal skin integrity and relief of perineal discomfort

NURSING PRIORITY NO. I   To assess causative/contributing factors:

- Identify client with condition(s) causing actual/potential for total incontinence as listed in
   Related Factors. *High-risk persons include frail elderly, women, presence of brain lesions/
   disease (e.g., stroke, cancer, Parkinson's disease, cerebral palsy, hydrocephalus, dementia);
   spinal cord injury (e.g., quadriplegia, paraplegia, herniated disk, pelvic crush injury); chronic
   neurological diseases (e.g., multiple sclerosis, child with myelomeningocele); pregnancy, prolonged
   labor, early postpartum period; genitourinary surgery/trauma (e.g., radical hysterectomy,
   abdominoperineal resection); peripheral neuropathy (e.g., diabetes mellitus, AIDS, poliomyelitis,
   Guillain-Barré syndrome); and lifestyle issues (e.g., certain medications, irritating foods, fluid
   intake, mobility limitations).*[1,2]

- Be aware of/note effect of global neurological impairment, neuromuscular trauma after surgery/radiation therapy or childbirth, or presence of fistula. *Injury to the nerves supplying the bladder can result in constant loss of urine because of loss of integrity of lower urinary tract function. Presence of vesicovaginal fistula may also cause incontinence.*[3]
- Determine if client is aware of incontinence. *Cognitive, developmental issues, or medical conditions can impair client's awareness and sensory perception of voiding need/process and incontinence.*[3]
- Check for perineal sensation and fecal impaction *to determine whether sensation and reflexes are impaired when neurological condition is present.*[1,4]
- Determine concomitant chronic retention (e.g., palpate bladder, scan/catheterize for urine volume and residual). *Rather than relaxing when the bladder contracts, the outlet contracts, leading to severe outlet obstruction and urine retention.*[3]
- Observe for overflow incontinence *due to chronic urinary retention or secondary to flaccid bladder associated with obstructive or neuropathic lesion.*[1,2] (Refer to ND overflow Incontinence for related interventions.)
- Carry out/assist with diagnostic procedures/tests (e.g., postvoid residual, urine flowmetry, pressure studies, cystoscopy, filling and voiding cystogram) *to establish diagnosis/identify needed interventions.*[1,5]

NURSING PRIORITY NO. 2 To assess degree of interference/disability:

- Have client/caregivers keep an incontinence chart. Note times of voiding and incontinence. *Determines pattern of urination and whether there is any control.*[1,4]
- Determine client's particular symptoms (e.g., continuous dribbling superimposed upon an otherwise normal voiding pattern, or high-volume urine loss that replaces any detectable pattern of bladder filling/storage/voiding). *Influences choice of interventions.*[11]
- Review past interventions *to ascertain cause for continence failure (e.g., client unable to sustain behavioral management of bladder training program, or medical conditions do not allow for success in voiding efforts.)*
- Ascertain effect of condition on lifestyle and self-esteem. *Incontinence is embarrassing and distressing and may severely affect the quality of life for the individual and even the family members.*[6]
- Inspect skin for areas of erythema/excoriation. *Constant loss of urine can abraid the skin, causing breakdown if not cared for frequently.*[5]

NURSING PRIORITY NO. 3 To assist in preventing/managing incontinence:

- Collaborate in treatment of underlying conditions (e.g., neurological disorders, prostate problems, chronic urinary tract infections, psychiatric disorders) *that contribute to incontinence.*
- Implement bladder training and/or incontinence management, as indicated:
  Provide ready access to bathroom, commode, bedpan, or urinal.
  Encourage adequate fluid and regulate time of intake *to ensure sufficient fluid intake and to prevent dehydration and promote a predictable voiding pattern where possible.*[4]
  Establish voiding/bladder emptying schedule by toileting at same time as recorded voidings and 30 minutes earlier than recorded time of incontinence. *Bladder training may be an effective strategy when neurological impairment is not extensive.*[6]
  Use condom catheter/other external collecting device during daytime and absorptive pads during the night if external device is not tolerated. *Maintains dry clothing and bedding, preventing skin irritation, odor with resultant embarrassment.*[4]

Nursing Diagnoses in Alphabetical Order

- Implement/instruct client/SO in techniques of clean intermittent self-catheterization (CISC) using small-lumen straight catheter (or Mitrofanoff continent urinary channel *for clients not able to catheterize themselves*), as indicated. *In the presence of neurological damage and when client is cognitively competent, these measures can assure a successful management program.*[8,9]

- Implement continuous urine collection (e.g., indwelling urethral or suprapubic catheter) when dictated by client's conditions (*e.g., severely impaired individual in whom other interventions [e.g., bladder training, self-catheterization] are not an option; or person lives alone and cannot provide own supportive care*).[2]

- Discuss/prepare for surgical intervention, when indicated. *Many forms of surgical repair have been developed, depending on underlying cause (e.g., to treat urethral hypermobility, to suspend the bladder, to repair vaginal walls, remove obstructions; provide artificial sphincter or bladder reservoir).*[7,10]

- Refer to ND functional/stress/reflex Urinary Incontinence for additional interventions specific to diagnosis.

NURSING PRIORITY NO. 4 To promote wellness (Teaching/Discharge Considerations):

- Assist client to identify regular period of time for bladder program *that meets individual physical and psychosocial needs.*[6,12]

- Suggest use of incontinence pads/adult briefs, as indicated (e.g., during social contacts/work hours, etc.). *Provides protection and enhances confidence when other measures have not been successful.*[7,12]

- Emphasize importance of pericare after voiding (using alcohol-free products) and application of oil-based emollient. *Protects the skin from irritation from the constant flow of urine.*[5]

- Instruct in proper care of catheter and clean technique. *Reduces risk of infection when client is using catheterization on a regular basis.*[6]

- Recommend use of silicone catheter. *When long-term/continuous placement is indicated after other measures/bladder training have failed, use of a silicone catheter has less problems with deterioration and infection than latex products.*[5]

- Encourage self-monitoring of catheter patency and avoidance of reflux of urine. *Reduces risk of infection.*[5]

- Suggest intake of acidifying juices, such as cranberry. *Discourages bacterial growth/adherence to bladder wall, preventing recurrent infections.*[5]

DOCUMENTATION FOCUS

Assessment/Reassessment

- Current elimination pattern.
- Assessment findings, including effect on lifestyle and self-esteem.

Planning

- Plan of care/interventions, including who is involved in planning.
- Teaching plan.

Implementation/Evaluation

- Response to interventions/teaching and actions performed.
- Attainment/progress toward desired outcome(s).
- Modifications to plan of care.

Cultural Collaborative Community/Home Care Diagnostic Studies Pediatric/Geriatric/Lifespan Medications

Discharge Planning

- Discharge plan/long-term needs and who is responsible for actions to be taken.
- Specific referrals made.

References

1. Guerrero, P., Sinert, R. (2002). Urinary incontinence. Accessed August 2007 at www.emedicine.com/emerg/topic791.htm.
2. Choe, J. M., Mardovin, W. Neurogenic bladder. Available at www.emedicine.com. Accessed September 2003.
3. Beers, M. H., Berkow, R. (eds). (1999). *The Merck Manual of Diagnosis and Therapy*. 17th ed. Whitehouse Station, NJ: Merck Research Laboratories.
4. ND: Urinary Incontinence. In Cox, H. C., et al. (2002). *Clinical Applications of Nursing Diagnosis: Adult, Child, Women's Psychiatric, Gerontic, and Home Health Considerations*. 4th ed. Philadelphia: F. A. Davis.
5. Doenges, M. E., Moorhouse, M. F., Geissler-Murr, A. C. (2002). *Nursing Care Plans: Guidelines for Individualizing Patient Care*. 6th ed. Philadelphia: F. A. Davis.
6. Newman, D. K., Palmer, M. H. (eds). (2003). The state of the science on urinary incontinence. *Am J Nurs, 293*, 3(suppl), 20.
7. Booth, C. (2002). Introduction to urinary incontinence. *Hospital Pharmacist*, 9(3), 65–68.
8. Understanding Female Urinary Incontinence. Patient UK. Family Doctor Series, pamphlet. (Update 2005). Accessed July 2007 at www.patient.co.uk/showdoc/23068768/.
9. Choe, J. M. (2003). Incontinence, urinary: Surgical therapies. Accessed July 2007 at www.emedicine.com/emerg/topic3084.htm.
10. Choe, J. M. (2002). Incontinence, urinary: Nonsurgical therapies. Accessed July 2007 at www.emedicine.com/emerg/topic3085.htm.
11. Gray, M. (2004). Stress urinary incontinence in women. *J Am Acad Nurse Pract*, 16(5), 188–190, 192–199.
12. Santos, A., Hunt, M. (2005). Managing incontinence: Once a cause of isolation and embarrassment, incontinence does not have to limit quality of life. From Paraplegia News, November 2005.

urge Urinary Incontinence

Definition: Involuntary passage of urine occurring soon after a strong sense of urgency to void

RELATED FACTORS
Decreased bladder capacity
Bladder infection; atrophic urethritis/vaginitis
Alcohol/caffeine intake; [increased fluids]
Use of diuretics
Fecal impaction
Detrusor hyperactivity with impaired bladder contractility

DEFINING CHARACTERISTICS

Subjective
Reports urinary urgency; involuntary loss of urine with bladder contractions/spasms; inability to reach toilet in time to avoid urine loss

Objective
Observed inability to reach toilet in time to avoid urine loss

Sample Clinical Applications: Abdominal trauma/surgery, PID, recurrent UTIs, brain injury/stroke, MS, Parkinson's disease, diabetes mellitus, dementia

DESIRED OUTCOMES/EVALUATION CRITERIA

Sample NOC linkages:

Urinary Continence: Control of elimination of urine from the bladder

Cognition: Ability to execute complex mental processes

Self-Care: Toileting: Ability to toilet self independently with or without assistive device

Client Will (Include Specific Time Frame)

- Verbalize understanding of condition.
- Demonstrate behaviors/techniques to control/correct situation.
- Report increase in interval between urge and involuntary loss of urine.
- Void every 3 to 4 hours in individually appropriate amounts.

ACTIONS/INTERVENTIONS

Sample NIC linkages:

Urinary Habit Training: Establishing a predictable pattern of bladder emptying to prevent incontinence for persons with limited cognitive ability who have urge, stress, or functional incontinence

Urinary Incontinence Care: Assistance in promoting continence and maintaining perineal skin integrity

Perineal Care: Maintenance of perineal skin integrity and relief of perineal discomfort

NURSING PRIORITY NO. 1   To assess causative/contributing factors:

- Note presence of conditions often associated with urgent voiding (e.g., stroke, MS, Parkinson's disease, spinal cord injury, Alzheimer's disease, obesity; pelvic inflammatory disease; abdominal/pelvic surgeries, recent/lengthy use of indwelling urinary catheter) *affecting bladder capacity, pelvic musculature tone, or innervation.*
- Ask client about urgency (more than just normal desire to void). *Urgency (also sometimes called overactive bladder syndrome) is a sudden compelling need to void that is difficult to defer and may be accompanied by leaking/incontinence.*[10,11]
- Note factors that may affect ability to respond to urge to void in timely manner. *Impaired mobility, use of sedation, or cognitive impairments may result in client not recognizing need to void or moving too slowly to make it to the bathroom, with subsequent loss of urine.*[3]
- Review client's medications/substance use (e.g., diuretics, antipsychotics, sedatives; caffeine, alcohol) *for agents that increase urine production or exert a bladder irritant effect.*[2]
- Assess for cloudy, odorous urine associated with acute, painful urgency symptoms. *Incontinence often leads to/or reflects urinary tract infections.*[1]
- Test urine for glucose. *Presence of glucose in urine causes polyuria, resulting in overdistention of the bladder and inability to hold urine until reaching the bathroom.*[4]
- Prepare for/assist with appropriate diagnostic testing (e.g., pre/postvoid bladder scanning; pelvic examination *for strictures, impaired perineal sensation or musculature;* urinalysis, uroflowmetry voiding pressures; cystoscopy, cystometrogram) *to determine anatomic and functional status of bladder and urethra.*[3–5,12]
- Assess for concomitant stress or functional incontinence. *Older women often have a mix of stress and urge incontinence, whereas individuals with dementia or disabling neurological disorders tend to have urge and functional incontinence.* (Refer to NDs stress/functional Urinary Incontinence for additional interventions.)

🌐 Cultural Ⓐ Collaborative 🏠 Community/Home Care ✎ Diagnostic Studies ∞ Pediatric/Geriatric/Lifespan ⚬ Medications

NURSING PRIORITY NO. 2 To assess degree of interference/disability:

- Measure amount of urine voided, especially noting amounts less than 100 cc or greater than 550 cc. *Bladder capacity may be impaired or bladder contractions facilitating emptying may be ineffective.*[6] (Refer to ND [acute/chronic] Urinary Retention.)
- Record frequency of voiding during a typical day and typical night. *Maintaining a voiding diary identifies degree of difficulty being experienced by client.*[7]
- Note length of warning time between initial urge and loss of urine. *Overactivity or irritability decreases the length of time between urge and loss and helps clarify the type of incontinence.*[2]
- Ascertain if client experiences triggers (e.g., sound of running water, putting hands in water, seeing a restroom sign, "key-in-the-lock" syndrome, etc.).[12]
- Ascertain effect on lifestyle (including daily activities, socialization, sexuality) and self-esteem. *There is a considerable reduction in the quality of life of individuals with an incontinence problem, affecting socialization and view of themselves as sexual beings and sense of self-esteem.*[4]

NURSING PRIORITY NO. 3 To assist in treating/preventing incontinence:

- Implement continence management interventions:
  Establish voiding schedule (habit and bladder training) based on client's usual voiding pattern. *Bladder retraining program is often successful in the control of urge incontinence.*[7,13]
  Recommend consciously delaying voiding by using distraction (e.g., slow, deep breathing); self-statements (e.g., "I can wait"); and contracting pelvic muscles when exposed to triggers. *Behavioral techniques for urge suppression.*[4,13,14]
  Encourage regular pelvic floor strengthening exercise (Kegel exercises) or use of vaginal cones. Combine activity with biofeedback, as appropriate. *Enhances effectiveness of training and success at controlling incontinence.*[7,13,15]
  Instruct client to tighten pelvic floor muscles before arising from bed. *Helps prevent loss of urine as abdominal pressure changes.*[7]
  Set alarm to awaken during night, if indicated. *May be necessary to continue voiding schedule.*[7]
  Increase fluid intake to 1500 to 2000 mL/day (or as indicated) *to prevent dehydration and promote good urine flow.*[7] *Note: Too much fluid can also increase bladder irritation, so amount of intake needs to be determined by individual response.*[19]
  Regulate liquid intake at prescheduled times, and limit fluids 2 to 3 hours prior to bedtime. *Promotes a predictable voiding pattern and can help limit nocturia.*[8]
  Modify diet, as indicated (e.g., reduce acidic/citrus juices, carbonated beverages, spicy foods, artificial sweetners, etc.), *to reduce bladder irritants.*[19]
  Suggest limiting intake of coffee/tea and alcohol *to reduce urge symptoms and nighttime incontinence.*[2,19]
  Manage bowel elimination *to prevent urinary problems associated with constipation/fecal impaction.*
- Offer assistance to cognitively impaired client (e.g., prompt client/or take to bathroom on regularly timed schedule) *to reduce frequency of incontinence episodes/promote comfort.*
- Provide assistance/devices, as indicated, for clients who are mobility impaired. *Providing means of summoning assistance, placing bedside commode, urinal, or bedpan within reach helps to avoid unintended loss of urine and promotes sense of control over situation.*[7]
- Collaborate in treating underlying cause. *Urgency symptoms may resolve with treatment of medical problem (e.g., infection, recovery from surgery, childbirth, or pelvic trauma) or may be resistant to resolution (e.g., incontinence associated with neurogenic bladder).*

- Refer to specialist/treament program, as indicated, for additional/specialized interventions (e.g., biofeedback, use of vaginal cones, electronic stimulation therapy). *Significant reduction in incontinence episodes is reported with use of combined therapies (e.g., electronic stimulation therapy plus pelvic muscle exercises).*[18]
- Administer medications (e.g., antibiotics, antimuscarinics [oxybutynin, tolterodine]) *to reduce incidence of urinary tract infections and reduce voiding frequency and urgency by blocking overactive detrusor contractions.*[10,16]
- Discuss possible surgical interventions to change position of/enlarge the bladder, add support to weakened pelvic muscles, replace the urinary sphincter, or implantation of a sacral nerve stimulator that acts as a bladder pacemaker. *When other options have failed, different surgical interventions have been developed to cure various forms of incontinence and minimize surgical trauma, thus decreasing the length of hospitalization.*[4,17]

NURSING PRIORITY NO. 4 To promote wellness (Teaching/Discharge Considerations):

- Encourage comfort measures (e.g., use of incontinence pads/undergarments, wearing loose-fitting or especially adapted clothing) *to prepare for/manage urge incontinence symptoms over the long-term as well as to enhance sense of security/confidence in abilities to be socially active.*[8]
- Emphasize importance of perineal care after each voiding. *Prevents skin irritation and reduces potential for bladder infection.*[9]
- Identify signs/symptoms indicating urinary complications and need for medical follow-up care. *Helps client be aware and seek intervention in a timely manner to prevent more serious problems from developing.*[7]

DOCUMENTATION FOCUS

Assessment/Reassessment

- Individual findings, including pattern of incontinence, effect on lifestyle and self-esteem.

Planning

- Plan of care/interventions and who is involved in planning.
- Teaching plan.

Implementation/Evaluation

- Response to interventions/teaching and actions performed.
- Attainment/progress toward desired outcome(s).
- Modifications to plan of care.

Discharge Planning

- Discharge needs/referrals and who is responsible for actions to be taken.
- Specific referrals made.

References

1. Wyman, J. F. (2003). Treatment of urinary incontinence in men and older women. In Newman, D. K., Palmer, M. H. (eds). The state of the science on urinary incontinence. *Am J Nurs,* 293, 3(suppl), 20.
2. What is urinary incontinence? Available at http://ourworld.compuserve.com/homepages/nacs/INCONT. HTM. Accessed September 2003.

3. Urinary incontinence. Penn State Health & Disease Information. Accessed August 2007 at www.hmc.psu.edu/healthinfo/uz/urinaryincontinence.htm.
4. Booth, C. (2002). Introduction to urinary incontinence. *Hosp Pharmacist,* 9(3), 65–68.
5. Beers, M. H., Berkow, R. (eds). (1999). *The Merck Manual of Diagnosis and Therapy.* 17th ed. Whitehouse Station, NJ: Merck Research Laboratories.
6. Doenges, M. E., Moorhouse, M. F., Geissler-Murr, A. C. (2004). *Nurse's Pocket Guide: Diagnoses, Interventions, and Rationales.* 9th ed. Philadelphia: F. A. Davis.
7. Newman, D. K., Palmer, M. H. (eds). (2003). The state of the science on urinary incontinence. *Am J Nurs,* 293, 3(suppl), 20.
8. Ford-Martin, P. A. (1999). Urinary incontinence. Gale Encyclopedia of Medicine. Gale Research. Accessed August 2007 at http://findarticles.com/p/articles/mi_g2601/is_0014/ai_2601001430/pg_3.
9. ND: Urinary Incontinence. In Cox, H. C., et al. (2002). *Clinical Applications of Nursing Diagnosis: Adult, Child, Women's, Psychiatric, Gerontic, and Home Health Considerations.* 4th ed. Philadelphia: F. A. Davis.
10. Gray, M. (2005). Assessment and management of urinary incontinence. *Nurse Practitioner: The American J of Primary Health Care,* 30(7), 32–43.
11. Gray, M. (2005). Overactive bladder: An overview. *Journal of Wound, Ostomy and Continence Nursing,* 32(3), Suppl, 1–5.
12. Newman, D. K. (2005). Assessment of the patient with an overactive bladder. *Journal of Wound, Ostomy and Continence Nursing,* 32(3) Suppl, 5–10.
13. Wyman, J. F. (2005). Behavioral interventions for the patient with overactive bladder. *Journal of Wound, Ostomy and Continence Nursing,* 32(3), Suppl, 11–15.
14. No author listed. (1995-2007). Urinary incontinence. The Merck Manual of Health & Aging (online), Section 3, Ch 57. Retrieved August 2007 at www.merck.com/pubs/mmanual_ha/sec3/ch57/ch57a.html.
15. Bump, R. C., Hurt, W. G., Fantl, J. A., et al. (1999). Assessment of Kegel pelvic muscle exercise performance after brief verbal instruction. *Am J Obstet Gynecol,* 165, 322–327.
16. Mauk, K. L. (2005). Medications for management of overactive bladder. ARN Network. June/July, 3–7.
17. Mayo Clinic. Surgical treatments for urinary incontinence. Retrieved August 2007 at www.mayoclinic.org/urinary-incontinence/surgery.html.
18. Incontinence—Biofeedback and electrical stimulation. (February 2007). Retrieved August 2007 at www.emedicinehealth.com/incontinence/page8_em.htm.
19. Incontinence—Nonsurgical treatment: Dietary measures. (February 2007). Retrieved August 2007 at www.emedicinehealth.com/incontinence/page6_em.htm.

risk for urge Urinary Incontinence

Definition: At risk for an involuntary loss of urine associated with a sudden, strong sensation or urinary urgency

RISK FACTORS

Effects of medications/caffeine/alcohol

Detrusor hyperreflexia (e.g., from cystitis, urethritis, tumors, renal calculi, CNS disorders above pontine micturition center)

Impaired bladder contractility; involuntary sphincter relaxation

Ineffective toileting habits

Small bladder capacity

NOTE: A risk diagnosis is not evidenced by signs and symptoms, as the problem has not occurred; rather, nursing interventions are directed at prevention.

Sample Clinical Applications: MS, BPH, recurrent UTIs, renal calculi, pelvic surgery/radiation, Guillain-Barré syndrome, dementia, major depression

DESIRED OUTCOMES/EVALUATION CRITERIA

Sample NOC linkages:

Urinary Continence: Control of elimination of urine from the bladder

Risk Control: Personal actions to prevent, eliminate, or reduce modifiable health threats

---

Neurological Status: Autonomic: Ability of the autonomic nervous system to coordinate visceral and hemostatic function

Client Will (Include Specific Time Frame)

- Identify individual risk factors and appropriate interventions.
- Demonstrate behaviors or lifestyle changes to prevent development of problem.

ACTIONS/INTERVENTIONS

Sample NIC linkages:

Urinary Habit Training: Establishing a predictable pattern of bladder emptying to prevent incontinence for persons with limited cognitive ability who have urge, stress, or functional incontinence

Self-Care Assistance: Toileting: Assisting another with elimination

Prompted Voiding: Promotion of urinary continence through the use of timed verbal toileting reminders and positive social feedback for successful toileting

NURSING PRIORITY NO. 1 To assess potential for developing incontinence:

- Note presence of diagnoses often associated with urgent voiding. *Such conditions as stroke, brain injury, multiple sclerosis, Parkinson's disease, spinal cord injury; delirium or dementias; pelvic inflammatory disease, abdominal/pelvic surgery; obesity/abdominal distention; acute bladder infection, kidney stones can affect bladder capacity, pelvic/bladder/urethral musculature tone, and/or innervation.*[1–3,10]
- Note factors that may affect ability to respond to urge to void. *Impaired mobility due to aging, chronic conditions, sedation, acute injuries, lack of access to toilet, impaired awareness (either cognition or sensation), or use of restraints can all affect client's ability to respond in a timely manner.*[2,4,10]
- Determine use/presence of bladder irritants. *A significant intake of alcohol or caffeine can result in increased output or concentrated urine and contribute to the possibility of incontinence.*[5]
- Review client's medications/other drugs that can affect bladder function, such as beta-blockers and cholinergic drugs *(can increase detrusor tone);* neuroleptics, antidepressants, sedatives, opiates *(can cause detrusor relaxation);* muscle relaxants and psychoactive drugs *(can cause sphincter relaxation);* diuretics *(can increase urine production).*[12]
- Measure amount of urine voided, especially noting amounts less than 100 mL or greater than 550 mL. *Provides information about amount of urine required to initiate desire to void, as well as potential for dehydration or excessive fluid loss if large voidings are frequent.*[6]
- Prepare for/assist with appropriate testing (e.g., urinalysis, noninvasive bladder scanning, urine culture, urine/serum glucose, voiding cystometrogram). *Accurate assessment and diagnosis can determine voiding pattern and identify pathology that may lead to the development of incontinence.*[2,4,13]

NURSING PRIORITY NO. 2 To prevent occurrence of problem:

- Assist in treatment of underlying conditions that may contribute to urge incontinence.
- Record intake and frequency/degree of urgency of voiding. *May reveal developing incontinence problem when need to void is more frequent and urgent in relation to normal fluid intake.*[7]

Cultural Collaborative Community/Home Care Diagnostic Studies Pediatric/Geriatric/Lifespan Medications

- Ascertain client's awareness/concerns about developing problem and whether lifestyle is affected (e.g., daily activities, socialization, sexual patterns). *Provides information regarding the degree of concern client is experiencing and need for preventive measures to be instituted.*[8]
- Regulate liquid intake at prescheduled times (with and between meals). *Promotes a predictable voiding pattern to establish a bladder-training program to prevent incontinence.*[5]
- Establish schedule for voiding (habit training) based on client's usual voiding pattern. *Can successfully reduce risk for incontinence.*[8]
- Provide assistance/devices, as indicated, for clients who are mobility impaired. *Providing means of summoning assistance and placing bedside commode, urinal, or bedpan within client's reach can promote sense of control in self-managing voiding.*[9]
- Encourage regular pelvic floor strengthening exercises (Kegel exercises or use of vaginal cones). *Can improve pelvic musculature tone and strength, preventing progression of incontinence problem.*[5]

NURSING PRIORITY NO. 3   To promote wellness (Teaching/Discharge Considerations):

- Provide information to client/SO about potential for urge incontinence and lifestyle measures to prevent development of incontinence, as individually indicated.
- Recommend limiting intake of coffee/tea and alcohol. *These substances have an irritating effect on the bladder and may contribute to incontinence.*[7]
- Suggest wearing loose-fitting or especially adapted clothing. *Facilitates response to voiding urge, especially in elderly or infirm individuals, enabling them to reach the toilet without loss of urine.*[10]
- Emphasize importance of perineal care after each voiding. *Reduces risk of ascending infection.*[11]

DOCUMENTATION FOCUS

Assessment/Reassessment
- Individual findings, including specific risk factors and pattern of voiding.

Planning
- Plan of care/interventions and who is involved in planning.
- Teaching plan

Implementation/Evaluation
- Response to interventions/teaching and actions performed.
- Attainment/progress toward desired outcome(s).
- Modifications to plan of care.

Discharge Planning
- Discharge needs/referrals and who is responsible for actions to be taken.
- Specific referrals made.

References

1. Guerrero, P., Sinert, R. (2002). Urinary incontinence. Accessed August 2007 at www.emedicine.com/emerg/topic791.htm.
2. Booth, C. (2002). Introduction to urinary incontinence. *Hosp Pharmacist,* 9(3), 65–68.
3. No author listed. (2000). Evidence-based clinical practice guideline—Continence for women. Washington: DC: Association of Women's Health, Obstetric and Neonatal Nurses (AWHONN). Available at http://guideline.gov. Accessed January 2004.
4. No author listed. (1996). Urinary incontinence. American Medical Directors Association (AMDA). Available at www.guidleine.gov. Accessed September 2003.

5. Newman, D. K., Palmer, M. H. (eds). (2003). The state of the science on urinary incontinence. *Am J Nurs*, 293, 3(suppl), 20.

6. Doenges, M. E., Moorhouse, M. F., Geissler-Murr, A. C. (2004). *Nurse's Pocket Guide: Diagnoses, Interventions, and Rationales*. 9th ed. Philadelphia: F. A. Davis.

7. What is urinary incontinence? Accessed September 2003 at http://ourworld.compuserve.com/homepages/nacs/INCONT.HTM.

8. Ford-Martin, P. A. (1999). Urinary incontinence. Gale Encyclopedia of Medicine. Gale Research. Accessed August 2007 at http://findarticles.com/p/articles/mi_g2601/is_0014/ai_2601001430/pg_3.

9. ND: Urinary Incontinence. In Cox, H. C., et al. (2002). *Clinical Applications of Nursing Diagnosis: Adult, Child, Women's, Psychiatric, Gerontic, and Home Health Considerations*. 4th ed. Philadelphia: F. A. Davis.

10. Wyman, J. F. (2003). Treatment of urinary incontinence in men and older women. In Newman, D. K., Palmer, M. H. (eds). The state of the science on urinary incontinence. *Am J Nurs*, 293, 3(suppl), 20.

11. Doenges, M. E., Moorhouse, M. F., Geissler-Murr, A. C. (2002). *Nursing Care Plans: Guidelines for Individualizing Patient Care*. 6th ed. Philadelphia: F. A. Davis.

12. Porter, R. S., Kaplan, J. L. (eds). (2003). The Merck Manuals Online Medical Library. Kidney and Urinary Tract Disorders: Urinary Incontinence. Accessed August 2007 at www.merck.com/mmhe/sec11/ch147/ch147a.html.

13. Newman, D. K. (2006). Using the BladderScan(r) for bladder volume assessment. Retrieved May 2007 at www.seekwellness.com/incontinence/using_the_bladderscan.htm.

[acute/chronic] Urinary Retention

Definition: Incomplete emptying of the bladder

RELATED FACTORS

High urethral pressure

Inhibition of reflex arc

Strong sphincter; blockage [e.g., benign prostatic hypertrophy-BPH, perineal swelling]

[Habituation of reflex arc]

[Infections; neurological diseases/trauma]

[Use of medications with side effect of retention (e.g., atropine, belladonna, psychotropics, antihistamines, opiates)]

DEFINING CHARACTERISTICS

Subjective
Sensation of bladder fullness

Dribbling

Dysuria

Objective
Bladder distention

Small/frequent voiding; absence of urine output

Residual urine [150 mL or more]

Overflow incontinence

[Reduced stream]

Sample Clinical Applications: BPH, prostatitis, cancer, perineal surgery/birth trauma, urethral calculi, MS, spinal cord compression, UTI, genital herpes

DESIRED OUTCOMES/EVALUATION CRITERIA

Sample NOC linkages:

Urinary Elimination: Collection and discharge of urine

Cultural　Collaborative　Community/Home Care　Diagnostic Studies　Pediatric/Geriatric/Lifespan　Medications

Symptom Control: Personal actions to minimize perceived adverse changes in physical and emotional functioning

Knowledge: Disease Process: Extent of understanding conveyed about a specific disease process

---

Client Will (Include Specific Time Frame)

- Verbalize understanding of causative factors and appropriate interventions for individual situation.
- Demonstrate techniques/behaviors to alleviate/prevent retention.
- Void in sufficient amounts with no palpable bladder distention; experience no postvoid residuals greater than 50 mL; have no dribbling/overflow.

ACTIONS/INTERVENTIONS

Acute retention
Sample NIC linkages:

Urinary Catheterization: Insertion of a catheter into the bladder for temporary or permanent drainage of urine

Fluid Monitoring: Collection and analysis of patient data to regulate fluid balance

NURSING PRIORITY NO. 1 To assess causative/contributing factors:

- Note presence of pathological conditions such as neurological injury/disease, kidney/bladder infection or stone formation, and reaction to medications, diagnostic dye, or anesthesia *that can cause mechanical obstruction, nerve dysfunction, ineffective contraction, or decompensation of detrusor musculature, resulting in ineffective emptying of the bladder and urine retention.*[1,7]
- Investigate reports of sudden loss of ability to pass urine/great difficulty passing urine, pain with urination, blood in urine. *May indicate urinary tract infection or obstruction.*[7]
- Review results of laboratory tests, such as urinalysis for presence of red/white blood cells, nitrates, glucose, bacteria, and cultures, as indicated; blood may be tested for infection, electrolyte imbalance, and (in men) prostate-specific antigen (PSA) *to determine presence of treatable conditions.*[3,4]
- Review medication regimen *for drugs that can cause/exacerbate retention (e.g., psychotropics, opiates, sedatives, alpha- and beta-blockers, anticholinergics, antihistamines, neuroleptics, anesthesia).*[2,7]
- Determine anxiety level. *Client may be too embarrassed to void in presence of others or talk about problem with care providers.*[2]
- Examine for fecal impaction, pelvic/perineal surgical site swelling, postpartal edema, vaginal or rectal packing, enlarged prostate, or other "mechanical" factors *that may produce a blockage of the urethra.*[2]
- Strain urine for presence of stones/calculi *that may be causing outlet obstruction, or to note when treatments are being effective in stone breakup/removal.*[1,7]

NURSING PRIORITY NO. 2 To determine degree of interference/disability:

- Ascertain if client can empty bladder completely, partially, or not at all, in spite of urge to urinate. *Signs of urinary retention caused by (1) blockage of the urethra or (2) disruption of complex system of nerves that connects the urinary tract with the brain. In men, blockage is*

---

most commonly caused by enlargement of the prostate, cancer, stones, and urethral stricture. Causes that can occur in both genders include scar tissue, injury, (as in car accident or fall), blood clots, infection, tumors, and stones (rare). Disruption of nerves, or nerve transmission, or interpretation of signals can be caused by injury (e.g., spinal cord injury or tumor, herniated disk, stroke), pelvic infections, surgery, and certain medications.[3,5,7]

- Determine if there has been any significant urine output in the previous 6 to 8 hours. *Small amount of urine may leak out of bladder, but generally not enough to relieve symptoms.*[3]
- Note recent amount/type of fluid intake. *Fluids may initially need to be restricted to prevent bladder distention until adequate urine flow is established.*[1]
- Palpate height of the bladder. Ascertain whether client has sensation of bladder fullness, level of discomfort. *Sensation and discomfort can vary, depending on underlying cause of retention. Most people with acute retention also feel pain in lower abdomen (pelvis). Back pain, fever, and painful urination may be present with retention if the cause is urinary tract infection.*[3]
- Catheterize/perform bladder scan/ultrasound for bladder residual after voiding *to determine presence/degree of urine retention.*[1]
- Review results of diagnostic tests. *Urine flow rate, bladder capacity, and postvoid residual scanning may be done. Ultrasound, CT scan, intravenous pyelogram (IVP) and cystoscopy can help locate the source of obstruction (e.g., lower or upper tract). Lumbar spine radiographs, CT scan, or MRI may be done when retention is thought to be due to an acute spinal problem (e.g., herniated disk, spinal cord disruption, infection).*[3,4,7,8]

NURSING PRIORITY NO. 3 To assist in treating/preventing retention:

- Assist in treatment to relieve mechanical obstruction (e.g., removal of blockage—vaginal packing, bowel impaction; application of ice *to reduce perineal swelling) that is restricting urinary flow.*[2]
- Administer medications as indicated (e.g., antibiotics, stool softeners, pain relievers) *to treat underlying cause, promote muscle relaxation.*[2]
- Provide privacy *to reduce retention caused by embarrassment/anxiety.*
- Assist client to sit upright on bedpan/commode or stand *to provide functional position of voiding.*[2]
- Encourage warm sitz bath or shower, voiding in tub/shower, if need be. *Warm water stimulates bladder to relax and may facilitate voiding.*[2]
- Use ice techniques, spirits of wintergreen, stroking inner thigh, running water in sink or warm water over perineum *to stimulate reflex arc.*[2]
- Teach client with mild or moderate obstructive symptoms to "double void" by urinating, resting on toilet for 3 to 5 minutes, and then making a second attempt to urinate. *Promotes more efficient bladder evacuation by allowing the detrusor to contract initially, then rest and contract again.*[5]
- Drain bladder with straight catheter per agency protocol or catheterize with intermittent or indwelling catheter *to resolve acute retention.*[2] *Note: References are mixed as to need for fractional drainage in increments of 200 mL at a time to prevent possibility of bladder spasm, syncope/hypotension.*[6]
- Provide adequate fluid intake, including use of acidifying fruit juices or ingestion of vitamin C/Mandelamine *to discourage bacterial growth and stone formation.*[2]
- Adjust fluid intake and timing if indicated, *to prevent bladder distention.*
- Prepare for more aggressive intervention (e.g., reconstructive surgery, lithotripsy, prostatectomy, etc.) as indicated *to remove source of obstruction, reconstruct sphincter, or provide for urinary diversion.*[2]

🌐 Cultural Ⓐ Collaborative 🏠 Community/Home Care ⬲ Diagnostic Studies ∞ Pediatric/Geriatric/Lifespan 💊 Medications

NURSING PRIORITY NO. 4 To promote wellness (Teaching/Discharge Considerations):

🏠 • Stress good voiding habits (e.g., 4 to 6 times/day). *Repeated holding of urination for prolonged periods can, over time, overstretch and weaken bladder muscles.*

🏠 • Encourage client to report problems immediately *so treatment can be instituted promptly.*[2]

🏠 • Emphasize need for adequate fluid intake.

Chronic Retention

Sample NIC linkages:

Urinary Retention Care: Assistance in relieving bladder distention

Exercise Therapy: Muscle Control: Use of specific activity or exercise protocols to enhance or restore controlled body movement

NURSING PRIORITY NO. 1 To assess causative/contributing factors:

• Review medical history for diagnoses, such as congenital defects, neurological disorders (e.g., MS, polio); prostatic hypertrophy/surgery; birth canal injury/scarring; spinal cord injury with lower motor neuron injury *that may cause detrusor muscle atrophy or chronic overdistention because of outlet obstruction.*[2,6]

• Determine presence of weak or absent sensory or motor impulses (as with CVAs, spinal injury, or diabetes) *that predispose client to compromised enervation or interpretation of sensory signals resulting in impaired urination.*[2]

• Evaluate customary fluid intake.

💊 • Assess client's medication regimen (e.g., psychotropic, antihistamines, atropine, belladonna) *to consult with primary care provider regarding client's continued use of drugs that are known to potentiate urinary retention.*[2]

NURSING PRIORITY NO. 2 To determine degree of interference/disability:

🏠 • Ascertain effect of condition on functioning/lifestyle. *Chronic urinary retention can limit client's desired lifestyle (e.g., daily activities, social functioning, etc.), and can lead to chronic incontinence and life-threatening complications (e.g., intractable urinary tract infections and kidney failure).*[3,9]

🏠 • Instruct client/SO to maintain voiding log noting frequency and timing of voiding, or dribbling *to determine severity of condition:*[5]

🏠 • Determine presence/severity (0 to 10 scale) of bladder spasms, pelvic pain, and other discomforts.

🧪 • Prepare for/assist with urodynamic testing (e.g., uroflowmetry to assess urine speed and volume, cystometrogram to measure bladder pressure and volume, bladder scan to measure retention or postvoid residual, leak point pressure).[7]

NURSING PRIORITY NO. 3 To assist in treating/preventing retention:

• Collaborate in treatment of underlying conditions (e.g., BPH, reduce/eliminate medications responsible for retention, repair perineal scarring/outlet obstruction, etc.), *which may correct/reduce severity of retention and associated overflow or total incontinence.*

🏠 • Instruct client/SO in management of voiding problems as indicated:

Attempt voiding in complete privacy *to reduce embarrassment and distractions.*[2]

Void on frequent, timed schedule *to maintain low bladder pressure/prevent overdistention of bladder.*[2]

Maintain consistent fluid intake *to wash out bacteria/avoid infections and limit bladder stone formation.*[9]

Adjust fluid amount and timing if indicated *to prevent bladder distention.*

Perform Credé's or Valsalva's maneuver if appropriate *to facilitate emptying of the bladder.*[2]

- Establish regular self-catheterization program, as indicated, *to prevent reflux and increased renal pressures, and to improve client's quality of life (e.g., ability to participate in desired/ needed activities and social interactions. Note: Clean intermittent catheterization (CIC) is a treatment option for individuals who can urinate but cannot completely empty their bladder.*[3,9]
- Consult with urologist/prepare for more aggressive intervention (e.g., reconstructive surgery, lithotripsy, prostatectomy, etc.) as indicated *to remove source of obstruction, reconstruct sphincter, or provide for urinary diversion.*[2]
- Refer for consideration of advanced/research-based therapies (e.g., implanted sacra/ tibial/pelvic electrical stimulating device) for long-term management of retention.[9]

NURSING PRIORITY NO. 4 To promote wellness (Teaching/Discharge Considerations):

- Establish regular schedule for bladder emptying whether voiding or using catheter.
- Instruct SO/caregiver(s) in clean intermittent catheterization techniques *so that more than one individual is able to assist the client in care of elimination needs.*[2]
- Instruct client/SO in care when client has indwelling (urethral or suprapubic catheter) or urinary diversion device (e.g., clean technique, emptying and cleaning of leg bag/drainage bag; irrigation and replacement, etc.) *to promote self-care, enhance independence, and prevent complications.*[2]
- Stress need for adequate fluid intake, including use of acidifying fruit juices or ingestion of vitamin C/Mandelamine *to discourage bacterial growth and bladder stone formation.*[2]
- Discuss appropriate use of herbal products *such as saw palmetto to improve symptoms of BPH.*
- Review signs/symptoms of complications *to promote timely contact with healthcare provider for evaluation/intervention.*

DOCUMENTATION FOCUS

Assessment/Reassessment

- Individual findings, including nature of problem, degree of impairment, and whether client is incontinent.

Planning

- Plan of care and who is involved in planning.
- Teaching plan.

Implementation/Evaluation

- Response to interventions.
- Attainment/progress toward desired outcome(s).
- Modifications to plan of care.

Discharge Planning

- Long-term needs/referrals and who is responsible for actions to be taken.
- Specific referrals made.

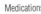

References

1. ND: Urinary Retention. In Doenges, M. E., Moorhouse, M. F., Geissler-Murr, A. C. (2002). *Nursing Care Plans: Guidelines for Individualizing Patient Care.* 6th ed. Philadelphia: F. A. Davis.
2. ND: Urinary Retention. In Doenges, M. E., Moorhouse, M. F., Murr, A. C. (2004). *Nurse's Pocket Guide: Diagnoses, Interventions, and Rationales.* 9th ed. Philadelphia: F. A. Davis.
3. Gaynes, S. M. (2001). Urinary Retention Inability to Urinate. Accessed August 2007 at www.emedicine.com/aaem/topic466.htm.
4. No author listed. (2003). The management of benign prostatic hyperplasia. Baltimore, MD: American Urological Association, Inc. Accessed August 2007 at www.guideline.com.
5. Gray, M. (2000). Urinary retention: Management in the acute care setting (part 2). *Am J Nurs,* 100(8), 36–44.
6. Policastro, M. A., Sinert, R., Guerrero, P. (2007). Urinary obstruction. Retrieved May 2007 at www.emedicine.com/emerg/topic624.htm.
7. Newman, D. K. (2005). Assessment of the patient with an overactive bladder. *Journal of Wound, Ostomy and Continence Nursing,* 32(3) Suppl, 5–10.
8. Albo, M., Richter, H. E. (2006). Urodynamic testing. Fact sheet for National Kidney and Urologic Diseases Information Clearinghouse. Retrieved August 2007 at http://kidney.niddk.nih.gov/kudiseases/pubs/urodynamic/index.htm.
9. Santos, A., Hunt, M. (2005). Managing incontinence: Once a cause of isolation and embarrassment, incontinence does not have to limit quality of life. *Paraplegia News,* 59(11). Retrieved August 2007 at www.pvamagazines.com/pnnews/magazine/article.php?art=1687.

impaired spontaneous Ventilation

Definition: Decreased energy reserves that results in an individual's inability to maintain breathing adequate to support life

RELATED FACTORS

Metabolic factors; [hypermetabolic state (e.g., infection), nutritional deficits/depletion of energy stores]

Respiratory muscle fatigue

[Airway size/resistance; inadequate secretion management]

DEFINING CHARACTERISTICS

Subjective
Dyspnea
Apprehension

Objective
Increased metabolic rate
Increased heart rate
Increased restlessness; decreased cooperation
Increased use of accessory muscles
Decreased tidal volume
Decreased PO_2/ SaO; increased PCO_2

Sample Clinical Applications: COPD, asthma, pulmonary embolus, acute respiratory distress syndrome, brain injury, chest trauma/surgery, Guillian-Barré syndrome, ALS

DESIRED OUTCOMES/EVALUATION CRITERIA

Sample NOC linkages:

Mechanical Ventilation Response: Adult: Alveolar exchange and tissue perfusion supported by mechanical ventilation

Respiratory Status: Ventilation: Movement of air in and out of the lungs
Endurance: Capacity to sustain activity

Client Will (Include Specific Time Frame)

- Reestablish/maintain effective respiratory pattern via ventilator, with absence of retractions/use of accessory muscles, cyanosis, or other signs of hypoxia; and with ABGs/SaO$_2$ within acceptable range.
- Participate in efforts to wean (as appropriate) within individual ability.

Sample NOC linkage:
Energy Conservation: Personal actions to manage energy for initiating and sustaining activity

Caregiver Will (Include Specific Time Frame)

- Demonstrate behaviors necessary to maintain client's respiratory function.

ACTIONS/INTERVENTIONS

Sample NIC linkages:
Ventilation Assistance: Promotion of an optimal spontaneous breathing pattern that maximizes oxygen and carbon dioxide exchange in the lungs
Mechanical Ventilation: Use of an artificial device to help patient breathe
Respiratory Monitoring: Collection and analysis of patient data to ensure airway patency and adequate gas exchange

NURSING PRIORITY NO. 1 To determine degree of impairment:

- Identify client with impending respiratory failure (e.g., developing apnea or slow, shallow breathing; declining mentation/obtunded with need for airway protection).[10]
- Assess spontaneous respiratory pattern, noting rate, depth, rhythm, symmetry of chest movement, and use of accessory muscles. *Tachypnea, shallow breathing, demonstrated/reports of dyspnea (using 0 to 10 scale); increased heart rate/dysrhythmias; pallor or cyanosis; and intercostal retractions/use of accessory muscles indicate increased work of breathing or gas exchange impairment.*[3,10]
- Auscultate breath sounds, noting presence/absence and equality of breath sounds, adventitious breath sounds (e.g., wheezing) *to evaluate presence/degree of ventilatory impairment.*
- Evaluate ABGs or pulse oximetry and capnography *to determine presence/degree of arterial hypoxemia (<55%) and hpercapnea (CO$_2$ >45%) resulting in impaired ventilation requiring support.*[11,12]
- Obtain/review results of pulmonary function studies (e.g., lung volumes, inspiratory and expiratory pressures, and forced vital capacity), as appropriate, *to assess presence/degree of respiratory insufficiency.*
- Investigate etiology of respiratory failure (e.g., exacerbation of COPD, pneumonia, pulmonary embolus, heart failure, trauma) *to determine client's ventilation needs/most appropriate type of ventilatory support.*[1]
- Review serial chest x-rays and imaging scans (e.g., MRI/CT) that may be performed *to diagnose disorder and monitor response to treatment.*
- Note response to current measures/respiratory therapy (e.g., bronchodilators, supplemental oxygen, IPPB treatments). *Client may already be receiving treatments to maintain airway*

patency and enhance gas exchange or may have respiratory failure associated with sudden event (e.g., severe trauma, sudden onset respiratory illness, surgery with complications).[1]
- Ascertain desires of client/SO(s) regarding plan for treatment of respiratory failure, as indicated. *Client may have advance directives, prior stated decisions about the level of therapy aggressiveness that he or she desires if situation is chronic/long-term. Family members may help in decision-making processes if client is a minor or is incapacitated.* [2]

NURSING PRIORITY NO. 2 To provide/maintain ventilatory support:

- Collaborate with physician, respiratory care practitioners regarding effective mode of ventilation (e.g., noninvasive oxygenation) or intubation and mechanical ventilation (e.g., continuous mandatory [CMV], assist control [ACV], intermittent mandatory [IMV], pressure support [PSV]). *Specific mode is determined by client's respiratory requirements, presence of underlying disease process, and the extent to which client can participate in ventilatory efforts.*
- Ensure effective ventilation:[1,4,8,12]
  Observe overall breathing pattern, distinguishing between spontaneous respirations and ventilator breaths. *Client may be completely dependent on the ventilator or able to take breaths but have poor oxygen saturation without the ventilator. The client on noncontrolled ventilation mode can still experience hyper/hypoventilation or "air hunger" and attempt to correct deficiency by overbreathing.*[1,12]
  Verify that client's respirations are in phase with the ventilator. *Decreases work of breathing, maximizes O_2 delivery when client is not fighting the ventilator.*
  Inflate tracheal/endotracheal tube cuff properly using minimal leak/occlusive technique *to ensure adequate ventilation/delivery of desired tidal volume.*
  Check cuff inflation periodically per facility protocol and whenever cuff is deflated/reinflated *to prevent risks associated with under/overinflation.*
  Check tubings for obstruction (e.g., kinking or accumulation of water) *that can impede flow of oxygen.* Drain tubing, as indicated; refrain from draining toward the client or back into the reservoir, *which can result in contamination/provide medium for growth of bacteria.*
  Check ventilator alarms for proper functioning. Do not turn off alarms, even for suctioning. Verify that alarms can be heard in the nurses' station by care providers *to ensure care provider is alerted to emergent situation/ventilator disconnect.*
  Suction, as needed, *to clear secretions if client is coughing excessively, has visible secretions, or is tripping high-pressure alarm on ventilator.*
  Remove from ventilator and ventilate manually *if source of ventilator alarm cannot be quickly identified and rectified.*
  Verify that oxygen line is in proper outlet/tank; monitor inline oxygen analyzer or perform periodic oxygen analysis *to deliver an acceptable oxygen percentage and saturation for client's specific needs.*
  Assess ventilator settings routinely and readjust, as indicated, *according to client's primary disease and results of diagnostic testing.*
  Verify tidal volume set to volume needed for individual situation and proper functioning of spirometer, bellows, or computer readout of delivered volume *to reduce risk of complications associated with alteration in lung compliance or leakage through machine/around tube cuff.*
  Monitor airway pressure for developing complications/equipment problems (e.g., increased airway resistance, retained secretions, decreased lung compliance, client out of phase/off ventilator).
  Promote periodic maximal ventilation of alveoli; check sigh rate intervals (usually 1 1/2 to 2 times tidal volume). *Reduces risk of atelectasis, helps mobilize secretions.*

Note inspired humidity and temperature; maintain hydration *to prevent excessive drying of mucosa/secretions.*

- Auscultate breath sounds periodically. Note frequent crackles or rhonchi that do not clear with coughing/suctioning. *May indicate developing complications (e.g., atelectasis, pneumonia, acute bronchospasm, pulmonary edema).*
- Note changes in chest symmetry. *May indicate improper placement of ET tube, development of barotrauma.*
- Keep resuscitation bag at bedside *to allow for manual ventilation whenever indicated (e.g., if client is removed from ventilator or troubleshooting equipment problems).*
- Administer and monitor response to medications that promote airway patency and gas exchange *to determine efficacy/need for change.*
- Administer sedation, as required, *to synchronize respirations and reduce work of breathing/energy expenditure.*
- Refer to NDs ineffective Airway Clearance, ineffective Breathing Pattern, and impaired Gas Exchange for related interventions.

NURSING PRIORITY NO. 3 To prepare for/assist with weaning process if appropriate:

- Determine client's physical/psychological readiness to wean. Weaning readiness testing should begin soon after intubation, whenever possible, *to limit complications associated with long-term mechanical ventilation.* Weaning parameters include (1) evidence for some reversal of the underlying cause of respiratory failure; (2) adequate oxygenation and normal pH; (3) hemodynamic stability; (4) capability and willingness to initiate inspiratory effort; (5) absence of excessive secretions; and (6) nutritional status sufficient *to maintain work of breathing.*[1,4–7,10]
- Determine mode for weaning. *Recent studies indicate that pressure support mode or multiple daily T-piece trials may be superior to IMV, low-level pressure support may be beneficial for unassisted breathing trials, and early extubation and institution of noninvasive positive pressure ventilation may have substantial benefits in alert, cooperative client.*[5,7,10]
- Explain to client/SO weaning activities/techniques, individual plan, and expectations. *Reduces fear of unknown, provides opportunities to deal with concerns, clarifies reality of fears, and helps reduce anxiety to a more manageable level.*[1,6,8,12]
- Engage client in specialized exercise program *to enhance respiratory muscle strength and general endurance.*
- Maximize weaning effort:
  Elevate head of bed/place in orthopedic chair, if possible, or position *to alleviate dyspnea and to facilitate oxygenation.*
  Coach client in "taking control" of breathing during weaning periods (e.g., to take slower, deeper breaths, practice abdominal/pursed-lip breathing, assume position of comfort) *to maximize respiratory function and reduce anxiety.*
  Instruct in/assist client to perform effective coughing techniques. *Necessary for secretion management after extubation.*
  Provide quiet environment, calm approach, and undivided attention of nurse. *Promotes relaxation, decreasing energy/oxygen requirements.*
  Involve family/SO(s), as appropriate. Provide diversionary activity. *Helps client focus on something other than breathing.*
  Instruct client in use of energy-saving techniques during care activities *to limit oxygen consumption and fatigue associated with work of breathing.*
- Acknowledge and provide ongoing encouragement for client's efforts. Communicate hope for successful weaning response (even partial). *Emotional support can enhance client's commitment to continue weaning activity, maximizing outcomes.*[1]

NURSING PRIORITY NO. 4 To prepare for discharge on ventilator when indicated:

- Ascertain plan for discharge placement (e.g., return home, short-term admission to subacute/rehabilitation center or permanent placement in extended-care facility). *Helps to determine care needs and fiscal impact of home care versus extended-care facility.*[8]

- Review layout of home, noting size of rooms, doorways, placement of furniture, number/type of electrical outlets *to identify necessary modifications/safety needs.*

- Determine specific equipment needs and resources for equipment/maintenance. Arrange for delivery before client discharge *to allow SO/caregivers to prepare for transfer.*

- Allow sufficient opportunity for SO(s)/family to practice new skills. Role-play potential crisis situations *to enhance confidence in ability to handle client's needs.*

- Demonstrate airway management techniques and proper equipment cleaning practices *to reduce risk of infection.*

- Instruct SO(s)/caregivers in other pulmonary physiotherapy measures (e.g., chest physiotherapy), as indicated. Refer for home respiratory therapy support, as needed.

- Provide positive feedback and encouragement for efforts of SO(s)/caregivers. *Promotes continuation of desired behaviors.*

- List names and phone numbers for identified contact persons/resources. *Can reduce sense of isolation and enhance likelihood of obtaining assistance/support when needed.*

- Review and provide written or audiovisual materials regarding proper ventilator management, maintenance, and safety for reference in home setting. *Provides information to enhance client's/SO's level of comfort with challenging tasks.*

- Identify signs/symptoms requiring prompt medical evaluation/intervention. *Timely treatment may prevent progression of problem/untoward complications.*

- Obtain no-smoking signs to be posted in home, and remind family members to refrain from smoking *to reduce risk of fire.*

- Have family/SO(s) notify utility company and fire department of presence of ventilator in home. *Client will be placed in high-risk list for follow-up in case of power outage or fire.*[9]

NURSING PRIORITY NO. 5 To promote wellness (Teaching/Discharge Considerations):

- Discuss impact of specific activities on respiratory status and problem-solve solutions *to maximize weaning effort or to reduce incidence of respiratory distress/failure.*

- Monitor health of visitors, persons involved in care *to protect client from sources of infection.*

- Encourage time-out/respite for caregivers *so they may attend to personal needs, wellness, and growth.* (Refer to ND risk for Caregiver Role Strain.)

- Provide opportunities for client/SO(s) to discuss advance directives. *Clarifies parameters for termination of therapy or other end-of-life decisions, as desired.*

- Recommend involvement in support group; introduce to other ventilator-dependent individuals who are successfully managing home ventilation, if desired, *to answer questions, provide role model, assist with problem-solving, and offer encouragement/hope for the future.*

DOCUMENTATION FOCUS

Assessment/Reassessment

- Baseline findings, subsequent alterations in respiratory function.
- Results of diagnostic testing.
- Individual risk factors/concerns.

Planning

• Plan of care and who is involved in planning.
• Teaching plan.

Implementation/Evaluation

• Client's/other's responses to interventions, teaching, and actions performed.
• Skill level/assistance needs of SO(s)/family.
• Attainment, progress toward desired outcome(s).
• Modifications to plan of care.

Discharge Planning

• Discharge plan, including appropriate referrals, action taken, and who is responsible for each action.
• Equipment needs and source.
• Resources for support persons/home-care providers.

References

1. CP: Ventilatory assistance (mechanical). In Doenges, M. E., Moorhouse, M. F., Geissler-Murr, A. C. (2002). *Nursing Care Plans: Guidelines for Individualizing Patient Care.* 6th ed. Philadelphia: F. A. Davis, pp. 167–179.
2. Campbell, M., Thill-Baharozian, M. (1994). Impact of the DNR therapeutic plan on patient care requirements. *Am J Crit Care,* 3, 202.
3. Gift, A., Narsavage, G. (1998). Validity of the numeric rating scale as a measure of dyspnea. *Am J Crit Care,* 7(3), 200.
4. Epstein, S. K. (2002). Weaning from mechanical ventilation. *Respir Care,* 47(4), 454–466.
5. MacIntyre, N. R., et al. (2001). Evidence-based guidelines for weaning and discontinuation of ventilatory support. (Collective task force facilitated by the American College of Chest Physicians; the American Association for Respiratory Care; and the American College of Critical Care Medicine) *Chest,* 120(6 suppl), 385S–484S.
6. Tasota, F. J., Dobbin, D. (2000). Weaning your patient from mechanical ventilation. *Nursing,* 30(10), 41.
7. Cook, D. J., et.al. (2000). Weaning from mechanical ventilation. For the McMaster Evidence-Based Practice Center. Agency for Healthcare Research and Quality. Available at www.chestnet.org. Accessed September 2003.
8. Lysaght, L. (2002). Ventilation, impaired spontaneous. In Ackley, B. J., Ladwig, G. B. *Nursing Diagnosis Handbook: A Guide to Planning Care.* 5th ed. St. Louis, MO: Mosby.
9. Humphrey, C. (1994). *Home Care Nursing Handbook.* 2d ed. Gaithersburg, MD: Aspen.
10. Sharma, S., Hayes, J. A. (2006). Hypoventilation syndromes. Retrieved May 2007 at www.emedicine.com/emerg/topic3470.htm.
11. D'Arcy, Y. (2007). Eye on capnography. *Men in Nursing,* 2(2), 25–29.
12. Amitai, A., Sinert, D. (2006). Ventilator management. Retrieved May 2007 at www.emedicine.com/emerg/topic788.htm.

dysfunctional Ventilatory Weaning Response

Definition: Inability to adjust to lowered levels of mechanical ventilator support that interrupts and prolongs the weaning process

RELATED FACTORS

Physiological
Ineffective airway clearance
Sleep pattern disturbance
Inadequate nutrition

Cultural Collaborative Community/Home Care Diagnostic Studies Pediatric/Geriatric/Lifespan Medications

Uncontrolled pain or discomfort
[Muscle weakness/fatigue, inability to control respiratory muscles; immobility]

Psychological

Knowledge deficit of the weaning process
Client's perceived inefficacy about the ability to wean
Decreased motivation/self-esteem
Anxiety; fear; insufficient trust in the nurse/[care provider]
Hopelessness; powerlessness
[Unprepared for weaning attempt]

Situational

Uncontrolled episodic energy demands
Inappropriate pacing of diminished ventilator support
Inadequate social support
Adverse environment (e.g., noisy, active environment; negative events in the room, low
    nurse-client ratio; unfamiliar nursing staff)
History of ventilator dependence >4 days
History of multiple unsuccessful weaning attempts

DEFINING CHARACTERISTICS

Mild DVWR

Subjective
Expressed feelings of increased need for O_2; breathing discomfort; fatigue, warmth
Queries about possible machine malfunction
Objective
Restlessness
Slight increase of respiratory rate from baseline
Increased concentration on breathing

Moderate DVWR

Subjective
Apprehension
Objective
Slight increase from baseline blood pressure (<20 mm Hg)/heart rate (<20 beats/min)
Baseline increase in respiratory rate (<5 breaths/min); slight respiratory accessory muscle
    use; decreased air entry on auscultation
Hypervigilance to activities; wide-eyed look
Inability to cooperate/respond to coaching
Diaphoresis
Color changes; pale, slight cyanosis

Severe DVWR

Objective
Agitation; decreased level of consciousness
Deterioration in arterial blood gases from current baseline
Increase from baseline BP (>20 mm Hg)/heart rate (>20 beats/min)
Respiratory rate that increases significantly from baseline; full respiratory accessory mus-
    cle use; shallow/gasping breaths; paradoxical abdominal breathing

Adventitious breath sounds, audible airway secretions
Asynchronized breathing with the ventilator
Profuse diaphoresis
Cyanosis

Sample Clinical Applications: Traumatic brain injury/stroke, substance overdose, COPD, crushing chest trauma, respiratory/cardiac arrest

DESIRED OUTCOMES/EVALUATION CRITERIA
Sample NOC linkages:
Mechanical Ventilation Weaning Response: Adult: Respiratory and psychological adjustment to progressive removal of mechanical ventilation
Respiratory Status: Ventilation: Movement of air in and out of the lungs
Respiratory Status: Gas Exchange: Alveolar exchange of carbon dioxide and oxygen to maintain arterial blood gas concentrations

Client Will (Include Specific Time Frame)

- Actively participate in the weaning process.
- Reestablish independent respiration with ABGs within client's normal range and be free of signs of respiratory failure.
- Demonstrate increased tolerance for activity/participate in self-care within level of ability.

ACTIONS/INTERVENTIONS

Sample NIC linkages:
Mechanical Ventilation: Use of an artificial device to assist a patient to breathe
Mechanical Ventilatory Weaning: Assisting the patient to breathe without the aid of a mechanical ventilator
Energy Management: Regulating energy use to treat or prevent fatigue and optimize function

NURSING PRIORITY NO. 1 To identify contributing factors/degree of dysfunction:

- Determine extent and nature of underlying disorders/factors (e.g., preexisting cardiopulmonary diseases, significant trauma, neuromuscular disorders; complications from surgical procedures, etc.) *that contribute to client's reliance on mechanical support, thus affecting weaning efforts.*[9]
- Note length of time client has been on ventilator. Review previous episodes of extubation/reintubation. *Previous unsuccessful weaning attempts (e.g., due to inability to protect airway or clear secretions; oxygen saturation <50% on room air, etc.) can influence weaning interventions. Although most individuals remain on the ventilator for 7 days or less, some require support for several weeks or more. Weaning is more difficult in those clients and may require multiple attempts.*[1,10]
- Complete Burns Weaning Assessment Program (BWAP) or similar checklist (e.g., stability of vital signs, factors that increase metabolic rate [e.g., sepsis, fever]; hydration status; need for/recent use of analgesia or sedation; nutritional state, muscle strength, and activity level) *to assess systemic parameters that may affect readiness for weaning.*[1-3,11,12]
- Ascertain client's alertness and understanding of weaning process, expectations, and concerns. *Client/SO may need specific and repeated instructions during process to allay fears and*

Cultural   Collaborative   Community/Home Care   Diagnostic Studies   Pediatric/Geriatric/Lifespan   Medications

enhance cooperation. Unrealistic expectations or unvoiced concerns can impair weaning process or willingness to participate.

- Determine psychological readiness, presence/degree of anxiety. *Weaning provokes anxiety regarding ability to breathe on own and likelihood of ventilator dependence. The client must be highly motivated, be able to actively participate in the weaning process, and be physically comfortable enough to work at weaning.*[4]
- Review laboratory studies, such as CBC, *to determine number/integrity of red blood cells for O_2 transport;* electrolytes; and nutritional markers, such as serum protein and albumin, *to determine if client has sufficient nutritional stores to meet demands of weaning.*[1,12]
- Review chest radiograph/pulse oximetry, ABGs, and/or capnometry. *Before weaning attempts, chest radiograph should show clear lungs or marked improvement in pulmonary congestion. ABGs should document satisfactory oxygenation on an FIO_2 of 40% or less.*[4] *Capnometry measures end-tidal carbon dioxide values and can be used to confirm correct placement of ET and monitor integrity of ventilation equipment, etc.*[5,10]

NURSING PRIORITY NO. 2 To support weaning process:

- Discuss with client/SO individual plan and expectations. *May reduce client's anxiety about process and ultimate outcome and support willingness to work at spontaneous breathing.*[1,2]
- Consult with dietitian, nutritional support team for adjustments in composition of diet prior to weaning *to prevent excessive production of CO_2, which could alter respiratory drive. Individuals on long-term ventilation may require tube-feeding through enteral feedings with high intake of carbohydrates, protein, and calories to improve respiratory muscle function.*[4,10]
- Collaborate in implementing weaning protocols and mode (e.g., spontaneous breathing trials with T-piece, partial client support [SIMV], or pressure support [PSV] during client's spontaneous breathing) *to determine if client can assume the full work of breathing and to provide support for spontaneous ventilation. Indeed, an increasing body of research suggests that the key to successful weaning lies not in the use of a particular method but, rather, through a coordinated approach by a skilled multidisciplinary team.*[6 9,12]
- Note response to activity/client care during weaning and limit, as indicated. Provide undisturbed rest/sleep periods. Avoid stressful procedures/situations or nonessential activities *to prevent excessive O_2 consumption/demand with increased possibility of weaning failure.*[4]
- Discuss impact of specific activities on respiratory status, and problem-solve solutions to maximize weaning effort.
- Time medications during weaning efforts *to minimize sedative effects.*
- Provide quiet room, calm approach, and undivided attention. *Enhances relaxation, thereby conserving energy.*
- Involve SO(s)/family, as appropriate (e.g., sit at bedside, provide encouragement, and help monitor client status).
- Provide diversionary activity (e.g., watching TV, reading aloud) *to focus attention away from breathing when not actively working at breathing exercises.*
- Acknowledge and provide ongoing encouragement for client's efforts.
- Minimize setbacks, focus client attention on gains and progress to date *to reduce frustration that may further impair progress.*
- Suspend weaning (take a "holiday") periodically as individually appropriate (e.g., initially may rest 45 or 50 minutes each hour, progressing to a 20-minute rest period every 4 hours, then weaning during daytime and resting during night).[9]

NURSING PRIORITY NO. 3 To prepare for discharge on ventilator when indicated:

- Prepare client/SO for alternative actions when client is unable to resume spontaneous ventilation (e.g., tracheostomy with long-term ventilation support in alternate care setting/home, palliative care/end-of-life procedures).[7]
- Ascertain that all needed equipment is in place, caregivers are trained, and safety concerns have been addressed (e.g., alternative power source, backup equipment, client call/alarm system) *to ease the transfer when client is going home on ventilator.*[4]
- Evaluate caregiver capabilities and burden when client requires long-term ventilator in the home *to determine potential or presence of skill-related problems or emotional issues (e.g., caregiver overload, burnout, or depression).*[8]
- Refer to ND impaired spontaneous Ventilation for additional interventions.

NURSING PRIORITY NO. 4 To promote wellness (Teaching/Discharge Considerations):

- Encourage client/SO(s) to evaluate impact of ventilatory dependence on their lifestyle and what changes they are willing or unwilling to make, when client is discharged on ventilator. *Quality-of-life issues must be examined/resolved by the ventilator-dependent client and SO(s); all parties need to understand that ventilatory support is a 24-hour job that ultimately affects everyone.*[4] *Findings may dictate alternate placement such as foster care or extended-care facility.*
- Discuss importance of time for self and identify appropriate sources for respite care. *Initially, caregivers have limited understanding of the magnitude of the demands on their time and energy. Knowing support is available enhances coping abilities.* (Refer to ND risk for Caregiver Role Strain.)
- Teach client/SO(s) to monitor health of visitors, persons involved in care; to avoid crowds during flu season; and to obtain immunizations, etc., *to protect client from sources of infection.*
- Engage in rehabilitation program *to enhance respiratory muscle strength and general endurance.*
- Encourage client/SO(s) to discuss advance directives. *Clarifies parameters for termination of therapy or other end-of-life decisions, as desired.*
- Recommend involvement in support group; introduce to other ventilator-dependent individuals who are successfully managing home ventilation, if desired, *to answer questions, provide role model, assist with problem-solving, and offer encouragement/hope for the future.*
- Identify conditions requiring immediate medical intervention *to treat developing complications/prevent respiratory failure.*

DOCUMENTATION FOCUS

Assessment/Reassessment

- Baseline findings and subsequent alterations.
- Results of diagnostic testing/procedures.
- Individual risk factors.

Planning

- Plan of care/interventions and who is involved in the planning.
- Teaching plan.

Cultural Collaborative Community/Home Care Diagnostic Studies Pediatric/Geriatric/Lifespan Medications

Implementation/Evaluation

- Client response to interventions.
- Attainment of/progress toward desired outcome(s).
- Modifications to plan of care.

Discharge Planning

- Status at discharge, long-term needs and referrals, indicating who is to be responsible for each action.
- Equipment needs/supplier.

References

1. Tasota, F. J., Dobbin, K. (2000). Weaning your patient from mechanical ventilation. *Nursing*, 30(10), 41.
2. No author listed. Weaning from mechanical ventilation: Protocols and beyond. Accessed August 2007 at www.ed4nurse.com/weaning.htm.
3. MacIntyre, N. R., et al. (2001). Evidence-based guidelines for weaning and discontinuation of ventilatory support. A collective task force facilitated by the American College of Chest Physicians; the American Association for Respiratory Care; and the American College of Critical Care Medicine. *Chest*, 120(6suppl), 385S–484S.
4. CP: Ventilatory assistance (mechanical). In Doenges, M. E., Moorhouse, M. F., Geissler-Murr, A. C. (2002). *Nursing Care Plans: Guidelines for Individualizing Patient Care.* 6th ed. Philadelphia: F. A. Davis, pp. 167–179.
5. Frakes, M. A. (2001). Measuring end-tidal carbon dioxide: Clinical applications and usefulness. *Crit Care Nurse*, 21(5), 23–35.
6. Henneman, E. A. (2001). Liberating patients from mechanical ventilation: A team approach. *Crit Care Nurse*, 21(3), 25–33.
7. Iregui, M., et al. (2002). Determinants of outcome for patients admitted to a long-term ventilator unit. *South Med J*, 95(3), 310–317.
8. Douglas, S. L., Daly, B. J. (2003). Caregivers of long-term ventilator patients: Physical and psychological outcomes. *Chest*, 123, 1073–1081.
9. Forrette, T. L. (2006). Transitioning from mechanical ventilation. Retrieved May 2007 at www.medscape.com/viewprogram/5230_pnt.
10. McLean, S. E., Jensen, L. A., Schroeder, D. G., et al. (2006). Improving adherence to a mechanical ventilation weaning protocol for critically ill adults: Outcomes after an implementation program. *Am J Crit Care*, 15(3), 299–309.
11. Burns, S. M. (2005). Mechanical ventilation of clients with acute respiratory distress syndrome and patents requiring weaning: The evidence guiding practice. *Crit Care Nurse*, 25(4), 14–24.
12. Epstein, C. D., Peerless, J. R. (2006). Weaning readiness and fluid balance in older critically ill surgical clients. *Am J of Crit Care*, 15(1), 54–64.

risk for [/actual] other-directed Violence

Definition: At risk for behaviors in which an individual demonstrates that he or she can be physically, emotionally, or sexually harmful to others

RISK FACTORS [/INDICATORS] FOR OTHER-DIRECTED VIOLENCE

History of:

Violence against others (e.g., hitting, kicking, scratching, biting, or spitting; throwing objects at someone; attempted rape, rape, sexual molestation; urinating/defecating on a person)

Threats (e.g., verbal threats against property/person, social threats, cursing, threatening notes/letters, threatening gestures, sexual threats)

Violent antisocial behavior (e.g., stealing, insistent borrowing, insistent demands for privileges, insistent interruption of meetings; refusal to eat/take medication, ignoring instructions)

Indirect violence (e.g., tearing off clothes, urinating/defecating on floor, stamping feet, temper tantrum, running in corridors, yelling, writing on walls, ripping objects off walls, throwing objects, breaking a window, slamming doors, sexual advances)

History of childhood abuse/witnessing family violence

Neurological impairment (e.g., positive EEG, CT, or MRI; neurological findings; head trauma; seizure disorders)

Cognitive impairment (e.g., learning disabilities, attention deficit disorder, decreased intellectual functioning); [organic brain syndrome]

Cruelty to animals; fire-setting

Prenatal/perinatal complications

History of substance abuse; pathological intoxication; [toxic reaction to medication]

Psychotic symptomatology (e.g., auditory, visual, command hallucinations; paranoid delusions; loose, rambling, or illogical thought processes); [panic states; rage reactions; catatonic/manic excitement]

Motor vehicle offenses (e.g., frequent traffic violations, use of a motor vehicle to release anger)

Suicidal behavior; impulsivity; availability of weapon(s)

Body language (e.g., rigid posture, clenching of fists and jaw, hyperactivity, pacing, breathlessness, threatening stances)

[Hormonal imbalance (e.g., premenstrual syndrome—PMS, postpartal depression/psychosis)]

[Expressed intent/desire to harm others directly or indirectly]

[Almost continuous thoughts of violence]

Sample Clinical Applications: Psychotic conditions (e.g., schizophrenia, paranoia), antisocial personality disorder, dementia, substance abuse (e.g., PCP, delirium tremens), postpartum psychosis, PMS, brain injured

risk for [actual/]self-directed Violence

Definition: At risk for behaviors in which an individual demonstrates that he or she can be physically, emotionally, or sexually harmful to self

RISK FACTORS [/INDICATORS] FOR SELF-DIRECTED VIOLENCE

Age 15 to 19; over 45

Marital status (single, widowed, divorced)

Employment problems (e.g., unemployed, recent job loss/failure); occupation (executive, administrator/owner of business, professional, semiskilled worker)

Conflictual interpersonal relationships

Family background (e.g., chaotic or conflictual, history of suicide)

Sexual orientation (bisexual [active], homosexual [inactive])

Physical health problems (e.g., hypochondriac, chronic or terminal illness)

Mental health problems (e.g., severe depression, [bipolar disorder] psychosis, severe personality disorder, alcoholism or drug abuse)

Emotional problems (e.g., hopelessness, [lifting of depressed mood], despair, increased anxiety, panic, anger, hostility); history of multiple suicide attempts; suicidal ideation; suicidal plan

Lack of personal resources (e.g., poor achievement, poor insight, affect unavailable and poorly controlled)

Lack of social resources (e.g., poor rapport, socially isolated, unresponsive family)

Verbal clues (e.g., talking about death, "better off without me," asking questions about lethal dosages of drugs)

Behavioral clues (e.g., writing forlorn love notes, directing angry messages at a significant other who has rejected the person, giving away personal items, taking out a large life insurance policy)

NOTE: A risk diagnosis is not evidenced by signs and symptoms, as the problem has not occurred; rather, nursing interventions are directed at prevention.

Sample Clinical Applications: Major depression, postpartum depression/psychosis, Munchausen syndrome, psychosis, substance abuse (e.g., PCP), abuse/neglect

DESIRED OUTCOMES/EVALUATION CRITERIA (FOR OTHER-/SELF-DIRECTED VIOLENCE)
Sample NOC linkages:

Aggression Self-Control: Self-restraint of assaultive, combative, or destructive behaviors toward others

Abusive Behavior Self-Restraint: Self-restraint of abusive and neglectful behaviors toward others

Impulse Self-Control: Self-restraint of compulsive or impulsive behaviors

Depression Self-Control: Personal actions to minimize melancholy and maintain interest in life events

Client Will (Include Specific Time Frame)

- Acknowledge realities of the situation.
- Verbalize understanding of why behavior occurs.
- Identify precipitating factors in individual situation.
- Express realistic self-evaluation and increased sense of self-esteem.
- Participate in care and meet own needs in an assertive manner.
- Demonstrate self-control as evidenced by relaxed posture, nonviolent behavior/verbalizations.
- Use resources and support systems in an effective manner.

ACTIONS/INTERVENTIONS (ADDRESSES BOTH "OTHER-" AND "SELF-DIRECTED")

Sample NIC linkages:

Anger Control Assistance: Facilitation of the expression of anger in an adaptive, nonviolent manner

Environmental Management: Violence Prevention: Monitoring and manipulation of the physical environment to decrease the potential for violent behavior directed toward self, others, or environment

Behavior Modification: Self-Harm: Assisting the patient to decrease or eliminate self-mutilating or self-abusive behavior (Addresses both "other-" and "self-directed")

NURSING PRIORITY NO. I To assess causative/contributing factors:

- Determine underlying dynamics as listed in Risk Factors.
- Identify conditions, such as acute/chronic brain syndrome, panic state, hormonal imbalance, PMS, postpartum psychosis, drug-induced psychotic states, postanesthesial/

postseizure confusion *that may interfere with ability to control own behavior and lead to violent episodes.*[1,13]

- Review laboratory findings (e.g., blood alcohol, blood glucose, ABGs, electrolytes, renal function tests). *Provides information about possible treatable sources of behavior.*[2,6]
- Ascertain client's perception of self/situation. Note use of defense mechanisms. *Individuals who are prone to violent behavior may see themselves as victims (denial), blaming others (projection), not following social norms, and impulsive.*[1]
- Observe/listen for early cues of distress/increasing anxiety. *Behaviors, such as irritability, lack of cooperation, demanding behavior, body posture/expression may signal escalating potential for violent behavior and need for immediate intervention.*[1,6]
- Observe for signs of suicidal/homicidal intent. *Perceived morbid or anxious feelings while with the client; warning from the client, "It doesn't matter," "I'd/They'd be better off dead"; mood swings; "accident-prone"/self-destructive behavior; possession of alcohol or other drug(s) in known substance abuser need to be noted, taken seriously, and treated appropriately.*[1,6,9] (Refer to ND risk for Suicide.)
- Note family history of suicidal/homicidal behavior. *Dynamics in family of origin/current family, parental deprivation or abuse in the early years of an individual's life may contribute to violent behavior in current situation as individual uses violence as a means of solving problems.*[1,9,10]
- Ask directly if the person is thinking of acting on thoughts/feelings. *Can determine reality and urgency of violent intent and importance of immediate intervention.*[6,11]
- Determine availability of suicidal/homicidal means. *Identifies urgency of situation and need to intervene by removing lethal means, possibly hospitalizing client, or instituting other measures to ensure safety of client and others.*[1,6,8]
- Assess client coping behaviors. *Client believes there are no alternatives other than violence and has been dealing with frustration and anger in unacceptable ways (yelling, hitting, other violent behaviors) and needs to learn alternative coping skills.*[1,9]
- Identify risk factors and assess for indicators of child abuse/neglect (e.g., unexplained/ frequent injuries, failure to thrive, and so forth). *Visible evidence of physical abuse/neglect makes it more easily recognized; however, behaviors of withdrawal, acting out may also signal the presence of abuse.*[6,9,12]
- Determine presence, extent, and acceptance of violence in the client's culture. *Youth violence has become a national concern with widely publicized school shootings and an increase in arrests of both boys and girls for violent crimes and weapons violations. Young people who are at risk for violence need to be identified, and positive programs aimed at promoting emotional wellness need to be instituted in schools, parent education meetings, churches, and community centers.*[3,7,12]

NURSING PRIORITY NO. 2 To assist client to accept responsibility for impulsive behavior and potential for violence:

- Develop therapeutic nurse-client relationship. Provide consistent caregiver when possible. *Promotes sense of trust, allowing client to discuss feelings openly and to begin to identify sources of anger and more acceptable ways of dealing with it.*[1,6]
- Maintain straightforward communication. *Avoids reinforcing manipulative behavior. Manipulation is used for management of powerlessness because of distrust of others, fear of loss of power/control, fear of intimacy, and search for approval.*[4,6]
- Discuss motivation for change (e.g., failing relationships, job loss, involvement with judicial system). *Crisis situation can provide impetus for change but requires timely therapeutic intervention to sustain efforts.*[7,8]

• Make time to listen to expressions of feelings. Acknowledge reality of client's feelings and that feelings are okay. (Refer to ND Self-Esteem, specify.) *Promotes understanding of how feelings lead to actions and that individual is responsible for controlling behavior in acceptable ways.*[5,6]

• Help client recognize that own actions may be in response to own fear (may be afraid of own behavior, loss of control), dependency, and feeling of powerlessness. *Promotes understanding of self and ability to deal with feelings in acceptable ways.*[6,14]

• Confront client's tendency to minimize situation/behavior. *Individuals often want to say that things "are not as bad" as portrayed or "It was just a small argument" and "I didn't think I hit her (or him) that hard." By confronting this minimalization, the reality of the situation can be brought out and discussed, leading to better understanding of the situation and changes in behavior.*[1,6,11]

• Identify feelings/events (e.g., individual/family, peer conflict, aggressive behavior, individual's view of self, hallucinations) involved in precipitating violent behavior. *By identifying the factors involved in current situation, an appropriate plan can be made to change actions to prevent future violent behavior.*[1,7,11]

• Discuss impact of behavior on others/consequences of actions. *Discussing these issues openly can help client to develop empathy and understand other person's reactions and begin to change behaviors that can lead to violence.*[5,8]

• Acknowledge reality of suicide/homicide as an option. Discuss consequences of actions if they were to follow through on intent. Ask how it will help client to resolve problems. *Acknowledging the reality of individual's thoughts provides opportunity to look at how actions would affect others, ability to control own behavior, and make choices to live and make a better life for self.*[6,12]

• Accept client's anger without reacting on emotional basis. Give permission to express angry feelings in acceptable ways and let client know that staff will be available to assist in maintaining control. *Promotes acceptance and sense of safety. Client's anger is usually directed at the situation and not at the caregiver, and by remaining separate, the therapist can be more helpful for resolution of the anger.*[6,9]

• Help client identify more appropriate solutions/behaviors. *Motor activities/exercise can lessen sense of anxiety and associated physical manifestations, thus diminishing feelings of anger.*[8]

• Provide directions for actions client can take, avoiding negatives, such as "do nots." *Discussing positive ideas to help client begin to look toward a better future can provide hope that violent behaviors can be changed, promoting feelings of self-worth and belief in control of own self.*[5,14]

NURSING PRIORITY NO. 3 To assist client in controlling behavior:

• Contract with client regarding safety of self/others. *Making a contract in which the individual agrees to refrain from any violent behavior for a specified period of time, from day one through the entire course of treatment, and written and signed by each party may help the client to follow through with therapy to find more effective ways of resolving conflict. Although there is little research on the effectiveness of these contracts, they are frequently used.*[6,7]

• Give client as much control as possible within constraints of individual situation. *Because control issues are a factor in violent behavior, giving client control in appropriate ways can enhance self-esteem, promote confidence in ability to change behavior.*[7]

• Be truthful when giving information and dealing with individual. *Builds trust, enhancing therapeutic relationship, and prevents manipulative behavior.*[5]

• Identify current/past successes and strengths. Discuss effectiveness of coping techniques used and possible changes. (Refer to ND ineffective Coping.) *Client is often not aware of positive aspects of life, and once recognized, they can be used as a basis for change.*[8]

Nursing Diagnoses in Alphabetical Order

- Give positive reinforcement for client's efforts. *Encourages continuation of desired behaviors.*[1]
- Assist client to distinguish between reality and hallucinations/delusions. *Violent behavior in clients with major mental disorders (schizophrenia, mania) may be in responce to command hallucinations and may require more aggressive treatment/hospitalization until behavior is under control.*[1,6]
- Approach in positive manner, acting as if the client has control and is responsible for own behavior. Be aware, though, that the client may not have control, especially if under the influence of drugs (including alcohol). *Individuals will often respond to a positive expectation, reducing threatening actions. Staff needs to be trained in management of this behavior and be prepared to take control of the situation if client is out of control.*[1,6]
- Maintain distance and do not touch client when situation indicates client does not tolerate such closeness. *Individuals who have experienced traumatic events, such as rape, or suffer from posttrauma response may fear close contact even with trusted persons.*[1,6]
- Remain calm and state limits on inappropriate behavior (including consequences) in a firm manner. *Calm manner enables client to de-escalate anger, and knowing what the consequences will be gives an opportunity to choose to change behavior and deal appropriately with situation. Consequences need to be decided beforehand and agreed to by client, or they may sound like punishment and be counterproductive.*[1,6,13]
- Direct client to stay in view of staff. *Intervention may be needed to maintain safety of client and others.*[1,6] (Refer to ND risk for Suicide.)
- Administer prescribed medications (e.g., antianxiety/antipsychotic), taking care not to oversedate client. *May be least restrictive way to help client control violent behaviors while learning new coping skills to handle anger and impulsive behavior. The chemistry of the brain is changed by early violence and has been shown to respond to serotonin as well as related neurotransmitter systems, which play a role in restraining aggressive impulses.*[1,6,9]
- Monitor for possible drug interactions, cumulative effects of drug regimen (e.g., anticonvulsants/antidepressants). *May be contributing factor in violent behavior.*[1,6]

NURSING PRIORITY NO. 4 To assist client/SO(s) to correct/deal with existing situation:

- Gear interventions to individual(s) involved, based on age, relationship, and so forth. *Conflict resolution skills can be learned by all age groups when age-appropriate materials are used.*[5,8]
- Maintain calm, matter-of-fact, nonjudgmental attitude. *Decreases defensive response, allowing individual to think about own responsibility in the conflict and choose positive behaviors instead of usual angry reaction.*[4,5,8]
- Notify potential victims in the presence of serious homicidal threat in accordance with legal/ethical guidelines. *The Tarasoff law requires that therapists/healthcare providers give notice when client expresses homicidal intent overtly or covertly in addition to helping the client realize that the proposed action is not wise or in his or her own best interest.*[1]
- Discuss situation with abused/battered person, providing accurate information about choices and effective actions that can be taken. *Promotes understanding of options, giving hope and support for planning for a violence-free future.*[2]
- Assist individual to understand that angry, vengeful feelings are appropriate in the situation and need to be expressed but not acted on. (Refer to ND Post-Trauma Syndrome, as psychological responses may be very similar.) *Helps client accept feelings as natural and begin to learn effective coping skills, and promotes sense of control over situation.*[2,11]
- Identify resources available for assistance (e.g., battered women's shelter, social services, financial). *Helps client to manage immediate needs such as food, shelter, and safety with a long-range goal of attaining/maintaining independence and violence-free life.*[2]

Cultural   Collaborative   Community/Home Care   Diagnostic Studies   Pediatric/Geriatric/Lifespan   Medications

NURSING PRIORITY NO. 5 To promote safety in event of violent behavior:

- Provide a safe, quiet environment and remove items from the client's environment that could be used to inflict harm to self/others. *Reducing stimuli can help client to calm down, and removing articles provides for safety of client and staff.*[1,5]
- Maintain distance from client who is striking out/hitting and take evasive/controlling actions, as indicated. *Staff safety is of prime importance, and avoiding physical confrontation until client regains control or takedown team is assembled can prevent injury.*[6]
- Call for additional staff/security personnel. *Having sufficient people available to handle the situation may defuse client's anger, allowing situation to calm down without further action. All personnel need to be trained in takedown techniques.*[6]
- Approach aggressive/attacking client from the front, just out of reach, in a commanding posture with palms down. *Safety is a prime concern, and these actions may defuse the situation.*[6]
- Tell client to *Stop* in a firm voice. *This may be sufficient to help client control own actions.*[6]
- Maintain direct/constant eye contact when appropriate. *Assists in identifying client's intentions and conveys sense of caring. Eye contact may be perceived as threatening, so it needs to be used cautiously.*[2,6]
- Speak in a low, commanding voice. *Tone of voice conveys message of control and concern, and can help to calm the client's anger.*[6]
- Provide client with a sense that caregiver is in control of the situation. *Client is feeling out of control, and seeing that staff are in control provides a feeling of safety.*[6]
- Maintain clear route for staff and client and be prepared to move quickly. *Safety for all is of prime importance, and staff may need to leave the room to regroup while continuing to protect the client. Takedown needs to be done quickly to gain control of the individual.*[6]
- Hold client, using restraints or seclusion when necessary until client regains self-control. *Brief period of physical restraint may be required until client regains control/other therapeutic interventions take effect.*[6]
- Administer medication, as indicated. *Client may require chemical restraint until control is regained.*[1,6]
- Discuss event with client after situation is calmed down and control is regained. *Helping client to understand how feelings of anger had gotten out of control and what can be done to prevent a recurrence can provide a learning opportunity for the individual.*[2,6]

NURSING PRIORITY NO. 6 To promote wellness (Teaching/Discharge Considerations):

- Promote client involvement in planning care within limits of situation, allowing for meeting own needs for enjoyment. *Individuals often believe they are not entitled to pleasure and good things in their lives and need to learn how to meet these needs in acceptable ways.*[6,14]
- Assist client to learn assertive behaviors. *Manipulative, nonassertive/aggressive behaviors lead to anger, which can result in violence. Learning assertiveness skills can facilitate change, increase self-esteem, and promote interpersonal relationships.*[1,4]
- Provide information about conflict-resolution skills and help client learn how to use them effectively. *Conflict is always present in human relationships, and learing how to manage conflict is one of the most important tools we can use to solve disagreements and improve relationships.*[4,5,8]
- Discuss reasons for client's behavior with SO(s). Determine desire/commitment of involved parties to sustain current relationships. *Family members may believe individual is purposefully behaving in angry ways, and understanding underlying reasons for behavior can defuse feelings of anger on their part, leading to willingness to resolve problems.*[1,4]

🏠 • Develop strategies to help parents learn more effective parenting skills. *Participating in parenting classes and learning appropriate ways of dealing with frustrations can improve family relationships and prevent angry interactions and the possibility of violent behavior.*[4,5]

🏠 • Identify support systems. *Presence of family/friends, clergy who can serve as mentors, listen to individual nonjudgmentally, can help client defuse angry feelings and learn appropriate ways of dealing with them.*[1] *Note: Not just the client needs help, but those around them need to learn how to provide positive role models and display a broader array of skills for resolving problems.*

🔗 • Refer to formal resources, as indicated. *May need individual/group psychotherapy, substance abuse treatment program, anger management class, social services, safe house to facilitate change.*[1]

🏠 • Promote violence prevention and emotional literacy programs in the schools and community. *These programs are based on the premise that intelligent management of emotions is critical to successful living. Aggressive youth lack skills in arousal management and nonviolent problem-solving, which can be learned in programs and reinforced by the adults in their lives.*[7,12,14]

• Refer to NDs impaired Parenting, family Coping, [specify]; Post-Trauma Syndrome.

DOCUMENTATION FOCUS

Assessment/Reassessment

• Individual findings, including nature of concern (e.g., suicidal/homicidal), behavioral risk factors, and level of impulse control, plan of action/means to carry out plan.
• Client's perception of situation, motivation for change.
• Family history of violence.
• Availability/use of resources.

Planning

• Plan of care and who is involved in the planning.
• Details of contract regarding violence to self/others.
• Teaching plan.

Implementation/Evaluation

• Actions taken to promote safety, including notification of parties at risk.
• Response to interventions/teaching and actions performed.
• Attainment/progress toward desired outcome(s).
• Modifications to plan of care.

Discharge Planning

• Long-range needs and who is responsible for actions to be taken.
• Available resources, specific referrals made.

References

1. Townsend, M. C. (2003). *Psychiatric Mental Health Nursing Concepts of Care.* 4th ed. Philadelphia: F. A. Davis.
2. Cox, H. C., et al. (2002). *Clinical Applications of Nursing Diagnosis.* 4th ed. Philadelphia: F. A. Davis.
3. Lipson, J. G., Dibble, S. L., Minarik, P. A. (1996). *Culture & Nursing Care: A Pocket Guide.* San Francisco: UCSF Nursing Press.
4. Gordon, T. (1989). *Teaching Children Self-Discipline: At Home and At School.* New York: Random House.
5. Gordon, T. (2000). Family Effectiveness Training Video. Solana Beach, CA: Gordon Training Intn'l.

6. Doenges, M. E., Townsend, M. C., Moorhouse, M. F. (1998). *Psychiatric Care Plans Guidelines for Individualizing Care*. 3d ed. Philadelphia: F. A. Davis.
7. Thomas, S. P. (2003). Identifying and intervening with girls at risk for violence. *J School Nurs*, 19(3), 130–139.
8. Porter-O'Grady, T. (2003). Managing conflict in the workplace. *NSNA/Imprint*, 48(4), 66–68.
9. Goleman, D. (October 3, 1995). Early Violence Leaves Its Mark on the Brain. *New York Times*. Retrieved August 2007 at www.cirp.org/library/psych/goleman/.
10. Society for Neuroscience. (2007). What Is Neuroscience. Retrieved August 2007 at www.sfn.org/index.cfm?pagename=whatIsNeuroscience.
11. Cooper, S. Sylvia's Inquiry into Violence and the Brain. Retrieved August 2007 at http://serendip.brynmawr.edu/local/suminst/bbi01/projects/cooper/.
12. Hyman, S. E. (August 3, 1998; updated 1999). Thinking about Violence in Our Schools, Discussion at the White House. National Institute of Mental Health. Retrieved August 2007 at www.medhelp.org/NIHlib/GF-376.html.
13. Eby, N., Car, M. (Spring 2004). Violence and Brain Injuries. *Quality Matters*. Retrieved August 2007 at Brain Injury Association of Montana. Available at www.biamt.org/publications/violence.htm.
14. Goleman, D. (2006). *Emotional Intelligence Why It Matters More Than IQ* (10th Anniversary ed). New York: Bantam Pub.

risk for [/actual] other-/self-directed Violence

NANDA has separated the diagnosis of Violence into its two elements: "directed at others" and "self-directed." However, the interventions in general address both situations and have been left in one block following the definition and supporting data of the two diagnoses.

impaired Walking

Definition: Limitation of independent movement within the environment on foot (Note: Specify level of independence using a standardized functional scale.)

RELATED FACTORS

Insufficient muscle strength; neuromuscular impairment; musculoskeletal impairment (e.g., contractures)

Limited endurance; deconditioning

Fear of falling; impaired balance

Impaired vision

Pain

Obesity

Depressed mood; cognitive impairment

Lack of knowledge

Environmental constraints (e.g., stairs, inclines, uneven surfaces, unsafe obstacles, distances, lack of assistive devices or persons, restraints)

DEFINING CHARACTERISTICS

Subjective or Objective

Impaired ability to walk required distances, walk on an incline/decline, walk on uneven surfaces, to navigate curbs, climb stairs

Sample Clinical Applications: Arthritis, obesity, amputation, brain injury/stroke, traumatic injury/fractures, chronic pain, peripheral vascular disease, spinal nerve compression, MS, cerebral palsy, Parkinson's disease, macular degeneration, dementia

DESIRED OUTCOMES/EVALUATION CRITERIA

Sample NOC linkages:

Ambulation: Ability to walk from place to place independently with or without assistive device

Mobility: Ability to move purposefully in own environment independently with or without assistive device

Balance: Ability to maintain body equilibrium

Client Will (Include Specific Time Frame)

- Be able to move about within environment as needed/desired within limits of ability or with appropriate adjuncts.
- Verbalize understanding of situation/risk factors and safety measures.

ACTIONS/INTERVENTIONS

Sample NIC linkages:

Exercise Therapy: Ambulation: Promotion and assistance with walking to maintain or restore autonomic and voluntary body functions during treatment and recovery from illness or injury

Body Mechanics Promotion: Facilitating the use of posture and movement in daily activities to prevent fatigue and musculoskeletal strain or injury

Exercise Therapy: Balance: Use of specific activities, postures, and movements to maintain, enhance, or restore balance

Refer also to NDs impaired Mobility [specify] for additional assessments and interventions.

NURSING PRIORITY NO. 1 To assess causative/contributing factors:

- Identify conditions/diagnoses (e.g., advanced age, vision impairments, pain, chronic fatigue, cognitive dysfunction, acute illness with weakness, *chronic illness* [e.g., cardiopulmonary disorders, cancer], musculoskeletal injuries [e.g., fractures, tendon/ligament injury, amputation], *balance problems* [e.g., inner ear infection/brain injury/stroke], *nerve disorders* [e.g., multiple sclerosis, Parkinson's disease, cerebral palsy], *spinal abnormalities* [disease, trauma, degeneration], *neuropathies* [e.g., peripheral, diabetic, alcoholic], *degenerative muscle disorders* [e.g., muscular dystrophy, myositis], *foot conditions* [e.g., plantar warts, bunions, ingrown toenails, pressure ulcers]) *that contribute to walking impairment and identify specific needs and appropriate interventions.*[1–10]
- Determine ability to follow directions and presence of emotional/behavioral responses *that may be affecting client's ability or desire to engage in activity.*
- Note client's particular symptoms (e.g., unable to bear weight, can't walk usual distance, limping, staggering, stiff leg, leg pain, shuffling, asymmetric or unsteady gait, etc.). *Influences choice of interventions.*[7,10,11]

NURSING PRIORITY NO. 2 To assess functional ability:

- Perform "Get-up and Go" test, as indicated, to assess client's basic ability to ambulate safely. Factors assessed include sitting balance, ability to transfer from sitting to standing and back to sitting, the pace and stability of ambulation, and the ability to turn without staggering. Additional testing is indicated for individuals requiring more than 20 seconds to complete test.[12]

- Determine muscle strength and tone, joint mobility, cardiovascular status, balance, endurance, and use of assistive device. *Identifies strengths and deficits (e.g., ability to ambulate with/without assistive devices) and may provide information regarding potential for recovery (e.g., client with severe brain injury may have permanent limitations because of impaired cognition affecting memory, judgment, problem-solving and motor planning, requiring more intensive inpatient and long-term care).*
- Note whether impairment is temporary or permanent. *Condition may be caused by reversible condition (e.g., weakness associated with acute illness or fractures/surgery with weight-bearing restrictions); or walking impairment can be permanent (e.g., congenital anomalies, amputation, severe rheumatoid arthritis).*[1,8]
- Assist with/review results of mobility testing (e.g., timing of walking over fixed distance, distance walked over set period of time [endurance], limb movement analysis, leg strength and speed of walking, ambulatory activity monitoring, etc.) *for differential diagnosis and to guide treatment interventions.*[11,12]
- Note emotional/behavioral responses of client/SO to problems of mobility. *Can negatively affect self-concept and self-esteem, autonomy, and independence. Social, occupational, and relationship roles can change, leading to isolation, depression, and economic consequences.*[8,9]

NURSING PRIORITY NO. 3 To promote safe, optimal level of independence in walking:

- Assist with treatment of underlying condition as needed/indicated by individual situation. *Treatment can often reverse or limit dysfunction.*
- Consult with PT/OT/rehabilitation team *to develop individual program (e.g., to improve general conditioning, coordination and balance, range-of-motion exercises, specific muscle strengthening, etc.), to instruct in specific tasks (e.g., stair-climbing or gait-training, etc.), and to identify/develop appropriate adjunctive devices (e.g., shoe insert, leg brace for proper foot alignment; customized cane, crutches, or walker).*[2]
- Monitor client's cardiopulmonary tolerance for walking. *Increased pulse rate, chest pain, breathlessness, irregular heartbeat is indicative of need to reduce level of activity.* (Refer to ND Activity Intolerance; decreased Cardiac Output for related interventions.)
- Encourage adequate rest and gradual increase in walking *to reduce fatigue or leg pain associated with walking and improve stamina.*[6,7] (Refer to NDs Fatigue; risk for Peripheral Neurovascular Dysfunction.)
- Administer medication, as indicated, *to manage pain and maximize level of functioning.* (Refer to NDs acute/chronic Pain.)
- Implement fall precautions for high-risk clients (e.g., frail or ill elderly, visually or cognitively impaired, person on multiple medications, presence of balance disorders, etc.) *to reduce risk of accidental injury.*[1,6] (Refer to NDs risk for Falls; risk for Disuse Syndrome for related interventions.)
- Instruct in proper application of prostheses, immobilizers (e.g., walking cast/boot), and braces before walking *to maintain joint stability or immobilization or to maintain alignment during movement.*[3,4]
- Demonstrate/remind client to properly use assistive devices (e.g., cane, crutches, walker) *prescribed to improve balance, reduce limb pain/dysfunction, and provide support during ambulation.*[2]
- Use adequate personnel and safety devices (e.g., gait belt, nonslip shoes, handrail) when ambulating *to prevent injury to client or caregivers.*[2,6]
- Limit distractions, provide safe environment. *Allows client to concentrate on walking activities or learning use of assistive devices.*[2]

Nursing Diagnoses in Alphabetical Order

- Provide cueing, as indicated. *Client may need reminders (e.g., lift foot higher, look where going, walk tall, etc.) to concentrate on/perform tasks of walking, especially when balance or cognition is impaired.*[5]
- Provide ample time to perform mobility-related tasks *to reduce risk of falling and manage fatigue or pain.*
- Provide positive, constructive feedback *to encourage continuation of efforts and enhance client's self-sufficiency.*[6]
- Assist client to obtain needed information, such as handicapped sticker for close-in parking, sources for mobility scooter, or special public transportation options, when indicated, *to deal with temporary or permanent disability access.*

NURSING PRIORITY NO. 4 To promote wellness (Teaching/Discharge Considerations):

- Evaluate client's home (or work) environment for barriers to walking (e.g., uneven surfaces, many steps, no ramps, long distances between places client needs to walk, etc.) *to determine needed changes, make recommendations for client safety.*
- Involve client/SO in problem-solving, assisting them to learn ways of managing deficits, *to enhance safety for client with long-term/permanent impairments.*
- Encourage participation in regular active and passive exercise program. Advance levels of exercise, as able, *to improve muscle tone/strength and increase stamina/endurance.*
- Discuss appropriate use of electric scooter, if indicated. *Enhances mobility, especially over distances to maintain independency and socialization.*
- Identify appropriate resources for obtaining and maintaining appliances, equipment, and environmental modifications *to promote safe mobility.*
- Instruct client/SO in safety measures in home, as individually indicated (e.g., maintaining safe travel pathway, proper lighting, wearing glasses, handrails on stairs, grab bars in bathroom, using walker instead of cane when sleepy or walking on uneven surface, etc.) *to reduce risk of falls.*
- Discuss need for emergency call/support system (e.g., Lifeline, HealthWatch) *to provide immediate assistance for falls, other home emergencies when client lives alone.*

DOCUMENTATION FOCUS

Assessment/Reassessment

- Individual findings, including level of function/ability to participate in specific/desired activities.
- Equipment/assistive device needs.

Planning

- Plan of care and who is involved in the planning.
- Teaching plan.

Implementation/Evaluation

- Responses to interventions/teaching and actions performed.
- Attainment/progress toward desired outcome(s).
- Modifications to plan of care.

Discharge Planning

- Discharge/long-range needs, noting who is responsible for each action to be taken.

- Specific referrals made.
- Sources of/maintenance for assistive devices.

References

1. ND: Walking impaired. In Doenges, M. E., Moorhouse, M. F., Geissler-Murr, A. C. (2002). *Nursing Care Plans: Guidelines for Individualizing Patient Care.* 6th ed. Philadelphia: F. A. Davis.
2. Kuang, T., Kedlaya, D. (2002, update 2007). Assistive devices to improve independence. Accessed August 2007. Available at www.emedicine.com/pmr/topic210.htm.
3. Teplicky, R., Law, M., Russell, D. (2002). The effectiveness of casts, orthotics, and splints for children with neurological disorders. *Infants & Young Children,* 15(1), 42–50.
4. Wilson, G. B. (1988). Progressive mobilization. In Sine, R. D., et al. (eds). *Basic Rehabilitation Techniques: A Self-Instructional Guide.* 3d ed. Gaithersburg, MD: Aspen.
5. Gee, Z. I., Passarella, P. M. (1985). *Nursing Care of the Stroke Patient: A Therapeutic Approach.* Pittsburgh, PA: AREN.
6. Jitramontree, N. (February 2001). Evidence-based protocol. Exercise promotion: Walking in elders. Iowa City, IA: University of Iowa Gerontological Nursing Interventions Research Center, Research Dissemination Core, 53.
7. Eberhardt, R. T. (2002). Editorial-Exercise for intermittent claudication: Walking for life? *J Cardiopulm Rehab,* 22(3), 199–200.
8. Mass, M. L. (1989). Impaired physical mobility. Unpublished manuscript. Cited in research article for National Institutes for Health.
9. Hogue, C. C. (1984). Falls and mobility late in life: An ecological model. *J Am Geriatr Soc,* 32, 858–861.
10. No author or pub date listed. Symptom: Walking symptoms. Accessed April 2007 at http://wrongdiagnosis.com/sym/walking_symptoms.htm.
11. Pearsen, O. R., Busse, M. E., van Deuresn, R. W. M., et al. (2004). Quantification of walking mobility in neruological disorders. *QJM: An International J of Medicine,* 97, 463–475.
12. Baer, H. R., Wolf, S. L. (2001). Modified Emory Functional Ambulation Profile: An outcome measure for the rehabilitation of poststroke gait dysfunction. *Stroke,* 32, 973. Retrieved August 2007 at http://stroke.ahajournals.org/cgi/content/full/32/4/973.

Wandering [specify sporadic or continual]

Definition: Meandering, aimless, or repetitive locomotion that exposes the individual to harm; frequently incongruent with boundaries, limits, or obstacles

RELATED FACTORS

Cognitive impairment (e.g., memory and recall deficits, disorientation, poor visuoconstructive or visuospatial ability, language defects); sedation

Cortical atrophy

Premorbid behavior (e.g., outgoing, sociable personality; premorbid dementia)

Separation from familiar environment; overstimulating environment

Emotional state (e.g., frustration, anxiety, boredom, depression, agitation)

Physiological state or need (e.g., hunger, thirst, pain, urination, constipation)

Time of day

DEFINING CHARACTERISTICS

Objective

Frequent/continuous movement from place to place, often revisiting the same destinations

Persistent locomotion in search of something; scanning/searching behaviors

Haphazard locomotion; fretful locomotion/pacing; long periods of locomotion without an apparent destination

Locomotion into unauthorized or private spaces; trespassing

Locomotion resulting in unintended leaving of a premise
Inability to locate significant landmarks in a familiar setting; getting lost
Locomotion that cannot be easily dissuaded; shadowing a caregiver's locomotion
Hyperactivity
Periods of locomotion interspersed with periods of nonlocomotion (e.g., sitting, standing, sleeping)

Sample Clinical Applications: Brain injury, dementias, developmental delays, major depression, substance abuse, amnesia, fugue

DESIRED OUTCOMES/EVALUATION CRITERIA
Sample NOC linkage:
Physical Injury Severity: Severity of injuries from accidents and trauma

Client Will (Include Specific Time Frame)

• Be free of injury, or unplanned exits.

Sample NOC linkages:
Risk Control: Personal actions to prevent, eliminate, or reduce modifiable health threats
Safe Home Environment: Physical arrangements to minimize environmental factors that might cause physical harm or injury in the home

Caregiver(s) Will (Include Specific Time Frame)

• Modify environment, as indicated, to enhance safety.
• Provide for maximal independence of client.

ACTIONS/INTERVENTIONS

Sample NIC linkages:
Elopement Precautions: Minimizing the risk of a patient leaving a treatment setting without authorization when departure presents a threat to the safety of patient or others
Area Restriction: Limitation of patient mobility to a specified area for purposes of safety or behavior management
Environmental Management: Safety: Manipulation of the patient's surroundings for therapeutic benefit

NURSING PRIORITY NO. 1   To assess degree of impairment/stage of disease process:

• Ascertain history of client's memory loss and cognitive changes.
• Review responses of collaborative diagnostic examinations (e.g., cognition, functional capacity, behavior, memory impairments, reality orientation, general physical health and quality of life). *A combination of tests is often needed to complete an evaluation of client's overall condition relating to chronic/irreversible condition. These tests include (but are not limited to) Mini-Mental State Examination (MMSE), Alzheimer's Disease Assessment Scale, cognitive subsection (ADAS-cog), Functional Assessment Questionnaire (FAQ), Clinical Global Impression of Change (CGIC), Neuropsychiatric Inventory (NPI).*[1]
• Evaluate client's past history (e.g., individual was very active physically and socially, or reacted to stress with physical activity rather than emotional reactions) *to help identify likelihood of wandering.*[2]

Cultural   Collaborative   Community/Home Care   Diagnostic Studies   Pediatric/Geriatric/Lifespan   Medications

- Determine presence of depression. *Research supports the idea that wandering develops more often in depressed client with Alzheimer's disease.*[2]
- Evaluate client's mental status during both daytime and nighttime, noting when client's confusion is most pronounced and when/how long client sleeps. *Information about cognition and behavioral habits can reveal circumstances under which client is likely to wander.*[3]
- Identify client's reason for wandering, if possible. Client may demonstrate searching behavior (e.g., looking for lost item, pursuing certain unattainable activity), inexhaustible drive to do things/remain busy, or be experiencing sensations (e.g., hunger, thirst, or discomfort) without ability to express the actual need.[2]
- Determine bowel/bladder elimination pattern, timing of incontinence, presence of constipation *for possible correlation to wandering behavior.*
- Note timing and pattern of wandering behavior. *Client attempting to leave at 5:00 p.m. every day may believe he is going home from work; client may be goal-directed (e.g., searching for person or object) or nongoal directed (wandering aimlessly). Knowledge of patterns can prompt caregivers to anticipate need for personal attention.*[3,6,8]
- Ascertain if client has delusions due to shadows, lights, and noises *to determine necessary changes to environment.*
- Evaluate usual travel patterns. *Activity may be (1) direct (from one location to another without diversion, (2) random (random direction with no obvious stopping point), (3) pacing (back and forth within limited area), or (4) lapping (circling large areas).*[2,6,7]
- Assist with/review results of specific testing (e.g., Algase Wandering Scale [AWS], Need-driven Dementia-compromised behavior [NDM]/similar tool), as indicated. *Researchers are using adjunct tools for clinical assessment, which quantify wandering in several domains (as reported by caregivers) to determine individual risks/safety needs.*[2,7]
- Monitor client's use/need for assistive devices, such as glasses, hearing aids, cane, safe walking shoes, comfortable clothing, etc. *Wandering client is at high risk for falls due to cognitive impairments and the fatigue related to functional decline, or forgetting necessary assistive devices or how to properly use them.*[4]

NURSING PRIORITY NO. 2 To assist client/caregiver to deal with situations:

- Provide a structured daily routine:
  Encourage participation in family activities and familiar routines, such as folding laundry, listening to music, or shared-walking time outdoors. *Activities and exercises may reduce anxiety, depression, and restlessness. Note: Repetitive activity (e.g., rocking, folding laundry, or paperwork) may help client with "lapping," wandering to reduce energy expenditure and fatigue.*[3]
  Offer food, fluids, toileting on a regular schedule when client is unable to verbalize, *as agitation, pacing, or wandering may be associated with these basic needs.*[3]
  Sit with client and talk *when client is socially gregarious, enjoys conversation, or reminiscence is calming.*
  Provide television/radio or music, *which may be more effective than talking or reading to decrease wandering.*[1]
  Monitor activities, loud conversations, number of visitors at one time *to prevent overstimulation/increased agitation.*
  Remove items from immediate environment (e.g., coat, hat, keys, etc.) *to reduce stimulus for leaving the site.*[3]
- Provide safe place for client to wander:
  Remove environmental safety hazards such as hot water faucets, knobs on kitchen stove; gate or block open stairways, etc.[1-3]

Keep area free of clutter, place comfortable furniture and other items against the wall/out of travel path *to accommodate safe walking and promote rest periods during times of continual lapping.*[1]

Install safety locks/latches on doors and windows; *door latches are complex and less accessible;* equip exits with alarms (that are always turned on).[1-3]

Provide for 24-hour supervision, as indicated. *Client can be awake at any time and fail to recognize day/night routines.*

🏠 • Register client with community/national resources such as SafeReturn Program administered by the Alzheimer's Association. *Program registers persons with dementia and operates a 24-hour help line to facilitate the return of lost persons. [800–272–3900].*[5,6]

• Monitor activity when hospitalized/admitted to facility:

Place in room near monitoring station; check client location on frequent basis.

Assign consistent staff as much as possible.

Create "Wanderer's lounge," or large safe walking area with inaccessible exits or outside gated area.[1-3]

Avoid overstimulation from activities or new partner/roommate during rest periods.

🏠 • Use technology to promote safety:

Provide pressure-sensitive bed/chair alarms *to alert caregivers of movement, especially when client frequently gets up at night or when no one is present.*

Provide client ID bracelet or necklace with updated photograph, client name, and emergency contact *to assist with identification efforts, particularly when progressive dementia produces marked changes in client's appearance.*[3,5]

Obtain electronic locator devices *to find client when there is the potential for client to get lost/go missing.*[4,5]

Install verbal door alarm system. *Voice command is more effective at redirecting client and less likely to increase agitation than loud sound.*[1]

🏠 • Use universal symbols, large-print signs, portraitlike photographs, or pictures and signs *to assist client in finding way, especially when client has diminished ability or has lost ability to read.*[3]

🏠 • Avoid using physical or chemical restraints (sedatives) to control wandering behavior. *May increase agitation, sensory deprivation, and falls, and can aggravate wandering behavior.*

NURSING PRIORITY NO. 3 To Promote Wellness (Teaching/Discharge Considerations):

🏠 • Identify problems that are remediable and assist client/SO to seek appropriate assistance and access resources. *Encourages problem-solving to improve condition rather than accept the status quo.*

🏠 • Notify neighbors about client's condition and request that they contact client's family or local police if they see client outside alone. *Community awareness can prevent/reduce risk of client being lost or hurt.*

🏠 • Help client/SO and family members develop plan of care when problem is progressive. *Client may initially need part-time assistance at home, progressing to enrollment in day-care program, then full-time home care or placement in care facility.*

🏠 • Refer to community resources, such as day-care programs, support groups, respite care, etc. *Caregiver(s) will require access to multiple kinds of assistance and opportunities to promote problem-solving, enhance coping, and obtain necessary respite.*

• Refer to NDs acute/chronic Confusion; impaired Environmental Interpretation Syndrome; risk for Falls; risk for Injury; disturbed Sensory Perception (specify); impaired Thought Processes.

🌐 *Cultural* 🅐 *Collaborative* 🏠 Community/Home Care 🧪 *Diagnostic Studies* ∞ *Pediatric/Geriatric/Lifespan* 💊 *Medications*

DOCUMENTATION FOCUS

Assessment/Reassessment

- Assessment findings, including individual concerns, family involvement, and support factors/availability of resources.

Planning

- Plan of care and who is involved in planning.
- Teaching plan.

Implementation/Evaluation

- Responses of client/SO(s) to plan interventions and actions performed.
- Attainment/progress toward desired outcome(s).
- Modifications to plan of care.

Discharge Planning

- Long-range needs and who is responsible for actions to be taken.
- Specific referrals made.

References

1. About Alzheimer's. (2003). Physicians and Care Professionals. Various Educational Materials. Accessed August 2007 at www.alz.org.
2. Futrell, M., Melillo, K. D. (2002). Evidence-based protocol. Wandering. Iowa City, IA: University of Iowa Gerontological Nursing Interventions Research Center, Research Dissemination Core. Accessed August 2007 at www.guideline.gov/summary/summary.aspx?doc_id=3250.
3. ND: Wandering. In Cox, H. C., et al. (2002). *Clinical Applications of Nursing Diagnosis: Adult, Child, Women's Psychiatric, Gerontic, and Home Health Considerations*. 4th ed. Philadelphia: F. A. Davis.
4. Brody, E., et al. (1984). Predictors of falls among institutionalized females with Alzheimer's disease. *J Am Geriatr*, 32, 877–882.
5. Rowe, M. A. (2003). People with dementia who become lost. *AJN*, 103(7), 32–39.
6. dbS Productions. (2000–2007). Alzheimer's disease and related disorders SAR research: Wandering overview. Excerpt from book in progress available at Source of Search & Rescue Research, Publications and Training. Retrieved August 2007 at www.dbs-sar.com/SAR_Research/wandering.htm.
7. Algase, D. L., Beel-Bates, C., Beattie, E. (2003). Wandering in long term care. Annals of Long-Term Care: *Clinical Care and Aging*, 11(1), 33–39.
8. Mayo Clinic Staff. (2005). Alzheimer's: Understand and control wandering. Retrieved May 2007 at www.mayoclinic.com/health/alzheimers/HQ00218.

Chapter 6

Health Conditions and Client Concerns with Associated Nursing Diagnoses

This chapter presents 850 disorders/health conditions and life situations reflecting all specialty areas, with associated nursing diagnoses written as client problem/need statements that include the "related to" and "evidenced by" components.

This section will facilitate and help validate the assessment and diagnosis steps of the nursing process. Because the nursing process is perpetual and ongoing, other nursing diagnoses may be appropriate based on changing individual situations. Therefore, the nurse must continually assess, identify, and validate new client needs and evaluate subsequent care.

To facilitate access to the health conditions/concerns and nursing diagnoses, the client needs have been listed alphabetically and coded to identify nursing specialty areas.

MS: Medical-Surgical
PED: Pediatric
OB/GYN: Obstetric/Gynecological
CH: Community/Home
PSY: Psychiatric/Behavioral

There is no separate category for geriatrics because concerns/conditions in this population are actually subsumed under the other specialty areas and because elderly persons are susceptible to the majority of these problems.

Abdominal hysterectomy **MS**
(Refer to Hysterectomy)

Abdominal perineal resection **MS**
(Also refer to Surgery, general)
   disturbed Body Image may be related to presence of surgical wounds possibly evidenced by verbalizations of feelings/perceptions, fear of reaction by others, preoccupation with change.
   risk for Constipation: risk factors may include decreased physical activity/gastric motility, abdominal muscle weakness, insufficient fluid intake, change in usual foods/eating pattern.
   risk for Sexual Dysfunction: risk factors may include altered body structure/function, radical resection/treatment procedures, vulnerability/psychological concern about response of significant other(s), and disruption of sexual response pattern (e.g., erection difficulty).

Abortion, elective termination **OB**
risk for decisional Conflict: risk factors may include unclear personal values/beliefs, lack of experience or interference with decision making, information from divergent sources, deficient support system.

deficient Knowledge [Learning Need] regarding reproduction, contraception, self-care, Rh factor may be related to lack of exposure/recall or misinterpretation of information possibly evidenced by request for information, statement of misconception, inaccurate follow-through of instructions, development of preventable events/complications.

risk for Spiritual Distress/moral Distress: risk factors may include perception of moral/ethical implications of therapeutic procedure, time contraints for decision making.

Anxiety [specify level] may be related to situational/maturational crises, unmet needs, unconscious conflict about essential values/beliefs possibly evidenced by increased tension, apprehension, fear of unspecific consequences, sympathetic stimulation, focus on self.

acute Pain/[Discomfort] may be related to aftereffects of procedure/drug effect possibly evidenced by verbal report, distraction behaviors, changes in muscle tone, autonomic responses/changes in vital signs.

risk for maternal Injury: risk factors may include surgical procedure, effects of anesthesia/medications.

Abortion, spontaneous termination OB

deficient Fluid Volume [isotonic] may be related to excessive blood loss, possibly evidenced by decreased pulse volume and pressure, delayed capillary refill, or changes in sensorium.

risk for Spiritual Distress: risk factors may include need to adhere to personal religious beliefs/practices, blame for loss directed at self or God.

deficient Knowledge [Learning Need] regarding cause of abortion, self-care, contraception/future pregnancy may be related to lack of familiarity with new self/healthcare needs, sources for support, possibly evidenced by requests for information and statement of concern/misconceptions, development of preventable complications.

Grieving related to perinatal loss, possibly evidenced by crying, expressions of sorrow, or changes in eating habits/sleep patterns.

risk for ineffective Sexuality Pattern: risk factors may include increasing fear of pregnancy or repeat loss, impaired relationship with significant other(s), self-doubt regarding own femininity.

Abruptio placentae   OB

(Also refer to Hemorrhage, prenatal)

deficient Fluid Volume [isotonic] may be related to excessive blood loss, possibly evidenced by hypotension, increased heart rate, decreased pulse volume and pressure, delayed capillary refill, or changes in sensorium.

Fear related to threat of death (perceived or actual) to fetus/self, possibly evidenced by verbalization of specific concerns, increased tension, sympathetic stimulation.

acute Pain may be related to collection of blood between uterine wall and placenta, possibly evidenced by verbal reports, abdominal guarding, muscle tension, or alterations in vital signs.

impaired fetal Gas Exchange may be related to altered uteroplacental O_2 transfer, possibly evidenced by alterations in fetal heart rate and movement.

Abscess, brain (acute)   MS

acute Pain may be related to inflammation, edema of tissues, possibly evidenced by reports of headache, restlessness, irritability, and moaning.

risk for Hyperthermia: risk factors may include inflammatory process/hypermetabolic state and dehydration.

acute Confusion may be related to physiological changes (e.g., cerebral edema/altered perfusion, fever), possibly evidenced by fluctuation in cognition/level of consciousness, increased agitation/restlessness, hallucinations.

Doenges Nursing Diagnosis Manual: Planning, Individualizing, and Documenting Client Care

risk for Suffocation/Trauma: risk factors may include development of clonic/tonic muscle activity and changes in consciousness (seizure activity).

Abscess, gingival   CH

impaired Dentition may be related to ineffective oral hygiene, access/economic barriers to professional care possibly evidenced by toothache, root caries, purulent drainage.

risk for imbalanced Nutrition: less than body requirements: risk factors may include decreased intake.

Abscess, skin/tissue   CH/MS

impaired Skin/Tissue Integrity may be related to immunological deficit/infection, possibly evidenced by disruption of skin, destruction of skin layers/tissues, invasion of body structures.

risk for Infection [spread]: risk factors may include broken skin/traumatized tissues, chronic disease, malnutrition, insufficient knowledge.

Abuse, physical   CH/PSY

(Also refer to Battered child syndrome)

risk for Trauma: risk factors may include vulnerable client, recipient of verbal threats, history of physical abuse.

Powerlessness may be related to abusive relationship, lifestyle of helplessness as evidenced by verbal expressions of having no control, reluctance to express true feelings, apathy, passivity.

chronic low Self-Esteem may be related to continual negative evaluation of self/capabilities, personal vulnerability, willingness to tolerate possible life-threatening domestic violence as evidenced by self-negative verbalization, evaluates self as unable to deal with events, rationalizes away/rejects positive feedback.

ineffective Coping may be related to situational or maturational crisis, overwhelming threat to self, personal vulnerability, inadequate support systems, possibly evidenced by verbalized concern about ability to deal with current situation, chronic worry, anxiety, depression, poor self-esteem, inability to problem-solve, high illness rate, destructive behavior toward self/others.

Sexual Dysfunction may be related to ineffectual/absent role model, vulnerability, physical abuse possibly evidenced by verbalizations, change in sexual behaviors/activities, inability to achieve desired satisfaction.

Abuse, psychological   CH/PSY

ineffective Coping may be related to situational or maturational crisis, overwhelming threat to self, personal vulnerability, inadequate support systems, possibly evidenced by verbalized concern about ability to deal with current situation, chronic worry, anxiety, depression, poor self-esteem, inability to problem-solve, high illness rate, destructive behavior toward self/others.

Powerlessness may be related to abusive relationship, lifestyle of helplessness as evidenced by verbal expressions of having no control, reluctance to express true feelings, apathy, passivity.

Sexual Dysfunction may be related to ineffectual/absent role model, vulnerability, psychological abuse (harmful relationship), possibly evidenced by reported difficulties, inability to achieve desired satisfaction, conflicts involving values, seeking confirmation of desirability.

Achalasia (cardiospasm)   MS

impaired Swallowing may be related to neuromuscular impairment, possibly evidenced by observed difficulty in swallowing or regurgitation.

imbalanced Nutrition: less than body requirements may be related to inability or reluctance to ingest adequate nutrients to meet metabolic demands/nutritional needs, possibly evidenced by reported/observed inadequate intake, weight loss, and pale conjunctiva and mucous membranes.

---

acute Pain may be related to spasm of the lower esophageal sphincter, possibly evidenced by reports of substernal pressure, recurrent heartburn, or gastric fullness (gas pains).

Anxiety [specify level]/Fear may be related to recurrent pain, choking sensation, altered health status, possibly evidenced by verbalizations of distress, apprehension, restlessness, or insomnia.

risk for Aspiration: risk factors may include regurgitation/spillover of esophageal contents.

deficient Knowledge [Learning Need] regarding condition, prognosis, self-care, and treatment needs may be related to lack of familiarity with pathology and treatment of condition, possibly evidenced by requests for information, statement of concern, or development of preventable complications.

Acidosis, metabolic   MS
(Refer to underlying cause/condition, e.g., Diabetic ketoacidosis; Renal dialysis)

Acidosis, respiratory   MS
(Also refer to underlying cause/condition)

impaired Gas Exchange may be related to ventilation perfusion imbalance (decreased oxygen-carrying capacity of blood, altered oxygen-supply, alveolar-capillary membrane changes) possibly evidenced by dyspnea with exertion, tachypnea, changes in mentation, irritability, tachycardia, hypoxia, hypercapnia.

Acne   CH/PED
impaired Skin Integrity may be related to secretion, infectious process as evidenced by disruptions of skin surface.

disturbed Body Image may be related to change in visual appearance as evidenced by fear of rejection of others, focus on past appearance, negative feelings about body, change in social involvement.

situational low Self-Esteem may be related to adolescence, negative perception of appearance as evidenced by self-negating verbalizations, expressions of helplessness.

Acoustic neuroma   MS
(Also refer to Surgery, general)

disturbed auditory Sensory Perception may be related to altered sensory reception (compression of eighth cranial nerve), possibly evidenced by unilateral sensorineural hearing loss/tinnitis.

risk for Falls: risk factors may include hearing difficulties, dizziness, sense of unsteadiness.

Acquired immune deficiency syndrome   CH
(Refer to AIDS)

Acromegaly   CH
chronic Pain may be related to soft tissue swelling, joint degeneration, peripheral nerve compression, possibly evidenced by verbal reports, altered ability to continue previous activities, changes in sleep pattern, fatigue.

disturbed Body Image may be related to biophysical illness/changes possibly evidenced by verbalization of feelings/concerns, fear of rejection or of reaction of others, negative comments about body, actual change in structure/appearance, change in social involvement.

risk for Sexual Dysfunction: risk factors may include altered body structure, changes in libido.

Acute respiratory distress syndrome   MS
(Refer to Respiratory distress syndrome, acute)

Adams-Stokes syndrome   CH
(Refer to Dysrhythmia)

ADD   **PEDS**
(Refer to Attention deficit disorder)

Addiction   **CH/PSY**
(Refer to specific substances; Substance dependence/abuse rehabilitation)

Addison's disease   **MS**
deficient Fluid Volume [hypotonic] may be related to vomiting, diarrhea, increased renal losses, possibly evidenced by delayed capillary refill, poor skin turgor, dry mucous membranes, report of thirst.
  decreased Cardiac Output may be related to hypovolemia and altered electrical conduction (dysrhythmias) or diminished cardiac muscle mass, possibly evidenced by alterations in vital signs, changes in mentation, and irregular pulse or pulse deficit.

CH
Fatigue may be related to decreased metabolic energy production, altered body chemistry (fluid, electrolyte, and glucose imbalance), possibly evidenced by unremitting overwhelming lack of energy, inability to maintain usual routines, decreased performance, impaired ability to concentrate, lethargy, and disinterest in surroundings.
  disturbed Body Image may be related to changes in skin pigmentation, mucous membranes, loss of axillary/pubic hair, possibly evidenced by verbalization of negative feelings about body and decreased social involvement.
  risk for impaired physical Mobility: risk factors may include neuromuscular impairment (muscle wasting/weakness) and dizziness/syncope.
  imbalanced Nutrition: less than body requirements may be related to glucocorticoid deficiency; abnormal fat, protein, and carbohydrate metabolism; nausea, vomiting, anorexia, possibly evidenced by weight loss, muscle wasting, abdominal cramps, diarrhea, and severe hypoglycemia.
  risk for impaired Home Maintenance: risk factors may include effects of disease process, impaired cognitive functioning, and inadequate support systems.

Adenoidectomy   **PED/MS**
Anxiety [specify level]/Fear may be related to separation from supportive others, unfamiliar surroundings, and perceived threat of injury/abandonment, possibly evidenced by crying, apprehension, trembling, and sympathetic stimulation (pupil dilation, increased heart rate).
  risk for ineffective Airway Clearance: risk factors may include sedation, collection of secretions/blood in oropharynx, and vomiting.
  risk for deficient Fluid Volume: risk factors may include operative trauma to highly vascular site/hemorrhage.
  acute Pain may be related to physical trauma to oronasopharynx, presence of packing, possibly evidenced by restlessness, crying, and facial mask of pain.

Adjustment disorder   **PED/PSY**
(Refer to Anxiety disorders—PED)

Adoption/loss of child custody   **PSY**
risk for complicated Grieving: risk factors may include actual loss of child, expectations for future of child/self, thwarted grieving response to loss.
  risk for Powerlessness: risk factors may include perceived lack of options, no input into decision process, no control over outcome.

Adrenal crisis, acute   **MS**
(Also refer to Addison's disease; Shock)

deficient Fluid Volume [hypotonic] may be related to failure of regulatory mechanism (damage to/suppression of adrenal gland), inability to concentrate urine, possibly evidenced by decreased venous filling/pulse volume and pressure, hypotension, dry mucous membranes, changes in mentation, decreased serum sodium.

acute Pain may be related to effects of disease process/metabolic imbalances, decreased tissue perfusion, possibly evidenced by reports of severe pain in abdomen, lower back, or legs.

impaired physical Mobility may be related to neuromuscular impairment, decreased muscle strength/control, possibly evidenced by generalized weakness, inability to perform desired activities/movements.

risk for Hyperthermia: risk factors may include presence of illness/infectious process, dehydration.

risk for ineffective Protection: risk factors may include hormone deficiency, drug therapy, nutritional/metabolic deficiencies.

Adrenalectomy   **MS**

altered Tissue Perfusion (specify) may be related to hypovolemia and vascular pooling of blood (vasodilation), possibly evidenced by diminished pulse, pallor/cyanosis, hypotension, and changes in mentation.

risk for Infection: risk factors may include inadequate primary defenses (incision, traumatized tissues), suppressed inflammatory response, invasive procedures.

deficient Knowledge [Learning Need] regarding condition, prognosis, self-care, and treatment needs may be related to unfamiliarity with long-term therapy requirements, possibly evidenced by request for information and statement of concern/misconceptions.

Adrenal insufficiency   **CH**
(Refer to Addison's disease)

Affective disorder   **PSY**
(Refer to Bipolar disorder; Depressive disorders, major)

Affective disorder, seasonal   **PSY**
(Also refer to Depressive disorders, major)

intermittent ineffective Coping may be related to situational crisis (fall/winter season), disturbance in pattern of tension relase, and inadequate resources available, possibly evidenced by verbalizations of inability to cope, changes in sleep pattern (too little or too much), reports of lack of energy/fatigue, lack of resolution of problem, behavioral changes (irritability, discouragement).

risk for imbalanced Nutrition: more/less than body requirements: risk factors may include eating in response to internal cues other than hunger, alteration in usual coping patterns, change in usual activity level, decreased appetite, lack of energy/interest to prepare food.

Agoraphobia   **PSY**
(Also refer to Phobia)

Anxiety [panic] may be related to contact with feared situation (public place/crowds), possibly evidenced by tachycardia, chest pain, dyspnea, gastrointestinal distress, faintness, sense of impending doom.

Agranulocytosis   **MS**

risk for infection: risk factors may include suppressed inflammatory response.

risk for impaired Oral Mucous Membrane: risk factors may include infection.

risk for imbalanced Nutrition: less than body requirements: risk factors may include inability to ingest food/fluids (lesions of oral cavity).

AIDS (acquired immunodeficiency syndrome) MS
(Also refer to HIV infection)

risk for Infection, [progression to sepsis/onset of new opportunistic infection]: risk factors may include depressed immune system, use of antimicrobial agents, inadequate primary defenses, broken skin, traumatized tissue, malnutrition and chronic disease processes.

risk for deficient Fluid Volume: risk factors may include excessive losses: copious diarrhea, profuse sweating, vomiting, hypermetabolic state or fever; and restricted intake (nausea, anorexia, lethargy).

acute/chronic Pain may be related to tissue inflammation/destruction: infections, internal/external cutaneous lesions, rectal excoriation, malignancies, necrosis, peripheral neuropathies, myalgias and arthralgias, possibly evidenced by verbal reports, self-focusing/narrowed focus, alteration in muscle tone, paresthesias, paralysis, guarding behaviors, changes in vital signs (acute), autonomic responses, and restlessness.

CH

imbalanced Nutrition: less than body requirements may be related to altered ability to ingest, digest, or absorb nutrients (nausea/vomiting, hyperactive gag reflex, intestinal disturbances); increased metabolic activity/nutritional needs (fever, infection), possibly evidenced by weight loss, decreased subcutaneous fat/muscle mass; lack of interest in food/aversion to eating, altered taste sensation; abdominal cramping, hyperactive bowel sounds, diarrhea, sore and inflamed buccal cavity.

Fatigue may be related to decreased metabolic energy production, increased energy requirements (hypermetabolic state), overwhelming psychological/emotional demands, altered body chemistry (side effects of medication, chemotherapy), possibly evidenced by unremitting/overwhelming lack of energy, inability to maintain usual routines, decreased performance, impaired ability to concentrate, lethargy/restlessness, and disinterest in surroundings.

ineffective Protection may be related to chronic disease affecting immune and neurological systems, inadequate nutrition, drug therapies, possibly evidenced by deficient immunity, impaired healing, neurosensory alterations, maladaptive stress response, fatigue, anorexia, disorientation.

PSY

Social Isolation may be related to changes in physical appearance/mental status, state of wellness, perceptions of unacceptable social or sexual behavior/values, physical isolation, phobic fear of others (transmission of disease), possibly evidenced by expressed feelings of aloneness/rejection, absence of supportive significant other(s) (SOs), and withdrawal from usual activities.

disturbed Thought Processes/chronic Confusion may be related to physiological changes (hypoxemia, central nervous system [CNS] infection by HIV, brain malignancies, or disseminated systemic opportunistic infection); altered drug metabolism/excretion, accumulation of toxic elements (renal failure, severe electrolyte imbalance, hepatic insufficiency), possibly evidenced by clinical evidence of organic impairment, altered attention span, distractibility, memory deficit, disorientation, cognitive dissonance, delusional thinking, impaired ability to make decisions/problem-solve, inability to follow complex commands/mental tasks, loss of impulse control and altered personality.

AIDS dementia   CH
(Also refer to Dementia, HIV)

impaired Environmental Interpretation Syndrome may be related to dementia, depression, possibly evidenced by consistent disorientation, inability to follow simple directions/instructions, loss of social functioning from memory decline.

ineffective Protection may be related to chronic disease affecting immune and neurological systems, inadequate nutrition, drug therapies, possibly evidenced by deficient immunity, impaired healing, neurosensory alterations, maladaptive stress response, fatigue, anorexia, disorientation.

Alcohol abuse/withdrawal   CH/MS/PSY
(Refer to Alcohol intoxication, acute; Delirium tremens; Substance dependency/abuse rehabilitation)

Alcohol intoxication, acute   MS
(Also refer to Delirium tremens)

acute Confusion may be related to substance abuse, hypoxemia, possibly evidenced by hallucinations, exaggerated emotional response, fluctuation in cognition/level of consciousness, increased agitation.

risk for ineffective Breathing Pattern: risk factors may include neuromuscular impairment/CNS depression.

risk for Aspiration: risk factors may include reduced level of consciousness, depressed cough/gag reflexes, delayed gastric emptying.

Alcoholism   CH
(Refer to Substance dependency/abuse rehabilitation)

Aldosteronism, primary   MS
deficient Fluid Volume [isotonic] may be related to increased urinary losses, possibly evidenced by dry mucous membranes, poor skin turgor, dilute urine, excessive thirst, weight loss.

impaired physical Mobility may be related to neuromuscular impairment, weakness, and pain, possibly evidenced by impaired coordination, decreased muscle strength, paralysis, and positive Chvostek's and Trousseau's signs.

risk for decreased Cardiac Output: risk factors may include hypovolemia and altered electrical conduction/dysrhythmias.

Alkalosis, metabolic   MS
(Refer to underlying cause/condition, e.g., Renal dialysis)

Alkalosis, respiratory   MS
(Also refer to underlying cause/condition)

impaired Gas Exchange may be related to ventilation perfusion imbalance (decreased oxygen-carrying capacity of blood, altered oxygen supply, alveolar-capillary membrane changes) possibly evidenced by dyspnea, tachypnea, changes in mentation, tachycardia, hypoxia, hypocapnia.

Allergies, seasonal   CH
(Refer to Hay fever)

Alopecia   CH
disturbed Body Image may be related to effects of illness/therapy or aging process, change in appearance, possibly evidenced by verbalization of feelings/concerns, fear of rejection/reaction of others, focus on past appearance, preoccupation with change, feelings of helplessness.

ALS   CH
(Refer to Amyotrophic Lateral Sclerosis)

Alzheimer's disease   CH
(Also refer to Dementia, presenile/senile)

risk for Injury/Trauma: risk factors may include inability to recognize/identify danger in environment, disorientation, confusion, impaired judgment, weakness, muscular incoordination, balancing difficulties, and altered perception.

chronic Confusion, related to physiological changes (neuronal degeneration), possibly evidenced by inaccurate interpretation of/response to stimuli, progressive/long-standing cognitive impairment, short-term memory deficit, impaired socialization, altered personality, and clinical evidence of organic impairment.

disturbed Sensory Perception (specify) may be related to altered sensory reception, transmission, or integration (neurological disease/deficit), socially restricted environment (homebound/institutionalized), sleep deprivation, possibly evidenced by changes in usual response to stimuli, change in problem-solving abilities, exaggerated emotional responses (anxiety, paranoia, hallucinations), inability to tell position of body parts, diminished/altered sense of taste.

Insomnia may be related to sensory impairment, changes in activity patterns, psychological stress (neurological impairment), possibly evidenced by wakefulness, disorientation (day/night reversal), increased aimless wandering, inability to identify need/time for sleeping, changes in behavior/performance, lethargy, dark circles under eyes, and frequent yawning.

ineffective Health Maintenance may be related to deterioration affecting ability in all areas, including coordination, communication, cognition, ineffective individual/family coping, possibly evidenced by reported or observed inability to take responsibility for meeting basic health practices, lack of equipment/financial or other resources, and impairment of personal support system.

PSY

risk for Stress Overload: risk factors may include inadequate resources, chronic illness, physical demands, threats of violence.

compromised family Coping/Caregiver Role Strain may be related to family disorganization, role changes, family/caregiver isolation, long-term illness/complexity and amount of home-care needs exhausting supportive/financial capabilities of family member(s), lack of respite, possibly evidenced by verbalizations of frustrations in dealing with day-to-day care, reports of conflict, feelings of depression, expressed anger/guilt directed toward client, and withdrawal from interaction with client/social contacts.

risk for Relocation Stress Syndrome: Risk factors may include little or no preparation for transfer to a new setting, changes in daily routine, sensory impairment, physical deterioration, separation from support systems.

Amenorrhea (secondary or pathological)   GYN
(Also refer to Anorexia nervosa)

imbalanced Nutrition: less than body requirements may be related to inability to ingest/digest food or absorb nutrients, possibly evidenced by verbal reports, aversion to eating, lack of interest in food, weight loss, excessive hair growth/lanugo, pale conjuntiva/mucous membranes, abnormal lab studies.

risk for Sexual Dysfunction: Risk factors may include altered body function.

Amphetamine abuse   PSY
(Refer to Stimulant abuse)

Amputation   MS

risk for ineffective peripheral Tissue Perfusion: risk factors may include reduced arterial/venous blood flow, tissue edema, hematoma formation, hypovolemia.

acute Pain may be related to tissue and nerve trauma, psychological impact of loss of body part, possibly evidenced by reports of incisional/phantom pain, guarding/protective behavior, narrowed/self-focus, and autonomic responses.

impaired physical Mobility may be related to loss of limb (primarily lower extremity), altered sense of balance, pain/discomfort, possibly evidenced by reluctance to attempt movement, impaired coordination; decreased muscle strength, control, and mass.

disturbed Body Image may be related to loss of a body part, possibly evidenced by verbalization of feelings of powerlessness, grief, preoccupation with loss, and unwillingness to look at/touch stump.

Amyotrophic lateral sclerosis (ALS)   MS

impaired physical Mobility may be related to muscle wasting/weakness, possibly evidenced by impaired coordination, limited range of motion, and impaired purposeful movement.

ineffective Breathing Pattern/impaired spontaneous Ventilation may be related to neuromuscular impairment, decreased energy, fatigue, tracheobronchial obstruction, possibly evidenced by shortness of breath, fremitus, respiratory depth changes, and reduced vital capacity.

impaired Swallowing may be related to muscle wasting and fatigue, possibly evidenced by recurrent coughing/choking and signs of aspiration.

PSY

Powerlessness [specify level] may be related to chronic/debilitating nature of illness, lack of control over outcome, possibly evidenced by expressions of frustration about inability to care for self and depression over physical deterioration.

Grieving may be related to perceived potential loss of self/physiopsychosocial well-being, possibly evidenced by sorrow, choked feelings, expression of distress, changes in eating habits/sleeping patterns, and altered communication patterns/libido.

CH

impaired verbal Communication may be related to physical barrier (neuromuscular impairment), possibly evidenced by impaired articulation, inability to speak in sentences, and use of nonverbal cues (changes in facial expression).

risk for Caregiver Role Strain: risk factors may include illness severity of care receiver, complexity and amount of home-care needs, duration of caregiving required, caregiver is spouse, family/caregiver isolation, lack of respite/recreation for caregiver.

Anaphylaxis   CH

(Also refer to Shock)

ineffective Airway Clearance may be related to airway spasm (bronchial), laryngeal edema, possibly evidenced by diminished/adventitious breath sounds, cough ineffective or absent, difficulty vocalizing, wide-eyed.

decreased Cardiac Output may be related to decreased preload—increased capillary permeability (third spacing) and vasodilation, possibly evidenced by tachycardia/palpitations, changes in BP, anxiety, restlessness.

Anemia   CH

Activity Intolerance may be related to imbalance between O_2 supply (delivery) and demand, possibly evidenced by reports of fatigue and weakness, abnormal heart rate or blood pressure (BP) response, decreased exercise/activity level, and exertional discomfort or dyspnea.

imbalanced Nutrition: less than body requirements may be related to failure to ingest/inability to digest food or absorb nutrients necessary for formation of normal red blood cells (RBCs), possibly evidenced by weight loss/weight below normal for age, height, body build; decreased triceps skinfold measurement, changes in gums/oral mucous membranes; decreased tolerance for activity, weakness, and loss of muscle tone.

deficient Knowledge [Learning Need] regarding condition, prognosis, self-care, and treatment needs may be related to inadequate understanding or misinterpretation of dietary/physiological needs, possibly evidenced by inadequate dietary intake, request for information, and development of preventable complications.

risk for delayed Surgical Recovery: Risk factors may include decreased O_2 delivery to tissues.

Doenges Nursing Diagnosis Manual: Planning, Individualizing, and Documenting Client Care

Anemia, iron-deficiency   **CH**

(Also refer to Anemia)

   risk for deficient Fluid Volume: risk factors may include active fluid loss/hemorrhage.

   risk for impaired Oral Mucous Membrane: risk factors may include dehydration, malnutrition, vitamin deficiency.

Anemia, pernicious   **CH**

(Also refer to Anemia)

   disturbed kinesthetic/visual Sensory Perception may be related to changes in reception/perception, possibly evidenced by paresthesia, inability to tell position of extremities (proprioception), loss of vibratory sensation, changes in sensory acuity (yellow-blue color blindness).

   risk for Constipation/Diarrhea: risk factors may include muscular weakness, changes in GI motility, neurological impairment.

   risk for Injury/Falls: risk factors may include generalized weakness, paresthesia of extremeties, loss of proprioception, ataxia.

Anemia, sickle cell   **MS**

impaired Gas Exchange may be related to decreased O_2-carrying capacity of blood, reduced RBC life span, abnormal RBC structure, increased blood viscosity, predisposition to bacterial pneumonia/pulmonary infarcts, possibly evidenced by dyspnea, use of accessory muscles, cyanosis/signs of hypoxia, tachycardia, changes in mentation, and restlessness.

   ineffective Tissue Perfusion (specify) may be related to stasis, vasoocclusive nature of sickling, inflammatory response, atrioventricular (AV) shunts in pulmonary and peripheral circulation, myocardial damage (small infarcts, iron deposits, fibrosis), possibly evidenced by signs and symptoms dependent on system involved; for example, renal: decreased specific gravity and pale urine in face of dehydration; cerebral: paralysis and visual disturbances; peripheral: distal ischemia, tissue infarctions, ulcerations, bone pain; cardiopulmonary: angina, palpitations.

CH

acute/chronic Pain may be related to intravascular sickling with localized vascular stasis, occlusion, infarction/necrosis and deprivation of O_2 and nutrients, accumulation of noxious metabolites, possibly evidenced by reports of localized, generalized, or migratory joint or abdominal/back pain; guarding and distraction behaviors (moaning, crying, restlessness), facial grimacing, narrowed focus, and autonomic responses.

   deficient Knowledge [Learning Need] regarding disease process, genetic factors, prognosis, self-care, and treatment needs may be related to lack of exposure/recall, misinterpretation of information, unfamiliarity with resources, possibly evidenced by questions, statement of concern/misconceptions, exacerbation of condition, inadequate follow-through of therapy instructions, and development of preventable complications.

   delayed Growth and Development may be related to effects of physical condition, possibly evidenced by altered physical growth and delay/difficulty performing skills typical of age group.

   compromised family Coping may be related to chronic nature of disease/disability, family disorganization, presence of other crises/situations impacting significant person/parent, lifestyle restrictions, possibly evidenced by significant person/parent expressing preoccupation with own reaction and displaying protective behavior disproportionate to client's ability or need for autonomy.

Anencephaly   **OB**

(Also refer to Fetal demise)

   Anxiety [specify level] may be related to situational crisis, threat of fetal death, interpersonal transmission/contagion, possibly evidenced by increased tension, apprehension, feelings of inadequacy, somatic complaints, difficulty sleeping.

risk for decisional Conflict [specify]: risk factors may include threat to value/belief system, multiple or divergent sources of information, support system deficit, feelings of guilt (particularly regarding ethical issues such as termination of pregnancy, organ donation).

Aneurysm, abdominal aortic   MS
(Refer to Aortic aneurysm, abdominal)

Aneurysm, cerebral   MS
(Refer to Cerebrovascular accident)

Aneurysm, ventricular   MS
decreased Cardiac Output may be related to altered stroke volume (decreased contractility, increased systemic vascular resistance), changes in heart rate/rhythm, possibly evidenced by dyspnea, adventitious breath sounds, S_3/S_4 heart sounds, changes in hemodynamic measurements, dysrhythmias.

ineffective Tissue Perfusion (specify) may be related to decreased arterial blood flow, possibly evidenced by BP changes, diminished pulses, edema, dyspnea, dysrhythmias, altered mental status, decreased renal function.

Activity Intolerance may be related to imbalance between oxygen supply and demand, possibly evidenced by weakness, fatigue, abnormal heart rate/BP response to activity, ECG changes (dysrhythmias, ischemia).

Angina pectoris   MS
acute Pain may be related to decreased myocardial blood flow, increased cardiac workload/O_2 consumption, possibly evidenced by verbal reports, narrowed focus, distraction behaviors (restlessness, moaning), and autonomic responses (diaphoresis, changes in vital signs).

decreased Cardiac Output may be related to inotropic changes (transient/prolonged myocardial ischemia, effects of medications), alterations in rate/rhythm and electrical conduction, possibly evidenced by changes in hemodynamic readings, dyspnea, restlessness, decreased tolerance for activity, fatigue, diminished peripheral pulses, cool/pale skin, changes in mental status, and continued chest pain.

Anxiety [specify level] may be related to situational crises, change in health status or threat of death, negative self-talk, possibly evidenced by verbalized apprehension, facial tension, extraneous movements, and focus on self.

CH
Activity Intolerance may be related to imbalance between O_2 supply and demand, possibly evidenced by exertional dyspnea, abnormal pulse/BP response to activity, and electrocardiogram (ECG) changes.

deficient Knowledge [Learning Need] regarding condition, prognosis, self-care, and treatment needs may be related to lack of exposure, inaccurate/misinterpretation of information, possibly evidenced by questions, request for information, statement of concern, and inaccurate follow-through of instructions.

risk for risk-prone health Behavior: Risk factors may include condition requiring long-term therapy/change in lifestyle, multiple stressors, assault to self-concept, and altered locus of control.

Anorexia nervosa   MS
imbalanced Nutrition: less than body requirements may be related to psychological restrictions of food intake or excessive activity, self-induced vomiting, laxative abuse, possibly evidenced by weight loss, poor skin turgor/muscle tone, denial of hunger, unusual hoarding or handling of food, amenorrhea, electrolyte imbalance, cardiac irregularities, hypotension.

risk for deficient Fluid Volume: risk factors may include inadequate intake of food and liquids, chronic/excessive laxative or diuretic use, self-induced vomiting.

PSY

disturbed Thought Processes may be related to severe malnutrition/electrolyte imbalance, psychological conflicts, possibly evidenced by impaired ability to make decisions, problem-solve, nonreality-based verbalizations, ideas of reference, altered sleep patterns, altered attention span/distractibility; perceptual disturbances with failure to recognize hunger, fatigue, anxiety, and depression.

disturbed Body Image/chronic low Self-Esteem may be related to altered perception of body, perceived loss of control in some aspect of life, unmet dependency needs, personal vulnerability, dysfunctional family system, possibly evidenced by negative feelings, distorted view of body, use of denial, feeling powerless to prevent/make changes, expressions of shame/guilt, overly conforming, dependent on others' opinions.

interrupted Family Processes may be related to ambivalent family relationships and ways of transacting issues of control, situational/maturational crises, possibly evidenced by enmeshed family, dissonance among family members, family developmental tasks not being met, family members acting as enablers.

Anthrax, cutaneous   MS/CH

impaired Skin/Tissue Integrity may be related to infectious agent, possibly evidenced by disruption of skin surface, damage to tissues.

[Discomfort] may be related to local edema, effects of circulating toxins, possibly evidenced by reports of headache, muscle aches, nausea, malaise.

risk for Infection [spread/sepsis]: risk factors may include broken skin, tissue destruction, lack of immunity, presence of infective agent.

Anthrax, gastrointestinal   MS

Anxiety [moderate to severe]/Fear may be related to situational crisis, change in health status/threat of death, interpersonal transmission/contagion, possibly evidenced by expressed concerns, apprehension, uncertainty, fearful, increased tension, restlessness, blocking of thought.

risk for deficient Fluid Volume: risk factors may include decreased intake (nausea), excessive loss (bloody vomit/diarrhea), hypermetabolic state.

imbalanced Nutrition: less than body requirements may be related to inability to ingest food/absorb nutrients, increased metabolic demands, possibly evidenced by reports of loss of appetite/nausea, abdominal pain, vomiting, diarrhea.

impaired Oral Mucous Membranes may be related to effects of infection, dehydration, possibly evidenced by oropharyngeal ulcerations, oral pain, difficulty swallowing.

Anthrax, inhalation (pulmonary)   MS

(Also refer to Ventilator assist/dependence)

[Discomfort] may be related to effects of inflammatory response, possibly evidenced by fever, malaise, weakness, fatigue, mild chest pain.

Anxiety [moderate to severe]/Fear may be related to situational crisis, change in health status/threat of death, interpersonal transmission/contagion, possibly evidenced by expressed concerns, apprehension, uncertainty, fearful, increased tension, restlessness, blocking of thought.

impaired Gas Exchange may be related to alveolar-capillary membrane changes (fluid collection/shifts into interstitial space/alveoli), possibly evidenced by dyspnea, restlessness, irritability, abnormal rate/depth of respirations, cyanosis, hypoxia, lethargy, confusion.

risk for impaired spontaneous Ventilation: risk factors may include problems with secretion management, mechanical compression of lungs (widening of mediastinum), depletion of energy stores.

Antisocial personality disorder   PSY

risk for other-directed Violence: risk factors may include contempt for authority/rights of others, inability to tolerate frustration, need for immediate gratification, easy agitation, vulnerable self-concept, inability to verbalize feelings, use of maladjusted coping mechanisms, including substance use.

ineffective Coping may be related to very low tolerance for external stress, lack of experience of internal anxiety (e.g., guilt/shame), personal vulnerability, unmet expectations, multiple life changes, possibly evidenced by choice of aggression and manipulation to handle problems/conflicts, inappropriate use of defense mechanisms (e.g., denial, projection), chronic worry, anxiety, destructive behaviors, high rate of accidents.

chronic low Self-Esteem may be related to lack of positive or repeated negative feedback, unmet dependency needs, retarded ego development, dysfunctional family system, possibly evidenced by acting-out behaviors (e.g., substance abuse, sexual promisicuity, feelings of inadequacy, nonparticipation in therapy.

compromised/disabled family Coping may be related to family disorganization/role changes, highly ambivalent family relationships, client providing little support in turn for the primary person(s), history of abuse/neglect in the home, possibly evidenced by expressions of concern or complaints, preoccupation of primary person with own reactions to situation, display of protective behaviors disproportionate to client's abilities or need for autonomy.

impaired Social Interaction may be related to inadequate personal resources (shallow feelings), immature interests, underdeveloped conscience, unaccepted social values possibly evidenced by difficulty meeting expectations of others, lack of belief that rules pertain to self, sense of emptiness/inadequacy covered by expressions of self-conceit/arrogance/contempt, behavior unaccepted by dominant cultural group.

Anxiety disorder, generalized   PSY

Anxiety [specify level]/Powerlessness may be related to real or perceived threat to physical integrity or self-concept (may or may not be able to identify the threat), unconscious conflict about essential values/beliefs and goals of life, unmet needs, negative self-talk, possibly evidenced by sympathetic stimulation, extraneous movements (foot shuffling, hand/arm fidgeting, rocking movements, restlessness), persistent feelings of apprehension and uneasiness, a general anxious feeling that client has difficulty alleviating, poor eye contact, focus on self, impaired functioning, free-floating anxiety, impaired functioning, and nonparticipation in decision making.

ineffective Coping may be related to level of anxiety being experienced by the client, personal vulnerability; unmet expectations/unrealistic perceptions, inadequate coping methods or support systems, possibly evidenced by verbalization of inability to cope/problem-solve, excessive compulsive behaviors (e.g., smoking, drinking), and emotional/muscle tension, alteration in societal participation, high rate of accidents.

Insomnia may be related to psychological stress, repetitive thoughts, possibly evidenced by reports of difficulty in falling asleep/awakening earlier or later than desired, reports of not feeling rested, dark circles under eyes, and frequent yawning.

risk for compromised family Coping: risk factors may include inadequate/incorrect information or understanding by a primary person, temporary family disorganization and role changes, prolonged disability that exhausts the supportive capacity of significant other(s).

impaired Social Interaction/Social Isolation may be related to low self-concept, inadequate personal resources, misinterpretation of internal/external stimuli, hypervigilance, possibly evidenced by discomfort in social situations, withdrawal from or reported change in pattern of interactions, dysfunctional interactions; expressed feelings of difference from others; sad, dull affect.

Anxiety disorders   PED/PSY

Anxiety [severe/panic] may be related to situational/maturational crisis, internal transmission/contagion, threat to physical integrity/self-concept, unmet needs, dysfunctional family system, independence conflicts, possibly evidenced by somatic complaints, nightmares, excessive psychomotor activity, refusal to attend school, persistent worry/fear of catastrophic doom to family/self.

ineffective Coping may be related to maturational crisis, multiple life changes/losses, personal vulnerability, lack of self-confidence, possibly evidenced by inability to problem-solve, persistent/overwhelming fears, inability to meet role expectations, social inhibition, panic attacks.

impaired Social Interaction may be related to excessive self-consciousness, inability to interact with unfamiliar people, altered thought processes possibly evidenced by verbalized/observed discomfort in social situations, inability to receive/communicate a satisfying sense of belonging/caring/interest, use of unsuccessful social interaction behaviors.

risk for Self-Mutilation/self-directed Violence: risk factors may include panic states, dysfunctional family, history of self-destructive behaviors, emotional disturbance, increasing motor activity.

compromised/disabled family Coping may be related to situational/developmental crisis (e.g., divorce, addition to family, midlife crisis), unrealistic parental expectations, frequent disruptions in living arrangements, high-risk family situations (neglect/abuse, substance abuse), possibly evidenced by SO reports of frustration with clinging behaviors, emotional lability, harsh/punitive response to tyrannical behaviors, disproportionate protective behaviors.

Anxiolytic abuse   PSY
(Refer to Depressant abuse)

Aortic aneurysm, abdominal (AAA)   MS

risk for ineffective peripheral Tissue Perfusion: risk factors may include interruption of arterial blood flow [embolus formation, spontaneous blockage of aorta].

risk for Infection: risk factors may include turbulent blood flow through arteriosclerotic lesion.

acute Pain may be related to vascular enlargement-dissection/rupture, possibly evidenced by verbal coded reports, guarding behavior, facial mask, change in abdominal muscle tone.

Aortic aneurysm repair, abdominal   MS
(Also refer to Surgery, general)

Fear related to threat of injury/death, surgical intervention, possibly evidenced by verbal reports, apprehension, decreased self-assurance, increased tension, changes in vital signs.

risk for deficient Fluid Volume: risk factors may include weakening of vascular wall, failure of vascular repair.

risk for ineffective renal/peripheral Tissue Perfusion: risk factors may include interruption of arterial blood flow, hypovolemia.

Aortic insufficiency   MS/CH
(Refer to Valvular heart disease)

Aortic stenosis   MS
(Also refer to Valvular heart disease)

decreased Cardiac Output may be related to structural changes of heart valve, left ventricular outflow obstruction, alteration of afterload (increased left ventricular end-diastolic pressure and systemic vascular resistance [SVR]), alteration in preload/increased atrial pressure and venous congestion, alteration in electrical conduction, possibly evidenced by fatigue, dyspnea, changes in vital signs/hemodynamic parameters, and syncope.

risk for impaired Gas Exchange: risk factors may include alveolar-capillary membrane changes/congestion.

CH

risk for acute Pain: risk factors may include episodic ischemia of myocardial tissues and stretching of left atrium.

Activity Intolerance may be related to imbalance between O_2 supply and demand (decreased/fixed cardiac output), possibly evidenced by exertional dyspnea, reported fatigue/weakness, and abnormal blood pressure or ECG changes/dysrhythmias in response to activity.

Aplastic anemia   CH
(Also refer to Anemia)

risk for ineffective Protection: risk factors may include abnormal blood profile (leukopenia, thrombocytopenia), drug therapies (antineoplastics, antibiotics, NSAIDs, anticonvulsants).

Fatigue may be related to anemia, disease states, malnutrition, possibly evidenced by verbalization of overwhelming lack of energy, inability to maintain usual routines/level of physical activity, tired, decreased libido, lethargy, increase in physical complaints.

Appendectomy   MS
(Also refer to Surgery, general)

risk for Infection: risk factors may include release of pathogenic organisms into peritoneal cavity (prior to or at time of surgery).

Appendicitis   MS
acute Pain may be related to distention of intestinal tissues by inflammation, possibly evidenced by verbal reports, guarding behavior, narrowed focus, and autonomic responses (diaphoresis, changes in vital signs).

risk for deficient Fluid Volume: risk factors may include nausea, vomiting, anorexia, and hypermetabolic state.

risk for Infection: risk factors may include release of pathogenic organisms into peritoneal cavity.

ARDS   MS
(Refer to Respiratory distress syndrome, acute)

Arrhythmia, cardiac   MS/CH
(Refer to Dysrhythmia, cardiac)

Arterial occlussive disease, peripheral CH
ineffective peripheral Tissue Perfusion may be related to decreased arterial blood flow, possibly evidenced by skin discolorations, temperature changes, altered sensation, claudication, delayed healing.

risk for impaired Walking: risk factors may include presence of circulatory problems, pain with activity.

risk for impaired Skin/Tissue Integrity: risk factors may include altered circulation/sensation.

Arthritis, gouty   CH
(Refer to Gout)

Arthritis, juvenile rheumatoid   PED/CH
(Also refer to Arthritis, rheumatoid)

risk for delayed Development: risk factors may include effects of physical disability and required therapy.

risk for Social Isolation: risk factors may include delay in accomplishing developmental task, altered state of wellness, and changes in physical appearance.

Arthritis, rheumatoid   CH

acute/chronic Pain may be related to accumulation of fluid/inflammatory process, degeneration of joint, and deformity, possibly evidenced by verbal reports, narrowed focus, guarding/protective behaviors, and physical and social withdrawal.

impaired physical Mobility may be related to musculoskeletal deformity, pain/discomfort, decreased muscle strength, possibly evidenced by limited range of motion, impaired coordination, reluctance to attempt movement, and decreased muscle strength/control and mass.

Self-Care Deficit [specify] may be related to musculoskeletal impairment, decreased strength/endurance and range of motion, pain on movement, possibly evidenced by inability to manage activities of daily living (ADLs).

disturbed Body Image/Role Performance, ineffective may be related to change in body structure/function, impaired mobility/ability to perform usual tasks, focus on past strength/function/appearance, possibly evidenced by negative self-talk, feelings of helplessness, change in lifestyle/physical abilities, dependence on others for assistance, decreased social involvement.

Arthritis, septic   CH

acute Pain may be related to joint inflammation, possibly evidenced by verbal/coded reports, guarding behaviors, restlessness, narrowed focus.

impaired physical Mobility may be related to joint stiffness, pain/discomfort, reluctance to initiate movement, possibly evidenced by limited range of motion, slowed movement.

Self-Care Deficit [specify] may be related to musculosketeal impairment, pain/discomfort, decreased strength, impaired coordination, possibly evidenced by inability to perform desired ADLs.

risk for Infection, spread: risk factors may include presence of infectious process, chronic disease states, invasive procedures.

Arthroplasty   MS

risk for Infection: risk factors may include breach of primary defenses (surgical incision), stasis of body fluids at operative site, and altered inflammatory response.

risk for deficient Fluid Volume [isotonic]: risk factors may include surgical procedure/trauma to vascular area.

impaired physical Mobility may be related to decreased strength, pain, musculoskeletal changes, possibly evidenced by impaired coordination and reluctance to attempt movement.

acute Pain may be related to tissue trauma, local edema, possibly evidenced by verbal reports, narrowed focus, guarded movement, and autonomic responses (diaphoresis, changes in vital signs).

Arthroscopy, knee   MS

deficient Knowledge [Learning Need] regarding procedure/outcomes and self-care needs may be related to unfamiliarity with information/resources, misinterpretations, possibly evidenced by questions and requests for information, misconceptions.

risk for impaired Walking: risk factors may include joint stiffness, discomfort, prescribed movement restrictions, use of assistive devices/crutches for ambulation.

Asbestosis   CH

impaired Gas Exchange may be related to alveolar-capillary membrane changes, ventilation perfusion imbalance, possibly evidenced by dyspnea, tachypnea, restlessness, clubbing of fingers, abnormal ABGs.

Activity Intolerance may be related to imbalance between oxygen supply/demand, possibly evidenced by exertional dyspnea, decreased exercise tolerance/abnormal cardiopulmonary response to activity.

ineffective Airway Clearance may be related to inflammatory response to inhaled foreign body (asbestos fibers), smoking/secondhand smoke, infection, possibly evidenced by dyspnea, adventitious breath sounds, increased sputum.

risk for Infection: risk factors may include decrease in ciliary action, stasis of body fluids, chronic disease, malnutrition, insufficient knowledge to avoid exposure.

acute Pain may be related to inflammation/irritation of the parietal pleura, possibly evidenced by verbal reports, guarding/distraction behaviors, self-focus, and autonomic responses (changes in vital signs).

Asperger's disorder   PED/PSY

impaired Social Interaction may be related to skill deficit about ways to enhance mutuality, communication barriers (poor pragmatic language skills), preoccupations/compulsions/repetitive motor mannerisms, possibly evidenced by observed discomfort in social situations, dysfunctional interactions with others, inability to receive/communicate satisfying sense of belonging.

risk for Injury: risk factors may include rituals/repetitive motor mannerisms, clumsiness/poor coordination, vulnerability to manipulation/peer pressure.

Aspiration, foreign body   CH

ineffective Airway Clearance may be related to presence of foreign body, possibly evidenced by dyspnea, ineffective cough, diminished or adventitious breath sounds.

Anxiety [specify] may be related to situational crisis, perceived threat of death, possibly evidenced by apprehension, anxiety, fearful, scared.

risk for Suffocation: risk for lack of safety education/precautions, eating large mouthfuls/pieces of food.

Asthma   MS

(Also refer to Emphysema)

ineffective Airway Clearance may be related to increased production/retained pulmonary secretions, bronchospasm, decreased energy/fatigue, possibly evidenced by wheezing, difficulty breathing, changes in depth/rate of respirations, use of accessory muscles, and persistent ineffective cough with or without sputum production.

impaired Gas Exchange may be related to altered delivery of inspired O_2/air trapping, possibly evidenced by dyspnea, restlessness, reduced tolerance for activity, cyanosis, and changes in ABGs and vital signs.

Anxiety [specify level] may be related to perceived threat of death, possibly evidenced by apprehension, fearful expression, and extraneous movements.

CH

Activity Intolerance may be related to imbalance between O_2 supply and demand, possibly evidenced by fatigue and exertional dyspnea.

risk for Contamination: risk factors may include presence of atmospheric pollutants, environmental contaminants in the home (e.g., smoking/secondhand tobacco smoke).

Atelectasis   MS

impaired Gas Exchange may be related to inflammatory process, stasis of secretions affecting O_2 exchange across alveolar membrane, and hypoventilation, possibly evidenced by restlessness/changes in mentation, dyspnea, tachycardia, pallor, cyanosis, and ABGs/oximetry evidence of hypoxia.

Atherosclerosis   **CH/MS**
(Refer to Coronary artery disease, Peripheral vascular disease)

Athlete's foot   **CH**
impaired *Skin Integrity* may be related to fungal invasion, humidity, secretions, possibly evidenced by disruption of skin surface, reports of painful itching.

    risk for Infection [spread]: risk factors may include multiple breaks in skin, exposure to moist/warm environment.

Atrial fibrillation   **CH**
(Also refer to Dysrhythmias)

    Activity Intolerance may be related to imbalance between oxygen supply/demand, possibly evidenced by dyspnea, dizziness, presyncope/syncopal episodes.

    risk for ineffective cerebral Tissue Perfusion: risk factors may include interruption of arterial flow (micro emboli).

Atrial flutter   **CH**
(Also refer to Dysrhythmias)

    Anxiety [specify] may be related to threat to/change in health status, possibly evidenced by expressed concerns, apprehension, awareness of physiological symptoms (palpitations, dizziness, presyncope/syncopal episodes), focus on self.

Atrial tachycardia   **CH**
(Refer to Dysrhythmias)

Attention deficit disorder   **PED/PSY**
ineffective Coping may be related to situational/maturational crisis, retarded ego development, low self-concept, possibly evidenced by easy distraction by extraneous stimuli, shifting between uncompleted activities.

    chronic low Self-Esteem may be related to retarded ego development, lack of positive/ repeated negative feedback, negative role models, possibly evidenced by lack of eye contact, derogatory self-comments, hesitance to try new tasks, inadequate level of confidence.

    deficient Knowledge regarding condition, prognosis, therapy may be related to misinformation/misinterpretations, unfamiliarity with resources, possibly evidenced by verbalization of problems/misconceptions, poor school performance, unrealistic expectations of medication regimen.

Autistic disorder   **PED/PSY**
impaired Social Interaction may be related to abnormal response to sensory input/inadequate sensory stimulation, organic brain dysfunction; delayed development of secure attachment/ trust, lack of intuitive skills to comprehend and accurately respond to social cues, disturbance in self-concept, possibly evidenced by lack of responsiveness to others, lack of eye contact or facial responsiveness, treating persons as objects, lack of awareness of feelings in others, indifference/aversion to comfort, affection, or physical contact; failure to develop cooperative social play and peer friendships in childhood.

    impaired verbal Communication may be related to inability to trust others, withdrawal into self, organic brain dysfunction, abnormal interpretation/response to or inadequate sensory stimulation, possibly evidenced by lack of interactive communication mode, no use of gestures or spoken language, absent or abnormal nonverbal communication; lack of eye contact or facial expression; peculiar patterns of speech (form, content, or speech production), and impaired ability to initiate or sustain conversation despite adequate speech.

    risk for Self-Mutilation: risk factors may include organic brain dysfunction, inability to trust others, disturbance in self-concept, inadequate sensory stimulation, or abnormal response to sensory input (sensory overload); history of physical, emotional, or sexual abuse; and response to demands of therapy, realization of severity of condition.

disturbed Personal Identity may be related to organic brain dysfunction, lack of development of trust, fixation at presymbiotic phase of development, possibly evidenced by lack of awareness of the feelings or existence of others, increased anxiety resulting from physical contact with others, absent or impaired imitation of others, repeating what others say, persistent preoccupation with parts of objects, obsessive attachment to objects, marked distress over changes in environment; autoerotic/ritualistic behaviors, self-touching, rocking, swaying.

compromised/disabled family Coping may be related to family members unable to express feelings; excessive guilt, anger, or blaming among family members regarding child's condition; ambivalent or dissonant family relationships, prolonged coping with problem exhausting supportive ability of family members, possibly evidenced by denial of existence or severity of disturbed behaviors, preoccupation with personal emotional reaction to situation, rationalization that problem will be outgrown, attempts to intervene with child are achieving increasingly ineffective results, family withdraws from or becomes overly protective of child.

Bacteremia   **MS**
(Refer to Sepsis)

Barbiturate abuse   **CH/PSY**
(Refer to Depressant abuse)

Battered child syndrome   **PED/CH**
(Also refer to Abuse)

risk for Trauma: risk factors may include dependent position in relationship(s), vulnerability (e.g., congenital problems/chronic illness), history of previous abuse/neglect, lack/nonuse of support systems by caregiver(s).

delayed Growth and Development may be related to inadequate caretaking/neglect, indifference, inconsistent responsiveness, environmental/stimulation deficiencies, possibly evidenced by delay/difficulty in performing age-appropriate skills, altered physical growth, loss of previously acquired skills, precocious/accelerated sexual awareness, flat affect, decreased responses.

interrupted Family Processes/impaired Parenting may be related to poor role model/identity, unrealistic expectations, presence of stressors, and lack of support, possibly evidenced by verbalization of negative feelings, inappropriate caretaking behaviors, and evidence of physical/psychological trauma to child.

PSY

chronic low Self-Esteem may be related to deprivation and negative feedback of family members, personal vulnerability, feelings of abandonment, possibly evidenced by lack of eye contact, withdrawal from social contacts, discounting own needs, nonassertive/passive, indecisive, or overly conforming behaviors.

Post-Trauma Syndrome may be related to sustained/recurrent physical or emotional abuse; possibly evidenced by acting-out behavior, development of phobias, poor impulse control, and emotional numbness.

Bedsores   **CH/MS**
(Refer to Ulcer, pressure)

Bed-wetting   **PED**
(Refer to Enuresis)

Benign prostatic hyperplasia   **CH/MS**
[acute/chronic] Urinary Retention/overflow Urinary Incontinence may be related to mechanical obstruction (enlarged prostate), decompensation of detrusor musculature, inability of bladder

to contract adequately, possibly evidenced by frequency, hesitancy, inability to empty bladder completely, incontinence/dribbling, nocturia, bladder distention, residual urine.

acute Pain may be related to mucosal irritation, bladder distention, colic, urinary infection, and radiation therapy, possibly evidenced by verbal reports (bladder/rectal spasm), narrowed focus, altered muscle tone, grimacing, distraction behaviors, restlessness, and autonomic responses.

risk for deficient Fluid Volume: risk factors may include postobstructive diuresis, endocrine/electrolyte imbalances.

Fear/Anxiety [specify level] may be related to change in health status (possibility of surgical procedure/malignancy); embarrassment/loss of dignity associated with genital exposure before, during, and after treatment, and concern about sexual ability, possibly evidenced by increased tension, apprehension, worry, expressed concerns regarding perceived changes, and fear of unspecific consequences.

Besnier-Boeck disease   **CH**
(Refer to Sarcoidosis)

Biliary calculus   **CH/MS**
(Refer to Cholelithiasis)

Biliary cancer   **MS**
(Also refer to Cancer)

imbalanced Nutrition: less than body requirements may be related to inability to ingest/absorb nutrients (anorexia, nausea, indigestion), abdominal discomfort, possibly evidenced by aversion to eating, observed lack of intake, muscle wasting, weight loss, and imbalances in nutritional studies.

risk for impaired Skin Integrity: risk factors may include accumulation of bile salts in skin, poor skin turgor, skeletal prominence.

death Anxiety may be related to lack of successful treatment options, poor prognosis, possibly evidenced by fear of the process of dying, leaving SO/family alone after death, negative death images, concern of overworking caregiver, deep sadness.

Binge-eating disorder   **PSY**
(Refer to Bulimia nervosa)

Bipolar disorders   **PSY**

risk for other-directed Violence: risk factors may include irritability, impulsive behavior; delusional thinking; angry response when ideas are refuted or wishes denied; manic excitement, with possible indicators of threatening body language/verbalizations, increased motor activity, overt and aggressive acts, hostility.

imbalanced Nutrition: less than body requirements may be related to inadequate intake in relation to metabolic expenditures, possibly evidenced by body weight 20% or more below ideal weight, observed inadequate intake, inattention to mealtimes, and distraction from task of eating; laboratory evidence of nutritional deficits/imbalances.

risk for Poisoning [lithium toxicity]: risk factors may include narrow therapeutic range of drug, client's ability (or lack of) to follow through with medication regimen and monitoring, and denial of need for information/therapy.

Insomnia may be related to psychological stress, lack of recognition of fatigue/need to sleep, hyperactivity, possibly evidenced by denial of need to sleep, interrupted nighttime sleep, one or more nights without sleep, changes in behavior and performance, increasing irritability/restlessness, and dark circles under eyes.

disturbed Sensory Perception (specify) [overload] may be related to decrease in sensory threshold, endogenous chemical alteration, psychological stress, sleep deprivation, possibly evidenced by increased distractibility and agitation, anxiety, disorientation, poor concentration, auditory/visual hallucination, bizarre thinking, and motor incoordination.

interrupted Family Processes may be related to situational crises (illness, economics, change in roles); euphoric mood and grandiose ideas/actions of client, manipulative behavior and limit-testing, client's refusal to accept responsibility for own actions, possibly evidenced by statements of difficulty coping with situation, lack of adaptation to change, or not dealing constructively with illness; ineffective family decision-making process, failure to send and receive clear messages, and inappropriate boundary maintenance.

Bladder cancer   MS
(Also refer to Cancer; Urinary diversion)

impaired Urinary Elimination may be related to presence of tumor, possibly evidenced by frequency, burning, dysuria.

acute/chronic Urinary Retention may be related to blockage of urethra, possibly evidenced by sensation of fullness, bladder distention, residual urine, dysuria.

Body dismorphic disorder   PSY
(Refer to Hypochondriasis)

Bone cancer   MS/CH
(Also refer to Myeloma, multiple; Amputation)

acute Pain may be related to bone destruction, pressure on nerves, possibly evidenced by verbal or coded report, protective behavior, autonomic responses.

risk for Trauma: risk factors may include increased bone fragility, general weakness, balancing difficulties.

Bone marrow transplantation   MS/CH
(Also refer to Transplantation, recipient)

risk for Injury: risk factors may include immune dysfunction/supression, abnormal blood profile, action of donor T cells.

Borderline personality disorder   PSY
risk for self/other-directed Violence/Self-Mutilation: risk factors may include use of projection as a major defense mechanism, pervasive problems with negative transference, feelings of guilt/need to "punish" self, distorted sense of self, inability to cope with increased psychological/physiological tension in a healthy manner.

Anxiety [severe to panic] may be related to unconscious conflicts (experience of extreme stress), perceived threat to self-concept, unmet needs, possibly evidenced by easy frustration and feelings of hurt, abuse of alcohol/other drugs, transient psychotic symptoms, and performance of self-mutilating acts.

chronic low Self-Esteem/disturbed Personal Identity may be related to lack of positive feedback, unmet dependency needs, retarded ego development/fixation at an earlier level of development, possibly evidenced by difficulty identifying self or defining self-boundaries, feelings of depersonalization, extreme mood changes, lack of tolerance of rejection or of being alone, unhappiness with self, striking out at others, performance of ritualistic self-damaging acts, and belief that punishing self is necessary.

Social Isolation may be related to immature interests, unaccepted social behavior, inadequate personal resources, and inability to engage in satisfying personal relationships, possibly evidenced by alternating clinging and distancing behaviors, difficulty meeting expectations of others, experiencing feelings of difference from others, expressing interests inappropriate to developmental age, and exhibiting behavior unaccepted by dominant cultural group.

Doenges Nursing Diagnosis Manual: Planning, Individualizing, and Documenting Client Care

Botulism (food borne)   **MS**

deficient Fluid Volume [isotonic] may be related to active losses (vomiting, diarrhea, decreased intake), nausea, dysphagia, possibly evidenced by reports of thirst; dry skin/mucous membranes, decreased BP and urine output, change in mental state, increased Hct.

impaired physical Mobility may be related to neuromuscular impairment, possibly evidenced by limited ability to perform gross/fine motor skills.

Anxiety [specify level]/Fear may be related to threat of death, interpersonal transmission, possibly evidenced by expressed concerns, apprehension, awareness of physiological symptoms, focus on self.

risk for impaired spontaneous Ventilation: risk factors may include neuromuscular impairment, presence of infectious process.

CH

Contamination may be related to lack of proper precautions in food storage/preparation as evidenced by gastrointestinal and neurological effects of exposure to biological agent.

Bowel obstruction   **MS**
(Refer to Ileus)

Bowel resection   **CH**
(Refer to Intestinal surgery [without diversion])

BPH   **CH/MS**
(Refer to Benign prostatic hyperplasia)

Brachytherapy (radioactive implants) MS

risk for Injury: risk factors may include radiation emitted by client (depending on type of procedure), accidental dislodgement or removal of radiation source.

risk for impaired physical Mobility: risk factors may include prescribed restrictions (48 hours for low-dose implants), reluctance to move (fear of dislodging implants), decreased strength/endurance, depressed mood.

Bradycardia   **CH**
(Refer to Dysrhythmia, cardiac)

Brain tumor   **MS**
(Also refer to Cancer)

acute Pain may be related to pressure on brain tissues, possibly evidenced by reports of headache, facial mask of pain, narrowed focus, and autonomic responses (changes in vital signs).

disturbed Thought Processes may be related to altered circulation to or destruction of brain tissue, possibly evidenced by memory loss, personality changes, impaired ability to make decisions/conceptualize, and inaccurate interpretation of environment.

disturbed Sensory Perception (specify) may be related to compression/displacement of brain tissue, disruption of neuronal conduction, possibly evidenced by changes in visual acuity, alterations in sense of balance/gait disturbance, and paresthesia.

risk for deficient Fluid Volume: risk factors may include recurrent vomiting from irritation of vagal center in medulla and decreased intake.

Self-Care Deficit [specify] may be related to sensory/neuromuscular impairment interfering with ability to perform tasks, possibly evidenced by unkempt/disheveled appearance, body odor, and verbalization/observation of inability to perform activities of daily living.

Breast cancer   **MS/CH**
(Also refer to Cancer)

Anxiety [specify level] may be related to change in health status, threat of death, stress, interpersonal transmission, possibly evidenced by expressed concerns, apprehension, uncertainty, focus on self, diminished productivity.

deficient Knowledge regarding diagnosis, prognosis, and treatment options may be related to lack of exposure/unfamiliarity with information resources, information misinterpretation, cognitive limitation/anxiety, possibly evidenced by verbalizations, statements of misconceptions, inappropriate behaviors.

risk for disturbed Body Image: risk factors may include significance of body part with regard to sexual perceptions.

risk for ineffective Sexual Patterns: risk factors may include health-related changes, medical treatments, concern about relationship with SO.

Bronchitis   CH

ineffective Airway Clearance may be related to excessive, thickened mucous secretions, possibly evidenced by presence of rhonchi, tachypnea, and ineffective cough.

Activity Intolerance [specify level] may be related to imbalance between O_2 supply and demand, possibly evidenced by reports of fatigue, dyspnea, and abnormal vital sign response to activity.

acute Pain may be related to localized inflammation, persistent cough, aching associated with fever, possibly evidenced by reports of discomfort, distraction behavior, and facial mask of pain.

Bronchogenic carcinoma   MS/CH
(Also refer to Cancer)

impaired Gas Exchange may be related to ventilation perfusion imbalance (bronchial narrowing with air trapping, atelectasis), presence of inflammatory exudate possibly evidenced by dyspnea, diminished/adventitious breath sounds, decreased chest expansion (depth of breathing), abnormal ABGs.

risk for ineffective Airway Clearance: risk factors may include retained secretions, inflammatory exudate, bronchial narrowing, pain, smoking/secondhand smoke, infection.

risk for Infection: risk factors may include stasis of body fluids, tissue destruction, chronic disease, malnutrition.

Bronchopneumonia   MS/CH
(Also refer to Bronchitis)

ineffective Airway Clearance may be related to tracheal bronchial inflammation, edema formation, increased sputum production, pleuritic pain, decreased energy, fatigue, possibly evidenced by changes in rate/depth of respirations, abnormal breath sounds, use of accessory muscles, dyspnea, cyanosis, effective/ineffective cough with or without sputum production.

impaired Gas Exchange may be related to inflammatory process, collection of secretions affecting O_2 exchange across alveolar membrane, and hypoventilation, possibly evidenced by restlessness/changes in mentation, dyspnea, tachycardia, pallor, cyanosis, and ABGs/oximetry evidence of hypoxia.

risk for Infection [spread]: risk factors may include decreased ciliary action, stasis of secretions, presence of existing infection.

Brown-Sequard syndrome   MS/CH
(Also refer to Paraplegia or Quadraplegia)

impaired physical Mobility may be related to neuromuscular and sensoriperceptual impairment, possibly evidenced by limited motion, weakness, or paralysis (hemiparaplegia).

disturbed kinesthetic/tactile Sensory Perception may be related to altered sensory transmission (e.g., neurological trauma, ischemia, inflammation, infection), possibly evidenced by reported change in sensory acuity—loss of touch, vibration, and position on one side of the body, loss of pain and temperature sensation on opposite side of body (hemianesthesia).

Buck's traction   MS
(Refer to Traction)

Buerger's disease   CH
(Refer to Peripheral vascular disease)

Bulimia nervosa   PSY/MS
(Also refer to Anorexia nervosa)

  impaired Dentition may be related to dietary habits, poor oral hygiene, chronic vomiting, possibly evidenced by erosion of tooth enamel, multiple caries, abraided teeth.

  impaired Oral Mucous Membrane may be related to malnutrition or vitamin deficiency, poor oral hygiene, chronic vomiting, possibly evidenced by sore, inflamed buccal mucosa; swollen salivary glands, ulcerations of mucosa, reports of constant sore mouth/throat.

  risk for deficient Fluid Volume: risk factors may include consistent self-induced vomiting, chronic/excessive laxative/diuretic use, esophageal erosion or tear (Mallory-Weiss syndrome).

  deficient Knowledge [Learning Need] regarding condition, prognosis, complication, treatment may be related to lack of exposure to/unfamiliarity with information about condition, learned maladaptive coping skills, possibly evidenced by verbalization of misconception of relationship of current situation and behaviors, distortion of body image, bingeing and purging behaviors, verbalized need for information/desire to change behaviors.

Bunion   CH
impaired Walking may be related to inflammation/degeneration of joint, inappropriate footwear, possibly evidenced by inability to walk required distances.

Bunionectomy   MS
(Also refer to Surgery, general; Postoperative recovery period)

  impaired Walking may be related to surgical intervention, restrictive therapy, possibly evidenced by inability to walk required distances, navigate curbs, climb stairs.

Burns (dependent on type, degree, and severity of the injury) MS/CH
risk for deficient Fluid Volume: risk factors may include loss of fluids through wounds, capillary damage and evaporation, hypermetabolic state, insufficient intake, hemorrhagic losses.

  risk for ineffective Airway Clearance: risk factors may include mucosal edema and loss of ciliary action (smoke inhalation), direct upper airway injury by flame, steam, chemicals.

  risk for Infection: risk factors may include loss of protective dermal barrier, traumatized/necrotic tissue, decreased hemoglobin, suppressed inflammatory response, environmental exposure/invasive procedures.

  acute/chronic Pain may be related to destruction of/trauma to tissue and nerves, edema formation, and manipulation of impaired tissues, possibly evidenced by verbal reports, narrowed focus, distraction and guarding behaviors, facial mask of pain, and autonomic responses (changes in vital signs).

  risk for imbalanced Nutrition: less than body requirements: risk factors may include hypermetabolic state in response to burn injury/stress, inadequate intake, protein catabolism.

  Post-Trauma Syndrome may be related to life-threatening event, possibly evidenced by reexperiencing the event, repetitive dreams/nightmares, psychic/emotional numbness, and sleep disturbance.

  ineffective Protection may be related to extremes of age, inadequate nutrition, anemia, impaired immune system, possibly evidenced by impaired healing, deficient immunity, fatigue, anorexia.

deficient Diversional Activity may be related to long-term hospitalization, frequent lengthy treatments, and physical limitations, possibly evidenced by expressions of boredom, restlessness, withdrawal, and requests for something to do.

　　risk for delayed Development: risk factors may include effects of physical disability, separation from SO(s), and environmental deficiencies.

Bursitis　　　　　　　　　　　　CH

acute/chronic Pain may be related to inflammation of affected joint, possibly evidenced by verbal reports, guarding behavior, and narrowed focus.

　　impaired physical Mobility may be related to inflammation and swelling of joint and pain, possibly evidenced by diminished range of motion, reluctance to attempt movement, and imposed restriction of movement by medical treatment.

CABG　　　　　　　　　　　　MS
(Refer to Coronary artery bypass surgery)

CAD　　　　　　　　　　　　CH/MS
(Refer to Coronary artery disease)

Calculi, urinary　　　　　　　CH/MS

acute Pain may be related to increased frequency/force of ureteral contractions, tissue distention/trauma and edema formation, cellular ischemia, possibly evidenced by reports of sudden, severe, colicky pains; guarding and distraction behaviors, self-focus, and autonomic responses.

impaired Urinary Elimination may be related to stimulation of the bladder by calculi, renal or ureteral irritation, mechanical obstruction of urinary flow, edema formation, inflammation, possibly evidenced by urgency and frequency; oliguria (retention); hematuria.

　　risk for deficient Fluid Volume: Risk factors may include stimulation of renal-intestinal reflexes causing nausea, vomiting, and diarrhea; changes in urinary output, postoperative diuresis; and decreased intake.

　　risk for Infection: risk factors may include stasis of urine.

　　deficient Knowledge [Learning Need] regarding condition, prognosis, self-care, and treatment needs may be related to lack of exposure/recall and information misinterpretation, possibly evidenced by requests for information, statements of concern, and recurrence/development of preventable complications.

Cancer　　　　　　　　　　　　MS
(Also refer to Chemotherapy; Radiation therapy)

　　Fear/death Anxiety may be related to situational crises, threat to/change in health/socioeconomic status, role functioning, interaction patterns; threat of death, separation from family, interpersonal transmission of feelings, possibly evidenced by expressed concerns, feelings of inadequacy/helplessness, insomnia; increased tension, restlessness, focus on self, sympathetic stimulation.

　　Grieving may be related to potential loss of physiological well-being (body part/function), perceived separation from SO(s)/lifestyle (death), possibly evidenced by anger, sadness, withdrawal, choked feelings, changes in eating/sleep patterns, activity level, libido, and communication patterns.

　　acute/chronic Pain may be related to the disease process (compression of nerve tissue, infiltration of nerves or their vascular supply, obstruction of a nerve pathway, inflammation), or side effects of therapeutic agents, possibly evidenced by verbal reports, self-focusing/narrowed focus, alteration in muscle tone, facial mask of pain, distraction/guarding behaviors, autonomic responses, and restlessness.

Fatigue may be related to decreased metabolic energy production, increased energy requirements (hypermetabolic state), overwhelming psychological/emotional demands, and altered body chemistry (side effects of medications, chemotherapy), possibly evidenced by unremitting/overwhelming lack of energy, inability to maintain usual routines, decreased performance, impaired ability to concentrate, lethargy/listlessness, and disinterest in surroundings.

impaired Home Maintenance may be related to debilitation, lack of resources, or inadequate support systems, possibly evidenced by verbalization of problem, request for assistance, and lack of necessary equipment or aids.

PED

compromised/disabled family Coping may be related to chronic nature of disease and disability, ongoing treatment needs, parental supervision, and lifestyle restrictions, possibly evidenced by expression of denial/despair, depression, and protective behavior disproportionate to client's abilities or need for autonomy.

readiness for enhanced family Coping may be related to the fact that the individual's needs are being sufficiently gratified and adaptive tasks effectively addressed, enabling goals of self-actualization to surface, possibly evidenced by verbalizations of impact of crisis on own values, priorities, goals, or relationships.

Candidiasis   CH
(Also refer to Thrush)

impaired Skin/Tissue Integrity may be related to infectious lesions, possibly evidenced by disruption of skin surfaces/mucous membranes.

acute Pain/[Discomfort] may be related to exposure of irritated skin/mucous membranes to excretions (urine/feces), possibly evidenced by verbal/coded reports, restlessness, guarding behaviors.

risk for Sexual Dysfunction: risk factors include presence of infectious process/vaginal discomfort.

Cannabis abuse   CH
(Refer to Depressant abuse)

Carbon monoxide poisoning   MS

impaired Gas Exchange may be related to altered oxygen-carrying capacity of blood, possibly evidenced by headache, confusion, somnolence, elevated CO levels.

Activity Intolerance may be related to imbalance between oxygen supply/demand, possibly evidenced by fatigue, exertional dyspnea.

risk for Injury: risk factors may include therapeutic intervention (hyperbaric oxygen therapy).

risk for Trauma/Suffocation: risk factors may include cognitive limitations/altered consciousness, loss of large- or small-muscle coordination (seizure).

CH

disturbed Thought Processes may be related to period of hypoxia/altered affinity of hemoglobin for oxygen, possibly evidenced by memory disturbances, difficulty concentrating.

Cardiac catheterization   MS

Anxiety [specify] may be related to threat to/change in health status, stress, family heredity, possibly evidenced by expressed concerns, apprehension, uncertainty, focus on self.

risk for decreased Cardiac Output: risk factors may include altered heart rate/rhythm (vasovagal response, ventricular dysrhythmias), decreased myocardial contractility (ischemia).

risk for ineffective Tissue Perfusion: risk factors may include mechanical reduction of arterial blood flow, local hematoma formation, thrombosis, emboli, allergic dye response.

Cardiac conditions, prenatal OB

risk for Cardiac Output [decompensation]: risk factors may include increased circulating volume, dysrhythmias, altered myocardial contractility, inotropic changes in the heart.

risk for excess Fluid Volume: risk factors may include increasing circulating volume, changes in renal function, dietary indiscretion.

risk for ineffective uteroplacental Tissue Perfusion: risk factors may include changes in circulating volume, right-to-left shunt.

risk for Activity Intolerance: risk factors may include presence of circulatory problems, previous episodes of intolerance, deconditioned status.

risk for maternal Infection: risk factors may include inadequate primary/secondary defenses, chronic condition, insufficient information to avoid exposure to pathogens.

Cardiac inflammatory disease MS

(Refer to Endocarditis; Myocarditis; Pericarditis)

Cardiac surgery MS/PED

Anxiety [specify level]/Fear may be related to change in health status and threat to self-concept/of death, possibly evidenced by sympathetic stimulation, increased tension, and apprehension.

risk for decreased Cardiac Output: risk factors may include decreased preload (hypovolemia), depressed myocardial contractility, changes in SVR (afterload), and alterations in electrical conduction (dysrhythmias).

deficient Fluid Volume [isotonic] may be related to intraoperative bleeding with inadequate blood replacement; bleeding related to insufficient heparin reversal, fibrinolysis, or platelet destruction; or volume depletion effects of intraoperative/postoperative diuretic therapy, possibly evidenced by increased pulse rate, decreased pulse volume/pressure, decreased urine output, hemoconcentration.

risk for impaired Gas Exchange: risk factors may include alveolar-capillary membrane changes (atelectasis), intestinal edema, inadequate function or premature discontinuation of chest tubes, and diminished oxygen-carrying capacity of the blood.

acute Pain[/Discomfort] may be related to tissue inflammation/trauma, edema formation, intraoperative nerve trauma, and myocardial ischemia, possibly evidenced by reports of incisional discomfort/pain in chest and donor site; paresthesia/pain in hand, arm, shoulder, anxiety, restlessness, irritability; distraction behaviors, and autonomic responses.

impaired Skin/Tissue Integrity related to mechanical trauma (surgical incisions, puncture wounds) and edema evidenced by disruption of skin surface/tissues.

Cardiogenic shock MS

(Refer to Shock, cardiogenic)

Cardiomyopathy CH/MS

decreased Cardiac Output may be related to altered contractility, possibly evidenced by dyspnea, fatigue, chest pain, dizziness, syncope.

Activity Intolerance may be related to imbalance between oxygen supply and demand, possibly evidenced by weakness/fatigue, dyspnea, abnormal heart rate/BP response to activity, ECG changes.

ineffective Role Performance may be related to changes in physical health, stress, demands of job/life, possibly evidenced by change in usual patterns of responsibility, role strain, change in capacity to resume role.

Carotid endarterectomy MS

(Also refer to Surgery, general)

risk for ineffective cerebral Tissue Perfusion: risk factors may include interruption of arterial flow (wound hematoma, emboli), pressure changes with edema formation (hyperperfusion syndrome).

Carpal tunnel syndrome   **CH/MS**

acute/chronic Pain may be related to pressure on median nerve, possibly evidenced by verbal reports, reluctance to use affected extremity, guarding behaviors, expressed fear of reinjury, altered ability to continue previous activities.

impaired physical Mobility may be related to neuromuscular impairment and pain, possibly evidenced by decreased hand strength, weakness, limited range of motion, and reluctance to attempt movement.

risk for Peripheral Neurovascular Dysfunction: risk factors may include mechanical compression (e.g., brace, repetitive tasks/motions), immobilization.

deficient Knowledge [Learning Need] regarding condition, prognosis, and treatment/safety needs may be related to lack of exposure/recall, information misinterpretation, possibly evidenced by questions, statements of concern, request for information, inaccurate follow-through of instructions/development of preventable complications.

Casts   **CH/MS**

(Also refer to Fractures)

risk for Peripheral Neurovascular Dysfunction: risk factors may include presence of fracture(s), mechanical compression (cast), tissue trauma, immobilization, vascular obstruction.

risk for impaired Skin Integrity: risk factors may include pressure of cast, moisture/debris under cast, objects inserted under cast to relieve itching, or altered sensation/circulation.

Self-Care Deficit [specify] may be related to impaired ability to perform self-care tasks, possibly evidenced by statements of need for assistance and observed difficulty in performing activities of daily living.

Cataract   **CH**

disturbed visual Sensory Perception may be related to altered sensory reception/status of sense organs, possibly evidenced by diminished acuity, visual distortions, and change in usual response to stimuli.

risk for Trauma: risk factors may include poor vision, reduced hand/eye coordination.

Anxiety [specify level]/Fear may be related to alteration in visual acuity, threat of permanent loss of vision/independence, possibly evidenced by expressed concerns, apprehension, and feelings of uncertainty.

deficient Knowledge [Learning Need] regarding ways of coping with altered abilities, therapy choices, lifestyle changes may be related to lack of exposure/recall, misinterpretation, or cognitive limitations, possibly evidenced by requests for information, statement of concern, inaccurate follow-through of instructions/development of preventable complications.

Cataract extraction (postoperative care)   **MS**

risk for Injury: risk factors may include increased intraocular pressure, intraocular hemorrhage, vitreous loss.

risk for Infection: risk factors may include invasive procedure/surgical manipulation, presence of chronic disease.

disturbed visual Sensory Perception may be related to altered sensory reception (use of eyedrops/cataract glasses), therapeutically restricted environment (surgical procedure, patching), possibly evidenced by visual distortions/blurring, visual confusion/change in depth perception.

Cat scratch disease   **CH**

acute Pain may be related to effects of circulating toxins (fever, headache, and lymphadenitis), possibly evidenced by verbal reports, guarding behavior, and autonomic response (changes in vital signs).

Hyperthermia may be related to inflammatory process, possibly evidenced by increased body temperature, flushed warm skin, tachypnea, and tachycardia.

Celiac disease   **CH**

imbalanced Nutrition: less than body requirements may be related to inability to absorb nutrients (mucosal damage, loss of villi, proliferation of crypt cells, shortened transit time through GI tract), possibly evidenced by weight loss, abdominal distention, steatorrhea, evidence of anemia/vitamin deficiencies.

Diarrhea may be related to irritation, malabsorption, possibly evidenced by abdominal pain, hyperactive bowel sounds, at least 3 loose stools per day.

risk for deficient Fluid Volume: risk factors may include mild to massive steatorrhea/diarrhea.

Cellulitis   **CH/MS**

risk for Infection [abscess, bacteremia]: risk factors may include broken skin, chronic disease, presence of pathogens, insufficient knowledge to avoid exposure to pathogens.

acute Pain[/Discomfort] may be related to inflammatory process, circulating toxins, possibly evidenced by reports of localized pain/headache, guarding behaviors, restlessness, autonomic responses.

impaired Tissue Integrity may be related to trauma, inflammation, or invasion of tissues by infectious bacterial agent, or altered circulation, possibly evidenced by redness, warmth, edema, tenderness/pain under the surface of skin or deep in tissues.

Cerebral embolism   **MS/CH**

(Refer to Cerebrovascular accident)

Cerebral palsy   **PED/CH**

(Refer to Palsy, cerebral [spastic hemiplegia])

Cerebrovascular accident   **MS**

ineffective cerebral Tissue Perfusion may be related to interruption of blood flow (occlusive disorder, hemorrhage, cerebral vasospasm/edema), possibly evidenced by altered level of consciousness, changes in vital signs, changes in motor/sensory responses, restlessness, memory loss; sensory, language, intellectual, and emotional deficits.

impaired physical Mobility may be related to neuromuscular involvement (weakness, paresthesia, flaccid/hypotonic paralysis, spastic paralysis), perceptual/cognitive impairment, possibly evidenced by inability to purposefully move involved body parts/limited range of motion; impaired coordination or decreased muscle strength/control.

impaired verbal [or written] Communication may be related to impaired cerebral circulation, neuromuscular impairment, loss of facial/oral muscle tone and control; generalized weakness/fatigue, possibly evidenced by impaired articulation, does not/cannot speak (dysarthria); inability to modulate speech, find or name words, identify objects, or inability to comprehend written/spoken language; inability to produce written communication.

Self-Care Deficit [specify] may be related to neuromuscular impairment, decreased strength/endurance, loss of muscle control/coordination, perceptual/cognitive impairment, pain/discomfort, and depression, possibly evidenced by stated/observed inability to perform ADLs, requests for assistance, disheveled appearance, and incontinence.

risk for impaired Swallowing: risk factors may include muscle paralysis and perceptual impairment.

risk for Unilateral Neglect: risk factors may include sensory loss of part of visual field with perceptual loss of corresponding body segment.

CH

impaired Home Maintenance may be related to condition of individual family member, insufficient finances/family organization or planning, unfamiliarity with resources, and inadequate support systems, possibly evidenced by members expressing difficulty in managing home in a comfortable manner/requesting assistance with home maintenance, disorderly surroundings, and overtaxed family members.

situational low Self-Esteem/disturbed Body Image/ineffective Role Performance may be related to biophysical, psychosocial, and cognitive/perceptual changes, possibly evidenced by actual change in structure or function, change in usual patterns of responsibility/physical capacity to resume role, and verbal/nonverbal response to actual or perceived change.

Cervix, dysfunctional   OB
(Refer to Dilation of Cervix, premature)

Cesarean birth   OB
(Also refer to Cesarean birth, unplanned/postpartal)

deficient Knowledge [Learning Need] regarding surgical procedure/expectation, postoperative routines/therapy, and self-care needs may be related to lack of information/misinterpretation, possibly evidenced by statements of concern, questions, and misconceptions.

risk for deficient Fluid Volume: risk factors may include restrictions of oral intake, blood loss.

risk for impaired parent/infant Attachment: risk factors may include separation, existing health conditions maternal/infant, lack of privacy.

Cesarean birth, postpartal   OB
(Also refer to Postpartal period)

risk for impaired parent/infant Attachment: risk factors may include developmental transition/gain of a family member, situational crisis (e.g., surgical intervention, physical complications interfering with initial acquaintance/interaction, negative self-appraisal).

acute Pain/[Discomfort] may be related to surgical trauma, effects of anesthesia, hormonal effects, bladder/abdominal distention, possibly evidenced by verbal reports (e.g., incisional pain, cramping/afterpains, spinal headache), guarding/distraction behaviors, irritability, facial mask of pain.

risk for situational low Self-Esteem: risk factors may include perceived "failure" at life event, maturational transition, perceived loss of control in unplanned delivery.

risk for Injury: risk factors may include biochemical or regulatory functions (e.g., orthostatic hypotension, development of PIH or eclampsia), effects of anesthesia, thromboembolism, abnormal blood profile (anemia/excessive blood loss, rubella sensitivity, Rh incompatibility), tissue trauma.

risk for Infection: risk factors may include tissue trauma/broken skin, decreased Hb, invasive procedures or increased environmental exposure, prolongs rupture of amniotic membranes, malnutrition.

Self-Care Deficit (specify) may be related to effects of anesthesia, decreased strength and endurance, physical discomfort, possibly evidenced by verbalization of inability to perform desired ADL(s).

Cesarean birth, unplanned   OB
(Also refer to Cesarean birth, postpartal)

deficient Knowledge [Learning Need] regarding underlying procedure, pathophysiology, and self-care needs may be related to incomplete/inadequate information, possibly evidenced by request for information, verbalization of concerns/misconceptions, and inappropriate/exaggerated behavior.

Anxiety [specify level] may be related to actual/perceived threat to mother/fetus, emotional threat to self-esteem, unmet needs/expectations, interpersonal transmission, possibly evidenced by increased tension, apprehension, feelings of inadequacy, sympathetic stimulation, and narrowed focus, restlessness.

Powerlessness may be related to interpersonal interaction, perception of illness-related regimen, lifestyle of helplessness, possibly evidenced by verbalization of lack of control, lack of participation in care or decision making, passivity.

risk for impaired fetal Gas Exchange: risk factors may include altered blood flow to placenta or through umbilical cord.

risk for acute Pain: risk factors may include increased/prolonged contractions, psychological reaction.

risk for Infection: risk factors may include invasive procedures, rupture of amniotic membranes, break in skin, decreased hemoglobin, exposure to pathogens.

Chemical dependence   PSY/CH
(Refer to specific agents; Substance dependency/abuse rehabilitation)

Chemotherapy   MS/CH
(Also refer to Cancer)

risk for deficient Fluid Volume: risk factors may include gastrointestinal losses (vomiting), interference with adequate intake (stomatitis/anorexia), losses through abnormal routes (indwelling tubes, wounds, fistulas), hypermetabolic state.

imbalanced Nutrition: less than body requirements may be related to inability to ingest adequate nutrients (nausea, stomatitis, and fatigue), hypermetabolic state, possibly evidenced by weight loss (wasting), aversion to eating, reported altered taste sensation, sore, inflamed buccal cavity; diarrhea or constipation.

impaired Oral Mucous Membrane may be related to side effects of therapeutic agents/radiation, dehydration, and malnutrition, possibly evidenced by ulcerations, leukoplakia, decreased salivation, and reports of pain.

disturbed Body Image may be related to anatomical/structural changes; loss of hair and weight, possibly evidenced by negative feelings about body, preoccupation with change, feelings of helplessness/hopelessness, and change in social environment.

ineffective Protection may be related to inadequate nutrition, drug therapy/radiation, abnormal blood profile, disease state (cancer), possibly evidenced by impaired healing, deficient immunity, anorexia, fatigue.

readiness for enhanced Hope may be related to expectations of therapeutic interventions, results of diagnostic procedures as evidenced by expressed desire to enhance belief in possibilities/sense of meaning to life.

Chickenpox   CH/PED
(Refer to Measles)

Chlamydia trachomatis infection   CH
(Refer to Sexually transmitted diseases)

Cholecystectomy   MS
acute Pain may be related to interruption in skin/tissue layers with mechanical closure (sutures/staples) and invasive procedures (including T-tube/nasogastric [NG] tube), possibly evidenced by verbal reports, guarding/distraction behaviors, and autonomic responses (changes in vital signs).

ineffective Breathing Pattern may be related to decreased lung expansion (pain and muscle weakness), decreased energy/fatigue, ineffective cough, possibly evidenced by fremitus, tachypnea, and decreased respiratory depth/vital capacity.

risk for deficient Fluid Volume: risk factors may include vomiting/NG aspiration, medically restricted intake, altered coagulation.

Cholelithiasis   CH

acute Pain may be related to inflammation and distortion of tissues, ductal spasm, possibly evidenced by verbal reports, guarding/distraction behaviors, and autonomic responses (changes in vital signs).

imbalanced Nutrition: less than body requirements may be related to inability to ingest/absorb adequate nutrients (food intolerance/pain, nausea/vomiting, anorexia), possibly evidenced by aversion to food/decreased intake and weight loss.

deficient Knowledge [Learning Need] regarding pathophysiology, therapy choices, and self-care needs may be related to lack of information, misinterpretation, possibly evidenced by verbalization of concerns, questions, and recurrence of condition.

Cholera   CH/MS

deficient Fluid Volume [isotonic] may be related to active volume loss (profuse watery diarrhea, vomiting), possibly evidenced by intense thirst, marked loss of tissue turgor, decreased urine output (oliguria/anuria), change in mental state, hemoconcentration.

risk for impaired Tissue Perfusion: risk factors may include hypovolemia, exchange problems (severe metabolic acidosis).

Christmas disease   CH
(Refer to Hemophilia)

Chronic obstructive lung disease   CH/MS

impaired Gas Exchange may be related to altered O_2 delivery (obstruction of airways by secretions/bronchospasm, air trapping) and alveoli destruction, possibly evidenced by dyspnea, restlessness, confusion, abnormal ABG values, and reduced tolerance for activity.

ineffective Airway Clearance may be related to bronchospasm, increased production of tenacious secretions, retained secretions, and decreased energy/fatigue, possibly evidenced by presence of wheezes, crackles, tachypnea, dyspnea, changes in depth of respirations, use of accessory muscles, cough (persistent), and chest radiograph findings.

Activity Intolerance may be related to imbalance between O_2 supply and demand, and generalized weakness, possibly evidenced by verbal reports of fatigue, exertional dyspnea, and abnormal vital sign response.

imbalanced Nutrition: less than body requirements may be related to inability to ingest adequate nutrients (dyspnea, fatigue, medication side effects, sputum production, anorexia), possibly evidenced by weight loss, reported altered taste sensation, decreased muscle mass/subcutaneous fat, poor muscle tone, and aversion to eating/lack of interest in food.

risk for Infection: risk factors may include decreased ciliary action, stasis of secretions, and debilitated state/malnutrition.

Circumcision   PEDS

deficient Knowledge [Learning Need] regarding surgical procedure, prognosis, and treatment may be related to lack of exposure, misinterpretation, unfamiliarity with information resources, possibly evidenced by request for information, verbalization of concern/misconceptions, inaccurate follow-through of instructions.

acute Pain may be related to trauma to/edema of tender tissues, possibly evidenced by crying, changes in sleep pattern, refusal to eat.

impaired urinary Elimination may be related to tissue injury/inflammation, or development of urethral fistula, possibly evidenced by edema, difficulty voiding.

risk for Injury [hemorrhage]: risk factors may include decreased clotting factors immediately after birth, previously undiagnosed problems with bleeding/clotting.

risk for Infection: risk factors may include immature immune system, invasive procedure/tissue trauma, environmental exposure.

Cirrhosis   MS

(Also refer to Substance Dependence/Abuse Rehabilitation; Hepatitis, acute viral)

risk for impaired Liver Function: risk factors may include viral infection, alcohol abuse.

risk for acute Confusion: risk factors may include alcohol abuse, increased serum ammonia level, and inability of liver to detoxify certain enzymes/drugs.

risk for Injury [hemorrhage]: risk factors may include abnormal blood profile (altered clotting factors), portal hypertension/development of esophageal varices.

CH

imbalanced Nutrition: less than body requirements may be related to inability to ingest/absorb nutrients (anorexia, nausea, indigestion, early satiety), abnormal bowel function, impaired storage of vitamins, possibly evidenced by aversion to eating, observed lack of intake, muscle wasting, weight loss, and imbalances in nutritional studies.

excess Fluid Volume may be related to compromised regulatory mechanism (e.g., syndrome of inappropriate antidiuretic hormone [SIADH], decreased plasma proteins/malnutrition) and excess sodium/fluid intake, possibly evidenced by generalized or abdominal edema, weight gain, dyspnea, BP changes, positive hepatojugular reflex, change in mentation, altered electrolytes, changes in urine specific gravity, and pleural effusion.

risk for impaired Skin Integrity: risk factors may include altered circulation/metabolic state, poor skin turgor, skeletal prominence, and presence of edema/ascites, accumulation of bile salts in skin.

situational low Self-Esteem/disturbed Body Image may be related to biophysical changes/altered physical appearance, uncertainty of prognosis, changes in role function, personal vulnerability, self-destructive behavior (alcohol-induced disease), possibly evidenced by verbalization of changes in lifestyle, fear of rejection/reaction of others, negative feelings about body/abilities, and feelings of helplessness/hopelessness/powerlessness.

Cleft lip/palate   PED/MS

(Also refer to Newborn, special needs)

ineffective Infant Feeding Pattern may be related to anatomical abnormality, possibly evidenced by inability to sustain an effective suck, inability to coordinate sucking/swallowing/breathing.

risk for Aspiration: risk factors may include impaired swallowing, regurgitation.

risk for impaired verbal Communication: risk factors may include anatomic defect, developmental delay.

risk for disturbed Body Image/Social Isolation: risk factors may include altered appearance/anatomic deficit, significance of body part (face).

Cocaine hydrochloride poisoning, acute   MS

(Also refer to Stimulant abuse; Substance dependence/abuse rehabilitation)

ineffective Breathing Pattern may be related to pharmacological effects on respiratory center of the brain, possibly evidenced by tachypnea, altered depth of respiration, shortness of breath, and abnormal ABGs.

risk for decreased Cardiac Output: risk factors may include drug effect on myocardium (degree dependent on drug purity/quality used), alterations in electrical rate/rhythm/conduction, preexisting myocardiopathy.

CH

risk for impaired Liver Function: risk factors may include cocaine abuse.

Coccidioidomycosis (San Joaquin/Valley Fever)   CH

acute Pain may be related to inflammation, possibly evidenced by verbal reports, distraction behaviors, and narrowed focus.

Fatigue may be related to decreased energy production; states of discomfort, possibly evidenced by reports of overwhelming lack of energy, inability to maintain usual routine, emotional lability/irritability, impaired ability to concentrate, and decreased endurance/libido.

deficient Knowledge [Learning Need] regarding nature/course of disease, therapy and self-care needs may be related to lack of information, possibly evidenced by statements of concern and questions.

Colectomy   MS
(Refer to Intestinal surgery [without diversion])

Colitis, ulcerative   MS
Diarrhea may be related to inflammation or malabsorption of the bowel, presence of toxins or segmental narrowing of the lumen, possibly evidenced by increased bowel sounds/peristalsis, urgency, frequent/watery stools (acute phase), changes in stool color, and abdominal pain/cramping.

acute/chronic Pain may be related to inflammation of the intestines/hyperperistalsis and anal/rectal irritation, possibly evidenced by verbal reports, guarding/distraction behaviors.

risk for deficient Fluid Volume: risk factors may include continued GI losses (diarrhea, vomiting, capillary plasma loss), altered intake, hypermetabolic state.

CH
imbalanced Nutrition: less than body requirements may be related to altered intake/absorption of nutrients (medically restricted intake, fear that eating may cause diarrhea) and hypermetabolic state, possibly evidenced by weight loss, decreased subcutaneous fat/muscle mass, poor muscle tone, hyperactive bowel sounds, steatorrhea, pale conjunctiva and mucous membranes, and aversion to eating.

ineffective Coping may be related to chronic nature and indefinite outcome of disease, multiple stressors (repeated over time), personal vulnerability, severe pain, inadequate sleep, lack of/ineffective support systems, possibly evidenced by verbalization of inability to cope, discouragement, anxiety; preoccupation with physical self, chronic worry, emotional tension; depression and recurrent exacerbation of symptoms.

risk for Powerlessness: risk factors may include unresolved dependency conflicts, feelings of insecurity/resentment, repression of anger and aggressive feelings; lacking a sense of control in stressful situations, sacrificing own wishes for others, and retreating from aggression or frustration.

Collagen disorders   CH
(Refer to Arthritis, rheumatoid/juvenile rheumatoid; Lupus erythematosus, systemic; Polyarteritis nodosa; Temporal arteritis)

Colorectal cancer   MS
(Refer to Cancer; Colostomy)

Colostomy   MS
risk for impaired Skin Integrity: risk factors may include absence of sphincter at stoma and chemical irritation from caustic bowel contents, reaction to product/removal of adhesive, and improperly fitting appliance.

risk for Diarrhea/Constipation: risk factors may include interruption/alteration of normal bowel function (placement of ostomy), changes in dietary/fluid intake, and effects of medication.

CH
deficient Knowledge [Learning Need] regarding changes in physiological function and self-care/treatment needs may be related to lack of exposure/recall, information misinterpretation, possibly

evidenced by questions, statement of concern, and inaccurate follow-through of instruction/development of preventable complications.

disturbed Body Image may be related to biophysical changes (presence of stoma; loss of control of bowel elimination) and psychosocial factors (altered body structure, disease process/associated treatment regimen, e.g., cancer, colitis), possibly evidenced by verbalization of change in perception of self, negative feelings about body, fear of rejection/reaction of others, not touching/looking at stoma, and refusal to participate in care.

impaired Social Interaction may be related to fear of embarrassing situation secondary to altered bowel control with loss of contents, odor, possibly evidenced by reduced participation and verbalized/observed discomfort in social situations.

risk for Sexual dysfunction: risk factors may include altered body structure/function, radical resection/treatment procedures, vulnerability/psychological concern about response of significant other(s), and disruption of sexual response pattern (e.g., erection difficulty).

Coma   MS

risk for Suffocation: risk factors may include cognitive impairment/loss of protective reflexes and purposeful movement.

risk for deficient Fluid Volume/imbalanced Nutrition: less than body requirements: risk factors may include inability to ingest food/fluids, increased needs/hypermetabolic state.

total Self-Care Deficit may be related to cognitive impairment and absence of purposeful activity, evidenced by inability to perform ADLs.

risk for ineffective Tissue Perfusion: cerebral: risk factors may include reduced or interrupted arterial/venous blood flow (direct injury, edema formation, space-occupying lesions), metabolic alterations, effects of drug/alcohol overdose, hypoxia/anoxia.

risk for Infection: risk factors may include stasis of body fluids (oral, pulmonary, urinary), invasive procedures, and nutritional deficits.

Coma, diabetic   MS

(Refer to Diabetic Ketoacidosis)

Compartment syndrome   MS

acute Pain may be related to increasing pressure within muscle, possibly evidenced by reports of progressing pain distal to injury unrelieved by routine analgesics.

ineffective peripheral Tissue Perfusion may be related to interruption of arterial blood flow/elevated tissue pressures, possibly evidenced by absent/diminished distal pulses, erythema, pain

risk for Peripheral Neurovascular dysfunction: risk factors may include reduction/interruption of blood flow (direct vascular injury, tissue trauma, excessive edema/elevated tissue pressures, hypovolemia).

Complex regional pain syndrome   CH

(Refer to Reflex sympathetic dystrophy)

Concussion of brain   CH

(Also refer to Postconcussion syndrome)

acute Pain may be related to trauma to/edema of cerebral tissue, possibly evidenced by reports of headache, guarding/distraction behaviors, and narrowed focus.

risk for deficient Fluid Volume: risk factors may include vomiting, decreased intake, and hypermetabolic state (fever).

risk for disturbed Thought Processes: risk factors may include trauma to/edema of cerebral tissue.

deficient Knowledge [Learning Need] regarding condition, treatment/safety needs, and potential complications may be related to lack of recall, misinterpretation, cognitive limitation, possibly evidenced by questions/statement of concerns, development of preventable complications.

Conduct disorder (childhood, adolescence)   PSY/PED

risk for self/other-directed Violence: risk factors may include retarded ego development, antisocial character, poor impulse control, dysfunctional family system, loss of significant relationships, history of suicidal/acting-out behaviors.

defensive Coping may be related to inadequate coping strategies, maturational crisis, multiple life changes/losses, lack of control of impulsive actions, and personal vulnerability, possibly evidenced by inappropriate use of defense mechanisms, inability to meet role expectations, poor self-esteem, failure to assume responsibility for own actions, hypersensitivity to slight or criticism, and excessive smoking/drinking/drug use.

disturbed Thought Processes may be related to physiological changes, lack of appropriate psychological conflict, biochemical changes, as evidenced by tendency to interpret the intentions/actions of others as blaming and hostile; deficits in problem-solving skills, with physical aggression the solution most often chosen.

chronic low Self-Esteem may be related to life choices perpetuating failure, personal vulnerability, possibly evidenced by self-negating verbalizations, anger, rejection of positive feedback, frequent lack of success in life events.

CH

compromised/disabled family Coping may be related to excessive guilt, anger, or blaming among family members regarding child's behavior; parental inconsistencies; disagreements regarding discipline, limit setting, and approaches; and exhaustion of parental resources (prolonged coping with disruptive child), possibly evidenced by unrealistic parental expectations, rejection or overprotection of child; and exaggerated expressions of anger, disappointment, or despair regarding child's behavior or ability to improve or change.

impaired Social Interaction may be related to retarded ego development, developmental state (adolescence), lack of social skills, low self-concept, dysfunctional family system, and neurological impairment, possibly evidenced by dysfunctional interaction with others (difficulty waiting turn in games or group situations, not seeming to listen to what is being said), difficulty playing quietly and maintaining attention to task or play activity, often shifting from one activity to another and interrupting or intruding on others.

Congestive heart failure   MS
(Refer to Heart Failure, chronic)

Conjunctivitis, bacterial   CH

acute Pain/[Discomfort] may be related to inflammation, ocular irritation, edema, possibly evidenced by verbal reports, irritability, guarding behavior.

risk for Infection [spread]: risk factors may include purulent discharge, insufficient knowledge to avoid spread.

risk for ineffective Therapeutic Regimen Management: risk factors may include length of therapy, perceived benefit.

Connective tissue disease   CH
(Refer to Arthritis, rheumatoid/juvenile rheumatoid; Lupus erythematosus, systemic; Polyarteritis nodosa; Temporal arteritis)

Conn's syndrome   MS/CH
(Refer to Aldosteronism, primary)

Constipation **CH**

Constipation may be related to weak abdominal musculature, GI obstructive lesions, pain on defecation, medications, diagnostic procedures, pregnancy, possibly evidenced by change in character/frequency of stools, feeling of abdominal/rectal fullness or pressure, changes in bowel sounds, abdominal distention.

acute Pain may be related to abdominal fullness/pressure, straining to defecate, and trauma to delicate tissues, possibly evidenced by verbal reports, reluctance to defecate, and distraction behaviors.

deficient Knowledge [Learning Need] regarding dietary needs, bowel function, and medication effect may be related to lack of information/misconceptions, possibly evidenced by development of problem and verbalization of concerns/questions.

Conversion disorder **PSY**
(Refer to Somatoform disorders)

Convulsions **CH**
(Refer to Seizure disorder)

COPD **CH**
(Refer to Chronic obstructive lung disease)

Corneal transplantation **MS**

risk for Injury: risk factors may include intraocular hemorrhage, edema/swelling, changes in visual acuity, increased intraocular pressure/glaucoma.

risk for Infection: risk factors may include surgical manipulation, use of corticosteroids, presence of chronic disease.

disturbed visual Sensory Perception may be related to altered sensory reception (use of eyedrops, edema/swelling), therapeutically restricted environment (patching), possibly evidenced by visual distortions/blurring, change in acuity.

Coronary artery bypass surgery **MS**

risk for decreased Cardiac Output: risk factors may include decreased myocardial contractility, diminished circulating volume (preload), alterations in electrical conduction, and increased SVR (afterload).

acute Pain may be related to direct chest tissue/bone trauma, invasive tubes/lines, donor site incision, tissue inflammation/edema formation, intraoperative nerve trauma, possibly evidenced by verbal reports, autonomic responses (changes in vital signs), and distraction behaviors/(restlessness), irritability.

disturbed Sensory Perception (specify) may be related to restricted environment (postoperative/acute), sleep deprivation, effects of medications; continuous environmental sounds/activities, and psychological stress of procedure, possibly evidenced by disorientation, alterations in behavior, exaggerated emotional responses, and visual/auditory distortions.

CH

ineffective Role Performance may be related to situational crises (dependent role)/recuperative process, uncertainty about future, possibly evidenced by delay/alteration in physical capacity to resume role, change in usual role or responsibility, change in self/others' perception of role.

Coronary artery disease **CH**

Activity Intolerance may be related to imbalance between oxygen supply/demand, sedentary lifestyle, possibly evidenced by exertional discomfort/pain, fatigue, abnormal heart rate response, ECG changes (dysrhythmias, ischemia).

risk for decreased Cardiac Output: risk factors may include altered heart rate/rhythm, altered contractility, increased peripheral vascular resistance.

Cor pulmonale   CH/MS
(Also refer to Heart failure, chronic; Chronic obstructive lung disease)

Activity Intolerance may be related to imbalance between O_2 supply/demand, generalized weakness, chest pain, possibly evidenced by exertional dyspnea, fatigue, cyanosis.

excess Fluid Volume may be related to compromised regulatory mechanism, possibly evidenced by shortness of breath, dependent edema, jugular vein distention, positive hepatojugular reflux, abnormal breath sounds, change in mental status.

impaired Gas Exchange may be related to ventilation perfusion imbalance (heart failure), possibly evidenced by dyspnea, restlessness, lethargy, cyanosis, abnormal ABG values (hypoxemia, hypercapnia, acidosis), polycythemia.

Cradle cap   CH
(Refer to Dermatitis, seborrheic)

Craniotomy   MS
(Also refer to Surgery, general)

risk for decreased Intracranial Adaptive Capacity: risk factors may include brain injuries/surgical procedure, systemic hypotension with intracranial hypertension.

disturbed Sensory Perception (specify) may be related to altered sensory reception, transmission or integration (neurological deficit), possibly evidenced by disorientation to time, place, person; motor incoordination, altered communication patterns, restlessness/irritability, change in behavior pattern.

risk for disturbed Thought Processes: risk factors may include trauma to/manipulation of brain tissue, changes in circulation/perfusion, increased intracranial pressure.

risk for Infection: risk factors may include traumatized tissues, broken skin, invasive procedures, nutritional deficits, altered integrity of closed system (CSF leak).

Creutzfeldt-Jakob disease   CH
impaired Memory may be related to neurological deficits, possibly evidenced by observed experiences of forgetting, inability to perform previously learned skills, inability to recall factual information or recent/past events.

Fear may be related to decreases in functional abilities, progressive deterioration, lack of treatment options, possibly evidenced by apprehension, irritability, defensiveness, suspiciousness, aggressive behavior, social isolation.

impaired Walking may be related to changes in muscle coordination/balance, visual changes, impaired judgment, myoclonic seizures, possibly evidenced by inability to walk desired distances, climb stairs, navigate uneven surfaces.

disturbed visual Sensory Perception may be related to altered sensory reception/integration (neurological disease), possibly evidenced by change in sensory acuity (visual field defects, diplopia, dimness/blurring, visual agnosia), change in usual response to stimuli.

total Self-Care Deficit may be related to cognitive decline, physical limitations, frustration over loss of independence, depression, possibly evidenced by impaired ability to perform ADLs, unkempt appearance/poor hygiene, apathy.

risk for Caregiver Role Strain: Risk factors may include illness severity of care receiver, duration of caregiving required, care receiver exhibiting deviant/bizarre behavior; family/caregiver isolation, lack of respite/recreation, spouse is caregiver.

Crohn's disease   MS/CH
(Also refer to Colitis, ulcerative)

imbalanced Nutrition: less than body requirements may be related to intestinal pain after eating and decreased transit time through bowel, possibly evidenced by weight loss, aversion to eating, and observed lack of intake.

Diarrhea may be related to inflammation of small intestines, presence of toxins, particular dietary intake, possibly evidenced by hyperactive bowel sounds, cramping, and frequent loose liquid stools.

deficient Knowledge [Learning Need] regarding condition, nutritional needs, and prevention of recurrence may be related to insufficient information/misinterpretation, unfamiliarity with resources, possibly evidenced by statements of concern/questions, inaccurate follow-through of instructions, and development of preventable complications/exacerbation of condition.

Croup   PED/CH

ineffective Airway Clearance may be related to presence of thick, tenacious mucus and swelling/spasms of the epiglottis, possibly evidenced by harsh/brassy cough, tachypnea, use of accessory breathing muscles, and presence of wheezes.

deficient Fluid Volume [isotonic] may be related to decreased ability/aversion to swallowing, presence of fever, and increased respiratory losses, possibly evidenced by dry mucous membranes, poor skin turgor, and scanty/concentrated urine.

Croup membranous   PED/CH
(Also refer to Croup)

risk for Suffocation: risk factors may include inflammation of larynx with formation of false membrane.

Anxiety [specify level]/Fear may be related to change in environment, perceived threat to self (difficulty breathing), and transmission of anxiety of adults, possibly evidenced by restlessness, facial tension, glancing about, and sympathetic stimulation.

C-Section   OB
(Refer to Cesarean birth, unplanned)

Cubital tunnel syndrome   CH

acute/chronic Pain may be related to pressure on ulnar nerve at elbow, possibly evidenced by verbal reports, reluctance to use affected extremity, guarding behaviors, expressed fear of reinjury, altered ability to continue previous activities.

impaired physical Mobility may be related to neuromuscular impairment and pain, possibly evidenced by decreased pinch/grasp strength, hand fatigue, and reluctance to attempt movement.

risk for Peripheral Neurovascular Dysfunction: risk factors may include mechanical compression (e.g., brace, repetitive tasks/motions), immobilization.

Cushing's syndrome   CH/MS

risk for excess Fluid Volume: risk factors may include compromised regulatory mechanism (fluid/sodium retention).

risk for Infection: risk factors may include immunosuppressed inflammatory response, skin and capillary fragility, and negative nitrogen balance.

imbalanced Nutrition: less than body requirements may be related to inability to utilize nutrients (disturbance of carbohydrate metabolism), possibly evidenced by decreased muscle mass and increased resistance to insulin.

Self-Care Deficit [specify] may be related to muscle wasting, generalized weakness, fatigue, and demineralization of bones, possibly evidenced by statements of/observed inability to complete or perform ADLs.

disturbed Body Image may be related to change in structure/appearance (effects of disease process, drug therapy), possibly evidenced by negative feelings about body, feelings of helplessness, and changes in social involvement.

Sexual Dysfunction may be related to loss of libido, impotence, and cessation of menses, possibly evidenced by verbalization of concerns or dissatisfaction with and alteration in relationship with significant other.

risk for Trauma [fractures]: risk factors may include increased protein breakdown, negative protein balance, demineralization of bones.

CVA   MS/CH
(Refer to Cerebrovascular accident)

Cyclothymic disorder   PSY
(Refer to Bipolar disorder)

Cystic fibrosis   CH/PED
ineffective Airway Clearance may be related to excessive production of thick mucus and decreased ciliary action, possibly evidenced by abnormal breath sounds, ineffective cough, cyanosis, and altered respiratory rate/depth.

risk for Infection: risk factors may include stasis of respiratory secretions and development of atelectasis.

imbalanced Nutrition: less than body requirements may be related to impaired digestive process and absorption of nutrients, possibly evidenced by failure to gain weight, muscle wasting, and retarded physical growth.

deficient Knowledge [Learning Need] regarding pathophysiology of condition, medical management, and available community resources may be related to insufficient information/misconceptions, possibly evidenced by statements of concern, questions; inaccurate follow-through of instructions, development of preventable complications.

compromised family Coping may be related to chronic nature of disease and disability, inadequate/incorrect information or understanding by a primary person, and possibly evidenced by significant person attempting assistive or supportive behaviors with less than satisfactory results, protective behavior disproportionate to client's abilities or need for autonomy.

Cystitis   CH
acute Pain may be related to inflammation and bladder spasms, possibly evidenced by verbal reports, distraction behaviors, and narrowed focus.

impaired Urinary Elimination may be related to inflammation/irritation of bladder, possibly evidenced by frequency, nocturia, and dysuria.

deficient Knowledge [Learning Need] regarding condition, treatment, and prevention of recurrence may be related to inadequate information/misconceptions, possibly evidenced by statements of concern and questions; recurrent infections.

Cytomegalic inclusion disease   CH
(Refer to Cytomegalovirus infection)

Cytomegalovirus (CMV) infection   CH
risk for disturbed visual Sensory Perception: risk factors may include inflammation of the retina.

risk for fetal Infection: risk factors may include transplacental exposure, contact with blood/body fluids.

D&C   **OB/GYN**
(Refer to Dilation and curettage)

Deep Vein Thrombosis   **CH/MS**
(Refer to Thrombophlebitis)

Degenerative disc disease   **CH/MS**
(Refer to Herniated nucleus pulposus)

Degenerative joint disease   **CH**
(Refer to Arthritis, rheumatoid)
   (Although this is a degenerative process versus the inflammatory process of rheumatoid arthritis, nursing concerns are the same.)

Dehiscence, abdominal wound   **MS**
impaired Skin Integrity may be related to altered circulation, altered nutritional state (obesity/malnutrition), and physical stress on incision, possibly evidenced by poor/delayed wound healing and disruption of skin surface/wound closure.
   risk for Infection: risk factors may include inadequate primary defenses (separation of incision, traumatized intestines, environmental exposure).
   risk for impaired Tissue Integrity: risk factors may include exposure of abdominal contents to external environment.
   Fear/Anxiety [severe] may be related to crises, perceived threat of death, possibly evidenced by fearfulness, restless behaviors, and sympathetic stimulation.
   deficient Knowledge [Learning Need] regarding condition/prognosis and treatment needs may be related to lack of information/recall and misinterpretation of information, possibly evidenced by development of preventable complications, requests for information, and statement of concern.

Dehydration   **PED**
deficient Fluid Volume [specify] may be related to etiology as defined by specific situation, possibly evidenced by dry mucous membranes, poor skin turgor, decreased pulse volume/pressure, and thirst.
   risk for impaired Oral Mucous Membrane: risk factors may include dehydration and decreased salivation.
   deficient Knowledge [Learning Need] regarding fluid needs may be related to lack of information/misinterpretation, possibly evidenced by questions, statement of concern, and inadequate follow-through of instructions/development of preventable complications.

Delirium tremens   **MS/PSY**
(Also refer to Alcohol intoxication, acute)
   Anxiety [severe/panic]/Fear may be related to cessation of alcohol intake/physiological withdrawal, threat to self-concept, perceived threat of death, possibly evidenced by increased tension, apprehension, fear of unspecified consequences; identifies object of fear.
   disturbed Sensory Perception (specify) may be related to exogenous (alcohol consumption/sudden cessation)/endogenous (electrolyte imbalance, elevated ammonia and blood urea nitrogen [BUN]) chemical alterations, sleep deprivation, and psychological stress, possibly evidenced by disorientation, restlessness, irritability, exaggerated emotional responses, bizarre thinking, and visual and auditory distortions/hallucinations.
   risk for decreased Cardiac Output: risk factors may include direct effect of alcohol on heart muscle, altered SVR, presence of dysrhythmias.
   risk for Trauma: risk factors may include alterations in balance, reduced muscle coordination, cognitive impairment, and involuntary clonic/tonic muscle activity.

imbalanced Nutrition: less than body requirements may be related to poor dietary intake, effects of alcohol on organs involved in digestion, interference with absorption/metabolism of nutrients and amino acids, possibly evidenced by reports of inadequate food intake, altered taste sensation, lack of interest in food, debilitated state, decreased subcutaneous fat/muscle mass, signs of mineral/electrolyte deficiency, including abnormal laboratory findings.

Delivery, precipitous/out of hospital OB
(Also refer to Labor, precipitous; Labor stages I–IV)

risk for deficient Fluid Volume: risk factors may include presence of nausea/vomiting, lack of intake, excessive vascular loss.

risk for Infection: risk factors may include broken/traumatized tissue, increased environmental exposure, rupture of amniotic membranes.

risk for fetal Injury: risk factors may include rapid descent/pressure changes, compromised circulation, environmental exposure.

Delusional disorder   PSY
risk for self/other-directed Violence: risk factors may include perceived threats of danger, increased feelings of anxiety, acting out in an irrational manner.

[severe] Anxiety may be related to inability to trust, possibly evidenced by rigid delusional system, frightened of other people and own hostility.

Powerlessness may be related to lifestyle of helplessness, feelings of inadequacy, interpersonal interaction, possibly evidenced by verbal expressions of no control/influence over situation(s), use of paranoid delusions, aggressive behavior to compensate for lack of control.

disturbed Thought Processes may be related to psychological conflicts, increasing anxiety/fear, possibly evidenced by interference with ability to think clearly/logically, fragmentation and autistic thinking, delusions, beliefs and behaviors of suspicion/violence.

impaired Social Interaction may be related to mistrust of others/delusional thinking, lack of knowledge/skills to enhance mutuality, possibly evidenced by discomfort in social situations, difficulty in establishing relationships with others, expression of feelings of rejection, no sense of belonging.

Dementia, HIV   CH/PSY
(Also refer to Dementia, presenile/senile)

acute/chronic Confusion may be related to direct CNS infection with HIV, disseminated systemic opportunistic infection, hypoxemia, brain malignancies, CVA, vasculitis, altered drug metabolism/excretion, electrolyte imbalance, sleep deprivation, possibly evidenced by fluctuation of cognition, progressive cognitive impairment, increased agitation, restlessness, altered interpretation/response to stimuli, clinical evidence of organic impairment.

[mild to severe] Anxiety may be related to threat to self-concept, unmet needs, perceived threat/change in health status, interpersonal transmission/contagion, possibly evidenced by reports of feeling scared, shaky, increased tension, loss of control/"going crazy," apprehension, increased wariness, extraneous movements/tremors, increased somatic complaints.

ineffective family Coping (specify) may be related to prolonged disease progression that exhausts the supportive capacity of SOs, highly ambivalent family relationship, sense of shame/guilt related to diagnosis, other crises SOs may be facing, possibly evidenced by intolerance, rejection, abandonment, neglectful relationships with other family members, SO preoccupied with personal reaction, distortion of reality of health problem.

Dementia, presenile/senile   CH/PSY
(Also refer to Alzheimer's disease)

impaired Memory may be related to neurological disturbances, possibly evidenced by observed experiences of forgetting, inability to determine if a behavior was performed, inability to perform previously learned skills, inability to recall factual information or recent/past events.

Fear may be related to decreases in functional abilities, public disclosure of disabilities, further mental/physical deterioration, possibly evidenced by social isolation, apprehension, irritability, defensiveness, suspiciousness, aggressive behavior.

Self-Care Deficit [specify] may be related to cognitive decline, physical limitations, frustration over loss of independence, depression, possibly evidenced by impaired ability to perform ADLs.

risk for Trauma: risk factors may include changes in muscle coordination/balance, impaired judgment, seizure activity.

risk for Caregiver Role Strain: risk factors may include illness severity of care receiver, duration of caregiving required, care receiver exhibiting deviant/bizarre behavior; family/caregiver isolation, lack of respite/recreation, spouse is caregiver.

Dementia, vascular   CH/PSY
(Refer to Alzheimer's disease)

Depersonalization disorder   PSY
(Refer to Dissociative disorders)

Depressant abuse   CH/PSY
(Also refer to Drug overdose, acute [depressants])

ineffective Denial may be related to weak underdeveloped ego, unmet self-needs, possibly evidenced by inability to admit impact of condition on life, minimizes symptoms/problem, refuses healthcare attention.

ineffective Coping may be related to weak ego, possibly evidenced by abuse of chemical agents, lack of goal-directed behavior, inadequate problem-solving, destructive behavior toward self.

imbalanced Nutrition: less than body requirements may be related to use of substance in place of nutritional food, possibly evidenced by loss of weight, pale conjunctiva and mucous membranes, electrolyte imbalances, anemias.

risk for Injury: risk factors may include changes in sleep, decreased concentration, loss of inhibitions.

Depression, major   PSY
risk for self-directed Violence: risk factors may include depressed mood and feelings of worthlessness and hopelessness.

[moderate to severe] Anxiety/disturbed Thought Processes may be related to psychological conflicts, unconscious conflict about essential values/goals of life, unmet needs, threat to self-concept, sleep deprivation, interpersonal transmission/contagion, possibly evidenced by reports of nervousness or fearfulness, feelings of inadequacy; agitation, angry/tearful outbursts, rambling/discoordinated speech, restlessness, hand rubbing or wringing, tremulousness; poor memory/concentration, decreased ability to grasp ideas, inability to follow/impaired ability to make decisions, numerous/repetitious physical complaints without organic cause, ideas of reference, hallucinations/delusions.

Insomnia may be related to biochemical alterations (decreased serotonin), unresolved fears and anxieties, and inactivity, possibly evidenced by difficulty in falling/remaining asleep, early morning awakening/awakening later than desired, reports of not feeling rested, physical signs (e.g., dark circles under eyes, excessive yawning); hypersomnia (using sleep as an escape).

Social Isolation/impaired Social Interaction may be related to alterations in mental status/thought processes (depressed mood), inadequate personal resources, decreased energy/inertia, difficulty engaging in satisfying personal relationships, feelings of worthlessness/low self-concept, inadequacy in or absence of significant purpose in life, and knowledge/skill deficit about social interactions, possibly evidenced by decreased involvement with others, expressed feelings of difference from others, remaining in home/room/bed, refusing invitations/suggestions of social involvement, and dysfunctional interaction with peers, family, or others.

interrupted Family Processes may be related to situational crises of illness of family member with change in roles/responsibilities, developmental crises (e.g., loss of family member/relationship), possibly evidenced by statements of difficulty coping with situation, family system not meeting needs of its members, difficulty accepting or receiving help appropriately, ineffective family decision-making process, and failure to send and to receive clear messages.

Depression, postpartum   OB/PSY
(Also refer to Depressive disorders)
risk for impaired parent/infant Attachment: risk factors may include anxiety associated with the parent role, inability to meet personal needs, perceived guilt regarding relationship with infant.

risk for other-directed Violence: risk factors may include hopelessness, increased anxiety, mood swings, despondency, severe depression/psychosis.

Depressive disorders   PSY
(Refer to Depression, major, Bipolar disorder, Premenstrual Dysphoric disorder)

de Quervain's syndrome   CH
acute/chronic Pain may be related to inflammation of tendon sheath at base of thumb, swelling, possibly evidenced by verbal reports, reluctance to use affected hand, guarding behaviors, expressed fear of reinjury, altered ability to continue previous activities.

impaired physical Mobility may be related to musculoskeletal impairment/swelling and pain, numbness of thumb/index finger, possibly evidenced by decreased grasp/pinch strength, weakness, limited range of motion of thumb, and reluctance to attempt movement.

Dermatitis, contact   CH
acute Pain/[Discomfort] may be related to cutaneous inflammation and irritation, possibly evidenced by verbal reports, irritability, and scratching.

impaired Skin Integrity may be related to exposure to chemicals/environmental allergens, pruritus, possibly evidenced by inflammation, epidermal edema, development of vesicles/bullae.

risk for Infection: risk factors may include broken skin and tissue trauma.

Social Isolation may be related to alterations in physical appearance, possibly evidenced by expressed feelings of rejection and decreased interaction with peers.

Dermatitis, seborrheic   CH
impaired Skin Integrity may be related to chronic inflammatory condition of the skin, possibly evidenced by disruption of skin surface with dry or moist scales, yellowish crusts, erythema, and fissures.

Developmental disorders, pervasive PED/PSY
(Refer to Autistic disorder; Rett's syndrome; Asperger's disorder)

Diabetes, gestational   OB
(Also refer to Diabetes mellitus)
risk for fetal Injury: risk factors may include elevated maternal serum glucose levels, changes in circulation.

risk for maternal Injury: risk factors may include changes in diabetic control, abnormal blood profile/anemia, tissue hypoxia, altered immune response.

deficient Knowledge [Learning Need] regarding diabetic condition, prognosis, self-care treatment needs may be related to lack of resources/exposure to information, misinformation, lack of recall, possibly evidenced by questions, statements of misconception, inaccurate follow-through of instructions, development of preventable complications.

Diabetes insipidus   MS/CH

deficient Fluid Volume [hypertonic] may be related to failure of regulatory mechanisms/hormone imbalance (e.g., brain injury, medication, sickle cell anemia, hypothyroidism), possibly evidenced by urinary frequency, thirst/polydipsia, dilute urine, dry skin/mucous membranes, decreased skin turgor, nocturia, increased serum sodium.

risk for ineffective Therapeutic Regimen Management: risk factors may include complexity of medication regimen, presence of side effects, economic difficulties, inadequate knowledge, perceived seriousness/benefits.

Diabetes, juvenile   PED

(Also refer to Diabetes mellitus)

risk for Injury: risk factors may include ineffective control/swings in serum glucose level, changes in mentation, developmental age, risk-taking behaviors.

ineffective Coping may be related to maturational crisis (desire to be like peers), inadequate level of perception of control, gender differences in coping strategies, possibly evidenced by use of forms of coping that impede adaptive behavior, inadequate problem-solving, risk-taking, destructive behavior toward self (loss of/inadequate diabetic control).

risk for ineffective Therapeutic Regimen Management: risk factors may include complexity/duration of treatmemt, perceived excessive demands made on individual, powerlessness, perceived susceptibility to complications.

Diabetes mellitus   CH/PED

deficient Knowledge [Learning Need] regarding disease process/treatment and individual care needs may be related to unfamiliarity with information/lack of recall, misinterpretation, possibly evidenced by requests for information, statements of concern/misconceptions, inadequate follow-through of instructions, and development of preventable complications.

risk for unstable blood Glucose: risk factors may include lack of adherence to diabetes management, medication management, indequate blood glucose monitoring, physical activity level, health status, stress, rapid growth periods.

imbalanced Nutrition: less than body requirements may be related to inability to utilize nutrients (imbalance between intake and utilization of glucose) to meet metabolic needs, possibly evidenced by change in weight, muscle weakness, increased thirst/urination, and hyperglycemia.

risk for risk-prone health Behavior: risk factors may include all-encompassing change in lifestyle, self-concept requiring lifelong adherence to therapeutic regimen and internal/altered locus of control.

risk for Infection: risk factors may include decreased leukocyte function, circulatory changes, and delayed healing.

risk for disturbed Sensory Perception (specify): risk factors may include endogenous chemical alteration (glucose/insulin or electrolyte imbalance).

compromised family Coping may be related to inadequate or incorrect information or understanding by primary person(s), other situational/developmental crises or situations the significant person(s) may be facing, lifelong condition requiring behavioral changes impacting family, possibly evidenced by family expressions of confusion about what to do, verbalizations that they are having difficulty coping with situation; family does not meet physical/emotional needs of its members; SO(s) preoccupied with personal reaction (e.g., guilt, fear), display protective behavior disproportionate (too little/too much) to client's abilities or need for autonomy.

Diabetes mellitus, intrapartum   OB
(Also refer to Diabetes mellitus)

risk for Trauma/impaired fetal Gas Exchange: risk factors may include inadequate maternal diabetic control, presence of macrosomia or intrauterine growth retardation (IUGR).

risk for maternal Injury: risk factors may include inadequate diabetic control (hypertension, severe edema, ketoacidosis, uterine atony/overdistention, dystocia).

[mild to moderate] Anxiety may be related to situational "crisis"/threat to health status (maternal or fetus), possibly evidenced by increased tension, apprehension, fear of unspecific consequences, sympathetic stimulation.

Diabetes mellitus, postpartum   OB

risk for imbalanced Nutrition: less than body requirements: risk factors may include inability to ingest/utilize nutrients appropriately, increased metabolic demands (recuperation, lactation).

risk for Injury: risk factors may include biochemical or regulatory complications (e.g., uterine hemorrhage, hypertension, hyperglycemia).

risk for impaired parent/infant Attachment: risk factors may include interruption in bonding process, physical illness/changes in physical abilities.

Diabetic ketoacidosis   CH/MS

deficient Fluid Volume [specify] may be related to hyperosmolar urinary losses, gastric losses, and inadequate intake, possibly evidenced by increased urinary output/dilute urine; reports of weakness, thirst; sudden weight loss, hypotension, tachycardia, delayed capillary refill, dry mucous membranes, poor skin turgor.

imbalanced Nutrition: less than body requirements that may be related to inadequate utilization of nutrients (insulin deficiency), decreased oral intake, hypermetabolic state, possibly evidenced by recent weight loss, reports of weakness, lack of interest in food, gastric fullness/abdominal pain, and increased ketones, imbalance between glucose/insulin levels.

unstable blood Glucose may be related to medication management, lack of diabetes management, inadequate blood glucose monitoring, presence of infection, possibly evidenced by elevated serum glucose level, presence of ketones in urine, nausea, weight loss, blurred vision, irritability.

Fatigue may be related to decreased metabolic energy production, altered body chemistry (insufficient insulin), increased energy demands (hypermetabolic state/infection), possibly evidenced by overwhelming lack of energy, inability to maintain usual routines, decreased performance, impaired ability to concentrate, listlessness.

risk for Infection: risk factors may include high glucose levels, decreased leukocyte function, stasis of body fluids, invasive procedures, alteration in circulation/perfusion.

Dialysis, general   CH
(Also refer to Dialysis, peritoneal; hemodialysis)

imbalanced Nutrition: less than body requirements may be related to inadequate ingestion of nutrients (dietary restrictions, anorexia, nausea/vomiting, stomatitis), loss of peptides and amino acids (building blocks for proteins) during procedure, possibly evidenced by reported inadequate intake, aversion to eating, altered taste sensation, poor muscle tone/weakness, sore/inflamed buccal cavity, pale conjunctiva/mucous membranes.

Grieving may be related to actual or perceived loss, chronic or fatal illness, and thwarted grieving response to a loss, possibly evidenced by verbal expression of distress/unresolved issues, denial of loss; altered eating habits, sleep and dream patterns, activity levels, libido; crying, labile affect; feelings of sorrow, guilt, and anger.

disturbed Body Image/situational low Self-Esteem may be related to situational crisis and chronic illness with changes in usual roles/body image, possibly evidenced by verbalization of changes in lifestyle, focus on past function, negative feelings about body, feelings of helplessness/powerlessness, extension of body boundary to incorporate environmental objects (e.g., dialysis setup), change in social involvement, overdependence on others for care, not taking responsibility for self-care/lack of follow-through, and self-destructive behavior.

Self-Care Deficit [specify] may be related to perceptual/cognitive impairment (accumulated toxins); intolerance to activity, decreased strength and endurance; pain/discomfort, possibly evidenced by reported inability to perform ADLs, disheveled/unkempt appearance, strong body odor.

Powerlessness may be related to illness-related regimen and healthcare environment, possibly evidenced by verbal expression of having no control, depression over physical deterioration, nonparticipation in care, anger, and passivity.

compromised/disabled family Coping may be related to inadequate or incorrect information or understanding by a primary person, temporary family disorganization and role changes, client providing little support in turn for the primary person, and prolonged disease/disability progression that exhausts the supportive capacity of significant persons, possibly evidenced by expressions of concern or reports about response of SO(s)/family to client's health problem, preoccupation of SO(s) with own personal reactions, display of intolerance/rejection, and protective behavior disproportionate (too little or too much) to client's abilities or need for autonomy.

Dialysis, peritoneal   MS/CH
(Also refer to Dialysis, general)

risk for excess Fluid Volume: risk factors may include inadequate osmotic gradient of dialysate, fluid retention (dialysate drainage problems/inappropriate osmotic gradient of solution, bowel distention), excessive PO/IV intake.

risk for Trauma: risk factors may include improper placement during insertion or manipulation of catheter.

acute Pain may be related to procedural factors (catheter irritation, improper catheter placement), presence of edema/abdominal distention, inflammation, or infection, rapid infusion/infusion of cold or acidic dialysate, possibly evidenced by verbal reports, guarding/distraction behaviors, and self-focus.

risk for Infection [peritonitis]: risk factors may include contamination of catheter/infusion system, skin contaminants, sterile peritonitis (response to composition of dialysate).

risk for ineffective Breathing Pattern: risk factors may include increased abdominal pressure with restricted diaphragmatic excursion, rapid infusion of dialysate, pain/discomfort, inflammatory process (e.g., atelectasis/pneumonia).

Diaper rash   PED
(Refer to Candidiasis)

Diaphragmatic Hernia   CH/MS
(Refer to Hernia, hiatal)

Diarrhea   PED/CH
deficient Knowledge [Learning Need] regarding causative/contributing factors and therapeutic needs may be related to lack of information/misconceptions, possibly evidenced by statements of concern, questions, and development of preventable complications.

risk for deficient Fluid Volume: Risk factors may include excessive losses through GI tract, altered intake.

acute Pain may be related to abdominal cramping and irritation/excoriation of skin, possibly evidenced by verbal reports, facial grimacing, and autonomic responses.

impaired Skin Integrity may be related to effects of excretions on delicate tissues, possibly evidenced by reports of discomfort and disruption of skin surface/destruction of skin layers.

DIC   MS
(Refer to Disseminated intravascular coagulation)

Diffuse axonal (brain) injury   MS
(Refer to Traumatic brain injury; Cerebrovascular accident)

Digitalis toxicity   MS/CH
decreased Cardiac Output may be related to altered myocardial contractility/electrical conduction, properties of digitalis (long half-life and narrow therapeutic range), concurrent medications, age/general health status, and electrolyte/acid-base balance, possibly evidenced by changes in rate/rhythm/conduction (development/worsening of dysrhythmias), changes in mentation, worsening of heart failure, elevated serum drug levels.

risk for imbalanced Fluid Volume: risk factors may include excessive losses from vomiting/diarrhea, decreased intake/nausea, decreased plasma proteins, malnutrition, continued use of diuretics; excess sodium/fluid retention.

deficient Knowledge [Learning Need] regarding condition/therapy and self-care needs may be related to information misinterpretation and lack of recall, possibly evidenced by inaccurate follow-through of instructions and development of preventable complications.

risk for disturbed Thought Processes: risk factors may include physiological effects of toxicity/reduced cerebral perfusion.

Dilation and Curettage   OB/GYN
(Also refer to Abortion, elective or spontaneous termination)

deficient Knowledge [Learning Need] regarding surgical procedure, possible postprocedural complications, and therapeutic needs may be related to lack of exposure/unfamiliarity with information, possibly evidenced by requests for information and statements of concern/misconceptions.

Dilation of Cervix, premature   OB
(Also refer to Preterm labor)

Anxiety [specify level] may be related to situational crisis, threat of death/fetal loss, possibly evidenced by increased tension, apprehension, feelings of inadequacy, sympathic stimulation, and repetitive questioning.

risk for maternal Injury: risk factors may include surgical intervention, use of tocolytic drugs.

risk for fetal Injury: risk factors may include premature delivery, surgical procedure.

Grieving may be related to perceived potential fetal loss, possibly evidenced by expression of distress, guilt, anger, choked feelings.

Dislocation/subluxation of joint   CH
acute Pain may be related to lack of continuity of bone/joint, muscle spasms, edema, possibly evidenced by verbal or coded reports, guarded/protective behaviors, narrowed focus, autonomic responses.

risk for Injury: risk factors may include nerve impingement, improper fitting of splint device.

impaired physical Mobility may be related to immobilization device/activity restrictions, pain, edema, decreased muscle strength, possibly evidenced by limited range of motion, limited ability to perform motor skills, gait changes.

Disruptive behavior disorder   PED/PSY
(Refer to Oppositional defiant disorder)

Disseminated intravascular coagulation   MS
risk for deficient Fluid Volume: risk factors may include failure of regulatory mechanism (coagulation process) and active loss/hemorrhage.

ineffective Tissue Perfusion (specify) may be related to alteration of arterial/venous flow (microemboli throughout circulatory system, and hypovolemia), possibly evidenced by changes in respiratory rate and depth, changes in mentation, decreased urinary output, and development of acral cyanosis/focal gangrene.

Anxiety [specify level]/Fear may be related to sudden change in health status/threat of death, interpersonal transmission/contagion, possibly evidenced by sympathetic stimulation, restlessness, focus on self, and apprehension.

risk for impaired Gas Exchange: risk factors may include reduced oxygen-carrying capacity, development of acidosis, fibrin deposition in microcirculation, and ischemic damage of lung parenchyma.

acute Pain may be related to bleeding into joints/muscles, with hematoma formation, and ischemic tissues with areas of acral cyanosis/focal gangrene, possibly evidenced by verbal reports, narrowed focus, alteration in muscle tone, guarding/distraction behaviors, restlessness, autonomic responses.

Dissociative disorders   PSY
[severe/panic] Anxiety/Fear may be related to a maladaptation or ineffective coping continuing from early life, unconscious conflict(s), threat to self-concept, unmet needs, or phobic stimulus, possibly evidenced by maladaptive response to stress (e.g., dissociating self/fragmentation of the personality), increased tension, feelings of inadequacy, and focus on self, projection of personal perceptions onto the environment.

risk for self/other-directed Violence: risk factors may include dissociative state/conflicting personalities, depressed mood, panic states, and suicidal or homicidal behaviors.

disturbed Personal Identity may be related to psychological conflicts (dissociative state), childhood trauma/abuse, threat to physical integrity/self-concept, and underdeveloped ego, possibly evidenced by alteration in perception or experience of the self, loss of one's own sense of reality/the external world, poorly differentiated ego boundaries, confusion about sense of self, purpose or direction in life; memory loss, presence of more than one personality within the individual.

compromised family Coping may be related to multiple stressors repeated over time, prolonged progression of disorder that exhausts the supportive capacity of significant person(s), family disorganization and role changes, high-risk family situation, possibly evidenced by family/SO(s) describing inadequate understanding or knowledge that interferes with assistive or supportive behaviors; relationship and marital conflict.

Diverticulitis   CH
acute Pain may be related to inflammation of intestinal mucosa, abdominal cramping, and presence of fever/chills, possibly evidenced by verbal reports, guarding/distraction behaviors, autonomic responses, and narrowed focus.

Diarrhea/Constipation may be related to altered structure/function and presence of inflammation, possibly evidenced by signs and symptoms dependent on specific problem (e.g., increase/decrease in frequency of stools and change in consistency).

deficient Knowledge [Learning Need] regarding disease process, potential complications, thera-peutic and self-care needs may be related to lack of information/misconceptions, possibly evidenced by statements of concern, request for information, and development of preventable complications.

risk for Powerlessness: risk factors may include chronic nature of disease process and recurrent episodes despite cooperation with medical regimen.

Down syndrome   PED/CH
(Also refer to Mental retardation)

delayed Growth and Development may be related to effects of physical/mental disability, possibly evidenced by altered physical growth; delay/inability in performing skills and self-care/self-control activities appropriate for age.

risk for Trauma: risk factors may include cognitive difficulties and poor muscle tone/coordination, weakness.

imbalanced Nutrition: less than body requirements may be related to poor muscle tone and protruding tongue, possibly evidenced by weak and ineffective sucking/swallowing and observed lack of adequate intake with weight loss/failure to gain.

interrupted Family Processes may be related to situational/maturational crises requiring incorporation of new skills into family dynamics, possibly evidenced by confusion about what to do, verbalized difficulty coping with situation, unexamined family myths.

risk for complicated Grieving: risk factors may include loss of "the perfect child," chronic condition requiring long-term care, and unresolved feelings.

risk for impaired parent/infant/child Attachment: risk factors may include ill infant/child who is unable to effectively initiate parental contact due to altered behavioral organization, inability of parents to meet the personal needs.

risk for Social Isolation: risk factors may include withdrawal from usual social interactions and activities, assumption of total child care, and becoming overindulgent/overprotective.

Dressler's syndrome   CH
acute Pain may be related to tissue inflammation and presence of effusion, possibly evidenced by verbal reports of chest pain affected by movement/position and deep breathing, guarding/distraction behaviors, self-focus, and autonomic responses (changes in vital signs).

Anxiety [specify level] may be related to threat to/change in health status, possibly evidenced by increased tension, apprehension, restlessness, and expressed concerns.

risk for ineffective Breathing Pattern: risk factors may include pain on inspiration.

risk for impaired Gas Exchange: risk factors may include ventilation perfusion imbalance (pleural effusion, pulmonary infiltrates).

Drug overdose, acute (depressants) MS/PSY
(Also refer to Substance dependence/abuse rehabilitation)

ineffective Breathing Pattern/impaired Gas Exchange may be related to neuromuscular impairment/CNS depression, decreased lung expansion, possibly evidenced by changes in respirations, cyanosis, and abnormal ABGs.

risk for Trauma/Suffocation/Poisoning: risk factors may include CNS depression/agitation, hypersensitivity to the drug(s), psychological stress.

risk for self/other-directed Violence: risk factors may include suicidal behaviors, toxic reactions to drug(s).

risk for Infection: risk factors may include drug injection techniques, impurities in injected drugs, localized trauma; malnutrition, altered immune state.

Drug withdrawal   CH/MS
disturbed Thought Processes may be related to substance abuse/cessation, sleep deprivation, malnutrition, possibly evidenced by inaccurate interpretation of environment, inappropriate/nonreality-based thinking, paranoia.

risk for Injury: risk factors may include CNS agitation (depressants).

risk for Suicide: risk factors may include alcohol/substance abuse, legal/disciplinary problems, depressed mood (stimulants).

acute Pain [/Discomfort] may be related to biochemical changes associated with cessation of drug use, possibly evidenced by reports of muscle aches, fever, diaphoresis, rhinorrhea/lacrimation, malaise.

Self-Care Deficit (specify) may be related to perceptual/cognitive impairment, therapeutic management (restraints), possibly evidenced by inability to meet own physical needs.

Insomnia may be related to cessation of substance use, fatigue, possibly evidenced by reports of insomnia/hypersomnia, decreased ability to function, increased irritability.

Fatigue may be related to altered body chemistry (drug withdrawal), sleep deprivation, malnutrition, poor physical condition, possibly evidenced by verbal reports of overwhelming lack of energy, inability to maintain usual level of physical activity, inability to restore energy after sleep, compromised concentration.

DTs   **MS/PSY**
(Refer to Delirium tremens)

Duchenne's muscular dystrophy   **PED/CH**
(Refer to Muscular dystrophy [Duchenne's])

Duodenal ulcer   **MS/CH**
(Refer to Ulcer, peptic)

DVT   **CH/MS**
(Refer to Thrombophlebitis)

Dysmenorrhea   **GYN**
acute Pain may be related to exaggerated uterine contractibility, possibly evidenced by verbal reports, guarding/distraction behaviors, narrowed focus, and autonomic responses (changes in vital signs).

risk for Activity Intolerance: risk factors may include severity of pain and presence of secondary symptoms (nausea, vomiting, syncope, chills), depression.

ineffective Coping may be related to chronic, recurrent nature of problem; anticipatory anxiety, and inadequate coping methods, possibly evidenced by muscular tension, headaches, general irritability, chronic depression, and verbalization of inability to cope, report of poor self-concept.

Dyspareunia   **GYN/PSY**
Sexual Dysfunction may be related to physical or psychological alteration in function (menopausal involution, allergy to contraceptive, abnormalities of genital tract, guilt, control issues), possibly evidenced by verbalization of problem, inability to achieve desired satisfaction, sexual aversion, alteration in relationship with significant other.

Anxiety [specify] may be related to situational crisis, stress, unconscious conflict about essential values, unmet needs, possibly evidenced by expressed concerns, distressed, feelings of inadequacy.

Dysrhythmia, cardiac   **CH/MS**
risk for decreased Cardiac Output: risk factors may include altered electrical conduction and reduced myocardial contractility.

Anxiety [specify level] may be related to perceived threat of death, possibly evidenced by increased tension, apprehension, and expressed concerns.

deficient Knowledge [Learning Need] regarding medical condition/therapy needs may be related to lack of information/misinterpretation and unfamiliarity with information resources, possibly evidenced by questions, statement of misconception, failure to improve on previous regimen, and development of preventable complications.

risk for Activity Intolerance: risk factors may include imbalance between myocardial O_2 supply and demand, and cardiac depressant effects of certain drugs (beta-blockers, antidysrhythmics).

risk for Poisoning [digitalis toxicity]: risk factors may include limited range of therapeutic effectiveness, lack of education/proper precautions, reduced vision/cognitive limitations.

Dysthymic disorder   PSY/CH
(Refer to Depression, major)

Dystocia   OB
(Also refer to Labor, stage I [latent/active phases])

risk for maternal Injury: risk factors may include alteration of muscle tone/contractile pattern, mechanical obstruction to fetal descent, maternal fatigue.

risk for fetal Injury: risk factors may include prolonged labor, fetal malpresentations, tissue hypoxia/acidosis, abnormalities of the maternal pelvis, CPD.

risk for deficient Fluid Volume: risk factors may include hypermetabolic state, vomiting, profuse diaphoresis, restricted oral intake, mild diuresis associated with oxytocin administration.

ineffective Coping may be related to situational crisis, personal vulnerability, unrealistic expectations/perceptions, inadequate/exhausted support systems, possibly evidenced by verbalizations and behavior indicative of inability to cope (loss of control, inability to problem-solve, or meet role expectations), irritability, reports of fatigue/tension.

Eating disorders   CH/PSY
(Refer to Anorexia nervosa; Bulimia nervosa)

Ebola   MS
(Also refer to Disseminated intravascular coagulation; Multiple organ dysfunction syndrome)

acute Pain [/Discomfort] may be related to infectious process, possibly evidenced by reports of headache, myalgia, abdominal or chest pain, sore throat, fever.

Hyperthermia may be related to inflammatory process, possibly evidenced by increased body temperature, flushes/warm skin, headache.

risk for deficient Fluid Volume: risk factors may include inadequate intake (nausea, painful swallowing, abdominal pain), increased losses (vomiting, diarrhea, hemorrhage/DIC), hypermetabolic state (fever).

risk for [spread of/secondary] Infection: risk factors may include mode of transmission, invasive monitoring/procedures, debilitated state, malnutrition, insufficient knowledge/resources to avoid exposure to pathogens.

acute Confusion may be related to infectious process, hypoxemia, possibly evidenced by fluctuations in cognition, agitation, change in level of consciousness (stupor/coma).

Eclampsia   OB
(Also refer to Pregnancy-Induced hypertension)

Anxiety [specify]/Fear may be related to situational crisis, threat of change in health status/death (self/fetus), separation from support system, interpersonal contagion, possibly evidenced by expressed concerns, apprehension, increased tension, decreased self-assurance, difficulty concentrating.

risk for maternal Injury: risk factors may include tissue edema/hypoxia, tonic-clonic convulsions, abnormal blood profile or clotting factors.

impaired physical Mobility may be related to prescribed bedrest, discomfort, anxiety, possibly evidenced by difficulty turning, postural instability.

risk for Self-Care Deficit (specify): risk factors may include weakness, discomfort, physical restrictions.

ECT   PSY
(Refer to Electroconvulsive therapy)

Ectopic pregnancy (tubal)   OB
(Also refer to Abortion, spontaneous termination)

acute Pain may be related to distention/rupture of fallopian tube, possibly evidenced by verbal reports, guarding/distraction behaviors, facial mask of pain, and autonomic responses (diaphoresis, changes in vital signs).

risk for deficient Fluid Volume [isotonic]: risk factors may include hemorrhagic losses and decreased/restricted intake.

Anxiety [specify level]/Fear may be related to threat of death and possible loss of ability to conceive, possibly evidenced by increased tension, apprehension, sympathetic stimulation, restlessness, and focus on self.

Eczema   CH
(Refer to Dermatitis, contact/seborrheic)

Pain [/Discomfort] may be related to cutaneous inflammation and irritation, possibly evidenced by verbal reports, irritability, and scratching.

risk for Infection: risk factors may include broken skin and tissue trauma.

Social Isolation may be related to alterations in physical appearance, possibly evidenced by expressed feelings of rejection and decreased interaction with peers.

Edema, pulmonary   MS

excess Fluid Volume may be related to decreased cardiac functioning, excessive fluid/sodium intake, possibly evidenced by dyspnea, presence of crackles (rales), pulmonary congestion on radiograph, restlessness, anxiety, and increased central venous pressure (CVP)/pulmonary pressures.

impaired Gas Exchange may be related to altered blood flow and decreased alveolar/capillary exchange (fluid collection/shifts into interstitial space/alveoli), possibly evidenced by hypoxia, restlessness, and confusion.

Anxiety [specify level]/Fear may be related to perceived threat of death (inability to breathe), possibly evidenced by responses ranging from apprehension to panic state, restlessness, and focus on self.

Elder abuse   CH/PSY
(Refer to Abuse, physical/psychological)

Electrical injury   MS
(Also refer to Burns)

risk for decreased Cardiac Output: risk factors may include altered heart rate/rhythm (ventricular fibrillation/asystole).

impaired [internal] Tissue Integrity may be related to thermal injury (along path of current), altered circulation (massive edema), possibly evidenced by damaged or destroyed tissue/necrosis.

risk for impaired peripheral Tissue Perfusion: risk factors may include reduction of venous/arterial blood flow (vein coagulation, muscle edema), increased tissue pressure (compartment syndrome).

risk for Trauma/Suffocation: risk factors may include muscle paralysis (CNS damage), loss of large- or small-muscle coordination (seizures).

Electroconvulsive therapy   PSY

decisional Conflict may be related to lack of relevant or multiple/divergent sources of information, mistrust of regimen/healthcare personnel, sense of powerlessness, support system deficit.

risk for Injury [effects of electroconvulsive therapy (ECT)]: risk factors may include effects of therapy on the cardiovascular, respiratory, musculoskeletal, and nervous systems, and pharmacological effects of anesthesia.

acute Confusion may be related to CNS effects of electric shock and medications/anesthesia, possibly evidenced by fluctuation in cognition, agitation.

impaired Memory may be related to neurological disturbance (electrical shock), possibly evidenced by reported/observed experiences of forgetting, difficulty recalling recent events/factual information.

Emphysema   CH/MS

impaired Gas Exchange may be related to alveolar capillary membrane changes/destruction, possibly evidenced by dyspnea, restlessness, changes in mentation, abnormal ABG values.

ineffective Airway Clearance may be related to increased production/retained tenacious secretions, decreased energy level, and muscle wasting, possibly evidenced by abnormal breath sounds (rhonchi), ineffective cough, changes in rate/depth of respirations, and dyspnea.

Activity Intolerance may be related to imbalance between O_2 supply and demand, possibly evidenced by reports of fatigue/weakness, exertional dyspnea, and abnormal vital sign response to activity.

imbalanced Nutrition: less than body requirements may be related to inability to ingest food (shortness of breath, anorexia, generalized weakness, medication side effects), possibly evidenced by lack of interest in food, reported altered taste, loss of muscle mass and tone, fatigue, and weight loss.

risk for Infection: risk factors may include inadequate primary defenses (stasis of body fluids, decreased ciliary action), chronic disease process, and malnutrition.

Powerlessness may be related to illness-related regimen and healthcare environment, possibly evidenced by verbal expression of having no control, depression over physical deterioration, nonparticipation in therapeutic regimen, anger, and passivity.

Encephalitis   MS

risk for ineffective cerebral Tissue Perfusion: risk factors may include cerebral edema altering/interrupting cerebral arterial/venous blood flow, hypovolemia, exchange problems at cellular level (acidosis).

Hyperthermia may be related to increased metabolic rate, illness, and dehydration, possibly evidenced by increased body temperature, flushed/warm skin, and increased pulse and respiratory rates.

acute Pain may be related to inflammation/irritation of the brain and cerebral edema, possibly evidenced by verbal reports of headache, photophobia, distraction behaviors, restlessness, and autonomic response (changes in vital signs).

risk for Trauma/Suffocation: risk factors may include restlessness, clonic/tonic activity, altered sensorium, cognitive impairment, generalized weakness, ataxia, vertigo.

Encopresis   PSY/PED

disturbed Body Image/chronic low Self-Esteem may be related to negative view of self, maturational expectations, social factors, stigma attached to loss of body function in public, family's belief condition is volitional, shame related to body odor, possibly evidenced by angry outbursts/oppositional behavior, verbalization of powerlessness, reluctance to engage in social activities.

Bowel Incontinence may be related to situational/maturational crisis, psychogenic factors (predisposing vulnerability, threat to physical integrity—child/sexual abuse), possibly evidenced by involuntary passage of stool at least once monthly, strong odor of feces on client, hiding soiled clothing in inappropriate places.

compromised/disabled family Coping may be related to inadequate/incorrect information or understanding of condition, belief that behavior is volitional, disagreement regarding treatment/coping strategies, possibly evidenced by attempts to intervene with child are increasingly ineffective, significant person describes preoccupation with personal reaction (excessive guilt, anger, blame regarding child's condition/behavior), overprotective behavior.

Endocarditis   MS

risk for decreased Cardiac Output: risk factors may include inflammation of lining of heart and structural change in valve leaflets.

Anxiety [specify level] may be related to change in health status and threat of death, possibly evidenced by apprehension, expressed concerns, and focus on self.

acute Pain may be related to generalized inflammatory process and effects of embolic phenomena, possibly evidenced by verbal reports, narrowed focus, distraction behaviors, and autonomic responses (changes in vital signs).

risk for Activity Intolerance: risk factors may include imbalance between O_2 supply and demand, debilitating condition.

risk for ineffective Tissue Perfusion (specify): risk factors may include embolic interruption of arterial flow (embolization of thrombi/valvular vegetations).

End of life care   CH
(Refer to Hospice care)

Endometriosis   GYN

acute/chronic Pain may be related to pressure of concealed bleeding/formation of adhesions, possibly evidenced by verbal reports (pain between/with menstruation), guarding/distraction behaviors, and narrowed focus.

Sexual Dysfunction may be related to pain secondary to presence of adhesions, possibly evidenced by verbalization of problem and altered relationship with partner.

deficient Knowledge [Learning Need] regarding pathophysiology of condition and therapy needs may be related to lack of information/misinterpretations, possibly evidenced by statements of concern and misconceptions.

Enteral feeding   MS/CH

risk for Infection: risk factors may include invasive procedure/surgical placement of feeding tube, malnutrition, chronic disease.

risk for Aspiration: risk factors may include presence of feeding tube, bolus tube feedings, increased intragastric pressure, delayed gastric emptying, medication administration.

risk for imbalanced Fluid Volume: risk factors may include active loss/failure of regulatory mechanisms (specific to underlying disease process/trauma), inability to obtain/ingest fluids.

Fatigue may be related to decreased metabolic energy production, increased energy requirements (hypermetabolic state, healing process), altered body chemistry (medications, chemotherapy), possibly evidenced by overwhelming lack of energy, inability to maintain usual routines/accomplish routine tasks, lethargy, impaired ability to concentrate.

Enteritis   MS/CH
(Refer to Colitis, ulcerative; Crohn's disease)

Enuresis   PSY/PED

impaired Urinary Elimination may be related to situational/maturational crisis, psychogenic factors (predisposing vulnerability, threat to physical integrity—child/sexual abuse), possibly evidenced by nocturnal/diurinal enuresis, strong odor of urine on client, hiding soiled clothing in inappropriate places.

disturbed Body Image/chronic low Self-Esteem may be related to negative view of self, maturational expectations, social factors, stigma attached to loss of body function in public, family's belief condition is volitional, shame related to body odor, possibly evidenced by angry outbursts/oppositional behavior, verbalization of powerlessness, reluctance to engage in social activities.

ineffective family Coping (specify) may be related to inadequate/incorrect information or understanding of condition, belief that behavior is volitional, disagreement regarding treatment/coping strategies, possibly evidenced by attempts to intervene with child are increasingly ineffective, significant person describes preoccupation with personal reaction (excessive guilt, anger, blame regarding child's condition/behavior), overprotective behavior.

Epididymitis   MS

acute Pain may be related to inflammation, edema formation, and tension on the spermatic cord, possibly evidenced by verbal reports, guarding/distraction behaviors (restlessness), and autonomic responses (changes in vital signs).

risk for Infection [spread]: risk factors may include presence of inflammation/infectious process, insufficient knowledge to avoid spread of infection.

deficient Knowledge [Learning Need] regarding pathophysiology, outcome, and self-care needs may be related to lack of information/misinterpretations, possibly evidenced by statements of concern, misconceptions, and questions.

Epilepsy   CH
(Refer to Seizure disorder)

Episiotomy   OB

acute Pain may be related to tissue trauma/edema, surgical incision, possibly evidenced by verbalizations, guarding behavior, self-focusing.

risk for Infection: risk factors may include broken skin, traumatized tissue, body excretions, inadequate hygiene.

risk for Sexual Dysfunction: risk factors may include recent childbirth, presence of incision.

Epistaxis   CH

[mild to moderate] Anxiety may be related to situational crisis, threat to health status, interpersonal transmission, possibly evidenced by expressed concerns, apprehension, anxiety.

risk for Aspiration: risk factors may include uncontrolled nasal bleeding.

risk for impaired Tissue Integrity: risk factors may include altered circulation/mechanical compression.

Epstein-Barr virus   CH
(Refer to Mononucleosis, infectious)

Erectile dysfunction   CH/PSY

Sexual Dysfunction may be related to altered body function, side effects of medication, possibly evidenced by reports of disruption of sexual response pattern, inability to achieve desired satisfaction.

situational low Self-Esteem may be related to functional impairment, perceived failure to perform satisfactorily, rejection of other(s), possibly evidenced by self-negating verbalizations, expressions of helplessness/powerlessness.

Esophageal reflux disease   CH
(Refer to Gastroesophageal reflux disease)

Esophageal varcies   CH/MS
(Refer to Varcies, esophageal)

Esophagitis   CH
(Refer to Gastroesophageal reflux disease; Achalasia)

ETOH withdrawal   MS/CH
(Refer to Alcohol intoxication, acute; substance dependence/abuse rehabilitation)

Evisceration   MS
(Refer to Dehiscence, abdominal)

Facial reconstructive surgery   MS/CH
(Also refer to Surgery, general; Intermaxillary fixation)
  risk for ineffective Airway Clearance: risk factors may include soft tissue edema, airway trauma, retained secretions.
  impaired Skin Integrity may be related to traumatic injury, surgical procedure (incisions/grafts), edema, altered circulation, possibly evidenced by disruption/destruction of skin layers.
  Fear/Anxiety may be related to situational crisis, memory of traumatic event, threat to self-concept (disfigurement), possibly evidenced by expressed concerns, apprehension, uncertainty, decreased self-assurance, restlessness.
  disturbed Body Image may be related to traumatic event, disfigurement, possibly evidenced by negative feelings about self, fear of rejection reaction by others, preoccupation with change, change in social involvement.
  risk for Social Isolation: risk factors may include change in physical appearance.

Failure to thrive, adult   CH/MS
adult Failure to Thrive may be related to depression, apathy, aging process, fatigue, degenerative condition, possibly evidenced by expressed lack of appetite, difficulty performing self-care tasks, altered mood state, inadequate intake, weight loss, physical decline.
  ineffective Protection may be related to inadequate nutrition, anemia, extremes of age, possibly evidenced by fatigue, weakness, deficient immunity, impaired healing, pressure sores.

Failure to thrive, infant/child   PED
imbalanced Nutrition: less than body requirements may be related to inability to ingest/digest/absorb nutrients (defects in organ function/metabolism, genetic factors), physical deprivation/psychosocial factors, possibly evidenced by lack of appropriate weight gain/weight loss, poor muscle tone, pale conjunctiva, and laboratory tests reflecting nutritional deficiency.
  delayed Growth and Development may be related to inadequate caretaking (physical/emotional neglect or abuse); indifference, inconsistent responsiveness, multiple caretakers; environmental and stimulation deficiencies, possibly evidenced by altered physical growth, flat affect, listlessness, decreased response; delay or difficulty in performing skills or self-control activities appropriate for age group.
  risk for impaired Parenting: risk factors may include lack of knowledge, inadequate bonding, unrealistic expectations for self/infant, and lack of appropriate response of child to relationship.
  deficient Knowledge [Learning Need] regarding pathophysiology of condition, nutritional needs, growth/development expectations, and parenting skills may be related to lack of information/misinformation or misinterpretation, possibly evidenced by verbalization of concerns, questions, misconceptions; or development of preventable complications.

Fat embolism syndrome   MS
(Refer to Pulmonary embolism; Respiratory distress syndrome, acute)

Fatigue syndrome, chronic   CH

Fatigue may be related to disease state, inadequate sleep, possibly evidenced by verbalization of unremitting/overwhelming lack of energy, inability to maintain usual routines, listlessness, compromised concentration.

   chronic Pain may be related to chronic physical disability, possibly evidenced by verbal reports of headache, sore throat, arthralgias, abdominal pain, muscle aches, altered ability to continue previous activities, changes in sleep pattern.

   Self-Care Deficit [specify] may be related to tiredness, pain/discomfort, possibly evidenced by reports of inability to perform desired ADLs.

   risk for ineffective Role Performance: risk factors may include health alterations, stress.

Febrile seizure   PED

Hyperthermia may be related to illness, dehydration, decreased ability to perspire, possibly evidenced by increase in body temperature, flushed/warm skin, seizures.

Fecal diversion   MS/CH
(Refer to Colostomy)

Fecal impaction   CH

Constipation may be related to irregular defecation habits, decreased activity, dehydration, abdominal muscle weakness, neurological impairment, possibly evidenced by inability to pass stool, abdominal distention/tenderness/pain, nausea/vomiting, anorexia.

Femoral popliteal bypass   MS
(Also refer to Surgery, general)

   risk for ineffective peripheral Tissue Perfusion: risk factors may include interruption of arterial blood flow, hypovolemia.

   risk for Peripheral Neurovascular Dysfunction: risk factors may include vascular obstruction, immobilization, mechanical compression/dressings.

   impaired Walking may be related to surgical incisions, dressings, possibly evidenced by inability to walk desired distance, climb stairs, negotiate inclines.

Fetal alcohol syndrome   PED

risk for Injury [CNS damage]: risk factors may include external chemical factors (alcohol intake by mother), placental insufficiency, fetal drug withdrawal in utero/postpartum and prematurity.

   disorganized Infant Behavior may be related to prematurity, environmental overstimulation, lack of containment/boundaries, possibly evidenced by change from baseline physiological measures, tremors, startles, twitches, hyperextension of arms/legs, deficient self-regulatory behaviors, deficient response to visual/auditory stimuli.

   risk for impaired Parenting: risk factors may include mental or physical illness, inability of mother to assume the overwhelming task of unselfish giving and nurturing, presence of stressors (financial/legal problems), lack of available or ineffective role model, interruption of bonding process, lack of appropriate response of child to relationship.

PSY

ineffective [maternal] Coping may be related to personal vulnerability, low self-esteem, inadequate coping skills, and multiple stressors (repeated over period of time), possibly evidenced by inability to meet basic needs/fulfill role expectations/problem-solve, and excessive use of drug(s).

   dysfunctional Family Processes: alcoholism may be related to lack of/insufficient support from others, mother's drug problem and treatment status, together with poor coping skills, lack of family stability/overinvolvement of parents with children and multigenerational addictive behaviors, possibly evidenced by abandonment, rejection, neglectful relationships with family members, and decisions and actions by family that are detrimental.

Fetal demise   OB

Grieving may be related to death of fetus/infant (wanted or unwanted), inability to meet personal expectations, possibly evidenced by verbal expressions of distress, anger, loss, crying, alteration in eating habits or sleep pattern.

situational low Self-Esteem may be related to perceived "failure" at a life event, possibly evidenced by negative self-appraisal in response to life event in a person with a previous positive self-evaluation, verbalization of negative feelings about the self (helplessness, uselessness), difficulty making decisions.

risk for ineffective Role Performance: risk factors may include stress, family conflict, inadequate support system.

risk for interrupted Family Processes: risk factors may include situational crisis, developmental transition [loss of child], family roles shift.

risk for Spiritual Distress: risk factors may include loss of loved one, blame for loss directed at self/God, alienation from other/support systems, challenged belief and value system (birth is supposed to be the beginning of life, not of death) and intense suffering.

Fetal transfusion syndrome   OB
(Refer to Twin-twin transfusion syndrome)

Fibrocytic breast disease   CH

[mild to moderate] Anxiety may be related to situational crisis, threat to health status, family heredity, interpersonal transmission, possibly evidenced by expressed concerns, apprehension, uncertainty, fearful, focus on self, increased tension.

acute/chronic Pain may be related to physical agents (edema formation, nerve irritation), possibly evidenced by verbal reports, guarded/protective behavior, expressive behavior, self-focusing.

risk for ineffective Coping: risk factors may include situational crisis, perceived high degree of threat, inadequate resources/social supports.

Fibroids, uterine   GYN
(Refer to Uterine myomas)

Fibromyalgia syndrome, primary   CH

acute/chronic Pain may be related to idiopathic diffuse condition, possibly evidenced by reports of achy pain in fibrous tissues (muscles, tendons, ligaments), muscle stiffness/spasm, disturbed sleep, guarding behaviors, fear of reinjury/exacerbation, restlessness, irritability, self-focusing, reduced interaction with others.

Fatigue may be related to disease state, stress, anxiety, depression, sleep deprivation, possibly evidenced by verbalization of overwhelming lack of energy, inability to maintain usual routines/level of physical activity, tired, feelings of guilt for not keeping up with responsibilities, increase in physical complaints, listlessness.

risk for Hopelessness: risk factors may include chronic debilitating physical condition, prolonged activity restriction (possibly self-induced), creating isolation, lack of specific therapeutic cure, prolonged stress.

Flail chest   MS
(Refer to Hemothorax; Pneumothorax)

Food poisoning   CH/MS
(Refer to Gastroenteritis)

Fractures   MS/CH
(Also refer to Casts; Traction)

risk for Trauma [additional injury]: risk factors may include loss of skeletal integrity/movement of skeletal fragments, use of traction apparatus.

acute Pain may be related to muscle spasms, movement of bone fragments, tissue trauma/edema, traction/immobility device, stress, and anxiety, possibly evidenced by verbal reports, distraction behaviors, self-focusing/narrowed focus, facial mask of pain, guarding/protective behavior, alteration in muscle tone, and autonomic responses (changes in vital signs).

risk for Peripheral Neurovascular Dysfunction: risk factors may include reduction/interruption of blood flow (direct vascular injury, tissue trauma, excessive edema, thrombus formation, hypovolemia).

impaired physical Mobility may be related to neuromuscular/skeletal impairment, pain/discomfort, restrictive therapies (bedrest, extremity immobilization), and psychological immobility, possibly evidenced by inability to purposefully move within the physical environment, imposed restrictions, reluctance to attempt movement, limited range of motion, and decreased muscle strength/control.

risk for impaired Gas Exchange: risk factors may include altered blood flow, blood/fat emboli, alveolar/capillary membrane changes (interstitial/pulmonary edema, congestion).

deficient Knowledge [Learning Need] regarding healing process, therapy requirements, potential complications, and self-care needs may be related to lack of exposure, misinterpretation of information, possibly evidenced by statements of concern, questions, and misconceptions.

Frostbite   MS/CH
impaired Tissue Integrity may be related to altered circulation and thermal injury, possibly evidenced by damaged/destroyed tissue.

acute Pain may be related to diminished circulation with tissue ischemia/necrosis and edema formation, possibly evidenced by verbal reports, guarding/distraction behaviors, narrowed focus, and autonomic responses (changes in vital signs).

risk for Infection: risk factors may include traumatized tissue/tissue destruction, altered circulation, and compromised immune response in affected area.

Fusion, cervical   MS
(Refer to Laminectomy, cervical)

Fusion, lumbar   MS
(Refer to Laminectomy, lumbar)

Gallstones   CH
(Refer to Cholelithiasis)

Gangrene, dry   MS
ineffective peripheral Tissue Perfusion may be related to interruption in arterial flow, possibly evidenced by cool skin temperature, change in color (black), atrophy of affected part, and presence of pain.

acute Pain may be related to tissue hypoxia and necrotic process, possibly evidenced by verbal reports, guarding/distraction behaviors, narrowed focus, and autonomic responses (changes in vital signs).

Gangrene, gas   MS
impaired Tissue Integrity may be related to trauma/surgery, infection, altered circulation, possibly evidenced by edema, brown/serous exudate, bronze or blackish green skin color, gas bubbles/crepitation, pain.

[severe] Anxiety/Fear may be related to situational crisis, interpersonal transmission, threat of death, possibly evidenced by expressed concerns, distress, apprehension, fearfulness, restlessness, irritability, focus on self.

risk for impaired renal Tissue Perfusion: risk factors may include effects of circulating toxins, altered circulation/shock.

risk for Injury: risk factors may include therapeutic intervention (hyperbaric oxygen therapy).

Gas, lung irritant   MS/CH

ineffective Airway Clearance may be related to irritation/inflammation of airway, possibly evidenced by marked cough, abnormal breath sounds (wheezes), dyspnea, and tachypnea.

risk for impaired Gas Exchange: risk factors may include irritation/inflammation of alveolar membrane (dependent on type of agent and length of exposure).

Anxiety [specify level] may be related to change in health status and threat of death, possibly evidenced by verbalizations, increased tension, apprehension, and sympathetic stimulation.

Gastrectomy, subtotal   MS

(Also refer to Surgery, general)

risk for imbalanced Nutrition: less than body requirements: risk factors may include restricted oral intake/early satiety, change in digestive process/malabsorption of nutrients, fear of complications (e.g., dumping syndrome, reactive hypoglycemia).

risk for Fatigue: risk factors may include malnutrition, anemia.

risk for Diarrhea: risk factors may include malabsorption.

Gastric partitioning   MS

(Refer to Gastroplasty)

Gastric resection   MS

(Refer to Gastrectomy, subtotal)

Gastric ulcer   MS/CH

(Refer to Ulcer, peptic)

Gastrinoma   MS/CH

(Refer to Zollinger-Ellison syndrome)

Gastritis, acute   MS

acute Pain may be related to irritation/inflammation of gastric mucosa, possibly evidenced by verbal reports, guarding/distraction behaviors, and autonomic responses (changes in vital signs).

risk for deficient Fluid Volume [isotonic]: risk factors may include excessive losses through vomiting and diarrhea, continued bleeding, reluctance to ingest/restrictions of oral intake.

Gastritis, chronic   CH

risk for imbalanced Nutrition: less than body requirements: risk factors may include inability to ingest adequate nutrients (prolonged nausea/vomiting, anorexia, epigastric pain).

deficient Knowledge [Learning Need] regarding pathophysiology, psychological factors, therapy needs, and potential complications may be related to lack of information/misinterpretation, possibly evidenced by verbalization of concerns, questions, misconceptions, and continuation of problem.

Gastroenteritis   CH/MS

Diarrhea may be related to toxins, contaminants, travel, infectious process, parasites, possibly evidenced by at least three loose liquid stools/day, hyperactive bowel sounds, abdominal pain.

       Doenges Nursing Diagnosis Manual: Planning, Individualizing, and Documenting Client Care

risk for deficient Fluid Volume: risk factors may include excessive losses (diarrhea, vomiting), hypermetabolic state (infection), decreased intake (nausea, anorexia), extremes of age/weight.

risk for Infection [transmission]: risk factors may include insufficient knowledge to prevent contamination (inappropriate handwashing and food handling).

Gastroesophageal reflux disease (GERD)   CH

acute/chronic Pain may be related to acidic irritation of mucosa, muscle spasm, recurrent vomiting, possibly evidenced by reports of heartburn, distraction behaviors.

impaired Swallowing may be related to GERD, esophageal defects, achalasia, possibly evidenced by reports of heartburn/epigastric pain, "something stuck" when swallowing, food refusal/volume limiting, nighttime coughing or awakening.

risk for imbalanced Nutrition: less than body requirements: risk factors may include limited intake, recurrent vomiting.

risk for Insomnia: risk factors may include nighttime heartburn, regurgitation of stomach contents.

risk for Aspiration: risk factors may include incompetent lower esophageal sphincter, regurgitation of gastric acid.

Gastrointestinal hemorrhage   MS

(Refer to Gastritis, acute or chronic; Ulcer, peptic; Colitis, ulcerative; Crohn's disease; Varices, esophageal)

Gastroplasty   MS

(Also refer to Surgery, general)

ineffective Breathing Pattern may be related to decreased lung expansion, pain, anxiety, decreased energy/fatigue, tracheobronchial obstruction, possibly evidenced by dyspnea, tachypnea, changes in respiratory depth, reduced vital capacity, wheezes, rhonchi, abnormal ABGs.

risk for ineffective peripheral Tissue Perfusion: risk factors may include diminished blood flow, hypovolemia, immobility/bedrest, interruption of venous blood flow (thrombus).

risk for deficient Fluid Volume: risk factors may include excessive gastric losses, nasogastric suction, diarrhea, reduced intake.

risk for imbalanced Nutrition: less than body requirements: risk factors may include decreased intake, dietary restrictions, early satiety, increased metabolic rate/healing, malabsorption of nutrients/impaired absorption of vitamins.

Diarrhea may be related to changes in dietary fiber/bulk, inflammation, irritation, malabsorption of bowel, possibly evidenced by loose/liquid stools, increased frequency, hyperactive bowel sounds.

Gender identity disorder   PSY

(For individuals experiencing persistent and marked distress regarding uncertainty about issues relating to personal identity, e.g., sexual orientation and behavior.)

Anxiety [specify level] may be related to unconscious/conscious conflicts about essential values/beliefs (ego-dystonic gender identification), threat to self-concept, unmet needs, possibly evidenced by increased tension, helplessness, hopelessness, feelings of inadequacy, uncertainty, insomnia and focus on self, and impaired daily functioning.

ineffective Role Performance/disturbed Personal Identity may be related to crisis in development in which person has difficulty knowing/accepting to which sex he or she belongs or is attracted, sense of discomfort and inappropriateness about anatomic sex characteristics, possibly evidenced by confusion about sense of self, purpose, or direction in life, sexual identification/preference, verbalization of desire to be/insistence that person is the opposite sex, change in self-perception of role, and conflict in roles.

ineffective Sexuality Pattern may be related to ineffective or absent role models and conflict with sexual orientation or preferences, lack of/impaired relationship with an SO, possibly evidenced by verbalizations of discomfort with sexual orientation/role, and lack of information about human sexuality.

risk for compromised/disabled family Coping: risk factors may include inadequate/incorrect information or understanding, significant other unable to perceive or to act effectively in regard to client's needs, temporary family disorganization and role changes, and client providing little support in turn for primary person.

readiness for enhanced family Coping may be related to individual's basic needs being sufficiently gratified and adaptive tasks effectively addressed to enable goals of self-actualization to surface, possibly evidenced by family member(s) attempts to describe growth/impact of crisis on own values, priorities, goals, or relationships; family member(s) moving in direction of health-promoting and enriching lifestyle that supports client's search for self; and choosing experiences that optimize wellness.

Genetic disorder   CH/OB

Anxiety may be related to presence of specific risk factors (e.g., exposure to teratogens), situational crisis, threat to self-concept, conscious or unconscious conflict about essential values and life goals, possibly evidenced by increased tension, apprehension, uncertainty, feelings of inadequacy, expressed concerns.

deficient Knowledge [Learning Need] regarding purpose/process of genetic counseling may be related to lack of awareness of ramifications of diagnosis, process necessary for analyzing available options, and information misinterpretation, possibly evidenced by verbalization of concerns, statement of misconceptions, request for information.

risk for interrupted Family Processes: risk factors may include situational crisis, individual/family vulnerability, difficulty reaching agreement regarding options.

Spiritual Distress may be related to intense inner conflict about the outcome, normal grieving for the loss of the perfect child, anger that is often directed at God/greater power, religious beliefs/moral convictions, possibly evidenced by verbalization of inner conflict about beliefs, questioning of the moral and ethical implications of therapeutic choices, viewing situation as punishment, anger, hostility, and crying.

Genital herpes   CH
(Refer to Herpes simplex; Sexually transmitted disease)

Genital warts (human papillomavirus) CH
(Refer to Sexually transmitted disease)

GERD   CH
(Refer to Gastroesophageal reflux disease)

GI bleeding   MS
(Refer to Gastritis, acute or chronic; Ulcer, peptic)

Gigantism   CH
(Refer to Acromegaly)

Gingivitis   CH
impaired Oral Mucous Membrane may be related to ineffective oral hygiene, ill-fitting dentures, decreased salivation, hormonal changes, possibly evidenced by edema, gingival bleeding, hyperplasia, oral pain.

Glaucoma   CH

disturbed visual Sensory Perception may be related to altered sensory reception and altered status of sense organ (increased intraocular pressure/atrophy of optic nerve head), possibly evidenced by progressive loss of visual field.

Anxiety [specify level] may be related to change in health status, presence of pain, possibility/reality of loss of vision, unmet needs, and negative self-talk, possibly evidenced by apprehension, uncertainty, and expressed concern regarding changes in life event.

Glomerulonephritis   PED

excess Fluid Volume may be related to failure of regulatory mechanism (inflammation of glomerular membrane inhibiting filtration), possibly evidenced by weight gain, edema/anasarca, intake greater than output, and blood pressure changes.

acute Pain may be related to effects of circulating toxins and edema/distention of renal capsule, possibly evidenced by verbal reports, guarding/distraction behaviors, and autonomic responses (changes in vital signs).

imbalanced Nutrition: less than body requirements may be related to anorexia and dietary restrictions, possibly evidenced by aversion to eating, reported altered taste, weight loss, and decreased intake.

deficient Diversional Activity may be related to treatment modality/restrictions, fatigue, and malaise, possibly evidenced by statements of boredom, restlessness, and irritability.

risk for disproportionate Growth: risk factors may include infection, malnutrition, chronic illness.

Gluten sensitive enteropathy   CH
(Refer to Celiac disease)

Goiter   CH

disturbed Body Image may be related to visible swelling in neck, possibly evidenced by verbalization of feelings, fear of reaction of others, actual change in structure, change in social involvement.

Anxiety may be related to change in health status/progressive growth of mass, perceived threat of death.

risk for imbalanced Nutrition: less than body requirements: risk factors may include decreased ability to ingest/difficulty swallowing.

risk for ineffective Airway Clearance: risk factors may include tracheal compression/obstruction.

Gonorrhea   CH
(Also refer to Sexually Transmitted Disease [STD])

risk for Infection [dissemination/bacteremia]: risk factors may include presence of infectious process in highly vascular area and lack of recognition of disease process.

acute Pain may be related to irritation/inflammation of mucosa and effects of circulating toxins, possibly evidenced by verbal reports of genital or pharyngeal irritation, perineal/pelvic pain, guarding/distraction behaviors.

deficient Knowledge [Learning Need] regarding disease cause/transmission, therapy, and self-care needs may be related to lack of information/misinterpretation, denial of exposure, possibly evidenced by statements of concern, questions, misconceptions, and inaccurate follow-through of instructions/development of preventable complications.

Gout   CH

acute Pain may be related to inflammation of joint(s), possibly evidenced by verbal reports, guarding/distraction behaviors, and autonomic responses (changes in vital signs).

impaired physical Mobility may be related to joint pain/edema, possibly evidenced by reluctance to attempt movement, limited range of motion, and therapeutic restriction of movement.

deficient Knowledge [Learning Need] regarding cause, treatment, and prevention of condition may be related to lack of information/misinterpretation, possibly evidenced by statements of concern, questions, misconceptions, and inaccurate follow-through of instructions.

Grand mal seizures   **CH/PED**
(Refer to Seizure disorder)

Grave's disease   **CH**
(Refer to Hyperthyroidism)

Guillain-Barré syndrome (acute polyneuritis) MS
risk for ineffective Breathing Pattern/Airway Clearance: risk factors may include weakness/paralysis of respiratory muscles, impaired gag/swallow reflexes, decreased energy/fatigue.

disturbed Sensory Perceptual (specify) may be related to altered sensory reception/transmission/integration (altered status of sense organs, sleep deprivation), therapeutically restricted environment, endogenous chemical alterations (electrolyte imbalance, hypoxia), and psychological stress, possibly evidenced by reported or observed change in usual response to stimuli, altered communication patterns, and measured change in sensory acuity and motor coordination.

impaired physical Mobility may be related to neuromuscular impairment, pain/discomfort, possibly evidenced by impaired coordination, partial/complete paralysis, decreased muscle strength/control.

Anxiety [specify level]/Fear may be related to situational crisis, change in health status/threat of death, possibly evidenced by increased tension, restlessness, helplessness, apprehension, uncertainty, fearfulness, focus on self, and sympathetic stimulation.

risk for Disuse Syndrome: Risk factors include paralysis and pain.

Gulf War syndrome   **CH/MS**
[chronic] Fatigue may be related to unknown environmental exposure, stress, anxiety, disease state, possibly evidenced by overwhelming lack of energy, inability to maintain usual routines/level of physical activity, lethargic, compromised concentration.

Anxiety [specify] may be related to exposure to toxins, change in health status, threat of death, change in role function/economic status, unmet needs, possibly evidenced by expressed concerns, apprehension, uncertainty, fear of unspecific consequences, sleep disturbance, irritability, preoccupation.

impaired Memory may be related to neurological disturbances, possibly evidenced by reported/observed experiences of forgetting, inability to recall recent events.

chronic Pain may be related to chronic physical condition, possibly evidenced by verbal reports of muscle/joint pain, headaches, altered ability to continue previous activities, fatigue, reduced interaction with others.

Diarrhea may be related to environmental exposure to toxins, high stress levels/anxiety, possibly evidenced by liquid stools, abdominal pain.

disturbed visual Sensory Perception may be related to altered sensory reception, possibly evidenced by blurred vision, photosensitivity.

Hallucinogen abuse   **CH/PSY**
(Also refer to Substance dependence/abuse rehabilitation)
disturbed Thought Processes may be related to physiological changes associated with drug use, impaired judgment, memory loss, possibly evidenced by inaccurate interpretation of

environment, bizarre thinking, disorientation, inability to make decisions, unpredictable behavior, distractibility, non-reality-based thinking.

Anxiety/Fear may be related to situational crisis, threat to/change in health status, perceived threat of death, inexperience/unfamiliarity with effects of drug, possibly evidenced by assumptions of "losing my mind/control," apprehension, preoccupation with feelings of impending doom, sympathetic stimulation.

Self-Care Deficit (specify) may be related to perceptual/cognitive impairment, therapeutic management (restraints), possibly evidenced by inability to meet own physical needs.

Hand-foot-mouth disease　　　PED/CH
(Also refer to Meningitis)

impaired Oral Mucous Membrane may be related to infection, dehydration, possibly evidenced by oral lesions/ulcers, pain, difficulty eating.

risk for Infection [transmission]: risk factors may include insufficient knowledge to avoid exposure to pathogens, inadequate acquired immunity.

risk for deficient Fluid Volume: risk factors may include deviations affecting intake (oral ulcers and pain), increased fluid needs (hypermetabolic state/fever).

Hansen's disease　　　CH
impaired Skin/Tissue integrity may be related to altered circulation, sensation, pigmentation and [invasion of tissues by bacterial infection], possibly evidenced by symmetric skin lesions lighter than normal color, nodules, plaques, thickened dermis with loss of sensation, and frequent involvement of the nasal mucosa resulting in nasal congestion and epistaxis.

risk for Infection [spread/transmission]: risk factors may include inadequate primary or secondary defenses, insufficient knowledge to avoid exposure to/early treatment of infectious bacterial [Mycobacterium leprae] agent.

impaired physical Mobility may be related to neuromuscular and sensoriperceptual impairments, possibly evidenced by muscular weakness or numbness/absence of sensation in hands, arms, legs, feet.

disturbed Body Image may be related to biophysical illness/trauma, possibly evidenced by permanent nerve damage, [cosmetic damage], actual change in structure, missing body part, fear of reaction/rejection by others.

Hantavirus　　　MS
(Refer to Hantavirus pulmonary syndrome)

Hantavirus pulmonary syndrome　　MS
(Also refer to Disseminated intravascular coagulation)

acute Pain [/Discomfort] may be related to inflammatory process/circulating toxins, possibly evidenced by reports of headache, myalgia, GI distress, fever.

impaired Gas Exchange may be related to alveolar-capillary membrane changes (fluid collection/shifts into interstitial space/alveoli), possibly evidenced by dyspnea, restlessness, irritability, abnormal rate/depth of respirations, lethargy, confusion.

[moderate to severe] Anxiety may be related to change in health status, threat of death, interpersonal transmission, possibly evidenced by expressed concerns, distressed, apprehension, extraneous movement.

risk for impaired spontaneous Ventilation: risk factors may include respiratory muscle fatigue, problems with secretion management.

Hashimoto's thyroiditis　　　CH
(Refer to Hypothyroidism; Goiter)

Hay fever   **CH**

acute Pain[/Discomfort] may be related to irritation/inflammation of upper airway mucous membranes and conjunctiva, possibly evidenced by verbal reports, irritability, and restlessness.

deficient Knowledge [Learning Need] regarding underlying cause, appropriate therapy, and required lifestyle changes may be related to lack of information, possibly evidenced by statements of concern, questions, and misconceptions.

Headache   **CH/MS**

(Also refer to Temporal arteritis)

acute/chronic Pain may be related to stress/tension, nerve irritation/pressure, vasospasm, increased intracranial pressure, possibly evidenced by verbal/coded reports, pallor, facial mask of pain, guarding/distraction behaviors, restlessness, self-focusing, changes in sleep pattern/appetite, preoccupation with pain.

risk for ineffective Coping: risk factors may include situational crisis, personal vulnerability, inadequate support systems, work overload/no vacations, inadequate relaxation, severe pain, overwhelming threat to self.

deficient Knowledge [Learning Need] regarding condition, prognosis, treatment needs may be related to lack of exposure/recall, unfamiliarity with information/resources, cognitive limitations, possibly evidenced by request for information, statement of misconceptions, inaccurate follow-through of instructions, development of preventable complications.

Head injury   **MS/CH**

(Refer to Traumatic brain injury)

Heart attack   **MS**

(Refer to Myocardial infarction)

Heart failure, chronic   **MS**

decreased Cardiac Output, may be related to altered myocardial contractility/inotropic changes; alterations in rate, rhythm, and electrical conduction; and structural changes (valvular defects, ventricular aneurysm), possibly evidenced by tachycardia/dysrhythmias, changes in blood pressure, extra heart sounds, decreased urine output, diminished peripheral pulses, cool/ashen skin, orthopnea, crackles; dependent/generalized edema and chest pain.

excess Fluid Volume may be related to reduced glomerular filtration rate/increased ADH production, and sodium/water retention, possibly evidenced by orthopnea and abnormal breath sounds, S_3 heart sound, jugular vein distention, positive hepatojugular reflex, weight gain, hypertension, oliguria, generalized edema.

risk for impaired Gas Exchange: risk factors may include alveolar-capillary membrane changes (fluid collection/shifts into interstitial space/alveoli).

CH

Activity Intolerance may be related to imbalance between O_2 supply/demand, generalized weakness, and prolonged bedrest/sedentary lifestyle, possibly evidenced by reported/observed weakness, fatigue; changes in vital signs, presence of dysrhythmias; dyspnea, pallor, and diaphoresis.

deficient Knowledge [Learning Need] regarding cardiac function/disease process, therapy and self-care needs may be related to lack of information/misinterpretation, possibly evidenced by questions, statements of concern/misconceptions; development of preventable complications or exacerbations of condition.

Heart transplantation   **MS/CH**

(Refer to Cardiac surgery; Transplantation, recipient)

Heat exhaustion   CH/MS

deficient Fluid Volume may be related to excessive losses (profuse sweating), hypermetabolic state (core temperature 101°F to 105°F/38.3°C to 40.6°C), lack of intake, extremes of age, possibly evidenced by weakness/fatigue, slow pulse/decreased BP, changes in mentation.

Heatstroke   MS

Hyperthermia may be related to prolonged exposure to hot environment/vigorous activity with failure of regulating mechanism of the body, possibly evidenced by high body temperature (greater than 105°F/40.6°C), flushed/hot skin, tachycardia, and seizure activity.

decreased Cardiac Output may be related to functional stress of hypermetabolic state, altered circulating volume/venous return, and direct myocardial damage secondary to hyperthermia, possibly evidenced by decreased peripheral pulses, dysrhythmias/tachycardia, and changes in mentation.

Hematoma, epidural   MS

acute Confusion may be related to head injury, possibly evidenced by fluctuation in cognition/level of consciousness.

risk for decreased Intracranial Adaptive Capacity: Risk factors may include brain injuries, decreased cerebral perfusion pressure, systemic hypotension with intracranial hypertension.

risk for ineffective Breathing Pattern: risk factors may include neuromuscular dysfunction (injury to respiratory center of brain), perception/cognitive impairment.

risk for deficient Fluid Volume: risk factors may include restricted oral intake, hypermetabolic state, loss of fluid through normal/abnormal routes.

Hematoma, subdural-acute   MS
(Refer to Traumatic brain injury)

Hematoma, subdural-chronic   CH

acute/chronic Pain may be related to physical agent (space-occupying clot), possibly evidenced by reports of increasing daily headache.

acute/chronic Confusion may be related to head injury, alcohol abuse, possibly evidenced by fluctuations in cognition, increased agitation/restlessness, misperceptions, inappropriate responses.

impaired physical Mobility may be related to neuromuscular impairment (hemiparesis), decreased muscle strength, cognitive impairment, possibly evidenced by limited ability to perform gross/fine motor skills, gait changes, postural instability.

Hemodialysis   MS/CH
(Also refer to Dialysis, general)

risk for Injury [loss of vascular access]: risk factors may include clotting/thrombosis, infection, disconnection/hemorrhage.

risk for deficient Fluid Volume: risk factors may include excessive fluid losses/shifts via ultrafiltration, hemorrhage (altered coagulation/disconnection of shunt), and fluid restrictions.

risk for excess Fluid Volume: risk factors may include excessive fluid intake, rapid IV, blood/plasma expanders/saline given to support BP during procedure.

ineffective Protection may be related to chronic disease state, drug therapy, abnormal blood profile, inadequate nutrition, possibly evidenced by altered clotting, impaired healing, deficient immunity, fatigue, anorexia.

Hemophilia   PED

risk for deficient Fluid Volume [isotonic]: risk factors may include impaired coagulation/hemorrhagic losses.

---

risk for acute/chronic Pain: risk factors may include nerve compression from hematomas, nerve damage or hemorrhage into joint space.

risk for impaired physical Mobility: risk factors may include joint hemorrhage, swelling, degenerative changes, and muscle atrophy.

ineffective Protection may be related to abnormal blood profile, possibly evidenced by altered clotting.

compromised family Coping may be related to prolonged nature of condition that exhausts the supportive capacity of significant person(s), possibly evidenced by protective behaviors disproportionate to client's abilities/need for autonomy.

Hemorrhage, postpartum   OB
deficient Fluid Volume [isotonic] may be related to excessive vascular loss, possibly evidenced by hypotension, tachycardia, dry skin/mucous membranes, decreased/concentrated urine, delayed capillary refill, change in mentation.

ineffective Tissue Perfusion may be related to hypovolemia, possibly evidenced by diminished arterial pulsations, cold extremities, changes in vital signs, changes in sensorium, decreased milk production.

[moderate] Anxiety may be related to situational crisis, threat of change in health status/death, interpersonal transmission/contagion, physiological response (catecholamine release), possibly evidenced by increased tension, apprehension, feelings of inadequacy/helplessness, sympathetic stimulation, self-focus.

risk for Infection: risk factors may include traumatized tissue, stasis of body fluids (lochia), decreased Hb, invasive procedures.

risk for impaired parent/infant Attachment: risk factors may include interruption in bonding process, physical condition, perceived threat to own survival.

Hemorrhage, prenatal   OB
deficient Fluid Volume [isotonic] may be related to excessive vascular loss, possibly evidenced by hypotension, increased pulse rate, decreased pulse pressure, decreased/concentrated urine, decreased venous filling, change in mentation.

ineffective uteroplacental Tissue Perfusion may be related to hypovolemia, possibly evidenced by changes in FHR or activity.

Fear may be related to threat of death [perceived or actual] to self/fetus, possibly evidenced by verbalizations of specific concerns, increased tension, sympathetic stimulation.

risk for maternal Injury: risk factors may include tissue/organ hypoxia, abnormal blood profile, impaired immune system.

acute Pain may be related to muscle contractions/cervical dilation, tissue trauma (fallopian tube rupture), possibly evidenced by reports, distraction behaviors, autonomic responses (change in BP/pulse).

Hemorrhagic fever, viral   MS
(Refer to Ebola; Hantavirus pulmonary syndrome)

Hemorrhoidectomy   MS/CH
acute Pain may be related to edema/swelling and tissue trauma, possibly evidenced by verbal reports, guarding/distraction behaviors, focus on self, and autonomic responses (changes in vital signs).

risk for Urinary Retention: risk factors may include perineal trauma, edema/swelling, and pain.

deficient Knowledge [Learning Need] regarding therapeutic treatment and potential complications may be related to lack of information/misconceptions, possibly evidenced by statements of concern and questions.

Hemorrhoids
CH/OB

acute Pain may be related to inflammation and edema of prolapsed varices, possibly evidenced by verbal reports and guarding/distraction behaviors.

Constipation may be related to pain on defecation and reluctance to defecate, possibly evidenced by frequency, less than usual pattern, and hard, formed stools.

Hemothorax
MS

(Also refer to Pneumothorax)

risk for Trauma/Suffocation: risk factors may include concurrent disease/injury process, dependence on external device (chest drainage system), and lack of safety education/precautions.

Anxiety [specify level] may be related to change in health status and threat of death, possibly evidenced by increased tension, restlessness, expressed concern, sympathetic stimulation, and focus on self.

Hepatitis, acute viral
MS/CH

impaired Liver Function related to viral infection as evidenced by jaundice, hepatic enlargement, abdominal pain, marked elevations in serum liver function tests.

Fatigue may be related to decreased metabolic energy production and altered body chemistry, possibly evidenced by reports of lack of energy/inability to maintain usual routines, decreased performance, and increased physical complaints.

imbalanced Nutrition: less than body requirements may be related to inability to ingest adequate nutrients (nausea, vomiting, anorexia); hypermetabolic state, altered absorption and metabolism, possibly evidenced by aversion to eating/lack of interest in food, altered taste sensation, observed lack of intake, and weight loss.

acute Pain/[Discomfort] may be related to inflammation and swelling of the liver, arthralgias, urticarial eruptions, and pruritus, possibly evidenced by verbal reports, guarding/distraction behaviors, focus on self, and autonomic responses (changes in vital signs).

risk for Infection: risk factors may include inadequate secondary defenses and immunosuppression, malnutrition, insufficient knowledge to avoid exposure to pathogens/spread to others.

risk for impaired Tissue Integrity: risk factors may include bile salt accumulation in the tissues.

risk for impaired Home Management: risk factors may include debilitating effects of disease process and inadequate support systems (family, financial, role model).

deficient Knowledge [Learning Need] regarding disease process/transmission, treatment needs, and future expectations may be related to lack of information/recall, misinterpretation, unfamiliarity with resources, possibly evidenced by questions, statement of concerns/misconceptions, inaccurate follow-through of instructions, and development of preventable complications.

Hepatorenal syndrome
MS

(Refer to Cirrhosis; Renal failure, acute)

Hernia, hiatal
CH

chronic Pain may be related to regurgitation of acidic gastric contents, possibly evidenced by verbal reports, facial grimacing, and focus on self.

deficient Knowledge [Learning Need] regarding pathophysiology, prevention of complications, and self-care needs may be related to lack of information/misconceptions, possibly evidenced by statements of concern, questions, and recurrence of condition.

Hernia, inguinal
MS

(Refer to Herniorrhaphy)

Herniated nucleus pulposus   CH/MS

acute/chronic Pain may be related to nerve compression/irritation and muscle spasms, possibly evidenced by verbal reports, guarding/distraction behaviors, preoccupation with pain, self/narrowed focus, and autonomic responses (changes in vital signs when pain is acute), altered muscle tone/function, changes in eating/sleeping patterns and libido, physical/social withdrawal.

impaired physical Mobility may be related to pain (muscle spasms), therapeutic restrictions (e.g., bedrest, traction/braces), muscular impairment, and depression, possibly evidenced by reports of pain on movement, reluctance to attempt/difficulty with purposeful movement, decreased muscle strength, impaired coordination, and limited range of motion.

deficient Diversional Activity may be related to length of recuperation period and therapy restrictions, physical limitations, pain and depression, possibly evidenced by statements of boredom, disinterest, "nothing to do," and restlessness, irritability, withdrawal.

Herniorrhaphy   MS/PED

acute Pain may be related to disruption of skin, tissue, and muscle integrity, possibly evidenced by verbal/coded reports, alteration in muscle tone, distraction/guarding behaviors, narrowed focus, and autonomic responses.

risk for Injury: risk factors may include surgical repair, insertion of graft, increased intra-abdominal pressure (straining at stool, heavy lifting, strenuous activity).

Heroin abuse   CH

risk for Infection: risk factors may include injection/reuse or sharing of needles, malnutrition, environmental exposure, insufficient knowledge/motivation to avoid pathogens.

imbalanced Nutrition: less than body requirements may be related to inadequate intake, possibly evidenced by anorexia, lack of food/methods to prepare food, economic difficulties, weight loss, poor muscle tone/decreased muscle mass.

risk for Trauma: risk factors may include personal vulnerability, cigarette smoking, lack of safety precautions, driving impaired/under the influence, high-crime neighborhood.

risk for ineffective Protection: risk factors may include effects of substance use, malnutrition, chronic disease, lifestyle choices, unhealthy environment.

Heroin withdrawal   CH/MS

acute Pain [/Discomfort] may be related to cessation of drug, muscle tremors/twitching, possibly evidenced by reports of muscle aches, hot/cold flashes, diaphoresis, lacrimation, rhinorrhea, drug cravings.

severe Anxiety may be related to CNS hyperactivity, possibly evidenced by apprehension, pervasive anxious feelings, jittery, restlessness, weakness, insomnia, anorexia.

risk for ineffective Therapeutic Regimen Management: risk factors may include protracted withdrawal, economic difficulties, family/social support deficits, perceived barriers/benefits.

Herpes simplex   CH

acute Pain may be related to presence of localized inflammation and open lesions, possibly evidenced by verbal reports, distraction behaviors, and restlessness.

risk for [secondary] Infection: risk factors may include broken/traumatized tissue, altered immune response, and untreated infection/treatment failure.

risk for ineffective Sexuality Pattern: risk factors may include lack of knowledge, values conflict, or fear of transmitting the disease.

Herpes zoster (shingles)   CH

acute Pain may be related to inflammation/local lesions along sensory nerve(s), possibly evidenced by verbal reports, guarding/distraction behaviors, narrowed focus, and autonomic responses (changes in vital signs).

deficient Knowledge [Learning Need] regarding pathophysiology, therapeutic needs, and potential complications may be related to lack of information/misinterpretation, possibly evidenced by statements of concern, questions, and misconceptions.

High altitude pulmonary edema (HAPE)   MS
(Also refer to Mountain sickness, acute)

impaired Gas Exchange may be related to ventilation perfusion imbalance, alveolar-capillary membrane changes, altered oxygen supply, possibly evidenced by dyspnea, confusion, cyanosis, tachycardia, abnormal ABGs.

excess Fluid Volume may be related to compromised regulatory mechanism, possibly evidenced by shortness of breath, anxiety, edema, abnormal breath sounds, pulmonary congestion.

High altitude sickness   MS
(Refer to Mountain sickness, acute; High altitude pulmonary edema)

High-risk pregnancy   OB
(Refer to Pregnancy, high-risk)

Hip replacement   MS
(Refer to Total joint replacement)

HIV infection   CH
(Also refer to AIDS)

risk-prone health Behavior may be related to life-threatening, stigmatizing condition/disease; assault to self-esteem, altered locus of control, inadequate support systems, incomplete grieving, medication side effects (fatigue/depression), possibly evidenced by verbalization of nonacceptance/denial of diagnosis, nonexistent or unsuccessful involvement in problem-solving/goal setting; extended period of shock and disbelief or anger; lack of future-oriented thinking.

deficient Knowledge [Learning Need] regarding disease, prognosis, and treatment needs may be related to lack of exposure/recall, information misinterpretation, unfamiliarity with information resources, or cognitive limitation, possibly evidenced by statement of misconception/request for information, inappropriate/exaggerated behaviors (hostile, agitated, hysterical, apathetic), inaccurate follow-through of instructions/development of preventable complications.

Hodgkin's disease   CH/MS
(Also refer to Cancer; Chemotherapy)

Anxiety [specify level]/Fear may be related to threat of self-concept and threat of death, possibly evidenced by apprehension, insomnia, focus on self, and increased tension.

deficient Knowledge [Learning Need] regarding diagnosis, pathophysiology, treatment, and prognosis may be related to lack of information/misinterpretation, possibly evidenced by statements of concern, questions, and misconceptions.

acute Pain [/Discomfort] may be related to manifestations of inflammatory response (fever, chills, night sweats) and pruritus, possibly evidenced by verbal reports, distraction behaviors, and focus on self.

risk for ineffective Breathing Pattern/Airway Clearance: risk factors may include tracheobronchial obstruction (enlarged mediastinal nodes or airway edema).

Hospice care   CH

acute/chronic Pain may be related to biological, physical, psychological agent, possibly evidenced by verbal/coded report, changes in appetite/eating, sleep pattern, protective behavior, restlessness, irritability.

Activity Intolerance/Fatigue may be related to generalized weakness, bedrest/immobility, pain, imbalance between oxygen supply and demand, possibly evidenced by inability to maintain usual routine, verbalized lack of desire/interest in activity, decreased performance, lethargy.

Grieving/death Anxiety may be related to anticipated loss of physiological well-being, perceived threat of death.

compromised/disabled family Coping/Caregiver Role Strain may be related to prolonged disease/disability progression, temporary family disorganization and role changes, unrealistic expectations, inadequate or incorrect information or understanding by primary person.

risk for moral Distress: risk factors may include conflict among decision makers, cultural conflicts, end-of-life decisions, loss of autonomy, physical distance of decision makers.

Huntington's disease   **CH**

Hopelessness may be related to chronic progressive debilitating condition, possibly evidenced by despondent verbalizations, withdrawal from environs, angry outbursts.

impaired Walking may be related to movement disorder (altered gait, ataxia, dystonia), possibly evidenced by inability to walk required distances, navigate curbs/uneven surfaces, climb stairs.

disturbed Thought Processes may be related to degenerative physiological changes, possibly evidenced by inaccurate interpretation of environment, cognitive dissonance, inappropriate social behavior.

imbalanced Nutrition: less than body requirements may be related to inability to ingest food (difficulty swallowing, cognitive decline), possibly evidenced by aversion to eating, inadequate food intake, weight loss, decreased subcutaneous fat/muscle mass.

total Self-Care Deficit may be related to neuromuscular impairment, cognitive decline, possibly evidenced by inability to perform desired ADLs.

risk for Caregiver Role Strain: risk factors may include progressive deterioration (physical and mental) of care receiver, duration of caregiving required, complexity/amount of caregiving tasks, caregiver's competing role commitments, family isolation, lack of respite/recreation for caregiver, bizarre behavior of care receiver.

Hydrocephalus   **PED/MS**

ineffective cerebral Tissue Perfusion may be related to decreased arterial/venous blood flow (compression of brain tissue), possibly evidenced by changes in mentation, restlessness, irritability, reports of headache, pupillary changes, and changes in vital signs.

disturbed visual Sensory Perception may be related to pressure on sensory/motor nerves, possibly evidenced by reports of double vision, development of strabismus, nystagmus, pupillary changes, and optic atrophy.

risk for impaired physical Mobility: risk factors may include neuromuscular impairment, decreased muscle strength, and impaired coordination.

risk for decreased Intracranial Adaptive Capacity: risk factors may include brain injury, changes in perfusion pressure/intracranial pressure.

CH

risk for Infection: risk factors may include invasive procedure/presence of shunt.

deficient Knowledge [Learning Need] regarding condition, prognosis, and long-term therapy needs/medical follow-up may be related to lack of information/misperceptions, possibly evidenced by questions, statement of concern, request for information, and inaccurate follow-through of instructions/development of preventable complications.

Hydrophobia   **CH/MS**
(Refer to Rabies)

Hyperactivity disorder   **PED/PSY**

defensive Coping may be related to mild neurological deficits, dysfunctional family system, abuse/neglect, possibly evidenced by denial of obvious problems, projection of blame/responsibility, grandiosity, difficulty in reality testing perceptions.

Doenges Nursing Diagnosis Manual: Planning, Individualizing, and Documenting Client Care

impaired Social Interaction may be related to retarded ego development, negative role models, neurological impairment, possibly evidenced by discomfort in social situations, interrupts/intrudes on others, difficulty waiting turn in games/group activities, difficulty maintaining attention to task.

disabled family Coping may be related to excessive guilt, anger, or blaming among family members, parental inconsistencies, disagreements regarding discipline/limit-setting/approaches, exhaustion of parental expectations, possibly evidenced by unrealistic parental expectations, rejection or overprotection of child, exaggerated expression of feelings, despair regarding child's behavior.

Hyperbilirubinemia   PED

risk for Injury [CNS involvement]: risk factors may include prematurity, hemolytic disease, asphyxia, acidosis, hyponatremia, and hypoglycemia.

risk for Injury [effects of treatment]: risk factors may include physical properties of phototherapy and effects on body regulatory mechanisms, invasive procedure (exchange transfusion), abnormal blood profile, chemical imbalances.

deficient Knowledge [Learning Need] regarding condition prognosis, treatment/safety needs may be related to lack of exposure/recall and information misinterpretation, possibly evidenced by questions, statement of concern, and inaccurate follow-through of instructions/development of preventable complications.

Hyperemesis gravidarum   OB

deficient Fluid Volume [isotonic] may be related to excessive gastric losses and reduced intake, possibly evidenced by dry mucous membranes, decreased/concentrated urine, decreased pulse volume and pressure, thirst, and hemoconcentration.

imbalanced Nutrition: less than body requirements may be related to inability to ingest/digest/absorb nutrients (prolonged vomiting), possibly evidenced by reported inadequate food intake, lack of interest in food/aversion to eating, and weight loss.

risk for ineffective Coping: risk factors may include situational/maturational crisis (pregnancy, change in health status, projected role changes, concern about outcome).

Hyperparathyroidism, primary   MS

risk for deficient Fluid Volume: risk factors may include excessive losses through normal routes (vomiting, diarrhea, gastric bleed).

impaired Urinary Elimination may be related to anatomical obstruction (renal calculi), possibly evidenced by decreased renal function.

risk for Trauma: risk factors may include decreased calcium levels/bone fragility.

Hypertension   CH

deficient Knowledge [Learning Need] regarding condition, therapeutic regimen, and potential complications may be related to lack of information/recall, misinterpretation, cognitive limitations, or denial of diagnosis, possibly evidenced by statements of concern/questions, and misconceptions, inaccurate follow-through of instructions, and lack of BP control.

risk-prone health Behavior may be related to condition requiring change in lifestyle, altered locus of control, and absence of feelings/denial of illness, possibly evidenced by verbalization of nonacceptance of health status change and lack of movement toward independence.

risk for Sexual Dysfunction: risk factors may include side effects of medication.

MS

risk for decreased Cardiac Output: risk factors may include increased afterload (vasoconstriction), fluid shifts/hypovolemia, myocardial ischemia, ventricular hypertrophy/rigidity.

acute Pain may be related to increased cerebrovascular pressure, possibly evidenced by verbal reports (throbbing pain located in suboccipital region, present on awakening and disappearing spontaneously after being up and about), reluctance to move head, avoidance of bright lights and noise, increased muscle tension.

Hypertension, intrapartum   **OB**
risk for imbalanced Fluid Volume: risk factors may include compromised regulatory mechanism/fluid shifts, excessive fluid intake, effects of drug therapy (oxytocin infusion).

risk for impaired fetal Gas Exchange: risk factors may include altered blood flow, vasospasms, prolonged uterine contractions.

impaired Urinary Elimination may be related to fluid shifts, hormonal changes, effects of medication, possibly evidenced by changes in amount/frequency of voiding, bladder distention, changes in urine specific gravity, presence of albumin.

risk for maternal Injury: risk factors may include tonic-clonic convulsions, altered clotting factors (release of thromboplastin from placenta).

acute Pain may be related to intensification of uterine activity, myometrial hypoxia, anxiety, possibly evidenced by verbalizations, altered muscle tone, distraction behaviors, autonomic responses, facial mask.

Hypertension, prenatal   **OB**
(Refer to Pregnancy-induced hypertension)

Hypertension, pulmonary   **CH/MS**
(Refer to Pulmonary hypertension)

Hyperthyroidism   **CH**
(Also refer to Thyrotoxicosis)
Fatigue may be related to hypermetabolic imbalance with increased energy requirements, irritability of CNS, and altered body chemistry, possibly evidenced by verbalization of overwhelming lack of energy to maintain usual routine, decreased performance, emotional lability/irritability, and impaired ability to concentrate.

Anxiety [specify level] may be related to increased stimulation of the CNS (hypermetabolic state, pseudocatecholamine effect of thyroid hormones), possibly evidenced by increased feelings of apprehension, overexcitement/distress, irritability/emotional lability, shakiness, restless movements, tremors.

risk for imbalanced Nutrition: less than body requirements: risk factors may include inability to ingest adequate nutrients for hypermetabolic rate/constant activity, impaired absorption of nutrients (vomiting/diarrhea), hyperglycemia/relative insulin insufficiency.

risk for impaired Tissue Integrity: risk factors may include altered protective mechanisms of eye related to periorbital edema, reduced ability to blink, eye discomfort/dryness, and development of corneal abrasion/ulceration.

Hypervolemia   **CH/MS**
excess Fluid Volume may be related to excess fluid/sodium intake, compromised regulatory mechanisms (renal failure, increased ADH), decreased plasma proteins, rapid/excessive administration of isotonic parenteral fluids, possibly evidenced by edema, abnormal breath sounds, S_3 heart sound, shortness of breath, positive hepatojugular reflex/elevated CVP, change in mental status.

Hypochondriasis   **PSY**
(Refer to Somatoform disorders)

Hypoglycemia   **CH**

disturbed Thought Processes may be related to inadequate glucose for cellular brain function and effects of endogenous hormone activity, possibly evidenced by irritability, changes in mentation, memory loss, altered attention span, and emotional lability.

risk for unstable blood Glucose: risk factors may include dietary intake, lack of adherence to diabetes management, inadequate blood glucose monitoring, medication management.

deficient Knowledge [Learning Need] regarding pathophysiology of condition and therapy/ self-care needs may be related to lack of information/recall, misinterpretations, possibly evidenced by development of hypoglycemia and statements of questions/misconceptions.

Hypoparathyroidism (acute)   **MS**

risk for Injury: risk factors may include neuromuscular excitability/tetany and formation of renal stones.

acute Pain may be related to recurrent muscle spasms and alteration in reflexes, possibly evidenced by verbal reports, distraction behaviors, and narrowed focus.

risk for ineffective Airway Clearance: risk factors may include spasm of the laryngeal muscles.

Anxiety [specify level] may be related to threat to, or change in, health status, physiological responses.

Hypophysectomy   **MS**

(Also refer to Surgery, general; Cancer)

Fear/Anxiety may be related to situational crisis (nature of diagnosis/procedure), change in health status, perceived threat of death, separation from support system, possibly evidenced by expressed concerns, apprehension, being scared, increased tension, extraneous movement, difficulty concentrating.

risk for deficient Fluid Volume: risk factors may include failure of regulatory mechanism (decreased ADH).

risk for Infection: risk factors may include traumatized tissue, invasive procedure, CSF leak.

Sexual Dysfunction may be related to altered body function (loss of anterior pituitary), possibly evidenced by sterility, decreased libido, impotence (male), infertility, atrophy of vaginal mucosa (female).

Hypothermia (systemic)   **CH**

(Also refer to Frostbite)

Hypothermia may be related to exposure to cold environment, inadequate clothing, age extremes (very young/elderly), damage to hypothalamus, consumption of alcohol/medications causing vasodilation, possibly evidenced by reduction in body temperature below normal range, shivering, cool skin, pallor.

deficient Knowledge [Learning Need] regarding risk factors, treatment needs, and prognosis may be related to lack of information/recall, misinterpretation, possibly evidenced by statement of concerns/misconceptions, occurrence of problem, and development of complications.

Hypothyroidism   **CH**

(Also refer to Myxedema)

impaired physical Mobility may be related to weakness, fatigue, muscle aches, altered reflexes, and mucin deposits in joints and interstitial spaces, possibly evidenced by decreased muscle strength/control and impaired coordination.

Fatigue may be related to decreased metabolic energy production, possibly evidenced by verbalization of unremitting/overwhelming lack of energy, inability to maintain usual routines, impaired ability to concentrate, decreased libido, irritability, listlessness, decreased performance, increase in physical complaints.

disturbed Sensory Perception (specify) may be related to mucin deposits and nerve compression, possibly evidenced by paresthesias of hands and feet or decreased hearing.

Constipation may be related to decreased peristalsis/physical activity, possibly evidenced by frequency less than usual pattern, decreased bowel sounds, hard dry stools, and development of fecal impaction.

Hypovolemia   CH/MS
deficient Fluid Volume may be related to active fluid loss (hemorrhage, vomiting/gastric intubation, diarrhea, burns, wounds/fistulas), regulatory failure (adrenal disease, recovery phase of ARF, DKA, HHNC, diabetes insipidus, sepsis), possibly evidenced by thirst, weight loss, poor skin turgor, dry mucous membranes, tachycardia, tachypnea, fatigue, decreased CVP.

Hysterectomy   GYN/MS
(Also refer to Surgery, general)

acute Pain may be related to tissue trauma/abdominal incision, edema/hematoma formation, possibly evidenced by verbal reports, guarding/distraction behaviors, and autonomic responses (changes in vital signs).

risk for perioperative-position Injury: risk factors may include immobilization/lithotomy position.

impaired Urinary Elimination/risk for [acute] Urinary Retention: risk factors may include mechanical trauma, surgical manipulation, presence of localized edema/hematoma, or nerve trauma with temporary bladder atony.

ineffective Sexuality Pattern/risk for Sexual Dysfunction: risk factors may include concerns regarding altered body function/structure, perceived changes in femininity, changes in hormone levels, loss of libido, and changes in sexual response pattern.

Ileal conduit   MS/CH
(Refer to Urinary diversion)

Ileocolitis   MS/CH
(Refer to Crohn's disease)

Ileostomy   MS/CH
(Refer to Colostomy)

Ileus   MS
acute Pain may be related to distention/edema and ischemia of intestinal tissue, possibly evidenced by verbal reports, guarding/distraction behaviors, narrowed focus, and autonomic responses (changes in vital signs).

Diarrhea/Constipation may be related to presence of obstruction/changes in peristalsis, possibly evidenced by changes in frequency and consistency or absence of stool, alterations in bowel sounds, presence of pain, and cramping.

risk for deficient Fluid Volume: risk factors may include increased intestinal losses (vomiting and diarrhea), and decreased intake.

Immersion foot   MS
impaired Skin/Tissue Integrity may be related to exposure to cold and wet environment (above freezing), altered circulation, presence of infection, possibly evidenced by tissue maceration, pain, soggy edema.

disturbed peripheral Sensory Perception may be related to altered sensory reception, possibly evidenced by paresthesia/numbness.

risk for ineffective Health Maintenance: risk factors may include lack of material resources, poor coping skills, inadequate knowledge of safety needs.

Impetigo   **PED/CH**

impaired Skin Integrity may be related to presence of infectious process and pruritus, possibly evidenced by open/crusted lesions.

acute Pain may be related to inflammation and pruritus, possibly evidenced by verbal reports, distraction behaviors, and self-focusing.

risk for [secondary] Infection: risk factors may include broken skin, traumatized tissue, altered immune response, and virulence/contagious nature of causative organism.

risk for Infection [transmission]: risk factors may include virulent nature of causative organism, insufficient knowledge to prevent infection of others.

Impotence   **CH**

(Refer to Erectile dysfunction)

Infant (at 4 weeks)   **PED**

readiness for enhanced Knowledge regarding infant care, developmental expectations, safety and well-being may be related to changing needs of infant, possibly evidenced by questions, expressed concerns/desire to learn more, behaviors congruent with expressed knowledge.

risk for acute Pain: risk factors may include accumulation of gas in confined space with cramping of intestinal musculature.

risk for Infection: risk factors may include immature immunological response, increased environmental exposure.

risk for sudden infant Death Syndrome: risk factors may include sleeping position, second-hand smoke exposure, type of bedding used.

risk for disturbed Sensory Perception: risk factors may include immature development of sensory organs, inappropriate/inadequate environmental stimuli, prenatal/intrapartal complications, postpartal course.

risk for imbalanced Nutrition: more than body requirements: risk factors may include obesity in one/both parents, rapid transition across growth percentiles.

Infant of addicted mother   **OB/PED**

risk for Injury [CNS damage]: risk factors may include prematurity, hypoxia, effects of medications/substance use/withdrawal, possible exposure to infectious agents (prenatal/intrapartal).

ineffective Airway Clearance/impaired Gas Exchange may be related to excess mucus production, depression of cough reflex and respiratory center, intrauterine asphyxia, possibly evidenced by tachypnea, tachycardia, cyanosis, nasal flaring, grunting respirations, hypoxia, acidosis.

risk for Infection: risk factors may include presence of maternal infections (GBS, STDs).

risk for imbalanced Nutrition: less than body requirements: risk factors may include inability to ingest/digest/absorb adequate nutrients to meet metabolic needs (e.g., poor/uncoordinated sucking and swallowing, frequent GI irritation with vomiting, diarrhea, repeated regurgitation, frequent hyperactivity).

risk for impaired Skin Integrity: risk factors may include mechanical factors (continual rubbing of face/knees against bedding, scratching face with hands), presence of excretions.

impaired Parenting may be related to lack of available or ineffective role model, unmet emotional maturation needs of parent, lack of support between/from SO, interruption in bonding process, lack of appropriate response of infant, possibly evidenced by reports of role inadequacy/inability to care for infant, inattention to infant needs, inappropriate caretaking behaviors, lack of parental attachment behaviors.

disabled family Coping may be related to significant person with chronically unexpressed feelings of guilt, anxiety, hostility, despair; dissonant discrepancy of coping styles, high-risk family situations, possibly evidenced by intolerance, rejection, abandonment/desertion, neglectful relationships between family members, neglectful care of infant, distortion of reality of parent's health problem/substance use.

Infant of HIV-positive mother   OB/PED
(Also refer to AIDS)
   risk for Infection: risk factors may include immature immune system, inadequate acquired immunity, suppressed inflammatory response, invasive procedures, malnutrition.
   imbalanced Nutrition: risk for less than body requirements: risk factors may include inability to ingest, digest, or absorb nutrients (e.g., impaired suck/swallow, GI infection, malabsorption, diarrhea).
   risk for delayed Growth and Development: risk factors may include separation from SO, inadequate caretaking, inconsistent responsiveness/multiple caretakers, environmental and stimulation deficiencies, effects of chronic condition/disabilities.
   deficient Knowledge [Learning Need] regarding condition, prognosis, treatment needs may be related to lack of exposure, misinterpretation, unfamiliarity with resources, lack of recall/interest in learning, possibly evidenced by questions, statements of misconceptions, inaccurate follow-through of instructions, development of preventable complications.

Infection, ear   PED
(Refer to Otitis media)

Infection, prenatal   OB
(Also refer to AIDS)
   risk for maternal/fetal Infection: risk factors may include inadequate primary defenses (e.g., broken skin, stasis of body fluids), inadequate secondary defenses (e.g., decreased hemoglobin, immunosuppression), inadequate acquired immunity, environmental exposure, malnutrition, rupture of amniotic membranes.
   deficient Knowledge regarding treatment/prevention, prognosis of condition may be related to lack of exposure to information or unfamiliarity with resources, misinterpretation, possibly evidenced by verbalization of problem, inaccurate follow-through of instructions, development of preventable complications/continuation of infectious process.
   [Discomfort] may be related to body response to infective agent, properties of infection (e.g., skin/tissue irritation, development of lesions), possibly evidenced by verbal reports, restlessness, withdrawal from social contacts.

Infection, puerperal   OB/CH
risk for Infection [spread/sepsis]: risk factors may include presence of infection, broken skin/traumatized tissues, high vascularity of involved area, invasive procedures/increased environmental exposure, anemia, chronic disease.
   acute Pain may be related to body response to infective agent/toxins, possibly evidenced by verbalizations, restlessness, guarding behavior, self-focusing, autonomic responses.
   imbalanced Nutrition: less than body requirements may be related to insufficient intake to meet metabolic demands (anorexia, nausea/vomiting, medical restrictions), possibly evidenced by aversion to eating, decreased/lack of oral intake, unanticipated weight loss.
   risk for impaired parent/infant Attachment: risk factors may include interruption in bonding process/separation, physical barriers, maternal fatigue/apathy.

Infection, wound   MS/CH
risk for Infection [sepsis]: risk factors may include presence of infection, broken skin, or traumatized tissues, stasis of body fluids, invasive procedures, or increased environmental exposure, chronic disease (e.g., diabetes, anemia, malnutrition), altered immune response, and untoward effect of medications (e.g., opportunistic/secondary infection).

impaired Skin/Tissue Integrity may be related to altered circulation, presence of infection, wound drainage, nutritional deficit, possibly evidenced by delayed healing, damaged tissues, invasion of body structures.

risk for delayed Surgical Recovery: risk factors may include presence of infection, activity restrictions/limitations, nutritional deficiency.

Infertility CH

situational low Self-Esteem may be related to functional impairment (inability to conceive), unrealistic self-expectations, sense of failure, possibly evidenced by self-negating verbalizations, expressions of helplessness, perceived inability to deal with situation.

chronic Sorrow may be related to perceived physical disability (inability to conceive), possibly evidenced by expressions of anger, disappointment, emptiness, self-blame, helplessness, sadness, feelings interfering with client's ability to achieve maximum well-being.

risk for Spiritual Distress: risk factors may include energy-consuming anxiety, low self-esteem, deteriorating relationship with SO, viewing situation as deserved/punishment for past behaviors.

Inflammatory bowel disease CH
(Refer to Colitis, ulcerative; Crohn's disease)

Influenza CH

acute Pain[/Discomfort] may be related to inflammation and effects of circulating toxins, possibly evidenced by verbal reports, distraction behaviors, and narrowed focus.

risk for deficient Fluid Volume: risk factors may include excessive gastric losses, hypermetabolic state, and altered intake.

Hyperthermia may be related to effects of circulating toxins and dehydration, possibly evidenced by increased body temperature, warm/flushed skin, and tachycardia.

risk for ineffective Breathing: risk factors may include response to infectious process, decreased energy/fatigue.

Inhalant intoxication/abuse CH/PSY
(Refer to Stimulant abuse)

Insomnia, acute CH

Insomnia may be related to daytime activity pattern, social/work schedule inconsistent with chronotype, travel across time zones, fatigue, life change, physical conditions (dyspnea, gastroesophageal reflux, night sweats), possibly evidenced by verbal reports of difficulties/not feeling well-rested, less than age-normed total sleep time, changes in behavior and performance, physical signs (dark circles under eyes, frequent yawning).

Insomnia, chronic CH

Sleep Deprivation may be related to sustained environmental stimulation, sustained circadian asynchrony, prolonged use of pharmacological/dietary antisoporifics, prolonged pain, sleep apnea, dementia, narcolepsy, possibly evidenced by daytime drowsiness, decreased ability to perform, lethargy, slowed reaction, apathy.

Insulin resistance syndrome CH
(Refer to Metabolic syndrome)

Insulin shock MS/CH
(Refer to Hypoglycemia)

Intermaxillary fixation MS/CH
(Also refer to Surgery, general)

risk for ineffective Airway Clearance: risk factors may include soft tissue trauma, retained secretions.

risk for Aspiration: risk factors may include facial trauma/surgery, wired jaws, difficulty swallowing.

impaired Tissue Integrity may be related to tissue trauma/damage, intraoperative manipulation, mechanical/fixation device, altered circulation, nutritional deficit, possibly evidenced by edema, hematoma/ecchymosis, erythema, inflammation, delayed healing.

impaired verbal Communication may be related to wiring of jaws, edema of mouth and surrounding structures, pain, possibly evidenced by inability/reluctance to talk.

risk for imbalanced Nutrition: less than body requirements: risk factors may include facial/tissue edema, inability to chew, difficulty swallowing, decreased appetite, increased metabolic needs.

Intervertebral disc excision   **MS**
(Refer to Laminectomy, cervical/lumbar)

Intestinal obstruction   **MS**
(Refer to Ileus)

Intestinal surgery (without diversion)   **MS**
(Also refer to Surgery, general)

risk for deficient Fluid Volume: risk factors may include excessive losses through normal routes (vomiting, diarrhea), excessive losses through abnormal routes (indwelling drains, NG/intestinal suctioning, hemorrhage), insufficient replacement, fever.

risk for Infection: risk factors may include chronic disease, malnutrition, opening of abdominal cavity/bowel, stasis of body fluids, altered peristalsis.

Constipation/Diarrhea may be related to effects of anesthesia, surgical manipulation, decreased dietary intake/bulk, physical inactivity, irritation, malabsorption, pain, effects of medication, possibly evidenced by change in bowel habits, change in stool characteristics, hyper/hypoactive bowel sounds, abdominal pain.

Intracranial infections   **MS**
(Refer to Abscess, brain [acute]; Encephalitis; Meningitis)

Irritable bowel syndrome   **CH**
acute Pain may be related to abnormally strong intestinal contractions, increased sensitivity of intestine to distention, hypersensitivity to hormones gastrin and cholecystokinin, skin/tissue irritation/perirectal excoriation, possibly evidenced by verbal reports, guarding behavior, expressive behavior (restlessness, moaning, irritability).

Constipation may be related to motor abnormalities of longitudinal muscles/changes in frequency and amplitude of contractions, dietary restrictions, stress, possibly evidenced by change in bowel pattern/decreased frequency, sensation of incomplete evacuation, abdominal pain/distention.

Diarrhea may be related to motor abnormalities of longitudinal muscles/changes in frequency and amplitude of contractions, stress, possibly evidenced by precipitous passing of liquid stool on rising or immediately after eating, rectal urgency/incontinence, bloating.

Kanner's syndrome   **PED/PSY**
(Refer to Autistic disorder)

Kaposi's sarcoma, AIDS-related   **CH/MS**
(Also refer to Chemotherapy)

disturbed Body Image may be related to widely disseminated lesions of varied color in skin/mucous membranes, possibly evidenced by verbalizations, fear of rejection/reaction of others, negative feelings about body, hiding body parts, change in social involvement.

risk for deficient Fluid Volume: risk factors may include extensive bleeding of visceral lesions.

Kawasaki disease   **PED**

Hyperthermia may be related to increased metabolic rate and dehydration, possibly evidenced by increased body temperature greater than normal range, flushed skin, increased respiratory rate, and tachycardia.

acute Pain may be related to inflammation and edema/swelling of tissues, possibly evidenced by verbal reports, restlessness, guarding behaviors, and narrowed focus.

impaired Skin Integrity may be related to inflammatory process, altered circulation, and edema formation, possibly evidenced by disruption of skin surface, including macular rash and desquamation.

impaired Oral Mucous Membrane may be related to inflammatory process, dehydration, and mouth breathing, possibly evidenced by pain, hyperemia, and fissures of lips.

risk for decreased Cardiac Output: risk factors may include structural changes/inflammation of coronary arteries and alterations in rate/rhythm or conduction.

Ketoacidosis   **CH**
(Refer to Diabetic ketoacidosis)

Kidney disease, polycystic   **CH**

risk for [urinary tract] Infection: risk factors may include inadequate primary defenses (traumatized tissue, stasis of body fluids); inadequate secondary defenses (suppressed inflammatory response); chronic disease.

acute/chronic Pain may be related to injuring agents—presence of cysts in kidneys/other organs, possibly evidenced by verbal report of back/lower side pain, headaches beyond tolerance, guarded/protective behavior, narrowed focus, sleep disturbance, distraction behaviors.

risk for excess Fluid Volume: risk factors may include compromised regulatory mechanism/kidney failure, possibly evidenced by oliguria, edema, abnormal breath sounds, jugular vein distention, hypertension.

Kidney failure, acute   **MS**
(Refer to Renal failure, acute)

Kidney failure, chronic   **CH/MS**
(Refer to Renal failure, chronic)

Kidney stone(s)   **CH**
(Refer to Calculi, urinary)

Knee replacement   **MS**
(Refer to Total joint replacement)

Kwashiorkor   **PED**

imbalanced Nutrition: less than body requirements may be related to financial/resource limitations, possibly evidenced by inadequate food intake less than recommended daily allowances, lack of food, weight loss, poor muscle tone, decreased subcutaneous fat/muscle mass, abnormal laboratory studies.

risk for Infection: risk factors may include malnutrition.

risk for disproportionate Growth: risk factors may include malnutrition, caregiver maladaptive feeding behaviors, deprivation/poverty, impaired insulin response, infection.

Labor, breech presentation   OB
Anxiety [specify level] may be related to situational crisis, threat to self/fetus, interpersonal transmission, possibly evidenced by increased tension, apprehension, fearfulness, restlessness, sympathetic stimulation.

risk for fetal Injury: risk factors may include entrapment of head, stretching of brachial plexus or spinal cord (nerve damage), hypoxia (brain damage).

Labor, dysfunctional   OB
(Refer to Dystocia)

Labor, induced/augmented   OB
deficient Knowledge [Learning Need] regarding procedure, treatment needs, and possible outcomes may be related to lack of exposure/recall, information misinterpretation, and unfamiliarity with information resources, possibly evidenced by questions, statement of concern/misconception, and exaggerated behaviors.

risk for maternal Injury: risk factors may include adverse effects/response to therapeutic interventions.

risk for impaired fetal Gas Exchange: risk factors may include altered placental perfusion/cord prolapse.

acute Pain may be related to altered characteristics of chemically stimulated contractions, psychological concerns, possibly evidenced by verbal reports, increased muscle tone, distraction/guarding behaviors, and narrowed focus.

Labor, precipitous   OB
Anxiety [specify level] may be related to situational crisis, threat to self/fetus, interpersonal transmission, possibly evidenced by increased tension; scared, fearful, restless/jittery; sympathetic stimulation.

risk for impaired Skin/Tissue Integrity: risk factors may include rapid progress of labor, lack of necessary equipment.

acute Pain may be related to occurrence of rapid, strong muscle contractions; psychological issues, possibly evidenced by verbalizations of inability to use learned pain-management techniques, sympathetic stimulation, distraction behaviors (e.g., moaning, restlessness).

Labor, preterm   OB/CH
Activity Intolerance may be related to muscle/cellular hypersensitivity, possibly evidenced by continued uterine contractions/irritability.

risk for Poisoning: risk factors may include dose-related toxic/side effects of tocolytics.

risk for fetal Injury: risk factors may include delivery of premature/immature infant.

Anxiety [specify level] may be related to situational crisis, perceived or actual threats to self/fetus, and inadequate time to prepare for labor, possibly evidenced by increased tension, restlessness, expressions of concern, and autonomic responses (changes in vital signs).

deficient Knowledge [Learning Need] regarding preterm labor treatment needs and prognosis may be related to lack of information and misinterpretation, possibly evidenced by questions, statements of concern, misconceptions, inaccurate follow-through of instruction, and development of preventable complications.

Labor, stage I (active phase)   OB
acute Pain[/Discomfort] may be related to contraction-related hypoxia, dilation of tissues, and pressure on adjacent structures combined with stimulation of both parasympathetic and

sympathetic nerve endings, possibly evidenced by verbal reports, guarding/distraction behaviors (restlessness), muscle tension, and narrowed focus.

impaired Urinary Elimination may be related to altered intake/dehydration, fluid shifts, hormonal changes, hemorrhage, severe intrapartal hypertension, mechanical compression of bladder, and effects of regional anesthesia, possibly evidenced by changes in amount/frequency of voiding, urinary retention, slowed progression of labor, and reduced sensation.

risk for ineffective [individual/couple] Coping: risk factors may include situational crises, personal vulnerability, use of ineffective coping mechanisms, inadequate support systems, and pain.

Labor, stage I (latent phase)   OB

deficient Knowledge [Learning Need] regarding progression of labor, available options may be related to lack of exposure/recall, information misinterpretation, possibly evidenced by questions, statements of misconceptions, inaccurate follow-through of instructions.

risk for mild Anxiety: risk factors may include situational crisis, unmet needs, stress.

risk for ineffective Coping: risk factors may include personal vulnerability, inadequate support systems or coping methods.

Labor, stage I (transition phase)   OB

acute Pain may be related to mechanical pressure of presenting part, tissue dilation/stretching and hypoxia, stimulation of parasympathetic and sympathetic nerves; emotional and muscular tension.

Fatigue may be related to discomfort/pain, overwhelming psychological emotional demands, increased energy requirements, decreased caloric intake, possibly evidenced by verbalizations, impaired ability to concentrate, emotional lability or irritability, lethargy, altered coping ability.

risk for ineffective [individual/couple] Coping: risk factors may include sense of "work overload," personal vulnerability, inadequate/exhausted support system.

risk for imbalanced Fluid Volume: risk factors may include reduced intake, excess fluid loss/hemorrhage, excess fluid retention, rapid fluid administration.

risk for decreased Cardiac Output: risk factors may include decreased venous return, hypovolemia, changes in systemic vascular resistence.

Labor, stage II (expulsion)   OB

acute Pain may be related to strong uterine contractions, tissue stretching/dilation, and compression of nerves by presenting part of the fetus, and bladder distention, possibly evidenced by verbalizations, facial grimacing, guarding/distraction behaviors (restlessness), narrowed focus, and autonomic responses (diaphoresis).

Cardiac Output [fluctuation] may be related to changes in SVR, fluctuations in venous return (repeated/prolonged Valsalva's maneuvers, effects of anesthesia/medications, dorsal recumbent position occluding the inferior vena cava and partially obstructing the aorta), possibly evidenced by decreased venous return, changes in vital signs (BP, pulse), urinary output, fetal bradycardia.

risk for impaired fetal Gas Exchange: risk factors may include mechanical compression of head/cord, maternal position/prolonged labor affecting placental perfusion, and effects of maternal anesthesia, hyperventilation.

risk for impaired Skin/Tissue Integrity: risk factors may include untoward stretching/lacerations of delicate tissues (precipitous labor, hypertonic contractile pattern, adolescence, large fetus) and application of forceps.

risk for Fatigue: risk factors may include pregnancy, stress, anxiety, sleep deprivation, increased physical exertion, anemia, humidity/temperature, lights.

Labor, stage III (placental expulsion)   OB

acute Pain may be related to tissue trauma, psychological response following delivery, possibly evidenced by verbalizations, changes in muscle tone, restlessness.

risk for deficient Fluid Volume: risk factors may include lack/restriction of oral intake, vomiting, diaphoresis, increased insensible water loss, uterine atony, lacerations of the birth canal, retained placental fragments.

risk for maternal Injury: risk factors may include positioning during delivery/transfers, difficulty with placental separation, abnormal blood profile.

risk for impaired parent/infant Attachment: risk factors may include physical barriers/separation, anxiety associated with the parent role.

Labor, stage IV (first 4 hr following delivery of placenta)   OB
Fatigue may be related to increased physical exertion, sleep deprivation, stress, environmental stimuli, hormonal changes, possibly evidenced by verbalization of overwhelming lack of energy, compromised concentration, listlessness.

acute Pain may be related to effects of hormones/medications, mechanical trauma/tissue edema, physical and psychological exhaustion, anxiety, possibly evidenced by reports of cramping (afterpains), muscle tremors, guarding/distraction behaviors, facial mask.

risk for deficient Fluid Volume: risk factors may include myometrial fatigue/failure of homeostatic mechanisms (e.g., continued uteroplacental circulation, incomplete vasoconstriction, effects of PIH).

risk for impaired parent/infant Attachment: risk factors may include maternal fatigue, physical barriers/separation, lack of privacy, anxiety associated with the parent role.

Laceration   CH
impaired Skin/Tissue Integrity may be related to trauma, possibly evidenced by disruption of skin layers, invasion of body structures.

risk for Infection: risk factors may include trauma, tissue destruction, increased environmental exposure.

Laminectomy, cervical   MS
(Also refer to Laminectomy, lumbar)

risk for perioperative-positioning Injury: risk factors may include immobilization, muscle weakness, obesity, advanced age.

risk for ineffective Airway Clearance: risk factors may include retained secretions, pain, muscular weakness.

risk for impaired Swallowing: risk factors may include operative edema, pain, neuromuscular impairment.

Laminectomy, lumbar   MS
(Also refer to Surgery, general)

ineffective Tissue Perfusion (specify) may be related to diminished/interrupted blood flow (dressing, edema/hematoma formation), hypovolemia, possibly evidenced by paresthesia, numbness; decreased range of motion, muscle strength.

risk for [spinal] Trauma: risk factors may include temporary weakness of spinal column, balancing difficulties, changes in muscle tone/coordination.

acute Pain may be related to traumatized tissues, localized inflammation, and edema, possibly evidenced by altered muscle tone, verbal reports, and distraction/guarding behaviors, autonomic changes.

impaired physical Mobility may be related to imposed therapeutic restrictions, neuromuscular impairment, and pain, possibly evidenced by limited range of motion, decreased muscle strength/control, impaired coordination, and reluctance to attempt movement.

risk for [acute] Urinary Retention: risk factors may include pain and swelling in operative area and reduced mobility/restrictions of position.

Laryngectomy   MS
(Also refer to Cancer; Chemotherapy)

ineffective Airway Clearance may be related to partial/total removal of the glottis, temporary or permanent change to neck breathing, edema formation, and copious/thick secretions, possibly evidenced by dyspnea/difficulty breathing, changes in rate/depth of respiration, use of accessory respiratory muscles, weak/ineffective cough, abnormal breath sounds, and cyanosis.

impaired Skin/Tissue Integrity may be related to surgical removal of tissues/grafting, effects of radiation or chemotherapeutic agents, altered circulation/reduced blood supply, compromised nutritional status, edema formation, and pooling/continuous drainage of secretions, possibly evidenced by disruption of skin/tissue surface and destruction of skin/tissue layers.

impaired Oral Mucous Membrane may be related to dehydration/absence of oral intake, poor/inadequate oral hygiene, pathological condition (oral cancer), mechanical trauma (oral surgery), decreased saliva production, difficulty swallowing and pooling/drooling of secretions, and nutritional deficits, possibly evidenced by xerostomia (dry mouth), oral discomfort, thick/mucoid saliva, decreased saliva production, dry and crusted/coated tongue, inflamed lips, absent teeth/gums, poor dental health and halitosis.

                                        CH

impaired verbal Communication may be related to anatomic deficit (removal of vocal cords), physical barrier (tracheostomy tube), and required voice rest, possibly evidenced by inability to speak, change in vocal characteristics, and impaired articulation.

risk for Aspiration: risk factors may include impaired swallowing, facial/neck surgery, presence of tracheostomy/feeding tube.

Laryngitis   CH/PED
(Refer to Croup)

Latex allergy   CH
latex Allergy Response may be related to no immune mechanism response, possibly evidenced by contact dermatitis—erythema, blisters; delayed hypersensitivity—eczema, irritation; hypersensitivity—generalized edema, wheezing/bronchospasm, hypotension, cardiac arrest.

Anxiety [specify level]/Fear may be related to threat of death, possibly evidenced by expressed concerns, hypervigilance, restlessness, focus on self.

risk for risk-prone health Behavior: risk factors may include health status requiring change in occupation.

Laxative abuse   CH
perceived Constipation may be related to health beliefs, faulty apprasial, impaired cognition/thought processes, possibly evidenced by expectation of daily bowel movement, expected passage of stool at same time every day.

Lead poisoning, acute   PED/CH
(Also refer to Lead poisoning, chronic)

Contamination may be related to flaking/peeling paint (young children), improperly lead-glazed ceramic pottery, unprotected contact with lead (e.g., battery manufacture/recycling, bronzing, soldering/welding), imported herbal products/medicinals, possibly evidenced by abdominal cramping, headache, irritability, decreased attentiveness, constipation, tremors.

risk for Trauma: risk factors may include loss of coordination, altered level of consciousness, clonic or tonic muscle activity, neurological damage.

risk for deficient Fluid Volume: risk factors may include excessive vomiting, diarrhea, or decreased intake.

deficient Knowledge [Learning Need] regarding sources of lead and prevention of poisoning may be related to lack of information/misinterpretation, possibly evidenced by statements of concern, questions, and misconceptions.

Lead poisoning, chronic   CH
(Also refer to Lead Poisoning, acute)

Contamination may be related to flaking/peeling paint (young children), improperly lead-glazed ceramic pottery, unprotected contact with lead (e.g., battery manufacture/recycling, bronzing, soldering/welding), imported herbal products/medicinals, possibly evidenced by chronic abdominal cramping, headache, personality changes, cognitive deficits, seizures, neuropathy.

imbalanced Nutrition: less than body requirements may be related to decreased intake (chemically induced changes in the GI tract), possibly evidenced by anorexia, abdominal discomfort, reported metallic taste, and weight loss.

disturbed Thought Processes may be related to deposition of lead in CNS and brain tissue, possibly evidenced by personality changes, learning disabilities, and impaired ability to conceptualize and reason.

chronic Pain may be related to deposition of lead in soft tissues and bone, possibly evidenced by verbal reports, distraction behaviors, and focus on self.

Legionnaires' disease   CH/MS

Hyperthermia may be related to illness/inflammatory process, possibly evidenced by increased body temperature, flushed/warm skin, chills.

acute Pain[/Discomfort] may be related to infectious agent/inflammatory response, effects of circulating toxins, possibly evidenced by reports of headache, myalgia, high fever, diaphoresis.

ineffective Airway Clearance may be related to tracheal bronchial inflammation, edema formation, increased sputum production, pleuritic pain, decreased energy, fatigue, possibly evidenced by changes in rate/depth of respirations, abnormal breath sounds, use of accessory muscles, dyspnea, cyanosis, effective/ineffective cough—with or without sputum production.

impaired Gas Exchange may be related to inflammatory process, collection of secretions affecting O_2 exchange across alveolar membrane, and hypoventilation, possibly evidenced by restlessness/changes in mentation, dyspnea, tachycardia, pallor, cyanosis, and ABGs/oximetry evidence of hypoxia.

Diarrhea may be related to infectious process, possibly evidenced by liquid stools, abdominal cramping.

risk for Infection [spread]: risk factors may include decreased ciliary action, stasis of secretions, presence of existing infection, improper disposal of contaminated materials.

Leprosy   CH
(Refer to Hansen's disease)

Leukemia, acute   MS
(Also refer to Chemotherapy)

risk for Infection: risk factors may include inadequate secondary defenses (alterations in mature white blood cells, increased number of immature lymphocytes, immunosuppression and bone marrow suppression), invasive procedures, and malnutrition.

Anxiety [specify level]/Fear may be related to change in health status, threat of death, and situational crisis, possibly evidenced by sympathetic stimulation, apprehension, feelings of helplessness, focus on self, and insomnia.

Activity Intolerance [specify level] may be related to reduced energy stores, increased metabolic rate, imbalance between O_2 supply and demand, therapeutic restrictions (bedrest)/effect of drug therapy, possibly evidenced by generalized weakness, reports of fatigue and exertional dyspnea, abnormal heart rate or BP response.

acute Pain may be related to physical agents (infiltration of tissues/organs/CNS, expanding bone marrow) and chemical agents (antileukemic treatments), possibly evidenced by verbal reports (abdominal discomfort, arthralgia, bone pain, headache); distraction behaviors, narrowed focus, and autonomic responses (changes in vital signs).

risk for deficient Fluid Volume: risk factors may include excessive losses (vomiting, hemorrhage, diarrhea), decreased intake (nausea, anorexia), increased fluid need (hypermetabolic state/fever), predisposition for kidney stone formation/tumor lysis syndrome.

Leukemia, chronic   CH

ineffective Protection may be related to abnormal blood profiles, drug therapy (cytotoxic agents, steroids), radiation treatments, possibly evidenced by deficient immunity, impaired healing, altered clotting, weakness.

Fatigue may be related to disease state, anemia, possibly evidenced by verbalizations, inability to maintain usual routines, listlessness.

imbalanced Nutrition: less than body needs may be related to inability to ingest nutrients, possibly evidenced by lack of interest in food, anorexia, weight loss, abdominal fullness/pain.

Lice, head   PED/CH
(Refer to Pediculosis capitis)

Lice, pubic   CH
(Refer to Pediculosis capitis)

Lightning injury   MS
(Also refer to Electrical injury)

risk for disturbed visual/auditory Sensory Perception: risk factors may include altered sensory reception (corneal laceration, retinal damage, development of cataracts, rupture of tympanic membrane).

acute Confusion may be related to CNS involvement, possibly evidenced by change in level of consciousness.

impaired Memory may be related to acute hypoxia, decreased cardiac output, electrolyte imbalance, neurological disturbance, possibly evidenced by inability to recall recent events, amnesia.

Liver failure   MS/CH
(Refer to Cirrhosis; Hepatitis, acute viral)

Liver transplantation   MS/CH
(Refer to Transplantation, recipient)

Lockjaw   MS
(Refer to Tetanus)

Long-term care   CH
(Also refer to condition requiring/contributing to need for facility placement)

Anxiety [specify level]/Fear may be related to change in health status, role functioning, interaction patterns, socioeconomic status, environment; unmet needs, recent life changes, and loss of friends/SO(s), possibly evidenced by apprehension, restlessness, insomnia, repetitive questioning, pacing, purposeless activity, expressed concern regarding changes in life events, and focus on self.

Grieving may be related to perceived/actual or potential loss of physiopsychosocial well-being, personal possessions and significant other(s), as well as cultural beliefs about aging/debilitation, possibly evidenced by denial of feelings, depression, sorrow, guilt; alterations in activity level, sleep patterns, eating habits, and libido.

risk for Poisoning [drug toxicity]: risk factors may include effects of aging (reduced metabolism, impaired circulation, precarious physiological balance, presence of multiple diseases/organ involvement) and use of multiple prescribed/OTC drugs.

disturbed Thought Processes may be related to physiological changes of aging (loss of cells and brain atrophy, decreased blood supply); altered sensory input, pain, effects of medications, and psychological conflicts (disrupted life pattern), possibly evidenced by slower reaction times, memory loss, altered attention span, disorientation, inability to follow, altered sleep patterns, and personality changes.

Insomnia may be related to internal factors (illness, psychological stress, inactivity) and external factors (environmental changes, facility routines), possibly evidenced by reports of difficulty in falling asleep/not feeling rested, interrupted sleep/awakening earlier than desired; change in behavior/performance, increasing irritability, and listlessness.

risk for ineffective Sexuality Pattern: risk factors may include biopsychosocial alteration of sexuality; interference in psychological/physical well-being, self-image, and lack of privacy/SO.

risk for Relocation Stress Syndrome: risk factors may include multiple losses, feeling of powerlessness, lack of/inappropriate use of support system, changes in psychosocial/physical health status.

LSD (lysergic acid diethylamide) intoxication MS/PSY
(Also refer to Hallucinogen abuse)

risk for Trauma: risk factors may include perceptual distortion, impaired judgment, dangerous decision making, changes in mood.

Anxiety [panic attack] may be related to drug side effects, possibly evidenced by severe apprehension, fear of unspecific consequences, CNS excitation, central autonomic hyperactivity.

Lung cancer   MS/CH
(Refer to Bronchogenic carcinoma)

Lung transplantation   MS/CH
(Also refer to Transplantation, recipient)

risk for impaired Gas Exchange: risk factors may include ventilation/perfusion mismatch, poor healing/stenosis of bronchial or tracheal anastomosis.

risk for Infection: risk factors may include medically induced immunosuppression, suppressed inflammatory response, antibiotic therapy, invasive procedures, effects of chronic/debilitating disease.

Lupus erythematosus, systemic   CH
Fatigue may be related to inadequate energy production/increased energy requirements (chronic inflammation), overwhelming psychological or emotional demands, states of discomfort, and altered body chemistry (including effects of drug therapy), possibly evidenced by reports of unremitting and overwhelming lack of energy/inability to maintain usual routines, decreased performance, lethargy, and decreased libido.

acute Pain may be related to widespread inflammatory process affecting connective tissues, blood vessels, serosal surfaces and mucous membranes, possibly evidenced by verbal reports, guarding/distraction behaviors, self-focusing, and autonomic responses (changes in vital signs).

impaired Skin/Tissue Integrity may be related to chronic inflammation, edema formation, and altered circulation, possibly evidenced by presence of skin rash/lesions, ulcerations of mucous membranes and photosensitivity.

disturbed Body Image may be related to presence of chronic condition with rash, lesions, ulcers, purpura, mottled erythema of hands, alopecia, loss of strength, and altered body function, possibly evidenced by hiding body parts, negative feelings about body, feelings of helplessness, and change in social involvement.

Lyme disease   CH/MS

acute/chronic Pain may be related to systemic effects of toxins, presence of rash, urticaria, and joint swelling/inflammation, possibly evidenced by verbal reports, guarding behaviors, autonomic responses, and narrowed focus.

Fatigue may be related to increased energy requirements, altered body chemistry, and states of discomfort evidenced by reports of overwhelming lack of energy/inability to maintain usual routines, decreased performance, lethargy, and malaise.

risk for decreased Cardiac Output: risk factors may include alteration in cardiac rate/rhythm/conduction.

Lymphedema   CH

disturbed Body Image may be related to physical changes (chronic swelling of lower extremity), possibly evidenced by verbalizations, fear of reaction of others, negative feelings about body, hiding body part, change in social involvement.

impaired Walking may be related to chronic/progressive swelling of lower extremity, possibly evidenced by difficulty walking required distances, climbing stairs, navigating uneven surfaces/declines.

risk for impaired Skin Integrity: risk factors may include altered circulation, significant edema, changes in sensation.

Macular degeneration   CH

disturbed visual Sensory Perception may be related to altered sensory reception, possibly evidenced by reported/measured change in sensory acuity, change in usual response to stimuli.

Anxiety [specify level]/Fear may be related to situational crisis, threat to or change in health status and role function, possibly evidenced by expressed concerns, apprehension, feelings of inadequacy, diminished productivity, impaired attention.

risk for impaired Home Maintenance: risk factors may include impaired cognitive functioning, inadequate support systems.

risk for impaired Social Interaction: risk factors may include limited physical mobility, environmental barriers.

Malaria   MS/CH

Hyperthermia may be related to illness/inflammatory process, possibly evidenced by increased body temperature (106°F), flushed/warm skin, tachycardia, headache, altered consciousness.

acute Pain[/Discomfort] may be related to infectious agent/inflammatory response, possibly evidenced by reports of headache, backache, myalgia, malaise, high fever, shaking chills, abdominal discomfort.

risk for deficient Fluid Volume: risk factors may include decreased intake (nausea, abdominal pain, prostration), excessive losses (vomiting, diarrhea), hypermetabolic state.

Fatigue may be related to disease state, anemia, lack of restful sleep, possibly evidenced by verbalization of unremitting/overwhelming lack of energy, inability to restore energy even after sleep, lethargy.

Mallory-Weiss syndrome   MS

(Also refer to Achalasia)

risk for deficient Fluid Volume [isotonic]: risk factors may include excessive vascular losses, presence of vomiting, and reduced intake.

deficient Knowledge [Learning Need] regarding causes, treatment, and prevention of condition may be related to lack of information/misinterpretation, possibly evidenced by statements of concern, questions, and recurrence of problem.

Malnutrition   CH

(Also refer to Anorexia nervosa)

adult Failure to Thrive may be related to depression, apathy, aging process, fatigue, degenerative condition, possibly evidenced by expressed lack of appetite, difficulty performing self-care tasks, altered mood state, inadequate intake, weight loss, physical decline.

ineffective Protection may be related to inadequate nutrition, anemia, extremes of age, possibly evidenced by fatigue, weakness, deficient immunity, impaired healing, pressure sores.

Marburg disease   MS

(Refer to Ebola)

Mastectomy   MS

impaired Skin/Tissue Integrity may be related to surgical removal of skin/tissue, altered circulation, drainage, presence of edema, changes in skin elasticity/sensation, and tissue destruction (radiation), possibly evidenced by disruption of skin surface and destruction of skin layers/subcutaneous tissues.

impaired physical Mobility may be related to neuromuscular impairment, pain, and edema formation, possibly evidenced by reluctance to attempt movement, limited range of motion, and decreased muscle mass/strength.

bathing/dressing Self-Care Deficit may be related to temporary loss/altered action of one or both arms, possibly evidenced by statements of inability to perform/complete self-care tasks.

disturbed Body Image may be related to loss of body part denoting femininity, possibly evidenced by not looking at/touching area, negative feelings about body, preoccupation with loss, and change in social involvement/relationship.

Mastitis   OB/GYN

acute Pain may be related to erythema and edema of breast tissues, possibly evidenced by verbal reports, guarding/distraction behaviors, self-focusing, autonomic responses (changes in vital signs).

risk for Infection [spread/abscess formation]: risk factors may include traumatized tissues, stasis of fluids, and insufficient knowledge to prevent complications.

deficient Knowledge [Learning Need] regarding pathophysiology, treatment, and prevention may be related to lack of information/misinterpretation, possibly evidenced by statements of concern, questions, and misconceptions.

risk for ineffective Breastfeeding: risk factors may include inability to feed on affected side/interruption in breastfeeding.

Mastoidectomy   PED/MS

risk for Infection [spread]: risk factors may include preexisting infection, surgical trauma, and stasis of body fluids in close proximity to brain.

acute Pain may be related to inflammation, tissue trauma, and edema formation, possibly evidenced by verbal reports, distraction behaviors, restlessness, self-focusing, and autonomic responses (changes in vital signs).

disturbed auditory Sensory Perception may be related to presence of surgical packing, edema, and surgical disturbance of middle ear structures, possibly evidenced by reported/tested hearing loss in affected ear.

Measles   CH/PED

acute Pain may be related to inflammation of mucous membranes, conjunctiva, and presence of extensive skin rash with pruritus, possibly evidenced by verbal reports, distraction behaviors, self-focusing, and autonomic responses (changes in vital signs).

Hyperthermia may be related to presence of viral toxins and inflammatory response, possibly evidenced by increased body temperature, flushed/warm skin, and tachycardia.

risk for [secondary] Infection: risk factors may include altered immune response and traumatized dermal tissues.

deficient Knowledge [Learning Need] regarding condition, transmission, and possible complications may be related to lack of information/misinterpretation, possibly evidenced by statements of concern, questions, misconceptions, and development of preventable complications.

Measles, German   PED/CH
(Refer to Rubella)

Melanoma, malignant   MS/CH
(Refer to Cancer; Chemotherapy)

Ménière's disease   CH
(Also refer to Vertigo)

disturbed auditory Sensory Perception may be related to altered state of sensory organ/ sensory reception, possibly evidenced by change in sensory acuity, tinnitus, vertigo.

Nausea may be related to inner ear disturbance, possibly evidenced by verbal reports, vomiting.

risk for total Self-Care Deficit: risk factors may include perceptual impairment, recurrent nausea, general weakness.

Meningitis, acute meningococcal   MS

risk for Infection [spread]: risk factors may include hematogenous dissemination of pathogen, stasis of body fluids, suppressed inflammatory response (medication-induced), and exposure of others to pathogens.

risk for ineffective cerebral Tissue Perfusion: risk factors may include cerebral edema altering/ interrupting cerebral arterial/venous blood flow, hypovolemia, exchange problems at cellular level (acidosis).

Hyperthermia may be related to infectious process (increased metabolic rate) and dehydration, possibly evidenced by increased body temperature, warm/flushed skin, and tachycardia.

acute Pain may be related to inflammation/irritation of the meninges with spasm of extensor muscles (neck, shoulders, and back), possibly evidenced by verbal reports, guarding/distraction behaviors, narrowed focus, photophobia, and autonomic responses (changes in vital signs).

risk for Trauma/Suffocation: risk factors may include alterations in level of consciousness, possible development of clonic/tonic muscle activity (seizures), and generalized weakness/prostration, ataxia, vertigo.

Meniscectomy   MS/CH

impaired Walking may be related to pain, joint instability, and imposed medical restrictions of movement, possibly evidenced by impaired ability to move about environment as needed/ desired.

deficient Knowledge [Learning Need] regarding postoperative expectations, prevention of complications, and self-care needs may be related to lack of information, possibly evidenced by statements of concern, questions, and misconceptions.

Menopause   GYN
ineffective Thermoregulation may be related to fluctuation of hormonal levels, possibly evidenced by skin flushed/warm to touch, diaphoresis, night sweats, cold hands/feet.

Fatigue may be related to change in body chemistry, lack of sleep, depression, possibly evidenced by reports of lack of energy, tired, inability to maintain usual routines, decreased performance.

risk for ineffective Sexuality Pattern: risk factors may include perceived altered body function, changes in physical response, myths/inaccurate information, impaired relationship with SO.

risk for stress urinary Incontinence: risk factors may include degenerative changes in pelvic muscles and structural support.

Health-Seeking Behaviors: Management of life-cycle changes may be related to maturational change, possibly evidenced by expressed desire for increased control of health practice, demonstrated lack of knowledge in health promotion.

Mental retardation   CH
(Also refer to Down Syndrome)

impaired verbal Communication may be related to developmental delay/impairment of cognitive and motor abilities, possibly evidenced by impaired articulation, difficulty with phonation, and inability to modulate speech/find appropriate words (dependent on degree of retardation).

risk for Self-Care Deficit [specify]: risk factors may include impaired cognitive ability and motor skills.

risk for imbalanced Nutrition: more than body requirements: risk factors may include decreased metabolic rate coupled with impaired cognitive development, dysfunctional eating patterns, and sedentary activity level.

impaired Social Interaction may be related to impaired thought processes, communication barriers, and knowledge/skill deficit about ways to enhance mutuality, possibly evidenced by dysfunctional interactions with peers, family, and/or SO(s), and verbalized/observed discomfort in social situation.

compromised family Coping may be related to chronic nature of condition and degree of disability that exhausts supportive capacity of SO(s), other situational or developmental crises or situations SO(s) may be facing, unrealistic expectations of SO(s), possibly evidenced by preoccupation of SO with personal reaction, SO(s) withdraw(s) or enter(s) into limited interaction with individual, protective behavior disproportionate (too much or too little) to client's abilities or need for autonomy.

impaired Home Maintenance may be related to impaired cognitive functioning, insufficient finances/family organization or planning, lack of knowledge, and inadequate support systems, possibly evidenced by requests for assistance, expression of difficulty in maintaining home, disorderly surroundings, and overtaxed family members.

risk for Sexual Dysfunction: risk factors may include biopsychosocial alteration of sexuality, ineffectual/absent role models, misinformation/lack of knowledge, lack of SO(s), and lack of appropriate behavior control.

Mesothelioma   CH/MS
(Also refer to Asbestosis; Cancer)

acute Pain may be related to tissue destruction, possibly evidenced by reports of chest pain (initially nonpleuritic), irritability, self-focusing, autonomic responses.

Activity Intolerance may be related to imbalance between oxygen supply/demand, possibly evidenced by dyspnea, fatigue.

Metabolic syndrome   CH

risk for unstable blood Glucose: risk factors may include dietary intake, weight gain, physical activity level.

sedentary Lifestyle may be related to deficient knowledge of health benefits of physical exercise, lack of interest/motivation or resources, possibly evidenced by verbalized preference for activities low in physical activity, choosing a daily routine lacking physical exercise.

risk for ineffective Tissue Perfusion (specify): risk factors may include arterial plaque formation (elevated triglycerides, low levels of HDL), prothrombotic state, proinflammatory state.

Migraine   CH/MS
(Refer to Headache)

Miscarriage   OB
(Refer to Abortion, spontaneous termination)

Mitral insufficiency   MS/CH
(Refer to Valvular heart disease)

Mitral stenosis   MS/CH

Activity Intolerance may be related to imbalance between O_2 supply and demand, possibly evidenced by reports of fatigue, weakness, exertional dyspnea, and tachycardia.

impaired Gas Exchange may be related to altered blood flow, possibly evidenced by restlessness, hypoxia, and cyanosis (orthopnea/paroxysmal nocturnal dyspnea).

decreased Cardiac Output may be related to impeded blood flow as evidenced by jugular vein distention, peripheral/dependent edema, orthopnea/paroxysmal nocturnal dyspnea.

deficient Knowledge [Learning Need] regarding pathophysiology, therapeutic needs, and potential complications may be related to lack of information/recall, misinterpretation, possibly evidenced by statements of concern, questions, inaccurate follow-through of instructions, and development of preventable complications.

Mitral valve prolapse (MVP)   CH
(Refer to Valvular heart disease)

Mononucleosis, infectious   CH

Fatigue may be related to decreased energy production, states of discomfort, and increased energy requirements (inflammatory process), possibly evidenced by reports of overwhelming lack of energy, inability to maintain usual routines, lethargy, and malaise.

acute Pain[/Discomfort] may be related to inflammation of lymphoid and organ tissues, irritation of oropharyngeal mucous membranes, and effects of circulating toxins, possibly evidenced by verbal reports, distraction behaviors, and self-focusing.

Hyperthermia may be related to inflammatory process, possibly evidenced by increased body temperature, warm/flushed skin, and tachycardia.

deficient Knowledge [Learning Need] regarding disease transmission, self-care needs, medical therapy, and potential complications may be related to lack of information/misinterpretation, possibly evidenced by statements of concern, misconceptions, and inaccurate follow-through of instructions.

Mood disorders   PSY
(Refer to Depression, major; Bipolar disorder, Premenstrual dysphoric disorder)

Mountain sickness, acute (AMS)   CH/MS

acute Pain may be related to reduced oxygen tension, possibly evidenced by reports of headache.

Fatigue may be related to stress, increased physical exertion, sleep deprivation, possibly evidenced by overwhelming lack of energy, inability to restore energy even after sleep, compromised concentration, decreased performance.

risk for deficient Fluid Volume: risk factors may include increased water loss (e.g., over-breathing dry air), exertion, altered fluid intake (nausea).

Multiple organ dysfunction syndrome MS

(Also refer to specific organs involved; Sepsis; Ventilator assist/dependence)

ineffective peripheral/renal/gastrointestinal Tissue Perfusion may be related to hypovolemia, selective vasoconstriction, microvascular embolization, possibly evidenced by cool skin, diminished pulses, oliguria/anuria, nausea, abdominal tenderness, hypoactive bowel sounds.

impaired Gas Exchange may be related to ventilation perfusion imbalance, alveolar hypoventilation, possibly evidenced by dyspnea, irritability, confusion, abnormal ABGs.

Activity Intolerance may be related to generalized weakness, bedrest, imbalance between oxygen supply/demand, pain, possibly evidenced by abnormal heart rate/BP response to activity, pallor, exertional discomfort, ECG changes (dysrhythmias, ischemia).

severe Anxiety/Fear may be related to situational crisis, change in health status, threat of death, possibly evidenced by expressed concerns, apprehension, increased tension, fearfulness, restlessness, decreased perceptual field.

imbalanced Nutrition: less than body requirements may be related to restricted intake, inability to digest food, increased metabolic demands, possibly evidenced by weight loss, poor muscle tone, decreased subcutaneous fat/muscle mass, abnormal laboratory studies.

risk for Infection: risk factors may include stasis of body fluids, immunosuppression, malnutrition, invasive devices/procedures, environmental exposure.

Multiple personality   PSY

(Refer to Dissociative Disorders)

Multiple sclerosis   CH

Fatigue may be related to decreased energy production/increased energy requirements to perform activities, psychological/emotional demands, pain/discomfort, medication side effects, possibly evidenced by verbalization of overwhelming lack of energy, inability to maintain usual routine, decreased performance, impaired ability to concentrate, increase in physical complaints.

disturbed visual/kinesthetic/tactile Sensory Perception may be related to delayed/interrupted neuronal transmission, possibly evidenced by impaired vision, diplopia, disturbance of vibratory or position sense, paresthesias, numbness, and blunting of sensation.

impaired physical Mobility may be related to neuromuscular impairment, discomfort/pain, sensoriperceptual impairments, decreased muscle strength, control or mass, deconditioning, as evidenced by limited ability to perform motor skills, limited range of motion, gait changes/postural instability.

Powerlessness/Hopelessness may be related to illness-related regimen and lifestyle of helplessness, possibly evidenced by verbal expressions of having no control or influence over the situation, depression over physical deterioration that occurs despite client compliance with regimen, nonparticipation in care or decision making when opportunities are provided, passivity, decreased verbalization/affect.

impaired Home Maintenance may be related to effects of debilitating disease, impaired cognitive or emotional functioning, insufficient finances, and inadequate support systems, possibly evidenced by reported difficulty, observed disorderly surroundings, and poor hygienic conditions.

compromised/disabled family Coping may be related to situational crises/temporary family disorganization and role changes, client providing little support in turn for SO(s), prolonged disease/disability progression that exhausts the supportive capacity of SO(s), feelings of guilt, anxiety, hostility, despair, and highly ambivalent family relationships, possibly evidenced by client expressing/confirming concern or report about SOs' response to client's illness, SO(s) preoccupied with own personal reactions, intolerance, abandonment, neglectful care of the client, and distortion of reality regarding client's illness.

Mumps   PED/CH

acute Pain may be related to presence of inflammation, circulating toxins, and enlargement of salivary glands, possibly evidenced by verbal reports, guarding/distraction behaviors, self-focusing, and autonomic responses (changes in vital signs).

Hyperthermia may be related to inflammatory process (increased metabolic rate) and dehydration, possibly evidenced by increased body temperature, warm/flushed skin, and tachycardia.

risk for deficient Fluid Volume: risk factors may include hypermetabolic state and painful swallowing, with decreased intake.

Muscular dystrophy (Duchenne's)   PED/CH

impaired physical Mobility may be related to musculoskeletal impairment/weakness, possibly evidenced by decreased muscle strength, control, and mass; limited range of motion; and impaired coordination.

delayed Growth and Development may be related to effects of physical disability, possibly evidenced by altered physical growth and altered ability to perform self-care/self-control activities appropriate to age.

risk for imbalanced Nutrition: more than body requirements: risk factors may include sedentary lifestyle and dysfunctional eating patterns.

compromised family Coping may be related to situational crisis/emotional conflicts around issues about hereditary nature of condition and prolonged disease/disability that exhausts supportive capacity of family members, possibly evidenced by preoccupation with personal reactions regarding disability and displaying protective behavior disproportionate (too little/too much) to client's abilities/need for autonomy.

Myasthenia gravis   MS

ineffective Breathing Pattern/Airway Clearance may be related to neuromuscular weakness and decreased energy/fatigue, possibly evidenced by dyspnea, changes in rate/depth of respiration, ineffective cough, and adventitious breath sounds.

impaired verbal Communication may be related to neuromuscular weakness, fatigue, and physical barrier (intubation), possibly evidenced by facial weakness, impaired articulation, hoarseness, and inability to speak.

impaired Swallowing may be related to neuromuscular impairment of laryngeal/pharyngeal muscles and muscular fatigue, possibly evidenced by reported/observed difficulty swallowing, coughing/choking, and evidence of aspiration.

Anxiety [specify level]/Fear may be related to situational crisis, threat to self-concept, change in health/socioeconomic status or role function, separation from support systems, lack of knowledge, and inability to communicate, possibly evidenced by expressed concerns, increased tension, restlessness, apprehension, sympathetic stimulation, crying, focus on self, uncooperative behavior, withdrawal, anger, and noncommunication.

CH

deficient Knowledge [Learning Need] regarding drug therapy, potential for crisis (myasthenic or cholinergic) and self-care management may be related to inadequate information/misinterpretation, possibly evidenced by statements of concern, questions, and misconceptions; development of preventable complications.

impaired physical Mobility may be related to neuromuscular impairment, possibly evidenced by reports of progressive fatigue with repetitive/prolonged muscle use, impaired coordination, and decreased muscle strength/control.

disturbed visual Sensory Perception may be related to neuromuscular impairment, possibly evidenced by visual distortions (diplopia) and motor incoordination.

Myelitis, transverse   **MS/CH**
(Refer to Paraplegia)

Myeloma, multiple   **MS/CH**
(Also refer to Cancer)
acute/chronic Pain may be related to destruction of tissues/bone, side effects of therapy, possibly evidenced by verbal or coded reports, guarding/protective behaviors, changes in appetite/weight, sleep; reduced interaction with others.

impaired physical Mobility may be related to loss of integrity of bone structure, pain, deconditioning, depressed mood, possibly evidenced by verbalizations, limited range of motion, slowed movement, gait changes.

risk for ineffective Protection: risk factors may include presence of cancer, drug therapies, radiation treatments, inadequate nutrition.

Myocardial infarction   **MS**
(Also refer to Myocarditis)
acute Pain may be related to ischemia of myocardial tissue, possibly evidenced by verbal reports, guarding/distraction behaviors (restlessness), facial mask of pain, self-focusing, and autonomic responses (diaphoresis, changes in vital signs).

Anxiety [specify level]/Fear may be related to threat of death, threat of change of health status/role functioning and lifestyle, interpersonal transmission/contagion, possibly evidenced by increased tension, fearful attitude, apprehension, expressed concerns/uncertainty, restlessness, sympathetic stimulation, and somatic complaints.

risk for decreased Cardiac Output: risk factors may include changes in rate and electrical conduction, reduced preload/increased SVR, and altered muscle contractility/depressant effects of some medications, infarcted/dyskinetic muscle, structural defects.

Myocarditis   **MS**
(Also refer to Myocardial Infarction)
Activity Intolerance may be related to imbalance in O_2 supply and demand (myocardial inflammation/damage) cardiac depressant effects of certain drugs, and enforced bedrest, possibly evidenced by reports of fatigue, exertional dyspnea, tachycardia/palpitations in response to activity, ECG changes/dysrhythmias, and generalized weakness.

risk for decreased Cardiac Output: risk factors may include degeneration of cardiac muscle.

deficient Knowledge [Learning Need] regarding pathophysiology of condition/outcomes, treatment, and self-care needs/lifestyle changes may be related to lack of information/misinterpretation, possibly evidenced by statements of concern, misconceptions, inaccurate follow-through of instructions, and development of preventable complications.

Myoclonus, nocturnal   **CH**
Sleep Deprivation may be related to periodic limb movement/irresistible urge to move legs to relieve uncomfortable sensations, possibly evidenced by decreased quality of sleep, daytime drowsiness, decreased ability to function, inability to concentrate.

Myofascial pain syndrome   **CH**
(Also refer to Fibromyalgia)

    acute/chronic Pain may be related to nocturnal bruxism (clenching/grinding teeth), possibly evidenced by reports of pain (temporomandibular region), headache, muscular tenderness to palpation, limitation in opening mouth.

    risk for impaired Dentition: risk factors may include bruxism, ineffective oral hygiene (limitations in opening mouth).

Myringotomy   **PED/MS**
(Refer to Mastoidectomy)

Myxedema   **CH**
(Also refer to Hypothyroidism)

    disturbed Body Image may be related to change in structure/function (loss of hair/thickening of skin, masklike facial expression, enlarged tongue, menstrual and reproductive disturbances), possibly evidenced by negative feelings about body, feelings of helplessness, and change in social involvement.

    imbalanced Nutrition: more than body requirements may be related to decreased metabolic rate and activity level, possibly evidenced by weight gain greater than ideal for height and frame.

    risk for decreased Cardiac Output: risk factors may include altered electrical conduction and myocardial contractility.

Narcolepsy   **CH**
Insomnia may be related to medical condition, possibly evidenced by hypersomnia, reports of unsatisfying nighttime sleep, vivid visual/auditory illusions/hallucinations at onset of sleep, sleep interrupted by vivid/frightening dreams.

    risk for Trauma: risk factors may include sudden loss of muscle tone/momentary paralysis (cataplexy), sudden inappropriate sleep episodes.

    risk for chronic low Self-Esteem: risk factors may include negative evaluation of self, personal vulnerability, chronic physical condition, impaired work/school performance, problems with social relationships, reduced quality of life.

Near drowning   **MS**
impaired Gas Exchange may be related to ventilation perfusion imbalance (patchy atelectasis), alveolar-capillary membrane changes, aspiration or acute reflex laryngospasm, possibly evidenced by severe hypoxia, pale/dusky skin, change in mentation (confusion to coma).

    risk for excess Fluid Volume: risk factors may include aspiration of fresh water.

    risk for Hypothermia: risk factors may include submersion in very cold water.

NEC   **PED**
(Refer to Necrotizing enterocolitis)

Necrotizing cellulitis/fasciitis   **MS**
(Also refer to Cellulitis; Sepsis)

    Hyperthermia may be related to inflammatory process, response to circulating toxins, possibly evidenced by body temperature above normal range, flushed/warm skin, tachycardia, altered mental status.

    impaired Tissue Integrity may be related to inflammation/edema (infection), ischemia, possibly evidenced by damaged or destroyed tissue/dermal gangrene.

Necrotizing enterocolitis   **PED**
(Also refer to Sepsis)

---

imbalanced Nutrition: less than body requirements may be related to inabililty to digest/ absorb nutrients (ischemia of bowel), possibly evidenced by abdominal pain/distention, gastric residuals after feedings, failure to gain weight.

risk for deficient Fluid Volume: risk factors may include vomiting, third-space fluid losses (bowel inflammmation, peritonitis), lack of oral intake.

Neglect/Abuse   CH/PSY
(Refer to Abuse, Battered child syndrome)

Nephrectomy   MS
acute Pain may be related to surgical tissue trauma with mechanical closure (suture), possibly evidenced by verbal reports, guarding/distraction behaviors, self-focusing, and autonomic responses (changes in vital signs).

risk for deficient Fluid Volume: risk factors may include excessive vascular losses and restricted intake.

ineffective Breathing Pattern may be related to incisional pain with decreased lung expansion, possibly evidenced by tachypnea, fremitus, changes in respiratory depth/chest expansion, and changes in ABGs.

Constipation may be related to reduced dietary intake, decreased mobility, GI obstruction (paralytic ileus), and incisional pain with defecation, possibly evidenced by decreased bowel sounds, reduced frequency/amount of stool, and hard/formed stool.

Nephrolithiasis   MS/CH
(Refer to Calculi, urinary)

Nephrotic syndrome   MS/CH
(Also refer to Renal failure, acute/chronic)

excess Fluid Volume may be related to compromised regulatory mechanism with changes in hydrostatic/oncotic vascular pressure and increased activation of the renin-angiotensin-aldosterone system, possibly evidenced by edema/anasarca, effusions/ascites, weight gain, intake greater than output, and BP changes.

imbalanced Nutrition: less than body requirements may be related to excessive protein losses and inability to ingest adequate nutrients (anorexia), possibly evidenced by weight loss/muscle wasting (may be difficult to assess due to edema), lack of interest in food, and observed inadequate intake.

risk for Infection: risk factors may include chronic disease and steroidal suppression of inflammatory responses.

risk for impaired Skin Integrity: risk factors may include presence of edema and activity restrictions.

Neuralgia, trigeminal   CH
acute Pain may be related to neuromuscular impairment with sudden violent muscle spasm, possibly evidenced by verbal reports, guarding/distraction behaviors, self-focusing, and autonomic responses (changes in vital signs).

deficient Knowledge [Learning Need] regarding control of recurrent episodes, medical therapies, and self-care needs may be related to lack of information/recall and misinterpretation, possibly evidenced by statements of concern, questions, and exacerbation of condition.

Neural tube defect   PED
(Refer to Spina bifida)

Neuritis   CH
acute/chronic Pain may be related to nerve damage usually associated with a degenerative process, possibly evidenced by verbal reports, guarding/distraction behaviors, self-focusing, and autonomic responses (changes in vital signs).

deficient Knowledge [Learning Need] regarding underlying causative factors, treatment, and prevention may be related to lack of information/misinterpretation, possibly evidenced by statements of concern, questions, and misconceptions.

Newborn, growth deviations   PED

(Also refer to Newborn, premature)

disproportionate Growth may be related to maternal nutrition, substance use/abuse, multiple gestation, prematurity, maternal conditions (e.g., PIH, diabetes), possibly evidenced by birth weight at or below tenth percentile/at or above 90th percentile (considering gestational age, ethnicity, etc.).

imbalanced Nutrition: less than body requirements may be related to decreased nutritional stores, increased insulin production/hyperplasia of pancreatic beta cells, possibly evidenced by weight deviation from expected, decreased muscle mass/fat stores, electrolyte imbalance.

risk for ineffective Tissue Perfusion: risk factors may include interruption of arterial/venous blood flow (hyperviscosity associated with polycythemia).

risk for Injury: risk factors may include altered growth, delayed CNS/neurological development, abnormal blood profile.

risk for disorganized Infant Behavior: risk factors may include functional limitations related to growth deviations (restricting neonate's opportunity to seek out, recognize, and interpret stimuli), electrolyte imbalance, psychological stress, low energy reserves, poor organizational ability, limited ability to control environment.

Newborn, normal   PED

risk for impaired Gas Exchange: risk factors may include prenatal or intrapartal stressors, excess production of mucus, or cold stress.

risk for imbalanced Body Temperature: risk factors may include large body surface in relation to mass, limited amounts of insulating subcutaneous fat, nonrenewable sources of brown fat and few white fat stores, thin epidermis with close proximity of blood vessels to the skin, inability to shiver, and movement from a warm uterine environment to a much cooler environment.

risk for impaired parent/infant Attachment: risk factors may include developmental transition (gain of a family member), anxiety associated with the parent role, lack of privacy (intrusive family/visitors).

risk for imbalanced Nutrition: less than body requirements: risk factors may include rapid metabolic rate, high-caloric requirement, increased insensible water losses through pulmonary and cutaneous routes, fatigue, and a potential for inadequate or depleted glucose stores.

risk for Infection: risk factors may include inadequate secondary defenses (inadequate acquired immunity, e.g., deficiency of neutrophils and specific immunoglobulins), and inadequate primary defenses (e.g., environmental exposure, broken skin, traumatized tissues, decreased ciliary action).

Newborn at 1 week   PED

(Also refer to Newborn, normal)

risk for Injury: risk factors may include physical (hyperbilirubinemia), environmental (inadequate safety precautions), chemical (drugs in breastmilk), psychological (inappropriate parental stimulation/interaction).

risk for Constipation/Diarrhea: risk factors may include type/amount of oral intake, medications or dietary intake of lactating mother, presence of allergies, infection.

risk for impaired Skin Integrity: risk factors may include excretions (ammonia formation from urea), chemical irritation from laundry detergent/diapering material, mechanical factors (e.g., long fingernails).

Newborn, postmature   PED

risk for impaired Gas Exchange: risk factors may include ventilation perfusion imbalances (meconium aspiration/pneumonitis).

Hypothermia may be related to decreased subcutaneous fat stores, poor metabolic reserves, exposure to cool environment, decreased ability to shiver, possibly evidenced by reduction in body temperature, cool skin, pallor.

risk for imbalanced Nutrition: less than body requirements: risk factors may include placental insufficiency, decreased subcutaneous fat stores, decreased glycogen stores at birth (neonatal hypoglycemia).

risk for impaired Skin Integrity: risk factors may include dry/peeling skin, long fingernails, absence of vernix caseous.

Newborn, premature   PED

impaired Gas Exchange may be related to alveolar-capillary membrane changes (inadequate surfactant levels), altered blood flow (immaturity of pulmonary arteriole musculature), altered O_2 supply (immaturity of central nervous system and neuromuscular system, tracheobronchial obstruction), altered O_2-carrying capacity of blood (anemia), and cold stress, possibly evidenced by respiratory difficulties, inadequate oxygenation of tissues, and acidemia.

ineffective Breathing Pattern may be related to immaturity of the respiratory center, poor positioning, drug-related depression and metabolic imbalances, decreased energy/fatigue, possibly evidenced by dyspnea, tachypnea, periods of apnea, nasal flaring/use of accessory muscles, cyanosis, abnormal ABGs, and tachycardia.

risk for ineffective Thermoregulation: risk factors may include immature CNS development (temperature regulation center), decreased ratio of body mass to surface area, decreased subcutaneous fat, limited brown fat stores, inability to shiver or sweat, poor metabolic reserves, muted response to hypothermia, and frequent medical/nursing manipulations and interventions.

risk for deficient Fluid Volume: risk factors may include extremes of age and weight, excessive fluid losses (thin skin, lack of insulating fat, increased environmental temperature, immature kidney/failure to concentrate urine).

risk for ineffective Infant Feeding Pattern: risk factors may include decreased energy/fatigue, poor positioning, drug-related depression, inability to coordinate sucking, swallowing, and breathing.

risk for disorganized Infant Behavior: risk factors may include prematurity (immaturity of CNS system, hypoxia), lack of containment/boundaries, pain, overstimulation, separation from parents.

risk for Injury [CNS damage]: risk factors may include tissue hypoxia, altered clotting factors, metabolic imbalances (hypoglycemia, electrolyte shifts, elevated bilirubin).

Newborn, small for gestational age PED
(Refer to Newborn, growth deviations)

Newborn, special needs   PED
(Also refer to specific condition)

parental/family Grieving may be related to perceived loss of the perfect child, alterations of future expectations, possibly evidenced by expression of distress at loss, sorrow, guilt, anger, choked feelings; interference with life activities, crying.

deficient parental Knowledge [Learning Need] regarding condition and infant care may be related to lack of/unfamiliarity with information resources, misinterpretation, possibly evidenced by questions, concerns, misconceptions, hesitancy or inadequate performance of activities.

risk for impaired parent/infant Attachment: risk factors may include delay/interruption in bonding process (separation, physical barriers), perceived threat to infant's survival, stressors (financial, family needs), lack of appropriate response of newborn, lack of support between/from SOs.

risk for ineffective family Coping: risk factors may include situational crises, temporary preoccupation of SO trying to manage emotional conflicts and personal suffering, being unable to perceive or act effectively in regards to infant's needs, temporary family disorganization.

risk for parental Social Isolation: risk factors may include perceived situational crisis, assuming sole/full-time responsibility for infant's care, lack of or inappropriate use of resources.

Nicotine abuse   CH

risk-prone health Behavior may be related to lack of motivation to change behavior, low state of optimism, absence of social/SO support for change, failure to intend to change behavior, possibly evidenced by denial of health problem, failure to take action, failure to achieve optimal sense of control.

risk for Injury: risk factors may include smoking habits (e.g., in bed, while driving, near combustible chemicals/O_2), children playing with cigarettes/matches.

risk for impaired Gas Exchange: risk factors may include progressive airflow obstruction, decreased oxygen supply (carbon monoxide).

risk for ineffective peripheral Tissue Perfusion: risk factors may include reduction of arterial/venous blood flow.

Nicotine withdrawal   CH

Health-Seeking Behaviors (smoking cessation) may be related to concern about health status, acceptance of deleterious effects of smoking, possibly evidenced by expressed concerns/desire to seek higher level of wellness.

risk for imbalanced Nutrition: more than body requirements: risk factors may include return of appetite, normalization of basal metabolic rate, eating in response to internal cues (substitution of food for activity of smoking).

risk for ineffective Therapeutic Regimen Management: risk factors may include economic difficulties, lack of support from SO/friends, continued enviromental exposure to secondhand smoke/smoking activity.

Nonketotic hyperglycemic-hyperosmolar coma   MS

deficient Fluid Volume may be related to excessive renal losses, inadequate oral intake, extremes of age, presence of infection, possibly evidenced by sudden weight loss, dry skin/mucous membranes, poor skin tugor, hypotension, increased pulse, fever, change in mental status (confusion to coma).

decreased Cardiac Output may be related to decreased preload (hypovolemia), altered heart rhythm (hyper/hypokalemia), possibly evidenced by decreased hemodynamic pressures (e.g., CVP), ECG changes/dysrhythmias.

imbalanced Nutrition: less than body requirements may be related to inadequate utilization of nutrients (insulin deficiency), decreased oral intake, hypermetabolic state, possibly evidenced by recent weight loss, imbalance between glucose/insulin levels.

risk for Trauma: risk factors may include weakness, cognitive limitations/altered consciousness, loss of large- or small-muscle coordination (risk for seizure activity).

Obesity   CH

imbalanced Nutrition: more than body requirements may be related to excessive intake in relation to metabolic needs, possibly evidenced by weight 20% greater than ideal for height and frame, sedentary activity level, reported/observed dysfunctional eating patterns, and excess body fat by triceps skinfold/other measurements.

Activity Intolerance may be related to imbalance between oxygen supply and demand, and sedentary lifestyle, possibly evidenced by fatigue or weakness, exertional discomfort, and abnormal heart rate/BP response.

    risk for Sleep Deprivation: risk factors may include sleep apnea.

    risk for ineffective Breathing Pattern: risk factors may include obesity.

PSY

disturbed Body Image/chronic low Self-Esteem may be related to view of self in contrast to societal values, family/subcultural encouragement of overeating; control, sex, and love issues, possibly evidenced by negative feelings about body, fear of rejection/reaction of others, feeling of hopelessness/powerlessness, and lack of follow-through with treatment plan.

    impaired Social Interaction may be related to verbalized/observed discomfort in social situations, self-concept disturbance, possibly evidenced by reluctance to participate in social gatherings, verbalization of a sense of discomfort with others, feelings of rejection, absence of/ineffective supportive SO(s).

Obesity-hypoventilation syndrome   CH
(Refer to Pickwickian syndrome)

Obsessive-Compulsive disorder   PSY
[severe] Anxiety may be related to earlier life conflicts, possibly evidenced by repetitive actions, recurring thoughts, decreased social and role functioning.

    risk for impaired Skin/Tissue Integrity: risk factors may include repetitive behaviors related to cleansing (e.g., handwashing, brushing teeth, showering).

    risk for ineffective Role Performance: risk factors may include psychological stress, health-illness problems.

Opioid abuse   CH/PSY
(Refer to Depressant abuse; Heroin abuse/withdrawal)

Oppositional defiant disorder   PED/PSY
ineffective Coping may be related to situational/maturational crisis, mild neurological deficits, retarded ego development, dysfunctional family system, negative role models, possibly evidenced by inability to meet age-appropriate role expectations, hostility toward others, defiant response to requests/rules, inability to delay gratification.

    impaired Social Interaction may be related to retarded ego development, dysfunctional family, negative role models, neurological impairment, possibly evidenced by discomfort in social situations, difficulty playing/interacting with others, aggressive behavior, bullies/bosses/others, refusal to comply with requests of others.

    chronic low Self-Esteem may be related to retarded ego development, lack of positive/repeated negative feedback, mild neurological deficits, negative role models, possibly evidenced by lack of eye contact, lack of self-confidence, physical risk-taking, distraction of others to cover up own failures, projection of blame.

    compromised/disabled family Coping may be related to anger, excessive guilt, blaming among family members regarding child's behavior, parental inconsistencies/disagreements regarding discipline and limit-setting, exhaustion of parental resources, possibly evidenced by unrealistic parental expectations, rejection/overprotection of child, exaggerated expressions of anger/disappointment/despair.

Organic brain syndrome   CH
(Refer to Alzheimer's disease)

Osgood-Schlatter disease   PED

acute Pain may be related to inflammation and swelling in region of patellar tendon, possibly evidenced by verbal reports, protective behavior, change in muscle tone.

impaired Walking may be related to inflammatory process (knee), possibly evidenced by impaired ability to walk desired distances, climb/descend stairs.

risk for ineffective Therapeutic Regimen Management: risk factors may include age (adolescent), perceived seriousness/benefit, competitive nature/peer pressure.

Osteitis deformans   CH
(Refer to Paget's disease)

Osteoarthritis (degenerative joint disease)   CH
(Refer to Arthritis, rheumatoid)

(Although this is a degenerative process versus the inflammatory process of rheumatoid arthritis, nursing concerns are the same.)

Osteomalacia   CH
(Refer to Rickets)

Osteomyelitis   MS/CH

acute Pain may be related to inflammation and tissue necrosis, possibly evidenced by verbal reports, guarding/distraction behaviors, self-focus, and autonomic responses (changes in vital signs).

Hyperthermia may be related to increased metabolic rate and infectious process, possibly evidenced by increased body temperature and warm/flushed skin.

ineffective bone Tissue Perfusion may be related to inflammatory reaction with thrombosis of vessels, destruction of tissue, edema, and abscess formation, possibly evidenced by bone necrosis, continuation of infectious process, and delayed healing.

risk for impaired Walking: risk factors may include inflammation and tissue necrosis, pain, joint instability.

deficient Knowledge [Learning Need] regarding pathophysiology of condition, long-term therapy needs, activity restriction, and prevention of complications may be related to lack of information/ misinterpretation, possibly evidenced by statements of concern, questions, and misconceptions, and inaccurate follow-through of instructions.

Osteoporosis   CH

risk for Trauma: risk factors may include loss of bone density/integrity increasing risk of fracture with minimal or no stress.

acute/chronic Pain may be related to vertebral compression on spinal nerve/muscles/ligaments, spontaneous fractures, possibly evidenced by verbal reports, guarding/distraction behaviors, self-focus, and changes in sleep pattern.

impaired physical Mobility may be related to pain and musculoskeletal impairment, possibly evidenced by limited range of motion, reluctance to attempt movement/expressed fear of reinjury, and imposed restrictions/limitations.

Otitis media   PED

acute Pain may be related to inflammation, edema/pressure, possibly evidenced by verbal/coded report, guarded behavior, restlessness, crying.

disturbed auditory Sensory Perception may be related to decreased sensory reception, possibly evidenced by reported change in sensory acuity, auditory distortions, change in usual response to stimuli.

---

risk for delayed Development: risk factors may include auditory impairment, frequent otitis media.

Ovarian cancer   MS
(Also refer to Cancer)

disturbed Body Image may be related to surgical change in reproductive organs/surgical menopause, loss of hair and weight, possibly evidenced by negative feelings about body/sense of mutilation, preoccupation with change, feelings of helplessness/hopelessness, and change in social involvement.

ineffective Sexuality Pattern/Sexual Dysfunction may be related to change in sexual organs, postoperative menopause, vulnerability, possibly evidenced by verbalizations of problem, inability in achieving desired satisfaction, alterations in relationship with SO.

Paget's disease, bone   CH
acute Pain may be related to compression/entrapment of nerves, joint degeneration, possibly evidenced by reports of headache, back/joint pain.

Fatigue may be related to disease state/hypermetabolic condition, possibly evidenced by overwhelming lack of energy, inability to maintain usual routines, tired.

disturbed Body Image may be related to physical deformities (enlarged skull, bowing of long bones), possibly evidenced by verbalization of feelings reflecting altered view of body, negative feelings about body, fear of rejection/reaction of others, change in social involvement.

disturbed auditory Sensory Perception may be related to altered sensory reception/transmission (nerve compression), possibly evidenced by decreased auditory acuity.

risk for impaired Walking: risk factors may include bowing of long bones, hobbling gait, joint stiffness/pain, paresis/paralysis.

risk for Injury/Falls: risk factors may include bone deformity/fragility, joint stiffness/pain, altered gait.

risk for decreased Cardiac Output: risk factors may include excessive circulatory demands (metabolically active and highly vascular nature of lesions).

Palliative care   CH
(Refer to Hospice Care)

Palsy, cerebral (spastic hemiplegia) PED/CH
impaired physical Mobility may be related to muscular weakness/hypertonicity, increased deep tendon reflexes, tendency to contractures, and underdevelopment of affected limbs, possibly evidenced by decreased muscle strength, control, mass, limited range of motion, and impaired coordination.

compromised family Coping may be related to permanent nature of condition, situational crisis, emotional conflicts/temporary family disorganization, and incomplete information/understanding of client's needs, possibly evidenced by verbalized anxiety/guilt regarding client's disability, inadequate understanding and knowledge base, and displaying protective behaviors disproportionate (too little/too much) to client's abilities or need for autonomy.

delayed Growth and Development may be related to effects of physical disability, possibly evidenced by altered physical growth, delay or difficulty in performing skills (motor, social, expressive), and altered ability to perform self-care/self-control activities appropriate to age.

Pancreas transplantation   MS/CH
(Refer to Transplantation, recipient)

Pancreatic cancer   MS
(Also refer to Cancer)

acute *Pain[/Discomfort]* may be related to pressure on surrounding organs/nerves, possibly evidenced by verbal reports, guarding/distraction behaviors, focus on self, and autonomic responses (changes in vital signs).

imbalanced *Nutrition: less than body requirements* may be related to inability to ingest/digest food, absorb nutrients, increased metabolic needs, possibly evidenced by inadequate food intake, anorexia, abdominal pain after eating, weight loss, cachexia.

risk for *Infection:* risk factors may include stasis of body fluids (biliary obstruction), malnutrition.

risk for impaired *Tissue Integrity:* risk factors may include poor skin turgor, skeletal prominence, presence of edema/ascites, bile salt accumulation in the tissues.

Pancreatitis   MS

acute *Pain* may be related to obstruction of pancreatic/biliary ducts, chemical contamination of peritoneal surfaces by pancreatic exudate/autodigestion, extension of inflammation to the retroperitoneal nerve plexus, possibly evidenced by verbal reports, guarding/distraction behaviors, self-focusing, grimacing, autonomic responses (changes in vital signs), and alteration in muscle tone.

risk for deficient *Fluid Volume:* risk factors may include excessive gastric losses (vomiting, nasogastric suctioning), increase in size of vascular bed (vasodilation, effects of kinins), third-space fluid transudation, ascites formation, alteration of clotting process, hemorrhage.

imbalanced *Nutrition: less than body requirements* may be related to vomiting, decreased oral intake as well as altered ability to digest nutrients (loss of digestive enzymes/insulin), possibly evidenced by reported inadequate food intake, aversion to eating, reported altered taste sensation, weight loss, and reduced muscle mass.

risk for *Infection:* risk factors may include inadequate primary defenses (stasis of body fluids, altered peristalsis, change in pH secretions), immunosuppression, nutritional deficiencies, tissue destruction, and chronic disease.

Panic disorder   PSY

Fear may be related to unfounded morbid dread of a seemingly harmless object/situation, possibly evidenced by physiological symptoms, mental/cognitive behaviors indicative of panic, withdrawal from or total avoidance of situations that place client in contact with feared object.

[severe to panic] Anxiety may be related to unidentified stressors, contact with feared object/situation, limitations placed on ritualistic behavior, possibly evidenced by attacks of immobilizing apprehension, physical/mental/cognitive behaviors indicative of panic, expressed feelings of terror/inability to cope.

Paralysis, infantile   PED
(Refer to Poliomyelitis)

Paranoid personality disorder   PSY

risk for other/self-directed *Violence:* risk factors may include perceived threats of danger, paranoid delusions, and increased feelings of anxiety.

[severe] Anxiety may be related to inability to trust (has not mastered tasks of trust versus mistrust), possibly evidenced by rigid delusional system (serves to provide relief from stress that justifies the delusion), frightened of other people and own hostility.

Powerlessness may be related to feelings of inadequacy, lifestyle of helplessness, maladaptive interpersonal interactions (e.g., misuse of power, force; abusive relationships), sense of severely impaired self-concept, and belief that individual has no control over situation(s), possibly evidenced by paranoid delusions, use of aggressive behavior to compensate, and expressions of recognition of damage paranoia has caused self and others.

---

disturbed Thought Processes may be related to psychological conflicts, increased anxiety, and fear, possibly evidenced by difficulties in the process and character of thought, interference with the ability to think clearly and logically, delusions, fragmentation, and autistic thinking.

compromised family Coping may be related to temporary or sustained family disorganization/role changes, prolonged progression of condition that exhausts the supportive capacity of SO(s), possibly evidenced by family system not meeting physical/emotional/spiritual needs of its members, inability to express or to accept wide range of feelings, inappropriate boundary maintenance; SO(s) describe(s) preoccupation with personal reactions.

Paranoid schizophrenia   PSY
(Refer to Schizophrenia)

Paraphilias   PSY
ineffective Sexuality Pattern may be related to conflict with sexual orientation or variant preferences, possibly evidenced by alterations in achieving sexual satisfaction, difficulty achieving desired satisfaction in socially acceptable ways.

chronic low Self-Esteem may be related to psychosocial factors (e.g., achievement of sexual satisfaction in deviant ways), substance use, possibly evidenced by expressions of shame/guilt, self-destructive behaviors, feelings of powerlessness, helplessness.

interrupted Family Processes may be related to situational crisis (e.g., revelation of sexual deviance/dysfunction), possibly evidenced by expressions of confusion about/difficulty dealing with situation, inappropriate boundary maintenance, family system does not meet emotional/security needs, failure to deal with traumatic experience constructively.

Paraplegia   MS/CH
(Also refer to Quadriplegia)
impaired Transfer Ability may be related to loss of muscle function/control, injury to upper extremity joints (overuse).

disturbed kinesthetic/tactile Sensory Perception may be related to neurological deficit with loss of sensory reception and transmission, psychological stress, possibly evidenced by reported/measured change in sensory acuity and loss of usual response to stimuli.

reflex urinary Incontinence/impaired Urinary Elimination may be related to loss of nerve conduction above the level of the reflex arc, possibly evidenced by lack of awareness of bladder filling/fullness, absence of urge to void, uninhibited bladder contraction, urinary tract infections (UTIs), kidney stone formation.

disturbed Body Image/ineffective Role Performance may be related to loss of body functions, change in physical ability to resume role, perceived loss of self/identity, possibly evidenced by negative feelings about body/self, feelings of helplessness/powerlessness, delay in taking responsibility for self-care/participation in therapy, and change in social involvement.

Sexual Dysfunction may be related to loss of sensation, altered function, and vulnerability, possibly evidenced by seeking of confirmation of desirability, verbalization of concern, alteration in relationship with SO, and change in interest in self/others.

Parathyroidectomy   MS
acute Pain may be related to presence of surgical incision and effects of calcium imbalance (bone pain, tetany), possibly evidenced by verbal reports, guarding/distraction behaviors, self-focus, and autonomic responses (changes in vital signs).

risk for excess Fluid Volume: risk factors may include preoperative renal involvement, stress-induced release of ADH, and changing calcium/electrolyte levels.

risk for ineffective Airway Clearance: risk factors may include edema formation and laryngeal nerve damage.

deficient Knowledge [Learning Need] regarding postoperative care/complications and long-term needs may be related to lack of information/recall, misinterpretation, possibly evidenced by statements of concern, questions, and misconceptions.

Parent-child relational problem   PED/PSY
impaired Parenting may be related to lack of/ineffective role model, lack of support between/from SO, interruption in bonding process, unrealistic expectations for self/child/partner, presence of stressors, lack of appropriate response of child to parent, possibly evidenced by frequent verbalization of disappointment in child, inability to care for/discipline child, lack of parental attachment behaviors, child abuse/abandonment.

chronic low Self-Esteem/ineffective Role Performance may be related to view self as "poor" or ineffective parent, belief that seeking help is an admission of defeat/failure, psychiatric/physical illness of the child, possibly evidenced by change in usual patterns/responsibility, expressions of lack of information, lack of follow-through of therapy, nonparticipation in therapy.

interrupted Family Process may be related to situational crisis of child/adolescent, maturational crisis (e.g., adolescence, midlife), possibly evidenced by expressions of confusion and difficulty coping with situation, family system not meeting physical/emotional/security needs of members, difficulty accepting help, parents not respecting each other's parenting practices.

compromised/disabled family Coping may be related to individual preoccupation with own emotional conflicts and personal suffering/anxiety about the crisis, temporary family disorganization, exhausted supportive capacity of members, highly ambivalent family relationships, possibly evidenced by detrimental decisions/actions, neglected relationships, intolerance, agitation, depression, hostility, aggression.

readiness for enhanced family Coping may be related to surfacing of self-actualization goals, possibly evidenced by expressing interest in making contact with another person experiencing a similar situation, moving in direction of health-promoting/enriching lifestyle, auditing/negotiating therapy program.

Parenteral feeding   MS/CH
risk for Infection: risk factors may include invasive procedure/surgical placement of feeding tube, malnutrition, chronic disease.

risk for Injury [multifactor]: risk factors may include catheter-related complications (air emboli, septic thrombophlebitis).

risk for imbalanced Fluid Volume: risk factors may include active loss/failure of regulatory mechanisms (specific to underlying disease process/trauma), complications of therapy—high glucose solutions/hyperglycemia (hyperosmolar nonketotic coma and severe dehydration), inability to obtain/ingest fluids.

Fatigue may be related to decreased metabolic energy production, increased energy requirements (hypermetabolic state, healing process), altered body chemistry (medications, chemotherapy), possibly evidenced by overwhelming lack of energy, inability to maintain usual routines/accomplish routine tasks, lethargy, impaired ability to concentrate.

Parkinson's disease   CH
impaired Walking may be related to neuromuscular impairment (muscle weakness, tremors, bradykinesia) and musculoskeletal impairment (joint rigidity), possibly evidenced by inability to move about the environment as desired, increased occurrence of falls.

impaired Swallowing may be related to neuromuscular impairment/muscle weakness, possibly evidenced by reported/observed difficulty in swallowing, drooling, evidence of aspiration (choking, coughing).

impaired verbal Communication may be related to muscle weakness and incoordination, possibly evidenced by impaired articulation, difficulty with phonation, and changes in rhythm and intonation.

risk for Stress Overload: risk factors may include inadequate resources, chronic illness, physical demands.

Caregiver Role Strain may be related to illness, severity of care receiver, psychological/cognitive problems in care receiver, caregiver is spouse, duration of caregiving required, lack of respite/recreation for caregiver, possibly evidenced by feeling stressed, depressed, worried; lack of resources/support, family conflict.

Passive-Aggressive personality disorder   PSY

[moderate to severe] Anxiety may be related to unconscious conflict, unmet needs, threat to self-concept, difficulty in asserting self directly, feelings of resentment toward authority figures, possibly evidenced by difficulty resolving feelings/trusting others, passive resistence to demands made by others, extraneous movements, irritability, argumentativeness.

ineffective Coping may be related to inadequate level of confidence in ability to cope/perception of control, uncertainty, high degree of threat, inadequate social support created by characteristics of relationships, disturbance in pattern of tension release, possibly evidenced by verbalizations or inability to cope/ask for help, lack of goal-directed behavior/resolution of problem, lack or assertive behavior, use of forms of coping that impede adaptive behavior, decreased use of social supports, risk-taking.

chronic low Self-Esteem may be related to retarded ego development, unmet dependency needs, early rejection by SO, lack of positive feedback, possibly evidenced by lack of self-confidence, feelings of inadequacy, fear of asserting self, dependency on others, directing frustrations toward others by using covert aggressive tactics, not accepting responsibility for what happens as a result of maladaptive behaviors, failing to work through negative feelings.

Powerlessness may be related to interpersonal interaction, lifestyle of helplessness, dependency feelings, difficulty connecting own passive-resistent behaviors with hostility or resentment, possibly evidenced by experiencing conscious hostility toward authority figures, releasing anger/hostility through others, getting back at others through aggravation.

PCP (phencyclidine) intoxication   MS/PSY

(Also refer to Hallucinogen abuse)

risk for self/other-directed Violence: risk factors may include drug abuse, psychotic symptomology, impulsivity.

risk for Trauma/Suffocation/Poisoning: risk factors may include clouded sensorium, increased muscle strength, myoclonic jerks/convulsions, ataxia, decreased pain perception, coma.

risk for ineffective cerebral Tissue Perfusion: risk factors may include alterations in blood flow (hypertensive crisis).

Pediculosis capitis   PED/CH

impaired Skin Integrity related to presence of nits, intense itching/scratching; possibly evidenced by redness, excoriation, disruption of skin surface.

risk for Infection [spread]: risk factors may include insufficient knowledge to avoid exposure/transmission of parasite.

impaired Home Maintenance may be related to lack of knowledge of vermin control or transmission, lack of care assistance or resources, possibly evidenced by poor hygiene practices, accumulation of dirt, unwashed clothing/linen or personal care item; presence of vermin.

Pediculosis pubis   CH

(Refer to Pediculosis capitis)

Pelvic inflammatory disease   OB/GYN/CH

risk for Infection [spread]: risk factors may include presence of infectious process in highly vascular pelvic structures, delay in seeking treatment.

acute Pain may be related to inflammation, edema, and congestion of reproductive/pelvic tissues, possibly evidenced by verbal reports, guarding/distraction behaviors, self-focus, and autonomic responses (changes in vital signs).

Hyperthermia may be related to inflammatory process/hypermetabolic state, possibly evidenced by increased body temperature, warm/flushed skin, and tachycardia.

risk for situational low Self-Esteem: risk factors may include perceived stigma of physical condition (infection of reproductive system).

deficient Knowledge [Learning Need] regarding cause/complications of condition, therapy needs, and transmission of disease to others may be related to lack of information/misinterpretation, possibly evidenced by statements of concern, questions, misconceptions, and development of preventable complications.

Periarteritis nodosa   MS/CH

(Refer to Polyarteritis [nodosa])

Pericarditis   MS

acute Pain may be related to tissue inflammation and presence of effusion, possibly evidenced by verbal reports of pain affected by movement/position, guarding/distraction behaviors, self-focus, and autonomic responses (changes in vital signs).

Activity Intolerance may be related to imbalance between O_2 supply and demand (restriction of cardiac filling/ventricular contraction, reduced cardiac output), possibly evidenced by reports of weakness/fatigue, exertional dyspnea, abnormal heart rate or BP response, and signs of heart failure.

risk for decreased Cardiac Output: risk factors may include accumulation of fluid (effusion), restricted cardiac filling/contractility.

Anxiety [specify level] may be related to change in health status and perceived threat of death, possibly evidenced by increased tension, apprehension, restlessness, and expressed concerns.

Perinatal loss/death of child   OB/CH

(Refer to Fetal demise)

Peripheral arterial occlusive disease   CH

(Refer to Arterial occlusive disease)

Peripheral vascular disease (atherosclerosis)   CH

ineffective peripheral Tissue Perfusion may be related to reduction or interruption of arterial/venous blood flow, possibly evidenced by changes in skin temperature/color, lack of hair growth, BP/pulse changes in extremity, presence of bruits, and reports of claudication.

Activity Intolerance may be related to imbalance between O_2 supply and demand, possibly evidenced by reports of muscle fatigue/weakness and exertional discomfort (claudication).

risk for impaired Skin/Tissue Integrity: risk factors may include altered circulation with decreased sensation and impaired healing.

Peritonitis   MS

risk for Infection [spread/septicemia]: risk factors may include inadequate primary defenses (broken skin, traumatized tissue, altered peristalsis), inadequate secondary defenses (immunosuppression), and invasive procedures.

deficient Fluid Volume [mixed] may be related to fluid shifts from extracellular, intravascular, and interstitial compartments into intestines or peritoneal space, excessive gastric losses (vomiting, diarrhea, NG suction), hypermetabolic state, and restricted intake, possibly evidenced by dry mucous membranes, poor skin turgor, delayed capillary refill, weak peripheral pulses, diminished urinary output, dark/concentrated urine, hypotension, and tachycardia.

acute Pain may be related to chemical irritation of parietal peritoneum, trauma to tissues, accumulation of fluid in abdominal/peritoneal cavity, possibly evidenced by verbal reports, muscle guarding/rebound tenderness, distraction behaviors, facial mask of pain, self-focus, autonomic responses (changes in vital signs).

risk for imbalanced Nutrition: less than body requirements: risk factors may include nausea/vomiting, intestinal dysfunction, metabolic abnormalities, increased metabolic needs.

Persian Gulf syndrome   CH/MS
(Refer to Gulf War syndrome)

Personality disorders   PSY
(Refer to Antisocial; Borderline; Obsessive-Compulsive; Passive-Aggressive; or Paranoid personality disorders)

Pertussis   PED
ineffective Airway Clearance may be related to retained secretions, excessive thick tenacious mucus, infection, possibly evidenced by dyspnea, adventitious breath sounds, hacking/paroxysmal cough.

deficient Fluid Volume may be related to decreased intake/anorexia, vomiting, increased insensible losses (fever/diaphoresis), possibly evidenced by decreased urine output/increased specific gravity, decreased BP, increased pulse rate, decreased skin/tongue turgor, dry skin/mucous membranes.

risk for Infection [transmission/secondary]: risk factors may include contagious nature of disease, stasis of body fluids, malnutrition, insufficient knowledge to avoid exposure to pathogens.

risk for imbalanced Nutrition: less than body requirements: risk factors may include inability to ingest food or absorb nutrients (anorexia, vomiting), increased metabolic demands.

risk for impaired Gas Exchange: risk factors may include compromised airways (tenacious mucus, inflammation), paroxysms of coughing, ventilation perfusion imbalance (atelectasis).

Pervasive developmental disorders PED/PSY
(Refer to Autistic disorder; Rett's syndrome; Asperger's disorder)

Pheochromocytoma   MS
Anxiety [specify level] may be related to excessive physiological (hormonal) stimulation of the sympathetic nervous system, situational crises, threat to/change in health status, possibly evidenced by apprehension, shakiness, restlessness, focus on self, fearfulness, diaphoresis, and sense of impending doom.

deficient Fluid Volume [mixed] may be related to excessive gastric losses (vomiting/diarrhea), hypermetabolic state, diaphoresis, and hyperosmolar diuresis, possibly evidenced by hemoconcentration, dry mucous membranes, poor skin turgor, thirst, and weight loss.

decreased Cardiac Output/ineffective Tissue Perfusion (specify) may be related to altered preload/decreased blood volume, altered SVR, and increased sympathetic activity (excessive secretion of catecholamines), possibly evidenced by cool/clammy skin, change in BP (hypertension/postural hypotension), visual disturbances, severe headache, and angina.

deficient Knowledge [Learning Need] regarding pathophysiology of condition, outcome, preoperative and postoperative care needs may be related to lack of information/recall, possibly evidenced by statements of concern, questions, and misconceptions.

Phlebitis   **CH**
(Refer to Thrombophlebitis)

Phobia   **PSY**
(Also refer to Anxiety Disorder, generalized)

Fear may be related to learned irrational response to natural or innate origins (phobic stimulus), unfounded morbid dread of a seemingly harmless object/situation, possibly evidenced by sympathetic stimulation and reactions ranging from apprehension to panic, withdrawal from/total avoidance of situations that place individual in contact with feared object.

impaired Social Interaction may be related to intense fear of encountering feared object/activity or situation and anticipated loss of control, possibly evidenced by reported change of style/pattern of interaction, discomfort in social situations, and avoidance of phobic stimulus.

Physical abuse   **CH/PSY**
(Refer to Abuse, physical; Battered child syndrome)

Pickwickian syndrome   **CH**
ineffective Breathing Pattern may be related to obesity, hypoventilation, possibly evidenced by decreased pulmonary function, hypercapnia, hypoxia, reduced effect of CO_2 in stimulating respirations.

PID   **GYN/OB/CH**
(Refer to Pelvic inflammatory disease)

Pinkeye   **CH**
(Refer to Conjunctivitis, bacterial)

Placenta previa   **OB**
risk for deficient Fluid Volume: risk factors may include excessive vascular losses (vessel damage and inadequate vasoconstriction).

impaired fetal Gas Exchange may be related to altered blood flow, altered oxygen-carrying capacity of blood (maternal anemia), and decreased surface area of gas exchange at site of placental attachment, possibly evidenced by changes in fetal heart rate/activity and release of meconium.

Fear may be related to threat of death (perceived or actual) to self or fetus, possibly evidenced by verbalization of specific concerns, increased tension, sympathetic stimulation.

risk for deficient Diversional Activity: risk factors may include imposed activity restrictions/bedrest.

Plague, bubonic   **MS**
Hyperthermia may be related to illness, dehydration, possibly evidenced by increased body temperature, tachycardia, chills, confusion.

acute Pain may be related to inflammatory process, enlarged lymph nodes, possibly evidenced by verbal/coded reports, expressive behavior, autonomic responses.

risk for deficient Fluid Volume: risk factors may include fever, decreased oral intake.

risk for impaired Skin Integrity: risk factors may include infectious process.

Plague, pneumonic   **MS**
risk for Infection [spread]: risk factors may include contagious nature of disease, close contact with others.

Hyperthermia may be related to illness, dehydration, possibly evidenced by increased body temperature, tachycardia, chills, severe headache, confusion.

impaired Gas Exchange may be related to alveolar-capillary membrane changes, possibly evidenced by tachypnea, dyspnea, stridor, hemoptysis, cyanosis.

deficient Fluid Volume may be evidenced by fever/hypermetabolic state, decreased intake, bleeding diathesis (DIC), possibly evidenced by weakness, decreased venous filling, decreased BP, decreased skin turgor, dry mucous membranes, change in mental state.

Plantar fasciitis   CH
acute/chronic Pain may be related to inflammation, possibly evidenced by report of stabbing, burning pain, guarding/protective behavior, change in posture/gait, altered ability to continue previous activities.

impaired Walking may be related musculoskeletal impairment, impaired balance, pain, possibly evidenced by impaired ability to walk required distances/climb stairs.

Pleural effusion   CH/MS
(Also refer to Hemothorax)

acute Pain may be related to inflammation/irritation of the parietal pleura, possibly evidenced by verbal reports, guarding/distraction behaviors, self-focus, and autonomic responses (changes in vital signs).

ineffective Breathing Pattern may be related to pain on inspiration, possibly evidenced by decreased respiratory depth, tachypnea, and dyspnea.

risk for impaired Gas Exchange: risk factors may include ventilation perfusion imbalance.

Pleurisy   CH
acute Pain may be related to inflammation/irritation of the parietal pleura, possibly evidenced by verbal reports, guarding/distraction behaviors, self-focus, and autonomic responses (changes in vital signs).

ineffective Breathing Pattern may be related to pain on inspiration, possibly evidenced by decreased respiratory depth, tachypnea, and dyspnea.

risk for Infection, [pneumonia]: risk factors may include stasis of pulmonary secretions, decreased lung expansion, and ineffective cough.

PMDD   GYN/PSY
(Refer to Premenstral dysphoric disorder)

PMS   GYN/PSY
(Refer to Premenstral dysphoric disorder)

Pneumoconiosis (black lung)   CH
(Refer to Pulmonary fibrosis)

Pneumonia   CH/MS
(Refer to Bronchitis; Bronchopneumonia)

Pneumonia, ventilator associated   CH
(Refer to Bronchopneumonia)

Pneumothorax   MS
(Also refer to Hemothorax)

ineffective Breathing Pattern may be related to decreased lung expansion (fluid/air accumulation), musculoskeletal impairment, pain, inflammatory process, possibly evidenced by dyspnea, tachypnea, altered chest excursion, respiratory depth changes, use of accessory muscles/nasal flaring, cough, cyanosis, and abnormal ABGs.

risk for decreased Cardiac Output: risk factors may include compression/displacement of cardiac structures.

acute Pain may be related to irritation of nerve endings within pleural space by foreign object (chest tube), possibly evidenced by verbal reports, guarding/distraction behaviors, self-focus, and autonomic responses (changes in vital signs).

Poliomyelitis   CH
(Also refer to Postpolio syndrome)

risk for/actual ineffective breathing pattern related to neuromuscular dysfunction/musculoskeletal [intercostal muscle] impairment, hypoventilation syndrome, possibly evidenced by dyspnea, decreased depth of breathing, altered chest excursion, respiratory failure.

impaired physical Mobility related to neuromuscular dysfunction/musculoskeletal impairment, decreased muscle strength/control or mass, contracture, decreased endurance, pain, prescribed movement restriction/bracing, possibly evidenced by limited ability to move, uncoordinated or jerky movements, gait changes, exaggerated lateral postural sway, postural instability.

Self-Care Deficit [specify] may be related to neuromuscular impairment, weakness, pain, fatigue, possibly evidenced by reported/observed inability to perform specified activities.

risk for Infection [transmission]: risk factors may include inadequate acquired immunity, malnutrition, or insufficient knowledge to avoid exposure to/transmission of pathogen.

Polyarteritis nodosa   MS/CH
ineffective Tissue Perfusion (specify) may be related to reduction/interruption of blood flow, possibly evidenced by organ tissue infarctions, changes in organ function, and development of organic psychosis.

Hyperthermia may be related to widespread inflammatory process, possibly evidenced by increased body temperature and warm/flushed skin.

acute Pain may be related to inflammation, tissue ischemia, and necrosis of affected area, possibly evidenced by verbal reports, guarding/distraction behaviors, self-focus, and autonomic responses (changes in vital signs).

Grieving may be related to perceived loss of self, possibly evidenced by expressions of sorrow and anger, altered sleep or eating patterns, changes in activity level, and libido.

Polycythemia vera   CH
Activity Intolerance may be related to imbalance between O_2 supply and demand, possibly evidenced by reports of fatigue/weakness.

ineffective Tissue Perfusion (specify) may be related to reduction/interruption of arterial/venous blood flow (insufficiency, thrombosis, or hemorrhage), possibly evidenced by pain in affected area, impaired mental ability, visual disturbances, and color changes of skin/mucous membranes.

Polyradiculitis   MS
(Refer to Guillain-Barré syndrome)

Postconcussion syndrome   CH
acute/chronic Pain may be related to neuronal damage, possibly evidenced by reports of headache.

disturbed Thought Processes may be related to head injury, possibly evidenced by memory deficit/problems, cognitive dissonance, distractibility.

Anxiety [specify level] may be related to situational crisis, change in health status/ongoing nature of disability, stress, unmet needs, possibly evidenced by expressed concerns, apprehension, uncertainty, feelings of inadequacy, focus on self, difficulty concentrating.

Postmaturity syndrome   PED
(Refer to Newborn, postmature)

Postmyocardial syndrome **CH**
(Refer to Dressler's syndrome)

Postoperative recovery period **MS**
ineffective Breathing Pattern may be related to neuromuscular and perceptual/cognitive impairment, decreased lung expansion/energy, and tracheobronchial obstruction, possibly evidenced by changes in respiratory rate and depth, reduced vital capacity, apnea, cyanosis, and noisy respirations.

risk for imbalanced Body Temperature: risk factors may include exposure to cool environment, effect of medications/anesthetic agents, extremes of age/weight, and dehydration.

disturbed Sensory Perception (specify)/disturbed Thought Processes may be related to chemical alteration (use of pharmaceutical agents, hypoxia), therapeutically restricted environment, excessive sensory stimuli and physiological stress, possibly evidenced by changes in usual response to stimuli, motor incoordination; impaired ability to concentrate, reason, and make decisions; and disorientation to person, place, and time.

risk for deficit Fluid Volume: risk factors may include restriction of oral intake, loss of fluid through abnormal routes (indwelling tubes, drains) and normal routes (vomiting, loss of vascular integrity, changes in clotting ability), extremes of age and weight.

acute Pain may be related to disruption of skin, tissue, and muscle integrity, musculoskeletal/bone trauma, and presence of tubes and drains, possibly evidenced by verbal reports, alteration in muscle tone, facial mask of pain, distraction/guarding behaviors, narrowed focus, and autonomic responses.

impaired Skin/Tissue Integrity may be related to mechanical interruption of skin/tissues, altered circulation, effects of medication, accumulation of drainage, and altered metabolic state, possibly evidenced by disruption of skin surface/layers and tissues.

risk for Infection: risk factors may include broken skin, traumatized tissues, stasis of body fluids, presence of pathogens/contaminants, environmental exposure, and invasive procedures.

Postpartum blues **OB/PSY**
(Refer to Depression, postpartum)

Postpartum period, 4 to 48 hours **OB/CH**
risk for impaired parent/infant Attachment/Parenting: risk factors may include lack of support between/from SO(s), ineffective or no role model, anxiety associated with the parental role, unrealistic expectations, presence of stressors (e.g., financial, housing, employment).

risk for deficient Fluid Volume: risk factors may include excessive blood loss during delivery, reduced intake/inadequate replacement, nausea/vomiting, increased urine output, and insensible losses.

acute Pain/[Discomfort] may be related to tissue trauma/edema, muscle contractions, bladder fullness, and physical/psychological exhaustion, possibly evidenced by reports of cramping (afterpains), self-focusing, alteration in muscle tone, distraction behaviors, and autonomic responses (changes in vital signs).

impaired Urinary Elimination may be related to hormonal effects (fluid shifts/continued elevation in renal plasma flow), mechanical trauma/tissue edema, and effects of medication/anesthesia, possibly evidenced by frequency, dysuria, urgency, incontinence, or retention.

Constipation may be related to decreased muscle tone associated with diastasis recti, prenatal effects of progesterone, dehydration, excess analgesia or anesthesia, pain (hemorrhoids, episiotomy, or perineal tenderness), prelabor diarrhea and lack of intake, possibly evidenced by frequency less than usual pattern, hard-formed stool, straining at stool, decreased bowel sounds, and abdominal distention.

Doenges Nursing Diagnosis Manual: Planning, Individualizing, and Documenting Client Care

Insomnia may be related to pain/discomfort, intense exhilaration/excitement, anxiety, exhausting process of labor/delivery, and needs/demands of family members, possibly evidenced by verbal reports of difficulty in falling asleep or staying asleep/not feeling well-rested, interrupted sleep, lack of energy.

Postpartum period, 4 to 6 weeks   OB/CH

disturbed Body Image may be related to unrealistic expectations of postpartum recovery, permanency of some changes, possibly evidenced by verbalization of negative feelings about body, feelings of helplessness, preoccupation with change, focus on past appearance, fear of rejection/reaction of others.

risk for Sexual Dysfunction: risk factors may include health-related transition, changes in body function (including lactation), lack of privacy, fear of pregnancy.

readiness for enhanced family Coping may be related to sufficiently meeting individual needs and adaptive tasks, possibly evidenced by family members moving in direction of health-promoting and enriching lifestyle.

readiness for enhanced Parenting may be related to sufficiently mastering skills/adapting to new responsibilities, possibly evidenced by expressed willingness to enhance parenting, physical and emotional needs of infant/children are met, bonding evident.

Postpartum period, postdischarge to 4 weeks OB/CH

risk for Fatigue: risk factors may include physical/emotional demands of infant and other family members, psychological stressors, continued discomfort.

Breastfeeding (specify) may be related to level of knowledge/support, previous experiences, infant gestational age, physical structure/characteristics of maternal breast, possibly evidenced by maternal verbalizations regarding level of satisfaction, observations of feeding process, infant response/weight gain.

risk for imbalanced Nutrition: less than body requirements: risk factors may include intake insufficient to meet metabolic demands/correct existing deficiencies (e.g., lactation, anemia/excessive blood loss, infection/excessive tissue trauma, desire to regain prenatal weight).

risk for Infection: risk factors may include tissue trauma/broken skin, decreased Hb, invasive procedures, increased environmental exposure, malnutrition.

risk for ineffective Coping: risk factors may include situational/developmental changes, temporary family disorganization/role changes, little support provided by partner/family members.

ineffective Role Performance may be related to situational crisis (addition and demands of new family member, changes in responsibilities of family members), possibly evidenced by change in usual patterns or responsibility, conflict in roles.

Postpolio syndrome   CH

Anxiety [specify]/Fear may be related to change in health status, progressive/debilitating disease, change in role function/economic status, possibly evidenced by expressed concerns, uncertainty, awareness of physiological symptoms, worried, sleep disturbance, forgetfulness.

Fatigue may be related to disease state, stress, anxiety, sleep deprivation, depression, possibly evidenced by overwhelming lack of energy, inability to maintain usual routines/level of physical activity, difficulty concentrating.

chronic Pain may be related to chronic physical disability, joint degeneration, possibly evidenced by reports of deep aching pain, altered ability to continue previous activities, change in sleep patterns, reduced interaction with others.

impaired Walking/physical Mobility may be related to neuromuscular impairment, decreased muscle strength/atrophy, decreased endurance, pain, inability to stand erect (flat back syndrome), possibly evidenced by gait disturbances, joint/postural instability, decreased ability to perform gross motor skills.

Sleep Deprivation may be related to sleep apnea (central and obstructive), chronic pain, possibly evidenced by daytime drowsiness, decreased ability to function, inability to concentrate.

impaired Swallowing may be related to neuromuscular impairment, pharyngeal muscle weakness, possibly evidenced by coughing, choking, recurrent pulmonary infections.

ineffective Airway Clearance may be related to neuromuscular dysfunction (muscle weakness/atrophy), retained secretions, possibly evidenced by diminished/adventitious breath sounds (chronic microatelectasis), poor cough (decreased pulmonary compliance, increased chest wall tightness).

Post-traumatic stress disorder   PSY

Post-Trauma Syndrome related to having experienced a traumatic life event, possibly evidenced by reexperiencing the event, somatic reactions, psychological/emotional numbness, altered lifestyle, impaired sleep, self-destructive behaviors, difficulty with interpersonal relationships, development of phobia, poor impulse control/irritability, and explosiveness.

risk for other-directed Violence: risk factors may include startled reaction, an intrusive memory causing a sudden acting out of a feeling as if the event were occurring; use of alcohol/other drugs to ward off painful effects and produce psychic numbing, breaking through the rage that has been walled off, response to intense anxiety or panic state, and loss of control.

ineffective Coping may be related to personal vulnerability, inadequate support systems, unrealistic perceptions, unmet expectations, overwhelming threat to self, and multiple stressors repeated over a period of time, possibly evidenced by verbalization of inability to cope or difficulty asking for help, muscular tension/headaches, chronic worry, and emotional tension.

complicated Grieving may be related to actual/perceived object loss (loss of self as seen before the traumatic incident occurred as well as other losses incurred in/after the incident), loss of physiopsychosocial well-being, thwarted grieving response to a loss, and lack of resolution of previous grieving responses, possibly evidenced by verbal expression of distress at loss, anger, sadness, labile affect; alterations in eating habits, sleep/dream patterns, libido; reliving of past experiences, expression of guilt, and alterations in concentration.

interrupted Family Processes may be related to situational crisis, failure to master developmental transitions, possibly evidenced by expressions of confusion about what to do and by family having difficulty coping, family system not meeting physical/emotional/spiritual needs of its members, not adapting to change or dealing with traumatic experience constructively, and ineffective family decision-making process.

Preeclampsia   OB

(Refer to Pregnancy-induced hypertension; Abruptio placentae)

Pregnancy, 1st trimester   OB/CH

risk for imbalanced Nutrition: less than body requirements: risk factors may include changes in appetite, insufficient intake (nausea/vomiting, inadequate financial resources and nutritional knowledge); meeting increased metabolic demands (increased thyroid activity associated with the growth of fetal and maternal tissues).

[Discomfort]/acute Pain may be related to hormonal influences, physical changes, possibly evidenced by verbal reports (nausea, breast changes, leg cramps, hemorrhoids, nasal stuffiness), alteration in muscle tone, restlessness, and autonomic responses (changes in vital signs).

risk for fetal Injury: risk factors may include environmental/hereditary factors and problems of maternal well-being that directly affect the developing fetus (e.g., malnutrition, substance use).

[maximally compensated] Cardiac Output may be related to increased fluid volume/maximal cardiac effort and hormonal effects of progesterone and relaxin (places the client at risk for hypertension and/or circulatory failure), and changes in peripheral resistance (afterload), possibly evidenced by variations in BP and pulse, syncopal episodes, presence of pathological edema.

readiness for enhanced family Coping may be related to situational/maturational crisis with anticipated changes in family structure/roles, needs sufficiently met and adaptive tasks effectively addressed to enable goals of self-actualization to surface, as evidenced by movement toward health-promoting and enriching lifestyle, choosing experiences that optimize pregnancy experience/wellness.

risk for Constipation: risk factors may include changes in dietary/fluid intake, smooth muscle relaxation, decreased peristalsis, and effects of medications (e.g., iron).

Fatigue/Insomnia may be related to increased carbohydrate metabolism, altered body chemistry, increased energy requirements to perform ADLs, discomfort, anxiety, inactivity, possibly evidenced by reports of overwhelming lack of energy/inability to maintain usual routines, difficulty falling asleep/dissatisfaction with sleep, decreased quality of life.

risk for ineffective Role Performance: risk factors may include maturational crisis, developmental level, history of maladaptive coping, absence of support systems.

deficient Knowledge [Learning Need] regarding normal physiological/psychological changes and self-care needs may be related to lack of information/recall and misinterpretation of normal physiological/psychological changes and their impact on the client/family, possibly evidenced by questions, statements of concern, misconceptions and inaccurate follow-through of instructions/development of preventable complications.

Pregnancy, 2nd trimester   OB/CH
(Also refer to Pregnancy, 1st trimester)

risk for disturbed Body Image: risk factors may include perception of biophysical changes, response of others.

ineffective Breathing Pattern may be related to impingement of the diaphragm by enlarging uterus, possibly evidenced by reports of shortness of breath, dyspnea, and changes in respiratory depth.

risk for [decompensated] Cardiac Output: risk factors may include increased circulatory demand, changes in preload (decreased venous return) and afterload (increased peripheral vascular resistance), and ventricular hypertrophy.

risk for excess Fluid Volume: risk factors may include changes in regulatory mechanisms, sodium/water retention.

ineffective Sexuality Pattern may be related to conflict regarding changes in sexual desire and expectations, fear of physical injury to woman/fetus, possibly evidenced by reported difficulties, limitations or changes in sexual behaviors/activities.

Pregnancy, 3rd trimester   OB/CH
(Also refer to Pregnancy, first and second trimesters)

deficient Knowledge [Learning Need] regarding preparation for labor/delivery, infant care may be related to lack of exposure/experience, misinterpretations of information, possibly evidenced by request for information, statement of concerns/misconceptions.

impaired Urinary Elimination may be related to uterine enlargement, increased abdominal pressure, fluctuation of renal blood flow, and glomerular filtration rate (GFR), possibly evidenced by urinary frequency, urgency, dependent edema.

risk for ineffective [individual/] family Coping: risk factors may include situational/maturational crisis, personal vulnerability, unrealistic perceptions, absent/insufficient support systems.

risk for maternal Injury: risk factors may include presence of hypertension, infection, substance use/abuse, altered immune system, abnormal blood profile, tissue hypoxia, premature rupture of membranes.

Pregnancy, adolescent   OB/CH
(Also refer to Pregnancy—prenatal period)

interrupted Family Processes may be related to situational/developmental transition (economic, change in roles/gain of a family member), possibly evidenced by family expressing confusion about what to do, unable to meet physical/emotional/spiritual needs of the members, family inability to adapt to change or to deal with traumatic experience constructively; does not demonstrate respect for individuality and autonomy of its members, ineffective family decision-making process, and inappropriate boundary maintenance.

Social Isolation may be related to alterations in physical appearance, perceived unacceptable social behavior, restricted social sphere, stage of adolescence, and interference with accomplishing developmental tasks, possibly evidenced by expressions of feelings of aloneness/rejection/difference from others, uncommunicative, withdrawn, no eye contact, seeking to be alone, unacceptable behavior, and absence of supportive SO(s).

disturbed Body Image/situational/chronic low Self-Esteem may be related to situational/maturational crisis, biophysical changes, and fear of failure at life events, absence of support systems, possibly evidenced by self-negating verbalizations, expressions of shame/guilt, fear of rejection/reaction of other, hypersensitivity to criticism, and lack of follow-through/nonparticipation in prenatal care.

deficient Knowledge [Learning Need] regarding pregnancy, developmental/individual needs, future expectations may be related to lack of exposure, information misinterpretation, unfamiliarity with information resources, lack of interest in learning, possibly evidenced by questions, statement of concern/misconception, sense of vulnerability/denial of reality, inaccurate follow-through of instruction, and development of preventable complications.

risk for impaired Parenting may be related to chronological age/developmental stage, unmet social/emotional/maturational needs of parenting figures, unrealistic expectation of self/infant/partner, ineffective role model/social support, lack of role identity, and presence of stressors (e.g., financial, social).

Pregnancy, high-risk   OB/CH
(Also refer to Pregnancy, 1st, 2nd, and 3rd trimesters)

Anxiety [specify level] may be related to situational crisis, threat of maternal/fetal death (perceived or actual), interpersonal transmission/contagion, possibly evidenced by increased tension, apprehension, feelings of inadequacy, somatic complaints, difficulty sleeping.

deficient Knowledge [Learning Need] regarding high-risk situation/preterm labor may be related to lack of exposure to/misinterpretation of information, unfamiliarity with individual risks and own role in risk prevention/management, possibly evidenced by request for information, statement of concerns/misconceptions, inaccurate follow-through of instructions.

risk of maternal Injury: risk factors may include preexisting medical conditions, complications of pregnancy.

risk for Activity Intolerance: risk factors may include presence of circulatory/respiratory problems, uterine irritability.

risk for ineffective Therapeutic Regimen Management: risk factors may include client value system, health beliefs/cultural influences, issues of control, presence of anxiety, complexity of therapeutic regimen, economic difficulties, perceived susceptibility.

Pregnancy-induced hypertension   OB/CH
(Also refer to Eclampsia)

deficient Fluid Volume [isotonic] may be related to a plasma protein loss, decreasing plasma colloid osmotic pressure allowing fluid shifts out of vascular compartment, possibly evidenced by edema formation, sudden weight gain, hemoconcentration, nausea/vomiting, epigastric pain, headaches, visual changes, decreased urine output.

decreased Cardiac Output may be related to hypovolemia/decreased venous return, increased SVR, possibly evidenced by variations in BP/hemodynamic readings, edema, shortness of breath, change in mental status.

ineffective [uteroplacental] Tissue Perfusion may be related to vasospasm of spiral arteries and relative hypovolemia, possibly evidenced by changes in fetal heart rate/activity, reduced weight gain, and premature delivery/fetal demise.

deficient Knowledge [Learning Need] regarding pathophysiology of condition, therapy, self-care/nutritional needs, and potential complications may be related to lack of information/recall, misinterpretation, possibly evidenced by statements of concern, questions, misconceptions, inaccurate follow-through of instructions/development of preventable complications.

Pregnancy, postmaturity   OB

Anxiety [specify level] may be related to situational crisis, threat to maternal/fetal health status (perceived or actual), interpersonal transmission/contagion, possibly evidenced by increased tension, apprehension, irritability, feelings of inadequacy, somatic complaints.

ineffective [uteroplacental] Tissue Perfusion may be related to placental involution/multiple infarcts and villous degeneration, possibly evidenced by decrease in fetal motion, meconium staining of amniotic fluid, intrauterine growth restriction, late decelerations on fetal monitor.

risk for maternal Injury: risk factors may include dysfunctional/prolonged labor.

risk for impaired fetal Gas Exchange: risk factors may include altered placental perfusion, cord compression (oligohydramnios).

risk for fetal Injury: risk factors may include prolonged labor (tissue hypoxia/acidosis), meconium aspiration.

Premature ejaculation   CH

Sexual Dysfunction may be related to altered body function, partner-related issues, possibly evidenced by reports of disruption of sexual response pattern, inability to achieve desired satisfaction.

situational low Self-Esteem may be related to functional impairment, perceived failure to perform satisfactorily, rejection of other(s), possibly evidenced by self-negating verbalizations, expressions of helplessness/powerlessness.

Premature infant   OB/PED

(Refer to Neonate, premature newborn)

Premenstrual dysphoric disorder   GYN/PSY

chronic Pain may be related to cyclic changes in female hormones affecting other systems (e.g., vascular congestion/spasms), vitamin deficiency, fluid retention, possibly evidenced by increased tension, apprehension, jitteriness, verbal reports, distraction behaviors, somatic complaints, self-focusing, physical and social withdrawal.

[moderate to panic] Anxiety may be related to cyclic changes in female hormones affecting other systems, possibly evidenced by feelings of inability to cope/loss of control, depersonalization, increased tension, apprehension, jitteriness, somatic complaints, and impaired functioning.

ineffective Coping may be related to personal vulnerability, threat to self-concept, multiple stressors (premenstrual symptoms) repeated over period of time, poor nutrition, possibly evidenced by verbalization of difficulty coping/problem-solving, inability to meet role expectation/seek help, emotional/muscular tension, chronic fatigue, insomnia, lack of appetite/overeating, high illness rate, decreased societal participation.

excess Fluid Volume may be related to abnormal alterations of hormonal levels, possibly evidenced by edema formation, weight gain, and periodic changes in emotional status/irritability.

deficient Knowledge [Learning Need] regarding pathophysiology of condition and self-care/treatment needs may be related to lack of information/misinterpretation, possibly evidenced by statements of concern, questions, misconceptions, and continuation of condition, exacerbating symptoms.

Premenstrual tension syndrome   GYN/PSY
(Refer to Premenstrual dysphoric disorder)

Prenatal substance abuse   OB
(Refer to Substance dependence/abuse, prenatal)

Pressure ulcer or sore   CH
(Also refer to Ulcer, decubitus)

ineffective peripheral Tissue Perfusion may be related to reduced/interrupted blood flow, possibly evidenced by presence of inflamed, necrotic lesion.

deficient Knowledge [Learning Need] regarding cause/prevention of condition and potential complications may be related to lack of information or misinterpretation, possibly evidenced by statements of concern, questions, misconceptions, and inaccurate follow-through of instructions.

Preterm labor   OB/CH
(Refer to Labor, preterm)

Prostate cancer   MS
(Also refer to Cancer; Prostatectomy)

[acute/chronic] Urinary Retention may be related to blockage of urethra, possibly evidenced by sensation of bladder fullness, dysuria, small/frequent voiding, residual urine, bladder distention.

acute Pain may be related to destruction of tissues, pressure on surrounding structures, bladder distention, possibly evidenced by verbal reports, restlessness, irritability, autonomic responses.

Prostatectomy   MS

impaired Urinary Elimination may be related to mechanical obstruction (blood clots, edema, trauma, surgical procedure, pressure/irritation of catheter/balloon) and loss of bladder tone, possibly evidenced by dysuria, frequency, dribbling, incontinence, retention, bladder fullness, suprapubic discomfort.

risk for deficient Fluid Volume: risk factors may include trauma to highly vascular area with excessive vascular losses, restricted intake, postobstructive diuresis.

acute Pain may be related to irritation of bladder mucosa and tissue trauma/edema, possibly evidenced by verbal reports (bladder spasms), distraction behaviors, self-focus, and autonomic responses (changes in vital signs).

disturbed Body Image may be related to perceived threat of altered body/sexual function, possibly evidenced by preoccupation with change/loss, negative feelings about body, and statements of concern regarding functioning.

CH

risk for Sexual Dysfunction: risk factors may include situational crisis (incontinence, leakage of urine after catheter removal, involvement of genital area) and threat to self-concept/change in health status.

    Doenges Nursing Diagnosis Manual: Planning, Individualizing, and Documenting Client Care

Prostatitis, acute   CH

(Also refer to Cystitis)

acute Pain[/Discomfort] may be related to inflammatory response, possibly evidenced by reports of low back/pelvic pain, arthralgia, myalgia.

impaired Urinary Elimination may be related to localized swelling, UTI, possibly evidenced by dysuria/burning on urination, frequency, urgency, nocturia, obstructed voiding.

Hyperthermia may be related to illness, possibly evidenced by high fever, flushed/warm skin, chills.

risk for ineffective Therapeutic Regimen Management: risk factors may include length of therapy, perceived seriousness/benefits.

Prostatitis, chronic   CH

(Also refer to Cystitis)

acute Pain[/Discomfort] may be related to inflammatory response, possibly evidenced by reports of back/pelvic/scrotal discomfort, low-grade fever.

impaired Urinary Elimination may be related to localized swelling, UTI, possibly evidenced by dysuria, frequency, urgency.

Pruritus   CH

acute Pain may be related to cutaneous hyperesthesia and inflammation, possibly evidenced by verbal reports, distraction behaviors, and self-focus.

risk for impaired Skin Integrity: risk factors may include mechanical trauma (scratching) and development of vesicles/bullae that may rupture.

Psoriasis   CH

impaired Skin Integrity may be related to increased epidermal cell proliferation and absence of normal protective skin layers, possibly evidenced by scaling papules and plaques.

disturbed Body Image may be related to cosmetically unsightly skin lesions, possibly evidenced by hiding affected body part, negative feelings about body, feelings of helplessness, and change in social involvement.

Psychological abuse   CH/PSY

(Refer to Abuse, psychological)

PTSD   PSY

(Refer to Post-traumatic stress disorder)

Pulmonary edema   MS

impaired Gas Exchange may be related to alveolar-capillary membrane changes (fluid collection/ shifts into interstitial space/alveoli), possibly evidenced by dyspnea, restlessness, irritability, abnormal rate/depth of respirations, lethargy, confusion.

[moderate to severe] Anxiety may be related to change in health status, threat of death, interpersonal transmission, possibly evidenced by expressed concerns, distressed, apprehension, extraneous movement.

risk for impaired spontaneous Ventilation: risk factors may include respiratory muscle fatigue, problems with secretion management.

Pulmonary edema, high altitude   MS

(Refer to High altitude pulmonary edema)

Pulmonary embolus   MS

ineffective Breathing Pattern may be related to tracheobronchial obstruction (inflammation, copious secretions or active bleeding), decreased lung expansion, inflammatory process, possibly evidenced by changes in depth or rate of respiration, dyspnea/use of accessory muscles, altered chest excursion, abnormal breath sounds (crackles, wheezes), and cough (with or without sputum production).

impaired Gas Exchange may be related to altered blood flow to alveoli or to major portions of the lung, alveolar-capillary membrane changes (atelectasis, airway/alveolar collapse, pulmonary edema/effusion, excessive secretions/active bleeding), possibly evidenced by profound dyspnea, restlessness, apprehension, somnolence, cyanosis, and changes in ABGs/pulse oximetry (hypoxemia and hypercapnia).

ineffective cardiopulmonary Tissue Perfusion may be related to interruption of blood flow (arterial/venous), exchange problems at alveolar level or at tissue level (acidotic shifting of the oxyhemoglobin curve), possibly evidenced by radiology/laboratory evidence of ventilation/perfusion mismatch, dyspnea, and central cyanosis.

Fear/Anxiety [specify level] may be related to severe dyspnea/inability to breathe normally, perceived threat of death, threat to/change in health status, physiological response to hypoxemia/acidosis, and concern regarding unknown outcome of situation, possibly evidenced by restlessness, irritability, withdrawal or attack behavior, sympathetic stimulation (cardiovascular excitation, pupil dilation, sweating, vomiting, diarrhea), crying, voice quivering, and impending sense of doom.

Pulmonary fibrosis   CH

impaired Gas Exchange may be related to alveolar-capillary membrane changes (inflammation, development of scar tissue), ventilation perfusion imbalance (retained secretions), possibly evidenced by dyspnea, adventitious breath sounds, nonproductive cough, cyanosis.

Anxiety [specify]/Fear may be related to situational crisis, change in health status, threat of death, interpersonal transmission, possibly evidenced by expressed concerns, apprehension, uncertainty, ruminations, increased tension.

Activity Intolerance may be related to imbalance between oxygen supply/demand, generalized weakness, possibly evidenced by exertional dyspnea, abnormal heart rate/BP response to activity, cyanosis.

risk for Infection: risk factors may include stasis of secretions, chronic disease, drug therapies (corticosteroids, cytotoxins).

Pulmonary hypertension   CH/MS

impaired Gas Exchange may be related to changes in alveolar membrane, increased pulmonary vascular resistance, possibly evidenced by dyspnea, irritability, decreased mental acuity, somnolence, abnormal ABGs.

decreased Cardiac Output may be related to increased pulmonary vascular resistance, decreased blood return to left side of heart, possibly evidenced by increased heart rate, dyspnea, fatigue.

Activity Intolerance may be related to imbalance between oxygen supply and demand, possibly evidenced by reports of weakness/fatigue, abnormal vital signs with activity.

[mild to moderate] Anxiety may be related to change in health status, stress, threat to self-concept, possibly evidenced by expressed concerns, uncertainty, anxiety, awareness of physiological symptoms, diminished productivity/ability to problem-solve.

Pulmonic insufficiency   MS/CH
(Refer to Valvular heart disease)

Pulmonic stenosis   MS/CH
(Refer to Valvular heart disease)

Purpura, idiopathic thrombocytopenic   CH

ineffective Protection may be related to abnormal blood profile, drug therapy (corticosteroids or immunosuppressive agents), possibly evidenced by altered clotting, fatigue, deficient immunity.

Activity Intolerance may be related to decreased oxygen-carrying capacity/imbalance between O$_2$ supply and demand, possibly evidenced by reports of fatigue/weakness.

deficient Knowledge [Learning Need] regarding therapy choices, outcomes, and self-care needs may be related to lack of information/misinterpretation, possibly evidenced by statements of concern, questions, and misconceptions.

Pyelonephritis   MS

acute Pain may be related to acute inflammation of renal tissues, possibly evidenced by verbal reports, guarding/distraction behaviors, self-focus, and autonomic responses (changes in vital signs).

Hyperthermia may be related to inflammatory process/increased metabolic rate, possibly evidenced by increase in body temperature, warm/flushed skin, tachycardia, and chills.

impaired Urinary Elimination may be related to inflammation/irritation of bladder mucosa, possibly evidenced by dysuria, urgency, and frequency.

deficient Knowledge [Learning Need] regarding therapy needs and prevention may be related to lack of information/misinterpretation, possibly evidenced by statements of concern, questions, misconceptions, and recurrence of condition.

Pyloric stenosis   PED

deficient Fluid Volume may be related to excessive projectile vomiting, possibly evidenced by decreased/concentrated urine, poor skin turgor, dry skin/mucous membranes, lethargy.

imbalanced Nutrition: less than body requirements may be related to inability to digest/absorb nutrients, possibly evidenced by weight loss, poor muscle tone, pale conjunctiva/mucous membranes.

Quadriplegia   MS/CH

(Also refer to Paraplegia)

ineffective Breathing Pattern may be related to neuromuscular impairment (diaphragm and intercostal muscle function), reflex abdominal spasms, gastric distention, possibly evidenced by decreased respiratory depth, dyspnea, cyanosis, and abnormal ABGs.

risk for Trauma [additional spinal injury]: risk factors may include temporary weakness/instability of spinal column.

Grieving may be related to perceived loss of self, anticipated alterations in lifestyle and expectations, and limitation of future options/choices, possibly evidenced by expressions of distress, anger, sorrow; choked feelings; and changes in eating habits, sleep, communication patterns.

total Self-Care Deficit related to neuromuscular impairment, evidenced by inability to perform self-care tasks.

Bowel Incontinence/Constipation may be be related to disruption of nerve innervation, perceptual impairment, changes in dietary/fluid intake, change in activity level, possibly evidenced by inability to evacuate bowel voluntarily, increased abdominal pressure/distention, dry/hard formed stool, change in bowel sounds.

impaired bed/wheelchair Mobility may be related to loss of muscle function/control.

risk for Autonomic Dysreflexia: risk factors may include altered nerve function (spinal cord injury at T6 or above), bladder/bowel/skin stimulation (tactile, pain, thermal).

impaired Home Maintenance may be related to permanent effects of injury, inadequate/absent support systems and finances, and lack of familiarity with resources, possibly evidenced by expressions of difficulties, requests for information and assistance, outstanding debts/financial crisis, and lack of necessary aids and equipment.

Rabies   **CH/MS**

Hyperthermia may be related to infection, possibly evidenced by fever, malaise.

risk for ineffective Airway Clearance: risk factors may include excessive salivation, muscle spasms (laryngeal/pharyngeal).

deficient Fluid Volume related to inability to drink (severe painful pharyngeal muscle spasms), excessive salivation, possibly evidenced by extreme thirst, decreased skin turgor, decreased output/concentrated urine.

risk for trauma: risk factors may include progressive restlessness, uncontrollable excitement, inability to utilize physical restraints for safety.

Radiation syndrome/poisoning   **MS**
(Dependent on dose and duration of exposure)

[severe] Anxiety/Fear may be related to situational crisis, threat of death, interpersonal transmission/contagion, unmet needs, possibly evidenced by expressed concerns, fearfulness, hoplessness, restlessness, agitation, anguish, increased tension, awareness of physiological symptoms.

deficient Fluid Volume may be related to intractable nausea, vomiting, diarrhea (GI tissue necrosis and atrophy), interference with adequate intake (stomatitis/anorexia), hemorrhagic losses (thrombocytopenia), possibly evidenced by dry skin/mucous membranes, poor skin turgor, decreased venous filling, reduced pulse volume/pressure, hypotension, weakness, change in mentation.

acute Confusion may be related to CNS inflammation, decreased circulation/hypotension, effects of circulating toxins, possibly evidenced by fluctuations in cognition/level of consciousness, agitation.

ineffective Protection may be related to effects of radiation, abnormal blood profile (leukopenia, thrombocytopenia, anemia), inadequate nutrition, possibly evidenced by neurosensory alterations, anorexia, deficient immunity, impaired healing, altered clotting, disorientation.

risk for Infection: risk factors may include inadequate primary defenses (traumatized/necrotic tissues, stasis of body fluids, altered peristalsis), inadequate secondary defenses (anemia, leukopenia).

Sexual Dysfunction may be related to altered body function, possibly evidenced by amenorrhea, decreased libido, infertility.

risk for disturbed visual Sensory Perception: risk factors may include altered sensory reception (development of cataracts).

Radiation therapy   **CH**
(Also refer to Brachytherapy; Cancer; Radiotherapy)

Nausea may be related to therapeutic procedure, irritation to GI system, possibly evidenced by verbal reports, vomiting, gastric stasis.

imbalanced Nutrition: less than body requirements may be related to inability to ingest adequate nutrients (nausea, stomatitis, and fatigue), hypermetabolic state, possibly evidenced by weight loss, aversion to eating, reported altered taste sensation, sore, inflamed buccal cavity, diarrhea.

impaired Oral Mucous Membrane may be related to side effects of radiation, dehydration, and malnutrition, possibly evidenced by ulcerations, leukoplakia, decreased salivation, and reports of pain.

ineffective Protection may be related to inadequate nutrition, radiation, abnormal blood profile, disease state (cancer), possibly evidenced by impaired healing, deficient immunity, anorexia, fatigue.

Radical neck surgery　　　　　　**MS**
(Refer to Laryngectomy)

Rape　　　　　　**CH**
deficient Knowledge [Learning Need] regarding required medical/legal procedures, prophylactic treatment for individual concerns (STDs, pregnancy), community resources/supports may be related to lack of information, possibly evidenced by statements of concern, questions, misconceptions, and exacerbation of symptoms.

Rape-Trauma Syndrome (acute phase) related to actual or attempted sexual penetration without consent, possibly evidenced by wide range of emotional reactions, including anxiety, fear, anger, embarrassment, and multisystem physical complaints.

risk for impaired Tissue Integrity: risk factors may include forceful sexual penetration and trauma to fragile tissues.

PSY

ineffective Coping may be related to personal vulnerability, unmet expectations, unrealistic perceptions, inadequate support systems/coping methods, multiple stressors repeated over time, overwhelming threat to self, possibly evidenced by verbalizations of inability to cope or difficulty asking for help, muscular tension/headaches, emotional tension, chronic worry.

Sexual Dysfunction may be related to biopsychosocial alteration of sexuality (stress of post-trauma response), vulnerability, loss of sexual desire, impaired relationship with SO, possibly evidenced by alteration in achieving sexual satisfaction, change in interest in self/others, preoccupation with self.

Raynaud's disease　　　　　　**CH**
acute/chronic Pain may be related to vasospasm/altered perfusion of affected tissues and ischemia/destruction of tissues, possibly evidenced by verbal reports, guarding of affected parts, self-focusing, and restlessness.

ineffective peripheral Tissue Perfusion may be related to periodic reduction of arterial blood flow to affected areas, possibly evidenced by pallor, cyanosis, coolness, numbness, paresthesia, slow healing of lesions.

deficient Knowledge [Learning Need] regarding pathophysiology of condition, potential for complications, therapy/self-care needs may be related to lack of information/misinterpretation, possibly evidenced by statements of concern, questions, and misconceptions; development of preventable complications.

Raynaud's phenomenon　　　　　　**CH**
(Refer to Raynaud's disease)

Reactive attachment disorder　　　　　　**PED/PSY**
(Refer to Anxiety disorders—PED)

Reflex sympathetic dystrophy　　　　　　**CH**
acute/chronic Pain may be related to continued nerve stimulation, possibly evidenced by verbal reports, distraction/guarding behaviors, narrowed focus, changes in sleep patterns, and altered ability to continue previous activities.

ineffective peripheral Tissue Perfusion may be related to reduction of arterial blood flow (arteriole vasoconstriction), possibly evidenced by reports of pain, decreased skin temperature and pallor, diminished arterial pulsations, and tissue swelling.

disturbed tactile Sensory Perception may be related to altered sensory reception (neurological deficit, pain), possibly evidenced by change in usual response to stimuli/abnormal sensitivity of touch, physiological anxiety, and irritability.

risk for ineffective Role Performance: risk factors may include situational crisis, chronic disability, debilitating pain.

risk for compromised family Coping: risk factors may include temporary family disorganization and role changes and prolonged disability that exhausts the supportive capacity of SO(s).

Regional Enteritis CH
(Refer to Crohn's disease)

Renal disease, end-stage CH/MS
(Also refer to Renal failure, chronic)

death Anxiety may be related to progressive debilitating disease, unmet needs, inadequate support system, personal vulnerability, past negative experiences, possibly evidenced by fear of the process of dying/loss of abilities, concerns of unfinished business, powerlessness/loss of control, denial of impending death.

Renal failure, acute MS
excess Fluid Volume may be related to compromised regulatory mechanisms (decreased kidney function), possibly evidenced by weight gain, edema/anasarca, intake greater than output, venous congestion, changes in BP/CVP, and altered electrolyte levels.

imbalanced Nutrition: less than body requirements may be related to inability to ingest/digest adequate nutrients (anorexia, nausea/vomiting, ulcerations of oral mucosa, and increased metabolic needs) in addition to therapeutic dietary restrictions, possibly evidenced by lack of interest in food/aversion to eating, observed inadequate intake, weight loss, loss of muscle mass.

risk for Infection: risk factors may include depression of immunological defenses, invasive procedures/devices, and changes in dietary intake/malnutrition.

disturbed Thought Processes may be related to accumulation of toxic waste products and altered cerebral perfusion, possibly evidenced by disorientation, changes in recent memory, apathy, and episodic obtundation.

Renal failure, chronic CH/MS
(Also refer to Dialysis, general)

risk for decreased Cardiac Output: risk factors may include fluid imbalances affecting circulating volume/myocardial workload/systemic vascular resistance, alterations in rate/rhythm/cardiac conduction (electrolyte imbalances, hypoxia), accumulation of toxins (urea), soft-calcification.

risk for ineffective Protection: risk factors may include abnormal blood profile (suppressed erythropoietin production/secretion, decreased RBC production/survival, altered clotting factors), increased capillary fragility, inadequate nutrition.

disturbed Thought Processes may be related to physiological changes—accumulation of toxins (e.g., urea, ammonia), metabolic acidosis, hypoxia, electrolyte imbalances, calcifications in brain, possibly evidenced by disorientation, memory deficit, altered attention span, decreased ability to grasp idea, impaired ability to make decisions/problem-solve, changes in sensorium, irritability, psychosis.

risk for impaired Skin Integrity: risk factors may include altered metabolic state/circulation (anemia with tissue ischemia)/sensation (peripheral neuropathy), decreased skin turgor, reduced activity/immobility, accumulation of toxins in the skin.

risk for impaired Oral Mucous Membrane: risk factors may include decreased/lack of salivation, fluid restrictions, chemical irritation (conversion of urea in saliva to ammonia).

Renal transplantation MS
(Also refer to Transplantation, recipient)

risk for excess Fluid Volume: risk factors may include compromised regulatory mechanism (implantation of new kidney requiring adjustment period for optimal functioning).

disturbed Body Image may be related to failure and subsequent replacement of body part and medication-induced changes in appearance, possibly evidenced by preoccupation with loss/change, negative feelings about body, and focus on past strength/function.

Fear may be related to potential for transplant rejection/failure and threat of death, possibly evidenced by increased tension, apprehension, concentration on source, and verbalizations of concern.

risk for Infection: risk factors may include broken skin/traumatized tissue, stasis of body fluids, immunosuppression, invasive procedures, nutritional deficits, and chronic disease.

CH

risk for ineffective Coping/compromised family Coping: risk factors may include situational crises, family disorganization and role changes, prolonged disease exhausting supportive capacity of SO/family, therapeutic restrictions/long-term therapy needs.

Repetitive motion injury   CH
(Refer to Carpal tunnel syndrome)

Respiratory distress syndrome, acute (ARDS)   MS
ineffective Airway Clearance may be related to loss of ciliary action, increased amount and viscosity of secretions, and increased airway resistance, possibly evidenced by presence of dyspnea, changes in depth/rate of respiration, use of accessory muscles for breathing, wheezes/crackles, cough with or without sputum production.

impaired Gas Exchange may be related to changes in pulmonary capillary permeability with edema formation, alveolar hypoventilation and collapse, with intrapulmonary shunting, possibly evidenced by tachypnea, use of accessory muscles, cyanosis, hypoxia per arterial blood gases (ABGs)/oximetry, anxiety and changes in mentation.

risk for deficient Fluid Volume: risk factors may include active loss from diuretic use and restricted intake.

risk for decreased Cardiac Output: risk factors may include alteration in preload (hypovolemia, vascular pooling, diuretic therapy, and increased intrathoracic pressure/use of ventilator/positive end-expiratory pressure [PEEP]).

Anxiety [specify level]/Fear may be related to physiological factors (effects of hypoxemia); situational crisis, change in health status/threat of death; possibly evidenced by increased tension, apprehension, restlessness, focus on self, and sympathetic stimulation.

risk for barotrauma Injury: risk factors may include increased airway pressure associated with mechanical ventilation (PEEP).

Respiratory distress syndrome (premature infant)   PED
(Also refer to Neonatal, premature newborn)
impaired Gas Exchange may be related to alveolar/capillary membrane changes (inadequate surfactant levels), altered oxygen supply (tracheobronchial obstruction, atelectasis), altered blood flow (immaturity of pulmonary arteriole musculature), altered oxygen-carrying capacity of blood (anemia), and cold stress, possibly evidenced by tachypnea, use of accessory muscles/retractions, expiratory grunting, pallor or cyanosis, abnormal ABGs, and tachycardia.

impaired Spontaneous Ventilation may be related to respiratory muscle fatigue and metabolic factors, possibly evidenced by dyspnea, increased metabolic rate, restlessness, use of accessory muscles, and abnormal ABGs.

risk for Infection: risk factors may include inadequate primary defenses (decreased ciliary action, stasis of body fluids, traumatized tissues), inadequate secondary defenses (deficiency of

---

neutrophils and specific immunoglobulins), invasive procedures, and malnutrition (absence of nutrient stores, increased metabolic demands).

risk for ineffective gastrointestinal Tissue Perfusion: risk factors may include persistent fetal circulation and exchange problems.

risk for impaired parent/infant Attachment: risk factors may include premature/ill infant who is unable to effectively initiate parental contact (altered behavioral organization), separation, physical barriers, anxiety associated with the parental role/demands of infant.

Respiratory syncytial virus   PED
impaired Gas Exchange may be related to inflammation of airways, ventilation perfusion imbalance (areas of consolidation), apnea, possibly evidenced by dyspnea, abnormal ABGs/hypoxia.

ineffective Airway Clearance may be related to infection, retained secretions, exudate in alveoli, inflammation of airways, possibly evidenced by dyspnea, adventitious breath sounds, cough.

risk for deficient Fluid Volume: risk factors may include increased insensible losses (fever/diaphoresis), decreased oral intake.

Restless leg syndrome   CH
(Refer to Myoclonus, nocturnal)

Retinal detachment   CH
disturbed visual Sensory Perception related to decreased sensory reception, possibly evidenced by visual distortions, decreased visual field, and changes in visual acuity.

[mild to moderate] Anxiety may be related to situational crisis, change in health status/role function, possibly evidenced by expressed concerns, apprehension, uncertainty, focus on self.

deficient Knowledge [Learning Need] regarding therapy, prognosis, and self-care needs may be related to lack of information/misconceptions, possibly evidenced by statements of concern and questions.

risk for impaired Home Maintenance: risk factors may include visual limitations/activity/restrictions.

Rett's syndrome   PED/PSY
(Also refer to Autistic disorder)

delayed Growth and Development may be related to effects of physical/mental disability, possibly evidenced by altered physical growth; delay/inability in performing skills and self-care/self-control activities appropriate for age.

impaired Walking/physical Mobility may be related to neuromuscular impairment, joint stiffness/contractures, disuse, possibly evidenced by limited range of motion, inability to perform gross motor skills/walk/reposition self.

risk for Trauma: risk factors may include cognitive deficits, lack of muscle tone/coordination, seizure activity.

imbalanced Nutrition: less than body requirements may be related to poor muscle tone, dependence on others/inability to meet own needs, possibly evidenced by weak and ineffective sucking/swallowing and observed lack of adequate intake with weight loss/failure to gain.

risk for complicated Grieving: risk factors may include loss of "the perfect child," chronic condition requiring long-term care, and unresolved feelings.

Reye's syndrome   PED
deficient Fluid Volume [isotonic] may be related to failure of regulatory mechanism (diabetes insipidus), excessive gastric losses (pernicious vomiting), and altered intake, possibly evidenced by increased/dilute urine output, sudden weight loss, decreased venous filling, dry mucous membranes, decreased skin turgor, hypotension, and tachycardia.

ineffective cerebral Tissue Perfusion may be related to diminished arterial/venous blood flow and hypovolemia, possibly evidenced by memory loss, altered consciousness, and restlessness/agitation.

risk for Trauma: risk factors may include generalized weakness, reduced coordination, and cognitive deficits.

ineffective Breathing Pattern may be related to decreased energy and fatigue, cognitive impairment, tracheobronchial obstruction, and inflammatory process (aspiration pneumonia), possibly evidenced by tachypnea, abnormal ABGs, cough, and use of accessory muscles.

Rheumatic fever   PED

acute Pain may be related to migratory inflammation of joints, possibly evidenced by verbal reports, guarding/distraction behaviors, self-focus, and autonomic responses (changes in vital signs).

Hyperthermia may be related to inflammatory process/hypermetabolic state, possibly evidenced by increased body temperature, warm/flushed skin, and tachycardia.

Activity Intolerance may be related to generalized weakness, joint pain, and medical restrictions/bedrest, possibly evidenced by reports of fatigue, exertional discomfort, and abnormal heart rate in response to activity.

risk for decreased Cardiac Output: risk factors may include cardiac inflammation/enlargement and altered contractility.

Rheumatic heart disease   PED/MS
(Also refer to Valvular heart disease)

Activity Intolerance may be related to imbalance between O_2 supply/demand, generalized weakness, and prolonged bedrest/sedentary lifestyle, possibly evidenced by reported/observed weakness, fatigue, changes in vital signs, presence of dysrhythmias, dyspnea, pallor.

risk-prone health Behavior may be related to health status requiring change in lifestyle/restriction of desired activities, unrealistic expectations, negative attitudes, possibly evidenced by denial of situation, demonstration of nonacceptance of health status, failure to achieve optimal sense of control.

risk for ineffective Therapeutic Regimen Management: risk factors may include complexity/duration of therapeutic regimen, imposed restrictions or limitations, economic difficulties, family patterns of healthcare, perceived seriousness/benefits.

risk for impaired Gas Exchange: risk factors may include alveolar-capillary membrane changes (fluid collection/shifts into interstitial space/alveoli).

Rhinitis, allergic   CH
(Refer to Hay fever)

Rickets   PED

delayed Growth and Development may be related to dietary deficiencies/indiscretions, malabsorption syndrome, and lack of exposure to sunlight, possibly evidenced by altered physical growth and delay or difficulty in performing motor skills typical for age.

deficient Knowledge [Learning Need] regarding cause, pathophysiology, therapy needs and prevention may be related to lack of information, possibly evidenced by statements of concern, questions, misconceptions, and inaccurate follow-through of instructions.

Ringworm, tinea   CH
(Also refer to Athlete's Foot)

impaired Skin Integrity may be related to fungal infection of the dermis, possibly evidenced by disruption of skin surfaces/presence of lesions.

deficient Knowledge [Learning Need] regarding infectious nature, therapy, and self-care needs may be related to lack of information/misinformation, possibly evidenced by statements of concern, questions, and recurrence/spread.

Rocky Mountain spotted fever   CH/MS
(Refer to Typhus)

RSD   CH
(Refer to Reflex sympathetic dystrophy)

RSV   PED
(Refer to Respiratory syncytial virus)

Rubella   PED/CH
acute Pain[/Discomfort] may be related to inflammatory effects of viral infection and presence of desquamating rash, possibly evidenced by verbal reports, distraction behaviors/restlessness.

deficient Knowledge [Learning Need] regarding contagious nature, possible complications, and self-care needs may be related to lack of information/misinterpretations, possibly evidenced by statements of concern, questions, and inaccurate follow-through of instructions.

Rubeola   PED/CH
(Refer to Measles)

Ruptured intervertebral disk   CH/MS
(Refer to Herniated nucleus pulposus)

Sarcoidosis   CH
(Also refer to Pulmonary fibrosis)
Fatigue may be related to disease state, anemia, possibly evidenced by lack of energy, lethargy, decreased performance, inability to maintain usual routines.

risk for disturbed visual Sensory Perception: risk factors may include altered sensory reception (e.g., inflammation of the eye, increased intraocular pressure).

risk for Injury: risk factors may include autoimmune dysfunction, abnormal blood profile (thrombocytopenia, leukopenia, anemia), sensory dysfunction.

SARS (Sudden acute respiratory syndrome)   MS
Hyperthermia may be related to inflammatory process, possibly evidenced by high fever, chills, rigors, headache.

acute Pain[/Discomfort] may be related to inflammation/circulating toxins, possibly evidenced by reports of myalgia, headache, malaise.

impaired Gas Exchange may be related to ventilation perfusion imbalance (interstitial infiltrates, areas of consolidation), possibly evidenced by dyspnea, changes in mentation/level of consciousness, restlessness, hypoxemia.

risk for impaired spontaneous Ventilation: risk factors may include hypermetabolic state/infection, depletion of energy stores, respiratory muscle fatigue.

risk for ineffective Protection: risk factors may include inadequate nutrition, abnormal blood profile (leukopnea, thrombocytopnia).

Scabies   CH
impaired Skin Integrity may be related to presence of invasive parasite and development of pruritus, possibly evidenced by disruption of skin surface and inflammation.

deficient Knowledge [Learning Need] regarding communicable nature, possible complications, therapy, and self-care needs may be related to lack of information/misinterpretation, possibly evidenced by questions and statements of concern about spread to others.

Scarlet fever   **PED**

Hyperthermia may be related to effects of circulating toxins, possibly evidenced by increased body temperature, warm/flushed skin, and tachycardia.

Pain/[Discomfort] may be related to inflammation of mucous membranes and effects of circulating toxins (malaise, fever), possibly evidenced by verbal reports, distraction behaviors, guarding (decreased swallowing), and self-focus.

risk for deficient Fluid Volume: risk factors may include hypermetabolic state (hyperthermia) and reduced intake.

Schizoaffective disorder   **PSY**

risk for other/self-directed Violence: risk factors may include depressed mood, feelings of worthlessness, hoplessness, unsatisfactory parent-child relationship, feelings of abandonment by SOs, anger turned inward/directed at the environment, punitive superego, irrational feeelings of guilt, numerous failures, misinterpretation of reality.

Social Isolation may be related to developmental regression, depressed mood, feelings of worthlessness, egocentric behaviors (offending others and discouraging relationships), delusional thinking, fear of failure, unresolved grief, possibly evidenced by sad/dull affect, absence of support systems, uncommunicative/withdrawn/catatonic behavior, absence of eye contact, preoccupation with own thoughts, repetitive/meaningless actions.

imbalanced Nutrition: less than body requirements may be related to energy expenditure in excess of intake, refusal/inability to take time to eat, lack of attention to/recognition of hunger cues, possibly evidenced by lack of interest in food, weight loss, pale conjunctiva and mucous membranes, poor muscle tone/skin turgor, amenorrhea, abnormal laboratory studies.

Schizophrenia (schizophrenic disorders)   **PSY**

disturbed Thought Processes may be related to disintegration of thinking processes, impaired judgment, presence of psychological conflicts, disintegrated ego boundaries, sleep disturbance, ambivalence and concomitant dependence, possibly evidenced by impaired ability to reason/problem-solve, inappropriate affect, presence of delusional system, command hallucinations, obsessions, ideas of reference, cognitive dissonance.

Social Isolation may be related to alterations in mental status, mistrust of others/delusional thinking, unacceptable social behaviors, inadequate personal resources, and inability to engage in satisfying personal relationships, possibly evidenced by difficulty in establishing relationships with others; dull affect, uncommunicative/withdrawn behavior, seeking to be alone, inadequate/absent significant purpose in life, and expression of feelings of rejection.

risk for self/other-directed Violence: risk factors may include disturbances of thinking/feeling (depression, paranoia, suicidal ideation), lack of development of trust and appropriate interpersonal relationships, catatonic/manic excitement, toxic reactions to drugs (alcohol).

ineffective Coping may be related to personal vulnerability, inadequate support system(s), unrealistic perceptions, inadequate coping methods, and disintegration of thought processes, possibly evidenced by impaired judgment/cognition and perception, diminished problem-solving/decision-making capacities, poor self-concept, chronic anxiety, depression, inability to perform role expectations, and alteration in social participation.

CH

interrupted Family Processes/disabled family Coping may be related to ambivalent family system/relationships, change of roles, and difficulty of family member in coping effectively with client's maladaptive behaviors, possibly evidenced by deterioration in family functioning, ineffective family decision-making process, difficulty relating to each other, client's expressions of despair at family's lack of reaction/involvement, neglectful relationships with client, extreme distortion regarding client's health problem, including denial about its existence/severity or prolonged overconcern.

ineffective Health Maintenance/impaired Home Maintenance may be related to impaired cognitive/emotional functioning, altered ability to make deliberate and thoughtful judgments, altered communication, and lack of/inappropriate use of material resources, possibly evidenced by inability to take responsibility for meeting basic health practices in any or all functional areas and demonstrated lack of adaptive behaviors to internal or external environmental changes, disorderly surroundings, accumulation of dirt/unwashed clothes, repeated hygienic disorders.

Self-Care Deficit [specify] may be related to perceptual and cognitive impairment, immobility (withdrawal/isolation and decreased psychomotor activity), and side effects of psychotropic medications, possibly evidenced by inability or difficulty in areas of feeding self, keeping body clean, dressing appropriately, toileting self, or changes in bowel/bladder elimination.

Sciatica   CH

acute/chronic Pain may be related to peripheral nerve root compression, possibly evidenced by verbal reports, guarding/distraction behaviors, and self-focus.

impaired physical Mobility may be related to neurological pain and muscular involvement, possibly evidenced by reluctance to attempt movement and decreased muscle strength/mass.

Scleroderma   CH
(Also refer to Lupus Erythematosus, Systemic [SLE])

impaired physical Mobility may be related to musculoskeletal impairment and associated pain, possibly evidenced by decreased strength, decreased range of motion, and reluctance to attempt movement.

ineffective Tissue Perfusion (specify) may be related to reduced arterial blood flow (arteriolar vasoconstriction), possibly evidenced by changes in skin temperature/color, ulcer formation, and changes in organ function (cardiopulmonary, GI, renal).

imbalanced Nutrition: less than body requirements may be related to inability to ingest/digest/absorb adequate nutrients (sclerosis of the tissues rendering mouth immobile, decreased peristalsis of esophagus/small intestines, atrophy of smooth muscle of colon), possibly evidenced by weight loss, decreased intake/food, and reported/observed difficulty swallowing.

risk-prone health Behavior may be related to disability requiring change in lifestyle, inadequate support systems, assault to self-concept, and altered locus of control, possibly evidenced by verbalization of nonacceptance of health status change and lack of movement toward independence/future-oriented thinking.

disturbed Body Image may be related to skin changes with induration, atrophy, and fibrosis, loss of hair, and skin and muscle contractures, possibly evidenced by verbalization of negative feelings about body, focus on past strength/function or appearance, fear of rejection/reaction by others, hiding body part, and change in social involvement.

Scoliosis   PED

disturbed Body Image may be related to altered body structure, use of therapeutic device(s), and activity restrictions, possibly evidenced by negative feelings about body, change in social involvement, and preoccupation with situation or refusal to acknowledge problem.

deficient Knowledge [Learning Need] regarding pathophysiology of condition, therapy needs, and possible outcomes may be related to lack of information/misinterpretation, possibly evidenced by statements of concern, questions, misconceptions, and inaccurate follow-through of instructions.

risk-prone health Behavior may be related to lack of comprehension of long-term consequences of behavior, possibly evidenced by minimizing health status change, failure to take action, and evidence of failure to improve.

Seasonal affective disorder   PSY
(Refer to Affective disorder, seasonal)

Sedative intoxication/abuse   CH/PSY
(Refer to Depressant abuse)

Seizure disorder   CH
deficient Knowledge [Learning Need] regarding condition and medication control may be related to lack of information/misinterpretations, scarce financial resources, possibly evidenced by questions, statements of concern/misconceptions, incorrect use of anticonvulsant medication, recurrent episodes/uncontrolled seizures.

chronic low Self-Esteem/disturbed Personal Identity may be related to perceived neurological functional change/weakness, perception of being out of control, stigma associated with condition, possibly evidenced by negative feelings about "brain"/self, change in social involvement, feelings of helplessness, and preoccupation with perceived change or loss.

impaired Social Interaction may be related to unpredictable nature of condition and self-concept disturbance, possibly evidenced by decreased self-assurance, verbalization of concern, discomfort in social situations, inability to receive/communicate a satisfying sense of belonging/caring, and withdrawal from social contacts/activities.

risk for Trauma/Suffocation: risk factors may include weakness, balancing difficulties, cognitive limitations/altered consciousness, loss of large- or small-muscle coordination (during seizure).

Separation anxiety disorder   PED/PSY
(Refer to Anxiety disorders—PED)

Sepsis   MS
(Also refer to Sepsis, Puerperal)
ineffective Tissue Perfusion (specify) may be related to changes in arterial/venous blood flow (selective vasoconstriction, presence of microemboli) and hypovolemia, possibly evidenced by changes in skin temperature/color, changes in blood/pulse pressure; changes in sensorium, and decreased urinary output.

risk for deficient Fluid Volume: risk factors may include marked increase in vascular compartment/massive vasodilation, vascular shifts to interstitial space, and reduced intake.

risk for decreased Cardiac Output: risk factors may include decreased preload (venous return and circulating volume), altered afterload (increased SVR), negative inotropic effects of hypoxia, complement activation, and lysosomal hydrolase.

Sepsis, puerperal   OB
risk for Infection [spread/septic shock]: risk factors may include presence of infection, broken skin, or traumatized tissues, rupture of amniotic membranes, high vascularity of involved area, stasis of body fluids, invasive procedures, or increased environmental exposure, chronic disease (e.g., diabetes mellitus, anemia, malnutrition), altered immune response, and untoward effect of medications (e.g., opportunistic/secondary infection).

Hyperthermia may be related to inflammatory process/hypermetabolic state, possibly evidenced by increase in body temperature, warm/flushed skin, and tachycardia.

risk for impaired parent/infant Attachment: risk factors may include interruption in bonding process, physical illness, perceived threat to own survival.

risk for ineffective peripheral Tissue Perfusion: risk factors may include interruption/reduction of blood flow (presence of infectious thrombi).

Septicemia   **MS**
(Refer to Sepsis)

Serum sickness   **CH**
acute Pain may be related to inflammation of the joints and skin eruptions, possibly evidenced by verbal reports, guarding/distraction behaviors, and self-focus.

deficient Knowledge [Learning Need] regarding nature of condition, treatment needs, potential complications, and prevention of recurrence may be related to lack of information/misinterpretation, possibly evidenced by statements of concern, questions, misconceptions, and inaccurate follow-through of instructions.

Severe acute respiratory syndrome   **MS**
(Refer to SARS)

Sexual desire disorder   **PSY**
Sexual Dysfunction may be related to boredom/conflict in relationship, depression, hormonal imbalance, harmful relationships/traumatic events in childhood, possibly evidenced by loss of sexual desire, disruption of sexual response pattern, alteration in relationship with SO.

Anxiety (specify) may be related to situational crisis, stress, unconscious conflict about essential values, unmet needs, possibly evidenced by expressed concerns, distress, feelings of inadequacy, fear of unspecific consequences.

situational low Self-Esteem may be related to perceived functional impairment, emotional insecurity, rejection by SO, possibly evidenced by expressions of helplessness, self-negating verbalizations, change in involvement with partner.

Sexual dysfunctions   **PSY**
(Refer to Dyspareunia; Erectile dysfunction; Sexual desire disorder; Vaginismus)

Sexually transmitted disease   **GYN/CH**
risk for Infection [transmission]: risk factors may include contagious nature of infecting agent and insufficient knowledge to avoid exposure to/transmission of pathogens.

impaired Skin/Tissue Integrity may be related to invasion of/irritation by pathogenic organism(s), possibly evidenced by disruptions of skin/tissue and inflammation of mucous membranes.

deficient Knowledge [Learning Need] regarding condition, prognosis/complications, therapy needs, and transmission may be related to lack of information/misinterpretation, lack of interest in learning, possibly evidenced by statements of concern, questions, misconceptions, inaccurate follow-through of instructions, and development of preventable complications.

Shingles   **CH**
(Refer to Herpes zoster)

Shock   **MS**
(Also refer to Shock, cardiogenic; Shock, hypovolemic/hemorrhagic; Sepsis)
ineffective Tissue Perfusion (specify) may be related to changes in circulating volume or vascular tone, possibly evidenced by changes in skin color/temperature and pulse pressure, reduced blood pressure, changes in mentation, and decreased urinary output.

Anxiety [specify level] may be related to change in health status and threat of death, possibly evidenced by increased tension, apprehension, sympathetic stimulation, restlessness, and expressions of concern.

Shock, cardiogenic   MS
(Also refer to Shock)

    decreased Cardiac Output may be related to structural damage, decreased myocardial contractility, and presence of dysrhythmias, possibly evidenced by ECG changes, variations in hemodynamic readings, jugular vein distention, cold/clammy skin, diminished peripheral pulses, and decreased urinary output.

    risk for impaired Gas Exchange: risk factors may include ventilation perfusion imbalance, alveolar-capillary membrane changes.

Shock, hypovolemic/hemorrhagic   MS
(Also refer to Shock)

    deficient Fluid Volume [isotonic] may be related to excessive vascular loss, inadequate intake/replacement, possibly evidenced by hypotension, tachycardia, decreased pulse volume and pressure, change in mentation, and decreased/concentrated urine.

Shock, septic   MS
(Refer to Sepsis)

Sicca syndrome   CH
(Refer to Sjögren syndrome)

Sick building syndrome   CH
Contamination may be related to presence of atmospheric/environmental contaminants in building (e.g., volatile organic compounds, carbon monoxide, asbestos, dust, fungi/molds, pollens, tobacco smoke), flooring surface (carpeted surfaces hold contaminant residue more than hard floor surfaces), poorly ventilated areas, lack of effective protection, possibly evidenced by headaches, eye/nose/throat irritation, dry cough, dry or itchy skin, dizziness, nausea, difficulty in concentrating, fatigue.

    Fatigue may be related to occupation/employment in a specific building or zone within a building as evidenced by reports of being tired, lethargic; decreased performance

Sick sinus syndrome   MS
(Also refer to Dysrhythmia, cardiac)

    decreased Cardiac Output may be related to alterations in rate, rhythm, and electrical conduction, possibly evidenced by ECG indication of dysrhythmias, reports of palpitations/weakness, changes in mentation/consciousness, and syncope.

    risk for Trauma: risk factors may include changes in cerebral perfusion with altered consciousness/loss of balance.

SIDS   PED
(Refer to Sudden infant death syndrome)

Sinusitis, chronic   CH
acute/chronic Pain may be related to inflammatory process, possibly evidenced by reports of headache/facial pain, irritability, change in sleep, fatigue.

    risk for Infection [spread]: risk factors may include chronic irritation/inflamed tissues, stasis of body fluids, improper handling of infectious material.

Sjögren syndrome   CH
impaired Oral Mucous Membrane related to decreased salivation, possibly evidenced by xerostomia (dry mouth), oral pain/discomfort, self-report of bad/diminished taste, difficulty eating/swallowing.

risk for impaired Tissue Integrity (cornea, mucous membranes): risk factors may include impaired fluid (e.g., tears/mucous) production.

risk for Infection: risk factors may include decreased secretions, tissue dryness/damage.

risk for disturbed visual Sensory Perception: risk factors may include altered sensory reception (light sensitivity, blurred vision, corneal ulcers).

Skin cancer   CH

impaired Skin Integrity may be related to invasive growth, surgical excision may be evidenced by disruption of skin surface, destruction of dermis.

risk for acute Pain: risk factors may include ulceration of skin, surgical incision.

risk for disturbed Body Image: risk factors may include skin lesion, surgical intervention.

deficient Knowledge [Learning Need] regarding condition, prognosis, treatment, prevention may be related to lack of information/misinterpretation, possibly evidenced by statements of concern, questions, misconceptions, inaccurate follow-through of instructions, and development of preventable complications/recurrence.

SLE   CH

(Refer to Lupus erythematosus, systemic)

Sleep apnea   CH

Sleep Deprivation may be related to sleep apnea (recurrent apneic episodes followed by gasping arousal), possibly evidenced by daytime drowsiness, tiredness, decreased ability to perform/slowed mentation.

impaired Gas Exchange may be related to altered oxygen supply (recurrent apneic episodes lasting 10 seconds to 2 minutes), possibly evidenced by morning headache, decreased mental acuity, abnormal ABGs (hypoxemia, hypercapnia), dysrhythmias (e.g., extreme bradycardia, ventricular tachycardia).

risk for ineffective Therapeutic Regimen Management: risk factors may include duration of therapy, associated discomfort, perceived seriousness/benefit.

Smallpox   MS

risk of Infection [spread]: risk factors may include contagious nature of organism, inadequate acquired immunity, presence of chronic disease, immunosuppression.

deficient Fluid Volume may be related to hypermetabolic state, decreased intake (pharyngeal lesions, nausea), increased losses (vomiting), fluid shifts from vascular bed, possibly evidenced by reports of thirst, decreased BP, venous filling and urinary output; dry mucous membranes, decreased skin turgor, change in mental state, elevated Hct.

impaired Tissue Integrity may be related to immunological deficit, possibly evidenced by disruption of skin surface, cornea, mucous membranes.

Anxiety [specify level]/Fear may be related to threat of death, interpersonal transmission/contagion, separation from support system, possibly evidenced by expressed concerns, apprehension, restlessness, focus on self.

CH

interrupted Family Processes may be related to temporary family disorganization, situational crisis, change in health status of family member, possibly evidenced by changes in satisfaction with family, stress-reduction behaviors, mutual support, expression of isolation from community resources.

ineffective community Coping may be related to human-made disaster (bioterrorism), inadequate resources for problem-solving, possibly evidenced by deficits of community participation, high illness rate, excessive community conflicts, expressed vulnerability/powerlessness.

Snake bite, venomous   **MS**

[severe] Anxiety/Fear may be related to situational crisis, threat of death, interpersonal transmission, possibly evidenced by expressed concerns, apprehension, irritability, jitteriness, increased tension, tremors.

acute Pain/[Discomfort] may be related to effects of toxins (edema formation, erythema, enlargement of lymph nodes, nausea, fever, diaphoresis, muscle fasciculations), possibly evidenced by reports of pain/paresthesias, guarded behavior, restlessness, autonomic responses.

impaired Skin Integrity may be related to trauma, inflammation, altered circulation, possibly evidenced by disruption of skin surface/destruction of skin layers (skin tense, discolored, necrosis around bite).

risk for deficient Fluid Volume: risk factors may include excessive losses (vomiting, edema formation, hemorrhage from mucous membranes).

Snow blindness   **CH**

disturbed visual Sensory Perception may be related to altered status of sense organ (irritation of the conjunctiva, hyperemia), possibly evidenced by intolerance to light (photophobia) and decreased/loss of visual acuity.

acute Pain may be related to irritation/vascular congestion of the conjunctiva, possibly evidenced by verbal reports, guarding/distraction behaviors, and self-focus.

Anxiety [specify level] may be related to situational crisis and threat to/change in health status, possibly evidenced by increased tension, apprehension, uncertainty, worry, restlessness, and focus on self.

Somatoform disorders   **PSY**

ineffective Coping may be related to severe level of anxiety that is repressed, personal vulnerability, unmet dependency needs, fixation in earlier level of development, retarded ego development, and inadequate coping skills, possibly evidenced by verbalized inability to cope/problem-solve, high illness rate, multiple somatic complaints of several years' duration, decreased functioning in social/occupational settings, narcissistic tendencies with total focus on self/physical symptoms, demanding behaviors, history of "doctor shopping," and refusal to attend therapeutic activities.

chronic Pain may be related to severe level of repressed anxiety, low self-concept, unmet dependency needs, history of self or loved one having experienced a serious illness, possibly evidenced by verbal reports of severe/prolonged pain, guarded movement/protective behaviors, facial mask of pain, fear of reinjury, altered ability to continue previous activities, social withdrawal, demands for therapy/medication.

disturbed Sensory Perception (specify) may be related to psychological stress (narrowed perceptual fields, expression of stress as physical problems/deficits), poor quality of sleep, presence of chronic pain, possibly evidenced by reported change in voluntary motor or sensory function (paralysis, anosmia, aphonia, deafness, blindness, loss of touch or pain sensation), la belle indifférence (lack of concern over functional loss).

impaired Social Interaction may be related to inability to engage in satisfying personal relationships, preoccupation with self and physical symptoms, altered state of wellness, chronic pain, and rejection by others, possibly evidenced by preoccupation with own thoughts, sad/dull affect, absence of supportive SO(s), uncommunicative/withdrawn behavior, lack of eye contact, and seeking to be alone.

Spina bifida   **PED**

(Also refer to Paraplegia; Newborn, special needs)

Bowel Incontinence/Constipation may be be related to disruption of nerve innervation, perceptual impairment, reduced activity level, possibly evidenced by inability to evacuate bowel voluntarily, increased abdominal pressure/distention, dry/hard formed stool, change in bowel sounds.

---

risk for impaired physical Mobility: risk factors may include neuromuscular impairment, developmental delay, musculoskeletal impairments (clubfoot, hip dislocation, joint deformities, kyphosis).

risk for decreased Intracranial Adaptive Capacity: risk factors may include structural changes (aqueductal stricture, malformation of brain stem).

risk for Infection: risk factors may include increased environmental exposure, invasive procedures, traumatized tissues (CSF leak).

Spinal cord injury (SCI)   MS/CH
(Refer to Paraplegia; Quadriplegia)

Splenectomy   MS/CH
(Refer to Surgery, general)

risk for Infection: risk factors may include inadequate secondary defenses (decreased antibody synthesis/reduced immunoglobin M), insufficient knowledge/motivation to avoid exposure to pathogens.

risk for ineffective Therapeutic Regimen Management: risk factors may include length of therapy, economic difficulties, perceived benefits.

Spongiform encephalopathy   CH
(Refer to Creutzfeldt-Jakob disease)

Sprain of ankle or foot   CH
acute Pain may be related to trauma to/swelling in joint, possibly evidenced by verbal reports, guarding/distraction behaviors, self-focusing, and autonomic responses (changes in vital signs).

impaired Walking may be related to musculoskeletal injury, pain, and therapeutic restrictions, possibly evidenced by reluctance to attempt movement, inability to move about environment easily.

Sprue, nontropical   CH
(Refer to Celiac disease)

Stapedectomy   MS
risk for Trauma: risk factors may include increased middle-ear pressure with displacement of prosthesis and balancing difficulties/dizziness.

risk for Infection: risk factors may include surgically traumatized tissue, invasive procedures, and environmental exposure to upper respiratory infections.

acute Pain may be related to surgical trauma, edema formation, and presence of packing, possibly evidenced by verbal reports, guarding/distraction behaviors, and self-focus.

Stasis dermatitis   CH
(Also refer to Venous insufficiency)

impaired Skin Integrity may be related to altered circulation, presence of edema, extremely fragile epidermis, pigmentation, possibly evidenced by erythema, scaling, brown discoloration, disruption of skin surface.

risk for Infection: risk factors may include circulatory stasis/edema formation (small-vessel vasoconstrictive reflexes) in lower extremities, persistent inflammation, tissue destruction.

STD   CH
(refer to Sexually transmitted disease)

Stillbirth   **OB**
(Refer to Fetal demise)

Stimulant abuse   **CH**
(Also refer to Cocaine hydrochloride poisoning, acute; Substance dependence/abuse rehabilitation)

imbalanced Nutrition: less than body requirements may be related to anorexia, insufficient/inappropriate use of financial resources, possibly evidenced by reported inadequate intake, weight loss/less than normal weight gain; lack of interest in food, poor muscle tone, signs/laboratory evidence of vitamin deficiencies.

risk for Infection: risk factors may include injection techniques, impurities of drugs; localized trauma/nasal septum damage, malnutrition, altered immune state.

Insomnia may be related to CNS sensory alterations/psychological stress, possibly evidenced by constant alertness, racing thoughts preventing rest, denial of need to sleep/reported inability to stay awake, initial insomnia then hypersomnia.

                                                  PSY
Fear/Anxiety [specify] may be related to paranoid delusions associated with stimulant use, possibly evidenced by feelings/beliefs that others are conspiring against or are about to attack/kill client.

ineffective Coping may be related to personal vulnerability, negative role-modeling, inadequate support systems; ineffective/inadequate coping skills with substitution of drug, possibly evidenced by use of harmful substance despite evidence of undesirable consequences.

disturbed Sensory Perception (specify) may be related to exogenous chemical, altered sensory reception/transmission/integration (hallucination), altered status of sense organs, possibly evidenced by responding to internal stimuli from hallucinatory experiences, bizarre thinking, anxiety/panic changes in sensory acuity (sense of smell/taste).

Stomatitis   **CH**
impaired Oral Mucous Membrane may be related to infection, vitamin deficiency, excessive alcohol/tobacco use, ill-fitting dentures, jagged teeth, orthodontic appliances, mouth breathing, nursing bottles with hard/too long nipples, possibly evidenced by oral pain, lesions/ulcers, white patches/plaques, sensitive tongue.

risk for deficient Fluid Volume: risk factors may include oral pain, difficulty swallowing.

Strep throat   **CH**
Hyperthermia may be related to illness/effects of toxins, inability to ingest sufficient fluids, possibly evidenced by body temperature above normal range, flushed dry skin, decreased urine output.

acute Pain may be related to injuring biological agent, possibly evidenced by report of throat, head, and abdominal pain, change in ability to eat, crying.

risk for Infection [transmission]: risk factors may include insufficient knowledge to avoid exposure to/transmission of pathogen.

Stress disorder, acute   **PSY**
(Refer to Post-traumatic stress disorder)

Substance dependence/abuse, prenatal   **OB**
imbalanced Nutrition: less than body requirements may be related to insufficient dietary intake to meet metabolic needs, inadequate/improper use of financial resources, possibly low-weight gain, decreased subcutaneous fat/muscle mass, reported altered taste sensation, lack of interest in food, protein/vitamin deficiencies.

---

ineffective Denial/Coping may be related to personal vulnerability, difficulty handling new situations, use of drugs for coping, inadequate support systems, possibly evidenced by denial, lack of acceptance of consequences of drug use, manipulation to avoid responsibility for self, impaired adaptive behaviors.

Powerlessness may be related to substance addiction, episodic compulsive indulgence, failed attempts at recovery, lifestyle of helplessness, possibly evidenced by statements of inability to stop behavior, continuous thinking about drug, alterations in personal/occupational/social life.

chronic low Self-Esteem may be related to social stigma attached to substance abuse, social expectation that one controls own behavior, continual negative evaluation of self, personal vulnerabilities, possibly evidenced by not taking responsibility for self, lack of follow-through, self-destructive behavior, denial that substance use is a problem.

compromised/disabled Family Coping may be related to codependency issues, situational crisis of pregnancy and drug abuse, family disorganization, exhausted supportive capacity of family members, possibly evidenced by denial or belief that all problems are due to substance use, financial difficulties, severely dysfunctional family, codependent behaviors.

Substance dependence/abuse rehabilitation   PSY/CH
(Following acute detoxification)

ineffective Denial/Coping may be related to personal vulnerability, difficulty handling new situations, learned response patterns, cultural factors, personal/family value systems, possibly evidenced by lack of acceptance that drug use is causing the present situation, use of manipulation to avoid responsibility for self, altered social patterns/participation, impaired adaptive behavior and problem-solving skills, employment difficulties, financial affairs in disarray, and decreased ability to handle stress of recent events.

Powerlessness may be related to substance addiction with/without periods of abstinence, episodic compulsive indulgence, attempts at recovery, and lifestyle of helplessness, possibly evidenced by ineffective recovery attempts, statements of inability to stop behavior/requests for help, continuous/constant thinking about drug or obtaining drug, alteration in personal/occupational and social life.

imbalanced Nutrition: less than body requirements may be related to insufficient dietary intake to meet metabolic needs for psychological/physiological/economical reasons, possibly evidenced by weight less than normal for height/body build, decreased subcutaneous fat/muscle mass, reported altered taste sensation, lack of interest in food, poor muscle tone, sore/inflamed buccal cavity, laboratory evidence of protein/vitamin deficiencies.

Sexual Dysfunction may be related to altered body function (neurological damage and debilitating effects of drug use), changes in appearance, possibly evidenced by progressive interference with sexual functioning; a significant degree of testicular atrophy, gynecomastia, impotence/decreased sperm counts in men; and loss of body hair, thin/soft skin, spider angiomas, and amenorrhea/increase in miscarriages in women.

dysfunctional Family Processes: alcoholism [substance abuse] may be related to abuse/history of alcoholism/drug use, inadequate coping skills/lack of problem-solving skills, genetic predisposition/biochemical influences, possibly evidenced by feelings of anger/frustration/responsibility for alcoholic's behavior, suppressed rage, shame/embarrassment, repressed emotions, guilt, vulnerability, disturbed family dynamics/deterioration in family relationships, family denial/rationalization, closed communication systems, triangulating family relationships, manipulation, blaming, enabling to maintain substance use, inability to accept/receive help.

OB

risk for fetal Injury: risk factors may include drug/alcohol use, exposure to teratogens.

deficient Knowledge [Learning Need] regarding condition/pregnancy, prognosis, treatment needs may be related to lack/misinterpretation of information, lack of recall, cognitive limitations/interference with learning, possibly evidenced by statements of concern, questions/misconceptions, inaccurate follow-through of instructions, development of preventable complications, continued use in spite of complications.

Sudden infant death syndrome   PED
complicated Grieving may be related to unexpected loss of child, lack of anticipatory grieving, possibly evidenced by expressions of distress, guilt, anger; idealization of child, reliving past with little reduction of intensity of grief, labile affect, crying, prolonged interference with life functioning, withdrawal.

risk for impaired Parenting: risk factors may include recent crisis, change in family unit, maladaptive coping strategies, sleep disruption, depression.

risk for interrupted Family Processes: risk factors may include situational crisis, loss of a family member.

risk for chronic Sorrow: risk factors may include death of a loved one, anniversary dates (birth, death, etc.), trigger events (e.g., infants on TV, at play).

Suicide attempt   MS
(Also refer to specific means, e.g., Drug overdose, acute; Wound, gunshot)

PSY
Hopelessness may be related to long-term stress, abandonment (actual or perceived), deteriorating physical/mental condition, challenged value/belief system, possibly evidenced by verbal cues, passivity, lack of involvement/withdrawal, angry outbursts.

risk for Suicide: risk factors may include prior/current attempt, marked changes in behavior/attitude/performance, impulsiveness, sudden euphoric recovery from major depression, living alone, loss of independence, economic instability, substance abuse, has a plan/available means.

chronic/situational low Self-Esteem may be related to losses, functional impairment, developmental changes, failures/rejection, possibly evidenced by evaluating self as unable to deal with events, expressions of helplessness/uselessness/shame/guilt, self-negating verbalizations.

compromised family Coping may be related to temporary family disorganization, role changes, prolonged disease/disability, situational/developmental crises, possibly evidenced by client expressing concern about SO's response to problems, SO confirms ineffective supportive behaviors, SO withdraws from client at the time of need.

Sunstroke   MS
(Refer to Heatstroke)

Surgery, general   MS
(Also refer to Postoperative recovery period)
deficient Knowledge [Learning Need] regarding surgical procedure/expectation, postoperative routines/therapy, and self-care needs may be related to lack of information/misinterpretation, possibly evidenced by statements of concern, questions, and misconceptions.

Anxiety [specify level]/Fear may be related to situational crisis, unfamiliarity with environment, change in health status/threat of death and separation from usual support systems, possibly evidenced by increased tension, apprehension, decreased self-assurance, fear of unspecific consequences, focus on self, sympathetic stimulation, and restlessness.

risk for perioperative-positioning Injury: risk factors may include disorientation, immobilization, muscle weakness, obesity/edema.

risk for ineffective Breathing Pattern: risk factors may include chemically induced muscular relaxation, perception/cognitive impairment, decreased energy.

risk for deficient Fluid Volume: risk factors may include preoperative fluid deprivation, blood loss, and excessive GI losses (vomiting/gastric suction).

Syndrome X   CH
(Refer to Metabolic syndrome)

Synovitis (knee)   CH
acute Pain may be related to inflammation of synovial membrane of the joint with effusion, possibly evidenced by verbal reports, guarding/distraction behaviors, self-focus, and autonomic responses (changes in vital signs).

impaired Walking may be related to pain and decreased strength of joint, possibly evidenced by reluctance to attempt movement, inability to move about environment as desired.

Syphilis, congenital   PED
(Also refer to Sexually Transmitted Disease [STD])
acute Pain may be related to inflammatory process, edema formation, and development of skin lesions, possibly evidenced by irritability/crying that may be increased with movement of extremities and autonomic responses (changes in vital signs).

impaired Skin/Tissue Integrity may be related to exposure to pathogens during vaginal delivery, possibly evidenced by disruption of skin surfaces and rhinitis.

delayed Growth and Development may be related to effect of infectious process, possibly evidenced by altered physical growth and delay or difficulty performing skills typical of age group.

deficient Knowledge [Learning Need] regarding pathophysiology of condition, transmissibility, therapy needs, expected outcomes, and potential complications may be related to caretaker/parental lack of information, misinterpretation, possibly evidenced by statements of concern, questions, and misconceptions.

Syringomyelia   MS
disturbed Sensory Perception (specify) may be related to altered sensory perception (neurological lesion), possibly evidenced by change in usual response to stimuli and motor incoordination.

Anxiety [specify level]/Fear may be related to change in health status, threat of change in role functioning and socioeconomic status, and threat to self-concept, possibly evidenced by increased tension, apprehension, uncertainty, focus on self, and expressed concerns.

impaired physical Mobility may be related to neuromuscular and sensory impairment, possibly evidenced by decreased muscle strength, control, and mass; and impaired coordination.

Self-Care Deficit [specify] may be related to neuromuscular and sensory impairments, possibly evidenced by statement of inability to perform care tasks.

Tarsal tunnel syndrome   CH
acute/chronic Pain may be related to pressure on posterior tibial nerve at ankle, possibly evidenced by verbal reports, reluctance to use affected extremity, guarding behaviors, expressed fear of reinjury, altered ability to continue previous activities.

impaired Walking may be related to neuromuscular impairment and increased pain with walking, possibly evidenced by inability to walk desired distances, climb stairs, navigate curbs/uneven surfaces.

Tay-Sachs disease   PED
delayed Growth and Development may be related to effects of physical condition, possibly evidenced by altered physical growth, loss of/failure to acquire skills typical of age, flat affect, and decreased responses.

disturbed visual Sensory Perception may be related to neurological deterioration of optic nerve, possibly evidenced by loss of visual acuity.

family Grieving may be related to expected eventual loss of infant/child, possibly evidenced by expressions of distress, denial, guilt, anger, and sorrow; choked feelings; changes in sleep/eating habits; and altered libido.

family Powerlessness may be related to absence of therapeutic interventions for progressive/ fatal disease, possibly evidenced by verbal expressions of having no control over situation/outcome and depression over physical/mental deterioration.

risk for Spiritual Distress: risk factors may include challenged belief and value system by presence of fatal condition with racial/religious connotations and intense suffering.

compromised family Coping may be related to situational crisis, temporary preoccupation with managing emotional conflicts and personal suffering, family disorganization, and prolonged/progressive disease, possibly evidenced by preoccupations with personal reactions, expressed concern about reactions of other family members, inadequate support of one another, and altered communication patterns.

TBI   MS/CH
(Refer to Traumatic brain injury)

Temporal arteritis   CH
acute Pain may be related to arterial inflammation, possibly evidenced by reports of severe headache, scalp tenderness, pain with chewing, myalgia.

risk for disturbed visual Sensory Perception: risk factors may include altered reception (arterial inflammation, ischemic optic neuropathy).

risk for ineffective Therapeutic Regimen Management: risk factors may include medication side effects, economic difficulties, perceived seriousness/benefits.

Temporomandibular joint syndrome   CH
chronic Pain may be related to pressure on nerves, possibly evidenced by reports of pain in TMJ area worsened with chewing, muscle tension headache.

risk for imbalanced Nutrition: less than body requirements: risk factors may include inability to ingest food (pain worsened by chewing, limited movement of joint).

risk for disturbed auditory Sensory Perception: risk factors may include altered sensory reception (tinnitus, occasionally deafness).

Tendonitis   CH
acute/chronic Pain may be related to inflammation, swelling of tendon, possibly evidenced by verbal reports, guarding/protective behavior, fear of reinjury, altered ability to continue previous activities.

impaired physical Mobility may be related to pain, joint stiffness, musculoskeletal impairment, prescribed movement restrictions, possibly evidenced by limited range of motion, limited ability to perform fine/gross motor skills.

risk for ineffective Role Performance: risk factors may include health alterations, fatigue, pain.

Testicular cancer   MS
(Also refer to Cancer)

disturbed Body Image may be related to surgical change in reproductive organs, loss of hair and weight, possibly evidenced by negative feelings about body/sense of mutilation, preoccupation with change, feelings of helplessness/hopelessness, and change in social environment.

Sexual Dysfunction may be related to change in sexual organs, postoperative impotence, vulnerability, possibly evidenced by verbalizations of problem, inability in achieving desired satisfaction, alterations in relationships.

Tetraplegia   **MS/CH**
(Refer to Quadriplegia)

Thoracotomy   **MS**
(Refer to Surgery, general; Hemothorax)

Thrombophlebitis   **CH/MS/OB**
ineffective peripheral Tissue Perfusion may be related to interruption of venous blood flow, venous stasis, possibly evidenced by changes in skin color/temperature over affected area, development of edema, pain, diminished peripheral pulses, slow capillary refill.

acute Pain[/Discomfort] may be related to vascular inflammation/irritation and edema formation (accumulation of lactic acid), possibly evidenced by verbal reports, guarding/distraction behaviors, restlessness, and self-focus.

Anxiety [specify level] may be related to change in health status, perceived/actual threat to self, situational crisis, interpersonal transmission, possibly evidenced by increased tension, apprehension, restlessness, sympathetic stimulation.

risk for impaired physical Mobility: risk factors may include pain and discomfort and restrictive therapies/safety precautions.

deficient Knowledge [Learning Need] regarding pathophysiology of condition, therapy/self-care needs, and risk of embolization may be related to lack of information/misinterpretation, possibly evidenced by statements of concern, questions, inaccurate follow-through of instructions, and development of preventable complications.

Thrombosis, venous   **MS**
(Refer to Thrombophlebitis)

Thrush   **CH**
impaired Oral Mucous Membrane may be related to presence of infection as evidenced by white patches/plaques, oral discomfort, mucosal irritation, bleeding.

risk for imbalanced Nutrition: less than body requirements: risk factors may include inability to ingest adequate amount of nutrients (oral pain).

Thyroidectomy   **MS**
(Also refer to Hyperthyroidism; Hypoparathyroidism, Hypothyroidism)

risk for ineffective Airway Clearance: risk factors may include hematoma/edema formation with tracheal obstruction, laryngeal spasms.

impaired verbal Communication may be related to tissue edema, pain/discomfort, and vocal cord injury/laryngeal nerve damage, possibly evidenced by impaired articulation, does not/cannot speak, and use of nonverbal cues/gestures.

risk for Injury [tetany]: risk factors may include chemical imbalance/excessive CNS stimulation.

risk for head/neck Trauma: risk factors may include loss of muscle control/support and position of suture line.

acute Pain may be related to presence of surgical incision/manipulation of tissues/muscles, postoperative edema, possibly evidenced by verbal reports, guarding/distraction behaviors, narrowed focus, and autonomic responses (changes in vital signs).

Thyrotoxicosis   **MS**
(Also refer to Hyperthyroidism)

risk for decreased Cardiac Output: risk factors may include uncontrolled hypermetabolic state increasing cardiac workload, changes in venous return and SVR; and alterations in rate, rhythm, and electrical conduction.

Anxiety [specific level] may be related to physiological factors/CNS stimulation (hypermetabolic state and pseudocatecholamine effect of thyroid hormones), possibly evidenced by increased feelings of apprehension, shakiness, loss of control, panic, changes in cognition, distortion of environmental stimuli, extraneous movements, restlessness, and tremors.

risk for disturbed Thought Processes: risk factors may include physiological changes (increased CNS stimulation/accelerated mental activity) and altered sleep patterns.

deficient Knowledge [Learning Needs] regarding condition, treatment needs, and potential for complications/crisis situation may be related to lack of information/recall, misinterpretation, possibly evidenced by statements of concern, questions, misconceptions, and inaccurate follow-through of instructions.

TIA   CH
(Refer to Transient ischemic attack)

Tic douloureux   CH
(Refer to Neuralgia, trigeminal)

TMJ syndrome   CH
(Refer to Temporomandibular joint syndrome)

Tonsillectomy   PED/MS
(Refer to Adenoidectomy)

Tonsillitis   PED
acute Pain may be related to inflammation of tonsils and effects of circulating toxins, possibly evidenced by verbal reports, guarding/distraction behaviors, reluctance/refusal to swallow, self-focus, and autonomic responses (changes in vital signs).

Hyperthermia may be related to presence of inflammatory process/hypermetabolic state and dehydration, possibly evidenced by increased body temperature, warm/flushed skin, and tachycardia.

deficient Knowledge [Learning Need] regarding cause/transmission, treatment needs, and potential complications may be related to lack of information/misinterpretation, possibly evidenced by statements of concern, questions, inaccurate follow-through of instructions, and recurrence of condition.

Total joint replacement   MS
risk for Infection: risk factors may include inadequate primary defenses (broken skin, exposure of joint), inadequate secondary defenses/immunosuppression (long-term corticosteroid use), invasive procedures/surgical manipulation, implantation of foreign body, and decreased mobility.

impaired physical Mobility may be related to pain and discomfort, musculoskeletal impairment, and surgery/restrictive therapies, possibly evidenced by reluctance to attempt movement, difficulty with purposefully moving within the physical environment, reports of pain/discomfort on movement, limited range of motion, and decreased muscle strength/control.

risk for ineffective peripheral Tissue Perfusion: risk factors may include reduced arterial/venous blood flow, direct trauma to blood vessels, tissue edema, improper location/dislocation of prosthesis, and hypovolemia.

acute Pain may be related to physical agents (traumatized tissues/surgical intervention, degeneration of joints, muscle spasms) and psychological factors (anxiety, advanced age), possibly evidenced by verbal reports, guarding/distraction behaviors, self-focus, and autonomic responses (changes in vital signs).

Tourette's syndrome   **CH**

chronic low Self-Esteem may be related to inherited disorder, continual negative evaluation of self/capabilities, personal vulnerability, possibly evidenced by self-negating verbalizations, expressed shame, exaggerated negative feedback about self, hesitancy to try new situations.

Social Isolation may be related to unaccepted social behaviors, inability to engage in satisfying personal relationships, rejection/ridicule by others.

risk for Injury: risk factors may include adverse side effects of medications, negative response of uneducated individuals.

Toxemia of pregnancy   **OB**

(Refer to Pregnancy-Induced Hypertension)

Toxic enterocolitis   **PED/MS**

(Also refer to Colostomy)

deficient Fluid Volume may be related to fulminating losses into the bowel, diarrhea, lack of intake evidenced by decreased/concentrated urine, dry mucous membranes, poor skin turgor, decreased venous filling, change in mentation.

risk for decreased Cardiac Output: risk factors may include decreased venous return, altered heart rate/rhythm.

Toxic megacolon   **MS**

(Refer to Toxic enterocolitis)

Toxic shock syndrome   **MS**

(Also refer to Sepsis)

Hyperthermia may be related to inflammatory process/hypermetabolic state and dehydration, possibly evidenced by increased body temperature, warm/flushed skin, and tachycardia.

deficient Fluid Volume [isotonic] may be related to increased gastric losses (diarrhea, vomiting), fever/hypermetabolic state, and decreased intake, possibly evidenced by dry mucous membranes, increased pulse, hypotension, delayed venous filling, decreased/concentrated urine, and hemoconcentration.

acute Pain may be related to inflammatory process, effects of circulating toxins, and skin disruptions, possibly evidenced by verbal reports, guarding/distraction behaviors, self-focus, and autonomic responses (changes in vital signs).

impaired Skin/Tissue Integrity may be related to effects of circulating toxins and dehydration, possibly evidenced by development of desquamating rash, hyperemia, and inflammation of mucous membranes.

Traction   **MS**

(Also refer to Casts; Fractures)

acute Pain may be related to direct trauma to tissue/bone, muscle spasms, movement of bone fragments, edema, injury to soft tissue, traction/immobility device, anxiety, possibly evidenced by verbal reports, guarding/distraction behaviors, self-focus, alteration in muscle tone, and autonomic responses (changes in vital signs).

impaired physical Mobility may be related to neuromuscular/skeletal impairment, pain, psychological immobility, and therapeutic restrictions of movement, possibly evidenced by limited range of motion, inability to move purposefully in environment, reluctance to attempt movement, and decreased muscle strength/control.

risk for Infection: risk factors may include invasive procedures (including insertion of foreign body through skin/bone), presence of traumatized tissue, and reduced activity with stasis of body fluids.

deficient Diversional Activity may be related to length of hospitalization/therapeutic intervention and environmental lack of usual activity, possibly evidenced by statements of boredom, restlessness, and irritability.

Transfusion reaction, blood   MS

(Also refer to Anaphylaxis)

risk for imbalanced Body Temperature: risk factors may include infusion of cold blood products, systemic response to toxins.

Anxiety [specify level] may be related to change in health status and threat of death, exposure to toxins, possibly evidenced by increased tension, apprehension, sympathetic stimulation, restlessness, and expressions of concern.

risk for impaired Skin Integrity: risk factors may include immunological response.

Transient ischemic attack   CH

ineffective cerebral Tissue Perfusion may be related to interruption of blood flow (e.g., vasospasm), possibly evidenced by altered mental status, behavioral changes, language deficit, change in motor/sensory response.

Anxiety [specify level]/Fear may be related to change in health status, threat to self-concept, situational crisis, interpersonal contagion, possibly evidenced by expressed concerns, apprehension, restlessness, irritability.

risk for ineffective Denial: risk factors may include change in health status requiring change in lifestyle, fear of consequences, lack of motivation.

Transplant, living donor   MS

(Also refer to Surgery, general; Nephrectomy)

decisional Conflict may be related to multiple/divergent sources of information, family system (demands/expectations/responsibilities to others), risk to self, possibly evidenced by verbalized uncertainty about choices, questioning personal values/beliefs, delayed decision making, increased tension.

[moderate to severe] Anxiety/Fear may be related to situational crisis, unconscious conflict about essential beliefs/values, familial association, threat to health status/death, possibly evidenced by expressed concerns, apprehension, uncertainty, increased tension, fear of failing family member (e.g., organ rejection), sympathetic stimulation.

Transplantation, recipient   MS

(Also refer to Surgery, general; Cardiac surgery)

Anxiety [specify level]/Fear may be related to unconscious conflict about essential values/beliefs, situational crisis, interpersonal contagion, threat to self-concept, threat of organ rejection/death, side effects of medication, possibly evidenced by increased tension, apprehension, uncertainty, expressed concerns, somatic complaints, sympathetic stimulation, insomnia.

risk for Infection: risk factors may include medically induced immunosuppression, suppressed inflammatory response, antibiotic therapy, invasive procedures, broken skin/traumatized tissue, effects of chronic/debilitating disease.

[Refer to specific conditions relative to compromise/failure of individual transplanted organ, e.g., Renal failure, acute, Heart failure, chronic; Pancreatitis.)

CH

ineffective Coping/compromised family Coping may be related to situational crisis, high degree of threat, uncertainty, family disorganization/role changes, prolonged disease exhausting supportive capacity of family/SO, possibly evidenced by verbalizations, sleep disturbance/fatigue, poor concentration, protective behaviors disproportionate to client's needs, SO describes preoccupation with personal reaction.

risk for ineffective Protection: risk factors may include drug therapies/compromised immune system, effects of debilitating disease.

readiness for enhanced Therapeutic Regimen Management may be related to desire to live life more fully, engage in healthy lifestyle, possibly evidenced by expressed desire to manage treatment and prevention of sequelae, reduction of risk factors, no unexpected sequelae.

risk for ineffective Therapeutic Regimen Management: risk factors may include complexity of therapeutic regimen and healthcare system, economic difficulties, family patterns of healthcare.

Transurethral resection of prostate   MS
(Refer to Prostatectomy)

Traumatic brain injury (TBI)   MS
risk for decreased Intracranial Adaptive Capacity: risk factors may include brain injuries, systemic hypotension with intracranial hypertension.

risk for ineffective Breathing Pattern: risk factors may include neuromuscular dysfunction (injury to respiratory center of brain), perception/cognitive impairment.

disturbed Sensory Perception (specify) may be related to altered sensory reception, transmission or integration (neurological trauma or deficit), possibly evidenced by disorientation to time, place, person; motor incoordination; altered communication patterns; restlessness/irritability; change in behavior pattern.

risk for Infection: risk factors may include traumatized tissues, broken skin, invasive procedures, decreased ciliary action, stasis of body fluids, nutritional deficits, altered integrity of closed system (CSF leak).

risk for imbalanced Nutrition: less than body requirements: risk factors may include altered ability to ingest nutrients (decreased level of consciousness), weakness of muscles for chewing/swallowing, hypermetabolic state.

CH

impaired physical Mobility may be related to perceptual/cognitive impairment, decreased strength/endurance, restrictive therapies/safety precautions, possibly evidenced by inability to purposefully move within physical environment—including bed mobility, transfer, ambulation, impaired coordination, limited range of motion, decreased muscle strength/control.

disturbed Thought Processes may be related to physiological changes, psychological conflicts, possibly evidenced by memory deficits, distractibility, altered attention span/concentration, disorientation to time, place, person, circumstances, or events; impaired ability to make decisions, problem-solve, reason or conceptualize; personality changes.

interrupted Family Processes may be related to situational transition and crisis, uncertainty about ultimate outcome/expectations, possibly evidenced by difficulty adapting to change, family not meeting needs of all members, difficulty accepting/receiving help, inability to express or to accept feelings of members.

Self-Care Deficit (specify) may be related to neuromuscular/musculoskeletal impairment, weakness, pain, perceptual/cognitive impairment, possibly evidenced by inability to perform desired/appropriate ADLs.

Trench foot   MS
(Refer to Immersion foot)

Trichinosis   CH
acute Pain may be related to parasitic invasion of muscle tissues, edema of upper eyelids, small localized hemorrhages, and development of urticaria, possibly evidenced by verbal reports, guarding/distraction behaviors (restlessness), and autonomic responses (changes in vital signs).

deficient Fluid Volume [isotonic] may be related to hypermetabolic state (fever, diaphoresis); excessive gastric losses (vomiting, diarrhea); and decreased intake/difficulty swallowing, possibly evidenced by dry mucous membranes, decreased skin turgor, hypotension, decreased venous filling, decreased/concentrated urine, and hemoconcentration.

ineffective Breathing Pattern may be related to myositis of the diaphragm and intercostal muscles, possibly evidenced by resulting changes in respiratory depth, tachypnea, dyspnea, and abnormal ABGs.

deficient Knowledge [Learning Need] regarding cause/prevention of condition, therapy needs, and possible complications may be related to lack of information, misinterpretation, possibly evidenced by statements of concern, questions, and misconceptions.

Tricuspid insufficiency   CH
(Refer to Valvular heart disease)

Tricuspid stenosis   CH
(Refer to Valvular heart disease)

Tubal pregnancy   OB
(Refer to Ectopic pregnancy)

Tuberculosis (pulmonary)   CH
risk for Infection [spread/reactivation]: risk factors may include inadequate primary defenses (decreased ciliary action/stasis of secretions, tissue destruction/extension of infection), lowered resistance/suppressed inflammatory response, malnutrition, environmental exposure, insufficient knowledge to avoid exposure to pathogens, or inadequate therapeutic intervention.

ineffective Airway Clearance may be related to thick, viscous, or bloody secretions; fatigue/poor cough effort, and tracheal/pharyngeal edema, possibly evidenced by abnormal respiratory rate, rhythm, and depth; adventitious breath sounds (rhonchi, wheezes), stridor and dyspnea.

risk for impaired Gas Exchange: risk factors may include decrease in effective lung surface, atelectasis, destruction of alveolar-capillary membrane, bronchial edema; thick, viscous secretions.

Activity Intolerance may be related to imbalance between O_2 supply and demand, possibly evidenced by reports of fatigue, weakness, and exertional dyspnea.

imbalanced Nutrition: less than body requirements may be related to inability to ingest adequate nutrients (anorexia, effects of drug therapy, fatigue, insufficient financial resources), possibly evidenced by weight loss, reported lack of interest in food/altered taste sensation, and poor muscle tone.

risk for ineffective Therapeutic Regimen Management: risk factors may include complexity of therapeutic regimen, economic difficulties, family patterns of healthcare, perceived seriousness/benefits (especially during remission), side effects of therapy.

TURP   MS
(Refer to Prostatectomy)

Twin-twin transfusion syndrome   OB
decreased Cardiac Output may be related to altered preload (hypovolemia, anemia) to donor fetus, possibly evidenced by oliguria/oliohydramnios.

excess Fluid Volume may be related to excess fluid intake (shunting of circulation) to recipient fetus, possibly evidenced by polyuria/polyhydramnios.

risk for disproportionate Growth: risk factors may include multiple gestation with imbalanced circulation/nutrition to both fetus.

Tympanoplasty   **MS**
(Refer to Stapedectomy)

Typhoid fever   **MS**
(Also refer to Sepsis)

risk for Infection [spread]: risk factors may include presence of bacteria in excretions, inadequate knowledge to avoid exposure to pathogen (food/water, fecally contaminated objects).

risk for deficient Fluid Volume [isotonic]: risk factors may include gastric irritation/ulcers.

imbalanced Nutrition: less than body requirements: risk factors may include inability to ingest/digest/absorb nutrients, hypermetabolic state, possibly evidenced by anorexia, abdominal pain, weight loss.

Typhus   **CH/MS**
Hyperthermia may be related to generalized inflammatory process (vasculitis), possibly evidenced by increased body temperature, warm/flushed skin, and tachycardia.

acute Pain may be related to generalized vasculitis and edema formation, possibly evidenced by verbal reports, guarding/distraction behaviors, self-focus, and autonomic responses (changes in vital signs).

ineffective Tissue Perfusion (specify) may be related to reduction/interruption of blood flow (generalized vasculitis/thrombi formation), possibly evidenced by reports of headache/abdominal pain, changes in mentation, and areas of peripheral ulceration/necrosis.

Ulcer, decubitus   **CH/MS**
impaired Skin/Tissue Integrity may be related to altered circulation, nutritional deficit, fluid imbalance, impaired physical mobility, irritation of body excretions/secretions, and sensory impairments, evidenced by tissue damage/destruction.

acute Pain may be related to destruction of protective skin layers and exposure of nerves, possibly evidenced by verbal reports, distraction behaviors, and self-focus.

risk for Infection: risk factors may include broken/traumatized tissue, increased environmental exposure, and nutritional deficits.

Ulcer, peptic (acute)   **MS/CH**
deficient Fluid Volume [isotonic] may be related to vascular losses (hemorrhage), possibly evidenced by hypotension, tachycardia, delayed capillary refill, changes in mentation, restlessness, concentrated/decreased urine, pallor, diaphoresis, and hemoconcentration.

risk for ineffective Tissue Perfusion (specify): risk factors may include hypovolemia.

Fear/Anxiety [specify level] may be related to change in health status and threat of death, possibly evidenced by increased tension, restlessness, irritability, fearfulness, trembling, tachycardia, diaphoresis, lack of eye contact, focus on self, verbalization of concerns, withdrawal, and panic or attack behavior.

acute Pain may be related to caustic irritation/destruction of gastric tissues, possibly evidenced by verbal reports, distraction behaviors, self-focus, and autonomic responses (changes in vital signs).

deficient Knowledge [Learning Need] regarding condition, therapy/self-care needs, and potential complications may be related to lack of information/recall, misinterpretation, possibly evidenced by statements of concern, questions, misconceptions; inaccurate follow-through of instructions, and development of preventable complications/recurrence of condition.

Ulcer, pressure   **CH/MS**
(Refer to Ulcer, decubitus)

Ulcer, venous stasis   **CH**
(Also refer to Venous insufficiency)

impaired Skin/Tissue Integrity may be related to altered venous circulation, edema formation, inflammation, decreased sensation, possibly evidenced by destruction of skin layers, invasion of body structures.

decreased peripheral Tissue Perfusion may be related to interruption of venous flow (small-vessel vasoconstrictive reflex), possibly evidenced by skin discoloration, edema formation, altered sensation, delayed healing.

Ulnar neuropathy   CH
(Refer to Cubital tunnel syndrome)

Unconsciousness   MS
(Refer to Coma)

Upper GI bleeding   MS
(Refer to Gastritis, acute or chronic; Ulcer, peptic)

Urinary diversion   MS/CH
risk for impaired Skin Integrity: risk factors may include absence of sphincter at stoma, character/flow of urine from stoma, reaction to product/chemicals, and improperly fitting appliance or removal of adhesive.

disturbed Body Image related factors may include biophysical factors (presence of stoma, loss of control of urine flow) and psychosocial factors (altered body structure, disease process/associated treatment regimen, such as cancer), possibly evidenced by verbalization of change in body image, fear of rejection/reaction of others, negative feelings about body, not touching/looking at stoma, refusal to participate in care.

acute Pain may be related to physical factors (disruption of skin/tissues, presence of incisions/drains), biological factors (activity of disease process, such as cancer, trauma), and psychological factors (fear, anxiety), possibly evidenced by verbal reports, self-focusing, guarding/distraction behaviors, restlessness, and autonomic responses (changes in vital signs).

impaired Urinary Elimination may be related to surgical diversion, tissue trauma, and postoperative edema, possibly evidenced by loss of continence, changes in amount and character of urine, and urinary retention.

Urinary tract infection   CH
(Refer to Cystitis)

Urolithiasis   MS/CH
(Refer to Calculi, urinary)

Uterine bleeding, dysfunctional   GYN/MS
Anxiety [specify level] may be related to perceived change in health status and unknown etiology, possibly evidenced by apprehension, uncertainty, fear of unspecified consequences, expressed concerns, and focus on self.

Activity Intolerance may be related to imbalance between oxygen supply and demand/decreased oxygen-carrying capacity of blood (anemia), possibly evidenced by reports of fatigue/weakness.

Uterine myomas   GYN
(Also refer to Anemia)
acute Pain/[Discomfort] may be related to growth/size/degeneration or twisting of tumors, possibly evidenced by reports of pressure, cramping, guarding behavior, irritability.

impaired Urinary Elimination may be related to uterine pressure on bladder, possibly evidenced by frequency, urgency.

risk for deficient Fluid Volume: risk factors may include excessive/chronic blood loss.

Uterus, rupture of, in pregnancy   OB

deficient Fluid Volume [isotonic] may be related to excessive vascular losses, possibly evidenced by hypotension, increased pulse rate, decreased venous filling, and decreased urine output.

decreased Cardiac Output may be related to decreased preload (hypovolemia), possibly evidenced by cold/clammy skin, decreased peripheral pulses, variations in hemodynamic readings, tachycardia, and cyanosis.

acute Pain may be related to tissue trauma and irritation of accumulating blood, possibly evidenced by verbal reports, guarding/distraction behaviors, self-focus, and autonomic responses (changes in vital signs).

Anxiety [specify level] may be related to threat of death of self/fetus, interpersonal contagion, physiological response (release of catecholamines), possibly evidenced by fearful/scared affect, sympathetic stimulation, stated fear of unspecified consequences, and expressed concerns.

UTI   CH
(Refer to Cystitis)

Vaginal hysterectomy   MS
(Refer to Hysterectomy)

Vaginismus   GYN/PSY

acute Pain may be related to muscle spasm and hyperesthesia of the nerve supply to vaginal mucous membrane, possibly evidenced by verbal reports, distraction behaviors, and self-focus.

Sexual Dysfunction may be related to physical or psychological alteration in function (severe spasms of vaginal muscles), possibly evidenced by verbalization of problem, inability to achieve desired satisfaction, and alteration in relationship with SO.

Vaginitis   GYN/CH

impaired Tissue Integrity may be related to irritation/inflammation and mechanical trauma (scratching) of sensitive tissues, possibly evidenced by damaged/destroyed tissue, presence of lesions.

acute Pain may be related to localized inflammation and tissue trauma, possibly evidenced by verbal reports, distraction behaviors, and self-focus.

deficient Knowledge [Learning Need] regarding hygienic/therapy needs and sexual behaviors/transmission of organisms may be related to lack of information/misinterpretation, possibly evidenced by statements of concern, questions, and misconceptions.

Vaginosis, bacterial   GYN

risk for impaired Tissue Integrity: risk factors may include vulvar/vaginal irritation, itching.

risk for [secondary] Infection: risk factors may include prescribed antibiotic therapy, insufficient knowledge to avoid exposure to pathogens.

Valvular heart disease   MS

decreased Cardiac Output may be related to alteration in preload/increased arterial pressure and venous congestion, increased afterload, changes in electrical conduction, possibly evidenced by variations in hemodynamic parameters, dysrhythmias/ECG changes, dyspnea, adventitious breath sounds, cyanosis/pallor, jugular vein distention, fatigue.

Activity Intolerance may be related to imbalance between oxygen supply and demand (decreased/fixed cardiac output), possibly evidenced by reports of fatigue/weakness, abnormal heart rate/BP in response to activity, exertional discomfort/dyspnea.

Anxiety may be related to threat to/change in health status (chronicity of disease), physiological effects, situational crisis (changes in lifestyle, hospitalization), possibly evidenced by expressed concerns, increased tension, apprehension, uncertainty, sympathetic stimulation, insomnia.

risk for excess Fluid Volume: risk factors may include increased sodium/water retention, changes in glomerular filtration.

risk for ineffective Tissue Perfusion (specify): risk factors may include interruption of arterial-venous flow (systemic emboli), venous thrombosis (venous stasis, decreased activity).

VAP   MS/CH
(Refer to Ventilator assist/dependence; Bronchopneumonia)

Varices, esophageal   MS
(Also refer to Ulcer, peptic [acute])

deficient Fluid Volume [isotonic] may be related to excessive vascular loss, reduced intake, and gastric losses (vomiting), possibly evidenced by hypotension, tachycardia, decreased venous filling, and decreased/concentrated urine.

Anxiety [specify level]/Fear may be related to change in health status and threat of death, possibly evidenced by increased tension/apprehension, sympathetic stimulation, restlessness, focus on self, and expressed concerns.

Varicose veins   CH
chronic Pain may be related to venous insufficiency and stasis, possibly evidenced by verbal reports.

disturbed Body Image may be related to change in structure (presence of enlarged, discolored tortuous superficial leg veins), possibly evidenced by hiding affected parts and negative feelings about body.

risk for impaired Skin/Tissue Integrity: risk factors may include altered circulation/venous stasis and edema formation.

Varicose Veins ligation/stripping   MS
risk for ineffective peripheral Tissue Perfusion: risk factors may include localized edema, vascular irritation, inadequate venous return, dressings.

impaired Skin Integrity may be related to surgical procedure, pressure dressings, tissue edema, vascular engorgement, possibly evidenced by incisions, development of complications (e.g., ulcerations).

Varicose veins sclerotherapy   MS
risk for impaired Skin Integrity: risk factors may include pressure wraps, extravasation of sclerosing agent.

risk for ineffective Therapeutic Regimen Management: risk factors may include perceived seriousness/benefit, required lifestyle/activity changes, postprocedure dressings.

Variola   MS
(Refer to Smallpox)

Vasculitis   CH
(Refer to Polyarteritis nodosa; Temporal arteritis)

Vasectomy   CH/MS
acute Pain[/Discomfort] may be related to manipulation of delicate tissues, edema/hematoma formation, possibly evidenced by verbal reports, guarding behavior, irritability.

deficient Knowledge regarding self-care, future expectations (issues of reproduction, safety/STDs) may be related to information misinterpretation, lack of recall, possibly evidenced by verbalizations, misconceptions, inaccurate follow-through of instructions.

Venereal disease   **CH**
(Refer to Sexually Transmitted Disease [STD])

Venous insufficiency   **CH**
(Also refer to Stasis dermatitis; Ulcer, venous stasis)

chronic Pain[/Discomfort] may be related to altered venous circulation, edema formation, possibly evidenced by reports of aching, fullness, tiredness of lower extremities with activity.

risk for risk-prone health Behavior: risk factors may include health status requiring change in lifestyle, lack of motivation to change behaviors.

risk for ineffective Therapeutic Regimen Management: risk factors may include economic difficulties, perceived seriousness/benefit, social support deficit.

Ventilator assist/dependence   **MS/CH**

ineffective Breathing Pattern/impaired spontaneous Ventilation may be related to neuromuscular dysfunction, respiratory muscle fatigue, spinal cord injury, hypoventilation syndrome, possibly evidenced by dyspnea, increased work of breathing/use of accessory muscles, reduced vital capacity/total lung volume, changes in respiratory rate, decreased PO_2/SaO_2, increased PCO_2.

ineffective Airway Clearance may be related to foreign body/artificial airway in trachea, inability to cough/ineffective cough, possibly evidenced by changes in rate/depth of respirations, abnormal breath sounds, anxiety/restlessness, cyanosis.

impaired verbal Communication may be related to physical barrier (artificial airway), neuromuscular weakness/paralysis, possibly evidenced by inability to speak.

Fear/Anxiety [specify] may be related to situational crisis, threat to self-concept, threat of death/dependency on machine, change in health status/socioeconomic status/role functioning, interpersonal transmission, possibly evidenced by increased muscle/facial tension, hypervigilance, restlessness, fearfulness, apprehension, expressed concerns, insomnia, negative self-talk.

risk for impaired Oral Mucous Membrane: risk factors may include inability to swallow oral fluids, decreased salivation, ineffective oral hygiene, presence of ET tube in mouth.

risk for imbalanced Nutrition: less than body requirements: risk factors may include inability to ingest nutrients, increased metabolic demands.

risk for dysfunctional Ventilatory Weaning Response: risk factors may include limited/insufficient energy stores, sleep disturbance, pain/discomfort, perceived inability to wean/decreased motivation, inadequate support/adverse environment, history of ventilator dependence greater than 1 week/unsuccessful weaning attempts.

Ventricular fibrillation   **MS**
(Also refer to Dysrhythmias)

decreased Cardiac Output may be related to altered electrical conduction and reduced myocardial contractility, possibly evidenced by absence of measurable cardiac output, loss of consciousness, no palpable pulses.

Ventricular tachycardia   **MS**
(Also refer to Dysrhythmias)

risk for decreased Cardiac Output: risk factors may include altered electrical conduction and reduced myocardial contractility.

Vertigo   **CH**

disturbed kinesthetic Sensory Perception may be related to altered status of sensory organ (middle/inner ear), altered sensory integration, possibly evidenced by visual distortions, altered sense of balance, falls.

risk for Falls: risk factors may include presence of postural hypotension, acute illness, medications, substance abuse.

West Nile Fever   CH/MS
Hyperthermia may be related to infectious process, possibly evidenced by elevated body temperature, skin flushed/warm to touch, tachycardia, increased respiratory rate.

acute Pain may be related to infectious process/circulating toxins, possibly evidenced by reports of headache, myalgia, eye pain, abdominal discomfort.

risk for deficient Fluid Volume: risk factors may include hypermetabolic state, decreased intake, anorexia, nausea, losses from normal routes (vomiting, diarrhea).

risk for impaired Skin Integrity: risk factors may include hyperthermia, decreased fluid intake, alterations in skin turgor, bedrest, circulating toxins.

Whooping cough   PED
(Refer to Pertussis)

Wilms' tumor   PED
(Also refer to Cancer; Chemotherapy)

Anxiety [specify level]/Fear may be related to change in environment and interaction patterns with family members and threat of death with family transmission and contagion concerns, possibly evidenced by fearful/scared affect, distress, crying, insomnia, and sympathetic stimulation.

risk for Injury: risk factors may include nature of tumor (vascular, mushy with very thin covering) with increased danger of metastasis when manipulated.

interrupted Family Processes may be related to situational crisis of life-threatening illness, possibly evidenced by a family system that has difficulty meeting physical, emotional, and spiritual needs of its members, and inability to deal with traumatic experience effectively.

deficient Diversional Activity may be related to environmental lack of age-appropriate activity (including activity restrictions) and length of hospitalization/treatment, possibly evidenced by restlessness, crying, lethargy, and acting-out behavior.

Withdrawal, drugs/alcohol   CH/MS
(Refer to Alcohol intoxication, acute; Drug overdose, acute; Drug withdrawal)

Wound, gunshot   MS
(Depends on site and speed/character of bullet)

risk for deficient Fluid Volume: risk factors may include excessive vascular losses, altered intake/restrictions.

acute Pain may be related to destruction of tissue (including organ and musculoskeletal), surgical repair, and therapeutic interventions, possibly evidenced by verbal reports, guarding/distraction behaviors, self-focus, and autonomic responses (changes in vital signs).

impaired Tissue Integrity may be related to mechanical factors (yaw of projectile and muzzle blast), possibly evidenced by damaged or destroyed tissue.

risk for Infection: risk factors may include tissue destruction and increased environmental exposure, invasive procedures, and decreased hemoglobin.

CH

risk for Post-Trauma Syndrome: risk factors may include nature of incident (catastrophic accident, assault, suicide attempt) and possibly injury/death of other(s) involved.

Zollinger-Ellison syndrome   MS/CH
(Also refer to Ulcer, peptic)

Diarrhea may be related to intestinal irritation (hypersecretion of gastric acid), possibly evidenced by at least three loose liquid stools/day, abdominal pain, change in bowel sounds.

risk for impaired Skin/Tissue Integrity: risk factors include frequent bowel movements, hyperacidity of liquid stools, esophageal regurgitation.

acute/chronic Pain may be related to acidic irritation of esophageal mucosa (GERD), muscle spasm, possibly evidenced by reports of heartburn, distraction behaviors.

risk for ineffective Therapeutic Regimen Management: risk factors may include length of therapy, economic difficulties, perceived susceptability.

Appendix

Definitions of Taxonomy II Axes

Axis 1 The Diagnostic Concept: The principal element or the fundamental and essential part, the root, of the diagnostic statement.

Axis 2 Subject of the diagnosis: The person(s) for whom a nursing diagnosis is determined. Values are:

Individual: A single human being distinct from others, a person.

Family: Two or more people having continuous or sustained relationships, perceiving reciprocal obligations, sensing common meaning, and sharing certain obligations toward others; related by blood or choice.

Group: A number of people with shared characteristics.

Community: A group of people living in the same locale under the same governance, such as neighborhoods, cities, census tracts.

When the unit of care is not explicity stated, it becomes the individual by default.

Axis 3 Judgment: A descriptor or modifier that limits or specifies the meaning of a nursing diagnosis. Values are:

Anticipatory: Realize beforehand, foresee.

Compromised: Damaged, made vulnerable.

Decreased: Lessened (in size, amount, or degree).

Defensive: Used or intended to defend or protect.

Deficient: Insufficient, inadequate.

Delayed: Late, slow, or postponed.

Disabled: Limited, handicapped.

Disorganized: Not properly arranged or controlled.

Disproportionate: Too large or too small in comparison with norm.

Disturbed: Agitated, interrupted, interfered with.

Dysfunctional: Not operating normally.

Effective: Producing the intended or desired effect.

Enhanced: Improved in quality, value, or extent.

Excessive: Greater than necessary or desirable.

Imbalanced: Out of proportion or balance.

Impaired: Damaged, weakened.

Ineffective: Not producing the intended or desired effect.

Interrupted: Having its continuity broken.

Low: below the norm.

Organized: Properly arranged or controlled.

Perceived: Observed through the senses.

Readiness for: In a suitable state for an activity or situation.

Situational: Related to a particular circumstance.

Axis 4 Location: Consists of parts/regions of the body or their related functions—all tissues, organs, anatomical sites or structures. Values are:

Auditory	*Olfactory*
Bladder	*Oral*
Cardiopulmonary	*Peripheral neurovascular*
Cerebral	*Peripheral vascular*
Gastrointestinal	*Renal*
Gustatory	*Skin*
Intracranial	*Tactile*
Kinesthetic	*Visual*
Mucous membranes	

Axis 5 Age: The age of the person who is the subject of the diagnosis. Values are:

Fetus	*School-age child*
Neonate	*Adolescent*
Infant	*Adult*
Toddler	*Older adult*
Preschool child	

Axis 6 Time: The duration of the diagnostic concept. Values are:

    Acute: Lasting less than 6 months.

    Chronic: Lasting more than 6 months.

    Intermittent: Stopping or starting again at intervals, periodic, cyclic.

    Continuous: Uninterrupted, going on without stop.

Axis 7 Status of the Diagnosis: The actuality or potentiality of the problem or related to the categorization of the diagnosis as a wellness/health promotion diagnosis. Values are:

Actual: Existing in fact or reality, existing at the present time.

Health Promotion: Behavior motivated by the desire to increase well-being and actualize human health potential.

Risk: Vulnerability, especially as a result of exposure to factors that increase the chance of injury or loss.

Wellness: The quality or state of being healthy.

Permission from NANDA International. (2007). *NANDA-I Nursing Diagnoses: Definitions & Classification 2007–2008*. Philadelphia: NANDA-1

Doenges & Moorhouse's Diagnostic Division Index

Neglect, unilateral, 461–465
Sensory perception, disturbed [specify
   type], 599–605
Stress overload, 657–660
Thought processes, disturbed, 698–703

PAIN/DISCOMFORT—*Ability to
   control internal/external environment
   to maintain comfort*
Comfort, readiness for enhanced, 140–145
Pain, acute, 494–499
Pain, chronic, 500–505

RESPIRATION—*Ability to provide and
   use oxygen to meet physiologic needs*
Airway clearance, ineffective, 49–54
Aspiration, risk for, 71–76
Breathing pattern, ineffective, 118–123
Gas exchange, impaired, 322–327
Ventilation, impaired spontaneous,
   763–768
Ventilatory weaning response,
   dysfunctional, 768–773

SAFETY—*Ability to provide safe,
   growth-promoting environment*
Allergy response, latex, 55–59
Allergy response, risk for latex, 59–62
Body temperature, risk for imbalanced,
   97–100
Contamination, 185–191
Contamination, risk for, 191–195
Death syndrome, risk for sudden infant,
   222–226
Environmental interpretation syndrome,
   impaired, 265–270
Falls, risk for, 274–278
Health maintenance, ineffective, 353–357
Home maintenance, impaired, 361–364
Hyperthermia, 372–376

Hypothermia, 376–381
Immunization status, readiness for
   enhanced, 384–388
Infection, risk for, 400–406
Injury, risk for, 406–410
Injury, risk for perioperative positioning,
   410–414
Mobility, impaired physical, 448–453
Poisoning, risk for, 508–513
Protection, ineffective, 536–538
Self-mutilation, 591–595
Self-mutilation, risk for, 595–599
Skin integrity, impaired, 614–620
Skin integrity, risk for impaired, 621–625
Suffocation, risk for, 661–665
Suicide, risk for, 665–670
Surgical recovery, delayed, 670–674
Tissue integrity, impaired, 703–709
Trauma, risk for, 721–727
Violence, risk for other-directed, 773–774
Violence, risk for self-directed, 774–781
Wandering [specify sporadic or continual],
   785–789

SEXUALITY—*[Component of Ego
   Integrity and Social Interaction]
   Ability to meet
   requirements/characteristics of
   male/female role*
Sexual dysfunction, 605–610
Sexuality patterns, ineffective, 610–614

SOCIAL INTERACTION—*Ability to
   establish and maintain relationships*
Attachment, risk for impaired
   parent/child, 76–80
Caregiver role strain, 130–136
Caregiver role strain, risk for, 136–140
Communication, impaired verbal, 145–151
Communication, readiness for enhanced,
   151–155

Conflict, parental role, 159–163
Coping, compromised family, 195–199
Coping, disabled family, 202–206
Coping, ineffective community, 211–214
Coping, readiness for enhanced
   community, 217–219
Coping, readiness for enhanced family,
   219–222
Family processes: alcoholism,
   dysfunctional, 278–283
Family processes, interrupted, 283–287
Family processes, readiness for enhanced,
   287–290
Loneliness, risk for, 438–441
Parenting, readiness for enhanced, 505–508
Role performance, ineffective, 562–566
Social interaction, impaired, 633–638
Social isolation, 638–642

TEACHING/LEARNING—*Ability
   to incorporate and use information to
   achieve health lifestyle/optimal
   wellness*
Development, risk for delayed, 236–240
Growth, risk for disproportionate, 343–347
Growth and development, delayed, 347–353
Health-seeking behaviors, 357–361
Knowledge, deficient [learning need]
   (specify), 423–428
Knowledge (specify), readiness for
   enhanced, 428–430
Noncompliance (specify), 465–470
Therapeutic regimen management:
   effective, 680–683
Therapeutic regimen management:
   ineffective, 683–686
Therapeutic regimen management
   ineffective community, 687–690
Therapeutic regimen management
   ineffective family, 690–692
Therapeutic regimen management:
   readiness for enhanced, 693–695

Nursing Diagnoses Index

Index

Buck's traction. *See* Traction
Buerger's disease. *See* Peripheral vascular disease
Bulimia nervosa, 815
Bunion, 815
Bunionectomy, 815
Burns, 815–816
Bursitis, 816

CABG. *See* Coronary artery bypass surgery
CAD. *See* Coronary artery disease
Calculi, urinary, 816
Cancer, 816–817. *See also specific types*
Candidiasis, 817
Cannabis abuse. *See* Depressant abuse
Carbon monoxide poisoning, 817
Cardiac catheterization, 817
Cardiac conditions, prenatal, 818
Cardiac inflammatory disease. *See* Endocarditis; Myocarditis; Pericarditis
Cardiac output, decreased, 123–129
  in Addison's disease, 795
  in anaphylaxis, 800
  in angina pectoris, 802
  in aortic stenosis, 805
  in cardiac catheterization, 817
  in cardiomyopathy, 817
  in coronary artery bypass surgery, 828
  definition of, 123
  in delirium tremens, 832
  in digitalis toxicity, 839
  documentation focus, 128–129
  in heart failure, 858
  in heatstroke, 859
  in mitral stenosis, 885
  in myocardial infarction, 888
  in myocarditis, 888
  NIC linkages, 124
  NOC linkages, 124
  in nonketotic hyperglycemic-hyperosmolar coma, 893
  nursing priorities, 124–128
  in Paget's disease, 896
  in pheochromocytoma, 902
  in pneumothorax, 904
  in pregnancy, 909
  in pregnancy-induced hypertension, 910–911
  in pulmonary hypertension, 914
  in renal failure, 918
  risk for
    in aldosteronism, 798
    in cardiac conditions, prenatal, 818
    in cardiac surgery, 818
    in cocaine poisoning, 824
    in coronary artery disease, 828
    in dysrhythmia, 842
    in electrical injury, 844
    in endocarditis, 846
    in hypertension, 865
    in labor, 875
    in Lyme disease, 881
    in myxedema, 889

  in pericarditis, 901
  in respiratory distress syndrome, 919
  in sepsis, 925
  in thyrotoxicosis, 936
  in toxic enterocolitis, 938
  in shock, 927
  in sick sinus syndrome, 927
  in twin-twin transfusion syndrome, 941
  in uterus, rupture of, 944
  in valvular heart disease, 944
  in ventricular aneurysm, 802
  in ventricular fibrillation, 946
Cardiac surgery, 818
Cardiogenic shock. *See* Shock, cardiogenic
Cardiomyopathy, 818
Caregiver role strain, 130–136
  in Alzheimer's disease, 799
  in amyotrophic lateral sclerosis, 800
  definition of, 130
  documentation focus, 135
  in hospice care, 864
  NIC linkages, 132
  NOC linkages, 132
  nursing priorities, 132–135
  in Parkinson's disease, 900
  risk for, 136–140
    in Creutzfeldt-Jakob disease, 829
    definition of, 136
    documentation focus, 139–140
    in Huntington's disease, 864
    NIC linkages, 137
    NOC linkages, 137
    nursing priorities, 137–139
Carotid endarterectomy, 818
Carpal tunnel syndrome, 819
Casts, 819
Cataract, 819
Cataract extraction, 819
Cat scratch disease, 819
Celiac disease, 820
Cellulitis, 820
Cerebral embolism. *See* Cerebrovascular accident
Cerebral palsy. *See* Palsy, cerebral
Cerebrovascular accident, 820–821
Cervix, dysfunctional. *See* Dilation of cervix, premature
Cesarean birth, 821
  postpartal, 821
  unplanned, 821–822
Chemotherapy, 822
Chickenpox. *See* Measles
Chlamydia trachomatis infection. *See* Sexually transmitted disease
Cholecystectomy, 822
Cholelithiasis, 823
Cholera, 823
Christmas disease. *See* Hemophilia
Chronic obstructive lung disease, 823
Circumcision, 823
Cirrhosis, 824
Cleft lip/palate, 824
Client care, mind mapping, 35–38
Client database, 23
Clients, interviewing, 23–24
Clinical Care Classification, 10

Cocaine hydrochloride poisoning, acute, 824
Coccidioidomycosis, 824–825
Code of Ethics for Nurses, 3
Colectomy. *See* Intestinal surgery
Colitis, ulcerative, 825
Collagen disorders. *See* Arthritis; Lupus erythematosus
Colorectal cancer. *See* Cancer; Colostomy
Colostomy, 825–826
Coma, 826
  diabetic. *see* Diabetic ketoacidosis
Comfort, readiness for enhanced, 140–145
  definition of, 140
  documentation focus, 144
  NIC linkages, 141
  NOC linkages, 141
  nursing priorities, 141–144
Communication, readiness for enhanced, 151–155
  definition of, 151
  documentation focus, 154–155
  NIC linkages, 152
  NOC linkages, 152
  nursing priorities, 152–154
Communication, impaired verbal, 145–151
  in amyotrophic lateral sclerosis, 800
  in autistic disorder, 809
  in cerebrovascular accident, 820
  definition of, 145
  documentation focus, 150
  in intermaxillary fixation, 871–872
  in laryngectomy, 877
  in mental retardation, 884
  in myasthenia gravis, 887
  NIC linkages, 146
  NOC linkages, 146
  nursing priorities, 146–150
  in Parkinson's disease, 900
  in thyroidectomy, 936
  readiness for enhanced, 151–155
    definition of, 151
    documentation focus, 154
    NIC linkages, 152
    NOC linkages, 152
    nursing priorities, 152–154
Compartment syndrome, 826
Complex regional pain syndrome. *See* Reflex sympathetic dystrophy
Concussion of brain, 826–827
Conduct disorder, 827
Conflict
  decisional [specify], 155–159
    in abortion, 791
    in anencephaly, 802
    definition of, 155
    documentation focus, 158
    NIC linkages, 156
    NOC linkages, 156
    nursing priorities, 156–158
    in transplant, 939
  parental role, 159–163
    definition of, 159
    documentation focus, 162
    NIC linkages, 160